Strandness's
Duplex Scanning in
Vascular Disorders

Strandness's Duplex Scanning in Vascular Disorders

FIFTH EDITION

Editors

R. Eugene Zierler, MD

Professor of Surgery, University of Washington School of Medicine
Medical Director, D. E. Strandness Jr Vascular Laboratory
University of Washington Medical Center and Harborview Medical Center
Seattle, Washington

David L. Dawson, MD

Professor, Department of Surgery
University of California, Davis
UC Davis Medical Center
Sacramento, California

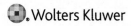 Wolters Kluwer

Philadelphia · Baltimore · New York · London
Buenos Aires · Hong Kong · Sydney · Tokyo

Acquisitions Editor: Keith Donnellan
Product Developmental Editor: Brendan Huffman
Production Project Manager: Marian Bellus
Design Coordinator: Teresa Mallon
Senior Manufacturing Manager: Beth Welsh
Marketing Manager: Dan Dressler
Prepress Vendor: SPi Global

5th Edition

Library of Congress Cataloging-in-Publication Data
Strandness's duplex scanning in vascular disorders / editors, R. Eugene Zierler, David L. Dawson. — Fifth edition.
      p. ; cm.
   Duplex scanning in vascular disorders
   Includes bibliographical references and index.
   ISBN 978-1-4511-8691-8 (hardback)
 I. Zierler, R. Eugene, editor. II. Dawson, David L., editor. III. Title: Duplex scanning in vascular disorders.
   [DNLM: 1. Vascular Diseases—ultrasonography. 2. Ultrasonography, Doppler, Duplex. WG 500]
   RC691.6.D87
   616.1'307543—dc23

                                                                        2014019552

DEDICATION

This fifth edition of *Strandness's Duplex Scanning in Vascular Disorders* is dedicated—
as Dr. Strandness would have wished—to the vascular technologists who serve our patients
and to the students, residents, and fellows who are the next generation of
vascular laboratory physicians.

It is also dedicated to our families who have provided love and encouragement
throughout our careers and especially to Brenda Zierler and Susie Dawson
whose support has been essential and profoundly appreciated.

R. Eugene Zierler
David L. Dawson

Aaron C. Baker, MD, MS
Clinical Fellow
Vascular and Endovascular Surgery
Mayo Clinic
Rochester, Minnesota

Dennis F. Bandyk, MD, FACS
Professor of Surgery
Chief, Vascular and Endovascular Surgery
Sulpizio Cardiovascular Center
University of California San Diego School of Medicine
San Diego, California

Kirk W. Beach, PhD, MD
Research Professor Emeritus
University of Washington
Seattle, Washington

Kari A. Campbell, BS, RVT
Registered Vascular Technologist
D. E. Strandness Jr Vascular Laboratory
University of Washington Medical Center
Seattle, Washington

Kim Cantwell-Gab, MN, ARNP, ACNP-BC, ANP-BC,
CVN, RVT, RDMS
Acute Care and Adult ARNP
Vascular Surgery and Vascular Medicine
Peace Health Thoracic and Vascular Surgery
Vancouver, Washington

Michael T. Caps, MD, MPH
Vascular Surgeon, Hawaii Permanente Medical Group
Moanalua Medical Center
Honolulu, Hawaii

Thais Coutinho, MD
Assistant Professor of Medicine
University of Ottawa
Staff Cardiologist
University of Ottawa Heart Institute
Ottawa, Ontario

David L. Dawson, MD, RVT, RPVI
Professor, Department of Surgery
University of California, Davis
UC Davis Vascular Center
Sacramento, California

David Del Pizzo, MHA, RVT
Chief Administrative Officer, Department of Radiology
University of California Davis Health System
Sacramento, California

Aaron Ebert, BS, RVT
Technical Director
Lake Washington Vascular Laboratories
Lake Washington Vascular Surgeons
Bellevue and Kirkland, Washington

Neal Futran, MD, DMD
Allison T. Wanamaker Professor and Chairman
Otolaryngology–Head and Neck Surgery
University of Washington School of Medicine
Seattle, Washington

Kathleen D. Gibson, MD
Lake Washington Vascular Surgeons
Bellevue and Kirkland, Washington

Holly M. Gray, BS, RVT
Senior Technologist, Vascular Laboratory
University of California Davis Health System
Sacramento, California

Jean Hadlock, BA, RVT (deceased)
Registered Vascular Technologist
D. E. Strandness Jr Vascular Laboratory
University of Washington Medical Center
Seattle, Washington

Ulrike M. Hamper, MD, MBA, FACR
Professor of Radiology, Urology and Pathology
Director, Division of Ultrasound
Russell H. Morgan Department of Radiology and
Radiological Science
The Johns Hopkins University, School of Medicine
Baltimore, Maryland

Nasim Hedayati, MD, RPVI
Assistant Professor, Department of Surgery
University of California, Davis
UC Davis Vascular Center
Sacramento, California

Kelley D. Hodgkiss-Harlow, MD, FACS
Clinical Assistant Professor of Surgery
Division of Vascular Surgery
Kaiser Permanente
San Diego, California

Misty Humphries, MD, RPVI
Assistant Professor, Department of Surgery
University of California, Davis
UC Davis Vascular Center
Sacramento, California

Ted R. Kohler, MD
Professor of Surgery
University of Washington
Chief, Peripheral Vascular Surgery
Veterans Affairs Puget Sound Healthcare System
Seattle, Washington

Iftikhar J. Kullo, MD
Professor of Medicine
Division of Cardiovascular Diseases and the Gonda Vascular
Center
Mayo Clinic
Rochester, Minnesota

Eugene S. Lee, MD, PhD, RPVI
Associate Professor, Department of Surgery
University of California, Davis
Northern California VA Health Care System
Mather, California

Daniel F. Leotta, PhD
Center for Industrial and Medical Ultrasound
Applied Physics Laboratory
University of Washington
Seattle, Washington

Kevin Lindholm, BS, RVT
Ultrasound Technologist/Clinical Research Associate
UC Davis Vascular Center
Sacramento, California

Melissa Loja, MD, MAS, RPVI
Senior Resident, Vascular Surgery
University of California Davis Health System
UC Davis Vascular Center
Sacramento, California

K. H. Kevin Luk, MD, MS
Assistant Professor
Division of Critical Care Medicine and Division of
Neuroanesthesiology and Perioperative Neurosciences
Department of Anesthesiology and Pain Medicine
University of Washington
Seattle, Washington

Mark H. Meissner, MD
Professor of Surgery
Department of Surgery
University of Washington School of Medicine
Seattle, Washington

Erica L. Mitchell, MD, MEd, SE
Associate Professor of Surgery
Program Director for Vascular Surgery
Vice-Chair of Quality, Department of Surgery
Division of Vascular Surgery
Oregon Health & Science University
Portland, Oregon

Nahush A. Mokadam, MD
Lester and Connie LeRoss Endowed Professorship in
Cardiovascular Surgery
Assistant Professor of Surgery
Division of Cardiothoracic Surgery
University of Washington Medical Center
Seattle, Washington

Gregory L. Moneta, MD
Professor and Chief
Division of Vascular Surgery
Oregon Health & Science University
Portland, Oregon

Bridget A. Mraz, BS, RVT, RDMS
Registered Vascular Technologist
D. E. Strandness Jr Vascular Laboratory
University of Washington Medical Center
Seattle, Washington

Derek P. Nathan, MD
Fellow
Division of Vascular Surgery
Department of Surgery, University of Washington
Seattle, Washington

Richard P. Rand, MD
Northwest Center for Aesthetic Plastic Surgery
Bellevue, Washington

Sheila M. Byrd-Raynor, PhD, RVT
Gryon, Switzerland

Margarita V. Revzin, MS, MD
Assistant Professor of Diagnostic Radiology
Section of Emergency Medicine and Ultrasound
Yale University School of Medicine
New Haven, Connecticut

Edward Ronningen, BS, RVT
Technical Director, Vascular Laboratory
University of California Davis Health System
Sacramento, California

Claudia Rumwell, RN, RVT, FSVU
Consultant and Instructor, Vascular Ultrasound
Division of Vascular Surgery
Oregon Health & Science University
Portland, Oregon

Leslie M. Scoutt, MD, FACR
Professor of Diagnostic Radiology and Vascular Surgery
Yale School of Medicine
Chief, Ultrasound Section
Medical Director, Non-Invasive Vascular Laboratory
Associate Program Director, Diagnostic Radiology
Yale-New Haven Hospital
New Haven, Connecticut

Deepak Sharma, MBBS, MD, DM
Associate Professor of Anesthesiology and Pain Medicine
Chief, Division of Neuroanesthesiology and Perioperative
Neurosciences
Program Director, Neuroanesthesiology Fellowship
Neuroanesthesiology Education Director
Adjunct Associate Professor, Department of Neurological
Surgery
University of Washington
Seattle, Washington

Sara M. Skjonsberg, BS, RVT
Registered Vascular Technologist
D. E. Strandness Jr Vascular Laboratory
University of Washington Medical Center
Seattle, Washington

Watson B. Smith, BA, RDMS, RVT
Registered Vascular Technologist
D. E. Strandness Jr Vascular Laboratory
University of Washington Medical Center
Seattle, Washington

Hjalti Thorisson, MD
Assistant Professor of Radiology, School of Medicine,
University of Iceland
Reykjavik, Iceland
Assistant Clinical Professor (adjunct), Yale School of Medicine
New Haven, Connecticut
Vascular and Interventional Radiologist, University Hospital
of Iceland and Röntgen Domus
Reykjavik, Iceland

Molly Zaccardi, MHA, RVT
Health Services Manager
D. E. Strandness Jr Vascular Laboratory
University of Washington Medical Center
Seattle, Washington

R. Eugene Zierler, MD, RPVI
Professor of Surgery
University of Washington School of Medicine
Medical Director, D. E. Strandness Jr Vascular Laboratory
University of Washington Medical Center and Harborview
Medical Center
Seattle, Washington

Robert M. Zwolak, MD, PhD
Professor of Surgery
Dartmouth Medical School
Section of Vascular Surgery
Dartmouth-Hitchcock Medical Center
Lebanon, New Hampshire

In order to properly treat disorders of the vascular system, it is necessary to make a correct diagnosis and precisely define the location and extent of involvement. The traditional history and physical examination are often followed by some form of angiography, which provides confirmation of the diagnosis and a precise delineation of the disease and its extent. This information is essential, particularly if some form of interventional therapy is planned. It is this approach that remains the mainstay of cardiovascular diagnosis.

While the invasive diagnostic methods provide important data, they do have serious drawbacks. They may produce discomfort to the patient and in some cases may be the cause of serious complications. More important, the information obtained tells us very little about the functional effects of the observed lesions. In addition, angiography is unable to provide information concerning the natural history of the disease. Due to the need for additional information, considerable effort has been expended in the development of suitable noninvasive methods that could provide both anatomic and functional information on the effects of vascular disorders. Most of the methods in current use do not provide precise information on the exact location and status of the disease. Nonetheless, the information on limb blood pressure and volume changes and flow has given us considerable insight as to how diseases of the vascular system affect function. The introduction of ultrasound as an imaging method and the employment of the Doppler principle to assess flow velocity began to change the field. While imaging and Doppler techniques have serious limitations when used separately, together the techniques overcome many problems. After the concept of duplex scanning was introduced in 1974, the entire field of noninvasive diagnosis took on new dimensions.

In one instrument—the ultrasonic duplex scanner—we now have the capability of examining every major artery and vein that is commonly affected by disease. This remarkable method is rapidly becoming the most commonly used diagnostic system in laboratories devoted to the study of vascular disease.

This book is a review of my approaches to the evaluation of vascular disease and the way in which duplex scanning plays a role in that evaluation. It is not intended to be an encyclopedia of past or present progress in the field. Since my experience has spanned the development and application of both the indirect and direct diagnostic methods, I am in a rather unique position to write on this subject. I was privileged to play a part in the development and testing of many of the methods in common use today. This is an exciting time for the physicians and technologists who work in this field. We not only have the ability to define vascular disease in more precise anatomic and physiologic terms, but we can also study the problem over time. It is no longer necessary to wonder if the treatment works; we can find out. In addition, the natural history of the diseases we treat can be studied for the first time.

This book will be of particular interest to vascular surgeons, radiologists, and those technologists who perform the tests. For residents and fellows with an interest in the vascular system, it should provide an overview of the diagnostic approaches that are available and are in use. While the views expressed are largely my own, I hope the content of this book will be of use to the reader.

D. Eugene Strandness Jr

Although it has only been a few years since the first edition, progress in the application of duplex scanning continues at a very rapid rate. Even though I am close to the laboratory, the technology, the technologists and the studies being done, I am continually amazed by what we can do. We provide services that are essential for proper patient care, and the laboratory is now accepted as the central place to have objective studies done.

As new information emerges about the role of vascular disease, our services will have to expand even further. For example, the clinical trials that have examined the place of carotid endarterectomy have shown how important the detection and grading of carotid artery stenosis can be. The vascular diagnostic service now has a clear mandate to provide the necessary screening tests for those patients who will need to proceed with arteriography and operation.

There have been concerns that duplex scanning may not be an accurate enough screening procedure, forcing the physician to resort to arteriography in selecting the patients who might be candidates for operation. This is not true, and it represents a step backward by subjecting patients to the hazards associated with this invasive procedure. Insisting on very high standards and quality control for our laboratories will allow us to maintain our standards and our important place in the medical community.

One step in this direction is the development of the Intersocietal Commission for the Voluntary Accreditation of Vascular Laboratories. This independent organization, supported by the major medical groups interested in ultrasound, is establishing guidelines for practice and performance that should go a long way in addressing concerns about our role.

The path to the future is very clear for all of us. The role of duplex scanning continues to increase. While there are other modalities in place that might be of value in this field, none of them can begin to satisfy or replace duplex scanning. This is the only technique that can be applied as frequently as necessary to monitor change. This is a very important point to understand.

D. Eugene Strandness Jr

This third edition has been considerably expanded to include the words and practice of my technologists at the University of Washington. Although my chapters relating to the applications of duplex scanning methods cover much of the background and progress in the field, I believe we all realize that this progress is only possible because of the technologists' excellent efforts. Just as a good surgical scrub nurse should hand the surgeon the correct instruments, the technologist must give the correct information to the referring physician. This is being accomplished in my laboratory because of the devotion of my technologists. I have often commented on the extraordinary role they play in our health care system. In fact, I cannot think of anyone not possessing a medical degree who has the same amount of responsibility to the patient, whose welfare and often whose outcome from an illness depend on the accuracy of the studies being done. This enormous responsibility is handled well by our technologists who willingly spend the necessary time to get the studies done accurately.

Progress continues on several fronts as evidenced by the new material in this book. Duplex scanning continues to make inroads on invasive tests, which, as will be shown, are now often avoided entirely, even to the point of taking the patient to the operating room on the basis of duplex scanning alone. This has been one of the major accomplishments in my lifetime and something only dreamed of when I started in this business.

Another major advance is the information that we can provide the patient. We no longer have to answer "I don't know" to a lot of questions. For example, based entirely on the long-term studies done with duplex scanning, we can now counsel patients on the risk of stroke depending on the degree of involvement found. We can tell them what the risk of stroke is likely to be and how often we should monitor the status of their disease. It is remarkable that in 1984, we knew—based on follow-up duplex studies—that a greater than 80% stenosis of the carotid bulb was particularly dangerous. The skeptics did not trust the data, but, 17 years later, they have to admit that the studies done with duplex in the long term turned out to be correct!

We are moving forward in many areas as evidenced by this volume. I hope that the detailed information provided by the technologists will complement my contributions and make this a useful bible for the vascular laboratory. Watching the technology grow and the technologists mature with these advances has been a great experience. What of the future? It is clear that quantitative three-dimensional imaging is going to play a key role in many areas. For example, with the advent of endovascular grafting of aortic aneurysms, the need for inexpensive long-term quantitative studies of outcome are essential. The need for this is obvious given the reports of spontaneous rupture in patients who were thought to have been successfully treated. We now have the capability of evaluating many aspects of these grafts and the changes that occur, not only with the grafts themselves but with the native aorta as well. The future will indeed be exciting for this field.

D. Eugene Strandness Jr

The first edition of *Duplex Scanning in Vascular Disorders* was written entirely by Dr. D. Eugene Strandness Jr, and was published in 1990. That book presented Dr. Strandness's personal approach to the diagnosis and follow-up of vascular disease, emphasizing the critical role of the vascular laboratory in providing both anatomic and physiologic information that could be applied in the clinical setting. This was the rationale for the original duplex concept of combining the ultrasound modalities of B-mode imaging and Doppler flow detection in a single instrument. Dr. Strandness spent his entire career at the University of Washington in Seattle, joining the faculty in 1962. His professional life spanned the development of the vascular laboratory from the first indirect physiologic techniques for evaluation of vascular disease to modern duplex scanning. Many of the diagnostic protocols and criteria that are in widespread use today, as well as numerous clinical research studies that have expanded the applications of duplex scanning, are products of the Strandness laboratory. In addition, Dr. Strandness trained many generations of vascular surgery fellows, scientists, and vascular technologists.

By the time the third edition of this book was published in 2002, duplex scanning was firmly established as a primary diagnostic method for carotid and peripheral artery disease, visceral vascular problems, and venous disorders. Duplex scanning had also been applied extensively to the follow-up of vascular interventions and studies on the natural history of various vascular disorders. Major clinical decisions were routinely being made based on the results of duplex scanning alone. The third edition was written by Dr. Strandness and the vascular technologists in his laboratory at the University of Washington. That book covered both the clinical applications and the techniques of duplex scanning—with Dr. Strandness providing the clinical chapters and the technologists writing separate chapters on the various technical scanning protocols. Dr. Strandness died on January 7, 2002, at the age of 73, just as the third edition was being published.

This new fourth edition, now titled *Strandness's Duplex Scanning in Vascular Disorders*, continues the tradition that Dr. Strandness initiated with the first three editions. Although this edition is expanded and reorganized, an effort has been made to preserve the character and focus of the earlier editions. This required the involvement of both physicians and vascular technologists, along with engineers, nurses, and others with expertise related to the vascular laboratory. Rather than divide the material into clinical and technical chapters, the topics have now been combined into single chapters organized by testing area. This provides in-depth and integrated discussions of clinical applications, diagnostic criteria, and technical protocols. In addition to the traditional applications of duplex scanning, there is coverage of specialized applications such as assessment of aortic endografts, follow-up of carotid and peripheral artery stents, and the role of duplex scanning in dialysis access procedures. There is also a background section on reporting, regulatory issues, and quality assurance, and a section that covers basic vascular physiology and physical principles of ultrasound. This book should serve as a resource for vascular surgeons, cardiologists, vascular medicine specialists, radiologists, vascular technologists, and other health care providers with an interest in the vascular laboratory.

Most of the chapter authors for this fourth edition are former trainees and colleagues of Dr. Strandness, and many of the chapters are the result of collaboration between physicians and technologists. Having worked with Dr. Strandness over the last 24 years of his life, I am certain he would agree on the importance of such collaborations. He often pointed out the extraordinary role that vascular technologists play in patient care and the high degree of responsibility they assume. It is my hope that this new edition will help preserve the legacy of Dr. Strandness and pass it on to future generations of vascular specialists.

R. Eugene Zierler
Seattle, Washington

Since the publication of the fourth edition of *Strandness's Duplex Scanning in Vascular Disorders* in 2010, vascular ultrasound has continued to grow and evolve with new applications, advances in instrumentation, and increasing numbers of sonographers and physicians dedicated to this field. Contrary to speculation that other diagnostic modalities—such as computed tomography and magnetic resonance imaging—would decrease the need for vascular laboratory services, the utilization of duplex ultrasound has actually increased, and the vascular laboratory remains firmly established as an important component of both vascular specialty practice and general medical care. The changes that are driving this growth are reflected in this updated fifth edition of the textbook originally written by Dr. D. Eugene Strandness Jr and first published in 1990.

Recent developments in vascular interventions, particularly endovascular techniques, have created challenges for sonographers and physicians with an interest in noninvasive vascular testing. These are covered in revised chapters on *Follow-up after Carotid Endarterectomy and Stenting*, *Follow-up after Peripheral Artery Angioplasty and Stenting*, and *Duplex Assessment of Aortic Endografts*. There has been renewed interest in interventions for venous disease, as reflected in an updated chapter on *Venous Ablation Procedures* and a new chapter on *Pelvic Venous Insufficiency*. New chapters have also been added on specialized aspects of vascular testing, including *Cardiovascular Risk Assessment in the Vascular Laboratory* and *Intravascular Imaging*. The expansion of ultrasound practice beyond the traditional dedicated diagnostic laboratory setting is discussed in a new chapter on *Vascular Applications in Point of Care Ultrasound*.

The growth in vascular sonography has prompted an increased emphasis on regulatory issues involving both personnel and facilities. The importance of standards for physicians who interpret vascular laboratory tests was highlighted in 2014 when the Vascular Surgery Board of the American Board of Surgery made the Registered Physician in Vascular Interpretation (RPVI) credential administered by the American Registry for Diagnostic Medical Sonography (ARDMS) a requirement for certification in Vascular Surgery. The Standards and Guidelines for accreditation of vascular testing facilities are updated regularly by the Intersocietal Accreditation Commission (IAC) Vascular Testing, and it is anticipated that by January 2017, all technical staff will be required to have an appropriate credential in vascular testing. These regulatory issues are covered in an updated chapter on *Credentialing and Accreditation*.

In addition to standards for personnel and facilities, the prominent role of the vascular laboratory in clinical practice has created a need for standards that can be applied to educational programs in vascular sonography and test interpretation. A new section on *Vascular Laboratory Education and Training* has been added as an Appendix, along with a detailed list of *Vascular Laboratory Testing Protocols*. With this additional material, the fifth edition can serve as the basis for a comprehensive vascular laboratory curriculum. It provides learners with specific *knowledge* in three domains: (1) patient and disease states; (2) physics and instrumentation; and (3) examination protocols and interpretation criteria. With this foundational knowledge, the vascular laboratory physician learns to provide a *patient care* service by interpreting vascular laboratory studies, ideally with the vascular laboratory organized to promote information exchange between technologists and physicians, as well as effective *communication* of the findings to the requesting provider. Other core competencies of *practice-based learning and improvement*, *professionalism*, and *systems-based practice* are addressed in the chapter on *Quality Assurance and Test Validation* and other chapters throughout the book.

The revised and new chapters in this fifth edition of *Strandness's Duplex Scanning in Vascular Disorders* maintain the general format of the fourth edition with a focus on the indications, techniques, interpretation, and applications of duplex scanning and other testing methods used in the vascular laboratory. Many chapters are again coauthored by physicians and vascular technologists in order to provide more integrated coverage of a particular topic, and the chapters are organized according to the major testing areas. Finally, since many of the chapter authors are former trainees and colleagues of Dr. Strandness, it is our hope that this fifth edition will continue Dr. Strandness's legacy and exemplify his spirit of innovation, investigation, collaboration, and dedication to patient care.

R. Eugene Zierler
Seattle, Washington

David L. Dawson
Sacramento, California

CONTENTS

SECTION I ■ LABORATORY ORGANIZATION

CHAPTER 1 ■ THE DIAGNOSTIC APPROACH TO THE VASCULAR PATIENT

KIM CANTWELL-GAB AND R. EUGENE ZIERLER

Dr. D. Eugene Strandness Jr, fondly referred to as "DES" (according to his initials and pronounced "dezz") by many who knew him, loved to teach about vascular disease. He believed in the traditional diagnostic process of beginning with a detailed history and complete physical examination and then choosing the physiologic or imaging tests that are best suited to answer the key clinical questions. There were many times when he would emerge from an examination room looking for surgery residents or medical students so he could show them something unique or interesting about the patient he was seeing. However, he did not limit his teaching to the residents and medical students; the vascular technologists and nurses were also important members of his team, and even the patient was often an active participant.

Patients loved Dr. Strandness and the personal interactions they had with him. We were fortunate to work alongside Dr. Strandness over many years in the vascular surgery clinic, the operating room, and on research projects, and he had a knack for remembering every patient's name and something personal about them. He would say, "Listen to your patients. At least 90% of your diagnosis is based on the history and physical examination. The other 10% depends on diagnostic tests." In this chapter, we discuss Dr. Strandness' approach to obtaining a patient's history and how he performed a vascular physical examination. In addition, we will include a few of his patient stories, because those are what many students, residents, fellows, and technologists fondly remember about their training with Dr. Strandness. The various diagnostic studies performed in each vascular testing area are covered in subsequent chapters.

Dr. Strandness was always quick to point out that patients traditionally enter the health care system only when their symptoms become significant enough for them to seek medical advice. Before performing any vascular laboratory tests, it is important to review the patient's presenting symptoms and risk factors and include that information with the request for diagnostic studies. This is important because it provides a specific indication for the test being done and assists the vascular technologist in determining the most appropriate diagnostic test to answer the clinical questions and establish a diagnosis.

PERIPHERAL ARTERIAL DISEASE

Atherosclerosis is a systemic disease that involves multiple arterial territories in the body, so the risk factors are generally the same regardless of where and how it presents. Atherosclerosis is also the most common cause of arterial disease of the lower extremities, and a variety of symptoms can occur depending upon the site and severity of the arterial lesions.[1] Peripheral arterial disease has been observed in 12% to 20% of the population, and the disorder affects men and women equally.[2] Well-known risk factors such as smoking, diabetes, hyperlipidemia, hypertension, and family history increase the incidence of the disease.[3] It is not entirely clear whether modification of these risk factors prevents the development of cardiovascular disease, but there is evidence that it may slow disease progression.[4]

The use of tobacco products appears to be one of the most important risk factors for the development of lower extremity atherosclerotic lesions. The amount of tobacco used is directly related to the extent of the disease, and cessation of tobacco use reduces the overall risk. Many other factors such as obesity, stress, and lack of exercise have been identified as contributing to the process.[5] C-reactive protein (CRP) is a sensitive marker of cardiovascular inflammation, both systemically and locally. Slight increases in serum CRP levels are associated with an increased risk of damage to the vasculature, especially if these increases are accompanied by other risk factors such as advanced age, hypertension, hypercholesterolemia, obesity, elevated blood glucose levels, smoking, or a positive history of cardiovascular disease.[6] Selvin and Erlinger[7] reported that 95% of the 2174 participants aged 40 years and older in the National Health and Nutrition Examination Survey had at least one or more cardiovascular risk factors out of a selected 15 traditional risk factors.

Arteries can become damaged or obstructed as a result of atherosclerotic plaque, thromboemboli, chemical or mechanical trauma, infections or inflammatory processes, vasospastic disorders, and congenital malformations. A sudden arterial occlusion typically causes profound and often irreversible tissue ischemia and tissue death. However, when arterial occlusions develop gradually, there is less risk of sudden tissue death because collateral circulation has time to develop and the tissues can adapt to the decreased blood flow.

Arterial Embolism and Thrombosis

Arterial emboli arise most commonly from thrombi that originate in the chambers of the heart as a result of atrial fibrillation, myocardial infarction, infective endocarditis, or chronic heart failure. When these thrombi become detached, they are carried from the left side of the heart into the arterial system where they lodge in and obstruct an artery that is smaller than the embolus. Emboli may also originate at sites of advanced aortic atherosclerosis when the atheromatous plaques become irregular or ulcerate.

The symptoms associated with arterial emboli depend primarily on the size of the embolus, the organ or tissue involved, and the state of the collateral vessels. The immediate effect is cessation of distal blood flow. Secondary vasospasm can contribute to the ischemia. The embolus can fragment or break apart, resulting in occlusion of more distal vessels. Emboli tend to lodge at arterial bifurcations and areas narrowed by atherosclerosis. Cerebral, mesenteric, renal, and coronary arteries can be involved in addition to the large arteries of the extremities.

Arterial thrombosis can also acutely occlude an artery. Acute arterial thrombosis frequently occurs in patients with preexisting symptoms of chronic ischemia. Thrombi often originate where the arterial wall has become damaged, generally as a result of atherosclerosis, but they can also develop where flow is relatively stagnant, such as in an arterial aneurysm. The manifestations of an acute thrombotic arterial occlusion are similar to those for embolic occlusion.

The signs and symptoms associated with an ischemic limb are usually described in terms of the six "Ps": pain, pallor, paresthesias, poikilothermia, pulselessness, and paralysis. Dr. Strandness also liked to add another "P" for the physician (although today he might use the term "provider" instead) who is the critical person in appreciating the significance of the presenting complaints. The symptoms of acute arterial occlusion in extremities with poor collateral flow are sudden severe pain and a gradual loss of sensory and motor function. Eventually, superficial veins may collapse because of decreased blood flow to the extremity. With severe ischemia, the part of the extremity distal to the occlusion is markedly colder and paler than the part proximal to the occlusion.

If the pain persists, it can be interpreted as a favorable sign, indicating that the nerves supplying the distal limb are still functioning. If the distal extremity is completely numb, the blood supply must be restored expeditiously if the nerves and other tissues are to survive. Dr. Strandness would emphasize to his students that the limb dies from the inside out—the nerves, then the muscles, and finally the skin. If it is suspected that the patient has limb-threatening ischemia, a prompt vascular consultation should be arranged, and diagnostic testing must be done without delaying the patient's trip to the interventional suite or operating room for definitive treatment.

Pulse deficits are invariably present in patients with embolism or thrombosis of major extremity arteries, with one important exception: when there have been extensive microemboli to the distal foot or hand. In this circumstance, the major arteries are usually patent and serve as conduits for the small atheroemboli that typically arise from ulcerated plaques or areas of thrombosis at some point proximal to the foot and toes (Figs. 1.1 and 1.2). Major pulse deficits provide information only on the most proximal site of occlusion; they provide no information on the possible distal extension of the thrombotic process.

A detailed history with regard to symptoms before the acute event is important. If the patient gives a history of

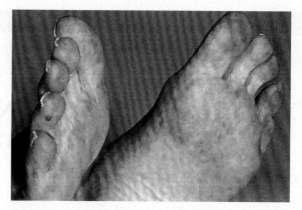

FIGURE 1.1. When patients develop microemboli that pass down to the plantar and digital arteries, the appearance of the foot may be a useful clue to the underlying process. This patient had embolized cholesterol crystals from ulcerated plaques to both feet. He presented with pain, coolness, and this very prominent livedo reticularis pattern of skin mottling. Transmetatarsal amputations were required to control the pain. The cholesterol crystals were seen by polarized light and were the cause of the arterial occlusion and ischemia.

intermittent claudication, this is evidence that the patient has chronic arterial occlusive disease, with the current acute episode representing a thrombosis in the region of a preexisting high-grade stenosis. In the course of the physical examination, look for the presence of an aortic, femoral, or popliteal artery aneurysm that could be the source of emboli or thrombosis as a cause of acute limb ischemia.

In patients who have palpable pulses to the level of the foot and appear to have microemboli as the cause of ischemia, listen for bruits from the level of the abdominal aorta to the popliteal fossa. Very few providers regularly listen over the superficial femoral and popliteal arteries for bruits, and Dr. Strandness would insist that this part of the physical examination be included in patients with suspected microemboli. The presence of a bruit indicates turbulent blood flow and a possible site of stenosis. Dr. Strandness told his residents that bruits are transmitted downstream from their site of origin, not upstream; "they go with the flow" was what he would say. Use a continuous wave (CW) Doppler to determine whether audible arterial flow is present in the tibial arteries. Dr. Strandness also considered ankle pressure measurement and calculation of the ankle-brachial index to be part of the routine vascular physical examination. He would often take

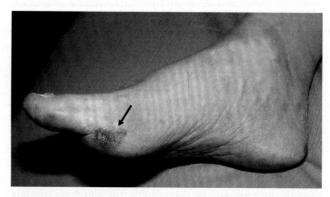

FIGURE 1.2. A focal area of skin infarction (*black arrow*) on the first metatarsal head caused by a small atheroembolus.

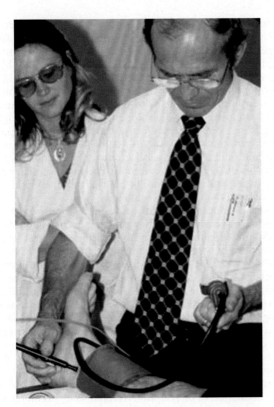

FIGURE 1.3. Dr. Strandness measuring an ankle pressure in the 1960s.

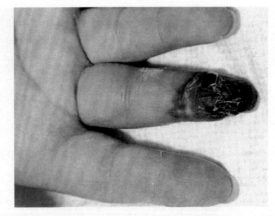

FIGURE 1.4. Patients with scleroderma may develop gangrene of the fingers. This is a result of thrombosis and occlusion of the digital arteries.

the time to perform this simple test himself, even when a vascular technologist was available (Fig. 1.3).

The causes of acute ischemia in the upper extremity are similar to those found in the lower extremity, but some differences can be noted. Atherosclerosis of the arteries supplying the arm tends to involve only the innominate artery and the first part of the subclavian artery. Thus, acute ischemia secondary to thrombosis of an atherosclerotic plaque is very unusual. The principal cause of acute upper extremity ischemia is emboli, which most often arise from the heart. An infrequent source of emboli is a lesion in the subclavian artery at the thoracic outlet. Chronic compression of the subclavian artery at that site can lead to intimal damage with subsequent thrombosis and release of emboli. These events typically occur in younger patients who are in good health. Therefore, in any patient who suddenly develops acute ischemia of the hand, suspect damage to the subclavian artery from repeated compression.

Other causes of acute hand ischemia are to be found among those disorders that include vasospasm, such as Raynaud's syndrome, Buerger's disease, scleroderma, and mixed connective tissue disorders, as discussed later in this chapter. Although vasospasm is usually a chronic problem, there are cases in which thrombosis of the digital and palmar arteries can lead to acute ischemia and gangrene. Dr. Strandness was known for his expertise in dealing with primary and secondary vasospastic disorders, and the most common underlying condition in his experience that was associated with this problem was scleroderma (Fig. 1.4). Many of the principles relating to the evaluation of acute ischemia of the hands are similar to those employed for the lower limb (see Chapters 12, 13, and 14).

Chronic Arterial Occlusion

The classic symptom of chronic peripheral arterial disease is intermittent claudication. This crampy muscular pain may be described by the patient as aching, fatigue, weakness, or even

numbness in the extremity. However, the key feature of claudication is that it is consistently produced by the same intensity of leg exercise or activity and relieved with a few minutes of rest. It may gradually improve or get worse over months and years, but it is relatively constant from day to day. The symptoms are caused by the inability of the diseased arteries and collateral vessels to provide adequate blood flow to the tissues in the face of increased demands for nutrients and oxygen during exercise. The sites of the responsible arterial lesions can be deduced from the location of claudication because the symptoms occur in muscle groups distal to the occlusive disease. As the arterial lesions progress, patients may notice that their comfortable walking distance is shorter, or they may experience increased pain with ambulation. McLafferty and coworkers[8] found that 50% to 70% of patients over 70 years of age with claudication perceived their discomfort to be a normal part of aging and did not report the symptoms to their providers.

Patients with unusual or atypical leg pain are commonly referred to a vascular specialist and the vascular laboratory for evaluation. These patients are often considered to have "pseudoclaudication" if no evidence of significant arterial occlusive disease is found. The most common nonvascular conditions responsible for such a presentation are neurospinal and orthopedic problems. The patient with pseudoclaudication frequently describes a walk-pain cycle that is not constant from day to day, for example, being able to walk a mile one day but limited to a few blocks the next day. In addition, the pain may be brought on by standing or sitting for prolonged periods of time, or the patient may have to lie down to obtain complete relief.

When arterial insufficiency becomes severe, the patient may have persistent pain in the distal foot and toes at rest. This "rest pain" indicates a critical state of ischemia, because it signifies that the tissue blood supply is inadequate at all times, not just during limb exercise. Rest pain is often worse at night and may interfere with sleep. Placing the limb in a dependent position typically reduces rest pain by producing a modest increase in distal limb blood flow. Changes resulting from chronic severe ischemia that can be noted on physical examination include loss of hair, brittle nails, dry or scaling skin, muscle atrophy, and ulcerations. Lower extremity edema may be apparent bilaterally or unilaterally and is usually caused by prolonged periods of dependency related to ischemic rest pain. Gangrenous changes or tissue necrosis appear after prolonged severe ischemia. In elderly patients who are inactive, gangrene may be the first sign of arterial occlusive disease (Fig. 1.5). These patients may have adjusted their lifestyle

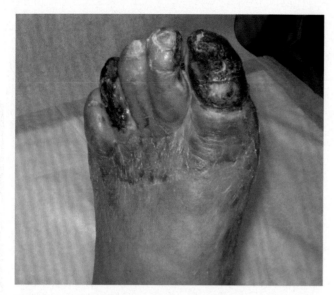

FIGURE 1.5. Necrosis or gangrene of several toes due to severe arterial occlusive disease in an elderly nonambulatory patient.

to accommodate the limitations imposed by their disease and may never walk far enough to develop symptoms of claudication. Although their circulation is severely impaired, this is not apparent until ulceration develops.

Arterial occlusive disease can reduce or obliterate pulsations in the extremities. The level of pulse deficit is a good marker for the most proximal level of involvement. Palpate pulses bilaterally and simultaneously, if possible, comparing both sides for symmetry in rate, rhythm, and quality. Palpation of pulses is subjective, and the examiner may mistake their own pulse for that of the patient. To prevent this, the examiner should apply light pressure and avoid using only the index finger for palpation because this finger has the strongest arterial pulsation of all the fingers. The thumb also has a strong intrinsic pulsation and should not be used for pulse palpation.

Dr. Strandness was insistent that all vascular patients should have a thorough evaluation of their feet for trophic changes, especially for evidence of emboli or ulcerations. One of Dr. Strandness' favorite stories was about a medical student who had been in to see a patient who had been followed for years in the clinic. The medical student gave his presentation and stated that the patient had normal lower extremity pulses bilaterally. Dr. Strandness did not say a word but went into the examination room with the medical student and pulled up the gentleman's trousers, noting that the patient still had his socks and shoes on, and asked the student how he was able to palpate pulses through the shoes. The next thing he did was ask the patient to remove his below-knee prosthetic limb so he could assess the patient's stump site. Dr. Strandness did not tell this story to make fun of the student (which the student clearly deserved), but rather to emphasize that all patients must have their socks and shoes removed for the physical examination.

Chronic arterial occlusive disease occurs less frequently in the upper extremities than in the lower extremities and causes less severe symptoms because the collateral circulation tends to be significantly better in the arms. The arms also have less muscle mass and are not subjected to the same heavy workload as the legs. As previously mentioned, upper extremity atherosclerotic lesions typically occur proximal to the origin of the vertebral artery, setting up the vertebral artery as a major contributor to collateral flow. When upper extremity arterial occlusive disease is symptomatic, the patient complains of arm fatigue and pain with exercise (arm claudication)

and inability to hold or grasp objects (e.g., painting, combing hair, using hand tools, placing objects on shelves above the head, and occasionally difficulty driving). Dr. Strandness would stress to the vascular technologists that they should ask the patient about the specific activities that produced his or her symptoms and try to perform an evaluation under similar conditions. Many patients with symptomatic upper extremity arterial occlusive disease do not present with classic claudication. This condition may cause vertebrobasilar symptoms such as vertigo, ataxia, syncope, or bilateral visual changes. Significant findings on physical examination include coolness and pallor of the affected extremity, decreased capillary refill of the digits, and a difference in brachial systolic blood pressures of more than 10 to 15 mm Hg.

One of Dr. Strandness' patients was a minister from a rural area who drove many miles daily visiting his parishioners. He initially presented to vascular surgery clinic for treatment of uncontrolled hypertension and renal artery stenosis. Once his renal artery disease had been treated and his blood pressure was under control, he began noticing that when driving and turning his head side to side he would become dizzy, and if he tilted his head, he developed severe vertigo. Duplex ultrasound evaluation showed that he had bilateral carotid artery disease and a subclavian artery occlusion. Physiologic noninvasive testing revealed that his upper extremity was stealing from his vertebrobasilar system when he drove long distances. What was most interesting about this patient was that when he was hypertensive, he appeared to have enough perfusion to his posterior circulation to be symptom free, but when his blood pressure was lowered to normal levels, he became symptomatic.

VASOSPASM

Patients who develop digital ischemia when their hands or feet are exposed to cold are often sent to the vascular laboratory for evaluation. This presentation is referred to as *Raynaud's syndrome* and can be divided into primary *Raynaud's phenomenon* and secondary *Raynaud's disease*. Raynaud's phenomenon is a common clinical disorder characterized by intermittent episodes of vasoconstriction of the small arteries of the hands and feet that cause dramatic color and temperature changes. Patients with Raynaud's phenomenon have a young age of onset (usually <30 years), and the episodes are associated with minimal pain and typically involve all digits in a bilateral and symmetrical fashion. In this primary benign form, the palmar and digital arteries remain patent without any demonstrable structural abnormalities. Epidemiologic studies indicate that the prevalence of Raynaud's phenomenon is between 6% and 20% in women and 3% and 13% in men. There is also a possible genetic susceptibility to the condition.[9]

By contrast, patients with Raynaud's disease have asymmetrical digit involvement and intense pain related to an underlying pathologic condition (Fig. 1.6). This secondary form is more serious because it is associated with intrinsic occlusive lesions in the digital arteries and a long list of systemic diseases, of which the collagen-vascular diseases are the most common. Secondary Raynaud's disease can also occur in the setting of arterial occlusions proximal to the wrist, hematologic syndromes, infectious diseases, and in patients with repetitive trauma from vibrating tools or anatomic abnormalities such as a cervical rib. Raynaud's disease is a form of intermittent arteriolar vasoconstriction that results in coldness, pain, and pallor of the fingertips or toes. Symptoms may result from a defect in basal heat production that eventually decreases the ability of cutaneous vessels to dilate. Episodes may be triggered by emotional factors or unusual sensitivity to cold.

The classic clinical picture consists of three phases and begins with pallor of the fingers or toes brought on by sudden

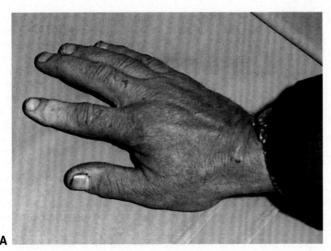
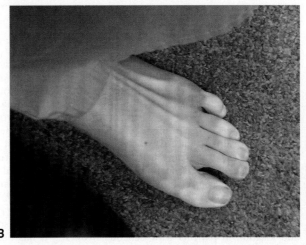

FIGURE 1.6. (*A*) This patient had secondary Raynaud's disease with digital artery occlusion and ischemia confined to the index finger of the right hand. (*B*) Another patient with Raynaud's disease and pallor involving the toes.

intense vasoconstriction. The skin then becomes bluish (cyanotic) due to pooling of deoxygenated blood in the tissues. The final phase occurs as vasospasm resolves and the small arteries vasodilate, producing a hyperemic state. This results in a reddish color (rubor) as oxygenated blood returns to the digits. The characteristic sequence of color changes in cold sensitivity of the Raynaud type is described as "*pallor*, *cyanosis*, and *rubor*" or "white, blue, and red." Numbness, tingling, and burning pain may occur as the colors change. The primary role of the vascular laboratory is to determine the anatomic status of the circulation to the digits and assess their response to cold exposure (see Chapter 14). The physical examination is usually not helpful unless digit ulceration is noted.

Buerger's disease is one of the systemic disorders associated with the development of cold sensitivity and vasospasm. It is regarded as an autoimmune vasculitis and occurs most often in men between 20 and 35 years of age. Considerable evidence indicates that heavy smoking or chewing of tobacco is a causative or aggravating factor.[10] The vasospastic manifestations of Buerger's disease are generally bilateral and symmetrical, with focal occlusive lesions in the small arteries. Pain is the outstanding symptom, and it is often aggravated by nicotine, cold exposure, or emotional disturbances.

ABDOMINAL AORTIC ANEURYSM

An aneurysm is a *permanent localized dilatation of an artery*. Symptoms are variable and depend on how rapidly the artery dilates and how the pulsating mass affects surrounding structures. Many patients are asymptomatic, and the aneurysm is found incidentally during a workup for some other problem. A history of smoking is the risk factor most strongly associated with an abdominal aortic aneurysm (AAA), but other factors such as having a first-degree relative with an AAA and having atherosclerosis are also independent risk factors.[11] Most aneurysms in the abdominal aorta occur below the level of the renal arteries. AAAs are more common among Caucasians, affecting men four to six times more often than women.[12] Some patients complain that they can feel their heart beating in their abdomen when lying down, or they may describe a "throbbing" feeling in their abdomen.

The most important diagnostic sign of an AAA is a palpable pulsatile mass in the epigastric area or upper abdomen. A systolic bruit may be auscultated over the mass. The physical examination should include palpation of the abdominal

aorta and the iliac, femoral, and popliteal arteries to determine whether there is a bounding pulse. As has been previously mentioned, if an AAA is present or suspected, evaluate the toes for evidence of embolization. When a small (3 to 4 cm in diameter) AAA is identified, serial ultrasound follow-up is often recommended at 6- to 12-month intervals until the aneurysm reaches a size at which intervention is justified—typically 5 to 6 cm in diameter. An aneurysm that shows rapid growth or becomes symptomatic warrants an urgent vascular consultation.

Aneurysms may also arise in the peripheral arteries. The most frequent site for peripheral aneurysms is the popliteal artery, but other arterial sites such as the subclavian, renal, or common femoral arteries can also be involved. Between 50% and 60% of popliteal aneurysms are bilateral and may be associated with AAAs. If a bounding popliteal pulse is palpated, perform a duplex ultrasound to rule out a popliteal artery aneurysm. Aortic and peripheral artery aneurysms are discussed further in Chapter 15, and point-of-care screening for AAA is covered in Chapter 27.

AORTIC DISSECTION

When an atherosclerotic aorta develops a tear in the intima or the media degenerates, a dissection may result. Arterial dissections are three times more frequent in men than in women and occur most commonly in the 50- to 70-year-old age group.[13] They are associated with poorly controlled hypertension, blunt chest trauma, and cocaine or methamphetamine use. A rupture may occur through the dissection flap back into the true lumen, allowing blood to reenter the main channel and resulting in a chronic dissection or causing occlusion of the branch arteries supplying the gastrointestinal tract, kidneys, spinal cord, or legs.

When aortic dissection occurs, onset of symptoms is usually sudden, with severe and persistent pain, often described as tearing or ripping. The location of the pain can include the anterior chest and shoulder region, interscapular area in the back, epigastric region, or abdomen, depending on the location and extent of the dissection. The patient may appear pale and sweaty, and tachycardia may be present. Blood pressure may be markedly different from one arm to the other if the dissection involves the orifice of the subclavian artery on one side. Because of the variable clinical picture associated with this condition, early diagnosis is usually difficult, and it may be mistaken for an acute myocardial infarction.

EXTRACRANIAL CEREBROVASCULAR DISEASE

In the United States, more than 790,000 strokes occur each year, of which about 185,000 are recurrent and 130,000 are fatal. One-quarter of the initial stroke survivors suffer a second stroke within 5 years.[14] Stroke remains the third most common cause of death in the Western world, with atheroembolism from the carotid artery accounting for as many as half of all these events. According to the Atherosclerosis Risk in Communities Study from the American Heart Association, approximately 83% of strokes are ischemic and 17% are hemorrhagic.[15] Most strokes occur in individuals older than 65 years, and women have 60,000 more strokes each year than men.[14] In the prospective Ischemic Stroke Genetics Study, there were no sex differences in stroke severity, stroke subtype, or infarct size and location in patients with ischemic strokes.[16] It has been shown that ethnic and racial minorities have an increased risk of stroke, and African Americans have almost twice as many strokes as Caucasians. African Americans of both sexes and women die at much higher rates than white men.[12]

Many risk factors for cerebrovascular disease are similar to those for atherosclerotic disease in other vascular territories; however, known coronary artery disease doubles stroke risk, and patients with atrial fibrillation have a risk five times greater. Hypertension (blood pressure >120/80 mm Hg) can double the lifetime risk of stroke.[14] Diabetes mellitus, or even prediabetes (impaired glucose tolerance), is an independent risk factor for an ischemic stroke or transient ischemic attack (TIA).[16] Additional risk factors associated with stroke are tobacco use, heavy alcohol consumption, hyperlipidemia, migraines, and pregnancy.[14,16]

Carotid atherosclerosis may reduce blood flow to the brain either by obstructing the lumen of the extracranial internal carotid artery or by embolizing to the intracranial arteries. The subtypes of arterial disease related to ischemic stroke are large-vessel disease, lacunar or small-vessel disease, and embolic stroke. In large-vessel disease, an atherosclerotic plaque can rupture, develop a thrombus, and give rise to an embolus that obstructs cerebral flow. Other large-vessel strokes may be caused by a severe stenosis or occlusion of the internal carotid artery, leading to ischemic injury downstream, also known as *watershed infarction*. Lacunar or small-vessel disease strokes usually involve small areas of infarction and have been associated with arteritis. Embolic strokes result from thrombi that form in the heart or elsewhere in the body, such as fat emboli related to long bone fractures or particulate emboli from intravenous drug abuse. In younger patients, strokes have also been attributed to arterial dissection, hypercoagulable states, sickle cell disease, and a patent foramen ovale (paradoxical embolism).[14]

Hemorrhagic strokes are associated with a higher mortality rate than ischemic strokes and are divided into two subtypes: intracranial hemorrhage and subarachnoid hemorrhage. Intracranial hemorrhage, defined as the presence of blood within the main cellular mass of the brain, accounts for 10% of all strokes and is associated with oral anticoagulant use and chronic hypertension. Subarachnoid hemorrhage accounts for 3% of all strokes and is more prevalent among middle-aged women, usually resulting from rupture of a cerebral aneurysm at a vessel bifurcation.[14] Headache, decreased level of consciousness, and vomiting are extremely common with hemorrhagic strokes. The Rotterdam study of over 4000 subjects followed for an average of 10 years found that a decreased glomerular filtration rate (GFR) was an independent risk factor for hemorrhagic but not for ischemic stroke.[17]

Strokes may be categorized by the vascular territory involved, with the common distributions being middle cerebral artery (MCA), anterior cerebral artery (ACA), posterior cerebral artery (PCA), brainstem, cerebellum, and strokes occurring in more than one vascular territory. Many providers simplify this scheme and refer to either anterior or posterior circulation strokes. Typical symptoms of an anterior circulation stroke include weakness, numbness, or tingling on one side of the body, expressive or receptive aphasia, transient monocular blindness (amaurosis fugax), and difficulty reading or writing. These symptoms generally originate in the MCA and ACA distributions. If a patient experiences double or blurred vision, vertigo that may or may not be positional, and syncopal episodes, the stroke is more likely to be related to the vertebrobasilar system or posterior circulation (PCA, brainstem, cerebellum). Light-headedness and dizziness are very nonspecific and, in the absence of other symptoms, cannot be attributed to carotid artery disease. One prospective study of over 2000 patients found that the most common stroke categories were MCA (50.8%) and small-vessel (12.8%) stroke.[18] This same study also found that patients with MCA and PCA strokes were older and those with strokes in multiple vascular beds were younger. The authors found no significant difference in the proportions of male to female patients with strokes in the various vascular territories.

Referrals to the vascular laboratory for a cerebrovascular duplex study include patients with neurologic symptoms, but many asymptomatic patients are referred after a bruit is found on physical examination. A bruit is only a sign that disease is present and cannot be used to determine the severity of the underlying arterial narrowing. Dr. Strandness was always quick to point out that a significant carotid stenosis can exist in the absence of a bruit. The physical examination should include evaluation of any neurologic deficit and palpation of carotid pulses to determine whether there is asymmetry, which would indicate a stenosis or occlusion. Auscultation should be done low in the neck, over the mid neck, and at the angle of the jaw to determine whether a carotid bruit is present. Auscultate the supraclavicular and infraclavicular spaces for bruits caused by lesions in the proximal aorta or the aortic arch branches. In addition, Dr. Strandness would stress the importance of listening for cardiac murmurs, especially if the symptoms suggested a possible embolic event. It is also important to measure the systolic blood pressure in both arms at the time the patient is first seen to determine whether subclavian steal syndrome is a possible diagnosis. In this setting, a high-grade stenosis or occlusion of one subclavian artery may result in reversal of flow in the ipsilateral vertebral artery, leading to posterior circulation symptoms. However, it must be pointed out that reversal of flow in the vertebral artery in and of itself is usually a benign finding.

RENOVASCULAR DISEASE

The clinical spectrum of chronic kidney disease (CKD) ranges from a mild decrease in GFR to end-stage renal failure. Stages of CKD are based on levels of estimated GFR, and most renal risk from atherosclerosis occurs at stage III CKD (estimated GFR <60 mL/min/1.73 m^2). It is estimated that renal artery stenosis is present in 2.1% of all new cases of end-stage renal failure.[12] Occlusive disease of the renal arteries may result in hypertension or ischemic nephropathy. Ischemic nephropathy is defined as a progressive decline in renal function secondary to global renal ischemia. CKD has effects that have been shown to harm the cardiovascular system, including inhibition of erythropoiesis and platelet function, induction of volume overload, dyslipidemia, hypertension, and vascular calcification.[17]

In evaluating claims data from over 1 million Medicare patients from 1999 to 2001, Kalra and colleagues[19] found that the prevalence of symptomatic atherosclerotic renovascular disease in the US Medicare population was approximately 0.5% overall and 5.5% in those with CKD. Since early 2000, atherosclerotic renovascular disease has been noted more commonly in older patients beginning dialysis therapy. The comorbid factors associated with a greater likelihood of atherosclerotic renovascular disease are peripheral arterial disease and atherosclerotic heart disease.[20] Other risk factors identified include hypertension, African American race, age older than 85 years, diabetes, obesity, excretory renal insufficiency, and low high-density lipoprotein (HDL) cholesterol level.[21] African American patients tend to develop end-stage renal failure a decade earlier than Caucasians and are less likely to have renal artery stenosis.[12]

As discussed in Chapter 24, the principal lesions associated with renal artery stenosis are atherosclerosis and fibromuscular dysplasia (FMD). Atherosclerotic lesions are usually ostial, involving the origin and proximal segments of the renal artery along with the adjacent aorta. Renal artery stenosis is present in approximately 5% to 10% of individuals aged 65 years or older, and the prevalence increases to 20% to 30% in high-risk subsets.[22] Atherosclerotic renal artery stenosis is a progressive disease that reduces blood flow to the kidneys and activates the renin-angiotensin-aldosterone system. This system preserves renal blood flow by the production of angiotensin II, resulting in renal arteriolar vasoconstriction and stimulation of sodium reabsorption, leading to increased blood flow through the kidney and maintenance of GFR.[23] Progression of renal artery disease leads to hypertension, renal dysfunction, and ultimately end-stage renal failure; it is most likely to occur in patients with preexisting high-grade renal artery stenosis, elevated systolic blood pressure, and diabetes mellitus.[24]

FMD is a nonatherosclerotic, noninflammatory arterial disease leading to segmental stenosis of the renal arteries. Three main types of FMD have been described: intimal, medial, and perimedial. The medial type is found in 85% of renal arteries with FMD.[25] The lesions tend to be multifocal with a "string-of-beads" appearance forming a long irregular stenosis. Unlike atherosclerotic lesions, stenoses due to FMD rarely affect the ostial or proximal segments of the renal artery but are typically found in the mid and distal segments, and they may involve the renal artery branches. In most series, FMD accounts for only 10% to 20% of renal artery lesions, with atherosclerosis being the most common cause of renal artery stenosis.[25] FMD is found mostly in women between 30 and 40 years of age, and it appears to have at least a partial genetic basis with an increased familial prevalence. Dr. Strandness had a special interest in renal artery FMD and followed three patients from the same family—two sisters and a brother—who all had this condition. The two sisters had renal, carotid, and mesenteric artery FMD, and the brother had renal and iliac artery involvement. He used these patients as teaching cases because the presence of FMD in more than one vascular territory is somewhat unusual, but he also considered them to be friends and loved to have them come into the clinic just to socialize.

The physical examination should include bilateral brachial stethoscope blood pressures to check for systolic and diastolic hypertension. Auscultation for midline abdominal or flank bruits should be part of every patient evaluation, especially if the patient presents with abrupt onset of flank pain, hematuria, or rapidly progressive hypertension, because there may be a renal artery dissection leading to renal infarction. Lower extremity edema, shortness of breath, or dyspnea on exertion may be indicative of volume overload due or congestive heart failure.

Reasons for referring a patient for a renovascular duplex evaluation include sudden onset of hypertension, abdominal bruits, uncontrolled hypertension in spite of a multiple drug antihypertensive regimen, sacral edema or bilateral lower extremity edema not relieved by diuretics, elevated creatinine, and acute azotemia during treatment with angiotensin-converting enzyme inhibitors. Labropoulos and associates[26] identified uncontrolled and controlled hypertension as the main reasons for referral to a university hospital vascular laboratory for renal duplex scanning.

MESENTERIC ARTERIAL DISEASE

Patients with a history of abdominal pain and weight loss may be referred to the vascular laboratory for evaluation of the mesenteric arteries. The finding of an abdominal bruit is another indication to examine the mesenteric arteries, along with the aorta and the renal and iliac arteries. It is commonly stated that symptoms of chronic mesenteric ischemia occur only when there is severe disease (>70% stenosis) in at least two of the three major mesenteric arteries (celiac, superior mesenteric, and inferior mesenteric). Furthermore, the superior mesenteric artery must be one of the involved vessels. The slow progression of atherosclerotic stenosis is such that collateral pathways usually have time to develop, so single-vessel mesenteric arterial disease rarely results in symptoms. In a population-based study using duplex ultrasound, 17.5% of a population over 65 years of age was found to have asymptomatic mesenteric artery stenosis.[27] However, if there is a sudden, complete occlusion of the superior mesenteric artery only, or if there is a superior mesenteric artery stenosis combined with previously interrupted collateral pathways, visceral ischemia may occur. In a retrospective study to identify factors affecting outcomes after surgical revascularization for chronic mesenteric ischemia, Mell and coworkers found that acute-on-chronic symptoms were present in 26% of patients. Presenting symptoms in these patients included postprandial pain (91%), weight loss (69%), and diarrhea (25%).[28]

The underlying pathophysiology of chronic mesenteric ischemia is failure to achieve hyperemic postprandial intestinal blood flow. In normal individuals, superior mesenteric artery blood flow increases after eating, with the maximum increase occurring at 30 to 90 minutes and the time interval to peak flow varying with the size and composition of the meal. Undiagnosed chronic mesenteric ischemia results in nutritional depletion. Dr. Strandness stressed to his students that you will never see an obese patient with symptomatic chronic mesenteric ischemia. In fact, he told us about a 350-pound woman who presented to the vascular surgery clinic for treatment of a celiac artery stenosis. The reason for referral was abdominal pain due to chronic mesenteric ischemia. While obtaining the history, the patient related to Dr. Strandness that she developed abdominal pain after eating large amounts of bacon and beans. She had not had any weight loss but had actually gained over 100 pounds in the previous 5 years.

The typical patient with symptomatic chronic mesenteric ischemia is a cachectic, middle-aged woman with a heavy smoking history who presents with postprandial abdominal pain and unintentional weight loss. The pain is usually located in the midepigastric region, occasionally radiates through to the back, and is often described as either dull or colicky. Postprandial pain can last from 1 to 3 hours and may be associated with nausea, vomiting, or diarrhea. Patients avoid certain types of food or almost stop eating altogether, resulting in weight loss. This specific behavior pattern is sometimes described as "food fear." In these patients, weight loss is due to inadequate nutritional intake rather than an absorption problem.

The Cardiovascular Health Study followed 533 participants for a mean of 6.5 years and found no statistically significant association between the presence of mesenteric artery stenosis and subsequent acute or chronic intestinal ischemia, gastrointestinal tract interventions, all-cause mortality, or cardiovascular events.[29] Duplex ultrasound is ideal for evaluating patients with an asymptomatic abdominal bruit, with median arcuate ligament compression of the celiac artery, or with suspected chronic mesenteric ischemia. However, it is less helpful in patients presenting with acute abdominal symptoms, because they are more likely to have technical limitations to abdominal ultrasound related to bowel gas. Mesenteric duplex scanning is discussed in Chapter 23.

VENOUS THROMBOSIS

Normal venous blood flow can be disrupted by a thrombus or thromboembolus obstructing the vein, incompetent venous valves, compression by adjacent structures, or a reduction in the effectiveness of the pumping action of the surrounding muscles. Decreased venous blood flow leads to increased venous pressure, a subsequent increase in capillary hydrostatic pressure, net filtration of fluid out of the capillaries into the interstitial space, and edema. Edematous tissues cannot receive adequate nutrition from the blood and, consequently, are more susceptible to injury, ulceration, and infection.

Lower extremity superficial veins, such as the great saphenous, are thick-walled vessels that lie just under the skin. Deep veins are thin walled and have a less muscular medial layer. As discussed in Chapter 6, normal deep and superficial veins have valves that maintain unidirectional flow back toward the heart. The valves are located at the base of a segment that is expanded into a sinus. This arrangement allows the valve leaflets to open without coming into contact with the wall of the vein, permitting rapid closure when the blood starts to flow backward. Perforating veins have valves that allow one-way blood flow from the superficial system to the deep system.

Three factors, known as *Virchow's triad*, are believed to play a significant role in the development of venous thrombosis, and these are stasis of blood, vessel wall injury, and altered blood coagulation. Venous stasis occurs when the flow rate is reduced and the blood remains in contact with the venous wall longer than normal. This happens in heart failure or shock and when skeletal muscle contraction is reduced, as in immobility, paralysis, or during anesthesia. Bedrest reduces blood flow in the legs by at least 50%.[1] Damage to the intimal lining of blood vessels creates a site for thrombus formation. Direct injury to the veins can result from fractures, blunt or penetrating trauma, and chemical irritation from intravenous medications. Increased blood coagulability occurs in patients who have had anticoagulant medications abruptly withdrawn and those with malignancies. Oral contraceptive use and a growing list of inherited conditions are also associated with hypercoagulability.

The annual incidence of deep vein thrombosis (DVT) is 1:10,000 but increases to 1:100 in patients over 70 years of age.[30] Upper extremity DVT accounts for approximately 4% of all cases of venous thromboembolic disease (see Chapter 20).[31] Exact figures for the annual number of deaths from pulmonary emboli are difficult to obtain because they come largely from autopsy statistics; however, autopsy series of hospitalized patients have shown that pulmonary embolism is the cause of 4% to 11% of deaths and only 1 in 4 of these patients had recent surgery.[32]

Risk factors for DVT have been studied in both surgical and medical patients. The Sirius study used a case-control design to assess clinical risk factors for DVT in outpatients, of whom 77.7% were medical patients. The factors that emerged as associated with DVT in the medical population are consistent with previous studies and include a history of venous thromboembolism, chronic venous insufficiency, heart failure, cancer, trauma, infectious diseases, pregnancy, and obesity. Immobilization, standing in one spot for more than 6 hours per day, long-distance travel, and a history of three or more pregnancies also emerged as factors associated with DVT.[32]

In general, upper extremity DVT is not as prevalent as lower extremity DVT. However, it is common in patients with central venous catheters and in those with an underlying disease that causes hypercoagulability such as cancer. Internal trauma to the veins may result from pacemaker leads, chemotherapy ports, dialysis catheters, or parenteral nutrition lines. Primary upper extremity DVT, which occurs in the absence of the aforementioned risk factors, has been found in approximately 30% of documented cases.[31] Martinelli and colleagues studied a series of patients with primary upper extremity DVT and found an adjusted odds ratio for upper extremity DVT of 6.2 for factor V Leiden, 5.0 for prothrombin G20210A, and 4.9 for anticoagulant protein deficiencies.[31] In women with factor V Leiden or prothrombin G20210A who were taking oral contraceptives, the odds ratio for upper extremity DVT increased to 13.6. In this same study, strenuous muscular effort with the affected arm was a common predisposing condition and was present in one-fourth of the patients.

Effort thrombosis is a disorder of the thoracic inlet in which chronic venous compression from repetitive overhead arm motion is thought to be the inciting factor leading to intimal damage and subsequent thrombosis. This is most likely to be seen in athletes such as swimmers, tennis players, and baseball pitchers. When subclavian-axillary vein thrombosis occurs, the arm becomes painful and swollen, and prominent superficial collateral veins may be visible over the shoulder area.[33] Dr. Strandness had numerous athletic patients with effort thrombosis. One such patient was an avid tennis player, a sport that Dr. Strandness also enjoyed and played several mornings every week before coming to the hospital. So it is not surprising that he found it extremely difficult to counsel the patient to give up a sport they both loved. However, the patient began taking golf lessons and found that it did not produce the same upper extremity discomfort caused by tennis. This patient eventually became as passionate about golf as he had been about tennis, and at each clinic visit, he would challenge Dr. Strandness to a game. It became quite the running argument between the two of them as to which sport required the most skill.

A major challenge associated with diagnosing lower extremity DVT is that the signs and symptoms are nonspecific. Despite this variability, clinical signs should always be investigated. Obstruction of the deep veins results in edema or swelling of the extremity because the outflow of venous blood is impeded. There may be limb discomfort, a feeling of heaviness, and functional impairment. In some instances, there may be an increase in the temperature of the limb, but this is extremely variable. Although Homans' sign (pain in the calf with passive dorsiflexion of the foot) has been used historically to assess for DVT, it is not a reliable or valid sign and has no clinical value in the diagnosis of lower extremity DVT. This was one of Dr. Strandness' pet peeves, and he made sure every medical student knew that most patients with leg symptoms from any cause will complain of pain when you sharply dorsiflex their foot. In only one situation is the clinical presentation, by itself, adequate to arrive at a diagnosis of lower extremity DVT. This is with iliofemoral venous thrombosis (phlegmasia cerulea dolens), which involves extensive thrombosis of the common iliac, external iliac, common femoral, and femoral veins (and sometimes, the inferior vena cava). When this occurs, the entire limb becomes acutely swollen and cyanotic with severe pain. No other disorder produces this dramatic clinical picture.

External compression of the left common iliac vein is frequently seen in the general population and can result in obstruction of venous outflow from the left leg and contribute to the development of DVT. When a patient presents with chronic left lower extremity edema, pain, varicosities, and acute DVT with no predisposing risk factors, external compression of the left common iliac vein may be present. This is known as May-Thurner syndrome or iliac compression syndrome and is due to the right common iliac artery compressing the left common iliac vein against the fifth lumbar vertebra, causing chronic injury and intimal fibrosis, spurs, and webs.[34]

Thrombosis of superficial veins produces pain, tenderness, redness, and warmth in the involved area—a condition referred to as *superficial thrombophlebitis*. These patients usually present with an erythematous, palpable cord. Dr. Strandness always emphasized the point that inflammation does not play a significant role in *deep* vein thrombosis, so the term "thrombophlebitis" should only be used to describe this combination of thrombosis and inflammation in the superficial veins. The risk of superficial venous thrombi becoming dislodged or fragmenting into clinically significant emboli is very low.

Postthrombotic Syndrome

One of every three to four patients with symptomatic lower extremity DVT will develop postthrombotic sequelae.[35] Chronic venous insufficiency can occur many years after an episode of venous thromboembolism, and up to 10% of patients develop leg ulcers.[36] In a population-based, case-control study in New Zealand, Walker and associates found that people with a history of DVT were almost three times more likely to have a leg ulcer and that the risk of developing a leg ulcer was more than twice as likely in people who were at high risk for venous thromboembolism.[36]

Venous insufficiency results from a combination of obstruction of the deep veins in the legs and reflux of blood through incompetent valves. This leads to failure of the calf musculovenous pump and ambulatory venous hypertension (see Chapters 6 and 21). Because the veins are relatively large, thin-walled structures, they distend readily when the venous pressure is elevated. In this state, the leaflets of the venous valves are stretched and prevented from closing completely, allowing reflux of blood back toward the periphery. This persistently elevated deep venous pressure eventually causes the signs and symptoms of the postthrombotic syndrome.

The clinical presentation may include brownish skin discoloration (hyperpigmentation), subcutaneous fibrosis (brawny induration), venous ectasia, pruritus, leg heaviness, and swelling. Severe cases can also show intractable edema and skin ulceration. The patient may be less symptomatic in the morning and more symptomatic in the evening after the legs have been dependent all day. The swelling always involves the ankle area

and may extend further up the limb, depending on the extent of the venous obstruction and valvular incompetence. However, if the edema also involves the dorsum of the foot, the clinical picture is more consistent with lymphedema. This is noteworthy because it is common to have patients referred to the vascular laboratory for venous studies when the underlying etiology is actually lymphatic obstruction. The region of hyperpigmentation is typically on the distal medial side of the calf and ankle, where the major perforating veins are found, but the ankle may be involved circumferentially (Fig. 1.7). The same pertains to the location of venous ulcers when they occur. The precise mechanism of venous stasis ulceration remains controversial, although it is generally accepted that chronic venous hypertension and incompetent perforating veins play a role.[37] Postthrombotic skin changes develop as a result of the rupture of small veins in the skin or extravasation of blood components through enlarged capillary pores. Red blood cells escape into the surrounding tissues and then break down, leaving brownish hemosiderin pigment. The skin becomes dry and cracked, and the subcutaneous tissues fibrose and atrophy. Venous ulcerations are typically large but shallow with irregular edges and located in the "gaiter area" of the medial or lateral malleoli (Fig. 1.8).

Studies have shown that well-fitting compression stockings decrease the incidence of mild to moderate postthrombotic symptoms from 47% to 20% and severe symptoms from 23% to 11%. In a randomized, controlled clinical trial of 180 consecutive patients with a first episode of symptomatic lower extremity DVT, over-the-counter 30- to 40-mm Hg below-knee compression stockings reduced the rate of postthrombotic sequelae by approximately 50%.[35]

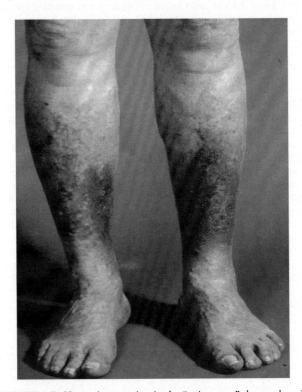

FIGURE 1.7. Hyperpigmentation in the "gaiter area" due to chronic venous insufficiency.

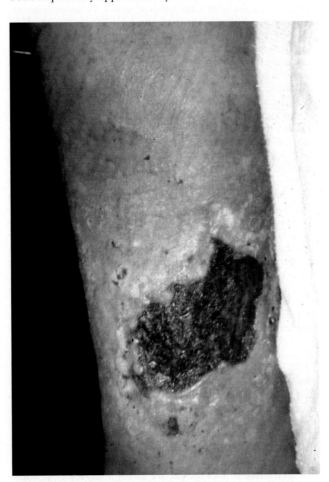

FIGURE 1.8. Venous stasis ulceration on the medial lower leg. Note the irregular border, shallow depth, and surrounding hyperpigmentation.

A less commonly recognized feature of the postthrombotic syndrome is venous claudication, which occurs when there is chronic proximal venous obstruction (usually involving the iliofemoral venous segments) in a patient who is very active physically. The patient experiences severe thigh and occasionally calf pain with increasing leg exercise, which is described as "bursting." Pain relief usually requires the patient to lie down and elevate the limb. The reason that venous claudication is not commonly recognized is that most patients with chronic venous obstruction do not exercise enough to become symptomatic. Venous claudication is caused by chronic obstruction of the venous outflow from the leg and is not due to valvular incompetence. Although the venous collaterals are adequate to maintain the limb free of edema while at rest or with moderate activity, the marked increase in limb blood flow that occurs with vigorous exercise cannot be accommodated, and the venous volume increases to the point of producing the bursting sensation and pain. It is only when the volume of blood on the venous side decreases that the pain will go away. Patients discover this early and find that elevation of the limb is beneficial in relieving the discomfort. Dr. Strandness had a patient with venous claudication who was a competitive skier. This young man was able to complete a race but was so symptomatic after each run that he had to lie on his back with his leg elevated and have his teammates massage his leg to promote venous drainage.

Varicose Veins

A common problem seen in the vascular surgery clinic is a patient who presents with varicose veins. Varicose veins are abnormally dilated, tortuous, superficial veins caused by incompetent venous valves. It is estimated that varicose veins occur in up to 30% of the adult population, with an increased incidence correlated with advancing age.[38] This condition is more common in women, people whose occupations require prolonged standing, and people who are obese. A hereditary weakness of the vein wall may contribute to the development of varicose veins, and the condition is commonly seen in several members of the same family. Varicose veins are rare before puberty. Pregnancy may predispose to varicosities because of hormonal effects related to venous distensibility, increased pressure from the gravid uterus, and increased blood flow.[38]

Varicose veins may be primary (without any associated abnormalities of the deep veins) or secondary (resulting from obstruction or reflux in the deep veins). If only the superficial veins are affected, the patient may have few or no symptoms, but she or he may be troubled by the appearance of their legs. Signs and symptoms in the legs may include dull aching, throbbing, or muscular cramps; increased muscle fatigue; ankle edema; itching over the veins; and a feeling of heaviness. Nocturnal cramps may be present. When deep venous obstruction results in secondary varicose veins, the patient may develop the signs and symptoms of chronic venous insufficiency or the postthrombotic syndrome.

Abdominal Venous Thrombosis

Abdominal venous thrombosis may present as Budd-Chiari syndrome (thrombosis of the hepatic veins) or splanchnic venous thrombosis (thrombosis of the portal, splenic, superior mesenteric, or inferior mesenteric veins). As with peripheral venous thrombosis, hereditary and acquired risk factors are implicated in the pathogenesis of abdominal venous thrombosis. The hereditary risk factors include the factor V Leiden gene mutation, prothrombin gene mutation, and deficiencies of protein C, protein S, and antithrombin III. Acquired causes include myeloproliferative disorders, malignancy, surgery, trauma, pregnancy,

oral contraceptives, and infection.[30,39] As with lower extremity DVT, it is widely accepted that abdominal venous thrombosis requires both a primary thrombophilic state and an additional factor that triggers pathologic thrombus formation.

Thrombosis of the abdominal veins may cause a wide spectrum of symptoms, depending on the involved segment of the venous system and the efficiency of compensatory mechanisms. In portal vein thrombosis, the hepatic artery dilates to stabilize liver function at normal levels during the acute stages. Within a few days after the obstruction, collateral vessels also rapidly develop into a cavernous transformation to bypass the obstructed portal vein segment. Similar collateral vessels develop when the inferior vena cava or hepatic veins are involved. With chronic portal venous obstruction, the liver has a gradual loss of mass, leading to liver dysfunction.[30] The clinical presentation can range from an asymptomatic patient to hematemesis, painless jaundice, abdominal pain, ascites, variceal bleeding, and pancytopenia due to hypersplenism, encephalopathy, hematochezia, or melena. In a study of 36 patients with abdominal venous thrombosis, abdominal pain was present in 44%, hepatomegaly in 11%, splenomegaly in 28%, and ascites in 36%.[39] The ultrasound findings associated with abdominal venous thrombosis are described in Chapter 22.

Hepatocellular carcinoma is the fifth most common neoplasm and the third most common cause of cancer-related death in the world; it is predicted to increase in prevalence over the next two decades in the United States owing to cirrhosis from hepatitis C infection.[40] Like many malignancies, hepatocellular carcinoma is associated with hemostatic activation, with a reported incidence of portal vein thrombosis ranging from 20% to 65%.[40] In a single-institution study of 194 patients with hepatocellular carcinoma by Connolly and coworkers, 31% were found to have portal vein thrombosis.[40] Factors associated with the development of portal vein thrombosis included advanced stage, major vessel involvement, higher Child-Turcotte-Pugh class, serum albumin level less than 3.5, and serum alpha-fetoprotein (AFP) greater than 400. These authors also found a higher rate of systemic venous thromboembolism compared with patients without portal vein thrombosis (11.5% vs. 4.4%).

CONCLUSION

The ability to diagnose and treat vascular disease has changed dramatically with advances in clinical research and evidence-based medicine and improvements in technology. What has not changed is the individual patient who presents with signs or symptoms of vascular disease and a question about his or her health. In this chapter, we have reviewed the traditional process of obtaining a vascular history and performing a focused physical assessment to guide initial vascular diagnostic testing. This systematic approach will result in optimal utilization of the vascular laboratory and the testing methods described throughout this book. It is also hoped that you have enjoyed some of Dr. Strandness' patient stories and will remember that he always put the patient first and expected them to be an active participant in their health care.

References

1. Lungstrom N, Emerson R. Alterations in blood flow. In Capstead L, Barasik J (eds). *Pathophysiology*, 3rd ed. St. Louis: Elsevier Saunders, 2005, p 398.
2. Hirsch AT, Gloviczki P, Drooz A, et al. Mandate for creation of a national peripheral arterial disease public awareness program: An opportunity to improve cardiovascular health. *Angiology* 2004;55:233-242.
3. Aboyans V, Criqui MH, Denenberg JO, et al. Risk factors for progression of peripheral arterial disease in large and small vessels. *Circulation* 2006;113:2623-2629.

4. Ostchega Y, Dillon CF, Hughes JP, et al. Trends in hypertension prevalence, awareness, treatment, and control in US adults: Data from the National Health and Nutrition Examination Survey 1988 to 2004. *J Am Geriatr Soc* 2007;55:1056-1065.
5. Bakhru A, Erlinger TP. Smoking cessation and cardiovascular disease risk factors: Results from the Third National Health and Nutrition Examination Survey. *PLoS Med* 2005;2:e160.
6. Shankar A, Jialian L, Nieto FJ, et al. Association between C-reactive protein level and peripheral arterial disease among US adults without cardiovascular disease, diabetes, or hypertension. *Am Heart J* 2007;154:495-501.
7. Selvin E, Erlinger TP. Prevalence of and risk factors for peripheral arterial disease in the United States: Results from the National Health and Nutrition Examination Survey 1999–2000. *Circulation* 2004;110:738-743.
8. McLafferty RB, Dunnington GL, Mattos MA, et al. Factors affecting the diagnosis of peripheral vascular disease before vascular surgery referral. *J Vasc Surg* 2000;31:870-879.
9. Bakst R, Merola JF, Franks AG Jr, et al. Raynaud's phenomenon: Pathogenesis and management. *J Am Acad Dermatol* 2008;59:633-653.
10. Puechal X, Fiessinger J-N. Thromboangiitis obliterans or Buerger's disease: Challenges for the rheumatologist. *Rheumatology* 2007;46:192-199.
11. Alund M, Mani K, Wanhainen A. Selective screening for abdominal aortic aneurysm among patients referred to the vascular laboratory. *Eur J Vasc Endovasc Surg* 2008;35:669-674.
12. Pasternak RC, Criqui MH, Benjamin EJ, et al. Atherosclerotic Vascular Disease Conference Writing Group I: Epidemiology. *Circulation* 2004;109:2605-2612.
13. Schermerhorn M, Cronenwett JL. Abdominal aortic and iliac aneurysms. In Rutherford R (ed). *Vascular Surgery*, 6th ed. Philadelphia: Elsevier Saunders, 2005, pp 1408-1445.
14. Fisher M. Stroke and TIA: Epidemiology, risk factors, and the need for early intervention. *Am J Manag Care* 2008;14(6 Suppl 2):S204-S211.
15. Cheanvechai V, Harthun NL, Graham LM, et al. Incidence of peripheral vascular disease in women: Is it different from that in men? *J Thorac Cardiovasc Surg* 2004;127:314-317.
16. Barrett KM, Brott TG, Brown RD Jr, et al. Sex differences in stroke severity, symptoms, and deficits after first-ever ischemic stroke. *J Stroke Cerebrovasc Dis* 2007;16:34-39.
17. Bos MJ, Koudstaal PJ, Hofman A, et al. Decreased glomerular filtration rate is a risk factor for hemorrhagic but not for ischemic stroke. The Rotterdam Study. *Stroke* 2007;38:3127-3132.
18. Ng YS, Stein J, Ning M, et al. Comparison of clinical characteristics and functional outcomes of ischemic strokes in different vascular territories. *Stroke* 2007;38:2309-2314.
19. Kalra PA, Guo H, Kausz A, et al. Atherosclerotic renovascular disease in the United States patients aged 67 years or older: Risk factors, revascularization, and prognosis. *Kidney Int* 2005;68:293-301.
20. Guo H, Kalra PA, Gilbertson DT, et al. Atherosclerotic renovascular disease in older US patients stating dialysis, 1996 to 2001. *Circulation* 2008;115:50-58.
21. Edwards MS, Hansen KJ, Craven TE, et al. Associations between renovascular disease and prevalent cardiovascular disease in the elderly: A population-based study. *Vasc Endovascular Surg* 2004;38:25-35.
22. Jaff MR. Conclusions. *J Hypertens* 2005;23(Suppl 3):S31-S33.
23. Wargo KA, Chong K, Chan ECY. Acute renal failure secondary to angiotensin II receptor blockade in a patient with bilateral renal artery stenosis. *Pharmacotherapy* 2003;23:1199-1204.
24. Caps MT, Perissinotto C, Zierler RE, et al. Prospective study of atherosclerotic disease progression in the renal artery. *Circulation* 1998;98:2866-2872.
25. Poulin P-F, Perdu J, La Batide-Alanore A, et al. Fibromuscular dysplasia. *Orphanet J Rare Dis* 2007;2:28. Retrieved http://www.OJRD.com/content/2/1/28. BioMed Central Open Access.
26. Labropoulos N, Ayuste B, Leon LR Jr. Renovascular disease among patients referred for renal duplex ultrasonography. *J Vasc Surg* 2007;46:731-737.
27. Hansen KJ, Wilson DB, Craven TE, et al. Mesenteric artery disease in the elderly. *J Vasc Surg* 2004;40:45-52.
28. Mell MW, Acher CW, Hoch JR, et al. Outcomes after endarterectomy for chronic mesenteric ischemia. *J Vasc Surg* 2008;48:1132-1138.
29. Wilson DB, Mostafavi K, Craven TE, et al. Clinical course of mesenteric artery stenosis in elderly Americans. *Arch Intern Med* 2006;166:2095-2100.
30. Bayraktar Y, Harmanci O. Etiology and consequences of thrombosis in abdominal vessels. *World J Gastroenterol* 2006;12:1165-1174.
31. Martinelli I, Battaglioli T, Bucciarelli P, et al. Risk factors and recurrent rate of primary deep vein thrombosis of the upper extremities. *Circulation* 2004;110:566-570.
32. Samama M-M. An epidemiologic study of risk factors for deep vein thrombosis in medical outpatients. *Arch Intern Med* 2000;160:3415-3420.
33. Shebel ND, Marin A. Effort thrombosis (Paget-Schroetter syndrome) in active young adults: Current concepts in diagnosis and treatment. *J Vasc Nurs* 2006;24:116-126.
34. Ludwig B, Han T, Amundson D. Postthrombotic syndrome complicating a case of May-Thurner syndrome despite endovascular therapy. Case report and review. *Chest* 2006;129:1382-1386.
35. Prandoni P, Lensing AWA, Prins MH, et al. Below-knee elastic compression stockings to prevent the post-thrombotic syndrome. *Ann Intern Med* 2004;141:249-256.
36. Walker N, Rodgers A, Birchall N, et al. Leg ulceration as a long-term complication of deep vein thrombosis. *J Vasc Surg* 2003;38:1331-1335.
37. Gohel MS, Barwell JR, Taylor M, et al. Long-term results of compression therapy alone versus compression plus surgery in chronic venous ulceration (ESCHAR): Randomised controlled trial. *BMJ* 2007;335:83. Available at www.bmj.com (accessed 3 January, 2009).
38. Bhutia SG, Balakrishnan A, Lees T. Varicose veins. *J Perioper Pract* 2008;18:346-352.
39. Dutta AK, Chacko A, George B, et al. Risk factors of thrombosis in abdominal veins. *World J Gastroenterol* 2008;14:4518-4522.
40. Connolly GC, Chen R, Hyrien O, et al. Incidence, risk factors and consequences of portal vein and systemic thromboses in hepatocellular carcinoma. *Thromb Res* 2008;122:299-306.

LABORATORY ORGANIZATION

CHAPTER 2 ■ PRELIMINARY AND FINAL REPORTS

R. EUGENE ZIERLER

In general terms, a vascular laboratory report is a document that describes a patient's vascular testing encounter and provides a formal record of the facts surrounding a visit to the laboratory. Depending on the circumstances, a report may be verbal, handwritten, typed, computer generated and printed, or electronic. The primary purpose of the report is to convey diagnostic information that can be used by the referring physician for the benefit of the patient. Quality patient care depends on accurate and timely communication between the vascular laboratory and health care providers. Vascular laboratory reports can be considered as either preliminary or final.

PRELIMINARY REPORTS

A vascular laboratory report is considered preliminary until it is reviewed, edited, and signed by an interpreting physician. In contrast to most other diagnostic imaging specialties, the use of preliminary reports generated directly by the examining technologist or sonographer is extremely common in the vascular laboratory. In both the 2000 and 2005 surveys of Registered Vascular Technologists conducted by the American Registry for Diagnostic Medical Sonography (ARDMS), approximately 90% of the respondents stated that they provided preliminary reports to referring physicians, either verbally or in writing.[1] Although this practice is so prevalent that it could be regarded as a standard in the United States, it remains controversial because the data in preliminary reports can be used to direct patient care without immediate input from an interpreting physician.

In order to carry out a complete and accurate examination, the technologist must rely on his or her knowledge of laboratory protocols and diagnostic criteria to document the key findings. This requires a certain level of interpretation, which forms the basis for the preliminary report. This report may be verbal, handwritten, or printed, but the preliminary status of the report must be clearly indicated so the referring health care provider will know that the results have not been reviewed by a physician. In many laboratories, a printed or electronic version of the preliminary report serves as a template for the final report. This typically includes the relevant patient information, indications for the test, a description of the test performed, a summary of the results, and a preliminary interpretation. The interpreting physician can then edit or add to this version to create the final report.

FINAL REPORTS

Whereas the preliminary and final versions of a vascular laboratory report may have much in common, the component that distinguishes a final from a preliminary report is an impression (or conclusion) that contains a physician's interpretation of the data gathered during the study. This requires that the interpreting physician review the original images and physiologic information (depending on the specific test performed). In those unusual cases in which there is a substantial difference between the preliminary and final reports that could affect patient care, the laboratory must have a mechanism for bringing this to the attention of the referring physician. Similarly, when an examination reveals a potentially urgent or life-threatening condition, there must be a mechanism for communicating these findings to the appropriate health care providers in a timely fashion.

The incidental identification of nonvascular abnormalities is common in the vascular laboratory. Examples of such findings include thyroid lesions, renal masses, and Baker's cysts. Unless the technologist and interpreting physician have expertise in nonvascular imaging, it is best not to render a detailed diagnosis in these cases, but rather to note the findings in the report and recommend additional imaging, as appropriate to the patient's circumstances.

Elements of a Final Report

The Intersocietal Accreditation Commission (IAC) Vascular Testing has published Standards for all aspects of vascular laboratory practice, including interpretation and reporting (see Chapter 3).[2] Table 2.1 lists the elements of a final report according to the IAC Standards. Although there is no single required format for final reports, they must include these basic elements. It is also important that interpretation and reporting be standardized within a particular laboratory. That is, all interpreting physicians in a laboratory must agree on and utilize consistent diagnostic criteria and a uniform report format. In general, diagnostic criteria

---

TABLE 2.1

ELEMENTS OF A FINAL VASCULAR LABORATORY REPORT[a]

Date of the examination
Clinical indications for the test
Description of the test performed
Overview of the results with pertinent normal and abnormal findings
Characterization of disease (if present) according to location, extent, severity, and etiology
Description of any incidental (nonvascular) findings
Reasons for technically limited or incomplete examinations
Comparison with previous studies, when appropriate
Summary of diagnostic findings (impression/conclusion)
Name of interpreting physician with signature or electronic verification (including date of signature/verification)
Note: The name of the technologist or sonographer performing the examination is not required on the final report, although it must be "part of the permanent record." However, many laboratories include this information in the final report.

[a]From the IAC Standards and Guidelines for Vascular Testing Accreditation (updated 15 June, 2013). For subsequent updates, see http://intersocietal.org/vascular/

---

must be available for interpretation of B-mode images, Doppler spectral waveforms and velocities, color Doppler images, and any other imaging or physiologic testing modalities used.

The physician interpretation must be available within 2 working days of the examination, and the final signed report should be available within 4 working days. All records related to the examination, including the final report, must be retained in accordance with local, state, and federal guidelines for medical records—generally 5 to 7 years for adult patients.

Reporting Terminology

It is stating the obvious to advocate the use of standard medical nomenclature and clear language in vascular laboratory reports, but achieving this goal requires effort by both technologists and physicians. For example, the terminology for describing the venous system in the lower limbs has been problematic.[3,4] Although many vascular laboratories use the historically correct term "superficial femoral vein" to describe the main deep vein of the thigh, experience has shown that some physicians are not aware that this is, in fact, a deep vein.[5] Therefore, they may not consider acute thrombosis of this vein as a serious problem requiring immediate treatment. In order to avoid errors in patient management related to this misunderstanding, it is now recommended that the superficial femoral vein be referred to simply as the *femoral vein*, along with the common femoral and deep femoral veins.

Other potential sources of confusion are abbreviations and eponyms. Nonvascular specialists may not be familiar with the common abbreviations used in the vascular laboratory, so it a good policy to provide definitions of any abbreviations used in a report. For the same reason, eponyms should be avoided. For example, the terms "Giacomini's vein" and "Leonardo's vein" sound erudite, but *posterior thigh circumflex vein* and *posterior accessory great saphenous vein* are more descriptive.

The physician's impression or conclusion should address the specific clinical indications for the test. If a patient is referred for workup of a neck bruit, then the final interpretation of the carotid examination should state whether or not a source for a bruit was identified. If the purpose of a venous evaluation is to look for evidence of chronic venous insufficiency, then it is not adequate to conclude that deep venous thrombosis is not identified—the presence or absence of reflux must also be noted. In addition, an effort should be made to avoid vague terms such as "moderate stenosis" or "functional occlusion" that have no standard definitions. Finally, after the interpreting physician has addressed the indications for the test, she or he should note how the findings compare with previous tests and offer recommendations for further follow-up, whenever possible.

SAMPLE REPORTS

Preliminary Reports

In many vascular laboratories, preliminary reports are either verbal or handwritten (or both). When a report is given verbally, it is important for the technologist to make a note documenting the person who received the report and the time of contact. Handwritten preliminary reports are often in the form of a "worksheet" that is used to record data at the time the study is performed. Figures 2.1 through 2.6 are examples of worksheets that can also serve as preliminary reports. Drawings done by the examining technologist can be very helpful when there are multiple abnormalities or unusual vascular anatomy. While worksheets such as these can be useful in the

Text continues on page 21

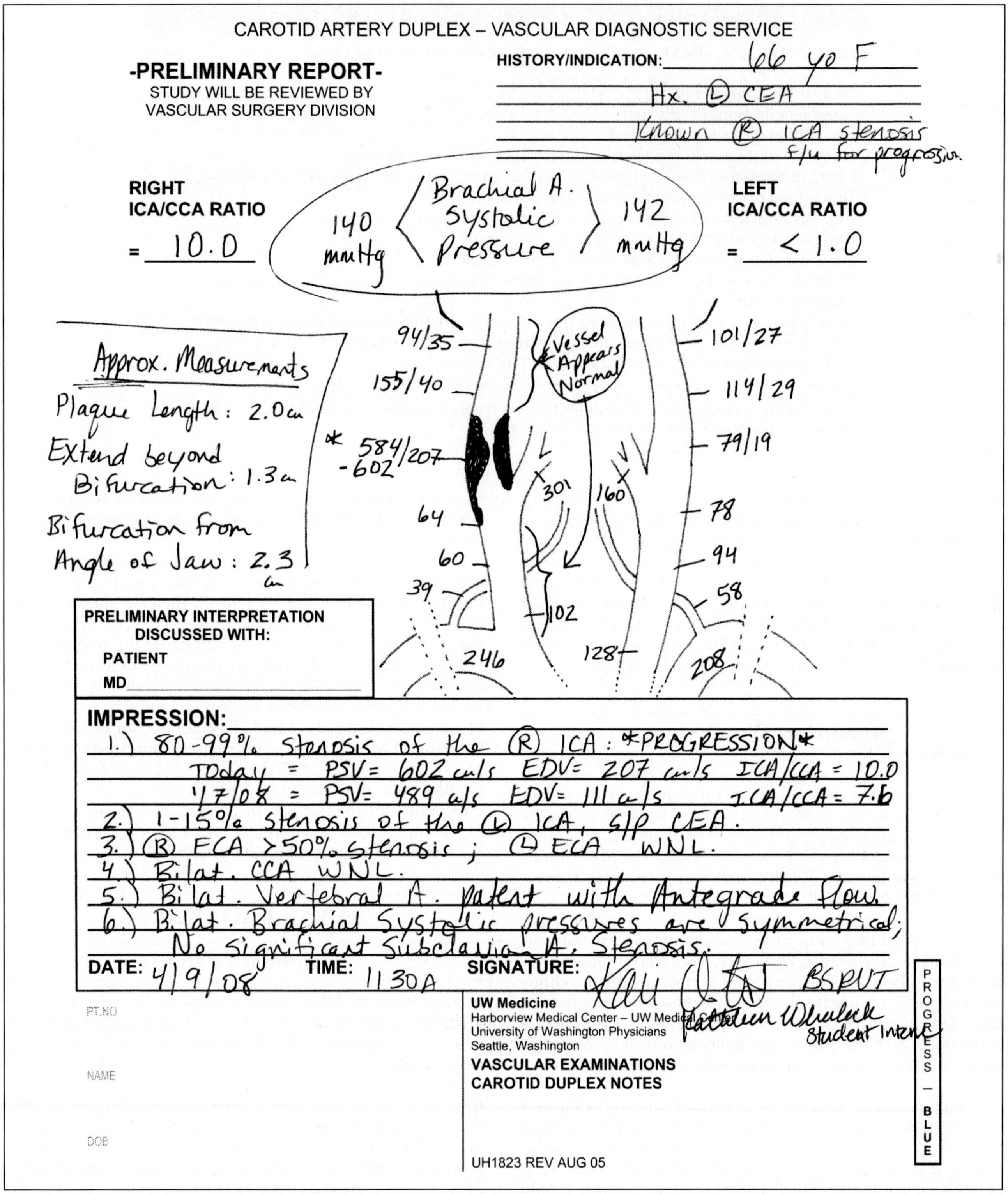

CAROTID ARTERY DUPLEX – VASCULAR DIAGNOSTIC SERVICE

-PRELIMINARY REPORT-
STUDY WILL BE REVIEWED BY
VASCULAR SURGERY DIVISION

HISTORY/INDICATION: _____ 66 yo F _____
_____ Hx. ⒧ CEA _____
_____ Known ⓡ ICA stenosis
f/u for progression.

**RIGHT
ICA/CCA RATIO**

= __10.0__

Brachial A.
Systolic
Pressure

140 mmHg   142 mmHg

**LEFT
ICA/CCA RATIO**

= __< 1.0__

Vessel Appears Normal

Approx. Measurements

Plaque Length: 2.0 cm

Extend beyond
Bifurcation: 1.3 cm

Bifurcation from
Angle of Jaw: 2.3 cm

94/35
155/40
* 584/207
- 602
64
60
39
301
160
102
246
128
208

101/27
114/29
79/19
78
94
58

**PRELIMINARY INTERPRETATION
DISCUSSED WITH:**

PATIENT

MD _____

IMPRESSION:

1.) 80-99% Stenosis of the ⓡ ICA : *PROGRESSION*
   Today = PSV= 602 cm/s EDV= 207 cm/s ICA/CCA = 10.0
   1/7/08 = PSV= 489 c/s EDV= 111 c/s ICA/CCA = 7.6
2.) 1-15% Stenosis of the ⒧ ICA, S/P CEA.
3.) ⓡ ECA >50% Stenosis ; ⒧ ECA WNL.
4.) Bilat. CCA WNL.
5.) Bilat. Vertebral A. patent with Antegrade flow.
6.) Bilat. Brachial Systolic pressures are symmetrical;
   No significant Subclavian A. Stenosis.

DATE: 4/9/08   **TIME:** 1130A   **SIGNATURE:** Kati C.W. BS RVT
                                                         Kathleen Whaleck
                                                         Student Intern

PT.NO

NAME

DOB

UW Medicine
Harborview Medical Center – UW Medical
University of Washington Physicians
Seattle, Washington

**VASCULAR EXAMINATIONS
CAROTID DUPLEX NOTES**

UH1823 REV AUG 05

PROGRESS – BLUE

FIGURE 2.1. Carotid duplex worksheet and preliminary report.

LOWER EXTREMITY ARTERIAL DUPLEX – VASCULAR DIAGNOSTIC SERVICE

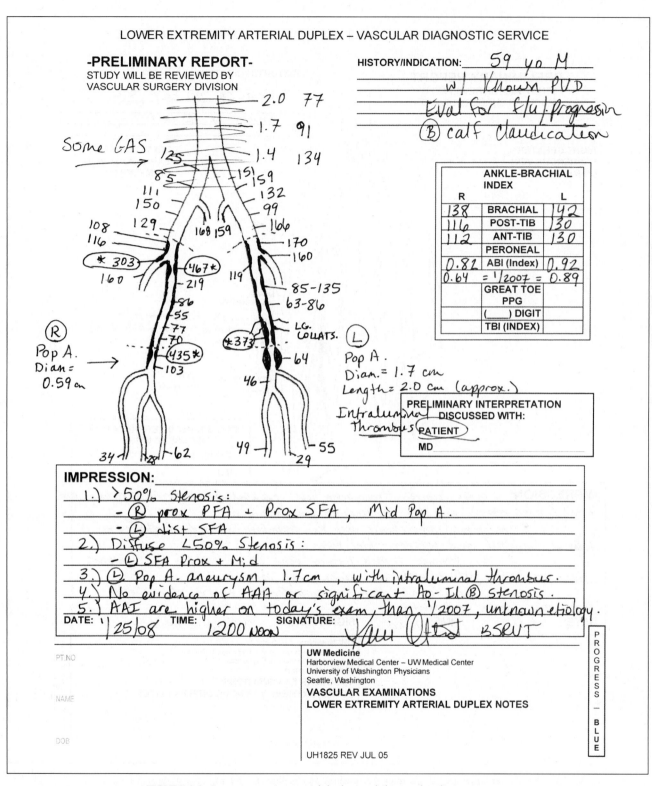

-PRELIMINARY REPORT-
STUDY WILL BE REVIEWED BY
VASCULAR SURGERY DIVISION

HISTORY/INDICATION: 59 yo M
w/ known PVD
Eval for f/u/progression
(B) calf claudication

Some GAS

2.0 77
1.7 91
1.4 134
125
85
111
150
108 129
116
* 303
160
467 *
168 159
219
86
55
77
70
435 *
103
R
Pop A.
Diam =
0.59 cm
15
159
132
99
166
170
160
119
85-135
63-86
LG. COLLATS. (L)
* 373
64
46
49 55
34 28 62 29

Pop A.
Diam = 1.7 cm
Length = 2.0 cm (approx.)
Intraluminal thrombus

ANKLE-BRACHIAL INDEX		
R		L
138	BRACHIAL	142
116	POST-TIB	130
112	ANT-TIB	130
	PERONEAL	
0.82	ABI (Index)	0.92
0.64 = ¹/2007 =		0.89
	GREAT TOE PPG	
	(___) DIGIT	
	TBI (INDEX)	

PRELIMINARY INTERPRETATION
DISCUSSED WITH:
PATIENT
MD

IMPRESSION:
1.) > 50% Stenosis:
   - (R) prox PFA + Prox SFA, Mid Pop A.
   - (L) dist SFA
2.) Diffuse <50% Stenosis:
   - (L) SFA Prox + Mid
3.) (L) Pop A. aneurysm, 1.7cm, with intraluminal thrombus.
4.) No evidence of AAA or significant Ao-Il. (B) stenosis.
5.) AAI are higher on today's exam than ¹/2007, unknown etiology.

DATE: 1/25/08   TIME: 1200 NOON   SIGNATURE: _____ BSRVT

PT.NO

NAME

DOB

UW Medicine
Harborview Medical Center – UW Medical Center
University of Washington Physicians
Seattle, Washington

VASCULAR EXAMINATIONS
LOWER EXTREMITY ARTERIAL DUPLEX NOTES

UH1825 REV JUL 05

P R O G R E S S — B L U E

FIGURE 2.2. Lower extremity arterial duplex worksheet and preliminary report.

LOWER EXTREMITY VENOUS DUPLEX – VASCULAR DIAGNOSTIC SERVICE

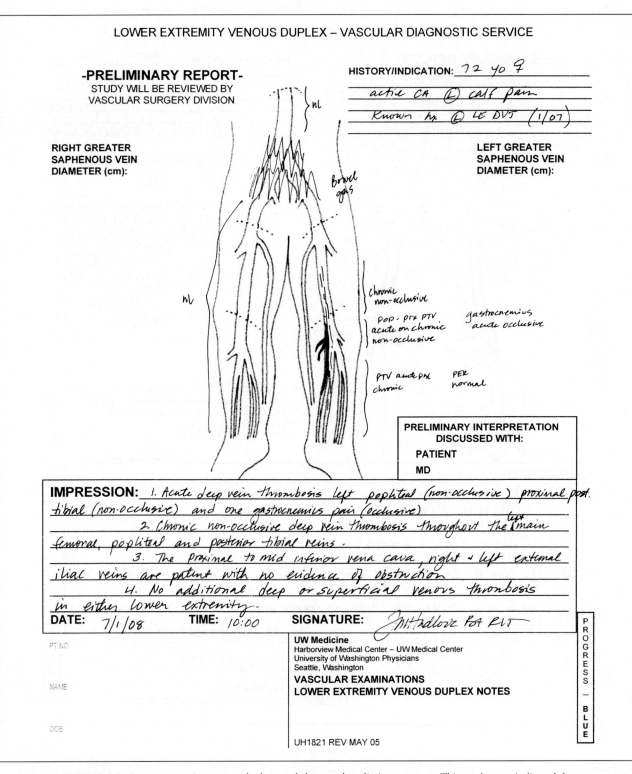

-PRELIMINARY REPORT-
STUDY WILL BE REVIEWED BY
VASCULAR SURGERY DIVISION

HISTORY/INDICATION: 72 yo ♀

active CA Ⓛ calf pain

Known hx Ⓛ LE DVT (1/07)

**RIGHT GREATER
SAPHENOUS VEIN
DIAMETER (cm):**

**LEFT GREATER
SAPHENOUS VEIN
DIAMETER (cm):**

nl

Bowel gas

nl

Chronic non-occlusive

Pop- prx PTV acute on chronic non-occlusive

gastrocnemius acute occlusive

PTV acute prx chronic

PER normal

**PRELIMINARY INTERPRETATION
DISCUSSED WITH:**

PATIENT

MD

IMPRESSION: 1. Acute deep vein thrombosis left popliteal (non-occlusive) proximal post. tibial (non-occlusive) and one gastrocnemius pair (occlusive)

2. Chronic non-occlusive deep vein thrombosis throughout the left main femoral, popliteal and posterior tibial veins.

3. The proximal to mid inferior vena cava, right & left external iliac veins are patent with no evidence of obstruction

4. No additional deep or superficial venous thrombosis in either lower extremity.

DATE: 7/1/08   **TIME:** 10:00   **SIGNATURE:** M. Hadlock PA RVT

FIGURE 2.3. Lower extremity venous duplex worksheet and preliminary report. This study was indicated for follow-up of a known deep vein thrombosis.

LABORATORY ORGANIZATION

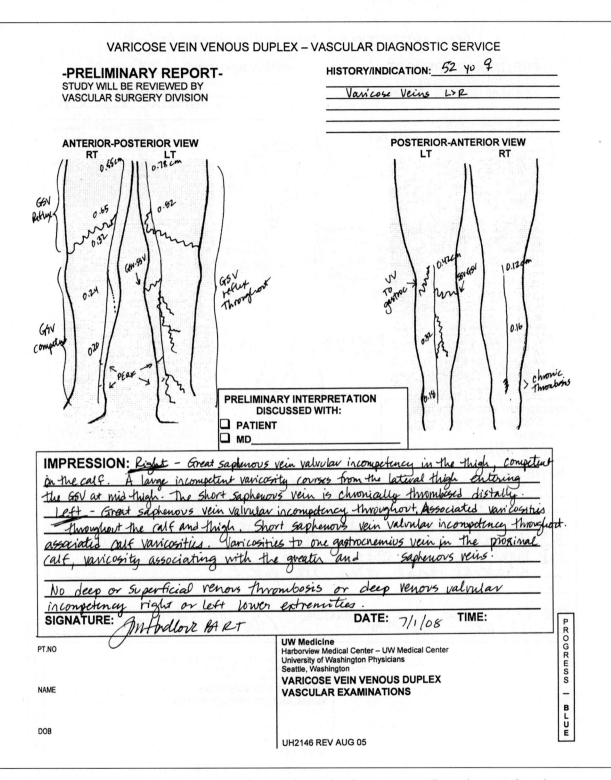

VARICOSE VEIN VENOUS DUPLEX – VASCULAR DIAGNOSTIC SERVICE

-PRELIMINARY REPORT-
STUDY WILL BE REVIEWED BY
VASCULAR SURGERY DIVISION

HISTORY/INDICATION: 52 yo ♀

Varicose Veins L>R

ANTERIOR-POSTERIOR VIEW
RT   LT

0.55cm   0.78 cm

GSV Reflux

0.65   0.82

0.32

GSV-SSV

0.24

GSV Competent

0.20

PERF

GSV reflux Throughout

POSTERIOR-ANTERIOR VIEW
LT   RT

UV to gastroc   0.42cm   SSV/GSV   0.12cm

0.32   0.16

0.10   chronic Thrombosis

**PRELIMINARY INTERPRETATION
DISCUSSED WITH:**
☐ PATIENT
☐ MD_____

IMPRESSION: Right – Great saphenous vein valvular incompetency in the thigh, competent on the calf. A large incompetent varicosity courses from the lateral thigh entering the GSV at mid thigh. The short saphenous vein is chronically thrombosed distally. Left – Great saphenous vein valvular incompetency throughout. Associated varicosities throughout the calf and thigh. Short saphenous vein valvular incompetency throughout, associated calf varicosities. Varicosities to one gastrocnemius vein in the proximal calf, varicosity associating with the greater and   saphenous veins.

No deep or superficial venous thrombosis or deep venous valvular incompetency right or left lower extremities.

SIGNATURE: JM Hodlox PA RT   DATE: 7/1/08   TIME:

PT.NO

NAME

DOB

UW Medicine
Harborview Medical Center – UW Medical Center
University of Washington Physicians
Seattle, Washington
**VARICOSE VEIN VENOUS DUPLEX
VASCULAR EXAMINATIONS**

UH2146 REV AUG 05

PROGRESS — BLUE

FIGURE 2.4. Lower extremity venous duplex worksheet and preliminary report. This study was performed to evaluate varicose veins.

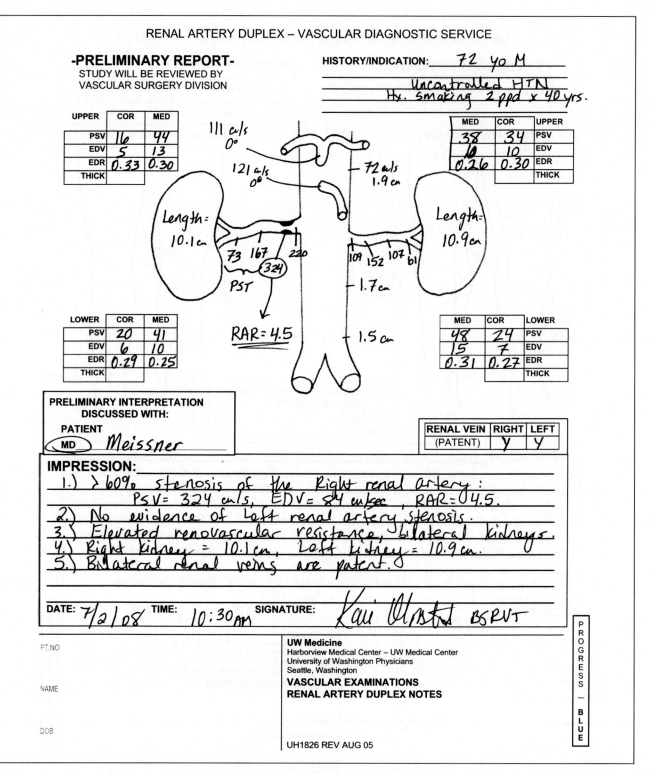

RENAL ARTERY DUPLEX – VASCULAR DIAGNOSTIC SERVICE

-PRELIMINARY REPORT-
STUDY WILL BE REVIEWED BY
VASCULAR SURGERY DIVISION

HISTORY/INDICATION: _72 yo M_
Uncontrolled HTN
Hx. smoking 2 ppd x 40 yrs.

UPPER	COR	MED
PSV	16	44
EDV	5	13
EDR	0.33	0.30
THICK		

MED	COR	UPPER
.38	.34	PSV
10	10	EDV
0.26	0.30	EDR
		THICK

111 cu/s 0°
121 cu/s 0°
72 cu/s 1.9 cm

Length = 10.1 cm
Length = 10.9 cm

73 167 220 (324)
PST
RAR = 4.5

109 152 107 61
1.7 cm
1.5 cm

LOWER	COR	MED
PSV	20	41
EDV	6	10
EDR	0.29	0.25
THICK		

MED	COR	LOWER
48	24	PSV
15	7	EDV
0.31	0.27	EDR
		THICK

PRELIMINARY INTERPRETATION DISCUSSED WITH:
PATIENT
(MD) _Meissner_

RENAL VEIN	RIGHT	LEFT
(PATENT)	Y	Y

IMPRESSION:
1.) >60% stenosis of the Right renal artery:
    PSV = 324 cu/s, EDV = 84 cu/sec, RAR = 4.5.
2.) No evidence of Left renal artery stenosis.
3.) Elevated renovascular resistance, bilateral kidneys.
4.) Right kidney = 10.1 cm. Left kidney = 10.9 cm.
5.) Bilateral renal veins are patent.

DATE: 7/2/08   TIME: 10:30 AM   SIGNATURE: _Kari Ulster_ BS RVT

PT.NO

NAME

DOB

UW Medicine
Harborview Medical Center – UW Medical Center
University of Washington Physicians
Seattle, Washington
VASCULAR EXAMINATIONS
RENAL ARTERY DUPLEX NOTES

UH1826 REV AUG 05

PROGRESS — BLUE

FIGURE 2.5. Renal duplex worksheet and preliminary report.

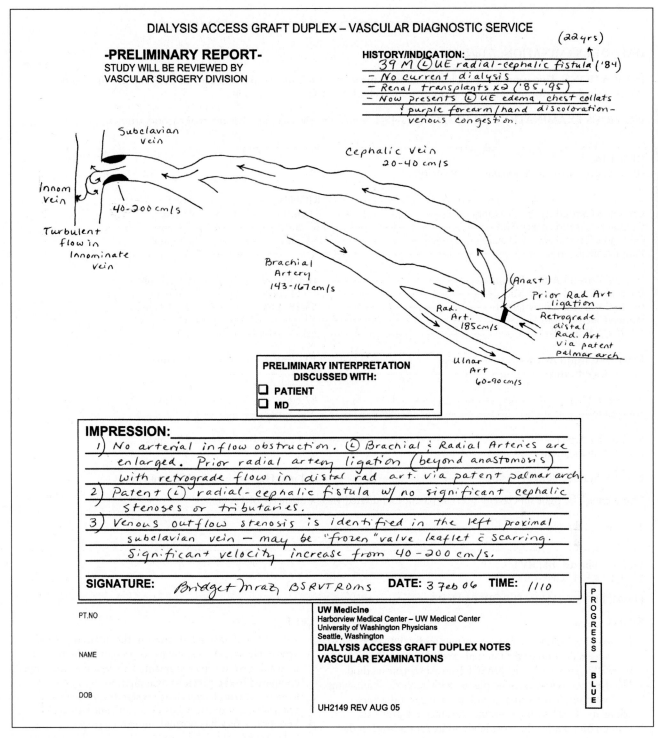

DIALYSIS ACCESS GRAFT DUPLEX – VASCULAR DIAGNOSTIC SERVICE

-PRELIMINARY REPORT-
STUDY WILL BE REVIEWED BY
VASCULAR SURGERY DIVISION

HISTORY/INDICATION:
(22 yrs)
39 M (L) UE radial-cephalic fistula ('84)
- No current dialysis
- Renal transplants x2 ('85, '95)
- Now presents (L) UE edema, chest collats
  + purple forearm/hand discoloration-
  venous congestion.

Subclavian Vein

Cephalic Vein
20-40 cm/s

Innom Vein

40-200 cm/s

Turbulent flow in Innominate vein

Brachial Artery
143-167 cm/s

(Anast)
Prior Rad Art ligation
Retrograde distal Rad. Art via patent palmar arch

Rad. Art.
185 cm/s

Ulnar Art
60-90 cm/s

PRELIMINARY INTERPRETATION
DISCUSSED WITH:
☐ PATIENT
☐ MD_____

IMPRESSION:_____
1) No arterial inflow obstruction. (L) Brachial + Radial Arteries are
   enlarged. Prior radial artery ligation (beyond anastomosis)
   with retrograde flow in distal rad art. via patent palmar arch.
2) Patent (L) radial-cephalic fistula w/ no significant cephalic
   stenoses or tributaries.
3) Venous outflow stenosis is identified in the left proximal
   subclavian vein — may be "frozen" valve leaflet c̄ scarring.
   Significant velocity increase from 40-200 cm/s.

SIGNATURE: Bridget Mraz BSRVT RDMS   DATE: 3 Feb 06   TIME: 1110

PT.NO

NAME

DOB

UW Medicine
Harborview Medical Center – UW Medical Center
University of Washington Physicians
Seattle, Washington
DIALYSIS ACCESS GRAFT DUPLEX NOTES
VASCULAR EXAMINATIONS

UH2149 REV AUG 05

PROGRESS — BLUE

LABORATORY ORGANIZATION

FIGURE 2.6. Dialysis access graft duplex worksheet and preliminary report.

clinical setting, they are not required, and some laboratories have stopped using worksheets in an effort to go "paperless."

Final Reports

Final reports must be typed, printed, or available in electronic form, and they must contain all the elements listed in Table 2.1. However, this still leaves room for considerable variation from one laboratory to another. For example, some final reports consist of complete sentences with a detailed patient history and description of the test performed, whereas others contain only short phrases and a list of findings. Some test data, such as blood pressures or flow velocities, are best presented in a tabular format. It is generally not necessary to include images or waveforms in a final report, although electronic archiving of images and report generation makes this possible. What is most appropriate for a particular laboratory will depend on the practice setting and the preferences of the technologists and physicians involved. Some examples of text from final reports are given in Figures 2.7 through 2.13.

Text continues on page 30

CAROTID ARTERY DUPLEX EVALUATION (COMPLETE)

DATE OF EXAMINATION: 7/18/2013

INDICATIONS: This is an 85-year-old female who presents with known carotid artery disease and asymptomatic bruits. We are asked to perform a follow-up examination to check for disease progression.

PREVIOUS EXAMINATION: 5/12/2009—16%-49% stenosis of the right and left internal carotid arteries.

RESULTS:
(Peak Systolic Velocity/End-Diastolic Velocity)

	RIGHT	LEFT
Common Carotid Artery Proximal	84 cm/s	48 cm/s
Common Carotid Artery Mid	67 cm/s	78 cm/s
Common Carotid Artery Distal	56 cm/s	67 cm/s
Plaque/Calcification	Y	Y
Internal Carotid Artery Proximal	163/53 cm/s	61/20 cm/s
Internal Carotid Artery Mid	83/24 cm/s	85/30 cm/s
Internal Carotid Artery Distal	55/19 cm/s	57/19 cm/s
Plaque/Calcification	Y	Y
ICA/CCA Ratio	2.4	1.1
External Carotid Artery	123 cm/s	57 cm/s
Plaque/Calcification	Y	Y
Vertebral Artery	82 cm/s	37 cm/s
Antegrade	Y	Y
Subclavian Artery	163 cm/s	222 cm/s
Plaque/Calcification	Y	Y
Brachial Systolic Blood Pressure	164 mm Hg	172 mm Hg

Comments: The right subclavian artery is patent and dilated with a diameter of 1.4 cm.

Y = Yes,   N = No

Kari A. Olmsted, BS, RVT
VASCULAR TECHNOLOGIST

FINAL PHYSICIAN INTERPRETATION:

RIGHT

1. Increased velocities are now consistent with 50%-79% diameter reduction of the internal carotid artery. This is less than 70% stenosis by the NASCET measurement method. Heterogeneous and calcified plaque with acoustic shadowing is present in the proximal to mid internal carotid artery segments. This lesion has progressed since the previous examination and is the most likely source for a bruit in the right neck.
2. Common carotid artery has no significant stenosis. Dense plaque is present in the distal common carotid segment and extends to the bifurcation.
3. External carotid artery has no significant stenosis.
4. Vertebral artery has normal, antegrade flow.
5. Subclavian artery is patent with less than 50% stenosis and dilation to 1.4 cm diameter.

LEFT

1. 16%-49% diameter reduction of the internal carotid artery. Heterogeneous plaque is present in the proximal internal carotid artery segment. This lesion is unchanged compared to the previous examination.
2. Common carotid artery has no significant stenosis.
3. External carotid artery has no significant stenosis.
4. Vertebral artery has normal, antegrade flow.
5. Subclavian artery has approximately 50% stenosis. This may be the source of a bruit in the left neck.

R. Eugene Zierler, MD
VASCULAR SURGERY ATTENDING
Finalized on 7/19/2013

FIGURE 2.7. Final report on a carotid duplex done for follow-up of known carotid disease and neck bruits.

LEFT CAROTID ARTERY DUPLEX EXAMINATION (LIMITED)

DATE OF EXAMINATION: 1/10/2013

INDICATIONS: This is a 58-year-old male with a history of radiation therapy involving the neck and known carotid artery stenosis. He is status post repeat stenting of the left common carotid artery on 1/9/2013.

PREVIOUS EXAMINATION: 12/13/2012 (prior to recent intervention)—Maximum velocities in the left common carotid artery are 410/164 cm/s.

RESULTS:
(Peak Systolic Velocity/End-Diastolic Velocity)

LEFT
Common Carotid Artery Proximal------------------------------------- 253/68 cm/s
Common Carotid Artery Mid-- 237/52 cm/s
Common Carotid Artery Distal---------------------------------------157/53 cm/s
Plaque/Calcification--- Y

Internal Carotid Artery Proximal------------------------------------ 106/34 cm/s
Internal Carotid Artery Mid-- 71/29 cm/s
Internal Carotid Artery Distal------------------------------------- 72/30 cm/s
Plaque/Calcification--N

External Carotid Artery---141 cm/s

Comments: The stents are visualized and appear widely patent with some wall thickening noted within the stented lumen.

Y = Yes, N = No

Watson B. Smith, RDMS, RVT
VASCULAR TECHNOLOGIST

FINAL PHYSICIAN INTERPRETATION:

LEFT

1. The common carotid artery stents are well visualized and patent. Peak systolic velocities are diffusely increased in the stented segment with no focal areas of stenosis identified, although they are decreased compared to the previous examination. It is recognized that flow velocities in widely patent carotid stents may be increased, and use of velocity criteria for native carotid arteries may result in overestimation of stenosis severity in the presence of a stent.

2. The internal and external carotid arteries are normal.

R. Eugene Zierler, MD
VASCULAR SURGERY ATTENDING
Finalized on 1/10/2013

FIGURE 2.8. Final report on a carotid duplex done for follow-up of a carotid stent.

LOWER EXTREMITY VENOUS DUPLEX EVALUATION (COMPLETE)

DATE OF EXAMINATION: 6/17/2013

INDICATIONS: This is a 57-year-old male who is post-op day #17 from a liver transplant. He has right lower extremity edema and pain.

PREVIOUS EXAMINATIONS: None

RESULTS:

DUPLEX OF INFERIOR VENA CAVA (IVC) AND BILATERAL ILIAC VEINS

The IVC and common iliac veins are poorly visualized due to bowel gas. Flow patterns in the right and left distal external iliac veins are spontaneous and phasic.

DUPLEX OF BILATERAL LOWER EXTREMITY VEINS

RIGHT

Deep System:
Intraluminal echoes and incomplete vein wall compression are found in the mid segment of the right common femoral vein. Spontaneous and weakly phasic Doppler flow was found throughout the proximal deep femoral, main thigh femoral, popliteal, paired posterior tibial, and paired peroneal veins. Complete vein wall compression is noted in the proximal deep femoral, main thigh femoral, popliteal, paired posterior tibial, and paired peroneal veins, as well as the gastrocnemius and soleal muscular veins.

Superficial System:
The right great saphenous vein has no detectable Doppler flow from the saphenofemoral confluence to mid calf level.

Incidentally, there is a 5.5 × 2.0 cm poorly circumscribed cystic mass superficial to the right proximal femoral vessels and deep to the surgical incision with no detectable Doppler flow.

LEFT

Deep System:
Doppler flow signals obtained in the left common femoral, proximal deep femoral, femoral vein throughout the thigh, popliteal, paired posterior tibial, and peroneal veins are normal (spontaneous, phasic, brisk augmentation). Vein wall compressibility is normal throughout these venous segments, including the gastrocnemius and soleal muscular veins.

Superficial System:
The left great saphenous vein is patent and compressible at the saphenofemoral confluence.

Watson B. Smith, RDMS, RVT
VASCULAR TECHNOLOGIST

FINAL PHYSICIAN INTERPRETATION:

1. Partial (nonocclusive) deep vein thrombosis is present in the right common femoral vein.
2. The right great saphenous vein has occlusive thrombus from the saphenofemoral confluence to mid calf level.
3. The right distal external iliac, proximal deep femoral, main thigh femoral, popliteal, paired posterior tibial, and paired peroneal veins are patent with no other evidence of deep vein thrombosis.
4. The left distal external iliac, common femoral, proximal deep femoral, main thigh femoral, popliteal, paired posterior tibial, paired peroneal, and great saphenous veins are normal with no evidence of deep vein thrombosis.
5. Incidentally, the 5.5-cm incisional cystic mass superficial to the right proximal femoral vessels is consistent with a hematoma.

R. Eugene Zierler, MD
VASCULAR SURGERY ATTENDING
Finalized on 6/17/2013

FIGURE 2.9. Final report on a lower extremity venous duplex done for postoperative lower extremity edema.

LOWER EXTREMITY ARTERIAL EVALUATION

DATE OF EXAMINATION: 9/13/2013

INDICATIONS: This is a 75-year-old male who is referred for noninvasive lower extremity arterial evaluation. He has symptoms of claudication in both legs. Risk factors include coronary artery disease, hypertension, high cholesterol, and diabetes.

PREVIOUS EXAMINATION: None

RESULTS:
ANKLE-BRACHIAL INDEX (mm Hg)

	RIGHT	LEFT
Brachial Artery	120	124
Posterior Tibial Artery	110	92
Anterior Tibial Artery	112	74
Ankle-Brachial Index	0.90	0.74

Continuous-wave Doppler waveforms were recorded:
Multiphasic tibial artery Doppler waveforms noted on the right.
Monophasic tibial artery Doppler waveforms noted on the left.

DUPLEX OF THE ABDOMINAL AORTA AND ILIAC ARTERIES (COMPLETE)

-All flow signals are obtained with a 60-degree Doppler angle, unless noted.
-Doppler flow velocities (cm/s) are reported as:
 Peak Systolic Velocity (PSV)/End Diastolic Velocity (EDV).
-Doppler Waveform Description: Triphasic (T), Biphasic (B),
-Monophasic (M), Monophasic-continuous (M/C), Poststenotic Turbulence (PST)

AORTA PROXIMAL	- diameter = 2.2 cm
AORTA MID	- diameter = 2.1 cm
AORTA DISTAL	- diameter = 2.1 cm

B-mode image: Poor image quality due to gas. Difficult to insonate and obtain Doppler arterial flow velocities.

	RIGHT	LEFT
COMMON ILIAC PROXIMAL	GAS	GAS
COMMON ILIAC MID	GAS	GAS
COMMON ILIAC DISTAL	GAS	GAS
HYPOGASTRIC	50 T	60 T

B-mode image: GAS

	RIGHT	LEFT
EXTERNAL ILIAC PROXIMAL	50 T	40 T
EXTERNAL ILIAC MID	51 T	41 T
EXTERNAL ILIAC DISTAL	52 T	70 T

B-mode image: unremarkable

DUPLEX OF THE LOWER EXTREMITY ARTERIES (COMPLETE)

	RIGHT	LEFT
COMMON FEMORAL PROXIMAL	55 T	39 T

B-mode image: Diffuse calcific plaque

	RIGHT	LEFT
PROFUNDA FEMORIS PROXIMAL	50 T	67 T

B-mode image: Diffuse plaque

(Continued)

LABORATORY ORGANIZATION

```
SUPERFICIAL FEMORAL PROXIMAL----------------------------------28--------------------19
SUPERFICIAL FEMORAL MID-----------------------------------------80--------------------22
SUPERFICIAL FEMORAL DISTAL-------------------------------------403--------------------25
```
B-mode image: Diffuse calcific plaque. Cannot rule out segmental occlusion on the left.

```
POPLITEAL PROXIMAL---------------------------------------------44 PST----------------25
POPLITEAL DISTAL-------------------------------------------------59--------------------25
TIBIO-PERONEAL TRUNK-------------------------------------------47--------------------22
```
B-mode image: Diffuse plaque

```
POSTERIOR TIBIAL DISTAL---------------------------------------- 20--------------------10
ANTERIOR TIBIAL DISTAL---------------------------------------- 20--------------------41
PERONEAL DISTAL-------------------------------------------------60--------------------48
```

Kari A. Olmsted, BS, RVT
VASCULAR TECHNOLOGIST

FINAL PHYSICIAN INTERPRETATION:

1. Resting ankle-brachial indices are borderline normal on the right at 0.90 and abnormal on the left at 0.74. Tibial artery Doppler flow waveforms are normally multiphasic on the right and abnormal monophasic on the left.
2. The abdominal aorta is patent. Unable to evaluate with Doppler due to dense gas. The bilateral common iliac arteries are not visualized.
3. The bilateral external and internal iliac arteries are patent with normal triphasic Doppler flow signals.
4. The bilateral common femoral and profunda femoris arteries are patent with calcific plaque and normal triphasic Doppler flow signals.
5. The right superficial femoral artery is patent with diffuse less than 50% stenosis and calcified plaque proximally. There is a focal, greater than 50% stenosis of the right distal superficial femoral artery.
6. The left superficial femoral artery has diffuse less than 50% stenosis and calcified plaque with decreased flow velocities throughout. Cannot rule out segmental occlusion or greater than 50% stenosis due to acoustic shadowing from calcified plaque.
7. The bilateral popliteal arteries are patent with abnormal monophasic Doppler flow signals and diffuse plaque.
8. The bilateral posterior tibial, anterior tibial, and peroneal arteries have calcified plaque and dampened, monophasic Doppler flow patterns at the ankle. Cannot rule out occlusion or greater than 50% stenosis due to acoustic shadowing.

R. Eugene Zierler, MD
VASCULAR SURGERY ATTENDING
Finalized on 9/14/2013

FIGURE 2.10. Final report on a lower extremity duplex done for symptoms of bilateral lower extremity claudication.

FEMORAL ARTERY DUPLEX EVALUATION—RULE OUT PSEUDOANEURYSM

DATE OF EXAMINATION: 6/16/02013

INDICATIONS: This is a 72-year-old male status-post right groin access on 6/12/2013 for cardiac catheterization who now presents with right groin swelling and pain.

PREVIOUS EXAMINATION: None

RESULTS:
ANKLE BRACHIAL INDEX (mm Hg)

	Right	Left
Brachial Artery	134	136
Posterior Tibial Artery	150	166
Anterior Tibial Artery	144	164
Ankle-Brachial Index	1.10	1.22

Distal tibial artery velocity waveforms are normally triphasic on the right and left.

DUPLEX OF FEMORAL ARTERY AND VEIN

Femoral Arteries: Normal Doppler waveforms and velocities are present in the right proximal femoral arteries.

Femoral Veins: Normal, spontaneous and phasic Doppler waveforms are present in the right proximal femoral veins.

A pseudoaneurysm measuring 2.8 × 2.1 × 4.3 cm is visualized arising from the distal right common femoral artery. The neck of the aneurysm is approximately 0.53 cm in length.

Jean Hadlock, BA RVT
VASCULAR TECHNOLOGIST

FINAL PHYSICIAN INTERPRETATION:

1. Ankle-brachial indices are normal at rest bilaterally: 1.10 on the right and 1.22 on the left. Distal tibial artery flow waveforms are normally triphasic bilaterally.
2. There is a pseudoaneurysm with an active flow cavity measuring 2.8 × 2.1 × 4.3 cm and a neck length of 0.53 cm originating from the distal right common femoral artery.
3. No evidence of arteriovenous fistula in the right proximal femoral area.
4. No evidence of venous injury or thrombus in the right groin vessels examined.

R. Eugene Zierler, MD
VASCULAR SURGERY ATTENDING
Finalized on 6/16/02013

FIGURE 2.11. Final report on a lower extremity duplex done for a suspected femoral artery pseudoaneurysm.

DUPLEX EVALUATION OF THE LOWER EXTREMITY ARTERIES AND BYPASS GRAFT SURVEILLANCE

DATE OF EXAMINATION: 4/8/2013

INDICATIONS: This is a 60-year-old male who is referred for noninvasive lower extremity arterial evaluation. He presents with a left femoral to distal popliteal artery bypass graft placed on 2/27/2013.

PREVIOUS EXAMINATIONS:
ABI: 2/18/2013 (Pre-op) Right 0.95, Left 0.36
ABI: 2/29/2013 (Post-op) Right 0.95, Left 0.59

RESULTS:

ANKLE-BRACHIAL INDEX (mm Hg)

	RIGHT	LEFT
Brachial Artery	120	118
Posterior Tibial Artery	112	86
Anterior Tibial Artery	98	84
Ankle-Brachial Index	0.93	0.74

Continuous-wave Doppler waveforms were recorded:
Multiphasic tibial artery Doppler waveforms noted on the right.
Monophasic/hyperemic tibial artery Doppler waveforms noted on the left.

--LEFT SIDE—(cm/s)

NATIVE INFLOW:
COMMON FEMORAL PROXIMAL---------------------------------- 156
COMMON FEMORAL DISTAL------------------------------------ 160
B-mode image: Mild diffuse plaque

PROFUNDA FEMORIS PROXIMAL---------------------------------- 123
PROFUNDA FEMORIS PROXIMAL-MID-------------------------- 100
B-mode image: Mild diffuse plaque

FEMORAL-DISTAL POPLITEAL ARTERY BYPASS GRAFT
PROXIMAL ANASTOMOSIS------------------------------------- 193
PROXIMAL THIGH GRAFT------------------------------------- 190-302**
PROXIMAL-MID THIGH GRAFT--------------------------------- 182
MID THIGH GRAFT(SITE 1*)--------------------------------147-191**
MID THIGH GRAFT(SITE 2*)--------------------------------119-174**
DISTAL THIGH GRAFT(SITE 3*)-----------------------------146-253**
PROXIMAL KNEE LEVEL GRAFT-------------------------------- 191
MID KNEE LEVEL GRAFT(SITE 4*)--------------------------- 114-297***
DISTAL KNEE LEVEL GRAFT---------------------------------- 121 PST
DISTAL ANASTOMOSIS--------------------------------------- 95

NATIVE OUTFLOW:
TIBIO-PERONEAL TRUNK PRE--------------------------------- 113
TIBIO-PERONEAL TRUNK AT---------------------------------- 289***
TIBIO-PERONEAL TRUNK POST-------------------------------- 164 PST
B-mode image: unremarkable

  * Velocity elevations at valve cusp sites. "SITE 4" may be at a
   valve cusp vs. ligated branch site.
 ** <50% stenosis
*** ≥50% stenosis

(*Continued*)

PST Poststenotic Turbulence

VASCULAR TECHNOLOGIST
Kari A. Olmsted, BS, RVT

FINAL PHYSICIAN INTERPRETATION:

1. The right resting ankle-brachial index is borderline normal at 0.93 and unchanged compared to the previous examinations.

2. The left resting ankle-brachial index remains abnormal at 0.72 but shows a borderline significant increase compared to the previous post-op examination. There has been a significant increase compared to the pre-op measurement of 0.36 (in general, changes in the ankle-brachial index are considered significant if they are 0.15 or more).

3. There are <50% stenoses at valve cusp sites in the thigh portion of the femoral to popliteal bypass graft, as described above.

4. There is ≥50% stenosis at a valve cusp site vs. ligated branch site in the femoral to popliteal bypass graft at the level of the knee.

5. There is ≥50% stenosis in the native outflow artery just beyond the distal bypass graft anastomosis.

6. The anastomotic sites of the femoral to popliteal bypass graft are widely patent.

VASCULAR SURGERY ATTENDING
R. Eugene Zierler, MD
Finalized on 4/9/2013

LABORATORY ORGANIZATION

FIGURE 2.12. Final report on a lower extremity duplex done for bypass graft surveillance.

RENAL ARTERY DUPLEX EVALUATION

DATE OF EXAMINATION: 7/1/2013

INDICATIONS:
This is a 76-year-old female with hypertension who presents for renal artery duplex evaluation.

PREVIOUS EXAMINATION: None

RESULTS:

Proximal Abdominal Aorta--- 120 cm/s; diameter = 1.7 cm
Mid Abdominal Aorta-- 116 cm/s; diameter = 1.9 cm

Renal Artery Velocities*--- Right---------------------- Left
Origin--- 50/0 cm/s------------------ 62/0 cm/s
Proximal-- 81/0 cm/s------------------ 80/0 cm/s
Mid-- 53/0 cm/s------------------ 75/0 cm/s
Distal-- 83/0 cm/s------------------ 54/0 cm/s
Renal/Aortic Ratio (RAR)--less than 1.0-------------- less than 1.0

*Velocities listed as Peak Systolic Velocity/End-Diastolic Velocity.

Markedly elevated vascular resistance noted throughout both renal arteries.

Kidney Length--- Right ---------------------- Left
--- 12.5 cm-------------------- 11.5 cm
Right renal cyst, lower pole: 1.2 × 1.2 cm

Parenchymal Doppler Flow--------------------------------------- Right ---------------------- Left
Medullary End Diastolic Ratio-- less than 0.20------------- less than 0.20
Parenchymal Velocities-- 8-15 cm/s------------------ 10-24 cm/s

Renal Vein Patency--- Right ----------------------- Left
--- Y ------------------------------ Y

Y = Yes, N = No

Kari A. Olmsted, BS, RVT
VASCULAR TECHNOLOGIST

FINAL PHYSICIAN INTERPRETATION:

RIGHT

1. No evidence of main renal artery stenosis. Markedly elevated vascular resistance noted in the flow waveforms.
2. Abnormally elevated renal parenchymal resistance.
3. Kidney Length: 12.5 cm, including a cyst in the lower pole.
4. Renal vein is patent.

R. Eugene Zierler, MD
VASCULAR SURGERY ATTENDING
Finalized on 7/2/2013

LEFT

1. No evidence of main renal artery stenosis. Markedly elevated vascular resistance is noted in the flow waveform.
2. Abnormally elevated renal parenchymal resistance.
3. Kidney length: 11.5 cm.
4. Renal vein is patent.

FIGURE 2.13. Final report on a renal duplex done for evaluation of hypertension.

References

1. ARDMS. 2005 Vascular Physical Principles & Instrumentation Survey Results. Available at http://www.ardms.org/downloads/Survey%20 Results%20and%20Summaries/2005VPIVTresults.htm (accessed 9 January, 2008).
2. The IAC Standards and Guidelines for Vascular Testing Accreditation. Available at http://intersocietal.org/vascular/main/vascular_standards.htm (updated 15 June, 2013).
3. Moses G, Gloviczki P. New discoveries in anatomy and new terminology of leg veins: Clinical implications. *Vasc Endovasc Surg* 2004;4:367-374.
4. Caggiati A, Bergan JJ, Glovickzi P, et al. Nomenclature of the veins of the lower limb: Extensions, refinements, and clinical applications. *J Vasc Surg* 2005;41:719-724.
5. Bundens WP, Bergan JJ, Halasz NA, et al. The superficial femoral vein: A potentially lethal misnomer. *JAMA* 1995;274:1296-1298.

CHAPTER 3 ■ CREDENTIALING AND ACCREDITATION

R. EUGENE ZIERLER

The modern vascular laboratory began in the 1960s with relatively simple physiologic tests performed with inexpensive equipment by vascular surgeons and their staff, usually in an office or clinic setting. Over the last 50 years, the field has expanded in scope to play a key role in the management of patients with vascular problems. As the clinical applications of vascular testing became more numerous and the complexity of the instrumentation increased, the vascular laboratory took on a unique professional identity. Individuals who performed vascular tests became known as "vascular technologists," and the Society of Non-Invasive Vascular Technology (SNIVT) was established in 1977 to develop and promote this field. In the 1980s, ultrasound imaging became the primary diagnostic method used in the vascular laboratory. Since ultrasound was also being used for a variety of nonvascular diagnostic applications, radiologists, cardiologists, neurologists, and other medical specialists started to take an interest in the vascular laboratory. In 1988, SNIVT changed its name to the Society of Vascular Technology (SVT), and it became the Society for Vascular Ultrasound (SVU) in 2002. The terms "vascular technologist" and "vascular sonographer" are now often used interchangeably.

One consequence of this tremendous growth was the recognition that a specific body of knowledge, training, and experience was required to perform and interpret vascular tests. There was also concern among those in the field that the lack of standards and accountability was resulting in poor-quality and inappropriate vascular testing. Therefore, it was inevitable that some type of regulation would be necessary. Credentialing of personnel and accreditation of vascular laboratory facilities are the two major regulatory processes for addressing these issues.

DEFINITIONS

Credentialing is a general term that describes a formal program for verifying professional knowledge, qualifications, and competence. The credentialing process for individuals includes both *certification* and *licensure*. Certification involves the application of private standards, while licensure is based on governmental or public standards. In some situations, the practical difference between certification and licensure may be small, particularly when licensure is based on certification status or passing a privately administered examination. In the United States, licensure is granted at the state level, and in those states with licensing statutes a license is mandatory for an individual to engage in the specified profession. Certification is common among healthcare professions and is well accepted for physicians, nurses, pharmacists, and many other allied health fields. Most certification organizations maintain a registry of individuals who have successfully completed their certification process in order to provide the public with information on appropriately qualified individuals. Licensure also applies to many healthcare professions, although licensure for sonographers is a relatively recent development. Several states now have sonography licensure, and many others are considering such requirements. Both certification and licensure are typically time-limited designations with specific requirements for maintaining credentialed status, such as continuing education or retesting. *Accreditation* can be considered as a form of credentialing, but it is applied to programs or facilities, rather than individuals.

The organizations offering credentialing and accreditation for the vascular laboratory are listed in Table 3.1. This chapter discusses the most widely recognized credentialing and accreditation pathways through the American Registry for Diagnostic Medical Sonography (ARDMS) and the Intersocietal Accreditation Commission (IAC) Vascular Testing.

THE AMERICAN REGISTRY FOR DIAGNOSTIC MEDICAL SONOGRAPHY

The ARDMS was incorporated in 1975 as an independent nonprofit organization to provide certification examinations in the various specialties of medical sonography. In addition to vascular technology, these now include abdomen, breast, neurosonology, obstetrics and gynecology, musculoskeletal sonography, and adult, pediatric, and fetal echocardiography (Table 3.2). The ARDMS has also developed a credential for physicians who interpret vascular laboratory tests—Registered Physician in Vascular Interpretation (RPVI). Although physicians can be eligible to take the examinations leading to the ARDMS sonography credentials, the RPVI is the first credential created specifically for physicians. As of late in 2013, the ARDMS has certified

TABLE 3.1

ORGANIZATIONS OFFERING CREDENTIALING AND ACCREDITATION FOR THE VASCULAR LABORATORY

Credentialing for Personnel
  American Registry for Diagnostic Medical Sonography (ARDMS)
  Cardiovascular Credentialing International (CCI)
  American Registry of Radiologic Technologists (ARRT)
  American Society of Neuroimaging (ASN)

Accreditation of Facilities
  Intersocietal Accreditation Commission (IAC)
    Vascular Testing
  American College of Radiology (ACR)

over 80,000 individuals, including more than 24,000 vascular technologists and about 2000 interpreting physicians. As a member of the National Commission for Certifying Agencies, the ARDMS examinations are required to be "practice based," that is, they must reflect current practice in diagnostic ultrasound. To make sure that this requirement is met, periodic "job task analysis" surveys are conducted to document the status of the various ultrasound specialties. These surveys are made available online to ARDMS registrants in a particular specialty and cover all aspects of ultrasound practice relevant to that specialty. The results of these surveys determine the topics covered and the content of the questions for the examination.[1-3]

Between 1975 and 1982, the ARDMS offered a certification examination in Peripheral Vascular Doppler. The Registered Vascular Technologist (RVT) examination was first administered in 1983, and through 2012 more than 24,000 individuals have obtained the RVT credential (Fig. 3.1). A survey conducted by the SNIVT in 1982, along with the 1988, 1994, 2000, 2005, and 2009 ARDMS vascular technology task surveys, documents the changes that have occurred in this specialty.

The 1982 SNIVT Survey

In 1982, ankle and segmental blood pressures were the most common examination methods for peripheral arterial disease, while continuous-wave Doppler and impedance plethysmography were the most widely used tests for deep vein thrombosis. Testing methods for extracranial carotid artery disease included phonoangiography, periorbital Doppler, and pressure or pulse delay oculoplethysmography. Patients were frequently subjected to multiple tests for a single vascular problem. B-mode or duplex imaging was used by less than 25% of the surveyed technologists and only for the diagnosis of carotid artery disease.[1]

The 1988 ARDMS Vascular Technology Task Survey

The most striking change in vascular technology between 1982 and 1988 was the growth of duplex scanning as a primary testing method.[2] According to the 1988 ARDMS survey, 96% of RVTs used duplex imaging; however, only 24% had access to color-flow instrumentation. The indirect testing methods were still widely used for peripheral arterial and venous disease, although 23% of RVTs were performing duplex scanning of the peripheral arteries and 75% of RVTs reported using duplex scanning for evaluation of lower extremity bypass grafts. Duplex scanning was the predominant technique for extracranial carotid artery testing, with only about one-half of RVTs still performing indirect cerebrovascular testing. Transcranial Doppler was being used by 17% of RVTs.

The 1994 ARDMS Vascular Technology Task Survey

The 1994 ARDMS survey indicated that 93% of RVTs utilized some form of duplex scanning with color-flow imaging.[3] While the use of indirect peripheral arterial tests declined

TABLE 3.2

SONOGRAPHY EXAMINATIONS AND CREDENTIALS OFFERED BY THE ARDMS

■ EXAMINATIONS		■ CREDENTIALS
■ PHYSICS	■ SPECIALTY	
SPI Sonography Principles & Instrumentation Examination	Abdomen (AB)	RDMS Registered Diagnostic Medical Sonographer
	Breast (BR)	
	Fetal Echocardiography (FE)	
	Neurosonology (NE)	
	Obstetrics and Gynecology (OB/GYN)	
	Adult Echocardiography (AE)	RDCS Registered Diagnostic Cardiac Sonographer
	Fetal Echocardiography (FE)	
	Pediatric Echocardiography (PE)	
	Vascular Technology (VT)	RVT Registered Vascular Technologist
MSK Musculoskeletal Sonography Examination		RMSK Registered in Musculoskeletal
PVI Physicians' Vascular Interpretation Examination		RPVI Registered Physician in Vascular Interpretation

Both the SPI and a specialty examination are required for the RDMS, RDCS, and RVT credentials. The RMSK and RPVI credentials require a single examination that includes some physics content.

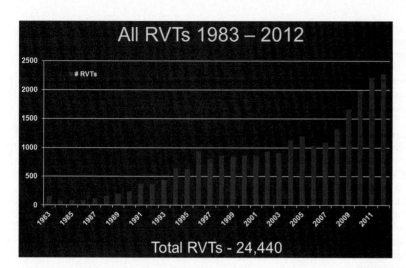

All RVTs 1983 – 2012

Total RVTs - 24,440

FIGURE 3.1. Annual numbers of individuals obtaining the RVT credential from 1983 through 2012.

slightly, arterial duplex scanning was used by 86% of RVTs. For venous testing, 95% of RVTs used duplex imaging for diagnosis of deep vein thrombosis, and 82% performed duplex saphenous vein mapping. Continuous-wave Doppler was still used by 69% of RVTs, but only about 10% reported using plethysmographic methods for venous disease. The indirect cerebrovascular tests continued to decline, with about 14% of RVTs using oculoplethysmography and 30% performing the periorbital Doppler test. Duplex scanning with color-flow imaging was used by 98% of RVTs for carotid evaluation. The use of transcranial Doppler among RVTs increased only slightly to 20%.

The 2000 ARDMS Vascular Technology Task Survey

In the fall of 1999, the ARDMS conducted its first "online" task survey for vascular technology. Among the responding RVTs, 41% were working in accredited vascular laboratories. It is noteworthy that approximately 90% of RVTs provided preliminary interpretations of examinations to referring physicians. Duplex imaging with color flow was used by 98% of RVTs for one or more applications. About 70% of RVTs measured segmental pressure gradients in the lower extremities, and 88% used duplex imaging to assess the lower extremity arteries. Mesenteric and renal artery duplex scanning were performed by 51% and 63% of RVTs, respectively. About 4% of RVTs reported using impedance plethysmography for lower extremity venous evaluation. For the extracranial carotid evaluation, less than 10% of RVTs still performed periorbital Doppler testing, while only about 2% used any type of oculoplethysmography. Duplex scanning with color-flow imaging was used by 98% of RVTs for carotid testing. The use of transcranial Doppler among RVTs remained around 20%. About 25% of RVTs performed some type of intraoperative monitoring by duplex scanning.

The 2005 ARDMS Vascular Technology Task Survey

The changes in the specialty between 2000 and 2005 were not as striking as were those noted in the prior periods.[4] In 2005, approximately 50% of the responding RVTs were working in accredited laboratories. When asked about the specialty of the physician who interpreted their test results, the responses included radiology in 43%, vascular surgery in 29%, and cardiology or vascular medicine in 14%. About 74% of RVTs

performed some nonvascular testing, such as general or cardiac ultrasound. As in the 2000 survey, 90% of RVTs provided preliminary interpretations to referring physicians. In 2005, essentially all RVTs used duplex instruments with color-flow imaging, and two-thirds had access to digital image storage. With regard to advanced applications of vascular imaging, 52% performed mesenteric duplex, 69% performed renal duplex, and 66% used duplex scanning for follow-up of endovascular aortic aneurysm repair. In addition, 85% of RVTs used duplex scanning to assess venous valvular incompetence.

The 2009 ARDMS Vascular Technology Task Survey

In late 2009, about 2000 RVTs were invited to complete an online task analysis, and 445 completed the survey for a response rate of 22%. The educational level of respondents was a Master's degree in 6%, Bachelor's degree in 31%, and an Associate degree in 28%. An MD degree was reported by 5%. When asked how many years they had been in a vascular technology practice, the response was 20 or more years in 18%, 16 to 20 years in 18%, 11 to 15 years in 18%, 6 to 10 years in 25%, and 0 to 5 years in 21%. Regarding workload, 40% performed up to 50 examinations per month and 29% performed 51 to 100 examinations per month. There were no major changes in the instrumentation used for testing or the types of tests performed between the 2005 and 2009 surveys.

The RVT Credential

Eligibility for the examinations leading to the RVT credential is determined by a set of prerequisites that are based on a candidate's education and ultrasound experience. These prerequisites are revised periodically to reflect ongoing changes in the field. The ARDMS sonography credentials (Registered Diagnostic Medical Sonographer [RDMS], Registered Diagnostic Cardiac Sonographer [RDCS], and RVT) require passing a physical principles examination and a specialty examination. In 2009, the separate physical principles examinations for the various sonography credentials were replaced by a single Sonography Principles and Instrumentation (SPI) examination (Table 3.2). This change recognizes that the basic principles of ultrasound are common to all the sonography specialties. It also makes it easier for sonographers to obtain multiple credentials, since they do not need to take different physical principles examinations for the RDMS,

RDCS, and RVT credentials. The SPI examination consists of approximately 120 questions and must be completed within 2 hours, while there are approximately 170 questions on the Vascular Technology examination that must be completed within 3 hours. ARDMS examinations are administered at testing centers located throughout the United States and Canada, as well as selected locations in Europe, Asia, and South America.

The specific topics covered in each ARDMS examination are based on the results of the job task analysis surveys that are performed every 3 to 5 years. Content outlines list the various topics and can serve as a study guide for those preparing to take the examinations. In 2010, a standard content outline format was adopted for all ARDMS examinations. This new format does not use the familiar major testing areas as main headings for the Vascular Technology examination, but divides the content into general "domains" that include Anatomy and Physiology, Pathology, Patient Care, Integration of Data, Protocols, Physics and Instrumentation, and Treatment. In this format, appropriate topics for each testing area (cerebrovascular, venous, peripheral arterial, and abdominal/visceral) are covered within the individual domains. For example, the Protocols domain constitutes 33% of the Vascular Technology examination and includes many tasks that vascular sonographers do on a daily basis, such as applying standards and guidelines for testing, measurement techniques, and physiologic testing. So although the new content outlines look quite different, this is mainly due to the way the material is organized. Tables 3.3 and 3.4 give the current content outlines for the SPI and Vascular Technology examinations.

The RPVI Credential

It is noteworthy that of the more than 24,000 individuals who have obtained the RVT credential, approximately 1800 are physicians (Fig. 3.2). The examinations leading to the RVT credential evaluate the knowledge and skills required to perform vascular tests, not the interpretive or diagnostic skills used by the physicians who interpret them. Furthermore, although credentialing of vascular technologists (or accreditation of vascular laboratories) is required for reimbursement by some insurance carriers, there are currently no such requirements for physicians. So why have so many physicians chosen to take the examinations and acquire the RVT credential? Presumably it is because they perceive that documenting their vascular laboratory expertise adds value to their practice.

TABLE 3.3

MAJOR HEADINGS IN THE CONTENT OUTLINE FOR THE SPI EXAMINATION[a]

Clinical Safety	4%
Physical Principles	10%
Ultrasound Transducers	7%
Pulse-Echo Instrumentation	35%
Doppler Instrumentation and Hemodynamics	35%
Quality Assurance	4%
Protocols	4%
New Technologies	1%

Percentages refer to the proportion of questions devoted to that content area.
[a]As of summer 2013.

TABLE 3.4

MAJOR HEADINGS IN THE CONTENT OUTLINE FOR THE VASCULAR TECHNOLOGY (VT) EXAMINATION[a]

Anatomy and Physiology	20%
Pathology	19%
Patient Care	4%
Integration of Data	10%
Protocols	33%
Physics and Instrumentation	5%
Treatment	7%
Other	2%

Percentages refer to the proportion of questions devoted to that content area.
[a]As of summer 2013.

This led the ARDMS to investigate the possibility of creating a credential specifically designed to evaluate what physicians actually do in the vascular laboratory.

In 2002, the ARDMS surveyed the Medical Staff of laboratories accredited by the Intersocietal Commission for the Accreditation of Vascular Laboratories (ICAVL) to assess their level of interest and support for a vascular laboratory physician credential. Of the 454 respondents, 38% were vascular surgeons, 26% were radiologists, 8% were cardiology/vascular medicine physicians, 4% were neurologists, and 24% did not report a specific specialty. All of the respondents (99%) interpreted vascular tests, while 33% performed some hands-on scanning. The majority (80%) spent 25% or less of their professional time interpreting vascular laboratory examinations. Although 43% considered the RVT credential to be appropriate for physicians, 51% indicated that there was a need for a separate physician credential, and 56% stated that they would be interested in obtaining such a credential.

Based on this survey, the ARDMS concluded that there was substantial interest in a credential for vascular laboratory physicians, so a committee was formed to develop and maintain the examination for this new credential with representatives from vascular surgery, vascular medicine/cardiology, radiology, and sonography. A task survey of vascular laboratory physician practice was carried out, and an appropriate content outline for the new examination was developed. As previously mentioned, this new credential is referred to as the RPVI, and the corresponding examination is the Physicians' Vascular Interpretation (PVI).

In contrast to the ARDMS sonography credentials, which require passing two separate examinations (physical principles and a specialty), the RPVI credential only requires one examination (Table 3.2). The examination consists of approximately 200 questions, many of which include still images or video clips, and it must be completed within 4 hours. There are multiple prerequisites for the PVI examination that recognize both formal and informal training in the vascular laboratory. A "pilot" examination was taken by about 60 applicants in late 2005 with a pass rate of 95%. The PVI examination was released to the medical community in January 2006, and as of late 2013, about 2000 physicians have obtained the RPVI credential (Fig. 3.3). There is no longer any reason for physicians to obtain the RVT credential unless they intend to work or function as technologists in a vascular laboratory.

The initial task analysis survey for the RPVI credential was carried out in 2005, and a second survey was done in 2011. For the 2011 survey, 2279 physicians were invited to

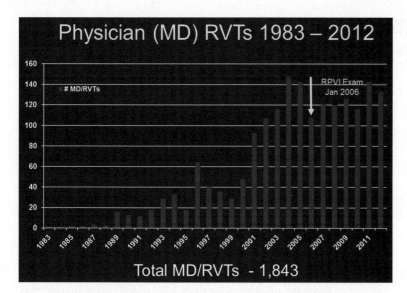

FIGURE 3.2. Annual numbers of physicians obtaining the RVT credential from 1983 through 2012. The RPVI credential was first offered in January 2006.

participate and 467 completed the online form for a response rate of 20%. The medical specialties represented included vascular/general surgery (41%), vascular medicine/cardiology (32%), radiology (12%), and other specialties (15%). Sixty-nine percent of the respondents interpreted more than 50 vascular examinations per month, with 23% interpreting more than 200 examinations per month. Experience as an interpreting physician was 5 years or less in 30%, 6 to 10 years in 30%, and more than 10 years in 40% of respondents. There did not appear to be any major changes in the testing areas or types of tests interpreted between the 2005 and 2011 RPVI surveys.

In 2012, the PVI examination content outline was revised to reflect the standard content outline format (Table 3.5). As with the Vascular Technology examination content outline, topics relating to the various testing areas (abdominal/visceral, cerebrovascular, peripheral arterial, and venous) are included within each major domain. The most important major domain for the PVI examination is Integration of Data, which accounts for 44% of the questions and covers a variety of tasks related to interpretation such as reporting on incidental findings, understanding clinical indications for testing, making comparisons with previous studies, analyzing

effects of anatomic or medical abnormalities, and recognizing technical limitations.

Recertification

Obtaining an ARDMS credential demonstrates "entry-level" competence at one point in time. However, a credential does not insure that an individual will remain competent over the span of a career. Recognizing this limitation, many healthcare professions have some continuing competency or recertification requirements following initial certification. These most commonly involve some combination of continuing medical education (CME) and reexamination. The ARDMS has a continuing competency requirement of 30 CME credits per 3-year cycle, with compliance monitored by random audits. In 2012, the ARDMS also started a formal recertification program. All ARDMS credentials will be valid for 10 years, and the recertification examination must be taken during the last 3 years of this period. The first recertification examinations will be given in 2019 and will be short (~50 questions), open book, and web based. Registrants with multiple credentials must take a separate recertification examination for each credential that they want to maintain.

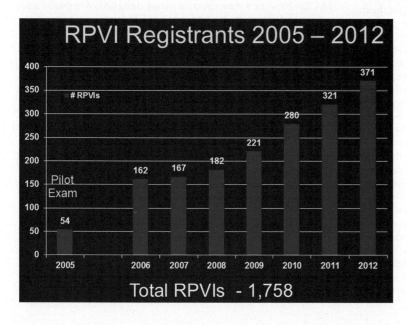

FIGURE 3.3. Annual numbers of physicians obtaining the RPVI credential from 2005 through 2012. A pilot examination was offered to a small number of qualified applicants in 2005, and the examination was made available to physicians in January 2006.

LABORATORY ORGANIZATION

TABLE 3.5

MAJOR HEADINGS IN THE CONTENT OUTLINE FOR THE PVI EXAMINATION[a]

Anatomy and Physiology	8%
Pathology	10%
Patient Care	8%
Integration of Data	44%
Protocols	16%
Physics and Instrumentation	10%
Other	4%

Percentages refer to the proportion of questions devoted to that content area.
[a]As of September 2012.

THE INTERSOCIETAL ACCREDITATION COMMISSION— VASCULAR TESTING

In 1989, leaders in the field of noninvasive vascular testing met to discuss growing concerns over the inappropriate use of vascular tests and the lack of standards for testing methods, diagnostic criteria, and quality assurance. This group understood that any regulatory actions that came from a single specialty would not be acceptable to all the specialties with a stake in the vascular laboratory, so they proposed an "intersocietal" model that included vascular surgeons, radiologists, neurologists, vascular medicine specialists, and vascular technologists. Support for the concept of vascular laboratory accreditation and financial sponsorship was obtained from a variety of professional societies, and the ICAVL was incorporated in 1990. The founding sponsors were The American Academy of Neurology (AAN), the American College of Radiology (ACR), the American Institute of Ultrasound in Medicine (AIUM), the North American Chapter of the International Society for Cardiovascular Surgery (ISCVS), the Society for Vascular Surgery (SVS), the Society for Vascular Medicine and Biology (SVMB), the Society of Diagnostic Medical Sonography (SDMS), and the SVT. The ICAVL Board included two representatives from each of the sponsoring organizations.

The initial meetings of the ICAVL Board were devoted to defining the scope of the accreditation process and establishing standards for all aspects of vascular laboratory practice. The overall goal was to establish a process for recognizing high-quality vascular diagnostic testing by peer review, issuing certificates of accreditation, and maintaining a registry of accredited laboratories. From the beginning, the ICAVL Standards and Guidelines were designed to be as inclusive as possible so they could be applied to all vascular laboratories regardless of size, clinical setting, or the medical specialties of the physicians involved. The general format of these standards was adapted from other accreditation programs such as the Joint Commission on Accreditation of Health Care Organizations. They addressed the basic laboratory resources of space, equipment, and personnel, as well as patient safety, reporting, and the qualifications of technical and medical staff. These aspects are covered in the Organization section of the Standards and Guidelines. Additional sections were devoted to each of the major testing areas: cerebrovascular, peripheral arterial, peripheral venous, and visceral vascular. The Standards and Guidelines for each testing area defined the primary instrumentation that was required and what methods were considered secondary or supplemental. Standards were

also created for indications, testing protocols, diagnostic criteria, and quality assurance. In 1996, the cerebrovascular testing section was divided into extracranial and intracranial cerebrovascular testing, and a separate section for vascular screening was added in 2005.

In 1991, 15 laboratories completed a pilot accreditation program, and 36 laboratories were granted formal ICAVL accreditation in 1992. As of August 2012, there were 1671 accredited vascular laboratories with 2486 testing sites. These accredited laboratories had the following distribution of testing areas: extracranial cerebrovascular 34%, peripheral arterial 28%, peripheral venous 27%, visceral vascular 8%, intracranial cerebrovascular 2%, and screening 1%. The average number of medical staff in accredited laboratories was four, with the following specialty distribution: radiology 37%, vascular surgery 32%, cardiology/vascular medicine 22%, neurology/neurosurgery 5%, and family medicine or other specialties 4%. Vascular surgery was the predominant specialty for medical directors, accounting for 44%, followed by cardiology/vascular medicine 34%, radiology 12%, neurology/neurosurgery 4%, and family medicine or other specialties 6%. ICAVL accreditation was limited to 3 years, and an application for reaccreditation was required to maintain accredited status. The standards and guidelines are reviewed and revised every 3 years.

The ICAVL added four additional sponsoring organizations in 1993: the American College of Cardiology, the American Society of Neuroimaging combined with the AAN, the Joint Section on Cerebrovascular Surgery/American Association of Neurological Surgeons and Congress of Neurological Surgeons, and the Society of Interventional Radiology. In 2000, the Society of Radiologists in Ultrasound was added, and in 2005 the American Society of Echocardiography became a sponsoring organization. The ACR withdrew sponsorship in 1996. The ISCVS and SVS merged into a single society in 2003, retaining the SVS name. The Society for Clinical Vascular Surgery was then added as a sponsor.

After it was incorporated in 1990, the ICAVL was joined by accrediting bodies devoted to four other diagnostic imaging specialties, all under the administrative authority of the IAC. These were the Intersocietal Commission for the Accreditation of Echocardiography Laboratories (ICAEL), the Intersocietal Commission for the Accreditation of Nuclear Medicine Laboratories (ICANL), the Intersocietal Commission for the Accreditation of Magnetic Resonance Laboratories (ICAMRL), and the Intersocietal Commission for the Accreditation of Computed Tomography Laboratories (ICACTL). In 2012, the IAC underwent a major restructuring designed to improve and streamline the accreditation process. The various accrediting bodies were renamed, with ICAVL becoming IAC Vascular Testing. The current sponsoring organizations of IAC Vascular Testing are listed in Table 3.6. The other IAC accrediting bodies included IAC Echocardiography, IAC Nuclear/PET, IAC MRI, IAC CT, and IAC Carotid Stenting.

THE ROLE OF CREDENTIALING AND ACCREDITATION

Until relatively recently, both credentialing of vascular technologists and accreditation of vascular laboratories were completely voluntary. However, the roles of credentialing and accreditation are changing along with many other aspects of medical practice. In order to promote quality in patient care and control costs, a number of state Medicare Carriers now require that noninvasive vascular diagnostic tests be performed by or under the direct supervision of credentialed vascular technologists to qualify for payment. Examples of appropriate technologist certification include the RVT credential granted by the ARDMS

TABLE 3.6

SPONSORING ORGANIZATIONS OF THE IAC—VASCULAR TESTING[a]

Vascular Surgery
Society for Vascular Surgery
Society for Clinical Vascular Surgery

Radiology
Society of Interventional Radiology
Society of Radiologists in Ultrasound

Cardiology
American College of Cardiology
American Society of Echocardiography

Vascular Medicine
Society for Vascular Medicine

Neurology/Neurosurgery
American Academy of Neurology/American Society of Neuroimaging
Joint Section on Cerebrovascular Surgery/American Association of Neurological Surgeons and Congress of Neurological Surgeons

Vascular Technology
Society for Vascular Ultrasound

Sonography
Society of Diagnostic Medical Sonography
American Institute of Ultrasound in Medicine

[a]As of January 2013.

and the RVS credential offered by Cardiovascular Credentialing International (CCI). Some carriers also accept laboratory accreditation by IAC or ACR as a qualification for reimbursement. Beginning in January 2003, all Technical Directors of accredited laboratories were required to have an appropriate credential in vascular testing. The IAC Vascular Testing Standards and Guidelines now state that starting in January 2017, credentialing will be required for all technical staff.

Although state licensure for sonographers or vascular technologists is still relatively uncommon, several states have instituted such requirements, and many others are considering various forms of sonography licensure. It is likely that sonography licensure will be based at least in part on credential status, since credentialing provides a standardized process for verifying entry level competence. Physicians must be licensed to practice medicine, but as of late 2013 there is no requirement

that a physician have the RPVI credential to receive payment for interpreting vascular laboratory tests. Although physician credentialing may be required for payment in the future, individual laboratories or institutions can still make the RPVI credential a requirement for local "interpreting privileges." The principal value of the RPVI credential is that it documents individual knowledge and expertise and provides a "common denominator" for evaluating vascular laboratory experience and training across multiple medical specialties. This is particularly important because interpretation of vascular laboratory tests is done in a variety of settings by physicians from diverse backgrounds. In June 2010, the Vascular Surgery Board of the American Board of Surgery announced that starting in 2014, all applicants for certification in vascular surgery will be required to possess the RPVI credential. This makes the RPVI credential a "prerequisite" for vascular surgery certification.

The process of applying for IAC Vascular Testing accreditation is detailed and lengthy; however, working through the application requires a thorough review of every aspect of the laboratory, and it is intended to be an educational and constructive project. This "self-evaluation" often identifies areas for improvement, such as incomplete diagnostic protocols, vague interpretation criteria, and lack of a quality assurance program. It also prompts a review of the available testing equipment, ongoing staff education, record keeping, and reporting practices. After all of the application documentation has been completed, the laboratory submits actual case studies performed by current staff members using current equipment. These case studies are carefully analyzed for compliance with the Standards and represent a key component of the application process.

Up-to-date information on issues in vascular laboratory credentialing and accreditation can be obtained from the sources below.

ARDMS
(800) 541-9754
www.ardms.org

IAC Vascular Testing
(800) 838-2110
www.intersocietal.org/vascular

References

1. Beach KW, Tyler AR, Martin DC, et al. Practices of peripheral vascular technologists revealed. *Bruit* 1982;6:29.
2. Anderson FA, Beach KW, Burnham CK, et al. The 1988 ARDMS survey on vascular technology. *J Vasc Technol* 1989;13:171.
3. Leers SA, Blackburn DR, Burnham SJ, et al. Vascular technology in evolution: Results of the 1994 ARDMS task survey. *J Vasc Technol* 1995;19:127.
4. ARDMS. 2005 Vascular Physical Principles & Instrumentation Survey Results. http://www.ardms.org/downloads/Survey%20Results%20and%20Summaries/2005VPIVTresults.htm (accessed on January 9, 2008).

CHAPTER 4 ■ QUALITY ASSURANCE AND TEST VALIDATION*

DAVID DEL PIZZO AND HOLLY M. GRAY

Ongoing improvement in imaging technologies provides sonographers and physicians with improved ability to assess vascular pathology, with better accuracy and more detail. Advances in clinical informatics provide new tools for data management in the vascular laboratory, including use of data for correlations to validate testing methods and interpretation standards.

Ensuring reliability of vascular laboratory reports is important, as there is increasing reliance on noninvasive examinations for clinical decision making. For example, venography is seldom used for diagnosis of deep vein thrombosis (DVT). Routine surveillance after aortic endograft procedures with duplex scanning is the norm in many centers. Critical clinical judgments, such as decisions about surgical interventions, the need for additional invasive studies, or treatment with anticoagulation therapy, are often based solely upon the results of ultrasound examinations. This reliance on the vascular laboratory makes it essential that testing and reporting are accurate and relevant. Therefore, vascular laboratories need ongoing quality programs to ensure complete, accurate, and high-quality results and reporting.[1]

Third-party payers, government agencies, and the public expect medical imaging facilities to document the reliability of their results. Regular reviews of laboratory processes, examination findings, and quality measures are essential parts of the process of good patient care and ensure the overall success of the vascular laboratory. Audit processes in the vascular laboratory may also confirm that testing is done for appropriate indications and in compliance with applicable standards for documentation of medical necessity. Additionally, it is important to the role of the vascular laboratory in the safe delivery of patient care. Laboratory protocols should incorporate standards that help meet established safety and outcomes priorities, such as National Patient Safety Goals (NPSGs) of The Joint Commission,[2] which include correct identification of patients, prevention of infections, and prevention of mistakes in surgery. Appropriate practices in the vascular laboratory, accurate reporting of results, and use of workflow practices to catch and correct errors will contribute to success in meeting NPSGs.

ELEMENTS OF QUALITY PROGRAMS

A comprehensive quality improvement (QI) program should include three components: quality control (QC), quality assurance (QA), and continuous quality improvement (CQI). All three components are required to be effective in ensuring safety, improving services, and enhancing the level of patient care.[3]

In the vascular laboratory, *quality control* generally relates to the calibration and maintenance of equipment. As part of the laboratory's QI program, there should be a standardized method of QC for all technology being used in the laboratory, thus minimizing the risk of inaccuracies arising from defective or uncalibrated equipment. Typically, manufacturers of ultrasound systems provide recommended QC schedules and specify the methods to be used to ensure proper equipment function. Equipment servicing and QC checks must be documented to provide a record of maintenance that can be referenced or audited.

Quality assurance is the systematic monitoring and evaluation of various aspects of a project, service, or facility to ensure that standards of quality are being met. The QA program in the vascular laboratory assesses compliance with established standards, policies, and protocols. QA programs also document the accuracy and outcomes of the testing procedures. Laboratory personnel should take into consideration current industry standards, published clinical research, evidence-based practice guidelines, and accepted thresholds when developing or updating their own QA policies, keeping in mind that some policies may be unique to their particular setting. It is important to ensure that the written technical protocols are followed by all members of the staff when performing examinations. Protocols should clearly define the scanning technique, the assessment of vessels and surrounding organs or tissues, what to document in a normal study, and how to evaluate and document any abnormalities. In addition, there need to be standardized diagnostic criteria for each examination that are applied in the same manner by all interpreting physicians. These

---

*Based on the chapter in the fourth edition authored by Cindy Weiland and Sandra L. Katanick.

criteria should be validated either by comparison to reports in the published literature or through validation procedures performed by the laboratory. Routine monitoring of these two aspects of laboratory practice—protocols and diagnostic criteria—will help ensure a systematic approach to the services provided by the laboratory and lead to improved standardization and more consistent test results.

Continuous quality improvement is the process by which a vascular laboratory becomes more successful overall. It is not a single activity; rather, it is an ongoing effort that addresses different aspects of the laboratory over time. Often, this component of the program is driven by the most urgent issues facing the laboratory. Data collection and analysis are most valuable if they address a current problem or are used to improve an already functional system.

Steps in organizing vascular laboratory quality programs include identifying (1) the individual(s) responsible for data collection, (2) where and how data will be obtained, (3) how often data collection will occur, (4) the format to be used to record the information, (5) how improvement will be measured, and (6) how the findings will be shared with laboratory staff. In addition, a dedicated forum is needed to review laboratory operations and the QA data; for example, monthly or quarterly meetings. These meetings should review the results of comparative studies, address discrepancies, discuss difficult cases, and address facility issues that affect quality of care. Minutes of these meetings should be documented.

The need for standards and accreditation of vascular laboratories was recognized early on, as vascular testing transitioned from a research tool to become a core element of vascular care.[4] Laboratories with a commitment to high-quality testing often seek accreditation or take measures to maintain the standards of accreditation. Accreditation specific to vascular laboratory testing is provided by the Intersocietal Accreditation Commission (IAC), which has several divisions (see Chapter 3). The first IAC division to be established was Vascular Testing, formerly known as the Intersocietal Commission for the Accreditation of Vascular Laboratories (ICAVL). As part of the process of applying for accreditation, facilities conduct a detailed self-evaluation using the *IAC Standards and Guidelines for Vascular Testing Accreditation.*[5] Description of a comprehensive, ongoing QI program is a mandatory component of the application.

The IAC standards state that:

- QI must be performed and there must be a written QI policy for all laboratory procedures.
- Results of studies must be correlated with other measurements; a log of these comparisons must be maintained, and for each area of testing, there must be greater than 70% accuracy agreement.

- QI meetings must be held to examine the results of comparative studies, review discrepancies, discuss difficult cases, and address facility issues.

DATA COLLECTION

Prospective gathering and organization of correlative data are essential to a successful quality program. The tracking methods used may be part of a commercial software package for vascular laboratory reporting, a radiology information system (RIS), or an electronic health record (EHR), or the method may be based on internally developed forms. Positive test results that could be expected to lead to clinical follow-up, another correlative examination, or surgical intervention should be tracked. The laboratory should have a method to maintain a log of patients with positive or unusual test findings. This may be as simple as a notebook kept in the testing rooms to catalog patients, but a secure electronic record consistent with the facilities documentation and information assurance policies is preferred. Electronic data collection may be a requirement in some large health systems, such as the Department of Veterans Affairs. The Picture Archiving and Communication System (PACS), RIS, or EHR used by the laboratory may include this capability. Using the lists created, assigned staff can gather information about treatment, further testing, or clinical outcomes, which can be compared with the findings of the noninvasive vascular examination.

Correlative information is obtained and logged (Table 4.1). It is generally easier if a log is kept for each type of test performed in the laboratory in order to streamline the data for analysis. The log should include testing dates, patient identifiers, noninvasive examination findings, and the results of any additional testing or follow-up (e.g., contrast angiography, magnetic resonance angiography [MRA], computed tomography angiography [CTA], or surgical intervention).

MEASURING ACCURACY WITH CORRELATIVE EXAMINATIONS

Specificity, sensitivity, and accuracy are used to describe the results of a diagnostic test in comparison with a standard examination (reference standard).[6] These measures express the quality of an examination in different ways. *Sensitivity* is the probability that a test will be positive when disease is present (true positive). *Specificity* is the probability that a test will be negative when disease is absent (true negative). These relationships are shown in Table 4.2. The *predictive value* of a

---

TABLE 4.1

SAMPLE QUALITY ASSURANCE LOG FOR CAROTID DUPLEX TESTING

DATE	PATIENT	DUPLEX FINDINGS RIGHT ICA	ANGIO-GRAPHY FINDINGS RIGHT ICA	RIGHT CORRELATION	DUPLEX FINDINGS LEFT ICA	ANGIO-GRAPHY FINDINGS	LEFT CORRELATION
2/5/13	J. Smith	1%–15%	30%	No	80%–99%	95%	Yes
2/5/13	M. Jones	Occlusion	Occlusion	Yes	80%–99%	70%	No
2/6/13	N. Bass	Normal	Normal	Yes	16%–49%	25%	Yes
2/7/13	M. Reynolds	80%–99%	99%	Yes	16%–49%	40%	Yes
2/9/13	R. Ricci	100%	Occlusion	Yes	Normal	Normal	Yes
2/9/13	S. Smith	50%–79%	60%	Yes	100%	99%	No
2/9/13	J. Ryan	50%–79%	75%	Yes	50%–79%	60%	Yes

TABLE 4.2

CALCULATING SPECIFICITY, SENSITIVITY, AND PREDICTIVE VALUES

	Disease Absent	Disease Present
Vascular Lab Test Is Negative	True Negative (TN)	False Negative (FN)
Vascular Lab Test Is Positive	False Positive (FP)	True Positive (TP)

Specificity = TN / (TN + FP)
Sensitivity = TP / (TP + FN)

Positive Predictive Value (PPV) = TP / (TP + FP) × 100
Negative Predictive Value (NPV) = TN / (FN + TN) × 100
Overall Accuracy = (TN + TP) / (TN + FN + FP + TP)

Disease absent or present is based on the gold standard test.

test is a measure of the number of times that the value obtained (positive or negative) is the true value. Thus, the percentage of all positive tests that are true positives is the *positive predictive value*, and the percentage of all negative tests that are true negatives is the *negative predictive value. Accuracy* is the number of correct findings whether a patient has disease or not. All of these measures are expressed as percentages. It is important to understand these definitions in order to precisely identify what the source of an overall low accuracy may be or to recognize trends that could potentially necessitate a change in one or more laboratory processes.

A matrix is generally the best method for calculating the overall accuracy of a test and identifying any outliers or inaccurate test results. To create a matrix, use the categories for reporting disease from the noninvasive vascular examination for both the x and the y axes. The results that correlate exactly will fall on the diagonal axis within the grid, which represents agreement between the vascular laboratory test and the standard test (Table 4.3). To complete the matrix, locate the category reported for the noninvasive vascular examination on the y axis on the far left of the matrix and indicate the correlative examination categories along the top x axis. Using the duplex findings, locate the appropriate category (row) and place the mark under the category located on the horizontal axis (column) representing the correlative examination findings. Keep in mind that the correlative examination findings often are not reported using the same categories as the vascular laboratory test, so the findings may need to be reclassified to fit into the matrix. Table 4.4 demonstrates a comparison of carotid duplex findings with angiographic findings. All occurrences of exact correlations are tallied within the yellow boxes falling along the diagonal axis within the grid, whereas those findings that do not correlate fall either to the left or to the right of the diagonal axis.

TABLE 4.3

SAMPLE MATRIX FOR CORRELATING RESULTS OF VASCULAR LAB TEST AND GOLD STANDARD TEST

		Gold Standard Imaging Findings				
		Normal	1%–49%	50%–69%	70%–99%	Occlusion
Vascular Lab Test	Normal	TN				
	1%–49%		A			
	50%–69%			B		
	70%–99%				C	
	Occlusion					D

1. Yellow cells falling along the diagonal axis indicate exact correlation
2. A, B, C, D indicate True Abnormal
3. TN = True Normal
4. Accuracy = (TN + A + B + C + D) / Total Tests

TABLE 4.4

SAMPLE MATRIX FOR CORRELATING RESULTS OF CAROTID DUPLEX WITH ANGIOGRAPHY

		Angiography Findings				
	Normal	1%–15%	16%–49%	50%–79%	80%–99%	Occlusion
Normal	6					
1%–15%		4				
16%–49%			15	1		
50%–79%			1	4		
80%–99%					3	
Occlusion					1	2

FALSE NEGATIVES

FALSE POSITIVES

Duplex Findings

1. False Positives = 2; False Negatives = 1
2. Overall Accuracy: $(34/37) \times 100 = 91.9\%$

Table 4.4 demonstrates two occurrences in which findings were overestimated by duplex ultrasound, falling to the left side of the diagonal as false positives. There was a single instance in which the duplex underestimated findings and is counted as a false negative along the right side of the diagonal axis. Both of these types of outliers affect not only the overall accuracy of the test but the sensitivity and specificity as well. In calculating the overall accuracy, the true normal and abnormal examinations (those on the diagonal axis of the matrix) are added together and then divided by the total number of entries within the matrix. Table 4.4 shows a total overall accuracy of 91.9%.

The accuracy of examinations that do not utilize criteria quantifying the severity of disease, but rather identify only the presence or absence of disease, such as peripheral venous duplex testing, can be tracked using a modified matrix. Inserting the examination results into this modified grid will identify the true positives, false positives, true negatives, and false negatives, as described in Table 4.2. This documentation will also provide the information needed to calculate the sensitivity, specificity, predictive values, and overall accuracy (Table 4.5).

WHEN CORRELATIVE EXAMINATIONS ARE NOT AVAILABLE

Historically, noninvasive vascular tests have been regularly correlated with imaging methods such as standard contrast angiography, digital subtraction angiography (DSA), and more recently, MRA and CTA. However, with advances in the technology of duplex ultrasound equipment and increased confidence in the ultrasound findings, patients are often treated based upon the noninvasive examination results alone; other imaging is not always performed. This is particularly true in peripheral venous testing for DVT in which ultrasound has become the "gold standard" and contrast venography or other imaging is rarely performed. In addition, patients regularly undergo carotid endarterectomy based on the carotid duplex findings alone.

Because of these changes in clinical practice, the number of alternative imaging examinations performed on patients undergoing vascular laboratory tests has decreased, and

TABLE 4.5

SAMPLE MATRIX FOR A TEST TO DETECT DVT

	Comparative Exam Findings	
Duplex Findings	**DVT Absent**	**DVT Present**
Negative for DVT	50	1
Positive for DVT	6	9

Specificity = 50 / (50 + 6) = 89%
Sensitivity = 9 / (9 + 1) = 90%

Positive Predictive Value (PPV) = 9 / (9 + 6) = 60%
Negative Predictive Value (NPV) = 50 / (50 + 1) = 98%
Overall Accuracy = (50 + 9) / 66 = 89%

This test only identifies the presence or absence of disease.

therefore, opportunities to correlate examination results have become less frequent. However, this increased confidence in ultrasound does not negate the need to monitor the accuracy of the noninvasive examination findings. In fact, when vascular laboratory tests are used in this way, it becomes even more imperative to regularly assess the image quality and the final interpretation. This can be accomplished through a variety of approaches that do not involve correlative examinations.

One method of assessing test validity is to compare the noninvasive examination findings with clinical outcomes or surgical findings. *Clinical correlation* refers to reviewing the treatment plan prescribed for the patient based on the noninvasive test results and the patient's subsequent management to see whether the clinical course was generally consistent with the vascular laboratory diagnosis. *Correlation with operative findings* involves reviewing the operative report and determining whether the severity of a lesion found at surgery was consistent with the noninvasive test findings. It is also possible to correlate the location of lesions or other abnormalities using this approach. Correlation with operative findings, however, can be imprecise, and there is a potential for reporting bias without independent, objective adjudication of the findings. Thus, IAC Vascular Testing now strongly discourages correlation with operative findings.

Another QA tool is the "over-reading" of the examination results by a second physician. This can be used as a method of QA that compares the final interpretation of each reader and ensures that conclusions are consistent among all of the interpreting physicians. Repeat testing by two separate examiners can provide valuable information regarding the technical consistency of the examination. After the first technologist completes the test, another technologist who is not provided with the findings of the initial test performs a second examination. The findings of the two examinations are compared for test accuracy and adherence to protocol. Although these approaches do not provide the information necessary to calculate detailed QA statistics, they do provide additional ongoing assessments of laboratory quality when correlative examinations are unavailable.

It is worth noting that analyses for correlation of vascular laboratory studies may be skewed by a selection bias. Patients with negative studies and benign clinical courses are less likely to have additional imaging performed. If correlations are available for only a selected cohort, calculated sensitivity and specificity for tests may be different than the values that would be obtained if all tested patients had correlative studies. Further, the predictive value of a test will be less if the test is performed for indications that are different than those used for validation studies.

PEER REVIEW

A system of peer review provides regular feedback that assists in improving or maintaining the consistency of the laboratory. The peer review process evaluates the quality of examinations and interpretations and should include all members of the medical and technical staff. A specified number of random cases for each staff member are collected at intervals stated in the laboratory policy (e.g., monthly or quarterly). The reviews for these cases should be anonymous whenever possible, and the anonymity maintained by the individual responsible for collecting the QA data. Discrepancies should be defined as minor or major, and discrepancy trends should be tracked. All inconsistencies are noted, forwarded to the appropriate personnel, and discussed at the laboratory QA meeting.

Physician Peer Review

The physician review will include a review of the examination findings and comparison with the final report by another member of the medical staff. Inconsistencies between the test findings and the final report should be documented. As well, the reports should be evaluated for adherence to the diagnostic criteria, report content and format, and timeliness of report availability. A worksheet can be developed that will aid in this process (Fig. 4.1).

Technologist/Sonographer Peer Review

The technologist or sonographer is primarily responsible for the performance of the examination and documentation of the test findings. They are trained to follow a laboratory protocol in order to obtain the most complete study possible for each patient. The technical staff review should consist of random case reviews completed by the technical director. This review should include assessment of examination completeness, adherence to protocol, and technical quality. As with the physician review, a worksheet to document and share the review findings should be developed (Fig. 4.2).

UTILIZING THE DATA

The data collected must be analyzed in order to develop plans for improvement. The information is of little value if it is not shared with staff and used as the basis for action plans. It is vitally important to the QA program that all staff members participate in the collection and assessment of the QA data in order to implement any changes required to correct the problems identified. It will then be necessary to collect follow-up data based on implementation of any new processes, protocols, or criteria. Once the QA information has been reviewed and discussed and the reasons for inconsistencies or inaccuracies identified, formulate a plan for action. One scenario of the steps taken when utilizing this approach follows.

Quality Assurance Data Review: Example Scenario

1. It is found that a laboratory's accuracy in carotid duplex testing is low, with most of the diagnostic errors from false-positive duplex findings in the 70% to 79% stenosis category, thus decreasing the overall accuracy to less than 70%.
2. The laboratory staff investigates to determine whether these misdiagnoses are due to one or more of the following:
   a. Technical errors by one or more technical staff members.
   b. Inappropriately applied diagnostic criteria by one or more medical staff members.
   c. Appropriately applied criteria that remain discordant with the alternative imaging diagnosis (e.g., possible inaccurate correlative imaging studies).
3. In this example, it is determined that the established diagnostic criteria were being applied incorrectly by some of the physicians interpreting the carotid duplex examinations.
4. A plan is implemented to routinely audit the final reports to ensure accurate application of the diagnostic criteria. The audit is continued for 6 months and is followed by a reevaluation of the correlation between the duplex scans and the alternative imaging. It was anticipated that the number of false-positive findings in the 70% to 79% category should decrease by 70%.

VASCULAR LABORATORY QUALITY ASSURANCE
Physician / Final Report Review

Type of Noninvasive Exam: _____

Physician i.d.: _____

Reviewer i.d.: _____

	Study #1 Date of Exam:	Study #2 Date of Exam:	Study #3 Date of Exam:
Interpretation			
Report			

Interpretation Scoring: No Discrepancies = 1 | Minor Discrepancies = 2 | Major Discrepancies = 3
Report Scoring: Accurate/Complete = 1 | Minor Inconsistencies = 2 | Major Inconsistencies = 3

REVIEW COMMENTS:
Study #1 _____
_____
_____

Study #2 _____
_____
_____

Study #3 _____
_____
_____
_____

FIGURE 4.1. Sample worksheet for physician peer review.

5. At the time of reevaluation, the overall accuracy had improved to 80% and the number of false-positive results in the 70% to 79% stenosis category had decreased by 72%. The results are communicated to all of the technical and medical staff of the laboratory and documented in the minutes of QA meeting.

QUALITY ASSURANCE MEETINGS

QA meetings should be held routinely and documented with minutes. Meetings may be weekly, monthly, or quarterly, based on the needs or unique qualities of the laboratory. Even small laboratories consisting of one or two physicians and technologists should hold formal meetings. All members of the technical and medical staff should be encouraged to participate. In addition, participation should be a part of the curriculum for trainees, including sonography students, as well as residents and fellows being trained in the interpretation of vascular laboratory studies. All staff members should be held to the processes, protocols, and criteria defined within the laboratory and should be given specific guidelines and expectations regarding their performance. If these specific expectations are not met by staff members, steps must be in place to hold them accountable.

Records of QA meetings are necessary, not just as a means for internal communication, but also to meet institutional requirements, for regulatory and accreditation standards, and for medico-legal legal purposes. Of note, information collected and used for QA purposes is generally protected from discovery in liability actions.

QUALITY ASSURANCE AND ACCREDITATION

Laboratories accredited by IAC Vascular Testing are required to maintain an ongoing QA program that includes a minimum of two QA meetings a year, a minimum number of required correlations for each type of testing performed in the laboratory, and an overall accuracy of 70% or greater for each area of testing. QA is considered necessary to ensure a commitment to high-quality patient care. When applying for accreditation or reaccreditation, the laboratory must submit at least the minimum number of correlations required, as documented in a log and accompanied by the appropriate QA matrix, demonstrating an acceptable level of overall accuracy.

CONCLUSION

No diagnostic test is correct 100% of the time, but variation and inconsistencies can be minimized. Inaccuracies in noninvasive diagnostic testing can result from improperly calibrated equipment; patient factors limiting the examination (bowel gas, body habitus, or movement), inadequately trained sonographers, and improper application of diagnostic criteria. Physicians and technologists should understand the factors that introduce uncertainties with noninvasive diagnostic testing procedures and take the necessary steps to monitor test accuracy and provide appropriate reporting of test findings.

VASCULAR LABORATORY QUALITY ASSURANCE
Technologist/Sonographer Exam Review

Type of Noninvasive Exam: _____
Date of Exam 1: _____ Date of Exam 2: _____ Date of Exam 3: _____
Technologist: _____

Criteria	Study #1	Study #2	Study #3
Type of Examination			
Adherence to protocol			
Exam is complete and thorough			
Waveform quality (CW Doppler, PW Doppler, PVR)			
Image quality (if applicable)			
Overall technical quality (system settings, accurate measurements and angle technique)			

Criteria Scoring: Exceeds = 1 | Meets = 2 | Some Deficiency = 3 | Unacceptable = 4

Review Comments:

Study #1 _____
_____
_____
_____

Study #2 _____
_____
_____
_____

Study #3 _____
_____
_____
_____

FIGURE 4.2. Sample worksheet for technologist/sonographer peer review.

References

1. Akbari CM, Stone L. Accreditation and credentialing in the vascular laboratory. *Semin Vasc Surg* 2002;15(3):178-181.
2. http://www.jointcommission.org/standards_information/npsgs.aspx (accessed February 16, 2014)
3. Christian PE, Waterstram-Rich KM (eds). *Nuclear Medicine and PET/CT Technologies and Techniques*, 6th ed. St. Louis: Mosby, 2007, pp 253-265.
4. Thiele BL. The vascular laboratory. Standards and certification. *Surg Clin North Am* 1990;70(1):1-11.
5. http://www.intersocietal.org/vascular/standards/IACVascular TestingStandards2013.pdf (accessed July 7, 2014)
6. Campbell MJ, Machin D, Walters SJ (eds). *Medical Statistics: A Textbook for the Health Sciences*, 4th ed. The Atrium, Southern Gate, Chichester, West Sussex: John Wiley & Sons, Ltd., 2007.

SECTION II ■ PRINCIPLES AND INSTRUMENTATION

CHAPTER 5 ■ HEMODYNAMICS OF NORMAL AND ABNORMAL ARTERIES

R. EUGENE ZIERLER

An in-depth understanding of the major diseases that affect the arterial system and the diagnostic methods that can be applied to them requires some knowledge of the basic principles that govern pressure and flow. The major mechanisms of arterial disease are obstruction of the lumen and disruption of the vessel wall. Arterial stenosis or occlusion may result from atherosclerosis, emboli, thrombi, fibromuscular dysplasia, trauma, or external compression. The clinical significance of a particular obstructive lesion depends on its location, severity, and duration, as well as the ability of the circulation to compensate by developing collateral pathways. Disruption of the arterial wall is typically caused by ruptured aneurysms or trauma. Because these pathologic mechanisms tend to involve the large and medium-sized arteries, the techniques for identification of arterial disease by duplex scanning have focused on these segments of the arterial system. Although some vascular disorders involve the small arteries and microcirculation, these are best examined by indirect physiologic tests.

When a patient with arterial disease first presents, the health care provider needs to answer certain questions, regardless of the underlying disorder. In the presence of arterial obstruction, it is important to know the overall severity of ischemia, as well as the location and relative severity of the responsible lesions. For aneurysmal disease, the key question usually relates to the size and location of the lesion. A combination of indirect physiologic tests and direct duplex imaging can provide the necessary diagnostic information for initial diagnostic and therapeutic decisions. Because duplex scanning assesses both vascular anatomy and flow characteristics at specific arterial sites, this approach is ideally suited for evaluation of the most common arterial problems.

PRESSURE AND FLOW IN NORMAL ARTERIES

Fluid Energy

Although pressure gradients are the most obvious forces involved, blood flows through the arterial system in response to differences in total fluid energy. The pressure in a fluid system is defined as force per unit area, with units such as dynes per square centimeter or millimeters of mercury (mm Hg). Intravascular arterial pressure (P) has three components: (1) dynamic pressure produced by cardiac contraction, (2) hydrostatic pressure, and (3) static filling pressure. Hydrostatic pressure depends on the specific gravity of blood and the height of the point of measurement above or below a specific reference level, generally considered to be the right atrium. The hydrostatic pressure is given by

$$P(\text{hydrostatic}) = -\rho g h \qquad [1]$$

where ρ is the specific gravity of blood (~1.056 g/cm^3), g is the acceleration due to gravity (980 cm/s^2), and h is the distance in centimeters above or below the right atrium. The magnitude of hydrostatic pressure may be relatively large. For example, in a man 5 feet 8 inches tall, the hydrostatic pressure at ankle level is approximately 90 mm Hg. The static filling pressure is usually in the range of 5 to 10 mm Hg and represents the residual pressure that exists in the absence of arterial flow; it is determined by the volume of blood and the elastic properties of the vessel wall.

Total fluid energy (E) consists of potential energy (E_p) and kinetic energy (E_k). The components of potential energy are intravascular pressure (P) and gravitational potential energy. Gravitational potential energy represents the ability of blood to do work because of its height above a specific reference level. The formula for gravitational potential energy is the same as that for hydrostatic pressure (Eq. 1) but with an opposite sign: $+\rho g h$. Because the static filling pressure is relatively low, and the gravitational potential energy and hydrostatic pressure usually cancel each other out, the predominant component of potential energy is the dynamic pressure of cardiac contraction. Potential energy can be expressed as

$$E_p = P + (\rho g h) \qquad [2]$$

Kinetic energy represents the ability of blood to do work on the basis of its motion. It is proportional to the specific gravity of blood and the square of blood velocity (v):

$$E_k = \tfrac{1}{2}\rho v^2 \qquad [3]$$

When fluid flows from one point to another, its total energy (E) remains constant, provided that flow is steady and there are no frictional energy losses. This is in accordance with the law of conservation of energy and constitutes Bernoulli's principle. In the horizontal diverging tube shown in Figure 5.1, steady flow

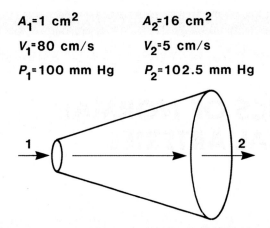

A_1=1 cm^2 A_2=16 cm^2

V_1=80 cm/s V_2=5 cm/s

P_1=100 mm Hg P_2=102.5 mm Hg

FIGURE 5.1. Effect of increasing cross-sectional area on pressure and velocity in an idealized frictionless fluid system. Flow is from left to right. While pressure increases between point 1 and point 2, total fluid energy remains constant as a result of a decrease in velocity. (Redrawn from Sumner DS. The hemodynamics and pathophysiology of arterial disease. In Rutherford RB (ed). *Vascular Surgery*. Philadelphia: WB Saunders, 1977.)

between point 1 and point 2 is accompanied by an increase in cross-sectional area and a decrease in flow velocity. The widening of the tube results in conversion of kinetic energy to potential energy in the form of pressure. Although the fluid moves against a pressure gradient of 2.5 mm Hg and therefore gains potential energy, the total fluid energy remains constant because of the decrease in velocity and a proportional loss of kinetic energy. The situation depicted in Figure 5.1 does not occur in human arteries because the required ideal flow conditions are not present. The fluid energy lost in moving blood through the arterial circulation is dissipated mainly in the form of heat.

Poiseuille's Law and Vascular Resistance

Energy losses in flowing blood occur either as viscous losses resulting from friction or as inertial losses related to changes in the velocity or direction of flow. The term *viscosity* describes the resistance to flow that arises because of the intermolecular attractions between fluid layers. Fluids with particularly strong intermolecular attractions offer a high resistance to flow and have high coefficients of viscosity. Because blood viscosity increases exponentially with increases in hematocrit, the concentration of red blood cells is the most important factor affecting the viscosity of whole blood. The viscosity of plasma is determined largely by the concentration of plasma proteins. Poiseuille's law describes the viscous energy losses that occur in an idealized flow model. This law states that the pressure gradient along a tube $(P_1 - P_2)$ is directly proportional to the mean flow velocity $(\bar{V})$ or volume flow (Q), the tube length (L), and the fluid viscosity (η) and is inversely proportional to either the second or the fourth power of the radius (r):

$$P_2 - P_2 = \bar{V}\frac{8L\eta}{r^4} = Q\frac{8L\eta}{\pi r^4} \qquad [4]$$

This equation is often simplified to: pressure = flow × resistance, where Q is flow and

$$R = \frac{8L\eta}{\pi r^4} \qquad [5]$$

is the resistance term. The hemodynamic resistance of an arterial segment increases as the flow velocity increases, provided

the lumen size remains constant. These additional energy losses are related to inertial effects or changes in kinetic energy and are proportional to the square of blood velocity (Eq. 3).

The strict application of Poiseuille's law requires steady laminar flow in a straight, rigid, cylindrical tube. Because these conditions seldom exist in the arterial circulation, Poiseuille's law can only estimate the minimum pressure gradient or viscous energy losses that may be expected in arterial flow. Energy losses due to inertial effects often exceed viscous energy losses, particularly in the presence of arterial disease. In the human circulation, approximately 90% of the total vascular resistance results from flow through the arteries and capillaries, whereas the remaining 10% results from venous flow. The arterioles and capillaries are responsible for over 60% of the total resistance, whereas the large and medium-sized arteries account for only about 15%.[1] Therefore, the arteries that are most commonly affected by atherosclerotic occlusive disease are normally very low resistance vessels.

Blood Flow Patterns

Laminar and Turbulent Flow

In the idealized flow conditions specified by Poiseuille's law, the flow pattern is *laminar*, with all flow streamlines moving parallel to the tube walls and the fluid arranged in a series of concentric layers or laminae like those shown in Figure 5.2. The velocity within each lamina remains constant, with the lowest velocity adjacent to the tube wall and increasing velocity toward the center of the tube. This results in a velocity profile that is parabolic in shape (Fig. 5.3).

In contrast to the linear streamlines of laminar flow, *turbulence* is an irregular flow state in which velocity varies at random with respect to space and time. These irregular velocity changes result in the dissipation of fluid energy as heat. When turbulence is the result of a stenotic arterial lesion, it generally occurs immediately downstream from the stenosis and may be present only over the systolic portion of the cardiac cycle when velocities are highest. Under conditions of turbulent flow, the velocity profile changes from the parabolic shape of laminar flow to a rectangular or blunt shape (see Fig. 5.3). Because of the random velocity changes, energy losses are much greater for a turbulent flow state than for a laminar flow state.

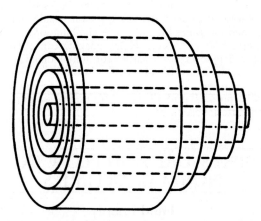

FIGURE 5.2. Laminar flow in a cylindrical tube. Concentric layers or laminae of fluid flow from left to right. The center laminae move more rapidly than do those near the periphery, and the flow profile is parabolic. (From Strandness DE, Sumner DS. Useful physical concepts. In Strandness DE, Sumner DS (eds). *Hemodynamics for Surgeons*. New York: Grune & Stratton, 1975, p 7.)

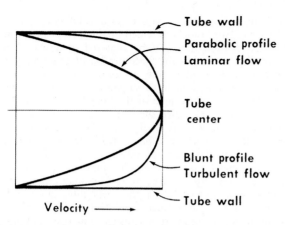

FIGURE 5.3. Velocity profiles of steady laminar and turbulent flow. Velocity is lowest adjacent to the tube wall and maximal in the center of the lumen. (From Sumner DS. The hemodynamics and pathophysiology of arterial disease. In Rutherford RB (ed). *Vascular Surgery*. Philadelphia: WB Saunders, 1977.)

Boundary Layer Separation

When fluid flows through a tube, the portion of fluid adjacent to the tube wall is referred to as the *boundary layer*. This layer is subject to both frictional interactions with the tube wall and viscous forces generated by the more rapidly moving fluid toward the center of the tube. When the tube geometry changes, such as at points of curvature, branching, or alteration in lumen diameter, small pressure gradients are created that cause the boundary layer to stop or reverse direction. This results in a complex, localized flow pattern known as an *area of flow separation* or *separation zone*.[2,3] Boundary layer separation has been observed in models of arterial anastomoses and bifurcations (Fig. 5.4).[3-5] In the diagram of a carotid bifurcation shown in Figure 5.5, the central rapid-flow stream of the common carotid artery is compressed along the inner wall of the bulb, producing a region of high shear stress, with an area of flow separation along the outer wall of the carotid bulb that includes helical flow patterns and flow reversal. The region of the carotid bulb adjacent to the separation zone is subject to relatively low shear stresses. Within the internal carotid artery distal to the bulb, flow reattachment occurs and a more laminar flow pattern is present (see Figs. 5.4 and 5.5).

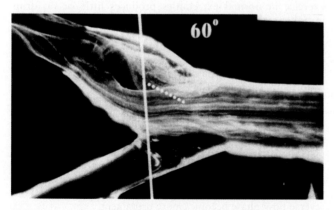

FIGURE 5.4. Flow visualization model of the normal carotid bulb using a pulsatile system and hydrogen bubbles as flow tracers. This frame was taken just after peak systole. The flow pattern seen in the outer (*top*) aspect of the model bulb is the region of flow separation; laminar flow is present along the flow divider. (From Ku DN, Giddens DP. Pulsatile flow in a model carotid bifurcation. *Arteriosclerosis* 1983;3:31-39, with permission.)

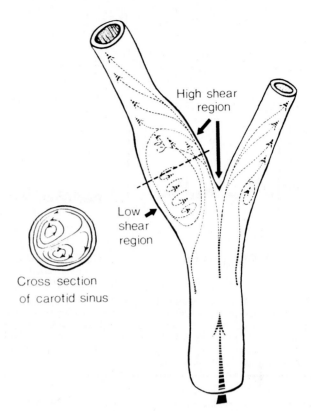

FIGURE 5.5. Carotid artery bifurcation shows an area of flow separation adjacent to the outer wall of the bulb. Rapid flow is associated with high shear stress, whereas the slower flow of the separation zone produces a region of low shear. (From Zarins CK, Giddens DP, Glagov S. Atherosclerotic plaque distribution and flow velocity profiles in the carotid bifurcation. In Bergan JJ, Yao JST (eds). *Cerebrovascular Insufficiency*. New York: Grune & Stratton, 1983.)

The complex flow patterns described in models of the carotid bifurcation have also been documented in human subjects by pulsed Doppler studies.[4,5] As shown in Figure 5.6, the Doppler spectral waveform obtained near the inner wall of a normal carotid bulb is typical of the forward, steady flow pattern found in the internal carotid artery. However, sampling of flow along the outer wall of the bulb demonstrates lower velocities with periods of both forward and reverse flow that are consistent with flow separation. Flow separation in the carotid bulb can also be seen with color-flow imaging, as shown in Figure 5.7. This is considered to be a normal finding and is particularly common in young individuals.[5] Wall thickening in the carotid bulb and alterations in arterial distensibility with increasing age make flow separation less prominent in older individuals.[6]

The clinical importance of boundary layer separation is that these localized flow disturbances may contribute to the formation of atherosclerotic plaques.[7] Examination of human carotid bifurcations, both at autopsy and during surgery, indicates that intimal thickening and atherosclerosis tend to occur along the outer wall of the carotid bulb, whereas the inner wall is relatively spared. These findings suggest that atherosclerotic lesions form near areas of flow separation and low shear stress.

Pulsatile Flow

In a pulsatile system, pressure and flow vary with time, and the velocity profile changes throughout the cardiac cycle. The hemodynamic principles that have been discussed are based on steady flow, and they cannot be applied to pulsatile flow

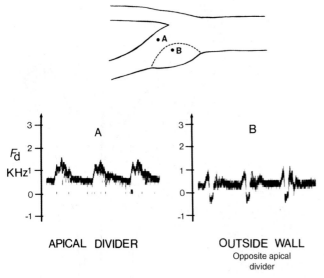

FIGURE 5.6. Flow separation in the normal carotid bulb shown by pulsed Doppler spectral waveform analysis. The flow pattern near the apical divider (*A*) is forward throughout the cardiac cycle, but near the outer wall of the bulb (*B*), the spectrum contains both forward (positive) and reverse (negative) flow components. The latter pattern indicates an area of flow separation.

in the arterial circulation; however, they can be used to determine the minimal energy losses that would be expected in a specific flow system. The resistance term of Poiseuille's law (Eqs. 4 and 5) estimates viscous energy losses in steady flow, but it does not account for the inertial effects, arterial wall elasticity, and wave reflections that influence pulsatile flow. The term *vascular impedance* is used to describe the resistance or opposition offered by a peripheral vascular bed to pulsatile blood flow.[8]

Bifurcations and Branches

Although the branches of the arterial system produce sudden changes in the flow pattern that are potential sources of energy loss, the effect of branching on the total pressure drop in normal arterial flow is relatively small. Arterial branches commonly take the form of bifurcations. Flow patterns in a bifurcation are determined mainly by the area ratio and the

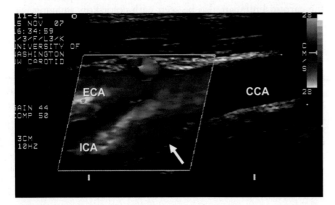

FIGURE 5.7. Color-flow image of a normal carotid bifurcation showing flow separation. As predicted by the model study shown in Figure 5.4, an area of flow separation is visualized along the outer wall of the carotid bulb (*white arrow*) as a blue region, indicating that the direction of flow in the separation zone is reversed. (CCA, common carotid artery; ICA, internal carotid artery; ECA, external carotid artery.)

branch angle. The area ratio is defined as the combined area of the secondary branches divided by the area of the primary artery. Bifurcation flow can be analyzed in terms of pressure gradient, velocity, and transmission of pulsatile energy. According to Poiseuille's law, an area ratio of 1.41 would allow the pressure gradient to remain constant along a bifurcation. If the combined area of the branches equals the area of the primary artery, then the area ratio is 1.0 and there is no change in the velocity of flow. For efficient transmission of pulsatile energy across a bifurcation, the vascular impedance of the primary artery should equal that of the branches, a situation that occurs with an area ratio of 1.15 for larger arteries and 1.35 for smaller arteries.[9] Human infants have a favorable area ratio of 1.11 at the aortic bifurcation, but the ratio gradually decreases with age. This decline in the area ratio of the aortic bifurcation leads to an increase in both the velocity of flow in the secondary branches and the amount of reflected pulsatile energy. For example, with an area ratio of 0.8, approximately 22% of the incident pulsatile energy is reflected back to the infrarenal aorta. This mechanism may play a role in the localization of atherosclerosis and aneurysms in this arterial segment.[10]

The curvature and angulation of an arterial bifurcation can also contribute to the development of flow disturbances and energy loss. As blood flows around a curve, the rapidly moving fluid in the center of the vessel tends to flow outward and be replaced by the slower fluid originally located near the arterial wall. This can result in complex helical flow patterns, such as those observed in the carotid bifurcation (see Fig. 5.4).[4] As the angle between the secondary branches of a bifurcation widens, the tendency to develop turbulent or disturbed flow increases. The average angle between the human iliac arteries is 54 degrees; however, with diseased or tortuous iliac arteries, this angle can approach 180 degrees, and flow disturbances are particularly likely to develop.

Pressure and Flow in Normal Limbs

As the arterial pressure pulse moves distally, the systolic pressure rises, the diastolic pressure falls, and the pulse pressure becomes wider. The decrease in mean arterial pressure between the heart and the ankle is normally less than 10 mm Hg. In normal individuals, the ratio of ankle systolic pressure to brachial systolic pressure (ankle-brachial index) has a mean value of 1.11 ± 0.10 in the resting state.[11] Moderate exercise in normal extremities produces little or no drop in ankle systolic pressure. Strenuous effort may be associated with a drop of several millimeters of mercury; however, pressures return rapidly to resting levels after cessation of exercise.

The velocity flow pattern in the major arteries of the leg is normally triphasic, as shown in Figure 5.8. An initial large forward-velocity phase resulting from cardiac systole is followed by a brief phase of flow reversal in early diastole and a third smaller phase of forward flow in late diastole. This triphasic pattern is modified by a variety of factors, including proximal arterial disease and changes in peripheral resistance. For example, body warming, which causes vasodilatation and decreased resistance, tends to eliminate the second phase of flow reversal; on exposure to cold, resistance increases and the reverse-flow phase becomes more prominent.

The average blood flow in the normal human leg is in the range of 300 to 500 mL/min under resting conditions.[8] Blood flow to the muscles of the lower leg is approximately 2.0 mL/100 g/min. With moderate exercise, total leg blood flow increases by a factor of 5 to 10, and muscle blood flow rises to around 30 mL/100 g/min. During strenuous exercise, muscle blood flow may reach 70 mL/100 g/min.

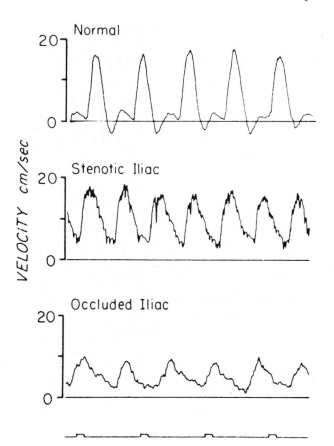

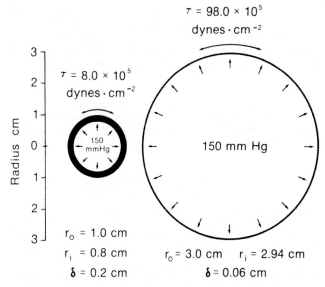

FIGURE 5.9. End-on view of a cylinder, 2 cm in diameter, that is expanded to 6 cm in diameter, while the wall area remains constant; τ, wall stress; δ, wall thickness; r_i, inside radius; r_o, outside radius. (From Sumner DS. The hemodynamics and pathophysiology of arterial disease. In Rutherford RB (ed). *Vascular Surgery*. Philadelphia: WB Saunders, 1977.)

FIGURE 5.8. Velocity flow waveforms obtained with a directional Doppler velocity detector from the femoral artery of a normal subject, a patient with external iliac stenosis, and a patient with common iliac occlusion. Note the normal triphasic velocity pattern and the abnormal dampened, monophasic velocity patterns. (From Strandness DE, Sumner DS. Blood flow to limbs. In *Hemodynamics for Surgeons*. New York: Grune & Stratton, 1975, p 257.)

Tangential Stress and Tension

When the structural components of the arterial wall are weakened, aneurysms may form. Rupture occurs when the tangential stress within the arterial wall becomes greater than the tensile strength. The tangential stress (τ) within the wall of a fluid-filled cylindrical tube can be expressed as

$$\tau = P\frac{r}{\delta} \qquad [6]$$

where P is the pressure exerted by the fluid, r is the internal radius, and δ is the thickness of the tube wall. Thus, tangential stress is directly proportional to pressure and radius but inversely proportional to wall thickness. Stress (τ) has the dimensions of force per unit area of tube wall (dynes per square centimeter). Equation 6 is similar to Laplace's law, which defines tangential tension (T) as the product of pressure and radius:

$$T = Pr \qquad [7]$$

Tension is given in units of force per tube length (dynes per centimeter). The terms *stress* and *tension* have different dimensions and describe the forces acting on the tube wall in different ways. Laplace's law can be used to characterize thin-walled structures such as soap bubbles; however, it is not suitable for describing the stresses in arterial walls.

Figure 5.9 shows a tube with an outside diameter of 2.0 cm and a wall thickness of 0.2 cm, dimensions similar to those of atherosclerotic aortas. If the internal pressure is 150 mm Hg, the tangential wall stress is 8.0×10^5 dynes/cm^2. Expansion of the tube to form an aneurysm with a diameter of 6.0 cm results in a decrease in wall thickness to 0.06 cm. The increased radius and decreased wall thickness increase the wall stress to 98.0×10^5 dynes/cm^2, assuming that the pressure remains constant. In this example, the diameter has been enlarged by a factor of 3, and the wall stress has increased by a factor of 12.

Although the tensile strength of collagen is very high, it constitutes only about 15% of the aneurysm wall.[12] Furthermore, the collagen fibers in an aneurysm are sparsely distributed and subject to fragmentation. The tendency of larger aneurysms to rupture is readily explained by the effect of increased radius on tangential stress (Eq. 6) and degenerative changes in the arterial wall. The relationship between tangential stress and blood pressure accounts for the contribution of hypertension to the risk of rupture. Another factor is that in about 55% of ruptured abdominal aortic aneurysms, the site of rupture is in the posterolateral aspect of the aneurysm wall.[13] The posterior wall of the aorta is relatively fixed against the spine, and repeated flexion in that area could result in structural fatigue and a localized area of weakness that might predispose to rupture.

HEMODYNAMICS OF ARTERIAL STENOSES

Energy Losses

According to Poiseuille's law (Eq. 4), the radius of a stenosis has a much greater effect on viscous energy losses than its length. Inertial energy losses, which occur at the entrance (contraction effects) and exit (expansion effects) of a stenotic segment, are proportional to the square of blood velocity (Eq. 3). Energy losses are also influenced by the geometry of a stenosis. A gradual vessel tapering results in less energy loss than an irregular or abrupt change in lumen size. The energy lost at the exit of a stenosis may be quite significant because of the sudden expansion of the flow stream and dissipation of kinetic energy in a zone of turbulence. Figure 5.10 illustrates the energy losses related to a 1-cm-long stenosis. The viscous energy losses are relatively small and occur within the stenotic segment. Inertial losses due to entrance and exit effects are much greater. Because most of the energy loss in this example results from inertial effects, the length of the stenosis is relatively unimportant.

Critical Arterial Stenosis

The extent of arterial narrowing required to produce a significant reduction in blood pressure or flow is called a *critical stenosis*. Because energy losses associated with a stenosis are inversely proportional to the fourth power of the radius (Eq. 4), there is an exponential relationship between pressure drop and reduction in lumen size. When this relationship is illustrated graphically (Fig. 5.11), the curves have a single sharp bend and further narrowing results in a rapid increase in the magnitude of the pressure drop.[14,15] In peripheral arteries with physiologic flow rates, the critical stenosis value is reached at approximately a 50% reduction in lumen diameter or a 75% reduction in cross-sectional lumen area.

Whereas lumen size is the most prominent feature of an arterial stenosis, blood flow velocity is also a major determinant of fluid energy losses, and the pressure drop across a stenosis varies with the flow rate. Consequently, a stenosis that is not significant at low or resting flow rates may become critical when flow rates are increased by reactive hyperemia or exercise. Because flow velocity depends on the distal vascular resistance, the critical stenosis value varies with the resistance of the runoff bed. In Figure 5.11, a system with a high flow velocity (low resistance) shows a reduction in pressure with less narrowing than a system with low flow

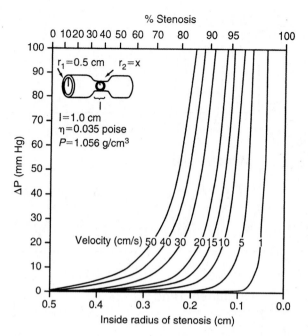

FIGURE 5.11. Relationship of pressure drop across a stenosis to the radius of the stenotic segment and the flow velocity. (From Strandness DE, Sumner DS. The effect of growth on arterial blood flow. In *Hemodynamics for Surgeons*. New York: Grune & Stratton, 1975, p 109.)

velocity (high resistance). The higher flow velocities produce curves that are less sharply bent, making the point of critical stenosis less distinct. The decrease in flow with progressive arterial narrowing is linearly related to the increase in pressure gradient as long as the peripheral resistance remains constant[15] In this situation, the curves for pressure drop and flow reduction are mirror images of each other, and

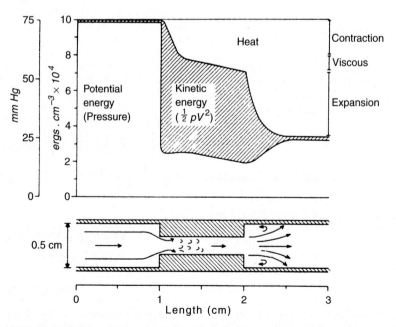

FIGURE 5.10. Energy losses resulting when blood flows steadily through a 1-cm-long stenosis. Inertial losses (contraction and expansion) are more significant than are viscous losses. (From Sumner DS. The hemodynamics and pathophysiology of arterial disease. In Rutherford RB (ed). *Vascular Surgery*. Philadelphia: WB Saunders, 1977.)

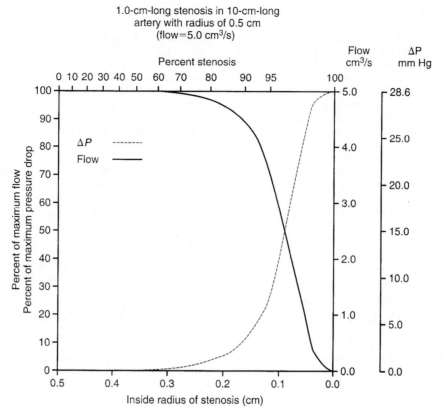

FIGURE 5.12. Effect of increasing stenosis on blood flow and pressure drop across the stenotic segment. Collateral and peripheral resistances are considered to be fixed. (From Strandness DE, Sumner DS. The effect of growth on arterial blood flow. In *Hemodynamics for Surgeons.* New York: Grune & Stratton, 1975, p 113.)

the critical stenosis value is the same for both (Fig. 5.12). Many vascular beds are able to maintain a constant level of blood flow over a wide range of perfusion pressures by the mechanism of autoregulation. This is achieved by constriction of resistance vessels in response to an increase in blood pressure and dilatation of resistance vessels when blood pressure decreases. For example, autoregulation permits the brain to maintain normal flow rates down to perfusion pressures in the range of 50 to 60 mm Hg.[16]

Stenosis Length and Multiple Stenoses

Poiseuille's law predicts that the radius of a stenosis has a much greater effect on viscous energy losses than its length (Eq. 4). Doubling the length of a stenosis results in a doubling of the associated viscous energy losses; however, reducing the radius by half increases energy losses by a factor of 16. Because inertial energy losses are primarily due to entrance and exit effects, they are independent of stenosis length (see Fig. 5.10). Therefore, separate short stenoses tend to be more significant than a single longer stenosis. It has been shown experimentally that when stenoses that are not significant individually are arranged in series, large reductions in pressure and flow can occur.[17] In other words, multiple subcritical stenoses may have the same effect as a single critical stenosis.

Collateral Circulation

The development of collateral circulation is one of the major mechanisms that compensates for the hemodynamic effects of an obstructed artery. The functional capacity of

a collateral system depends on the level and extent of the occlusive lesions. For example, the profunda-geniculate network can compensate to a large degree for an isolated superficial femoral artery occlusion; however, the addition of an iliac lesion severely limits collateral flow. A collateral system consists of three components: (1) stem arteries, which are large distributing branches, (2) a midzone of smaller intramuscular channels, and (3) reentry vessels that join the major artery distal to the point of obstruction.[8] Collateral vessels are preexisting pathways that enlarge when flow through the parallel major artery is reduced. The main stimuli for collateral development are an abnormal pressure gradient across the collateral system and increased velocity of flow through the midzone vessels.

Collateral vessels are smaller, longer, and more numerous than the major arteries that they replace. Although considerable enlargement may occur in the midzone vessels, collateral resistance is always greater than that of the original unobstructed artery. In addition, the acute changes in collateral resistance during exercise are minimal.[18] Therefore, the resistance of a collateral system can be considered as fixed. Unlike collateral resistance, the resistance of the peripheral runoff bed is quite variable. Vascular resistance in the lower limb can be divided into segmental and peripheral components. Segmental resistance consists of the relatively fixed parallel resistances of the major normal or diseased artery and the bypassing collateral vessels. Peripheral resistance includes the highly variable resistances of the distal arterioles and cutaneous circulation. The total vascular resistance of the limb can be estimated by adding the segmental and the peripheral resistances.

Normally, the resting segmental resistance is very low and the peripheral resistance is relatively high. Using the superficial femoral artery and profunda-geniculate collateral system as an example, the pressure drop across a normal femoropopliteal arterial segment is minimal. With exercise, the peripheral resistance falls and flow through the segmental arteries increases by a factor of up to 10, with little or no pressure drop. With moderate arterial disease, such as an isolated superficial femoral artery occlusion, the segmental resistance is increased as a result of collateral flow, and an abnormal pressure drop is present across the thigh. Because of a compensatory decrease in peripheral resistance, the total resistance of the limb and the resting blood flow often remain in the normal range.[19] During exercise, the segmental resistance remains high and fixed, whereas the peripheral resistance decreases further. However, the capacity of the peripheral circulation to compensate for a high segmental resistance is limited, and exercise flow is less than normal. In this situation, exercise is associated with a still larger pressure drop across the diseased arterial segment, and the clinical consequence is calf muscle ischemia and claudication.

Pressure and Flow in Limbs with Arterial Occlusive Disease

If an arterial lesion is hemodynamically significant at resting flow rates, there is a measurable reduction in distal blood pressure. In general, limbs with a lesion at one anatomic level have ankle-brachial indices between 0.90 and 0.50, whereas limbs with lesions at multiple levels have indices less than 0.50.

The ankle-brachial index also correlates to some extent with the clinical severity of disease; in limbs with intermittent claudication, the index has a mean value of 0.59 ± 0.15; in limbs with ischemic rest pain, 0.26 ± 0.13; and in limbs with impending gangrene, 0.05 ± 0.08.[11] Because of the increased segmental vascular resistance in limbs with arterial occlusive disease, the ankle systolic pressure falls dramatically during leg exercise. The extent and duration of the pressure drop are proportional to the severity of the arterial lesions (Figs. 5.13 and 5.14).[20] When blood flows through an arterial stenosis or a high-resistance collateral bed, the distal pulse pressure is reduced to a greater extent than the mean pressure.[21] This suggests that the systolic pressure beyond a lesion is a more sensitive indicator of hemodynamic significance than the mean pressure. It is well known that palpable pedal pulses in patients with superficial femoral artery stenosis can disappear after leg exercise. This occurs when increased flow through high-resistance vessels causes a reduction in pulse pressure.

Resting leg or calf blood flow in most patients with intermittent claudication is not significantly different from values obtained in normal individuals. However, the capacity to increase limb blood flow during exercise is quite limited, and pain occurs in the muscles that have been rendered ischemic. As the occlusive process becomes more severe, the decrease in peripheral vascular resistance can no longer compensate, and resting flow is less than normal. When this occurs, signs and symptoms of ischemia at rest appear. With increasing degrees of disease, the hyperemia that follows exercise becomes more prolonged, and the peak calf blood flow is both decreased and delayed.[20]

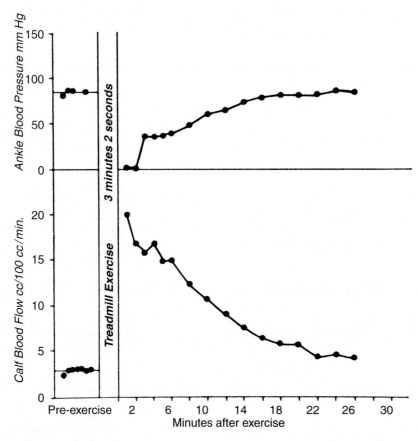

FIGURE 5.13. Preexercise and postexercise ankle blood pressure and calf blood flow in a patient with severe stenosis of the superficial femoral artery. (From Sumner DS, Strandness DE Jr. The relationship between calf blood flow and ankle blood pressure in patients with intermittent claudication. *Surgery* 1969;65:763-771.)

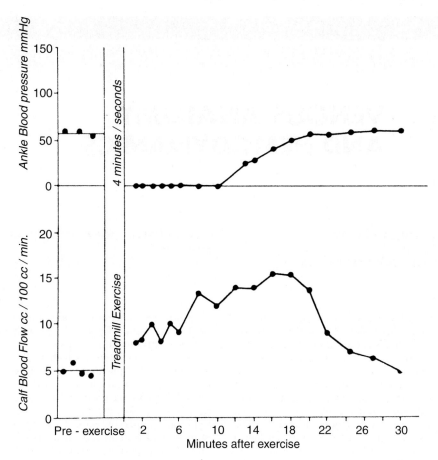

FIGURE 5.14. Preexercise and postexercise ankle blood pressure and calf blood flow in a patient with iliac stenosis and superficial femoral artery occlusion. (From Sumner DS, Strandness DE Jr. The relationship between calf blood flow and ankle blood pressure in patients with intermittent claudication. *Surgery* 1969;65:763-771.)

PRINCIPLES AND INSTRUMENTATION

Changes in the velocity flow pattern are also useful in the evaluation of arterial occlusive disease. Whereas the peak pressure normally increases, the peak flow velocity decreases as blood flows toward the periphery. Because a stenotic lesion is accompanied by a compensatory decrease in peripheral resistance, one of the earliest changes noted distal to a stenosis is the disappearance of the reverse-flow phase (see Fig. 5.8). As a stenosis becomes more severe, the distal flow pattern becomes monophasic, with a slow rise, a rounded peak, and a gradual decline toward the baseline in diastole. The characteristics of the flow pulse proximal to an arterial obstruction are variable and depend on the capacity of the collateral circulation.

References

1. Burton AC (ed). *Physiology and Biophysics of the Circulation*, 2nd ed. St. Louis: Mosby-Year Book, 1972.
2. Gutstein WH, Schneck DJ, Marks JO. In vitro studies of local blood flow disturbance in a region of separation. *J Atheroscler Res* 1968;8: 381-388.
3. Logerfo FW, Soncrant T, Teel T, et al. Boundary layer separation in models of side-to-end arterial anastomoses. *Arch Surg* 1979;114:1364-1373.
4. Ku DN, Giddens DP, Phillips DJ, et al. Hemodynamics of the normal human carotid bifurcation—In vitro and in vivo studies. *Ultrasound Med Biol* 1985;1:13-26.
5. Phillips DJ, Greene FM Jr, Langlois Y, et al. Flow velocity patterns in the carotid bifurcations of young, presumed normal subjects. *Ultrasound Med Biol* 1983;1:39-49.
6. Reneman RS, van Merode T, Hick P, et al. Flow velocity patterns in and distensibility of the carotid artery bulb in subjects of various ages. *Circulation* 1985;71:500-509.
7. Fox JA, Hugh AE. Localization of atheroma: A theory based on boundary layer separation. *Br Heart J* 1966;28:388-394.
8. Strandness DE Jr, Sumner DS (eds). *Hemodynamics for Surgeons*. New York: Grune & Stratton, 1975.
9. McDonald DA. Steady flow of a liquid in cylindrical tubes. In *Blood Flow in Arteries*, 2nd ed. London: Edward Arnold, 1974, pp 17-54.
10. Lalleman RC, Gosling RG, Newman DL. Role of the bifurcation in atheromatosis of the abdominal aorta. *Surg Gynecol Obstet* 1973;137:987-990.
11. Yao JST. Hemodynamic studies in peripheral arterial disease. *Br J Surg* 1970;57:761-766.
12. Sumner DS, Hokanson DE, Strandness DE Jr. Stress–strain characteristics and collagen-elastin content of abdominal aortic aneurysms. *Surg Gynecol Obstet* 1970;130:459-466.
13. Darling RC. Ruptured arteriosclerotic abdominal aortic aneurysms—A pathologic and clinical study. *Am J Surg* 1970;119:397-401.
14. Berguer R, Hwang NHC. Critical arterial stenosis—A theoretical and experimental solution. *Ann Surg* 1974;180:39-50.
15. May AG, Van de Berg L, DeWeese JA, et al. Critical arterial stenosis. *Surgery* 1963;54:250-259.
16. James IM, Millar RA, Purves MY. Observations on the intrinsic neural control of cerebral blood flow in the baboon. *Circ Res* 1969;25: 77-93.
17. Flanigan DP, Tullis JP, Streeter VL, et al. Multiple subcritical arterial stenosis: Effect on poststenotic pressure and flow. *Ann Surg* 1977;186: 663-668.
18. Ludbrook J. Collateral artery resistance in the human lower limb. *J Surg Res* 1966;6:423-434.
19. Sumner DS, Strandness DE Jr. The effect of exercise on resistance to blood flow in limbs with an occluded superficial femoral artery. *Vasc Surg* 1970;4:229-237.
20. Sumner DS, Strandness DE Jr. The relationship between calf blood flow and ankle blood pressure in patients with intermittent claudication. *Surgery* 1969;65:763-771.
21. Keitzer WF, Fry WT, Kraft RO, et al. Hemodynamic mechanism for pulse changes seen in occlusive vascular disease. *Surgery* 1965;57:163-174.

CHAPTER 6 ■ VENOUS ANATOMY AND HEMODYNAMICS

MARK H. MEISSNER

LOWER EXTREMITY VENOUS ANATOMY
VENOUS HEMODYNAMICS
THE DETERMINANTS OF AMBULATORY VENOUS
   PRESSURE

VENOUS HYPERTENSION AND THE MICROCIRCULATION
SUMMARY

The hemodynamics of the lower extremity venous system is in many respects more complicated and less well understood than it is for the arterial system. The central return of blood in the upright position depends on complex interactions between the heart, respiratory changes in venous pressure, the peripheral muscle pumps, and a multiply interconnected series of valved conduits. Failure of these components leads to a spectrum of chronic venous disorders ranging from uncomplicated telangiectasias and varicose veins to venous ulceration. The signs and symptoms may result from either primary degenerative causes or from secondary disorders, most commonly acute deep venous thrombosis (DVT). Regardless of etiology, the ultimate clinical and hemodynamic manifestations are similar. The more severe skin manifestations of chronic venous disease, termed *chronic venous insufficiency*, are specifically associated with ambulatory venous hypertension, or the failure to adequately reduce venous pressure with exercise.[1]

LOWER EXTREMITY VENOUS ANATOMY

Any description of lower extremity venous hemodynamics requires a clear understanding of venous anatomy. The nomenclature of the lower extremity veins was updated in 2002, clarifying many definitions and eliminating most eponyms.[2] The venous system of the lower extremities includes the deep veins, which lie beneath the muscular fascia and drain the lower extremity muscles; the superficial veins, which are above the deep fascia and drain the cutaneous microcirculation; and the perforating veins that penetrate the muscular fascia and connect the superficial and deep veins. Communicating veins connect veins of the same anatomic type.[2] However, it has been more recently emphasized that the lower extremity veins actually lie in three compartments—the deep veins in the compartment below the muscular fascia (N3), the great and small saphenous veins enveloped by the thin saphenous fascia (N2 compartment), and the saphenous tributaries within the epifascial (N1) compartment.[3]

The deep veins of the lower extremity follow the course of the associated arteries, with the number of valves increasing from proximal to distal. The muscular venous sinuses are the principal collecting system of the calf muscle pump. The gastrocnemius veins collect blood from the medial and lateral heads of the gastrocnemius muscle and drain into the popliteal vein, while the large soleus veins are of greatest

numeric importance and usually drain into the posterior tibial or peroneal veins. These veins play an important role in the muscle pump function of the calf.

The superficial veins, which include the great saphenous vein and small saphenous vein, drain the skin and subcutaneous tissue. The principle veins of the superficial system of the medial thigh are the great saphenous vein and the anterior and posterior accessory great saphenous veins, all of which may be important sources of reflux. There are usually two main saphenous tributaries in the calf, an anterior branch and the posterior arch (Leonardo's) vein, which begins behind the medial malleolus and joins the great saphenous vein just below the knee. The intersaphenous vein (vein of Giacomini) connects the small saphenous and great saphenous veins. The superficial venous system is completed by the lateral subdermic plexus formed by a network of small veins located laterally above and below the knee.[4] Reflux in the lateral subdermic plexus is particularly associated with telangiectasias around the lateral knee.

Perforating veins may empty directly into the axial deep veins (direct perforators) or into the venous sinuses of the calf (indirect perforators). Although perforating veins are numerous and variable, four groups are of clinical significance—those of the foot, the medial calf, the lateral calf, and the thigh. Although net flow is from superficial to deep in the calf and thigh, the foot perforators are unique in directing flow toward the superficial veins.[5,6] The medial calf perforators include the paratibial perforators joining the main great saphenous vein or its branches and the posterior tibial perforators that originate in the posterior arch vein. The perforators of the femoral canal connect the great saphenous vein with the distal femoral or proximal popliteal vein.

VENOUS HEMODYNAMICS

The lower extremity venous system functions both as a reservoir to facilitate cardiovascular homeostasis through volume shifts and to ensure the efficient return of blood to the heart. The elliptical cross-section of the lower extremity veins allows large volume shifts to be accommodated with minimal change in pressure over a range of 5 to 25 mm Hg. Veins are collapsible tubes and exhibit nonlinear volume-pressure relationships such that an increase in volume initially causes a "bending" of the wall associated with an increase in cross-sectional area without changes in pressure or perimeter (Fig. 6.1). Once a circular configuration is reached, the vein wall enters

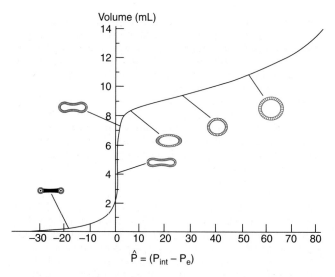

Volume (mL)

$\hat{P} = (P_{int} - P_e)$

FIGURE 6.1. Pressure-volume relationships in collapsible tubes. During the "bending" phase of venous distension, large changes in volume are accommodated without significant changes in pressure. As the vein becomes elliptical and enters the "stretching" phase, pressures rise and increase further as the vein becomes circular. (Adapted from Katz AI, Chen Y, Moreno AH. Flow through a collapsible tube: Experimental analysis and mathematical model. *Biophysical J* 1969;9:1261–1279.) Ref. (56)

a "stretching" phase, where further increases in volume are associated with increases in both perimeter and pressure.[7] This arrangement allows large acute volume shifts to be accommodated by expansion or contraction of the venous reservoir.

Despite the importance of this reservoir capacity, the primary function of the venous circulation is to return blood to the heart. Lower extremity venous return is determined by the interaction of the dynamic pressure gradient between the lower extremities and the right atrium, respiratory-dependent changes in intra-abdominal and intrathoracic pressure (the respiratory pump), and the skeletal muscle pumps. In the resting supine position, the pressure is 12 to 18 mm Hg at the venous end of the capillary and falls steadily toward atrial pressures of 4 to 7 mm Hg.[1] In the supine position, this dynamic pressure gradient is augmented by the effects of the respiratory pump. Although venous return is usually regarded

as being augmented during inspiration, the situation is complex and depends on breathing mechanics.[8] With diaphragmatic breathing, femoral venous return is abolished during inspiration and augmented during expiration (Fig. 6.2). This pattern is dictated by changes in intra-abdominal pressure rather than other factors such as constriction of the inferior vena cava at the diaphragmatic hiatus. In contrast, femoral venous blood flow is always positive during ribcage breathing, being slightly augmented during inspiration. The capacitance of the thigh veins appears to be the most important contributor to augmentation of venous flow induced by respiration.

In the upright position, the physiological effects of gravity and hydrostatic pressure oppose venous return. Resting venous pressure in the upright position rises by approximately 0.8 mm Hg per centimeter below the right atrium and reaches 80 to 100 mm Hg at the ankle, varying with height, weight, and calf muscle volume.[9,10] At rest, arterial inflow is balanced by the action of the respiratory pump, and pressure in the deep and superficial veins is equal. However, as arterial inflow rises with activity, effective venous return requires the interaction of the peripheral venous pumps and competent venous valves.[11–15] Despite the importance of the skeletal muscle pumps, there continues to be some respiratory modulation of venous return during exercise.[8]

The valves function to divide the hydrostatic column of blood into segments and to insure unidirectional, antegrade venous flow. The superficial, deep, and most perforating veins contain bicuspid valves consisting of folds of endothelium supported by a thin layer of connective tissue. Although often believed to be oriented parallel to the skin, the angle between the free edges of adjacent valves averages 84 degrees in the great saphenous vein and 88 degrees in the femoral vein.[16] The offsetting of adjacent valves likely induces rotational momentum and helical flow in the veins, a strategy that limits flow instability and decreases energy dissipation elsewhere in the circulation. The valve cups lie within the valve sinus, which is always wider than the adjacent vein. The valve sinus enlarges and assumes a more spherical shape at the time of valve closure.[17] Distension of the valve sinus separates the commissures, tightening the edge of the cusps and resulting in valve closure.

Within the deep venous system, there are an average of 5 venous valves between the inguinal ligament and popliteal fossa, although the number varies from 2 to 9.[18] These valves are usually 3 to 5 cm apart and tend to be consistently positioned at major venous junctions.[16] Their arrangement is

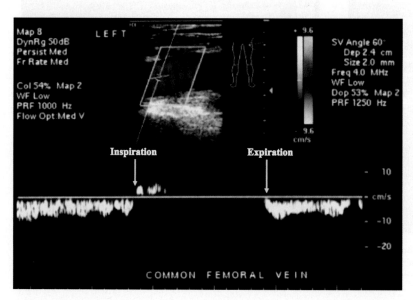

COMMON FEMORAL VEIN

FIGURE 6.2. Common femoral Doppler waveform with quiet breathing in the supine position. With diaphragmatic breathing, unobstructed venous flow (displayed below the baseline) in the lower extremities decreases or ceases as abdominal pressure rises during inspiration and increases with expiration.

variable elsewhere, but in general, the inferior vena cava and common iliac veins have no valves; the external iliac and common femoral veins above the saphenofemoral junction have one valve at most; the femoral vein above the adductor canal has three or more valves; the distal femoral and popliteal veins have one or two valves; and the tibial/peroneal veins have numerous valves spaced at approximately 2 cm intervals.[6,18] Although the muscle venous sinusoids are valveless, they frequently empty into profusely valved draining veins.[18] Within the superficial venous system, a valve is present at the saphenofemoral junction in 94% to 100% of individuals[19] and there are usually one or two subterminal valves within 2 cm of the terminal valve.[4] The great saphenous vein usually has at least 6 valves, while the small saphenous vein has 7 to 10 closely spaced valves.[6] Although the perforating veins of the calf generally direct flow from superficial to deep, most evidence suggest that only the larger perforating veins have valves.[6,20]

The valves of the lower extremity veins open and close at a cycle frequency of 34 to 36 per minute in the supine position and 19 to 20 per minute in the standing position.[21] Knowledge regarding the mechanism of valve closure is largely derived from duplex observations of valves in response to nonphysiological provocative maneuvers such as Valsalva's maneuver or distal calf compression. Under such conditions, valve closure is initiated by reversal of the normal, antegrade transvalvular pressure gradient during the relaxation or diastolic phase after calf muscle compression.[22] As this pressure gradient reversal gradually increases, there is initially a short period of retrograde flow until the gradient becomes sufficient to cause valve closure. Rather than simple cessation of antegrade flow, valve closure under these artificial conditions requires retrograde flow at a velocity of at least 30 cm/s. Under such conditions, reverse flow duration is less than 0.5 seconds in 95% of normal valves.

Recent ultrasound observations under physiologic conditions, without augmentation or provocative maneuvers, suggest a different mechanism of valve closure.[17,21] The valve cycle can be divided into four phases: opening, equilibrium, closing, and closed. At equilibrium, the valves are open but not apposed to the venous wall, causing a luminal narrowing of approximately 35% in comparison to the distal vein (Fig. 6.3A and B). This relative stenosis causes flow acceleration at the valve cusp with flow separation at the leading edge producing a vortex in the valve sinus. According to Bernoulli's

law, pressure decreases as velocity increases. Therefore, as luminal velocity increases at the end of the equilibrium phase, luminal pressure accordingly decreases, causing the valve to close when the vortex pressure behind the cusp exceeds the luminal pressure (Fig. 6.4). Among 12 normal subjects examined at rest in the upright position, flow reversal during valve closure occurred in only 1 subject. In this setting, cusp closure is initiated by an increase in forward flow velocity that is followed by a dilation of the valve sinus and subsequent valve closure. In distinct contrast to the mechanism of valve closure under the artificial conditions of a provocative maneuver, reverse flow is not necessary under normal physiologic conditions, and valve closure occurs despite ongoing antegrade flow.

Approximately 90% of the venous return in the lower extremities is via the deep veins through the action of the foot, calf, and thigh muscles pumps.[23] The action of these valved pumps is dependent on normally functioning muscle groups, a full range of joint mobility, and the deep fascia of the leg which constrains the muscles during contraction and allows high pressures to be generated within the muscular compartments.[24] Among these, the calf muscle pump is the most important as it is the most efficient, has the largest capacitance, and generates the highest pressures.[5,13] The normal calf pump ejects over 40% to 60% of the venous volume with a single contraction.[12,13,25] The thigh muscle pump, which has an ejection fraction of only 15%, is thought to be substantially less important, while compression of the plantar venous plexus likely functions to prime the calf muscle pump.[15]

With contraction of the calf muscle (systole), pressure in the posterior compartment rises to as high as 250 mm Hg[13] and the gastrocnemius and soleus veins are emptied of blood. With subsequent muscle relaxation (diastole), resting venous pressure is lowered as the valves prevent retrograde flow. Efficient function of the calf muscle pump requires not only the presence of competent valves but, as importantly, the presence of distal conduits, which have normal compliance and collapse as blood is ejected forward, thereby reducing pressure as the valves close.[7] Pressure in the posterior tibial veins accordingly decreases from 80 to 100 mm Hg to less than 30 mm Hg. The degree to which venous pressure is reduced increases with a more rapid pace and decreases with restricted mobility of the knee and ankle.[10] The reduction in deep venous pressure during calf muscle diastole favors flow from the superficial to the deep system through the perforating veins. In contrast to

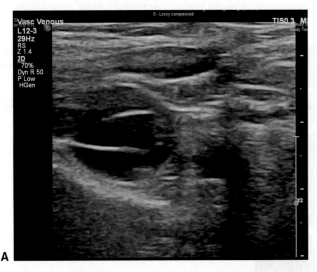
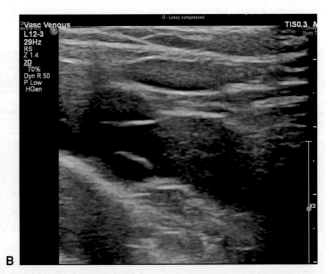

A   **B**

FIGURE 6.3. Cross-sectional (*A*) and longitudinal (*B*) B-mode images of a venous valve during the equilibrium phase of the valve cycle. During equilibrium, the valve cusps are open, but not fully opposed to the wall. This results in a relative stenosis at the leading edge of the valve cusps.

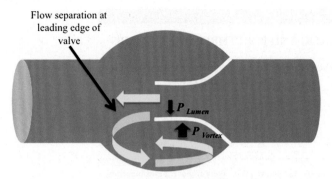

Flow separation at leading edge of valve

$\downarrow P_{Lumen}$

$\uparrow P_{Vortex}$

FIGURE 6.4. Mechanism of venous valve closure. The relative stenosis produced by the leading edge of the valve cusps leads to flow separation and vortex formation in the valve sinus. As luminal flow velocity changes at the end of the equilibrium phase of valve closure, vortex pressure exceeds luminal pressure resulting in valve closure. (Adapted from Lurie F, Kistner RL, Eklof B, et al. Mechanism of venous valve closure and role of the valve in circulation: A new concept. *J Vasc Surg* 2003;38:955–961.) Ref. (21)

the ambulatory pressure reduction in the superficial and calf veins, pressure in the femoral and popliteal veins does not fall, producing an ambulatory pressure gradient between the thigh and calf veins of approximately 35 mm Hg.[9] However, retrograde flow into the calf is prevented by competent valves, with capillary inflow causing a slow return of pressure in the calf veins to resting levels.

THE DETERMINANTS OF AMBULATORY VENOUS PRESSURE

The clinical manifestations of chronic venous insufficiency result from ambulatory venous hypertension, or the failure to adequately reduce venous pressure with activity (Fig 6.5). Ambulatory venous pressure (AVP) can be determined using a

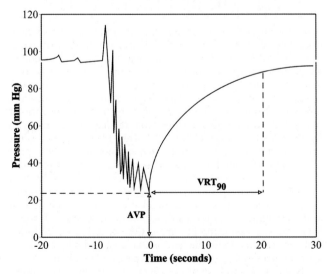

FIGURE 6.5. Ambulatory venous pressure measured from cannulation of a dorsal foot vein. In the normal limb, pressure declines with plantar flexion. Ambulatory venous pressure (AVP) at the end of ten tiptoe maneuvers is less than 30 mm Hg in normal limbs. The time required for return to baseline is measured as the 90% venous refilling time (VRT). Limbs with hemodynamically significant reflux have an elevated AVP and rapid 90% VRT.

21-gauge needle inserted into a dorsal foot vein to measure the response to 10 tiptoe movements, usually at a rate of 1 per second. The AVP is the lowest pressure achieved at the end of this exercise. Under normal circumstances, lower extremity venous pressure is reduced from approximately 100 mm Hg (depending on individual height) to a mean of 22 mm Hg within 7 to 12 steps.[14] Chronic venous insufficiency is associated with elevated AVPs as well as shortened refilling times after exercise ceases. The severity of chronic venous disease is closely related to the magnitude of venous hypertension. Ulceration usually does not occur at AVPs of less than 30 mm Hg, while the incidence is 100% at pressures greater than 90 mm Hg.[26]

Although commonly attributed to venous reflux, ambulatory venous hypertension may result from failure of any component of the lower extremity venous system—valvular incompetence, venous outflow obstruction, skeletal muscle pump failure, or limited range of ankle motion.[9,27,28] Reflux, or pathologic retrograde flow, occurs when the valves are absent or rendered incompetent by degenerative processes (primary venous disease) or an episode of DVT (secondary venous disease). Under these circumstances, retrograde flow during calf muscle relaxation prevents the usual reduction in pressure and rapid venous refilling occurs. While reflux in asymptomatic and mildly symptomatic patients is usually isolated and segmental, that in patients with skin changes and ulceration is usually multisegmental and frequently involves the deep, superficial, and perforating veins.[29] Approximately two-thirds of patients with ulcers have multisystem venous disease.[30] Although reflux in superficial and distal deep veins appears to be important in the pathogenesis of venous ulceration, it is likely the axial reflux volume, rather than the precise localization that is of greatest hemodynamic importance.[9]

Despite its importance, reflux is hardly the sole determinant of ambulatory venous hypertension. For any given volume of reflux, AVP will be higher in the presence of venous obstruction.[31] Postthrombotic limbs with edema, hyperpigmentation, or ulceration are more likely to have a combination of reflux and residual obstruction than either abnormality alone (Table 6.1).[31,32] However, despite these observations, reflux has, in the past, often been regarded as more important than obstruction. This is likely related to the observation that the hemodynamic effects of chronic venous obstruction are difficult to quantify. Although acute venous obstruction can be detected using a variety of plethysmographic techniques, chronically obstructed limbs have a larger residual volume and are well collateralized, often with near normal venous outflow. Thus, there are no reliable physiologic tests for diagnosis of a hemodynamically significant chronic venous obstruction.

The clinical consequences of venous obstruction are highly related to location, with the effects of iliofemoral venous obstruction being substantially worse than femoropopliteal obstruction. Among 41 limbs in 37 patients followed for a mean of 5 years after iliofemoral venous thrombosis, 71% of limbs had advanced venous disease (CEAP class C3-C6) and 44% of patients had symptoms of venous claudication.[33] Iliofemoral DVT is also among the strongest predictors of the postthrombotic syndrome.[34] In contrast, femoral venous obstruction is much better tolerated. Among 61 patients undergoing femoral vein harvest for aortic reconstruction, mild edema was seen in only 31% of limbs, and none developed skin changes or ulceration.[35] This is likely related to robust collaterals between the profunda femoris and popliteal veins, both remnants of the axial limb vein, leading to what has been termed "axial transformation of the profunda."[36]

Although patients with greater than 50% stenosis of the iliac vein have been shown to benefit from stenting, defining a critical degree of venous stenosis has been elusive.[37] Arterial concepts of "critical" stenosis, defined as the degree of stenosis associated with sharp declines in pressure and flow, are

TABLE 6.1

ULTRASOUND FINDINGS IN ASYMPTOMATIC AND POSTTHROMBOTIC LIMBS

	■ ASYMPTOMATIC LEGS (%)	■ POSTTHROMBOTIC LEGS (%)
Normal	18	3
Reflux only	35	18
Obstruction only	12	15
Reflux + obstruction	35	65

Postthrombotic limbs with edema, hyperpigmentation, or ulceration are more likely to have a combination of reflux and residual obstruction than either abnormality alone. Adapted from, Johnson BF, Manzo RA, Bergelin RO, et al. Relationship between changes in the deep venous system and the development of the postthrombotic syndrome after an acute episode of lower limb deep vein thrombosis: A one- to six-year follow-up. *J Vasc Surg* 1995;21:307–313.

not directly applicable to the venous circulation, as the critical parameter is upstream pressure rather than downstream perfusion.[38] The determinants of such a "critical" stenosis are far more complex than in the arterial circulation, with some of the components including the degree of outflow stenosis, the inflow volume, the Starling (tissue or intra-abdominal) pressure, and the left atrial pressure. The effects of these components on upstream pressure are not additive, but tend to be dominated by the component with the highest pressure.

Experimental models suggest that the Starling pressure has a significant influence on the degree of stenosis that increases upstream pressure. At very low Starling pressures, corresponding to low intra-abdominal pressure, stenoses of as little as 10% cause a sharp rise in upstream pressure. In contrast, the degree of stenosis has relatively little effect on upstream pressure at high Starling pressures. Increases in intra-abdominal pressure alone, both experimentally and in the obese, can increase venous pressure in the lower extremities.[39] Therefore, lesser degrees of stenosis may be more symptomatic in patients with lower intraabdominal pressures. Regardless, it is clear that chronic iliac vein obstruction occurs more frequently than previously recognized and is at least as important as reflux in the pathogenesis of chronic venous insufficiency. Correction of any underlying iliac vein obstruction often results in symptomatic improvement that is independent of the presence of uncorrected reflux or changes in AVP.[31,40]

Abnormal calf muscle pump function is also associated with higher noninvasive indices of venous pressure.[41] Although the relationship with disease severity has not been consistent, the calf muscle pump ejection fraction is lowest in limbs with active ulceration (35%), followed by limbs with healed ulcers (49%), and those without ulceration but with duplex evidence of reflux (53%).[12,29,42,43] This observation may be related to a progressive decrease in ankle range of motion with increasing severity of disease.[41] Several structural and metabolic abnormalities have also been identified in the gastrocnemius muscles of patients with chronic venous disease, implying failure of the contractile function of the calf muscles themselves.[24]

The role of the perforating veins in chronic venous insufficiency remains controversial. Normal perforating veins have been traditionally considered to direct flow from the superficial to the deep system. Cockett accordingly described the blowout syndrome, whereby high venous pressures developing during muscle contraction were hypothesized to be transmitted from the deep to superficial system via incompetent perforating veins.[9] However, such theories are not entirely consistent with more recent observations. Incompetent perforators are more often associated with superficial venous reflux than with deep venous reflux.[44] Although inward flow toward the deep veins predominates, it is also clear that bidirectional flow can occur

in normal perforating veins.[9,20] Furthermore, although outward flow is most common in incompetent perforating veins, bidirectional flow can also been seen, particularly with less severe venous disease (CEAP clinical classes 1–3).[44]

At least some evidence suggests that the direction of flow within the perforating veins may be more a reflection of local hemodynamics than of the perforating veins themselves, consistent with the observation that small perforators lack valves.[20] The question remains as to whether perforating veins function normally to equalize pressure between the deep and superficial systems, whether they function pathologically to transmit high venous pressures from the deep to superficial systems, or both. This is reflected in recent guidelines that specifically distinguish incompetent from pathologic perforators.[45] Pathologic perforators are defined as perforating veins located beneath an active or healed ulcer that are greater than 3 mm in diameter with outward flow persisting for greater than 0.5 seconds after a provocative maneuver.

VENOUS HYPERTENSION AND THE MICROCIRCULATION

Venous hypertension ultimately leads to reduced microcirculatory flow and shear. The endothelium is particularly sensitive to wall shear stress, and there is increasing evidence that the microcirculatory effects of venous hypertension ultimately lead to a chronic inflammatory process (Fig. 6.6).[46] Early observations suggested that leukocytes were sequestered in the dependent lower extremities as demonstrated by a reduction in the ratio of white cells to red cells returning from the legs of patients with chronic venous insufficiency.[47–49] This phenomenon occurs early in the course of chronic venous disease and has been observed both in limbs with varicose veins and lipodermatosclerosis.[50–52] According to the "white cell trapping" hypothesis of chronic venous insufficiency, reduced flow and shear in the postcapillary venules leads to endothelial activation, white blood cell margination, and reversible leukocyte adhesion.[48] Trapped leukocytes subsequently become activated, increasing endothelial permeability, migrating extravascularly, and releasing toxic oxygen metabolites, proteolytic enzymes, and cytokines.

Notably, compression stockings, one of the key components in the management of chronic venous insufficiency, appear to increase shear stress in the calf veins.[53] Increased shear may be responsible for the increased levels of tissue factor pathway inhibitor[54] and reduced levels of inflammatory cytokines[55] associated with compression, potentially accounting for at least some of the beneficial effects of compression in acute and chronic venous disease.

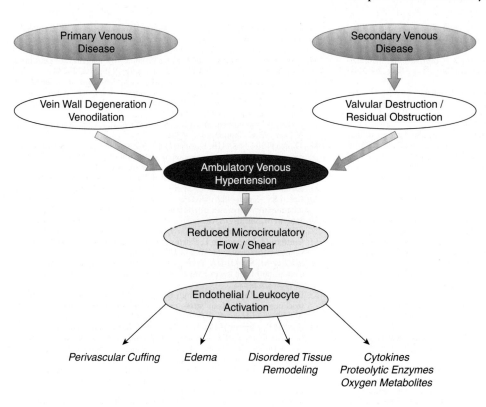

FIGURE 6.6. Pathophysiology of chronic venous insufficiency. Regardless of etiology, ambulatory venous hypertension is the final common pathway responsible for the clinical manifestations of chronic venous insufficiency. A reduction in microcirculatory flow and shear associated with venous hypertension ultimately leads to a cascade of chronic inflammatory processes.

SUMMARY

Venous hemodynamics is, in many respects, more complex than arterial hemodynamics, depending on multiple interactions between hydrostatic pressure, a series of valved conduits, and the respiratory and muscular pumps. Failure of any component of the lower extremity venous system and its associated pumps leads to ambulatory venous hypertension or a failure to lower venous pressure with exercise. Some contributing factors, such as the role of reflux secondary to valvular incompetence, are well understood. However, others, such as the origins of calf muscle pump dysfunction, the hemodynamic consequences of venous obstruction, and the role of incompetent perforating veins, are poorly understood and constitute fertile ground for further research.

References

1. Meissner MH, Moneta G, Burnand K, et al. The hemodynamics and diagnosis of venous disease. *J Vasc Surg* 2007;46(Suppl S):4S–24S.
2. Caggiati A, Bergan JJ, Gloviczki P, et al. Nomenclature of the veins of the lower limbs: An international interdisciplinary consensus statement. *J Vasc Surg* 2002;36:416–422.
3. Zygmunt J. What is new in duplex scanning of the venous system? *Perspect Vasc Surg Endovasc Ther* 2009;21(2):94–104.
4. Hamper UM, DeJong MR, Scoutt LM. Ultrasound evaluation of the lower extremity veins. *Radiol Clin North Am* 2007;45:525–547, ix.
5. Burnand KG. The physiology and hemodynamics of chronic venous insufficiency of the lower limb. In Gloviczki P, Yao JST (eds). *Handbook of Venous Disorders Guidelines of the American Venous Forum*, 2nd ed. London: Arnold, 2001, pp 49–57.
6. Mozes G, Carmichael SW, Gloviczki P. Development and anatomy of the venous system. In Gloviczki P, Yao JST (eds). *Handbook of Venous Disorders*, 2nd ed. London: Arnold, 2001, pp 11–24.
7. Raju S, Green AB, Fredericks RK, et al. Tube collapse and valve closure in ambulatory venous pressure regulation: Studies with a mechanical model. *J Endovasc Surg* 1998;5:42–51.
8. Miller JD, Pegelow DF, Jacques AJ, et al. Skeletal muscle pump versus respiratory muscle pump: Modulation of venous return from the locomotor limb in humans. *J Physiol* 2005;563:925–943.
9. Recek C. Conception of the venous hemodynamics in the lower extremity. *Angiology* 2006;57:556–563.
10. Kugler C, Strunk M, Rudofsky G. Venous pressure dynamics of the healthy human leg. Role of muscle activity, joint mobility and anthropometric factors. *J Vasc Res* 2001;38:20–29.
11. Alimi YS, Barthelemy P, Juhan C. Venous pump of the calf: A study of venous and muscular pressures. *J Vasc Surg* 1994;20:728–735.
12. Araki CT, Back TL, Padberg FT, et al. The significance of calf muscle pump function in venous ulceration. *J Vasc Surg* 1994;20:872–877.
13. Ludbrook J. The musculovenous pumps of the human lower limb. *Am Heart J* 1966;71:635–641.
14. Pollack AA, Wood EH. Venous pressure in the saphenous vein at the ankle in man during exercise and changes in posture. *J Appl Physiol* 1949;1:649–662.
15. White JV, Katz ML, Cisek P, et al. Venous outflow of the leg: Anatomy and physiologic mechanism of the plantar venous plexus. *J Vasc Surg* 1996;24:819–824.
16. Lurie F, Kistner RL. The relative position of paired valves at venous junctions suggests their role in modulating three-dimensional flow pattern in veins. *Eur J Vasc Endovasc Surg* 2012;44:337–340.
17. Lurie F, Kistner RL, Eklof B. The mechanism of venous valve closure in normal physiologic conditions. *J Vasc Surg* 2002;35:713–77.
18. Negus D. The surgical anatomy of the veins of the lower limb. In Dodd H, Cockett FB (eds). *The Pathology and Surgery of the Veins of the Lower Limb*, 2nd ed. Edinburgh: Churchill Livingstone, 1976, pp 18–49.
19. Leu HJ, Vogt M, Pfrunder H. Morphological alterations of non-varicose and varicose veins. (A morphological contribution to the discussion on pathogenesis of varicose veins.) *Basic Res Cardiol* 1979;74:435–444.
20. Sarin S, Scurr J, Coleridge Smith P. Medial calf perforators in venous diseases: The significance of outward flow. *J Vasc Surg* 1992;16:40–46.
21. Lurie F, Kistner RL, Eklof B, et al. Mechanism of venous valve closure and role of the valve in circulation: A new concept. *J Vasc Surg* 2003;38:955–961.
22. van Bemmelen PS, Beach K, Bedford G, et al. The mechanism of venous valve closure. *Arch Surg* 1990;125:617–619.
23. Goldman MP, Fronek A. Anatomy and pathophysiology of varicose veins. *J Dermatol Surg Oncol* 1989;15:138–145.
24. Qiao T, Liu C, Ran F. The impact of gastrocnemius muscle cell changes in chronic venous insufficiency. *Eur J Vasc Endovasc Surg* 2005;30:430–436.
25. Christopoulos DG, Nicolaides AN, Szendro G, et al. Air-plethysmography and the effect of elastic compression on venous hemodynamics of the leg. *J Vasc Surg* 1987;5:148–159.
26. Nicolaides AN, Hussein MK, Szendro G, et al. The relationship of venous ulceration with ambulatory venous pressure measurements. *J Vasc Surg* 1993;17:414–419.
27. Nicolaides AN. Investigation of chronic venous insufficiency: A consensus statement (France, March 5–9, 1997). *Circulation* 2000;102:E126–E163.
28. Hosoi Y, Zukowski A, Kakkos SK, et al. Ambulatory venous pressure measurements: New parameters derived from a mathematic hemodynamic model. *J Vasc Surg* 2002;36:137–142.
29. Labropoulos N, Giannoukas AD, Nicolaides AN, et al. The role of venous reflux and calf muscle pump function in nonthrombotic chronic venous insufficiency. Correlation with severity of signs and symptoms. *Arch Surg* 1996;131:403–446.

PRINCIPLES AND INSTRUMENTATION

30. Hanrahan LM, Araki CT, Rodriguez AA, et al. Distribution of valvular incompetence in patients with venous stasis ulceration. *J Vasc Surg* 1991;13:805–811.

31. Neglen P, Thrasher TL, Raju S. Venous outflow obstruction: An underestimated contributor to chronic venous disease. *J Vasc Surg* 2003;38:879–885.

32. Johnson BF, Manzo RA, Bergelin RO, et al. Relationship between changes in the deep venous system and the development of the postthrombotic syndrome after an acute episode of lower limb deep vein thrombosis: A one- to six-year follow-up. *J Vasc Surg* 1995;21:307–313.

33. Delis KT, Bountouroglou D, Mansfield AO. Venous claudication in iliofemoral thrombosis: Long-term effects on venous hemodynamics, clinical status, and quality of life. *Ann Surg.* 2004;239:118–126.

34. Kahn SR, Shrier I, Julian JA, et al. Determinants and time course of the postthrombotic syndrome after acute deep venous thrombosis. *Ann Intern Med* 2008;149:698–707.

35. Valentine RJ, Clagett GP. Aortic graft infections: Replacement with autogenous vein. *Cardiovasc Surg* 2001;9:419–425.

36. Raju S, Fountain T, Neglen P, et al. Axial transformation of the profunda femoris vein. *J Vasc Surg* 1998;27:651–659.

37. Neglen P, Hollis KC, Olivier J, et al. Stenting of the venous outflow in chronic venous disease: Long-term stent-related outcome, clinical, and hemodynamic result. *J Vasc Surg* 2007;46:979–990.

38. Raju S, Kirk O, Davis M, et al. Hemodynamics of "critical" venous stenosis. *J Vasc Surg Venous Lymphat Disord* 2014;2:52–59.

39. Willenberg T, Clemens R, Haegeli LM, et al. The influence of abdominal pressure on lower extremity venous pressure and hemodynamics: A human in-vivo model simulating the effect of abdominal obesity. *Eur J Vasc Endovasc Surg* 2011;41:849–855.

40. Raju S, Neglen P. High prevalence of nonthrombotic iliac vein lesions in chronic venous disease: A permissive role in pathogenicity. *J Vasc Surg* 2006;44:136–143.

41. Back TL, Padberg FT Jr, et al. Limited range of motion is a significant factor in venous ulceration. *J Vasc Surg* 1995;22:519–523.

42. Cordts PR, Hartono C, LaMorte WW, et al. Physiologic similarities between extremities with varicose veins and with chronic venous insufficiency utilizing air plethysmography. *Am J Surg* 1992;164:260–264.

43. van Bemmelen PS, Mattos MA, Hodgson KJ, et al. Does air plethysmography correlate with duplex scanning in patients with chronic venous insufficiency? *J Vasc Surg* 1993;18:796–807.

44. Labropoulos N, Mansour MA, Kang SS, et al. New insights into perforator vein incompetence. *Eur J Vasc Endovasc Surg* 1999;18:228–234.

45. Gloviczki P, Comerota AJ, Dalsing MC, et al. The care of patients with varicose veins and associated chronic venous diseases: Clinical practice guidelines of the Society for Vascular Surgery and the American Venous Forum. *J Vasc Surg* 2011;53:2S–48S.

46. Bergan JJ, Schmid-Schonbein GW, Smith PD, et al. Chronic venous disease. *N Engl J Med* 2006;355:488–498.

47. Thomas PRS, Nash GB, Dormandy JA. White cell accumulation in dependent legs of patients with venous hypertension: A possible mechanism for trophic changes in the skin. *Br Med J* 1988;296:1693–1695.

48. Coleridge Smith PD, Thomas P, Scurr JH, et al. Causes of venous ulceration: A new hypothesis. *Br Med J (Clin Res Ed)* 1988;296:1726–1727.

49. Coleridge Smith PD. Update on chronic-venous-insufficiency-induced inflammatory processes. *Angiology* 2001;52(Suppl 1):S35–S42.

50. Saharay M, Shields DA, Georgiannos SN, et al. Endothelial activation in patients with chronic venous disease. *Eur J Vasc Endovasc Surg* 1998;15:342–349.

51. Ciuffetti G, Mannarino E, Paltriccia R, et al. Leucocyte activity in chronic venous insufficiency. *Int Angiol* 1994;13:312–316.

52. Saharay M, Shields DA, Porter JB, et al. Leukocyte activity in the microcirculation of the leg in patients with chronic venous disease. *J Vasc Surg* 1997;26:265–273.

53. Downie SP, Raynor SM, Firmin DN, et al. Effects of elastic compression stockings on wall shear stress in deep and superficial veins of the calf. *Am J Physiol Heart Circ Physiol* 2008;294:H2112–H2120.

54. Arcelus JI, Caprini JA, Hoffman KN, et al. Modifications of plasma levels of tissue factor pathway inhibitor and endothelin-1 induced by a reverse Trendelenburg position: Influence of elastic compression—preliminary results. *J Vasc Surg* 1995;22:568–572.

55. Beidler SK, Douillet CD, Berndt DF, et al. Inflammatory cytokine levels in chronic venous insufficiency ulcer tissue before and after compression therapy. *J Vasc Surg* 2009;49:1013–1020.

56. Katz AI, Chen Y, Moreno AH. Flow through a collapsible tube: Experimental analysis and mathematical model. *Biophysical J* 1969;9:1261–1279.

DANIEL F. LEOTTA AND KIRK W. BEACH

PRINCIPLES AND INSTRUMENTATION

Ultrasonic duplex scanning, the combination of two-dimensional (2D) ultrasound B-mode imaging and single-gate pulse Doppler blood velocimetry with spectral waveform analysis, is the most successful and widely used noninvasive method available for the examination and classification of vascular disease. This chapter focuses on the physics and instrumentation behind these ultrasound methods for the examination of blood vessels. This is not a comprehensive reference, but rather a review of selected topics in order to emphasize their importance or to offer a different perspective from those found in standard physics texts.

ULTRASOUND PROPAGATION THROUGH TISSUE

Linear Mechanics of Longitudinal Waves

The basis of all ultrasound imaging methods is the propagation of sound waves through tissue. Sound waves are *mechanical waves*. Two common types of mechanical waves are transverse waves and longitudinal waves. For a *transverse wave*, particle motion is perpendicular to the direction of wave propagation. For a *longitudinal wave*, particle motion is parallel to the direction of wave propagation. In tissue, transverse waves are attenuated in short distances, converting all of the wave energy into heat. However, ultrasound does not travel through tissue as a transverse wave; it passes through tissue as a longitudinal

wave, with regions of tissue compression and regions of tissue decompression. The pressure increase and decrease as an ultrasound wave passes can be several times the atmospheric pressure. Although the motion of the tissue as the ultrasound wave passes is just a few nanometers, the maximum molecular velocities are near 1 cm/s, and the accelerations are nearly 1000 times the acceleration of gravity.

The physical principles of ultrasound transmission can be derived from Newton's equations using a model of masses (representing molecules) and springs (representing chemical bonds) (Fig. 7.1):

$$\text{Force} = \text{mass} \times \text{acceleration, } and$$
$$\text{Force} = \text{stiffness} \times \text{compression}$$

When these equations are applied to molecules in a material, the compression force is set equal to the acceleration force:

$$\text{Molecular force} = \text{density} \times \text{molecular acceleration}$$
$$= \text{stiffness} \times (\text{compression change with distance})$$

Ultrasound wave mechanics are derived from this equation. If u is the distance of each molecule from its resting position, y is distance along the direction that the wave is traveling, and t is time, the previous equations become

$$\text{Molecular force} = \text{density} \times d^2u/dt^2 = \text{stiffness} \times d^2u/dy^2$$

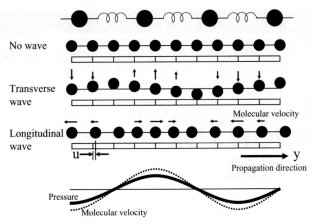

FIGURE 7.1. Mass and spring model for tissue mechanics. The ultrasound transmission properties of tissue can be derived by considering the tissue to be assembled from masses (representing tissue density) and springs (representing tissue stiffness). *No wave*: At rest, with no wave present, the masses are equally distributed in the tissue. *Transverse wave*: If a transverse wave passes through the tissue, the displacement of the tissues can be seen, like the lateral displacement as a wave passes along a rope. *Longitudinal wave*: Ultrasound passes through tissue as a longitudinal wave, with regions of tissue compression and regions of tissue decompression. *Pressure fluctuation and molecular velocity*: The pressure fluctuation and the molecular velocity are in phase; the ratio of pressure fluctuation to molecular velocity is the tissue impedance. The acceleration is $1/4$ cycle ahead of the molecular velocity and the displacement is $1/4$ cycle delayed.

where the second derivatives d^2u/dt^2 and d^2u/dy^2 represent tissue acceleration and tissue distortion, respectively. These equations can be solved by assuming that molecular displacement u is dependent on the variable group $(y + C \times t)$ having units of centimeters; C has units of centimeters per second (cm/s). The previous derivatives can then be expressed as

$$d^2u/dy^2 = u'' \quad and \quad d^2u/dt^2 = C^2 \times u''$$

and the equation becomes

$$density \times C^2 \times u'' = stiffness \times u''$$

Therefore, for *any* waveshape of u, the equation is correct if $C^2 =$ (stiffness/density). In this equation, C^2 is positive, but the value of C can be either positive or negative, and it is the *speed* of the ultrasound wave.

The meaning of C is further understood by looking at Figure 7.2. The wave has different locations at different times. As time advances (from top to bottom), the wave moves from left to right. The line marked "wave speed" shows a place on the wave near a crest where the value $(y + C \times t)$ is constant. In Figure 7.2, C is negative; thus, as time increases, y must also increase to keep $(y + C \times t)$ constant. The expression $(y + C \times t)$ provides the relationship between advancing time and advancing location, which is speed. The wave period T (the time it takes to change from one peak to the next) and the wavelength λ (the distance it takes to change from one peak to the next) are related by C, the wave speed:

$$C = (wave\ length)/(wave\ period) = \lambda/T$$

Wave period (T) is the inverse of frequency (F), so that

$$C = \lambda \times F$$

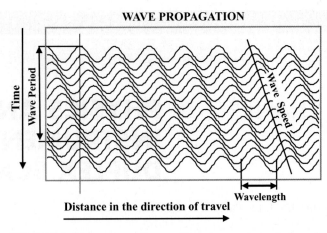

WAVE PROPAGATION

FIGURE 7.2. Wave propagation over time. As a wave travels through a medium, the wave length (λ) and the wave period (T = 1/F) are related by the wave speed (C = λ/T = λ × F). The wave function is dependent on the variable (y – C × t) where y is the distance along the direction of travel and t is time.

The following equation is also an important relationship to remember for any longitudinal mechanical (sound) wave traveling through a material:

$$C = \sqrt{(\kappa/\rho)}$$

where κ is stiffness and ρ is density. Of course, both stiffness and density depend on temperature; thus, C will vary with temperature.

The speed of sound in typical soft tissue is 1540 m/s or 1.54 mm/µs, whereas the speed of sound in air is 331 m/s. These are determined by the density and stiffness of the materials. Typical sound and ultrasound wavelengths are presented in Table 7.1.

Ultrasound Frequencies and Wavelength

Frequency is measured in hertz, which is an expression of cycles of compression and decompression per second. Medical ultrasound frequencies are measured in millions of cycles per second, or megahertz (MHz). Wavelength is related to the spatial resolution of an ultrasound image. Because your ears are about 15 cm apart, you cannot tell where a 20-Hz sound (15-m wavelength in air) is coming from, but you can identify where a 2-kHz sound (15-cm wavelength in air) is coming from. By using 5-MHz ultrasound in tissue (0.3-mm wavelength), it is possible to resolve objects that are a few millimeters apart.

TABLE 7.1

SOUND WAVELENGTHS FOR DIFFERENT FREQUENCIES

■ SOUND FREQUENCY	■ WAVELENGTH IN AIR (FOR C = 300 m/s)	■ WAVELENGTH IN TISSUE (FOR C = 1500 m/s)
20 Hz	15 m	75 m
1 kHz	30 cm	1.5 m
20 kHz	15 mm	7.5 cm
1 MHz	0.3 mm	1.5 mm
10 MHz	0.03 mm	0.15 mm

C, wave speed (see text).

Impedance and Wave Speed

As a sound pulse (or wave) travels through tissue, zones of high pressure and low pressure are created. The high-pressure regions occur where the molecules are squeezed together, and the low-pressure regions occur where the molecules are spread apart. The pressure elevation or depression from atmospheric pressure is called *pressure fluctuation* (p). Pressure fluctuation is equal to the stiffness (κ) times du/dy. As a sound pulse travels through tissue, the molecules oscillate in the direction of the sound wave. The instantaneous molecular velocity (v) of the oscillating molecules is du/dt, and because u is dependent on (y + C × t), du/dt = C × du/dy. Therefore, v/C = p/κ, or

$$Z = p/v = \kappa/C = \sqrt{\kappa \times \rho} = \rho \times C$$

Z is called the *acoustic impedance* of the tissue. In physical terms, impedance is the ratio between the pressure fluctuation that the tissue feels as a wave passes and the molecular velocity of the molecules as the wave passes. Be sure to avoid confusing the molecular velocity of the molecules (v) with the wave speed (C). The molecular velocity (v) oscillates in the positive and negative directions during ultrasound wave passage at the ultrasound frequency; v is greater when the wave intensity is greater. C is the speed at which the wave passes and does not change with wave intensity, as long as the intensity is low. If the intensity is high, the "linear" model of springs and masses in Figure 7.1 does not hold. The "nonlinear" waves at higher intensities cause harmonics, which are the basis of harmonic imaging (discussed later in this chapter).

It is important to remember that impedance (Z), like wave speed (C), is dependent on the density and the stiffness (1/elasticity) of the tissue. Just as wave speed changes with temperature, impedance changes with temperature because temperature affects both stiffness and density.

Amplitude and Phase

In addition to the wavelength (in units of distance) and period (in units of time), each wave has two other properties: the *amplitude* and the *phase* (Fig. 7.3). All of the information in

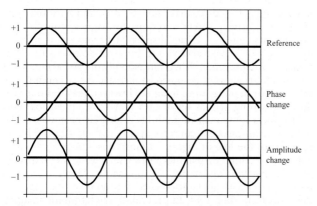

FIGURE 7.3. Wave phase and amplitude. Two parameters define a wave of a particular frequency: the amplitude and the phase. The amplitude of a wave is taken as the peak difference of a parameter from ambient conditions. In ultrasound, the parameter is usually pressure fluctuation from atmospheric pressure, but could be molecular velocity, acceleration, or displacement. Amplitude of the ultrasonic echo is used for B-mode imaging. The phase is the time difference of a wave feature from the same feature on a reference wave. Therefore, phase is always represented as a difference. That difference could be in time or in distance along the propagation direction.

a wave is encoded in the amplitude and phase. Ultrasound B-mode imaging displays the echo amplitude, and Doppler velocity information is acquired from the phase. These two kinds of information are independent: one can change while the other remains constant.

The amplitude of a sound wave can be measured in many different ways, but each method measures properties experienced by the molecules of the material through which the sound is traveling. Each molecule experiences a pressure fluctuation, which is a displacement back and forth along the direction of wave travel associated with a molecular velocity and acceleration. The displacement, velocity, and acceleration are like the displacement, velocity, and acceleration of a swing or a pendulum.

Frequency and phase are closely related. When a 5-MHz Doppler looks at an approaching blood velocity of 75 cm/s, the Doppler echo has a frequency of 5.005 MHz. The frequency is increased by 0.1% or 1/1000 of the transmit frequency. Another way to think of this is that the phase becomes more advanced with every cycle: for every 1000 cycles, the phase has advanced 1 cycle. After the first 10 cycles, the phase has advanced 1/100 of a cycle. Because one cycle is 360 degrees, after 10 cycles, the phase has advanced 3.6 degrees, and after 100 cycles, the phase has advanced 36 degrees. It can be convenient to think about the Doppler shift as a continuing change in phase rather than a frequency shift.

Pressure Fluctuation and Molecular Velocity, Displacement, and Acceleration

Molecular velocity, displacement, acceleration, and pressure are related to ultrasound intensity. These four measured values are ways to look at the mechanical "shaking" that the molecules experience as an ultrasound wave passes through the tissue. First, ultrasound intensity is related to energy:

$$\text{Energy} = \text{force} \times \text{distance}$$

$$\text{Power} = \text{energy/time} = \text{force} \times \text{distance/time}$$

$$\begin{aligned}\text{Intensity} &= \text{power/area} \\ &= \text{force/area} \times \text{distance/time} \\ &= \text{pressure fluctuation} \times \text{molecular velocity}\end{aligned}$$

As discussed earlier, the *pressure fluctuation* is the fluctuation of the pressure in the tissue due to the passing of an ultrasound wave; the *molecular velocity* is the velocity of molecules in the tissue due to the passing of the ultrasound wave.

As shown previously, in the solution to Newton's equations, the ratio of tissue pressure fluctuation to molecular velocity fluctuation represents the *tissue impedance* (Z):

$$Z = (\text{pressure fluctuation})/(\text{molecular velocity})$$

By substitution:

$$\begin{aligned}\text{Intensity} &= (\text{pressure fluctuation})^2/Z \\ &= Z \times (\text{molecular velocity})^2\end{aligned}$$

If the ultrasound is continuous wave (CW), the average intensity is the average of the sine wave amplitude squared. That average is half of the squared maximum value:

$$\begin{aligned}\text{Average intensity} &= (\text{maximum pressure fluctuation})^2/2 \times Z \\ &= Z/2 \times (\text{molecular velocity})^2\end{aligned}$$

This is also true within an ultrasound pulse. The temporal peak intensity is computed from this same expression.

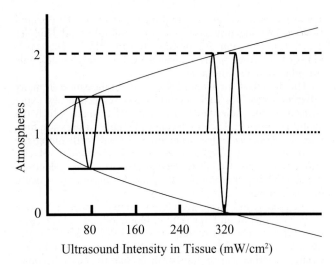

FIGURE 7.4. Tissue pressure fluctuation versus medical ultrasound intensity. Intensity is equal to one-half of the square of the peak pressure fluctuation divided by the tissue impedance. Using the impedance of water, which is near the impedance of human tissues, at an intensity of 320 mW/cm^2 (SPTP), the pressure fluctuation equals 1 atm.

A graph of the pressure fluctuations versus CW intensity (Fig. 7.4) indicates that a physical problem occurs within the range of diagnostic ultrasound intensities: at temporal peak intensities greater than 320 mW/cm^2, the pressure fluctuation becomes greater than 1 atm. Therefore, the minimum pressure theoretically becomes negative. This is impossible according to the physical laws of thermodynamics. Thus, the linear equation for compressibility, which is based on thermodynamics, does not apply for these conditions. The wave becomes nonlinear (Fig. 7.5) and gives rise to harmonics.

Nonlinear Mechanics

With nonlinear mechanics, the linear equations presented earlier no longer apply. The relationship between pressure and displacement, which is based on the nature of molecular bonds, does not hold for large fluctuations in pressure.

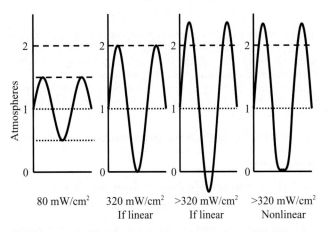

FIGURE 7.5. Ultrasound waveshape changes with nonlinear propagation. As an ultrasound sine wave propagates through tissue, the shape of the wave changes: the peaks increase in height and sharpness, and the valleys become blunted. This effect is greater at higher intensities. This change in shape is due to nonlinear stiffness of the tissue, which causes the wave velocity to be higher when the pressure is at the peaks and the wave velocity to be lower when the minimum pressure is at or below zero.

The nonlinear relationship between compression and force is shown in Figure 7.6. In the central region, stiffness is linear, but when compression becomes too great or too small, the effective stiffness changes. When the wave intensity is very large, during compression, the stiffness is increased, causing an increase in the wave speed and an increase in the wave impedance. Likewise, during decompression, the stiffness is decreased, causing decreases in both the wave "speed" and "impedance." Speed and impedance are in quotation marks in these cases because their definitions become less useful in these nonlinear conditions than in the linear conditions.

Harmonics and Ultrasound Contrast Agents

The flattened valleys and the enhanced peaks of the waveshape in Figure 7.5 (*right*) can be represented as a combination of sine waves (Fig. 7.7). In this example, a sine wave at the original frequency and a sine wave at two times the original frequency are shown. The wave at the original frequency is called the *fundamental*; the wave at two times the frequency is called a *harmonic*. The wave at two times the fundamental frequency is called by different names: it is called the "first harmonic" by some people and the "second harmonic" by others. Both groups agree on the name "first overtone" for that frequency. Harmonics occur at two times, three times, or any integer multiple of the fundamental. Any periodic (repeating) waveshape can be formed from a series of sine wave harmonics of the fundamental by selecting the phase and the amplitude of each harmonic. This is the Fourier theorem and is the basis of the Fourier transform. The *lower curve* in Figure 7.7 shows the combination of the fundamental and the harmonic.

Harmonics are present in all diagnostic ultrasound echoes. If the transmitted intensity is increased, the intensity of the harmonics increases as more of the power from the fundamental frequency is converted to the harmonics. The attenuation of ultrasound is proportional to frequency; thus, the harmonics are attenuated more rapidly than the fundamental. Some of that attenuation is due to absorption (conversion to heat), so that if the ultrasound intensity is doubled, the amount of ultrasound converted to heat more than doubles because of the conversion to harmonics and the subsequent conversion to heat.

The subject of harmonics has been recognized for decades but was not often discussed until recently, and harmonic displays are relatively recent additions to diagnostic ultrasound instruments. Interest in the display of harmonics is primarily a result of a general desire to improve detection of ultrasound contrast agents. When ultrasound contrast agents were introduced, they were designed to increase the strength of the echo signals in ultrasound images. However, they did not produce the strong echoes on images that were hoped for. This led to the development of methods to display harmonics. The bubbles in ultrasound contrast agents will change the linear portions of the line in Figure 7.6 and cause the generation of harmonics. Thus, displaying harmonic echoes was expected to show contrast agents more prominently. However, tissues without contrast agents also reflect harmonic echoes back to the transducer (Fig. 7.8). In general, tissue harmonic imaging improves the lateral resolution and image contrast.

To generate a harmonic image using a 3-MHz transducer, it is logical to transmit at 3 MHz and receive at 6 MHz, but this cannot be done because a transducer is not sensitive at even multiples of the frequency. The 3-MHz transducer must have a "damping" material to make it "broadband," so that it will operate between 1.5 and 4.5 MHz. Then, for harmonic imaging, it is possible to reduce the transmit frequency to 2 MHz and increase the receive frequency to select 4-MHz echoes to generate the harmonic image.

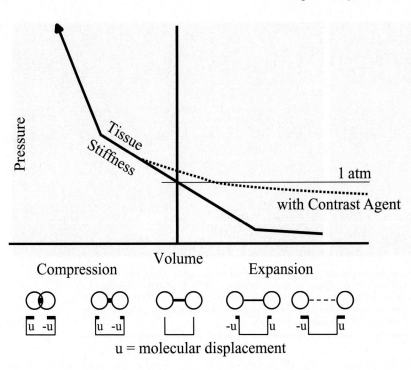

FIGURE 7.6. Nonlinear behavior of tissue stiffness. Near atmospheric pressure, the compressional force is linearly related to the change in dimension of the tissue, but at higher or lower pressures, the force significantly deviates from linear. The addition of an acoustic contrast agent consisting of bubbles expands the tissue and increases the nonlinearity.

Transmitted Ultrasound

Continuous Wave

CW ultrasound is used for Doppler applications. The instruments are generally inexpensive and often provide nondirectional audible output. However, CW Doppler instruments can provide directional information, and they can also produce spectral waveforms. The transmitted ultrasound is "narrowband" because only one ultrasound frequency is transmitted. Because the transmission is continuous, no information about the depth of the detected flow is available.

Burst and Pulse

The terms pulse and burst have similar meanings. *Pulse* refers to the shortest burst of ultrasound that can be sent into tissue with the transducer available. *Burst* refers to an intentionally prolonged transmit oscillation. For most diagnostic imaging applications, the transmitted ultrasound pulse is on for a short period of time (Fig. 7.9), less than a microsecond, and off for 100 μs. For most pulsed Doppler applications, a burst of ultrasound lasting 1 μs is sent into tissue. For transcranial Doppler applications, the transmitted burst may last 15 μs. Long transmit bursts are narrowband, so they define the Doppler frequency with precision and they are resistant to noise. For B-mode imaging, a short (broadband) transmit pulse is used to ensure the best

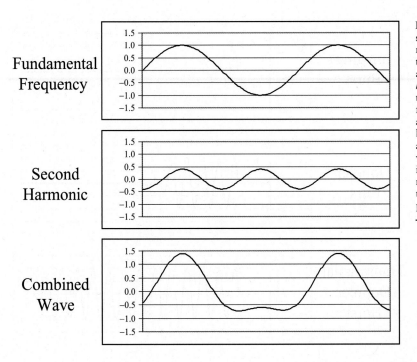

FIGURE 7.7. Harmonic components of nonsinusoidal waves. Any periodic repeating wave can be represented by a series of sine waves starting with the fundamental and adding wave frequencies that are multiples of the fundamental. These waves are *harmonics*. The first harmonic is the fundamental, the second harmonic has a frequency twice that of the fundamental, and so on. Each harmonic has a unique amplitude and phase that it contributes to the combined wave. Here, 1.5 cycles of the fundamental (*top*) are added to 3 cycles of the second harmonic (*middle*) with a phase that causes the peaks to align, producing a wave with blunted minimums and enhanced maximums (*bottom*). The combined wave is similar to the wave in Figure 7.5 that resulted from nonlinear propagation in tissue.

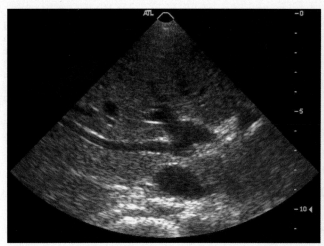
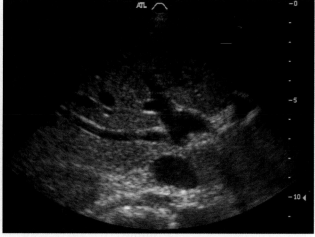

FIGURE 7.8. Harmonic image of liver without contrast agent. In typical medical ultrasound imaging, the SPTP intensities are much higher than 320 mW/cm^2, so nonlinear wave propagation and the formation of harmonics are common. An image formed by showing the amplitude of the fundamental frequency echo (*left*) looks different from an image of the same tissue formed by transmitting a lower frequency and forming an image based on the strength of the second harmonic of the transmitted frequency (*right*).

(smallest) depth resolution. This allows the visualization of small structures in the depth direction, like the intima-media thickness.

During the "off" period, the receiver is accepting echoes from successively deeper locations. This period lasts between 40 and 400 μs. An ultrasound instrument computes the depth of the echo reflector by measuring the time from the transmit pulse to the echo, assuming an ultrasound speed of 1.54 mm/μs. Echoes from shallow structures (1 cm deep) return soon after the transmit pulse (about 13 μs); echoes from deeper structures (3 cm deep) return later after the transmit pulse (about 40 μs); echoes from the deepest structures (25 cm deep) return latest (about 325 μs) (Table 7.2).

Duty Factor

The *duty factor* (DF; or *duty cycle*) is a measure of the fraction of time that the ultrasound instrument is transmitting. In a CW instrument, the system is always transmitting, and

the DF is 1.0, or 100%. In a pulse-echo B-mode ultrasound instrument imaging a maximum depth of 19 cm, the transmit pulse is 1 μs, and the pulse repetition period (PRP; time between pulses) is 250 μs. Thus, the DF is 1/250, or 0.004, or 0.4%. The concept of DF also applies to a home heating system. To heat a home on a cool day, the furnace might be on for 15 minutes out of every hour (DF = 25%), but on a cold day, the furnace might be on for 30 minutes out of every hour (DF = 50%). The DF is an important part of the computation of ultrasound intensities.

Power and Intensity

There is a great deal of confusion in ultrasound physics literature about power and intensity. Here is the reason for the confusion. Power is a measure of energy per time and has units of watts. As an ultrasonic wave passes through tissue, the power

FIGURE 7.9. Burst length of ultrasound pulses. For B-mode imaging, short (broadband) ultrasound bursts are transmitted into tissue (*top*) to get the best depth resolution. For Doppler, medium-length ultrasound bursts are transmitted into tissue (*middle*). For transcranial Doppler, in which the echoes are greatly attenuated and the transmitted burst energy must be high while limiting the SPTP intensity, long (narrowband) ultrasound bursts are transmitted into tissue (*bottom*).

Imaging Burst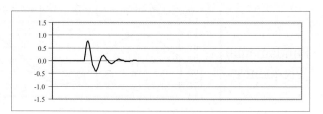

Doppler Burst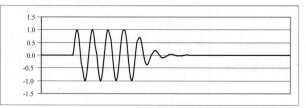

Transcranial Doppler Burst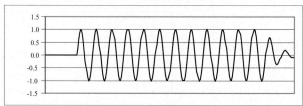

PRINCIPLES AND INSTRUMENTATION

TABLE 7.2

TIME REQUIRED FOR AN ECHO TO RETURN FROM A KNOWN DEPTH

DEPTH (cm)	TIME (MINIMUM POSSIBLE PRI) (μs)	MAXIMUM POSSIBLE PRF (kHz)
1	13	60
2	26	40
3	39	20
5	65	12
10	130	6
15	195	5
20	260	4
25	325	3

PRF, pulse repetition frequency; PRI, pulse repetition interval.

is distributed over the cross-sectional area of the ultrasound beam pattern. Power divided by the cross-sectional area is equal to the intensity. The intensity is easily measured with an ultrasound transducer called a *hydrophone* and determines whether the ultrasound propagation is linear or nonlinear. Intensity is related to pressure fluctuation and is therefore the quantity usually discussed in ultrasound physics. Intensity is dependent on both the ultrasound power in the beam pattern and the cross-sectional area of the beam pattern. Changes in intensity due to changes in cross-sectional area of the beam pattern can easily be confused with changes in intensity due to changes in ultrasound power. It is important to keep the two factors separate.

In tissue, ultrasound power decreases with distance as the wave propagates. The decrease in power is due to attenuation in the tissue. *Attenuation* has two factors: (1) conversion of the ultrasound power to heat (absorption) and (2) scattering of the ultrasound power in directions other than the direction of the ultrasound beam. The attenuation (both absorption and scattering) of ultrasound in tissue is dependent on the tissue type and the ultrasound frequency.

Measures of Ultrasound Intensity

There are six common measures of ultrasound intensity:

- Spatial average temporal average (SATA)
- Spatial peak temporal average (SPTA)
- Spatial average pulse average (SAPA)
- Spatial peak pulse average (SPPA)
- Spatial average temporal peak (SATP)
- Spatial peak temporal peak (SPTP)

Between 1980 and 1990, the number of measures was changed from four to six, and the naming of the measures changed. The new measures are *pulse average* values, which were previously called "temporal peak." *Temporal peak* now refers to an instantaneous peak value rather than a value averaged over the pulse. Two of the six measures (SATA and SPTA) are used for computing heating effects; the rest are used for considering ultrasonic cavitation and nonlinear effects of ultrasound.

All of these are measures of an ultrasound transmit beam and depend on two factors: (1) the beam power and (2) the beam area. The initial power of the beam is selected by applying the proper voltage to the ultrasound transducer based on the transducer thickness, the damping material on the back of the transducer, the area of the face of the

transducer, and the efficiency of coupling to the body tissues under examination:

$$\text{Initial beam power} = (\text{transducer voltage})^2 \times (\text{transducer area}) \times (\text{coupling to tissue})/\text{damping}$$

As the ultrasound pulse proceeds into tissue, the beam power decreases owing to attenuation:

$$\text{Beam power} = \text{initial beam power} \times (\text{attenuation rate})^{\text{depth}}$$

The beam area is dependent on the focal character of the transducer. Intensity is the ratio of beam power to beam area:

$$\text{Intensity} = \text{beam power/beam area} = \text{W/cm}^2$$

The beam power can be expressed as a maximum or as a temporal average.

The most widely accepted method of measuring the ultrasound beam is to begin with a measurement of the total beam power. Beam power is measured by directing the beam onto a submerged weighing pan of a standard balance. When the ultrasound beam strikes the pan, a force appears. The force is equal to

$$\text{Force} = 2 \times \text{power/C}$$

In water, where the speed of sound is 148,000 cm/s, a 1-W temporal average ultrasound beam generates a force equal to the weight of a 1.38-mg mass. This force can be demonstrated by imaging water in a tank. By turning up the gain, particles suspended in the water can be seen. As the transmit power is increased, the suspended particles can be seen on the ultrasound image rushing away from the ultrasound scanhead because of the ultrasound force. By measuring the ultrasound beam with a hydrophone, the beam diameter and area can be determined. From these measurements, the SATA intensity can be determined:

$$\text{SATA} = \text{power/area}$$

A look at the interrelationships of the six intensity terms listed above can provide a more complete picture of tissue exposure. The intensity measures are related by combinations of four factors: (1) duty factor (Fig. 7.10), (2) beam factor (Fig. 7.11), (3) pulse factor (Fig. 7.12), and (4) image factor (Fig. 7.13). These four factors all have the same range: maximum = 1, minimum = 0. Using a hydrophone and an oscilloscope (which traces the voltage in time that is generated by the hydrophone),

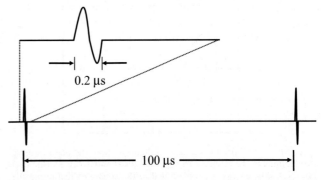

FIGURE 7.10. Duty factor. The duration of an ultrasound transmit burst (*top*) is short compared with the time interval separating bursts (*bottom*). The ratio of burst length to interval is called the *duty factor*.

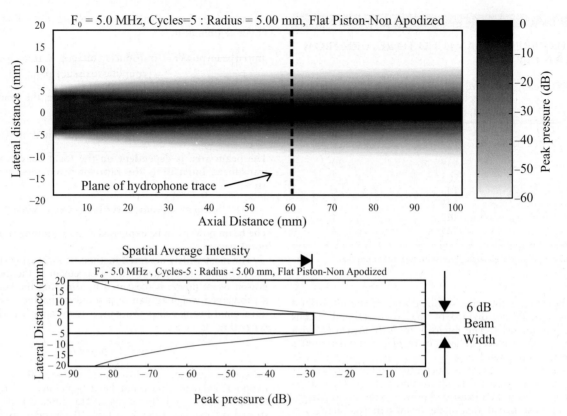

FIGURE 7.11. Beam factor. *Top,* The beam pattern of a flat circular transducer extends from the face of the transducer into tissue. Near the transducer in the Fresnel zone is a complex area of varying intensity formed by diffraction, which is the constructive and destructive interference of the waves from the transducer face. Far from the transducer in the Fraunhofer zone, the beam pattern becomes much smoother. *Bottom,* A profile of the maximum pressure fluctuation taken across the beam at the transition zone between the Fresnel and the Fraunhofer zones shows the intensity peak. A *box* is drawn that shows the width of the central portions of the beam where intensities are at least 25% (>6 dB) of the peak. The spatial average intensity across that beam width is between one-half and one-third of the central peak intensity.

the factors shown in Figures 7.10 to 7.13 can be determined. Then, the intensities can be computed:

SPTA = SATA/beam factor
SAPA = SATA/DF
SATP = SATA/DF/pulse factor
SPPA = SATA/beam factor/DF
SPTP = SATA/beam factor/DF/pulse factor

Different ultrasound modes have different DFs (Table 7.3). In some examinations, the ultrasound beam is held stationary (A-mode, M-mode, and pulsed Doppler). For 2D imaging, however, the scanhead sweeps the ultrasound beam across a plane of tissue, penetrating each element of tissue only once per image frame for 2D B-mode, and typically eight times

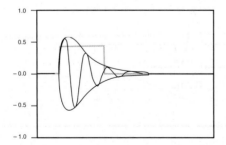

FIGURE 7.12. Pulse factor. The oscillations show the acoustic pressure applied to the tissue, with a gradual onset and decay. During each half-cycle, the energy is proportional to the square of the amplitude, indicated by the envelope of the pulse. The square pulse is a simplified model of the ultrasound burst power showing the temporal average power for the duration of the pulse. The pulse average power is less than the instantaneous temporal peak power of the pulse.

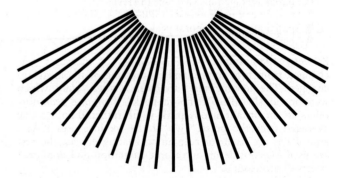

FIGURE 7.13. Image factor. The 2D B-mode image is formed from more than 100 pulse-echo lines. Therefore, the average intensity exposure of tissue on any one line is equal to the exposure computed for repeat exposures if all pulses were delivered along a single line, divided by the number of lines in the image.

TABLE 7.3

TRANSMIT PARAMETERS FOR ULTRASOUND EXAMINATION METHODS

■ METHOD	■ F (MHz)	■ IF	■ PRF (kHz)	■ PRP (μs)	■ PD (μs)	■ DF
Continuous-wave Doppler	5	1	—	—	—	1.00
Transcranial pulsed Doppler	2	1	5	200	10	0.05
Cardiovascular pulsed Doppler	5	1	10	100	1	0.01
M-mode imaging	5	1	1	1000	0.5	0.0005
2D B-mode imaging	5	0.01	5	200	0.5	0.000025
2D color-flow imaging	5	0.05	5	200	1	0.00025

DF, duty factor (dimensionless); F, ultrasound frequency; IF, image factor = 1/number of ultrasound lines in an image (dimensionless); PD, pulse duration = length of transmit pulse or burst (s); PRF, pulse repetition frequency = number of transmitted pulses per second (Hz); PRP, pulse repetition period = 1/PRF (s); 2D, two-dimensional.

per image for 2D color Doppler. Thus, in 2D imaging, the *image factor* must be included in exposure computations for a voxel (a small volume) of tissue, indicating the number of ultrasound scan lines per image that are acquired from other locations in tissue. This allows an increase in the energy in each transmit burst, because only one ultrasound pulse passes through each voxel of tissue in each frame. The frame rate is usually about 30 images/s; thus, only 30 pulses/s heat each segment of tissue. However, because the bursts have higher energy, they have high peak positive and negative pressures, which thereby increase the chance of cavitation in the tissue.

Theoretical Intensities versus Actual Intensities

Unknown factors, such as the attenuation of overlying tissue and refractive spreading of the ultrasound beam, make correct theoretical computations of the ultrasound intensities impossible. Experimental investigations of ultrasound intensities must be performed if accurate values are to be known. Unfortunately, properly mimicking the conditions of an examination and then placing a calibrated hydrophone at the location of maximum intensity (a location that is unknown within the depths of tissue) to determine the maximum intensity is either difficult or impossible. Almost any conceivable arrangement is seriously flawed. Thus, we are left with a few general conclusions:

1. The computed intensities and, consequently, the computed heating effects are generally more severe than any actually achieved in the body tissues.
2. Caution demands that ultrasound examinations be limited to minimum transmit powers (and therefore maximum receiver gain settings) consistent with achieving diagnostic data.
3. Caution also demands that ultrasound image acquisition be limited to the shortest possible time and that for demonstrations and discussions, the freeze frame and cine functions on the system be used whenever possible.
4. Examiner training should begin with learning about the proper use of the instrumentation so that the recommendations in conclusions 2 and 3 above can be followed.

Attenuation

As an ultrasound wave passes farther and farther into tissue, the energy in the ultrasound pulse decreases because of the conversion of that energy into other forms of energy, including heat, and into scattered ultrasound. Conversion can also occur from one ultrasound frequency into another, forming harmonics of the fundamental frequency. Attenuation computations can be easily understood by using the concept of the half-value layer (or half-energy layer). A *half-value layer* is a layer of tissue thick enough to convert half of the energy in an incoming ultrasound pulse into heat and scattered ultrasound, leaving the remaining half of the ultrasound energy in the pulse as it passes out of the layer. All other attenuation computations can be derived from this concept. Each tissue type has an attenuation rate that can be expressed as a half-value layer (Table 7.4). For most tissues, attenuation increases with ultrasound frequency, so the half-value layer for 2-MHz ultrasound is half as thick as a half-value layer for 1-MHz ultrasound. The wavelength of 2-MHz ultrasound is half as long as the wavelength of 1-MHz ultrasound; therefore, it is most convenient to express the thickness of the half-value layer in wavelengths.

Attenuation can also be expressed as decibels and nepers. Half-value layers and decibels are defined in units of energy, power, or intensity; nepers are defined in units of amplitude. All are based on the exponential curve, which is the mathematic function that describes the decay of the ultrasound power or energy as ultrasound passes through attenuating tissue. Here, an example using units of *half-value layers in wavelengths* (HVLW) is presented to simplify understanding.

Imagine that a 15-MHz ultrasound burst with an energy of 64 ergs is sent into a layer of fat that is 0.5 cm thick. The wavelength of the 15-MHz ultrasound in fat is about 0.1 mm [(1.5 mm/μs)/(15 cycles/μs)]. The fat layer is 50 wavelengths thick, that is, 1 HVLW thick. When the burst emerges from the other side, the remaining energy in the burst is 32 ergs. If the burst passes through another 1-HVLW layer, the energy would be 16 ergs. After passing through a third 1-HVLW layer, the burst contains energy of 8 ergs. Every HVLW layer converts half of the energy into heat and scattered ultrasound, leaving half in the remaining beam. After three HVLW layers, only $(1/2)^3$ of

TABLE 7.4

HALF-VALUE LAYERS FOR DIFFERENT TISSUES

■ TISSUE	■ HALF-VALUE LAYER (λ)
Plasma	700
Blood	250
Brain	75
Fat	50
Liver	30
Kidney	20
Muscle	15
Bone	0.1

FIGURE 7.14. Half-value layer. As ultrasound is attenuated by any tissue layer, a fraction of the incoming ultrasound is converted to heat. The fraction passing out of the layer is dependent on the thickness and the material. For any material, there is a thickness that will attenuate the ultrasound to a value that is one-half of the incoming energy. The decay in intensity is logarithmic (*upper curve*). If the log of the energy is displayed on the vertical axis, the decay forms a linear plot (*lower curve*). In this figure, the vertical axis is plotted as intensity and associated pressure fluctuation amplitude. Intensity is valid only if the beam cross-sectional area remains constant.

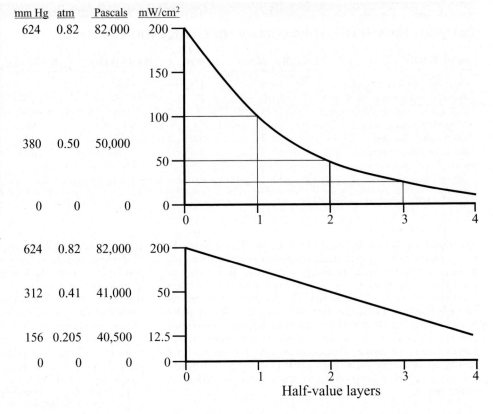

the energy remains. Thus, to compute the remaining energy in a burst,

$$\text{Remaining energy} = \text{initial energy} \times \left(\frac{1}{2}\right)^{T/\lambda/HVLW}$$

where T is the thickness of the tissue and HVLW is the number of half-value layers through which the ultrasound has passed. A logarithmic plot of the ratio of the remaining to the initial energy versus distance will give a linear (straight line) graph (Fig. 7.14).

Scattering

The use of ultrasound in medicine spans the range from active tissue ablation to passive acoustic thermography. Between these extremes lies pulse-echo diagnostic ultrasound (Table 7.5). As ultrasound passes through tissue, it crosses boundaries between tissues having different impedances. At each boundary, some ultrasound is reflected, but most passes through the boundary.

A voxel is the smallest resolvable volume of tissue and must be analyzed as a single unit; the volume of a voxel is usually about a cubic millimeter. Typically, there are 1,000,000 cells in each voxel of tissue, and within the voxel, the boundaries are the cell walls. Reflections from each of the boundaries travel in a different direction. This is called *scattering*. Incident ultrasound is scattered in all directions from each voxel. The scattered ultrasound that goes back along the direction of the incident ultrasound beam to the transducer is called *backscatter*.

The backscattered ultrasound from each voxel along the ultrasound beam is the signal that is used to create the ultrasound image and Doppler waveform. That signal must be greater than the natural ultrasound noise emitted from the tissue. Tissues emit ultrasound because they are warm. The intensity of the "thermal noise" from tissue is about 10/1,000,000,000,000,000 W/cm^2. This is more easily expressed in scientific notation as 10×10^{-15} W/cm^2 or 10 femtowatts/cm^2. This can also be expressed in decibels. Decibels always need a reference value; in this case, the maximum SPTA transmit intensity 100 mW/cm^2 will be used as

TABLE 7.5

ULTRASOUND INTENSITIES IN THE HUMAN BODY

■ APPLICATION	■ COMMENT	■ INTENSITIES	■ EFFECT IN TISSUE
Arterial cautery	Pressures > systolic blood pressure	>10,000,000 mW/cm^2	25 °C rise/s
Surgical	Neural ablation	>10,000 mW/cm^2	46 °C-54 °C in 20 min
Medical	Metabolic injury	1000 mW/cm^2	43 °C-44 °C in 60 min
Therapeutic	Tissue heating	1000 mW/cm^2	40 °C-45 °C in 10 min
Diagnostic	Transmitted	100 mW/cm^2	39 °C in 1 min
Diagnostic	Maximum echo	0.1 mW/cm^2	—
Diagnostic	Minimum echo	10^{-8} mW/cm^2	—
Thermography	Acoustic noise	0.4×10^{-10} mW/cm^2	—

a reference. Thermal noise is 10^{-13} times the reference, or 13 bels or 130 dB below the reference. The backscatter reflectivity of most tissue voxels is less than 0.1% (30 dB) of the incident ultrasound.

Backscatter for different tissue types is compared in the following example. If an ultrasound burst reaches a voxel of interest after passing through 6.5 half-value layers, the ultrasound is attenuated to 1% (0.01) of the original energy in the burst. If the voxel of interest contains liver or muscle cells, about 0.1% of the ultrasound will be reflected back to the transducer as backscatter. If the voxel contains the surface of a bone or a metal surgical clip, 100% (1.0) of the ultrasound will be returned as backscatter. If the voxel contains blood, 0.0001% (60 dB below bone) of the ultrasound will be returned to the transducer as backscatter. As the backscatter passes back along the ultrasound beam pattern to the transducer, it will pass back through 6.5 half-value layers, attenuating the backscattered echo to 1% of the backscattered energy. Reviewing the path of the ultrasound from the voxel of interest: Burst attenuation is 1% (0.01, or 20 dB), reflection from liver produces echo energy of 0.1% (0.001, or 30 dB), and backscatter attenuation is 1% (0.01, or 20 dB) for a total echo strength of (20 + 30 + 20) = 70 dB, compared with the echo that would be produced by a metal plate in contact with the transducer backscattering all of the incident ultrasound. Summarizing for different possible tissues in the voxel of interest, a bone surface echo is 40 dB down, liver is 70 dB down, and blood is 100 dB down.

For an acceptable ultrasound image, the strength of the backscattered echo must be about 100 times (20 dB) greater than the thermal noise. Therefore, if you want the moving speckles of blood in your image to appear brighter than the noise, you need a transmit intensity (100 + 20) = 120 dB greater than thermal noise or $(10^{-14}$ W/cm^2 × $10^{+12}) = 10^{-2}$ W/cm^2 = 10 mW/cm^2. If you use a lower transmit intensity, blood in the voxel of interest will look like noise on the image, and the Doppler spectral waveform will look like noise. If for this example the tissue between the ultrasound transducer is muscle, 6.5 HVLW is about 100 wavelengths (15 cm for 1-MHz ultrasound and 3 cm for 5-MHz ultrasound). If you want to see deeper with 5-MHz ultrasound, you must use a higher transmit intensity (power/area).

Reflection

Some tissue interfaces in the body are large and flat with great impedance changes, such as the diaphragm-pleura interface above the liver. Such interfaces act like mirrors, reflecting entire images into false locations. It is not unusual to see images of liver parenchyma that appear to be located above the diaphragm, where the lung is actually located. It is also easy to view a mirror image of the subclavian artery reflected in the pleura, appearing to be at a depth within the lung. Vascular walls can cause such reflections as well. However, these reflected images are usually displayed at a lower echo intensity than a direct image. Mirror images are more likely to appear in color Doppler imaging than in B-mode imaging because color Doppler is designed to show full brightness even if the signal is weak, whereas B-mode brightness decreases if the echo is weak.

Resolution

One goal in ultrasound B-mode imaging is to achieve the best depth (axial) resolution possible. To ensure that the depth resolution is as small as possible (able to resolve small structures), the shortest possible ultrasound transmit pulse is used (see Fig. 7.9). One factor in resolution is that the burst-echo ultrasound path is folded, so that tissue voxels spaced at 1-mm intervals in depth add 2 mm per voxel to the roundtrip ultrasound path length, and the roundtrip path length is measured by the ultrasound system to determine depth. The ultrasound burst length is the smallest possible resolution division of the roundtrip ultrasound path. Therefore, the voxel dimension along the beam path should be equal to half of the burst length. If the burst length is 2 cycles of ultrasound, then the voxel length should be equal to the wavelength of the ultrasound. *Resolution* is defined as the closest that two objects can be and still be recognized as separate. Therefore, resolution is the distance between the centers of two bright voxels that have a third, dim voxel between them. The middle low-echo voxel shows that the reflections are separate. Thus, the depth resolution is about equal to the burst length.

This is superior to the lateral resolution, which is about equal to the ultrasound beam pattern width. The beam pattern width is greater than the value of the wavelength times depth divided by aperture. Because depth is almost always greater than aperture, the lateral resolution is poorer than the depth resolution. In a typical case, the focal depth is 80 mm, and the transducer diameter (aperture) is 10 mm. The lateral resolution is greater than eight times the wavelength of the ultrasound. The result is that a small reflecting sphere in the image, which should appear as a bright dot, instead appears as a horizontal dash. If imaged with 5-MHz ultrasound, the dash will appear to be about 0.3 mm deep and 3 mm wide.

Sound Speed Errors

The exact time for an echo to return cannot be determined from the depth of the reflector alone; the time also depends on the speed of travel of the ultrasound in tissue:

$$\text{Time} = \text{roundtrip distance} / \text{speed} = 2 × \text{depth} / \text{speed}$$
$$= \text{cm} / \text{cm} / \text{s} = \text{s}$$

It is a common assumption that ultrasound travels at a speed of 1540 m/s in soft tissue (or 154,000 cm/s, or 1.54 mm/µs); however, the speed is quite variable (Table 7.6). Thus, if the ultrasound passed only through fat on the way to and from the reflector, the reflector would appear to be 6% deeper than the actual depth because the echo returned 6% later than expected because the speed of ultrasound through the fat is 6% slower than the value assumed. Therefore, the thickness of a layer of fat (speed = 145,000 cm/s) that appears to be 1 cm thick on the ultrasound image is actually 0.94 cm thick (1 × 145,000/154,000 = 0.94). If the overlying tissue were muscle, the reflector would appear to be 3% shallower than the actual depth. When using a biopsy probe, these sound speed errors can contribute to the uncertainty of the expected location of the probe.

TABLE 7.6

ULTRASOUND WAVE SPEED IN DIFFERENT TISSUES

■ TISSUE	■ ULTRASOUND SPEED (mm/ms)
Bone	3.50
Cartilage	1.67
Muscle	1.58
Blood	1.57
Liver	1.55
Fat	1.45

Refraction

A common problem in ultrasound imaging is refractive distortion. The pulse-echo ultrasound imaging process assumes that the ultrasound beam passes into tissue and returns from a straight line along which the transducer is pointed. However, because of the range of speeds of ultrasound propagation, the ultrasound beam may bend, causing structures to appear in the wrong lateral location. This does not affect the depth location. The effect is most obvious when it results in apparent duplication of an object. This has been reported in early pregnancy (25% of women appear to have twins in the 5th week of gestation) and in the appearance of double aortic valves. The duplicate pregnancy images are due to refraction in the rectus abdominis muscles, and the duplicated aortic valve images are due to refraction in the parasternal cartilage. Refraction also distorts all other lateral measurements, including fetal bone length and the measured cross-sectional widths of blood vessels.

Whenever ultrasound scan lines pass from a material with one ultrasound speed into another material with a different ultrasound speed (see Table 7.6), the chance of refractive distortion is present. If the ultrasound beam is perpendicular to the interface, no deflection occurs, but if the ultrasound beam approaches the interface at a grazing angle, angular deflections of more than 45 degrees can occur, causing lateral displacement of the images of all objects deeper than that refracting interface. The maximum refraction angle passing from one tissue to another and back (Table 7.7) can be computed from Snell's law of refraction, which can be found in almost any physics book.

In principle, length measurements due to sound speed errors can be removed by substituting the proper speed into the measurement for the "average" soft tissue ultrasound speed of 154,000 cm/s. In contrast, lateral measurements all have great uncertainty because of refractive bending of the ultrasound beams. The errors in lateral measurements cannot be removed or corrected because it is impossible to determine the refraction that has been introduced into the ultrasound beam by the tissue. Thus, lateral measurements and cross-sectional area measurements cannot be made with full confidence from ultrasound images.

Best Ultrasound Frequency for Doppler Evaluation of Blood Flow

The best choice of ultrasound frequency for imaging depends on a balance between obtaining the best lateral and depth resolution and obtaining signals from the deepest tissues of interest. High ultrasound frequencies allow superior lateral and depth resolution but are strongly attenuated by tissue, limiting the ability to penetrate to great depths. As a general rule, those tissues that scatter ultrasound more strongly also attenuate ultrasound more strongly. In decreasing order of scattering and attenuation, we have calcium, muscle, fat, blood, and urine. It is difficult to obtain ultrasound echoes from tissues located under calcium.

The selection of the best ultrasound frequency for Doppler measurements can be objectively determined. Red blood cells are 8 μm in diameter. Ultrasound waves are 300 μm long (5 MHz). When the reflectors scattering a wave (red blood cells) are much smaller than the wavelength, the scatterers are called *Rayleigh scatterers*. The relationship between the scattering of ultrasound by blood cells (which are smaller than the wavelength of ultrasound) and the ultrasound frequency is

$$R = B \times F^4$$

where R is the fraction of the ultrasound scattered back to the transducer by the red blood cells, B is the reflection coefficient, and F is the ultrasound frequency. The penetration of ultrasound in tissue is

$$P = 10^{-T \times F \times (\alpha/10)}$$

where P is the fraction of the ultrasound energy that is still present after traveling through tissue of thickness T with attenuation coefficient α. The attenuation coefficient is in dB/MHz/cm; it is divided by 10 to convert dB (decibels) to bels. The power returning to the transducer is the fraction of power arriving at the reflector (P) times the fraction of power scattered back toward the transducer (R) times the fraction of power returning from the reflector (P), or

$$P \times R \times P = 10^{-T \times F \times (\alpha/10)} \times B \times F^4 \times 10^{-T \times F \times (\alpha/10)}$$

Using calculus, the ultrasound frequency that will give the greatest Doppler echo strength can be determined by setting the derivative with respect to frequency to zero and solving for frequency. The result is the ultrasound frequency (F) that gives the strongest echo from blood when the blood is under an overlying tissue of thickness (T) and attenuation coefficient (α):

$$F = 2/T \times 1/(\alpha/10) \times 1/\ln(10)$$

The effect of different overlying tissues on an examination of a blood vessel is presented in Table 7.8.

Intravascular catheter Doppler systems may penetrate 1 mm to 1 cm of blood to obtain the necessary signals. Based on Table 7.8, an ultrasound frequency greater than 50 MHz will give the strongest Doppler signal from blood using an intravascular catheter. If instead the examination is performed through a 0.2-cm (2-mm) arterial wall with muscle fibers transverse to the ultrasound beam, 13-MHz ultrasound gives the strongest signal. Through 0.2 cm of skull with transcranial Doppler, the strongest Doppler signal is achieved at 2.2 MHz. Examination of a carotid artery through 2 cm of muscle and fat with a Doppler ultrasound frequency near 5 MHz gives the

TABLE 7.7

TABLE 7.7

MAXIMUM ANGLE OF REFRACTION (IN DEGREES) FOR SOUND PASSING FROM ONE TISSUE TO ANOTHER AND BACK

	■ CARTILAGE	■ MUSCLE	■ BLOOD	■ LIVER	■ FAT
Cartilage	0	37	39	43	59
Muscle	37	0	13	22	47
Blood	39	13	0	18	45
Liver	43	22	18	0	41
Fat	59	47	45	41	0

TABLE 7.8

ULTRASOUND FREQUENCY FOR THE STRONGEST DOPPLER SIGNAL FROM BLOOD IN VESSELS VIEWED THROUGH DIFFERENT TISSUES

| | | | OVERLYING TISSUE | | |
| | | | MUSCLE | | |
	■ BLOOD	■ FAT	■ LONGITUDINAL	■ TRANSVERSE	■ BONE
Attenuation (dB/cm/MHz)	0.18	0.63	1.2	3.3	20
DEPTH (cm)					
0.2	241 MHz	69 MHz	36 MHz	13 MHz	2.2 MHz
0.5	97 MHz	28 MHz	14 MHz	5 MHz	0.9 MHz
2	24 MHz	7 MHz	4 MHz	1.3 MHz	0.2 MHz
5	10 MHz	3 MHz	1.4 MHz	0.5 MHz	0.1 MHz
8	6 MHz	2 MHz	0.9 MHz	0.3 MHz	—
15	3 MHz	1 MHz	0.5 MHz	0.2 MHz	—

strongest signal. Examination of the aortic valve at a depth of 10 cm through 1 or 2 cm of muscle with fibers oriented transverse to the ultrasound beam requires 2- or 3-MHz ultrasound for the strongest signal. Examination of the renal arteries or fetal arteries at a depth of 10 cm under muscle and fat may require an ultrasound frequency of 1 MHz to achieve the strongest signal.

ULTRASOUND TRANSDUCERS AND SCANHEADS

PZT and PVDF

Ultrasound transducers are wafers of piezoelectric material that are coated on the top and bottom with an electrical conductor. The two materials commonly used for transducers are lead (Pb) zirconate (Z) titanate (Ti), which is a ceramic, abbreviated PZT, and polyvinylidene fluoride, which is a soft plastic, abbreviated PVDF. The two materials are similar in that they can have piezoelectric properties if polarized. *Piezoelectric* means that when a voltage is applied to the electrodes so that an electric field is present across the thickness, the transducer tends to expand (or if the polarity is reversed, the transducer tends to contract). This is the conversion of electrical energy to mechanical energy. Alternatively, if the transducer is squeezed or stretched in its thickness dimension, a voltage will appear between the electrodes. Conversion of electrical to mechanical energy is used to transmit ultrasound, and conversion of mechanical to electrical energy is used to receive ultrasound.

The two materials differ in several respects. PZT is a brittle ceramic with very high acoustic impedance. When in contact with the body, which has low impedance, most of the ultrasound energy generated in the transducer is reflected back into the transducer, "trapping" the energy and making the transducer "ring" at a single frequency determined by the transducer thickness. An acoustic matching layer is required between the transducer and the body to allow efficient transmission of the ultrasound between the transducer and the body. This layer has an impedance midway between PZT and the body, and a thickness of one-fourth of a wavelength. In contrast, PVDF is a soft plastic with ultrasound impedance near that of tissue. When placed in contact with tissue, the ultrasound energy flows between the body tissues and the PVDF without reflection. Therefore, the PVDF does not resonate at a single frequency, making it a broadband transducer.

Thickness and Frequency

For a transducer to produce a vibration with a long duration and a narrow frequency band, it must retain the energy for many cycles rather than transmitting the energy into tissue or into an absorbing material on the back of the transducer, called a *backing material*. It is therefore easy to make a narrowband transducer with PZT by not using either a matching layer to couple it with tissue or a backing material. Such a transducer is shown in Figure 7.15. Notice that the PZT transducer is most efficient at an ultrasound frequency at which the transducer thickness is equal to half a wavelength (in PZT). This is called the *fundamental frequency*. This frequency is a "natural" frequency of vibration because the impedance changes at the surfaces cause most of the ultrasound to reflect back into the transducer, trapping energy in the transducer for many cycles.

To create high-frequency ultrasound transducers, thin wafers of piezoelectric material are used; conversely, to create low-frequency ultrasound transducers, thick wafers of piezoelectric material are used. The thickness of the transducer is equal to half the wavelength of the ultrasound in the PZT material. A transducer that oscillates or rings at a single frequency is called a *narrowband transducer*. This relationship is also true for PVDF transducers, but because of the impedance similarity between tissue and PVDF, energy is not trapped in the PVDF; thus, it does not oscillate like PZT. Therefore, PVDF transducers are not narrowband, they are wideband. In ultrasound, a wideband transducer emits a short ultrasound burst if excited by a short electrical pulse.

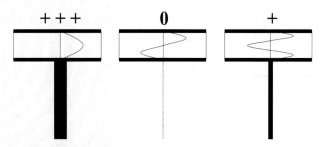

FIGURE 7.15. Sensitivity of ultrasound transducers. An ultrasound transducer is sensitive to odd harmonics of the fundamental frequency. Even harmonics (*center*) have a region of compression opposed by a region of decompression. The transducer has one-third of the voltage sensitivity to the third harmonic (*right*) as to the fundamental (*left*).

The transducer is not sensitive (able to receive ultrasound) when the wavelength is equal to the thickness (twice the fundamental frequency) because the compression voltage of the first (positive) half-cycle cancels the decompression voltage of the second (negative) half-cycle (see Fig. 7.15). At triple the fundamental frequency, the transducer is one-third as sensitive because the voltage generated by the first (positive) half-cycle of ultrasound is canceled by the second (negative) half-cycle, leaving only the third (positive) half-cycle to contribute to the voltage on the transducer not canceled. This is equally true for PZT and PVDF.

Single Element

From the earliest days of medical ultrasound in the 1950s to the advent of electronic switching in about 1985, pulse-echo ultrasound systems used a single transducer for both transmitting and receiving, whereas CW Doppler systems used one transducer for transmitting and one for receiving. Single-element transducers can both transmit and receive because the transmit process (requiring between 10 and 400 V to create enough ultrasound intensity) is separated from the receive process (which generates microvolts) by time. The transmit burst lasts less than 1 μs, and echoes are received for the following 100 μs (if the maximum depth of observation is 75 mm). It often takes a few microseconds for the transducer to settle down after transmitting to begin receiving well; this recovery period causes a blank zone in the shallowest few millimeters of the image.

Aperture Shapes

Each ultrasound beam pattern is determined by two design factors: (1) the ultrasound wavelength (determined by the ultrasound frequency and the tissue that conducts the ultrasound beam) and (2) the shape of the aperture or transducer forming the ultrasound beam. The shape of the ultrasound beam pattern is determined by diffraction of the beam through the aperture. Most ultrasound systems use transducer apertures that are circular or rectangular in shape.

Ultrasound Beam Patterns

The diameter or width of a diagnostic ultrasound transducer is always greater than several times the wavelength of ultrasound. When the echo from a point reflector located near the transducer face reaches the transducer face, some regions of the transducer face experience compression and others experience decompression (rarefaction) (Fig. 7.16). The echo from a point reflector located far from the transducer face intersects the transducer surface with only a single compression or rarefaction zone at a time. Reflectors that are near the transducer causing mixed compressions and rarefactions on the transducer face are in the Fresnel zone, or the near field; reflectors that are far from the transducer causing nearly uniform compression or expansion of the transducer are in the Fraunhofer zone, or far field. There is a difference between the image speckle seen in the Fresnel zone and that seen in the Fraunhofer zone. Speckle in the Fresnel zone has a fine structure in both the depth direction and the lateral direction; speckle in the Fraunhofer zone has a fine structure in the depth direction but a coarse structure in the lateral direction, making the speckles look like transverse dashes.

An echo from the near field compresses a part of the transducer and expands another part. Therefore, the resultant voltage, which is some average of the positive and negative effects, is less than it would be had the transducer been expanded or compressed together because the negative portions "subtract" from the positive portions. At some positions, the net effect of an echo will be positive, and nearby, the net effect will be negative. A transition from a net positive voltage to a net negative voltage can occur if the reflector is moved a distance of one-fourth of a wavelength. Either a net positive voltage or a net negative voltage is displayed as a white spot at a picture element (or *pixel*) on the ultrasound image corresponding to the location of the reflector causing the voltage. If the magnitude is great (either positive or negative), the white

FIGURE 7.16. Near and far field of an ultrasound transducer. The Fresnel zone is separated from the Fraunhofer zone by the transition zone, which is the closest distance that the transducer can come to a point source and be subjected only to compression or decompression (*top group*). For a concave focused transducer (*bottom group*), at the best focus of the transducer, there are times when the entire transducer face is exposed to maximum compression or decompression; this never happens to a flat transducer. The concentric rings show the expansion of spherical waves from a point origin; not shown is the decrease in intensity and pressure amplitude with distance from the central origin.

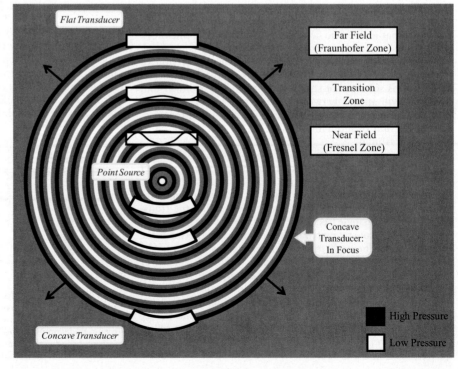

pixel will be bright; if the magnitude is small (either positive or negative), the pixel will be dim. Only if the voltage is zero will the spot be black. Thus, one reflector in tissue may cause a bright pixel on the screen, and a similar reflector, located one-fourth of a wavelength away, may cause a dark pixel on the screen. This process produces *speckle* on the ultrasound image. Speckle is not tissue texture, and it cannot be used for identification of tissue type. The combination of positive and negative waves that cancel each other, providing a zero result, is called *destructive interference*; the combination of positive and positive waves or negative and negative waves to create a larger result is called *constructive interference*.

In contrast, an echo from a reflector in the far field serves to compress all points on the transducer surface in unison, causing improved sensitivity. Of course, the reflectors in the far field are so far away that the echoes are weak both because of attenuation and because the reflected ultrasound is spreading as it returns from the reflector.

At the boundary of the near and far fields, there is a natural region of greatest ultrasound intensity and greatest transducer sensitivity. This zone is about half the width of a flat transducer, representing the natural focal zone of a flat transducer. This boundary between the Fresnel zone (near field) and the Fraunhofer zone (far field) is called the *transition zone*. The smooth central lobe of the beam pattern in the Fraunhofer zone differs markedly from the variable pattern in the Fresnel zone (see Fig. 7.11). The transition zone can be moved to a greater depth by increasing the width of the transducer. The transducer may be focused by making the transducer concave (or by placing a converging lens in the ultrasound beam path), which pulls the transition zone and far field closer to the transducer, thereby reducing the beam width at the focus.

Diffraction and Side Lobes

Every transducer generates side lobes because of wave diffraction. A flat disk sends most of the ultrasound energy along the central axis of the beam pattern. This axis is called the *central lobe* or *main lobe* of the beam pattern. The direction of the central lobe is not dependent on wavelength (or frequency).

In addition to the central lobe, wavelength-dependent portions of the beam pattern are formed by diffraction effects (Fig. 7.17). These *side lobes* are formed by constructive interference of ultrasound waves at acute angles to the transducer face. By what is known as the *principle of reciprocity*, the transducer beam pattern is the same for both transmit and receive. Therefore, the transducer not only transmits power in the direction of the side lobes but is also sensitive to echoes returning at the angles of the side lobes.

Focusing

Fixed Mechanical Focus

If the transducer is concave, a reflector at the center of curvature, equidistant from all points on the transducer surface, experiences compression or rarefaction from the entire transducer surface at once. The transducer, in turn, receives only compression or rarefaction on its entire surface at a given time from a reflector at that point (see Fig. 7.16). This is the *focal zone* of the transducer. To focus effectively, the focal zone must be within the Fresnel zone of an equivalent unfocused (planar) transducer.

Electronic Focus: Annular Array

A transducer with a concave shape or a converging lens has a well-defined, fixed mechanical focus; to change the focus to a different depth requires constructing a new transducer. A transducer can be divided into elements (segments) that can be electronically controlled so that all points on the transducer face no longer need to operate in unison. By operating the elements near the edge about a hundred nanoseconds early and the elements near the center a hundred nanoseconds later, the focal zone can be brought nearer to the transducer face.

One way to divide the transducer into elements is to form a series of concentric rings called an *annular array*. This transducer can be focused electronically, but the beam must be steered (pointed) electronically. The advantage of electronic focusing is flexibility. The focus can be changed in milliseconds

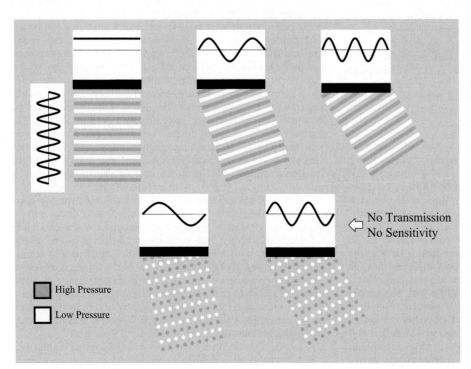

FIGURE 7.17. Side lobes from a flat transducer. The main lobe of the ultrasound beam pattern from a flat transducer is along the axis of the transducer (*upper left*). For beam angles in which 3/2 cycles (*upper center*) or 5/2 cycles (*upper right*) intersect the transducer face, the transducer is also sensitive. Between the side lobes are nulls in which the area of the transducer face under compression always equals the area of decompression as a wave travels from that angle toward the transducer (*bottom*). By the principle of reciprocity, the receive beam pattern sensitivity and the transmit beam pattern intensity are identical.

No Transmission
No Sensitivity

High Pressure

Low Pressure

by the ultrasound system. This allows the system to be focused at 3 cm deep 40 μs after pulse transmission when echoes from 3 cm are returning and to be focused at 6 cm deep 80 μs after pulse transmission when echoes from 6 cm are returning.

Electronic Focus: Linear Array

Another type of segmented transducer array used for electronic focusing is the *linear array*, which has rectangular elements arranged in rows. Linear *sequential* arrays and linear *phased* arrays are the extremes of a continuum of arrays. All consist of a straight row of rectangular transducers. Often, the array includes 64 or 128 transducers. The simplest sequential arrays use one transducer at a time to create an ultrasound pulse and receive the echoes from that pulse; phased arrays use all elements in the array to create each pulse and to receive the echoes from that pulse. Between those extremes, an array might use 16 elements at a time to transmit and receive, moving to a new group for the next pulse echo. The group of 16 elements is called an *aperture*. Individual transducers in the array are called *elements*.

In these arrays, *mechanical* focusing (usually by an acoustic lens) is used in the "thickness" or "elevation" direction perpendicular to the line of transducers, and *electronic* focusing is used in the direction parallel to the line of the transducers. Transmit focusing from an aperture of the array requires forming a concave wavefront, which converges on the focal zone. This is achieved by transmitting first from the elements at the edges of the aperture, then successively from elements closer to the center of the aperture. The time between the transmissions from successive elements is the time required for the ultrasound to travel a fraction of a wavelength from the prior element. For 5-MHz ultrasound, each ultrasound cycle takes 200 ns, so the time delay is a fraction of that, ranging from 0 to 40 ns, depending on the distance to the focal point. Time delays are also applied on receive to compensate for the differences in arrival time across the array.

Transmit Focusing

Because an ultrasound pulse is transmitted once for all depths along a particular ultrasound scan line, only one focal depth can be selected for transmission. That focal depth is operator selectable and is usually marked on the side of the ultrasound image. Some ultrasound instruments with electronic focusing allow multiple transmit focuses. In those cases, a separate pulse-echo cycle is used for each transmit depth. Multiple transmit depths are indicated by multiple marks on the side of the ultrasound image. Because of the extra transmit pulses required, the frame rate decreases as focal zones are added.

Receive Focusing

In contrast to transmit focusing, which allows only one focal depth per pulse-echo cycle, in receive mode, there is ample time to adjust the electronic focus during the time intervals between depths. In a pulse-echo cycle, transmission typically lasts for 0.5 μs (2.5 cycles of 5-MHz ultrasound), whereas receive lasts between 40 and 200 μs (13 μs for each centimeter of depth). During the receive period, echoes consisting of curved wavefronts coming from a focal region arrive first at the center of the aperture and a few nanoseconds later at the margins of the aperture. Those echoes can be aligned in time by electronically delaying the echoes arriving at the central transducers by enough nanoseconds to align with the echoes arriving at the elements near the aperture margins. During a typical receive period, every additional 13 μs after the transmit pulse (corresponding to echoes coming from an additional centimeter in depth), the electronic delays for the elements in the aperture are adjusted to focus at the corresponding depth.

If the ultrasound image spans depths from 0 to 8 cm, the receive focus will be adjusted eight times during the receive period. This is called *dynamic focus*. In instruments which use this method, dynamic receive focus is always active. Dynamic focus improves lateral resolution at all depths.

Because focusing at deeper depths requires larger apertures, transducer elements will often be added to the aperture during the later portion of the 200-μs receive period. This is called *dynamic aperture*.

Beam Direction

Mechanical Beam Steering

If the diameter of an ultrasound transducer is much greater than the wavelength of the ultrasound, the ultrasound beam will be directed into tissue in a direction perpendicular to the face of the transducer. By tilting an ultrasound transducer so that its axis points in the desired direction, a particular line of tissue can be examined. Before 1975, most beam pointing was done by hand. The sonographer would manually "scan" the ultrasound beam across a plane in tissue to form an image. However, around 1975, real-time 2D mechanical scanners were introduced, with the transducer driven by a motor to tilt the transducer in a sequence of directions to automatically form a real-time sector scan. Typically, an automatic scan takes 50 ms to complete. Therefore, a 2D image can be formed at 20 images/s.

Within a mechanically steered scanhead, the transducer is often mounted on a hinge pin and motor-driven to tilt to the left and right to create a sector (fan-shaped) scan. An alternative to angular oscillations is to mount transducers on a rotating wheel. A scan of parallel beams (rectangular scan) can also be formed mechanically. Rather than tilting the transducer, the transducer is translated across the entire width of the field of view.

Linear Sequential Arrays

Mechanical systems that scan by moving a transducer from location to location or angle to angle are limited by inertia. To work well, the ultrasound beam pattern (scan line) must move from one location to another in a few microseconds and must be stable at the new location during the period of the pulse-echo cycle. An alternative is to use one transducer (or group of transducers) for every ultrasound scan line in the image and electronically turn on the appropriate transducer when needed. This allows rapid switching from one scan line to the next. Arrays that scan by switching between array elements are known as *linear sequential arrays*; they are commonly referred to simply as *linear arrays*. There is no physical limit to how quickly the electronic switching can be done or how far the previous line is from the next. In today's world, electronic reliability is much greater than mechanical reliability; thus, the elimination of mechanical parts reduces the chance of future equipment failure. However, the cost of electronic systems is often greater than that of mechanical systems.

The original linear arrays used a single element for each line in an image; these are known as *low-density* linear arrays. A rectangular scan is obtained by placing a series of identical transducers in a line with the transducers aimed along parallel lines. This linear array scanhead must have a length equal to the width of the field of view of the image. To control each ultrasound beam, the width of each transducer must be much greater than the wavelength of the ultrasound. Thus, for 5-MHz ultrasound with a wavelength of 0.03 cm, the width of each transducer must be at least 0.15 cm; to form an image with 50 scan lines requires a scanhead 7.5 cm wide.

Low-density linear arrays have limited lateral resolution. *Lateral resolution* is defined as the ability to see two objects closely spaced side by side in the image as separate objects. To achieve this, three ultrasound scan lines are required. In addition to two scan lines, one providing reflections from each of the two objects, a third ultrasound beam must pass between the objects without reflections to show the space between. Thus, with transducers spaced at 0.15 cm, the pair of objects must be separated by at least 0.3 cm to have one transducer receive a reflection from one, a second transducer pass an unreflected beam between them, and a third transducer receive a reflection from the other. In addition, the ultrasound beam pattern of the middle scan line must be narrow enough to pass between the two objects without reflection. To make the focal region of a beam pattern narrow requires a large aperture. This aperture is often 10 times as wide as the focal region. However, to image at the focal depth, the spacing between the beam patterns should be equal to the focal width. This requires overlapping the apertures for adjacent lines.

Newer linear array scanheads are *high-density* linear arrays, with the transducer divided into segments about 0.05 cm wide. These small apertures are too narrow to be able to point the ultrasound beam pattern to form a narrow focal zone. To transmit and receive ultrasound along a single scan line, five or more elements are operated together, giving an effective aperture width of 0.25 cm and a narrowest beam (transition zone) at a depth of 0.5 cm while allowing the adjacent ultrasound lines to be spaced at 0.05 cm. If a larger group is selected, say 10 together, the transition zone occurs at a depth of 2 cm, near the depth of the carotid artery. If delays are applied to the transducer elements in the aperture to focus the ultrasound beam in the near field, a narrow focus can be formed to improve the lateral resolution at depths near the focal region. A wide effective transducer aperture is required to achieve good focusing. The use of overlapping groups of transducer segments allows closely spaced scan lines and wide transducer apertures, which produce good ultrasound beam control and narrow focal zones.

Curvilinear Arrays

A variation of the standard linear array places the transducers on a curved surface, convex to the ultrasound field. This is known as a curved linear array or *curvilinear array*. As adjacent groups of transducers are used, the beams not only originate from adjacent locations but also point in diverging directions, creating a sector scan rather than a rectangular scan.

Phased Arrays

Just as electronic methods can be used to focus the ultrasound beam from multiple transducer elements, electronic methods can also be used to tilt the ultrasound beam originating from a group of transducer elements. Electronic beam steering uses a segmented transducer with the segments aligned in a row as in a linear sequential array. However, unlike a linear sequential array, each segment is much thinner than the wavelength of sound; when operated together, the 32, 64, or 128 segments form an aperture much wider than the wavelength of sound. This is known as a *linear phased array* or more simply a *phased array*.

In a linear sequential array, ultrasound is transmitted from an aperture consisting of a part of the array; the echoes from all depths are received over a period of 100 µs by the elements in the aperture. A new pulse is then transmitted from a new aperture. This sequentially moves the scan line in the lateral direction and creates a rectangular image. In a phased array scanhead, the aperture always includes all of the transducers in the array. Each ultrasound scan line is formed by transmitting the beam pattern at a different angle from the same aperture. The angle of the transmitted beam pattern is selected by applying a slight time delay (nanoseconds) to each element in the array during the formation of the transmit burst. By applying similar delays to the echoes received by each element, the received beam pattern angle can also be selected to align with the transmitted pattern. The combination of all angles creates a sector image.

Suppose that a 5-MHz (0.03-cm wavelength) phased array scanhead has 128 segments, each 0.01 cm wide; the group is 1.28 cm wide. Transmitting from each segment in turn, starting with transducer element #1 and ending with #128, waiting just 0.01 µs between transmissions would take 1.28 µs to complete the transmission. The ultrasound transmitted from transducer element #1 has traveled 0.197 cm (over six wavelengths) in that time (0.128 µs × 0.154 cm/µs). The result is to tilt the ultrasound beam toward the direction of element #128. The angle of tilt, θ, can be determined by trigonometry with $\mathrm{Sin}\,\theta = 0.197\,\mathrm{cm}/1.28\,\mathrm{cm}$, so $\theta = 9$ degrees.

On receive, the echoes coming from an angle of 9 degrees tilted toward element #128 reach element #128 first. It will take 1.28 µs for the echo wavefront to sweep from element #128 to element #1. If the receiving system is coordinated with the expected sweep of echoes from an angle of 9 degrees, echoes from that angle will be selectively enhanced; other echoes from other angles that do not progressively sweep across the elements at a rate of 0.01 µs/element will be suppressed. Thus, by properly timing the transmission, the outgoing ultrasound beam is directed at a specified angle. Also, by properly adjusting the incoming ultrasound for its timing (phase), the echoes from the chosen angle can be detected while ultrasound noise coming from all other angles is rejected.

One of the problems with a phased array system is that some of the ultrasound always propagates into tissue in the wrong direction. Some ultrasound goes straight into the tissue without being tilted; other parts of the ultrasound enter in selected directions depending on the ultrasound wavelength and the spacing of the transducers. These unwanted (grating lobe) beams create "ghost" images of tissue structures that are displayed in the wrong location in the image. One way to control this problem is to use an array with more segments that are more closely spaced. Manufacturers have moved from 16 to 32 to 64 to 128 elements to improve beam steering and to suppress grating lobe artifacts. Each element requires a set of wires, a transmitter, and a receiver. This group (transmitter, wire, transducer, receiver) is called a *channel*. The more channels, the better control over beam steering and the higher the complexity and cost.

Combined Sequential and Phased Arrays

Most linear arrays now combine sequencing and phasing to direct the ultrasound beam. When the full aperture of an array is not needed for steering, the aperture origin of the ultrasound beam can be translated from location to location along the array and the beam can be steered from that aperture to the available range of angles (Fig. 7.18). This allows flexibility in adjusting both the beam origin and its angle. Combined sequencing and phasing allows such features as the creation of a trapezoidal or parallelogram image format, real-time compound imaging, and steering of the color box in color Doppler imaging.

Multidimensional Arrays

1.5-Dimensional Arrays

Some of the literature on evaluating vascular B-mode images suggests that the image is a tomogram providing a thin section that if passed through the vessel in a longitudinal plane would

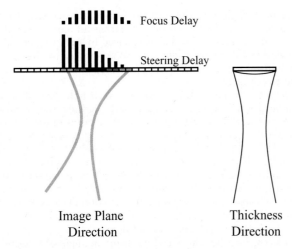

FIGURE 7.18. Linear array transducer with sequencing and phasing. This linear array has 28 elements. The length of each element in the lateral image direction is half a wavelength, the length of the entire array is 14 wavelengths, and the width of the active 10-element aperture is 5 wavelengths. The width of the elements in the image thickness direction is 4 wavelengths. Electronic delay of the cycles in the transmit and receive paths on the left side of the aperture steer the ultrasound beam to the left. Additional delays shift the focal zone close to the transducer array. In the image thickness direction, the fixed aperture and a lens provide a fixed focus in the thickness direction.

show only the superficial and deep portions of the vessel wall. Between the lines representing the wall, only intraluminal material would appear (Fig. 7.19, *left*). The ultrasound beam, however, has considerable thickness in the direction perpendicular to the image plane. The effect of this thickness can be seen when there is an extraluminal calcified region present in the lateral arterial wall. This calcium is a good reflector of ultrasound and lies at a depth between the superficial and the deep walls of the vessel in the image. The reflections from this extraluminal calcium structure will be excluded from a thin image, but included in a thick image at a location between

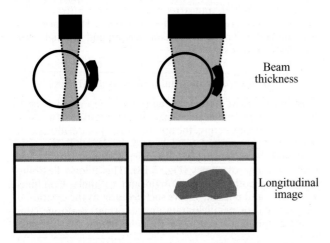

FIGURE 7.19. Effect of image thickness on the ultrasound image. A thin image plane (*top left*) images the superficial and deep arterial walls and the lumen between (*bottom left*). An image of the same vessel using a scanhead with a thick image plane (*top right*) includes objects that are located in the lateral vessel walls (*bottom right*). The focus in the beam thickness direction can vary from 2 mm to greater than 1 cm. Therefore, objects that are on the lateral vessel walls may appear to be in the vessel lumen. Cross-sectional views may help to identify those structures that are not within the lumen.

the deep and the superficial wall (see Fig. 7.19, *right*). Thus, a thick image plane can show tissue pathology as intraluminal echoes when they are in fact from extraluminal sources.

Thin image planes are generated by mechanical sector scanheads that have circular transducers. This is because the lateral focus and the thickness focus are identical for circular transducers. Fixed focused circular transducers generate thin images at the focal depth but thicker images both shallow and deep to the focus. Circular annular arrays generate the thinnest image planes because electronic focusing can be applied over a range of depths. Thick image planes are generated by both linear array and phased array scanheads. Lateral resolution and image plane thickness are completely independent of each other in linear and phased array scanheads because of the asymmetric (rectangular) apertures used.

To reduce the slice thickness of the ultrasound image, focusing must be applied in the slice thickness direction. With standard linear and phased arrays, a fixed lens is used to focus the slice thickness at one depth. In order to allow dynamic receive focus and selectable transmit focus in the thickness direction, the transducer array must be divided in the thickness direction in addition to the divisions in the lateral direction. Because steering is not done in the thickness direction, only five or seven elements are required in that direction. This is known as a rectangular array or a *1.5-dimensional array*.

For a 1.5D array, the electronic focusing is symmetric in the thickness direction (about the center image plane). Therefore, if five elements are present, only three wires are needed: the corresponding elements on opposite sides from the center are connected together. An array with 128 elements in the lateral direction and three channels (five elements) in the thickness direction requires 3×128, or 384, channels.

2D Arrays

Manufacturers are now producing three-dimensional (3D) real-time imaging systems that are able to sweep an ultrasound beam in any direction from a 2D phased array transducer. A square array divided into 32 elements in one direction and 32 elements in the other direction yields 1024 possible channels in all. The ultrasound beam sweeps out a pyramidal volume in the tissue. Computer methods can be used to display the volume data in a number of formats, including surface rendering as solids, transparent views through the tissues, and 2D slices in three perpendicular directions (orthogonal slices). The main current application of 2D arrays is in cardiac imaging, for which there is interest in acquiring 3D ultrasound images at high volume rates. A volume rate is similar to a frame rate, except it is 3D rather than 2D.

ECHO DEMODULATION AND IMAGING

All pulse-echo ultrasound instruments from a simple A-mode system to a 2D color-flow system are based on the same building blocks: a system clock, a timer that sets the pulse repetition interval (PRI) and, therefore, the pulse repetition frequency (PRF = 1/PRI) given a maximum depth, a transmit-receive switch, a transducer in contact with the patient, a time-gain compensation (TGC) system to adjust the signal amplitude to compensate for attenuation, and a demodulator-display system to provide the diagnostic information. CW Doppler systems differ from this in that they have no timer, transmit-receive switch, or TGC system and have two transducers rather than one.

Pulse-echo systems differ in (1) how the ultrasound beam is moved across the body during an examination, (2) how the echoes are demodulated (amplitude or phase), and (3) how the results are assembled for display. *Demodulation* extracts the information of interest for a particular examination mode from the returned ultrasound echoes. After demodulation, commonly displayed data include the echogenicity of structures at different locations under the transducer, the motions of tissue over time during the cardiac cycle, and the speed of blood during the cardiac and respiratory cycle. The extracted information is generally formatted as a 2D image showing the depth and lateral dimension of anatomy (2D B-mode), reflector depth versus time (M-mode), or velocity versus time (spectral waveform). Quantitative dimensional and temporal measurements can be made from these displays. Lengths and areas can be measured from 2D B-mode and M-mode, displacement over time can be measured from M-mode, and velocity changes can be measured from spectral waveforms. Color can be added to 2D images to show blood velocity with anatomy (color flow).

2D B-Mode

To create an amplitude-demodulated B-mode (brightness mode) image, a short pulse of ultrasound is transmitted into tissue. Echoes that return after 26.8 μs from a depth of 2 cm are amplified a small amount by the TGC system to compensate for the effects of ultrasound attenuation by 2 cm of tissue to and from the depth of the echo source. Echoes that return after 67 μs from a depth of 5 cm are amplified more by the TGC to compensate for the attenuation of the greater thickness of tissue traversed to obtain the echo. The amplified echo, in the form of an electrical oscillation, is then amplitude demodulated by inverting the negative excursions and sending the result into a filter that selects the peaks for measurement of the amplitude.

The signal amplitudes are determined by the echogenicities of the corresponding tissues represented in the image. If attenuation has been properly compensated by the TGC, the image brightness corresponds to tissue type. The weakest echoes in the image are caused by clear fluid, the next brightest by blood; stronger echoes are generated by fat and muscle and organ parenchyma; the strongest echoes are caused by bone, metal clips, and other "hard" structures. The difference in echogenicity between blood and bone is 60 dB for 5-MHz ultrasound. This is the same as saying that calcium reflects 1 million times more ultrasound energy than blood.

Doppler Methods

In pulse-echo imaging, the brightness of each point on the 2D B-mode image screen is associated with the strength or amplitude of the echo returning from the corresponding depth in the direction that the ultrasound beam is pointed. Doppler data, corresponding to the speed of blood flowing through the tissue, use phase information (rather than amplitude information) in the echo (see Fig. 7.3). Although the amplitude information obtained from a single pulse is sufficient to determine the echogenicity of the tissue (ability to generate a strong echo), the phase from a single pulse is not sufficient to determine the speed of moving blood. To determine the speed of the tissue, a series of pulse-echo cycles is required along the same ultrasound beam. The change in phase from pulse to pulse corresponds to the change in distance from the reflector to the transducer; a change in phase of one-fourth of an ultrasound wave represents a motion of one-eighth of the wavelength of ultrasound in tissue.

If a new pulse of 5-MHz ultrasound is sent into the patient's body every 500 μs and if, during the interval between the pulses, the phase shifts by one-fourth of a wave (corresponding to motion of the blood toward the transducer of 0.0393 mm), the speed at which the blood approaches the transducer can be computed:

$$\text{Speed of approach} = 0.00393\,\text{cm}/0.0005\,\text{s} = 7.85\,\text{cm/s}$$

Phase changes that are much smaller or larger can also be measured. The maximum practical measurable phase change is half a wave (180 degrees). Larger changes cause aliasing, an ambiguity in the velocity measurement. The smallest practical measurable phase change is less than 1 degree (0.006 waves). Using 5-MHz ultrasound with a wavelength near 320 μm, the maximum phase change is equivalent to a motion of tissue of 80 μm, and the smallest measurable phase change is equivalent to a motion of 0.04 μm, which is about the size of a large molecule.

The phase change between pulses (measured in waves) divided by the time between pulses is called the *Doppler frequency*:

$$\text{Doppler frequency} = \text{phase change between pulses/time difference between pulses} = \text{hertz}$$

The time between pulses is usually so short that the phase change is less than half of a wave or a cycle. A typical time between ultrasound pulses is 100 μs (0.1 ms). Using the numbers just given for tissue motion, the maximum measurable speed is (80 μm/100 μs), or 0.8 m/s; the smallest is (0.04 μm/100 μs), or 0.0004 m/s. This is the same as 80 cm/s for the maximum and 0.04 cm/s for the minimum speed detectable.

The expression given earlier for Doppler frequency (f) is a form of the Doppler equation. The rate of phase change between pulses is equal to twice the speed at which the reflector approaches the ultrasound transducer (S) divided by the wavelength of sound (λ).

$$f = 2 \times S/\lambda = \text{Hz} = \text{cycles/s} = \text{cm/s/cm/cycles}$$

Unfortunately, the Doppler equation is rarely written like this. There seems to be a preference to compute the wavelength (λ) from the speed of ultrasound in tissue (C) and the ultrasound frequency (F):

$$\lambda = C/F = \text{cm/cycle} = \text{cm/s/cycles/s}$$

Substituting the wavelength into the Doppler equation yields

$$f = 2 \times S \times F/C$$

To continue beyond this requires knowing the angle of the velocity vector representing the blood flow. If the angle θ between the blood flow velocity and the ultrasound beam is known (Fig. 7.20), the following expression:

$$\cos\theta = \text{length of adjacent side/length of hypotenuse} = S/V$$

yields the conventional Doppler equation:

$$f = 2 \times F \times V \times \cos\theta/C$$

which can be inverted to yield velocity, as follows:

$$V = f \times C/F \times 2 \times \cos\theta$$

Testing the Doppler Equation

Although the substitution of ultrasound speed divided by frequency for wavelength is harmless, the substitution of $(V \times \cos\theta)$ for the speed of approach (S) introduces an unfortunate variability in the Doppler results. The final version of the Doppler

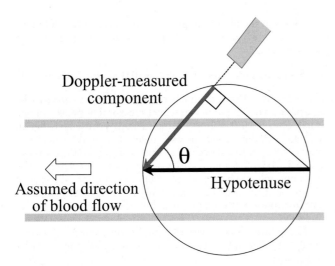

FIGURE 7.20. Doppler examination angle. The Doppler equation is written to describe the right triangle that is formed from the blood velocity vector and the ultrasound beam. The blood velocity is the hypotenuse of the right triangle. A right triangle can be fitted into a circle with the hypotenuse as the diameter.

equation suggests that the blood velocity magnitude (blood speed) can be determined if the Doppler angle is known. Blood speed would be useful for computing volume flow rates and pressure differences. Examiners often substitute into this equation the angle between the axis of the blood vessel and the Doppler ultrasound beam measured on the ultrasound B-mode image during duplex scanning. All manufacturers recommend this method. Over a wide range of angles, this method should yield a single value of peak systolic velocity for a blood vessel.

A simple attempt to validate this relationship in the common carotid artery yielded higher values of angle-adjusted velocity at an examination angle of 50 degrees than at an angle of 44 degrees (Fig. 7.21); the values measured at 60 degrees were even higher. Thus, for the same blood flow in the same vessel, changing the Doppler examination angle causes a change in the value of the velocity measurement. This angle-dependent variability occurs in most arteries and veins. It does not depend on instrument manufacturer or the type of transducer.

The reason for this problem does not rest in ultrasound physics. The problem lies with an incorrect assumption about the nature of blood flow. When blood or any fluid flows (1) at a constant rate (2) along a straight pipe (3) over long distances, the flow finally settles to a parabolic profile, with all velocity vectors parallel to the tube axis. However, blood flow in arteries is (1) pulsatile, not constant, (2) often through curved vessels, and (3) divided in short segments and, therefore, does not flow along velocity vectors parallel to the vessel axis. In general, normal blood flow is helical and converges into stenoses. Setting a Doppler cursor parallel to the vessel axis does not mean that the cursor is parallel to the velocity vectors. Although the component of velocity parallel to the vessel axis is needed to compute the volume flow along the vessel, the magnitude of the velocity vector in the helical direction is needed to compute the kinetic energy if the Bernoulli equation is to be used. Thus, the meaning of velocity is obscure.

The effect of Doppler angle-dependent variability can be demonstrated by measuring the angle-adjusted velocity at a series of angles in two different arteries: the common carotid artery and the distal superficial femoral artery (Table 7.9). The common carotid artery is short and curved proximal to the location of measurement; the distal superficial femoral artery is long and straight proximal to the location of measurement. Table 7.9 demonstrates a nearly constant angle-adjusted velocity in the distal superficial femoral artery, indicating

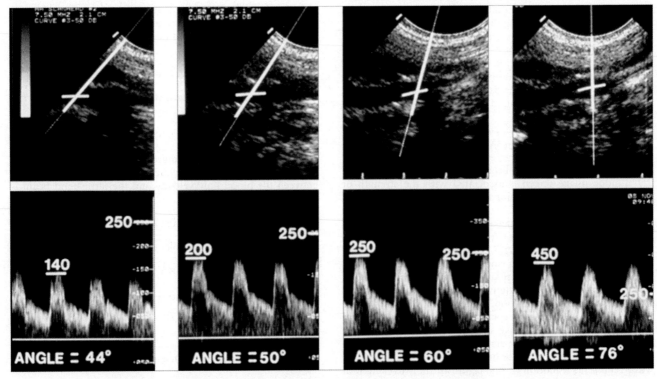

FIGURE 7.21. Angle-adjusted blood velocity in the common carotid artery. A test of the Doppler equation in the carotid artery at different angles shows that the computed velocity is not independent of the Doppler examination angle. Instead, the computed velocity is higher if the Doppler examination angle is closer to 90 degrees.

TABLE 7.9

MEASURED DOPPLER FREQUENCY AND ANGLE-ADJUSTED VELOCITY IN CAROTID AND FEMORAL ARTERIES

DOPPLER EXAMINATION ANGLE (DEGREES)	COMMON CAROTID ARTERY		DISTAL SUPERFICIAL FEMORAL ARTERY	
	DOPPLER FREQUENCY (kHz)	VELOCITY (cm/s)	DOPPLER FREQUENCY (kHz)	VELOCITY (cm/s)
40	4.732	97	3.561	73
50	4.299	105	2.906	71
60	3.726	117	2.292	72
70	3.180	146	1.524	70

velocities parallel to the vessel axis, but a progressive increase of measured velocity values at angles closer to 90 degrees in carotid arteries.

Because of this systematic progression of angle-adjusted velocity values with increasing Doppler examination angle, a consistent Doppler examination angle should be used in every examination to minimize this source of variability. In addition, the examination angle should always be entered into data reports along with each measured Doppler frequency or velocity. In a long, straight vessel, far from a bifurcation, the effect does not occur; thus, in those cases, the conventional use of angle-adjusted velocities may be appropriate.

Aliasing

The phase changes between ultrasound pulses are used to determine the Doppler frequency. Phase changes that exceed one-half of a wave between pulses cause confusion because a phase change increase of five-eighths of a wave is identical

to a phase change decrease of three-eighths of a wave ($^5/_8 - 1 = -^3/_8$). If the phase change between pulses in the positive or negative direction is greater than one-half of a wave, the smallest possible change is assumed to be correct in the absence of other evidence (Figs. 7.22 and 7.23). This error in direction and magnitude of the frequency shift measurement is called *aliasing*. Aliasing can often be prevented by keeping the time between pulses short. If the data are being taken from great depths, the instrument must wait a long time after transmitting a pulse for the echo to return before transmitting a new pulse; therefore, the time between pulses may be long enough to introduce aliasing. The aliasing frequency (Nyquist frequency) is determined by the maximum depth of Doppler analysis (Table 7.10).

In most Doppler systems, the PRF and the Nyquist limit are lower than those listed in Table 7.10 to ensure that there is adequate time between the echoes from the deepest depths and the next transmit pulse. If the speed of the blood is sufficient to produce Doppler signals of a higher frequency than the Nyquist limit, the frequency detected and displayed by a

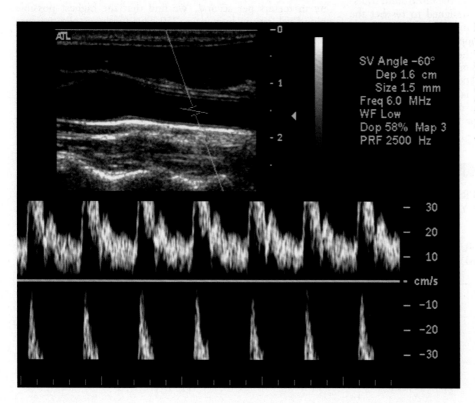

FIGURE 7.22. Aliasing of the arterial velocity waveform. This carotid arterial waveform shows peak systole disconnected from the onset of systole. This "aliased" peak systolic velocity display occurs because the Doppler pulse repetition frequency (PRF) sample rate was lower than half of the peak systolic Doppler frequency shift (Nyquist limit).

PRINCIPLES AND INSTRUMENTATION

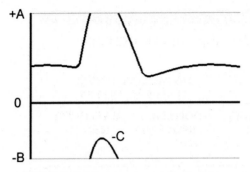

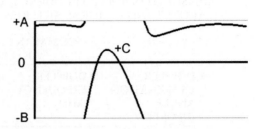

FIGURE 7.23. Computation of the peak frequency or velocity during aliasing. When the spectral waveform is aliased, the peak frequency (PF) can be calculated as PF = A − B + C. *On the left*, note that A is positive and B and C are negative. *On the right*, note that A and C are positive and B is negative.

pulsed Doppler on a spectral waveform is in the wrong direction and of the wrong frequency. Thus, whenever possible, the highest PRF should be used.

CW Doppler

Doppler systems are often divided into *CW* systems and *pulsed* systems. It is useful to think of the CW Doppler and the pulsed Doppler as the extremes of a range of choices. All Doppler systems measure the speed of blood along the axis of the ultrasound beam, and all Doppler systems can be used to measure the peak component of the velocity vector along the ultrasound beam axis. The differences between pulsed and CW Doppler are the size of the active sample volume and the range of Doppler frequency shifts that can be measured without ambiguity.

Pulsed Doppler systems usually use a single ultrasound transducer for both transmitting and receiving. In a CW system, the transmitting transducer is always in use, so a second receiving transducer adjacent to the transmitting transducer is required. The width of the active Doppler sample volume is determined by the focal characteristics of the ultrasound transducer. The ultrasound transducer is designed to restrict the insonated region to a pencil-sized beam. The two transducers (transmitter and receiver) in CW Doppler each have a beam pattern. The active sample volume is the volume of overlap of the two beams. Because the two beam patterns are angled with respect to each other and cross at mid depth, the active sample volume is widest at mid depth and narrow at both shallow and deep depths where the overlap is not so great. In pulsed Doppler, using a single transducer for both transmitting and

receiving, the transmitting and the receiving beam patterns overlap throughout their length. Therefore, the width of the beam pattern is narrow at mid depths where the narrow focal region is located.

In CW Doppler systems, the length (in the direction of the ultrasound beam) of the active sample volume within the beam is determined by the region of overlap between the beam patterns of the transmitting transducer and the receiving transducer. In pulsed systems, the active sample volume is determined by the duration of the transmitted ultrasound burst and the duration of the receiver gate. The location of the sample volume is determined by the time between the transmit burst and the opening of the receiver gate to accept echo signals from the selected depth. Thus, CW Doppler systems have longer active sample volumes than do pulsed Doppler systems.

An upper limit for Doppler frequency detection can be estimated. The highest blood velocity possible in humans can be computed by substituting the highest systolic blood pressure (225 mm Hg) into the Bernoulli equation:

$$p = 4 \times V^2$$

where p is pressure in millimeters of mercury and V is velocity in meters per second. We find that the highest possible blood velocity in humans is 750 cm/s (with systolic pressure of 144 mm Hg, V_{max} = 600 cm/s). From this, the maximum possible Doppler shift in humans can be calculated. Assuming a zero Doppler examination angle, the resultant Doppler shift is dependent on the ultrasound frequency. Using a 10-MHz Doppler, a blood velocity of 750 cm/s produces a Doppler frequency shift of 100 kHz (f = 2 × S × F/C = 2 × 750 cm/s × 10,000 kHz/150,000 cm/s = 100 kHz).

Although CW Doppler is capable of detecting the highest Doppler shifts possible in humans (100 kHz), these audio signals cannot be heard because this frequency is beyond the limit of human hearing. In addition, although modern instruments perform electronic analysis of the Doppler shift frequencies, most analyzers sample the audio signal and perform a digital frequency analysis. At a typical sample frequency of 50 kHz, the highest Doppler frequency that can be displayed without aliasing is 25 kHz. Thus, if these signals are analyzed with a digital spectrum analyzer, the resultant waveform will probably alias.

Pulsed Doppler

In pulsed Doppler, every time the system transmits a burst of ultrasound and receives an echo back from the depth of interest, the phase of the echo is measured. This measurement is called a *sample*, and the sample rate is equal to the PRF. The sample rate of a pulsed Doppler is limited by the depth to the

TABLE 7.10

MAXIMUM PULSE REPETITION FREQUENCY AND NYQUIST (ALIASING) FREQUENCY FOR DOPPLER AT DIFFERENT DEPTHS

■ DEPTH (cm)	■ ECHO RETURN TIME (μs)	■ MAXIMUM PRF (kHz)	■ NYQUIST FREQUENCY (kHz)
3	40	25.0	12.5
5	67	15.0	7.5
10	134	7.6	3.8
15	200	5.0	2.5
20	268	3.8	1.9

PRF, pulse repetition frequency.

selected Doppler sample volume because the Doppler ultrasound system must wait until the echo from the selected depth is received before transmitting again. If the system does not wait, the echo from the desired depth will arrive at the same time as stronger echoes from more recent transmissions reflecting from tissues at shallower depths. These shallow echoes will obscure the phase measurement from the depth of interest. Of course, when receiving the echo from the selected depth, echoes from deeper depths may also be present, but these have been attenuated and, therefore, are small enough to have little effect on the phase measurement. The depth of the expected Doppler sample volume (E) is found by the following equation:

$$E = C \times t/2$$

where t is the time between the transmit pulse and the receiver gate opening and C is the speed of ultrasound in tissue. Additional sample volumes along the ultrasound beam will be spaced at intervals of G from the shallowest volume:

$$G = C/(2 \times PRF)$$

The shallowest Doppler sample volume is located at a depth less than G; thus, E < G because PRF is always selected to be below 1/t. In a typical example with a PRF of 12.8 kHz, the first Doppler sample volume must be at a depth of less than 6 cm [G = 154,000 cm/s/(2 × 12,800 cycles/s)]. If the Doppler sample volume is set at a depth of 4 cm, other sample volumes will exist at 10 cm (4 + 6), 16 cm (10 + 6), 22 cm (16 + 6), and at deeper 6-cm intervals. The length (size) of the Doppler sample volume is often adjustable with the front panel controls on a duplex scanner. The sample volume length can be increased by increasing the duration of the transmit burst (Tt) or the duration of the receiver gate (Tr). The sample volume length (SL) is

$$SL = C \times (Tt + Tr)/2$$

By increasing the ultrasound transmit duration and the receive duration, the length of the sample volume can become nearly equal to the depth of the sample volume.

Pulsed Doppler Aliasing

Sample volumes at deeper depths require lower PRFs because the system must wait for the return of the echoes. In Doppler, the low PRF may result in aliasing. As an example, if high Doppler shift frequencies are obtained from a sample volume at 9 cm, aliasing may occur. For the first sample volume to be located at 9 cm, a PRF as low as 8 kHz is required [PRF = C/(2 × depth) = 154,000 cm/s/(2 × 9 cm) = 8.56 kHz]. Aliasing will occur at Doppler shift frequencies exceeding the Nyquist limit of 4 kHz (8 kHz/2).

Frequency Analysis

During a Doppler examination, an experienced examiner can recognize the sounds of the high Doppler frequencies associated with stenoses and the hissing sounds associated with spectral broadening. However, because of the need for documentation and quantitative measurement, images representing the Doppler signal are also generated. These images are based on a frequency analysis of the Doppler shift. Although a few systems combine the Doppler data from systole with those from diastole, most Doppler frequency analysis systems display a waveform allowing analysis of the systolic frequencies separately from the diastolic frequencies. The displays can be divided into those that determine the complete spectrum of the Doppler frequencies representing all of the velocities in the sample volume and those that determine only a single characteristic Doppler frequency as representative of the blood velocities.

Spectrum Analyzers

A number of methods are available to rapidly determine the spectrum of Doppler frequencies in a signal and to display the successive spectra over time as a spectral waveform. The fast Fourier transform (FFT) method is the most popular; however, other methods, such as the time compression analyzer, the parallel filter analyzer, and the chirp Z analyzer, work equally well. For the user, the difference between these systems rests in the cost and availability; the displays are identical. Common features of the data analysis in these analyzers are discussed here.

The Doppler signal is analyzed in sections about 10 ms (0.01 s) long. Each analysis produces a spectrum, so that the spectral waveform consists of a display of 100 spectra/s. During each analysis of 10 ms, the instrument records the Doppler signal and analyzes it. The recording is done in digital form, taking 25,600 samples/s. If the system takes 25,600 samples/s for 0.01 s, it has 256 samples to analyze. In the analysis, a test will be made for the strength of each of 128 frequencies in the signal (256/2). The number of samples is divided by 2 because of the Nyquist sampling theorem, which states that at least two samples are needed per cycle to identify the presence of a frequency in a signal. The results are then displayed, usually as a gray-scale spectrum.

The number and choice of frequencies tested in the signal analysis are determined by the time and sample rate. The lowest Doppler frequency in the display and the spacing between frequencies are equal to the number of spectra per second. A typical spectrum analyzer takes 0.01 s of Doppler data for each analysis: The lowest Doppler frequency is 100 Hz (cycles/s). Other frequencies tested are 200, 300, 400 Hz, and so forth. The highest frequency tested is equal to half of the sample rate. If the Doppler sample rate is 25,600 Hz, the highest frequency tested is 12,800 Hz. Thus, a total of 128 frequency tests will be done on 256 data points.

The frequency resolution of the spectrum analyzer is related to the time resolution of the spectrum analyzer; the frequency range is related to the Doppler sample volume depth. There is no agreement on the required or optimal frequency resolution. One manufacturer may have a frequency resolution of 50 Hz because each spectrum takes 0.02 s; another has a poorer frequency resolution of 125 Hz because each spectrum takes 0.008 s. However, there is agreement that it is best to use the highest allowable sample frequency (or PRF) in order to avoid aliasing. PRF is determined by the depth of the vessel under examination rather than by the instrument manufacturer (see Table 7.10).

With some instruments, it is possible to perform the Doppler examination at a depth greater than the normal maximum examination depth dictated by the PRF. This is called *high pulse repetition Doppler*. The trick is to use a higher PRF than is allowed by the depth of the sample volume. The result is that the desired Doppler signal is acquired not from the shallowest active Doppler sample volume but from a second or third sample volume in depth. Because of attenuation of ultrasound in tissue, the instrument is less sensitive to the deeper Doppler sample volumes than to the shallower. Thus, if moving blood is present in the associated shallow sample volume, the velocity in the shallow sample volume will dominate the signal.

Characteristic Frequency Analyzers

The first frequency analyzers used in ultrasonic Doppler diagnostic systems measured and displayed a single Doppler frequency as a function of time. These systems were used because they were electronically simple and thus inexpensive at the time. Three instantaneous characteristic frequencies could be used as the Doppler frequency: the mean, the mode, and the median. The instantaneous average frequency (properly called the *mean*) is rarely used because the average is so sensitive to noise. If 90% of the Doppler power is between 500 Hz and 600 Hz, the average should be near 550 Hz, but if 10% of the power is noise at 10,000 Hz, the average frequency is 1495 Hz. The *mode* (most intense) frequency is resistant to noise; if 90% of the Doppler signal power is between 500 and 600 Hz, the mode is likely to be present between 500 and 600 Hz. Noise at 10,000 Hz will not affect the mode, although the exact value of the mode is still subject to noise. The *median* is also very resistant to noise; half of the signal power is at frequencies lower than the median, and half of the power is at frequencies above the median.

Single descriptive values can also be extracted from spectral waveforms. The value most often selected from the Doppler spectral waveform for diagnostic purposes is the highest value during systole, from the upper envelope of the waveform. The *upper envelope* is the series of highest frequency values from each spectrum in the waveform; each value has power at least 1/100 of the mode frequency (20 dB down from the mode).

Color Doppler Imaging

In color Doppler imaging, each Doppler frequency is assigned a color. Once the Doppler shift is computed for a region in the image, the color corresponding to the Doppler shift is displayed at the corresponding image location. This allows only one frequency to be displayed for the Doppler signal in each Doppler sample volume. The color may represent the mode, the median, or the average instantaneous Doppler frequency. The frequency for color Doppler at each depth is identified by one of three methods: averaging the frequencies of an FFT spectrum, averaging the phase changes between pulses in the Doppler signal (lambda processor), or averaging the phase changes between pulses weighted by the strength of the signal (pulse-pair covariance).

In a typical *FFT analysis* for color Doppler, the pulsed Doppler system acquires 16 phase samples in time from 16 pulse-echo cycles for each sample volume in depth. A Fourier transform is used to create a spectrum showing the intensity of eight frequency ranges in the forward direction and eight in the reverse direction. The ranges with low intensity are thought to contain noise and are set to zero. An average of the remaining adjacent frequencies is computed. A color is selected based on the result. Gathering the 16 pulse-echo cycles for a 4-cm depth takes less than 1 ms.

In a typical *lambda processor*, at each sample depth, the six phase changes occurring in the six intervals between seven pulse-echo cycles in sequence are averaged to determine the average frequency shift. If the sample volume is located in moving blood far from solid tissues, this system works well. If, however, there are strong echoes from nearby stationary solid structures mixed with the changing signals from moving blood, the lambda processor detects no Doppler frequency shift, even though an FFT analysis would. Thus, the lambda processor leaves gaps in the color display between the color indicating blood flow in the center of an artery and the echogenic vascular wall. This system was used on the first duplex color Doppler imaging system.

In a typical *pulse-pair covariance* or *autocorrelation processor*, echoes from the first two (initializing) pulse-echo cycles of each sample volume are obtained to determine the phase and amplitude (intensity) of echoes from strong stationary reflectors. The phase and amplitude changes of subsequent echoes from each sample volume are compared with the initializing pulses, and the weighted average is taken; phase angle changes associated with strong differences from the initializing echo samples are weighted heavily because they are considered to be less likely to contain noise. Seven or eight pulse-echo cycles (taking about 0.5 ms) are required to determine the Doppler frequency and assign the appropriate color to the Doppler sample volume. This method is used in most color Doppler imaging systems.

In color Doppler systems, multiple sample volumes are processed at the same time along the length of a Doppler line. The number of samples is determined by the depth of the image and the size of the color Doppler pixels. As a typical example, if each pixel (sample volume) represents 1 mm in depth and the depth of the image is 6.4 cm, 64 sample volumes are needed. Because these systems are pulsed Doppler systems, all are subject to aliasing under the same conditions as conventional single-gate pulsed Doppler.

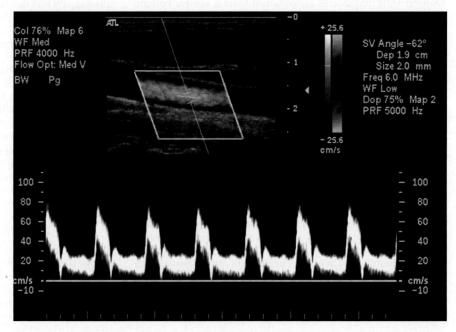

FIGURE 7.24. Comparison of velocity values in color Doppler and spectral Doppler. The color Doppler image (captured at peak systole) shows a maximum velocity of approximately 26 cm/s; this is an average velocity without angle correction. The spectral display, which includes adjustment for the Doppler angle, indicates that the maximum peak systolic velocity is approximately 80 cm/s, with an average peak systolic velocity of approximately 60 cm/s.

Color Doppler versus Spectral Waveform Doppler

The phase measurement in Doppler processing often contains considerable noise; more than two pulse-echo cycles are required to average out the noise. The average phase change over a series of 8 to 32 pairs of pulse-echo cycles is used to determine the Doppler frequency in each sample volume in color Doppler instruments. Each color represents the average Doppler frequency shift from the corresponding sample volume in tissue. In conventional single-gate pulsed Doppler with spectral waveform analysis, each spectrum in the spectral waveform is generated using 256 pulse-echo cycles. This allows the display of more than one Doppler frequency. Each spectrum in the waveform includes data on the strength of each of the frequencies present, rather than reporting only a single average frequency. During the measurement of the spectral waveform, the highest frequencies are usually reported; these are higher than the frequencies resulting from the averaging process in the color image. In addition, color Doppler images do not include correction for the Doppler angle. Thus, velocity values reported from a conventional pulsed Doppler study are higher than the corresponding values reported from a color Doppler examination (Fig. 7.24). If the lower color-flow value were used for diagnosis, clinically significant arterial stenoses might be missed or underreported.

Suggested Readings

1. Evans DH, McDicken WN. *Doppler Ultrasound: Physics, Instrumentation and Signal Processing*, 2nd ed. Chichester: Wiley, 2000.
2. Health Canada. *Guidelines for the Safe Use of Diagnostic Ultrasound*. Ottawa: Public Works and Government Services Canada, 2001.
3. Hedrick WR, Hykes DL, Starchman DE. *Ultrasound Physics and Instrumentation*, 4th ed. St. Louis: Elsevier Mosby, 2005.
4. Kremkau FW. *Diagnostic Ultrasound: Principles and Instruments*, 7th ed. Philadelphia: WB Saunders, 2005.
5. Nelson TR, Pretorius DH. Three-dimensional ultrasound imaging. *Ultrasound Med Biol* 1998;24:1243-1270.
6. Oates C. *Cardiovascular Haemodynamics and Doppler Waveforms Explained*. London: Greenwich Medical Media, 2001.
7. Zagzebski JA. *Essentials of Ultrasound Physics*. St. Louis: Mosby, 1996.

PRINCIPLES AND INSTRUMENTATION

SECTION III ■ CEREBROVASCULAR

CHAPTER 8 ■ EXTRACRANIAL CAROTID AND VERTEBRAL ARTERIES

GREGORY L. MONETA, ERICA L. MITCHELL AND CLAUDIA RUMWELL

This chapter provides an overview of extracranial carotid duplex scanning technique and the ultrasound criteria used for grading carotid artery stenosis. The clinical relevance of duplex scanning in the management of symptomatic and asymptomatic carotid artery disease is also discussed. Topics related to intracranial cerebrovascular ultrasound testing are covered in Chapters 9 and 11.

TECHNICAL POINTS

A complete carotid duplex examination, including the vertebral and subclavian arteries, generally requires 15 to 60 minutes to complete. This time is dependent on examiner experience and skill, severity of disease, and patient cooperation. The indication for the examination is recorded along with the appropriate International Classification of Diseases, 9th edition (ICD-9) code. Carotid and subclavian arteries should be auscultated bilaterally to evaluate for bruits. The presence or absence of carotid and radial artery pulses is also recorded, and brachial systolic and diastolic blood pressures are measured bilaterally. The duplex portion of the examination includes the bilateral carotid and vertebral arteries. Flow characteristics in one carotid artery may be influenced significantly by the status of the contralateral carotid artery; therefore, bilateral examinations are indicated in all cases.[1]

Instrumentation

Any duplex ultrasound system that includes high-resolution B-mode imaging, pulsed Doppler, and spectral waveform analysis is adequate for performing a complete carotid examination. The common carotid artery (CCA) bifurcation is located 2 to 3 cm deep to the skin surface, whereas the most proximal CCA or vertebral artery and the distal internal carotid artery (ICA) may be slightly deeper. Depth is, therefore, not a major issue when selecting a scan head to perform the examination, and transducer frequencies from 5 to 12 MHz are used. High-frequency transducers (7.5 to 12 MHz) provide better B-mode images of the bifurcation region, whereas scan heads with 5-MHz transducer frequencies may be needed for the distal ICA, the origin of the CCA, and the vertebral arteries. Modern scan heads have multiple imaging frequencies and allow the examiner to change frequencies without having to change scan heads.

Pulsed Doppler and B-mode imaging frequencies may be the same or different during the examination. The pulsed Doppler frequency should be between 4.5 and 10 MHz, but most spectral waveform criteria for carotid stenosis were derived using a 5-MHz Doppler frequency, so that frequency should be used whenever possible. If a pulsed Doppler frequency other than 5 MHz is used to generate spectral waveforms for classification of stenosis, some published interpretation criteria may not apply.

Mechanical sector, linear array, or phased array scan head designs can all be utilized. A linear array imaging format is particularly useful for the mid and distal CCA and the bifurcation region, where the vessels are approximately parallel to the skin surface. With a linear array scan head, manipulations with "heel-and-toe maneuvers" may be necessary to obtain perpendicular B-mode imaging angles because the vessel curves away from the transducer. The sector-type imaging formats of a curved array or the smaller footprint phased array may be successfully used in the regions of the distal ICA and for vessels in the supraclavicular region.

Patient Preparation and Positioning

The patient is positioned supine with her or his head resting flat on the bed in a foam donut or with a rolled-up towel under the neck for support. The use of a pillow is discouraged unless the patient has difficulty breathing or cannot lie flat because of preexisting back problems. A pillow may raise the head excessively, which creates less flexibility of movement and shortens the length of the neck, both of which interfere with obtaining the optimal imaging windows. A towel or a tissue is tucked into the patient's clothing for protection from the ultrasound gel, or a patient gown may be provided.

The technologist is seated at the head of the bed with the scanner to the left, near enough so that the operator may easily reach the most frequently used controls. The technologist should be seated slightly lower than the bed, with the elbow of the scanning arm resting on the bed for support and the last two fingers of the scanning hand resting gently on the patient's shoulder. This position decreases the stress on the technologist's back and arm during the examination. A stable scanning position for the arm is essential when trying to make fine adjustments in scan head orientation and obtaining Doppler signals from small vessels. The patient's chin is slightly hyperextended and turned

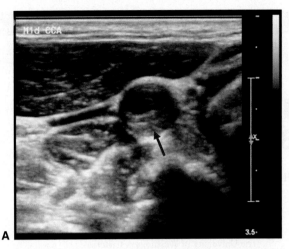
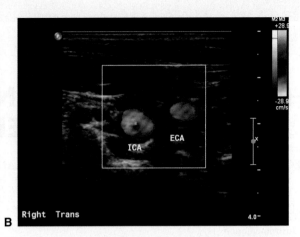

FIGURE 8.1. Transverse or cross-sectional images. *A*, B-mode image shows an eccentric plaque in the mid common carotid artery (CCA; *arrow*). *B*, Color-flow image of the carotid bifurcation shows the internal carotid artery (ICA) is larger in caliber than the external carotid artery (ECA).

toward the contralateral side at about a 45-degree angle from the midline. This head position may be changed as the examination proceeds to access the best imaging windows.

Examination Technique

The carotid duplex examination includes both longitudinal and transverse scans of the vessels. A transverse (or cross-sectional) scan, starting at the most proximal CCA, is helpful to gain orientation when beginning the examination. This view helps the technologist determine the proper position of the scan head relative to the arteries and become familiar with the patient's anatomy, especially in the area of the bifurcation and the distal ICA where tortuosity is common. Transverse views also often provide the most revealing images of eccentric plaques (Fig. 8.1). Several imaging windows may be necessary to obtain optimal cross-sectional views. The longitudinal view is suboptimal for visualizing plaque. Carotid artery plaque is usually eccentric; therefore, one longitudinal view will show only a portion of the plaque. Rotating the scan head around the long axis of the artery or sliding the scan head side to side with small movements will help to document the complex nature of the plaque. Caliper measurements of the lumen from either longitudinal or transverse views in complex

disease are fraught with problems and, in general, should be discouraged as a means of accurately predicting diameter reduction. Velocity waveforms should never be obtained from a transverse view. The Doppler angles in such orientations are either unknown or close to perpendicular to the flow direction, resulting in useless Doppler velocity information. Color Doppler images of vessels in cross section can be deceiving for the same reasons.

Most of the carotid duplex scan is accomplished using a longitudinal view, which permits the most favorable Doppler angles for recording velocity data and for color Doppler imaging. Using the longitudinal orientation, the pulsed Doppler sample volume is swept continuously throughout the length of the vessels, especially in the area of the bifurcation, searching for areas of increased velocity or flow disturbance. Spot-checking velocity information or sampling sporadically from random locations is poor technique and should be avoided. Neither the B-mode nor the color Doppler image will reliably pinpoint the area of maximal velocity or flow disturbance. Gray-scale and color or power Doppler images alert the examiner to the presence of plaque in the arterial wall that may preclude penetration of the vessel by ultrasound (Fig. 8.2). Color Doppler and B-mode images are helpful primarily for localizing a particular area of interest that needs more specific, in-depth investigation with the pulsed Doppler sample volume (Fig. 8.3).

FIGURE 8.2. Calcific plaque in the arterial wall (*arrow*) precludes penetration of the vessel by ultrasound in this power Doppler image, resulting in acoustic shadowing and a "color void." In some cases, it may be possible to obtain a Doppler signal by varying the angle of the scan head. Some information on the possible presence of stenosis in the area of a color void can also be obtained by analysis of the Doppler spectral waveforms immediately proximal and distal to the shadowed segment.

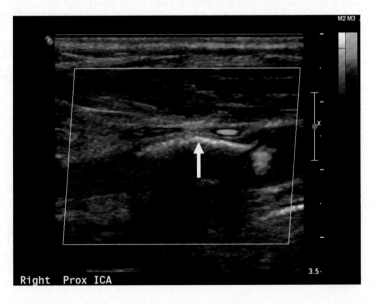

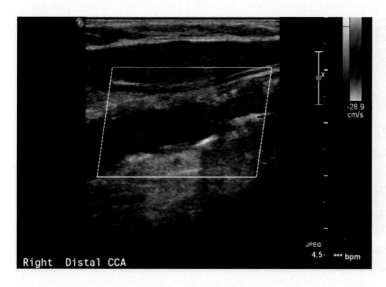

Right Distal CCA

FIGURE 8.3. Color Doppler clearly indicates compromise of the arterial lumen in this common carotid artery (CCA) but is generally not as accurate as spectral waveform analysis in quantifying the degree of stenosis.

The value of detailed characterization of carotid plaque composition and surface features by gray-scale imaging in routine clinical practice is controversial. It is common for interpreting physicians to comment on the ultrasound characteristics and surface features of a significant carotid plaque. Retrospective analyses suggest that plaques that are predominantly echolucent or irregular are more likely to be associated with neurologic symptoms than predominately echo-dense or smooth plaques.[2-5] However, thus far, this research is largely qualitative, and although advances in imaging technology can now provide very detailed gray-scale images (Figs. 8.4 and 8.5), there are still no definite therapeutic recommendations that can be made based on ultrasound plaque characteristics alone.

Ultrasound beam angles for optimal B-mode images are different from those required for obtaining Doppler spectral waveforms. Maximal ultrasound reflection occurs when the ultrasound beam is perpendicular to the surface being imaged. The optimal B-mode imaging angle is therefore 90 degrees to the surface of the artery. The angle that produces the highest Doppler frequency shift is 0 degrees or parallel to the direction of flow. However, it is difficult to achieve Doppler angles parallel to flow in the cervical cerebrovascular vessels, and angles up to 60 degrees between the vessel axis and the Doppler beam are acceptable. Angles greater than 60 degrees introduce errors into measuring Doppler frequency shifts that may be clinically significant and should be avoided. Therefore, the same view

used to obtain an optimal Doppler signal may not yield the highest resolution B-mode image. The physical principles of vascular imaging with ultrasound are discussed in detail in Chapter 7. Most ultrasound instruments have fixed B-mode imaging elements with a steerable Doppler beam, and the operator manipulates the scan head to individually optimize the angles for each modality. Some ultrasound instruments allow the operator to electronically steer the B-mode image and Doppler beam independently, allowing optimization of both modalities simultaneously. Every effort should be made to create the optimal angles for B-mode imaging and Doppler spectral waveform analysis.

CAROTID FLOW PATTERNS

Normal Common and Internal Carotid Arteries

Doppler spectral waveforms are obtained from the CCA, ICA, the origin of the external carotid artery (ECA), and the proximal vertebral artery. As previously mentioned, a continuous or "point-to-point" sampling technique should be used to examine the CCA and ICA. Spectral waveforms are also obtained from any site of suspected abnormality suggested by

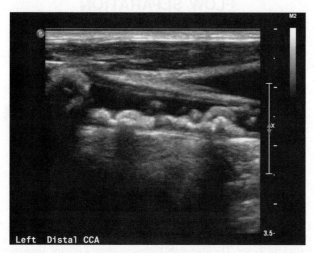

Left Distal CCA

FIGURE 8.4. This gray-scale image demonstrates bulky plaque with irregular surface characteristics in the distal common carotid artery (CCA).

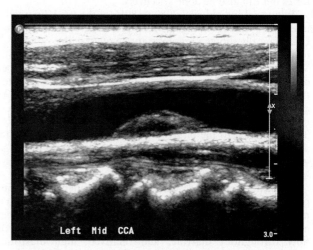

Left Mid CCA

FIGURE 8.5. This gray-scale image shows a heterogeneous plaque in the mid common carotid artery (CCA) with an echolucent center and generally smooth surface.

CEREBROVASCULAR

FIGURE 8.6. Normal common carotid artery (CCA) color Doppler image and spectral waveform, with a rapid systolic upstroke and forward flow throughout diastole. There is also a clear "window" under the systolic peak, indicating laminar or non-disturbed flow. The relatively high diastolic flow velocity represents the low resistance of the internal carotid circulation, whereas the transient low-velocity "valley" (near the baseline) in late systole is a feature of the normal external carotid flow pattern. Peak systolic velocity is 110 cm/s.

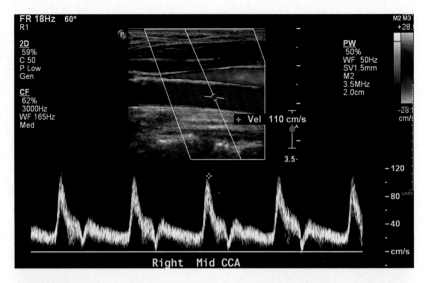

FIGURE 8.7. Normal mid internal carotid artery (ICA) color Doppler image and spectral waveform, with a rapid systolic upstroke, continued forward flow throughout diastole, and relatively high diastolic velocities. As in the normal CCA (see Fig. 8.6), there is a clear "window" under the systolic peak, indicating laminar flow. This is a typical low-resistance arterial flow pattern. Peak systolic velocity (PSV) is 72 cm/s, with end-diastolic velocity (EDV) of 26 cm/s.

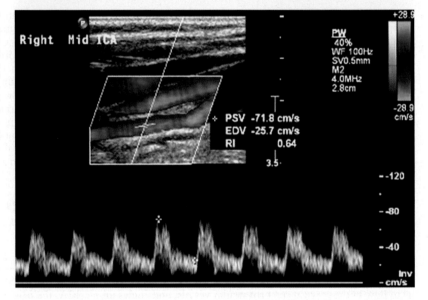

gray-scale or color Doppler images. Evaluation of the subclavian arteries, as discussed in Chapter 14, is performed as a routine component of the carotid duplex scan in many laboratories but can also be done selectively.

In normal individuals, 70% to 80% of the CCA flow volume enters the low-resistance ICA, and therefore, flow in the CCA typically shows a low-resistance pattern with a rapid systolic upstroke and forward flow throughout diastole (Fig. 8.6). When evaluating the CCA, a spectral waveform should be obtained from the most proximal CCA segment accessible to the scan head. For calculating velocity ratios between the ICA and the CCA (ICA/CCA ratio), the CCA peak systolic velocity (PSV) should be measured in the mid-neck approximately 3 cm proximal to the bifurcation where the vessel is straight and free of significant occlusive disease. Comparison of CCA waveforms from the two sides of the neck should reveal similar PSV and end-diastolic flow velocities.

Spectral waveforms are recorded routinely from the proximal, mid, and distal cervical ICA segments. The normal ICA flow pattern is characteristic of a low-resistance artery, with a rapid systolic upstroke, continued forward flow throughout diastole, and relatively high diastolic velocities (Fig. 8.7). The normal proximal ICA often includes a dilation or "bulb" of variable size that tapers gradually toward the mid and distal segments (Fig. 8.8). The

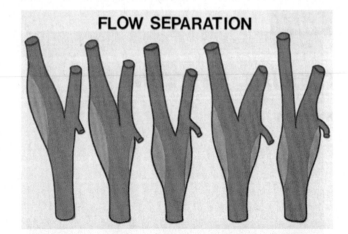

FIGURE 8.8. Illustration of variations in the location and extent of the carotid bulb. The most common configurations are the two at the *left* of the figure. The *blue areas* represent regions of flow separation (see text).

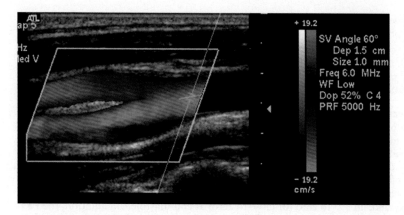

FIGURE 8.9. Color Doppler image of a normal CCA bifurcation. The area of flow reversal (*dark blue*) along the outer wall of the bulb is a normal finding and indicates an absence of plaque. This is referred to as an area of flow separation (see text).

unidirectional flow pattern described previously is normally found in the carotid bulb along the flow divider of the bifurcation. However, there is transient reversal of flow at peak systole near the center stream and at the outer wall opposite the flow divider. This area of reversed flow is often seen in color Doppler images (Fig. 8.9). As discussed in Chapter 5, this complex flow pattern is referred to as an area of *boundary layer separation* or *flow separation*. Flow velocities along the outer wall in the separation zone may drop to zero at the end of diastole (Fig. 8.10). These normal flow patterns are used in conjunction with the absence of visible plaque on the B-mode image to identify a normal carotid bulb. Flow patterns in the carotid bulb may extend to the mid-ICA and can be apparent in waveforms obtained at that level. The distal ICA includes the segment at least 3 cm above the carotid bifurcation. Atherosclerosis usually develops within 2 cm of the bifurcation and rarely is limited to the distal ICA. However, there are a few conditions, such

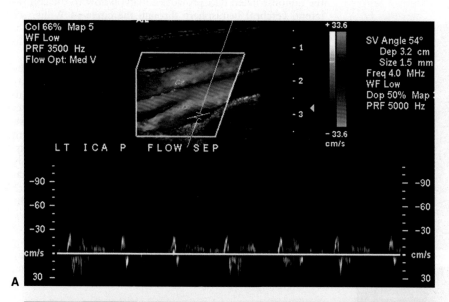

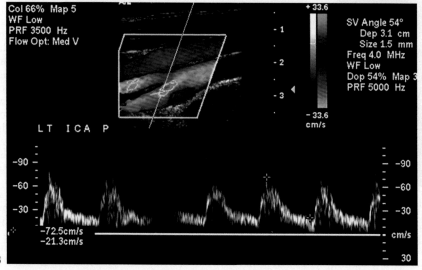

FIGURE 8.10. *A,* Color Doppler image and spectral waveform of a normal carotid bulb with the sample volume placed near the outer wall in the region of flow separation. The spectral waveform shows relatively low velocities with periods of forward and reverse flow during the cardiac cycle. *B,* The sample volume has been moved to a location near the inner wall or flow divider where there are higher velocities and a unidirectional flow pattern, typical of a normal internal carotid artery (ICA) (see Fig. 8.7).

CEREBROVASCULAR

as fibromuscular dysplasia, in which velocity increases are localized to the distal ICA without the presence of proximal ICA plaque (Fig. 8.11).[6]

Flow Patterns with Carotid Stenosis

Detecting carotid stenosis with Doppler spectral waveforms focuses on three areas: the prestenotic region, the site of stenosis, and the poststenotic region. Although the most important Doppler findings are observed by sampling at the stenotic site, the pre- and poststenotic regions also provide valuable diagnostic information (Fig. 8.12). Complete characterization of carotid stenosis involves a combination of Doppler spectral waveform analysis, color Doppler, gray-scale (B-mode) imaging, and, in selected cases, power Doppler. However, spectral analysis is the predominant modality for quantification of carotid stenosis. In most cases, color Doppler imaging is not the primary means for assessing the severity of an ICA stenosis. An exception is in distinguishing ICA occlusion from a high-grade stenosis, in which color or power Doppler may identify very low velocity flow in the area of the stenosis that cannot be detected by conventional pulsed Doppler.

The pulsed Doppler spectral waveforms and color Doppler findings should be cross-checked for concordance. If there is disagreement between the impressions obtained with the color

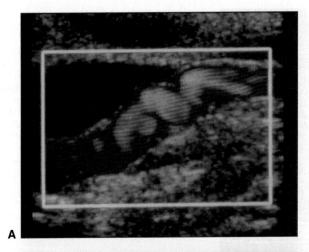

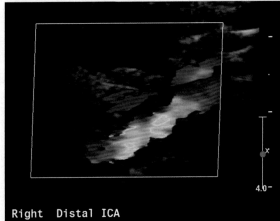

FIGURE 8.11. *A*, Power Doppler image of the distal cervical ICA in a patient with fibromuscular dysplasia. *B*, Color Doppler image of the distal cervical internal carotid artery (ICA) in another patient with fibromuscular dysplasia. In both images, there is localized irregularity of the arterial wall, resulting in focal areas of velocity increase.

and the pulsed Doppler examinations (i.e., color Doppler suggests high-grade stenosis but velocities are only moderately elevated), the findings of both should be reviewed to resolve the discrepancy.

Common Carotid Artery

In the majority of cases, carotid stenosis or occlusion occurs in the proximal ICA. Consequently, the CCA exhibits flow patterns typical of a prestenotic region. In the presence of a very high-grade ICA stenosis or occlusion, outflow is primarily through the high-resistance ECA circulation. In this situation, the CCA spectral waveform takes on the high-resistance flow characteristics of the ECA (Fig. 8.13), with flow velocity going to zero (or close to zero) at end-diastole.[7] In addition, the PSV and the overall flow velocity may be substantially lower than normal owing to reduced flow volume in the CCA. By observing these changes in the CCA flow pattern, one can often predict the presence of high-grade stenosis or occlusion of the ICA. For this and other reasons, it is good practice to begin the interpretation of carotid ultrasound studies by comparing the CCA Doppler spectral waveforms side to side.

The CCA contralateral to a high-grade ICA stenosis or occlusion may demonstrate an increased flow velocity with particular elevation of the end-diastolic velocity (EDV). These changes represent a compensatory increase in blood flow as the nonobstructed ICA provides collateral flow to the contralateral cerebral hemisphere through the circle of Willis (see Chapter 9). This compensatory increase in flow can be substantial, and flow velocities related to a stenosis may be artificially elevated on the side with high-volume flow.[1]

In the presence of a significant stenosis at the origin of the CCA or innominate artery, the ipsilateral CCA waveform may be dampened, with low overall PSV and a slower rise to peak systole when compared with the contralateral CCA waveform (Fig. 8.14). In such cases, the cervical CCA represents the poststenotic region, rather than the prestenotic region as occurs with ICA stenosis. It is very important to recognize the CCA flow pattern caused by a proximal stenosis, because it is often the only indication of clinically significant carotid occlusive disease that may be treatable. The CCA waveform changes associated with proximal stenosis are also important diagnostically because the overall reduction in flow velocity may artificially lower velocities in an ipsilateral ICA stenosis, leading to underestimation of the severity of that lesion. In some cases of proximal CCA or innominate artery stenosis, the ipsilateral CCA waveform may exhibit poststenotic turbulence low in the neck, representing disturbed flow distal to the more proximal stenosis.

Internal Carotid Artery

The normal ICA spectral waveform is indicative of high-volume flow in a low-resistance vascular bed. The systolic upstroke is rapid, PSV is less than 125 cm/s, and forward flow is maintained throughout diastole.[8] In the absence of plaque, there is generally a clear "window" under the systolic peak of the spectral waveform because there is little turbulent flow, as shown in Figure 8.7. On color Doppler, the presence of color shifts, indicating high-velocity flow, and color mosaics, indicating poststenotic turbulence, aids in selecting potential areas for examination with the pulsed Doppler. Lack of diastolic flow in an ICA indicates distal cervical ICA high-grade stenosis or intracranial stenosis or occlusion (Fig. 8.15).

Hemodynamic quantification of ICA stenosis severity is primarily achieved by analysis of Doppler spectral waveforms and measurements of PSV and EDV, or comparisons of PSV in the ICA with those in the CCA (ICA/CCA ratio). As a stenosis develops, the PSV becomes elevated first, making PSV the principal measure of stenosis severity. The increase in EDV

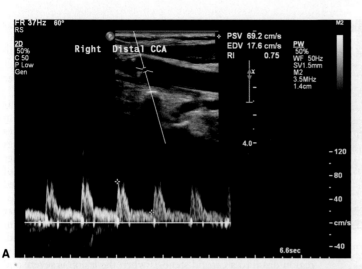

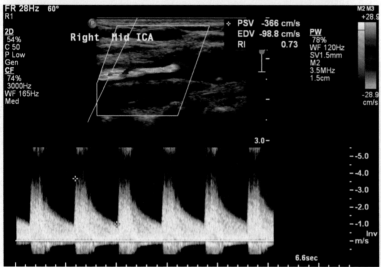

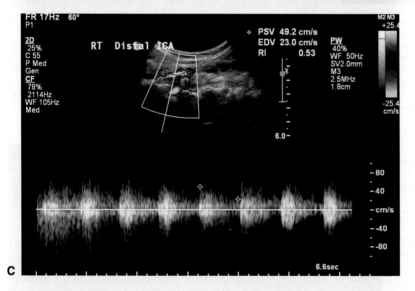

FIGURE 8.12. Information on the presence and severity of a carotid stenosis is obtained by sampling flow from the prestenotic region, the site of stenosis, and the poststenotic region. *A*, The flow pattern proximal to a severe stenosis depends on the intervening branches and collaterals. This spectral waveform from a distal common carotid artery (CCA) proximal to a stenotic internal carotid artery (ICA) shows a relatively low peak systolic velocity (PSV) of 69 cm/s, but the flow pattern is otherwise normal due to the patent ipsilateral ECA. *B*, The PSV within the mid ICA stenosis is increased to 366 cm/s. *C*, The poststenotic spectral waveform taken from the distal ICA shows turbulent flow (spectral broadening) with a decreased PSV of 49 cm/s.

lags behind PSV as stenosis severity progresses, but EDV rises rapidly as the stenosis becomes severe (diameter reductions of ≥60%). Thus, elevation of EDV is a good marker for high-grade ICA stenosis (Fig. 8.16).[9] The ICA/CCA ratio is also a very important measure of stenosis severity.[10] Because it is a ratio, it compensates for abnormally high- and low-flow states that may skew the PSV and EDV upward or downward.

To accurately measure flow velocity and classify stenosis severity, the pulsed Doppler sample volume must be placed within the area of greatest stenosis. Color Doppler imaging has demonstrated that the orientation of the stenotic jet within a stenosis is frequently not parallel to the longitudinal axis of the vessel. This finding has resulted in controversy with regard to the proper technique of Doppler angle adjustment

CEREBROVASCULAR

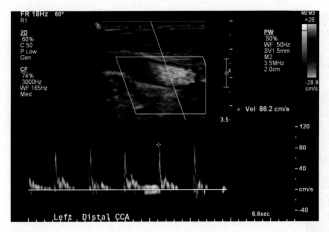

FIGURE 8.13. Distal left common carotid artery (CCA) waveform in a patient with left ICA occlusion. When the ICA is occluded, the CCA waveform takes on the high-resistance flow pattern of an ECA. There may be a phase of reversed flow in late systole/early diastole and flow to, or nearly to, the zero flow baseline at end-diastole.

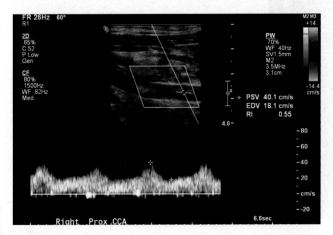

FIGURE 8.14. Right common carotid artery (CCA) waveform in a patient with a high-grade innominate artery stenosis. In the presence of a significant stenosis at the origin of the CCA or in the innominate artery, the ipsilateral CCA waveform may be dampened, with low peak velocities and a slower rise to peak systole than those found in the contralateral CCA waveform. This waveform is severely dampened with a decreased PSV of 40 cm/s.

FIGURE 8.15. This internal carotid artery (ICA) spectral waveform shows a high-resistance pattern with absent diastolic flow in a patient with a left hemispheric stroke and acute occlusion of the ipsilateral anterior and middle cerebral arteries.

for obtaining velocity waveforms at sites of stenosis. In areas of mild to moderate stenosis, a Doppler angle of 60 degrees to the long axis of the vessel is recommended. However, in areas of more severe stenosis, the Doppler angle of 60 degrees should be defined by the long axis of the stenotic flow jet, as demonstrated by color Doppler.

The pulsed Doppler sample volume size should be kept as small as possible, usually 1.5 mm, to detect discrete changes in flow velocity. This is important because the highest velocities may be localized to a small area in the flow jet that emanates from the stenosis. A large sample volume that incorporates flow from many points within the vessel in the generation of spectral waveforms may give the false impression of disturbed flow, potentially leading to the misdiagnosis of moderate disease in an otherwise normal vessel. In practice, the sonographer identifies the area of stenosis and carefully sweeps a small sample volume through until the point of highest velocity is found.

Damping of Doppler spectral waveforms may be seen in the region distal to a carotid stenosis when the lesion is severe and flow reducing. The most common waveform abnormality seen distal to a carotid stenosis is spectral broadening caused by disturbed blood flow or frank turbulence. At best, a poststenotic flow disturbance is a qualitative measure of arterial stenosis; nevertheless, its detection is important. With proper gain settings, spectral broadening or "filling-in" of the Doppler spectral waveform generally indicates the presence of carotid stenosis with a diameter reduction of at least 50%. However, this level of disturbed flow occasionally can be seen with nonstenotic disease. Diagnostically, the most significant poststenotic flow disturbance produces simultaneous forward and reverse spectral waveform components, accompanied by poor definition of the upper spectral waveform border. Such disturbed flow implies the presence of severe carotid stenosis. Severely disturbed flow distal to a highly calcified plaque may be the only substantial evidence for the presence of clinically significant stenosis if calcification prevents direct insonation of the stenotic site.

Vertebral Artery

On rare occasions, a stenosis may be found in the cervical portion of the vertebral artery associated with cervical osteoarthritis. However, the origin of the vertebral from the subclavian artery is by far the most common site of disease in the vertebral artery. The vertebral artery origin lies deep in the base of the neck and may be difficult to access with ultrasound. Mean vertebral artery diameter is about 4 mm, but the vertebral arteries are frequently asymmetrical in size with one (most commonly the left) being larger than the other.

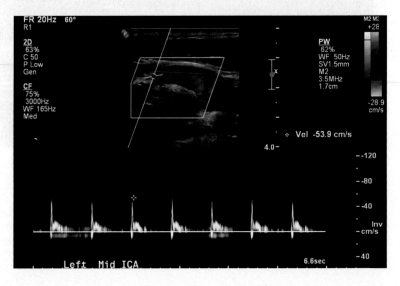

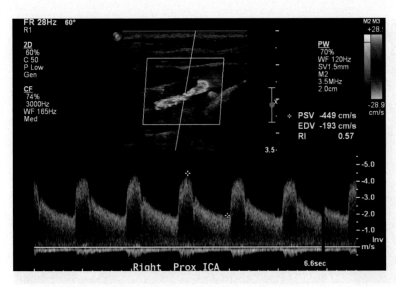

FIGURE 8.16. Color Doppler image and spectral waveform from a severe, 80% to 99% internal carotid artery (ICA) stenosis. The color shifts indicate a high velocity jet and the spectral waveform shows an increased peak systolic velocity (PSV) of 449 cm/s and markedly elevated end-diastolic velocity (EDV) of 193 cm/s. See Table 8.1 for velocity criteria.

The vertebral artery is most commonly interrogated with ultrasound farther distally in the neck, from an anteroposterior window, as it passes through the transverse processes of the cervical spine. The transverse processes serve as a reference to ensure that the vertebral artery is actually under examination, as illustrated in Figure 8.17. The artery is usually visualized deeper but adjacent to the vertebral vein. Color Doppler is helpful to locate the vessel. A spectral waveform from the vertebral artery in the mid-neck provides information about direction of flow, waveform shape, and velocity, but it does not always rule out stenotic disease at the origin. The normal vertebral artery waveform is similar to that of the ICA, with PSV in the range of 20 to 40 cm/s and diastolic flow well above the baseline.[11] However, velocities up to 80 to 90 cm/s are frequently seen without apparent clinical importance and may represent collateral flow through a dominant vertebral artery or a small but otherwise normal vertebral artery. Evaluation of disturbed flow distally may help determine which elevated velocities are associated with a vertebral artery stenosis and which are not. Velocity patterns are usually similar in the two vertebral arteries, but systolic and diastolic velocities may differ if vertebral artery diameters are asymmetrical. For this reason, if there is concern for stenosis based on an elevated PSV in a vertebral artery, recording of vertebral artery diameters is important.

Flow in the vertebral artery is normally antegrade (toward the brain) with a rapid systolic upstroke and a low-resistance pattern with continuous diastolic flow (Fig. 8.17). A so-called resistive vertebral artery waveform with low diastolic or no diastolic flow (Fig. 8.18) indicates a more distal stenosis or occlusion of the vertebral artery, a vertebral artery that ends in a small intracranial vessel, or a hypoplastic vertebral artery. Overall, about 50% of the time a resistive vertebral artery waveform is associated with major vertebrobasilar disease; however, in some cases, a resistive vertebral artery waveform is not associated with any clear anatomic abnormality.[12]

In cases of anatomic subclavian steal, color Doppler provides an important initial clue to the diagnosis, because flow in the vertebral artery will be retrograde and in the same direction as flow in the accompanying vein. Doppler spectral waveforms must still be used to verify arterial flow and will demonstrate reversed or bidirectional flow in cases of subclavian steal (Fig. 8.19).

External Carotid Artery

The ECA is smaller in diameter than the ICA at the level of the carotid bulb but similar in diameter beyond the bulb. It has little clinical significance in most cases but can serve as an

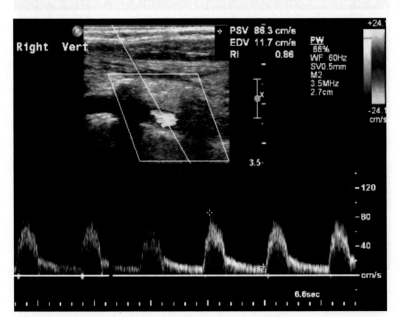

FIGURE 8.17. Color Doppler image and spectral waveform from a normal vertebral artery showing the "color voids" secondary to the transverse processes of the cervical vertebrae that serve as a reference to ensure that the vertebral artery is the vessel under examination. The spectral waveform shows a low-resistance flow pattern with a peak systolic velocity (PSV) of 88 cm/s.

CEREBROVASCULAR

FIGURE 8.18. This vertebral artery spectral waveform shows abnormal "resistive" flow. A high-resistance flow pattern in a vertebral artery (diastolic flow to or near the zero baseline) is suggestive of a more distal stenosis or occlusion of the vertebral artery, a hypoplastic vertebral artery, or a vertebral artery that ends in a small intracranial artery.

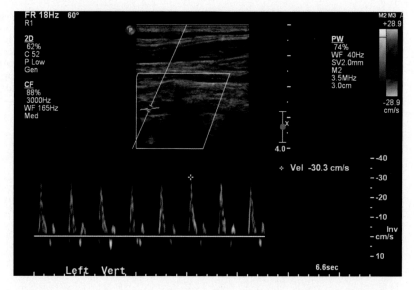

FIGURE 8.19. *A,* Color Doppler image and spectral waveform showing completely reversed flow in a left vertebral artery in a patient with left subclavian artery occlusion. The *color image* indicates flow away from the brain (toward the arm), and the spectral waveform shows reversed flow below the zero baseline. *B,* This patient has a high-grade innominate artery stenosis with almost complete reversal of flow in the right vertebral artery.

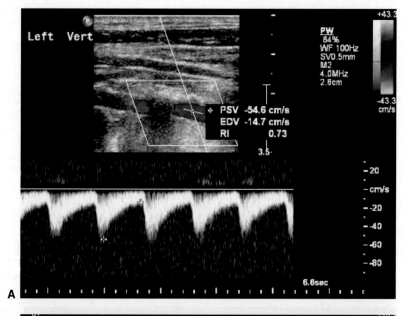

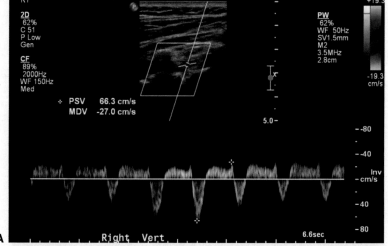

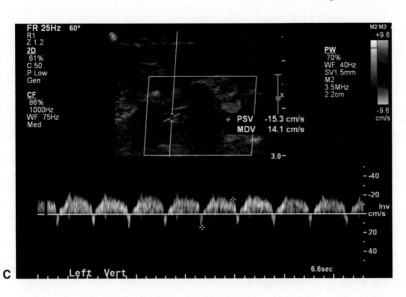

FIGURE 8.19. (*Continued*) *C,* In some cases of subclavian or innominate artery stenosis, flow in the vertebral artery exhibits a "to and fro" pattern above and below the baseline rather than total reversal of flow.

important source of collateral flow to the brain in the presence of high-grade stenosis or occlusion of the ICA. The ECA may also serve as a conduit for emboli to the brain in the setting of ICA occlusion, so-called carotid "stump syndrome."[13]

The normal ECA spectral waveform has a sharp systolic upstroke, a prominent phase of reversed flow in late systole or early diastole, and velocity that is near or at the zero baseline at end-diastole (Fig. 8.20A). This flow pattern is equivalent to that of other peripheral arteries supplying a relatively high-resistance vascular bed. The PSV of the ECA is normally higher than that of the ICA. The ECA may adopt the flow characteristics of the ICA in end-diastole as the resistance in the face and scalp decreases with temperature changes or when the ECA serves as a source of extracranial to intracranial collateral flow.

The "temporal tap" is a technique for identifying the ECA that relies on the fact that the superficial temporal artery (STA) is a branch of the ECA. Rapid compressions of the ipsilateral STA while monitoring the waveform in the suspected ECA can produce audible oscillations in the Doppler signal. These oscillations are also visible on the spectral waveform if the vessel

in the neck being insonated is the ECA (Fig. 8.20B). No oscillations should be noted if the vessel is the ICA. This technique may be used to distinguish the ICA from the ECA, but it is not always accurate, and there are conditions in which the STA tap can be misleading. These include (1) ECA collateralization in the presence of a chronic occlusive lesion in the ICA; (2) The ICA as well as the ECA may respond to the compressions if the back pressure of the oscillations is strong enough; and (3) The STA may not be adequately compressed. Therefore, the STA tap maneuver can be useful in selected cases, but it should not serve as the only means of distinguishing the ICA from the ECA.

CLASSIFYING CAROTID STENOSIS

The University of Washington Criteria

Duplex ultrasound criteria for quantifying carotid artery stenosis were originally developed in the late 1970s and early 1980s by comparing duplex-derived spectral waveforms and

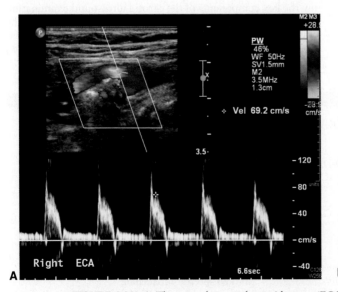

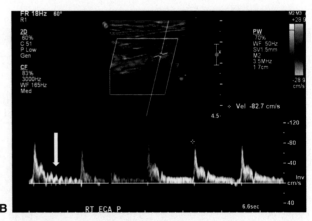

FIGURE 8.20. *A,* The normal external carotid artery (ECA) spectral waveform has a sharp systolic upstroke, and there is often a prominent phase of reversed flow in late systole or early diastole. Velocity at the end of diastole is at or near the zero baseline. *B,* Oscillations in the ECA spectral waveform can be induced by rapid digital compressions of the ipsilateral STA—the so-called "temporal tap." The presence of these oscillations (*arrow*) indicates that the spectral waveform does indeed originate from the ECA.

contrast arteriograms. The resulting duplex categories of stenosis were relatively broad, and sensitivities and specificities for detecting an ICA stenosis of 50% to 99% diameter reduction were in the range of 90% to 95%. There are now a variety of spectral criteria for classifying carotid artery disease. Some focus on categories of stenosis, whereas others focus on threshold levels of stenosis. One of the most widely accepted classification schemes for categories of ICA stenosis was developed at the University of Washington under the direction of Dr. D. Eugene Strandness, Jr. These criteria have been useful both for studying the natural history of carotid atherosclerosis and in clinical practice. In the University of Washington criteria, spectral waveform analysis and velocity measurements are used to classify ICA lesions into the following categories of angiographic stenosis: Normal, 1% to 15%, 16% to 49%, 50% to 79%, 80% to 99%, and occlusion (Table 8.1). Prospective validation of these criteria has demonstrated an overall agreement of 82% with contrast angiography. The ability of the criteria to detect carotid disease is 99% sensitive, and the ability of the criteria to recognize normal arteries is 84% specific.[8]

These duplex criteria for classifying carotid artery stenosis have undergone reevaluation to remain relevant to current clinical practice. This reevaluation was stimulated in large part by the randomized trials testing the efficacy of carotid endarterectomy (CEA) that were reported in the 1990s (Table 8.2).[14-18] These trials have had a profound impact on validating the indications for CEA in patients with carotid bifurcation atherosclerosis. The trials identified significant benefit in terms of stroke reduction for CEA in patients with specific levels of ICA stenosis. In particular, patients with symptomatic ICA stenosis of 70% to 99% had dramatic benefit from CEA. Patients with symptomatic ICA stenosis of 50% to 69% and patients with asymptomatic ICA stenosis between 60% and 99% also benefited from CEA, although to a lesser degree.

In the major North American trials of CEA in Table 8.2 (North American Symptomatic Carotid Endarterectomy Trial [NASCET][14] and Asymptomatic Carotid Atherosclerosis Study [ACAS][17]), stenosis severity was calculated from arteriograms by comparing the diameter of the minimal residual ICA lumen at the stenotic site with the diameter of the normal distal cervical ICA.[19] This approach to measuring the severity of stenosis is often referred to as the "NASCET method." The categories of carotid stenosis in the University of Washington criteria were developed long before the CEA trials by comparing the diameter of the residual ICA lumen at its narrowest point with an estimate of the diameter of the normal ICA bulb. Because the bulb has a greater diameter than the distal ICA, the two methods of measuring stenosis do not give the same calculated percentage of angiographic stenosis for the same lesion. Calculations of angiographic stenosis using the distal ICA as the reference vessel result in lower stenosis percentages than calculations using the bulb as the reference site. This effect is particularly striking for lesions in the middle of the stenosis range.

In a review of 1001 carotid angiograms, 34% of the ICAs were classified as having a 70% to 99% stenosis using the bulb as the reference vessel, but when the distal cervical ICA was used as the reference site, only 16% of the ICAs were classified as 70% to 99% stenosis.[20] More than 99% of stenosis measurements based on the distal ICA were less than the corresponding bulb-based measurement. Thus, the duplex stenosis criteria using the bulb as the reference vessel are not directly applicable to the results of the major clinical trials evaluating CEA.

Other Criteria for Internal Carotid Stenosis

Since the randomized CEA trials were completed, additional duplex criteria have been developed by comparing duplex scan results to angiographic ICA stenosis as determined by the NASCET measurement method. Such criteria are considered more useful in selection of patients for carotid intervention because they are directly applicable to the threshold levels of carotid stenosis addressed in the CEA trials. The initial studies addressing the issue of duplex criteria relevant to the CEA trials were performed at the Oregon Health & Science University (OHSU).[10,21] Subsequent publications from many different institutions proposed different criteria for the identification of clinically relevant threshold levels of ICA stenosis.[22-27]

Recognizing that duplex criteria from different centers differed from the threshold levels of angiographic stenosis determined by the CEA trials, a panel of authorities from a variety of medical specialties assembled in 2002 to review the carotid ultrasound literature. The panel developed a consensus regarding the key components of the carotid ultrasound examination and reasonable criteria for stratification of ICA stenosis.[28] The consensus committee recommended that all carotid examinations be performed with gray-scale imaging, color Doppler,

---

TABLE 8.1

UNIVERSITY OF WASHINGTON VELOCITY AND SPECTRAL WAVEFORM CRITERIA FOR CLASSIFICATION OF ICA DISEASE

◾ ARTERIOGRAPHIC DIAMETER REDUCTION	◾ PEAK SYSTOLIC VELOCITY	◾ END-DIASTOLIC VELOCITY	◾ SPECTRAL WAVEFORM CHARACTERISTICS
0% (normal)	<125 cm/s	—	Minimal or no spectral broadening; boundary layer separation present in the carotid bulb
1%-15%	<125 cm/s	—	Spectral broadening during deceleration phase of systole only
16%-49%	<125 cm/s	—	Spectral broadening throughout systole
50%-79%	≥125 cm/s	<140 cm/s	Marked spectral broadening
80%-99%	≥125 cm/s	≥140 cm/s	Marked spectral broadening
100% (occlusion)	—	—	No flow signal in the ICA; decreased diastolic flow in the ipsilateral CCA

Diameter reduction is based on arteriographic methods that compared the residual ICA lumen diameter to the estimated diameter of the carotid bulb. Velocity criteria are based on the angle-adjusted velocity using a Doppler angle of ≤60 degrees.

TABLE 8.2

MAJOR RANDOMIZED TRIALS ASSESSING THE EFFICACY OF CEA

SYMPTOMATIC STENOSIS
North American Symptomatic Carotid Endarterectomy Trial (NASCET)[14]
European Carotid Surgery Trial (ECST)[15]
VA Cooperative Study # 309[16]

ASYMPTOMATIC STENOSIS
Asymptomatic Carotid Atherosclerosis Study (ACAS)[17]
Asymptomatic Carotid Surgery Trial (ACST)[18]

and Doppler spectral waveforms. Examinations should be performed by a credentialed vascular technologist in accordance with the standards of one of the recognized accrediting bodies, as discussed in Chapter 3. Doppler waveforms should be obtained with an insonation angle as close to 60 degrees as possible, but not exceeding 60 degrees, and the sample volume should be placed within the area of maximal stenosis. The panelists recommended the consistent use of relatively broad categories to classify the degree of ICA stenosis. The panel also concluded that Doppler is relatively inaccurate for subcategorizing ICA stenoses of less than 50% diameter reduction and recommended that these lesions be reported under a single less than 50% stenosis category and that subcategories for minor degrees of stenosis not be used.

The consensus panel noted that PSV is generally easy to obtain. However, the data suggested that reproducibility of PSV, even among experienced vascular technologists, is a significant problem, and PSV should not be used as a continuous variable in classifying carotid disease. Even so, the degree of stenosis determined by ICA PSV and the degree of narrowing of the ICA lumen seen on gray-scale and color Doppler imaging should correlate with PSV as the primary parameter for determining ICA stenosis. Additional parameters such as ICA/CCA ratio and ICA EDV are secondary parameters and should be employed as internal checks; they are especially useful when ICA PSV may not be representative of the extent of disease. After their discussions, the consensus panel recommended criteria stratifying ICA stenosis into specific categories relevant to the CEA trials (Table 8.3). For example, the threshold for a 70% or greater ICA stenosis as determined by the NASCET measurement method is a PSV of 230 cm/s or a ICA/CCA ratio of 4.0. It is important to point out that these criteria have not been subjected to much in the way of retrospective or prospective evaluation and do not represent the results of any one laboratory or study. They are not meant to serve as a substitute for continuous quality assurance in individual laboratories (see Chapter 4).

Special Cases of Internal Carotid Velocities and Waveforms

Bilateral high-grade ICA stenosis: Doppler-derived flow velocities from the ICA contralateral to an ICA occlusion or high-grade stenosis may indicate a higher degree of narrowing than is observed angiographically.[1] This is likely due to compensatory collateral flow. In this situation, overestimation of stenosis by duplex scanning is more common in less severe categories of stenosis than in higher severity categories.[29]

Carotid dissection: In cases of dissection of the CCA or ICA dissection flaps can be readily visible within the vessel lumen (Fig. 8.21) and can, in acute cases, be seen to flutter within the lumen. Spectral waveforms may exhibit a bidirectional or "to-and-fro" flow pattern with flow above and below the baseline reflecting flow in the true and false lumens (Fig. 8.22).

Carotid string sign: When the ICA is very severely narrowed over a relatively long distance, the ICA velocities may be depressed rather than elevated (Fig. 8.23).

Carotid artery aneurysms: Carotid artery aneurysms are rare. They become lined with thrombosis and place the patient at risk for stroke from either thrombosis or embolization (Fig. 8.24).

Heart failure/cardiac support devices: Severe heart failure results in dramatic decreases in cardiac output. In such cases, the ICA waveform is dramatically blunted with a delayed upstroke and depressed velocity (Fig. 8.25). Conversely, balloon pump support of a failing heart results in "spiked" internal carotid waveforms (Fig. 8.26).

TABLE 8.3

CONSENSUS PANEL RECOMMENDATIONS FOR CLASSIFICATION OF INTERNAL CAROTID ARTERY STENOSIS

Normal: ICA PSV < 125 cm/s and no visible plaque or intimal thickening. Normal arteries should also have an ICA/CCA ratio < 2.0 and ICA EDV < 40 cm/s.

ICA stenosis < 50%: ICA PSV < 125 cm/s with visible plaque or intimal thickening. Such arteries should also have an ICA/CCA ratio < 2.0 and an ICA EDV < 40 cm/s.

ICA stenosis of 50% to 69%: ICA PSV is 125-230 cm/s and there is visible plaque. Such arteries should also have an ICA/CCA ratio of 2.0-4.0 and an ICA EDV of 40-100 cm/s.

ICA stenosis ≥ 70%-99% but less than near occlusion: ICA PSV > 230 cm/s and visible plaque with lumen narrowing on gray-scale and color Doppler imaging. The higher the PSV, the more likely it is (higher positive predictive value) that there is severe disease. Such stenoses should also have an ICA/CCA ratio > 4.0 and an ICA EDV > 100 cm/s.

Near occlusion of the ICA: The velocity parameters may not apply. "Preocclusive" lesions may be associated with high, low, or undetectable velocity measurements. The diagnosis of near occlusion is therefore established primarily by demonstration of a markedly narrowed lumen with color Doppler. In some near-occlusive lesions, color or power Doppler can distinguish between near occlusion and occlusion by demonstrating a thin wisp of flow traversing the lesion.

Occlusion: There is no detectable patent lumen on gray-scale imaging and no flow with pulsed Doppler, color Doppler, or power Doppler. Near-occlusive lesions may be misdiagnosed as occlusions when only gray-scale ultrasound and pulsed Doppler spectral waveforms are used.

CCA, common carotid artery; EDV, end-diastolic velocity; ICA, internal carotid artery; ICA/CCA ratio, maximal ICA PSV divided by the maximal CCA PSV; PSV, peak systolic velocity.
From Grant EG, Benson CB, Moneta GL, et al. Carotid artery stenosis: Gray-scale and Doppler US diagnosis—Society of Radiologists in Ultrasound Consensus Conference. *Radiology* 2003;229:340-346.

CEREBROVASCULAR

FIGURE 8.21. A dissection flap (*arrow*) is visible in the lumen of the proximal common carotid artery (CCA) in this B-mode image.

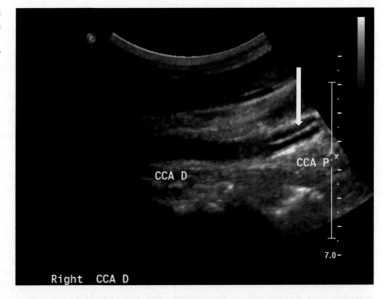

FIGURE 8.22. In the presence of a carotid dissection, spectral waveforms may exhibit a "to-and-fro" pattern with flow above and below the baseline, reflecting flow in the true and false lumens.

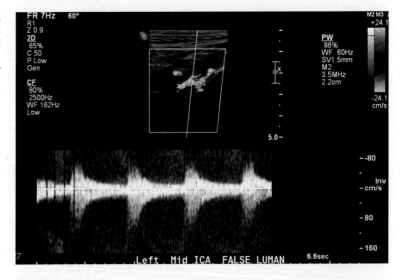

FIGURE 8.23. When the internal carotid artery (ICA) is very severely narrowed over a long segment (a carotid "string sign"), the peak velocities may be decreased rather than significantly elevated. In this example, a narrow flow channel is present with a PSV of 110 cm/s.

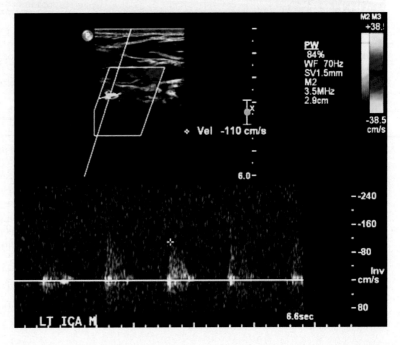

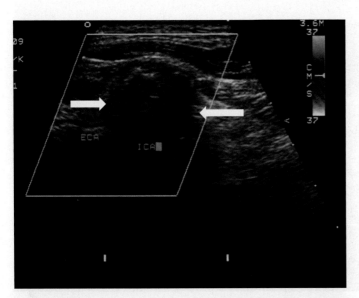

FIGURE 8.24. A transverse or cross-sectional color-flow image of an internal carotid artery (ICA) aneurysm: The walls of the aneurysm are indicated by the *arrows*. The aneurysm is almost completely filled with thrombus resulting in a dramatically narrowed central lumen. The external artery (ECA) lumen is also indicated on the color-flow image.

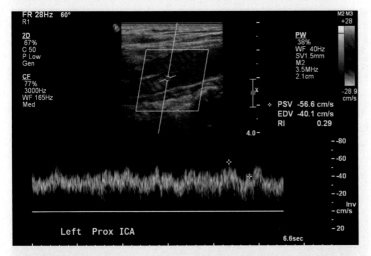

FIGURE 8.25. In patients with severe heart failure, the internal carotid artery (ICA) waveform is dramatically dampened with a delayed upstroke and decreased peak velocity. With some cardiac support devices, flow may be relatively continuous.

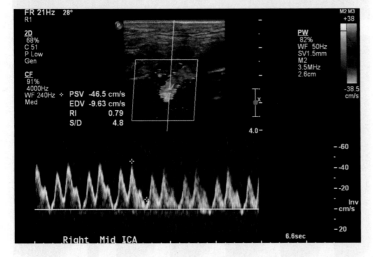

FIGURE 8.26. An intra-aortic balloon pump produces "spiked" internal carotid artery (ICA) spectral waveforms.

Stented carotid arteries: Duplex ultrasound criteria developed for the native ICA appear to be not strictly applicable to stented carotid arteries, especially for less severe degrees of in-stent stenosis. With rare exceptions, the number of patients in reported follow-up studies that have actually had in-stent restenosis is small, and no study has correlated the degree of stenosis or increase in ICA velocities with clinical symptoms or outcomes. These studies have also not evaluated the effect of the stented carotid artery on the contralateral nonstented artery. Currently, it appears that for more modest lesions, a higher PSV threshold than the usual 125 cm/s will be needed to identify a 50% or greater stenosis in a stented ICA, whereas criteria to detect high-grade stenosis in native ICAs still work reasonably well to identify high-grade stenosis in stented ICAs (Fig. 8.27).[30] This topic is more fully addressed in Chapter 10.

CEREBROVASCULAR

FIGURE 8.27. Duplex images of a high-grade carotid in-stent stenosis. *A,* The metallic stent is visualized within the common carotid artery (CCA) lumen on B-mode imaging. *B,* Color Doppler image shows the stent and narrowed CCA lumen. *C,* Spectral waveform with the Doppler sample volume positioned in the high-velocity jet. The peak systolic velocity (PSV) is 485 cm/s, with EDV of 249 cm/s.

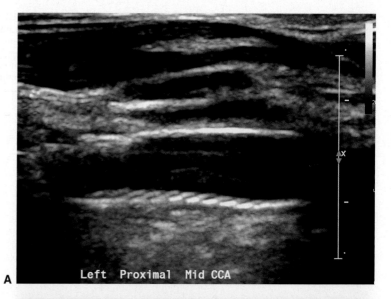

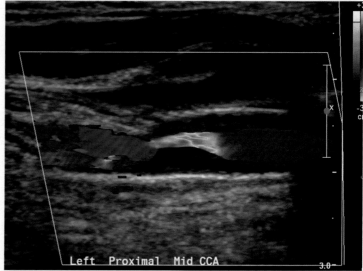

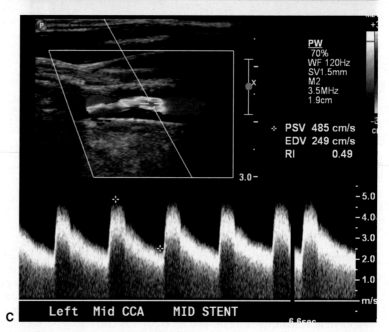

Common Carotid and External Carotid Stenosis

The criteria used for classifying disease in the ICA cannot be directly applied for lesions in the ECA or the CCA. However, as with the ICA, relative degrees of stenosis may be determined by the presence of plaque on B-mode imaging, disturbances in color Doppler flow, and spectral waveforms that show broadening and increases in PSV. Stenosis of more than 50% can be inferred by the presence of a focally increased PSV followed by poststenotic turbulence. Normally, the CCA spectral waveform has attributes of both the ICA and the ECA waveforms. Therefore, the CCA waveform will take on the features of the "normal" vessel (ICA or ECA) when the other is occluded. If there is a proximal CCA (or innominate artery) high-grade stenosis or occlusion, the ipsilateral CCA Doppler flow waveform will be dampened, with low PSV as compared with the contralateral side. Poststenotic turbulence also may be seen. There are no widely employed validated criteria that provide categories of diameter reduction for stenosis in the CCA or ECA. A focal increase in PSV at the origin of the ECA to greater than about 200 cm/s is often considered as indicative of a 50% or greater stenosis. A recent comparison of carotid duplex scans and CT angiography from 115 common carotid arteries in 62 patients concluded that a common carotid PSV of ≥182 cm/s identified a CCA stenosis of 50% or greater with a sensitivity of 64% and a specificity of 88%.[31]

CONCLUSION

Carotid duplex scanning is safe, efficient, and highly accurate. Inevitably, the interpretation of ultrasound studies has changed somewhat since the pioneering work of Dr. Strandness and his laboratory at the University of Washington. However, despite advances in alternative noninvasive imaging of the carotid arteries, duplex ultrasound remains the dominant noninvasive method for assessing the extracranial carotid and vertebral arteries.

References

1. Abou-ZamZam AM Jr, Moneta GL, Edwards JM, et al. Is a single preoperative duplex scan sufficient for planning bilateral carotid endarterectomy? *J Vasc Surg* 2000;31:282-288.
2. Goes E, Janssens W, Maillet B, et al. Tissue characterization of atheromatous plaques: Correlation between ultrasound image and histological findings. *J Clin Ultrasound* 1990;18:611-617.
3. Gray-Weale AC, Graham JC, Burnett JR, et al. Carotid artery atheroma: Comparison of pre-operative B-mode ultrasound appearance with carotid endarterectomy specimen. *J Cardiovasc Surg* 1988;29:115-123.
4. Bock RW, Lusby RJ. Carotid plaque morphology and interpretation of echolucent lesion. In Labs KH, et al (eds). *Diagnostic Vascular Ultrasound*. London: Edward Arnold, 1992, pp 225-236.
5. El-Barghouty N, Geroulakos G, Nicolaides A, et al. Computer assisted carotid plaque characterization. *Eur J Vasc Endovasc Surg* 1995;9:389-393.
6. Effeney DJ, Ehrenfeld WK, Stoney RJ, et al. Fibromuscular dysplasia of the internal carotid artery. *World J Surg* 1979;3:179-184.
7. Roederer GO, Langlois YE, Chan AT, et al. Ultrasonic duplex scanning of the extracranial carotid arteries: Improved accuracy using new features from the carotid artery. *J Cardiovasc Ultrasonogr* 1982;1:373-380.
8. Strandness DE Jr. Extracranial arterial disease. In *Duplex Scanning in Vascular Disorders*. New York: Raven, 1990, pp 92-120.
9. Roederer GO, Langlois YE, Jager KA, et al. A simple spectral parameter for accurate classification of severe carotid artery disease. *Bruit* 1989;3:174-178.
10. Moneta GL, Edwards JM, Chitwood RW, et al. Correlation of North American Symptomatic Carotid Endarterectomy Trial (NASCET): Angiographic definition of 70% to 90% internal carotid artery stenosis with duplex scanning. *J Vasc Surg* 1993;17:152-159.
11. Bendick PJ, Glover JL. Hemodynamic evaluation of the vertebral arteries by duplex ultrasound. *Surg Clin North Am* 1990;70:235-244.
12. Kim ESH, Thompson M, Nacion KM, et. al. Radiologic importance of a high-resistance vertebral artery Doppler waveform on carotid duplex ultrasonography. *J Ultrasound Med* 2010;29:1161-1165.
13. Kumar SM, Wang JC, Barry MC, et al. Carotid stump syndrome: Outcome from surgical management. *Eur J Vasc Endovasc Surg* 2001;21:214-219.
14. North American Symptomatic Carotid Endarterectomy Trial (NASCET) Collaborators. Beneficial effect of carotid endarterectomy in patients with high-grade carotid stenosis. *N Engl J Med* 1991;325:445-453.
15. European Carotid Surgery Trialists' Collaborative (ECST) Group. MRC European Carotid Surgery Trial: Interim results for symptomatic patients with severe (70-99%) or with mild (0-29%) carotid stenosis. *Lancet* 1996;347:1591-1593.
16. Mayberg MR, Wilson SE, Yatsu F, et al. Carotid endarterectomy and prevention of cerebral ischemia in symptomatic carotid stenosis: Veterans Affairs Cooperative Studies Program 309 Trialist Group. *JAMA* 1991;266:3289-3294.
17. Executive Committee for Asymptomatic Carotid Atherosclerosis Study. Endarterectomy for asymptomatic carotid artery stenosis. *JAMA* 1995;273:1421-1428.
18. MRC Asymptomatic Carotid Surgery Trial (ACST) Collaborative Group. Prevention of disabling and fatal strokes by successful carotid endarterectomy in patients without recent neurological symptoms: Randomized controlled trial. *Lancet* 2004;363:1491-1502.
19. North American Symptomatic Carotid Endarterectomy Trial (NASCET) Steering Committee. North American Symptomatic Carotid Endarterectomy Trial: Methods, patient characteristics, and progress. *Stroke* 1991;22:711-720.
20. Rothwell PM, Gibson RJ, Slattery J, et al. Equivalence of measurements of carotid stenosis: A comparison of three methods on 1001 angiograms. *Stroke* 1994;25:2435-2439.
21. Moneta GL, Edwards JM, Papanicolaou G, et al. Screening for asymptomatic internal carotid artery stenosis: Duplex criteria for discriminating 60% to 99% stenosis. *J Vasc Surg* 1995;21:989-994.
22. AbuRahma AF, Robinson PA, Stickler DL, et al. Proposed new duplex classification for threshold stenoses used in various symptomatic and asymptomatic carotid endarterectomy trials. *Ann Vasc Surg* 1998;12:349-358.
23. Carpenter JP, Lexa FJ, Davis JT. Determination of duplex Doppler ultrasound criteria appropriate to the North American Symptomatic Carotid Endarterectomy Trial. *Stroke* 1996;27:695-699.
24. Hood DB, Mattos MA, Mansour A, et al. Prospective evaluation of new duplex criteria to identify 70% internal carotid artery stenosis. *J Vasc Surg* 1996;23:254-261.
25. Carpenter JP, Lexa FJ, Davis JT. Determination of 60% or greater carotid artery stenosis by duplex Doppler ultrasonography. *J Vasc Surg* 1995;22:97-703.
26. Browman MW, Cooperberg PL, Harrison PB, et al. Duplex ultrasonography criteria for internal carotid stenosis of more than 70% diameter: Angiographic correlation and receiver operating characteristic curve analysis. *Can Assoc Radiol J* 1995;46:291-295.
27. Neale ML, Chambers JL, Kelly AT, et al. Reappraisal of duplex criteria to assess significant carotid stenosis with special reference to reports from the North American Symptomatic Carotid Endarterectomy Trial and the European Carotid Surgery Trial. *J Vasc Surg* 1994;20:642-649.
28. Grant EG, Benson CB, Moneta GL, et al. Carotid artery stenosis: Grayscale and Doppler US diagnosis—Society of Radiologists in Ultrasound Consensus Conference. *Radiology* 2003;229:340-346.
29. Fujitani RM, Mills JL, Wang LM, et al. The effect of unilateral internal carotid arterial occlusion upon contralateral duplex study: Criteria for accurate interpretation. *J Vasc Surg* 1992;16:459-467.
30. Setacci C, Chisci E, Setacci F, et al. Grading carotid intra-stent re-stenosis: A six-year follow-up study. *Stroke* 2008;30:1189-1196.
31. Slovut DP, Romero JM, Hannon KM, et al. Detection of common carotid artery stenosis using duplex ultrasonography: A validation study with computed tomographic angiography. *J Vasc Surg* 2010;51:65-70.

CEREBROVASCULAR

CHAPTER 9 ■ TRANSCRANIAL DUPLEX IMAGING

SHEILA M. BYRD-RAYNOR AND WATSON B. SMITH

The aim of this chapter is to review the role of transcranial duplex imaging (TCI) in the routine vascular laboratory setting. TCI is an advanced ultrasound technique typically used in association with extracranial carotid and vertebral duplex scanning (see Chapter 8). This chapter discusses the hemodynamic consequences of carotid stenosis on the cerebral circulation and how these pertain to TCI examination findings. Illustrative diagrams of the cerebral circulation are introduced to assist both the new and the experienced user in the understanding of collateral flow patterns. Advanced ultrasound scanning techniques and tips for performing the study are also covered.

INDICATIONS AND APPLICATIONS

Although the brain has a high metabolic rate, neurons do not store significant energy reserves. Therefore, the brain is critically dependent on constant blood flow through the cerebral arteries to maintain normal activity. The brain is so intolerant of ischemia that an interruption of cerebral blood flow (CBF) can result in loss of consciousness in as little as 5 seconds. Hence, adequate CBF must be maintained throughout a variety of physiologic conditions, including a circulatory crisis. In this situation, the maintenance of flow to the brain is the number-one priority. Whereas the usual cardiovascular response is widespread vasoconstriction, the cerebral regulating vessels dilate. For these important reasons, there is clinical interest in assessing the cerebral circulation with noninvasive techniques such as transcranial Doppler ultrasound.

Vascular laboratories commonly receive requests to perform carotid duplex examinations on patients who have experienced a transient ischemic attack (TIA) or stroke. This is done to evaluate the extracranial common carotid artery (CCA) and its branches for atherosclerosis and other causes of neurologic symptoms. A high-grade stenosis or occlusion in the internal carotid artery (ICA) can act as a source of emboli to the brain and also produce hemodynamic impairment.[1,2] Although such lesions are often symptomatic, there is a chance that no symptoms will occur and CBF could be virtually unaffected, even in the case of a total ICA occlusion. It is for these reasons that clinicians may request further information about the cerebral circulation based on TCI in order to determine the best management for an individual patient. In a simple statement, Dr. D. Eugene Strandness Jr, once reminded us that "In order to properly treat disorders of the vascular system, it is necessary to make a correct diagnosis and precisely define the location and extent of involvement."

A routine carotid duplex scan can identify disease in the extracranial arteries to the brain, but it cannot predict the downstream effects on the cerebral circulation. To determine the effects of carotid disease on the brain for any individual, a transcranial Doppler examination (TCD) or TCI may be utilized. These tests directly measure flow velocities in the large arteries of the brain and define collateral flow patterns that can be useful for planning treatment. Unfortunately, many anatomic variations of the hemodynamically complete and well-balanced circle of Willis are commonly observed. Based on more than 50 radiologic and anatomic studies, Lippert and Pabst[3] found that in about 50% of the population, at least one artery in the circle of Willis is either absent or hypoplastic. These anatomic variations reduce the collateral potential and increase the risk of stroke in patients with severe stenosis in an ICA.[4] The circle of Willis behaves as a pressure equalizer and, therefore, takes part in the regulation of CBF before vasodilatation of the resistance arteries is involved. Consequently, knowledge of the compensatory capacity of the circle of Willis is crucial for neurosurgeons, vascular surgeons, and other specialists when a procedure in the intracranial or extracranial cerebral arteries is to be attempted.[5] Such procedures include carotid endarterectomy and carotid angioplasty with stenting. In addition, TCI can provide an indirect assessment of the status of the distal cerebral vascular bed with regard to vasodilatation or vasoconstriction.[6] In combination with a carotid duplex study, TCI constitutes a complete noninvasive cerebrovascular examination and can provide additional valuable information about a patient's hemodynamic status. However, as mentioned previously, TCI is a targeted, advanced ultrasound examination—it should be used on selected patients and is not necessary in every individual who is referred for a carotid duplex scan.

ANATOMY OF THE INTRACRANIAL ARTERIES

The middle cerebral artery (MCA), anterior cerebral artery (ACA), posterior cerebral artery (PCA), and the basilar artery (BA) are considered the basal cerebral vessels. These are conducting vessels of the intracranial circulation and are muscular by nature. Compared with the aorta, which is approximately 25 mm in diameter, the basal cerebral vessels are small and range between 2 and 4 mm in diameter. The basal cerebral circulation sits within the relatively rigid bony structure of the cranium at the base of the brain. The intracranial contents are incompressible, and therefore, any increase in the volume of one component (brain tissue, blood, or cerebral spinal fluid) must be associated with a corresponding decrease in another. In contrast to the blood supply to many other organs, CBF must be kept within a narrow range, which averages approximately 55 mL/100 g of brain tissue/min.[7] On the basis of studies on cerebral cortical slices by both K.A.C. Elliott (1903–1986) in Montreal and Henry McIlwain (1912–1992) in London, it was estimated that the majority of the oxidative metabolism of the brain is devoted to the support of neural conduction and transmission. It has been established that the brain stores no oxygen and has no significant stores of glycogen. Thus, failure of CBF due to vascular occlusion can cause irreversible damage after about 8 minutes. Similar damage will occur after about 90 minutes of severe hypoglycemia.

Blood flow is delivered to the brain via four main arteries in the neck—two ICAs and two vertebral arteries. For the purposes of this chapter, we refer to these extracranial vessels as *inflow vessels* to the brain because they carry blood flow to the cerebral circulation. At the base of the brain, the ICAs bifurcate to form the MCA and ACA. These vessels are commonly referred to as the *anterior circulation*. They are mainly responsible for delivering blood flow to the temporal, parietal, and frontal regions of the brain if there is no disease or anatomic anomaly. The two vertebral arteries join to form the BA after they have entered the foramen magnum. The BA courses toward the level of the anterior circulation vessels and then divides into the right and left PCAs. This system is referred to as *posterior circulation* and delivers blood to the region of the brainstem.[8]

The intracranial vessels are referred to as *outflow* vessels because they directly supply the brain parenchyma. This terminology provides a simple way to relate the effects of extracranial arterial disease to the downstream effects measured in the cerebral circulation. Figure 9.1 presents the *inflow/outflow* concept as a stylized map of the extracranial and intracranial circulations, so the complete network can be easily visualized. The distinction between *inflow* and *outflow* vessels is drawn at the angle of the jaw. This level was chosen because it is approximately the point at which the extracranial carotid duplex examination ends and the TCI begins.

Circle of Willis

The anterior and posterior circulations are linked together by small connecting vessels, the single anterior communicating artery (ACoA) and a posterior communicating artery (PCoA) on each side; this unique structure is called the *circle of Willis*. These small connecting vessels form a link between separate flow systems in the brain—the anterior and posterior circulations via the PCoAs and the right and left hemispheres via the ACoA. This arrangement provides backup blood flow delivery should one or more of the contributing arteries become diseased. Although the circle of Willis appears to be an effective system for maintaining constant blood flow, less

than half of the human population has a complete circle of Willis.[3] The communicating arteries are frequently hypoplastic or absent, so the shunting of blood flow from one artery to another may be ineffective in times of need. It is difficult to determine the completeness and the capacity of the circle of Willis to supply collateral flow without carotid compression maneuvers; therefore, it is rarely assessed without a compelling indication.

Flow rates in the communicating arteries are normally small but sufficient to keep these vessels active. The flows arise from pressure phase delays between the right and left sides of the circle of Willis, which are the consequence of the asymmetry introduced by the brachiocephalic artery. Because the volume flow rates along these arteries are normally about two orders of magnitude smaller than the volume outflow rates in the other cerebral arteries,[9] even magnetic resonance angiography (MRA) techniques may not be able to detect the presence of the communicating arteries in subjects with a complete circle of Willis or with anatomic variations involving these arteries. The most frequent anatomic variations reported in Lippert and Pabst[3] are shown in Figure 9.2.

INTERPRETATION

Step 1. Goals of the Examination

For patients with extracranial carotid stenosis, the main goals of the TCI examination are to detect the presence or absence of collateral flow, determine the pathways of collateral flow (this may prove important for surgical planning or intervention), comment on the symmetry of the MCA velocities between hemispheres, and in some cases, relate the findings to established normal ranges. The TCI examination can also identify significant stenoses in the intracranial cerebral arteries. This information is meant to give the clinician an indication of how well the patient is or is not compensated for the inflow disease. Whether intracranial collateral flow is present or absent is largely determined by the hemodynamic effects of the extracranial carotid stenosis.

Step 2. Flow Velocities

There are well-established normal values for TCD flow velocities in the basal cerebral vessels, as listed in Table 9.1.[10-13] These cerebral vessels have a consistent flow velocity relationship to each other. The MCA velocity is usually the highest because the majority of blood from the ICA flows directly into the MCA territory. The ACA and PCA supply less brain tissue, so their flow velocities are lower. This results in the important relationship of MCA > ACA > PCA = BA for the relative flow velocities. Recognizing this relationship is the first step in the interpretation of TCI studies. Mean Doppler flow velocities (time-averaged peak velocities) are generally used in TCI. These are often provided directly by the ultrasound machine, but they can also be calculated from peak systolic velocity (PSV) and end-diastolic velocity (EDV) using a simple equation similar to that for mean arterial blood pressure.

$$\text{Mean velocity} = (\text{PSV} - \text{EDV})/3 + \text{EDV}$$

Flow velocities show a consistent decrease with increasing age.[14] These findings correlate well with age-related studies of CBF.[15] This supports the validity and sensitivity of TCD to estimate changes in CBF based on velocity data.

In nonimaging TCD studies, velocities are acquired at a zero-degree Doppler angle. However, because of the tortuosity of the intracranial vessels and the lack of an image, this

**DEFINITION OF INFLOW VESSELS
AND
OUTFLOW VESSELS**

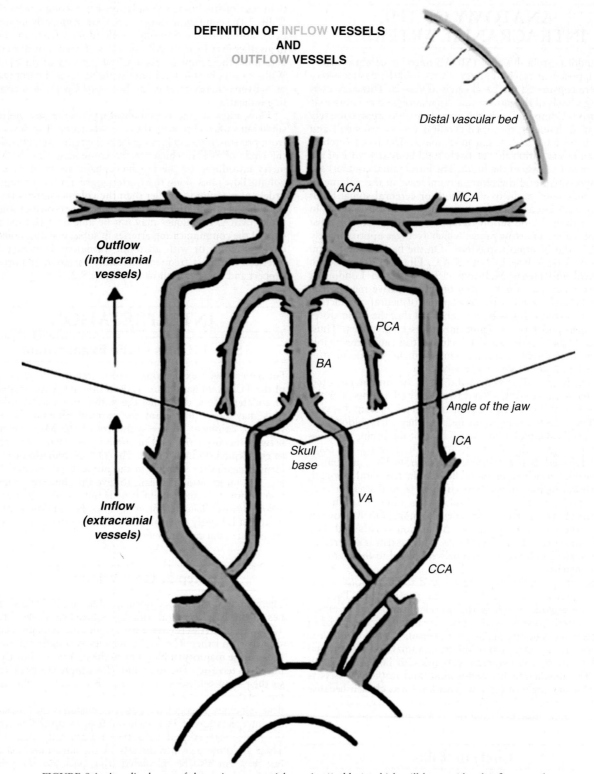

FIGURE 9.1. A stylized map of the main extracranial arteries (*in blue*), which will be considered *inflow* vessels, and the intracranial vessels (*in green*), which will be considered *outflow* vessels for the purposes of this chapter. (Copyright © Sheila Raynor.)

angle is only an assumption, and measurements are realistically acquired between 0 and 30 degrees. Because nonimaging TCD was the original study method in the 1980s, the majority of published data are based on these assumptions with regard to Doppler angle. When TCI became available, the technologist had the option to angle correct. Although this is a topic of ongoing debate, many vascular laboratories using TCI continue to leave the Doppler angle set at zero degree so their results can be compared with data reported in the literature.

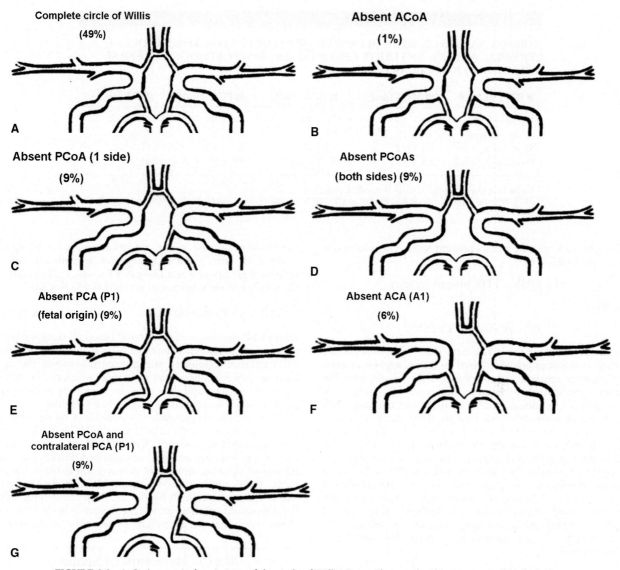

Complete circle of Willis

(49%)

A

Absent ACoA

(1%)

B

Absent PCoA (1 side)

(9%)

C

Absent PCoAs

(both sides) (9%)

D

Absent PCA (P1)

(fetal origin) (9%)

E

Absent ACA (A1)

(6%)

F

**Absent PCoA and
contralateral PCA (P1)**

(9%)

G

FIGURE 9.2. *A-G*, Anatomical variations of the circle of Willis. For each case, the absent artery and its frequency are indicated, according to Lippert H, Pabst R. *Arterial Variations in Man: Classification and Frequency.* Munich: JF Bergmann, 1985 (depicted on only one side, but it can also be absent on the other side).

Step 3. Side-to-Side Comparisons

Although it is useful to compare TCI findings from a specific patient with published values, the most helpful comparisons are often within an individual. Comparison of the right and left MCAs, right and left ACAs, and right and left PCAs often gives a better idea of what the "normal" values are for that individual, because heart rate, blood pressure, and cardiac output are all matched. A patient referred for a TCI examination will often have extracranial pathology that affects interpretation of the intracranial findings. For example, in unilateral extracranial ICA stenosis, the downstream effects of a diseased side can be compared with a normal side.

Step 4. Hemodynamics and Indices

Before beginning a TCI examination, it is helpful to know whether to expect evidence of collateral flow based on simple hemodynamic principles. Figure 9.3 reviews the dynamics of an arterial stenosis. In a mild or moderate stenosis, there is

a slight increase in velocity (*dashed white line*) through the stenosis but then a normalization of velocity distal to the stenosis, because very little energy is lost. If we look at the corresponding change in pressure (*dashed green line*), there is a mild decrease through the stenosis but a recovery of pressure distally. In effect, this indicates that the *inflow* to the cerebral circulation should be relatively unaffected by mild or moderate stenoses. In this situation, a TCI examination may not demonstrate any collateral flow patterns.

Some clinicians have questioned whether TCI adds any valuable information at lower levels of carotid stenosis. However, even at lower levels of stenosis, it can be useful to evaluate the symmetry or asymmetry between the right and the left hemispheres, because there may already be vasodilatory mechanisms activated to maintain CBF at a constant level. In this case, measuring a parameter such as pulsatility index (PI), resistance index (RI), or mean RI may show subtle changes that would otherwise go undetected. Indices have indeed been a major part of TCD interpretation in the past. They are thought to provide indirect information about the small regulatory vessels that are inaccessible by TCI but play an important

TABLE 9.1

NORMAL VALUES OF MEAN BLOOD FLOW VELOCITY FOR THE MIDDLE CEREBRAL ARTERY, ANTERIOR CEREBRAL ARTERY, POSTERIOR CEREBRAL ARTERY, AND BASILAR ARTERY[a]

■ REFERENCE	■ MCA (cm/s)	■ ACA (cm/s)	■ PCA (cm/s)	■ BA (cm/s)
Aaslid et al[10]	62 ± 12	51 ± 12	44 ± 11	48 mean
Hennerici et al[11]	58 ± 12	53 ± 10	37 ± 10	36 ± 12
Ringelstein et al[12]	55 ± 12	49 ± 9	40 ± 10	41 ± 10
Harders[13]	65 ± 17	50 ± 13	40 ± 9	39 ± 9

[a]Values are given as mean velocity ± standard deviation.
ACA, anterior cerebral artery; BA, basilar artery; MCA, middle cerebral artery; PCA, posterior cerebral artery.

role in maintaining CBF at a constant level. The two major historical indices: PI[16]

$$PI = (PSV - EDV)/\text{mean velocity}$$

and RI[17]

$$RI = (PSV - EDV)/PSV$$

are found throughout the literature on TCD.[18] The introduction of these indices was originally based on the assumption of interplay between resistance and compliance of the vascular bed. The accuracy and tendency of these two indices are nearly identical in most clinical applications, and both indices seem to change with alterations in vasomotor tone seen in vasomotor reserve testing.[19] Because the cerebral conduit vessels such as the MCA are relatively stiff, we assume that the cerebral arterial compliance is practically negligible, and therefore, the indices must represent changes in resistance. The problem with using PI or RI is that changes in resistance are often small and can be overshadowed by changes in cardiovascular factors such as blood pressure. Therefore, subtle changes in central factors may influence the PI or RI without the investigator being aware of such influence.

A recently derived parameter, the mean RI, could also prove useful.[20]

$$\text{Mean resistance index} = \text{mean blood pressure (mmHg)}/\\ \text{mean blood flow velocity (cm/s)}$$

This index includes one of the major cardiovascular influences (blood pressure) in conjunction with flow velocity. Although systemic blood pressure is not often recorded during TCI examinations, it should become a more common part of the examination because it can aid in interpretation of relative changes. Of note, mean RI should not be confused with the term *cerebral vascular resistance* (CVR), which is calculated as the ratio of cerebral perfusion pressure (CPP) to CBF:

$$CVR = CPP\,(mmHg)/CBF\,(mL/100\ g\ brain/min)$$

where CPP equals the mean arterial blood pressure minus the intracranial pressure. This ratio cannot be calculated from TCD ultrasound velocity measurements; however, the mean RI is an indicator of cerebral resistance, which can be derived from velocity data and does consider the effects of changes in mean arterial blood pressure on the flow velocities.

These indices are generally calculated only on the most distal velocity measurement taken from the MCA trunk in order to look for indirect evidence of vasodilatation or vasoconstriction of the downstream distal vascular bed. Indices are a useful way of showing differences in waveform shape in numeric terms. For example, if the PI for the MCA on the unaffected side is 1.0 whereas the PI for the MCA on the stenotic side is 0.5, this would reflect an important difference in the waveform shape and indicate an asymmetry between the hemispheres.

Step 5. Detection of Stenosis

As with stenosis in the extracranial carotid arteries, intracranial arterial stenosis is associated with characteristic changes in the normal flow pattern: a focal velocity increase, localized turbulence, and a poststenotic decrease in velocity (Fig. 9.4). Slow systolic acceleration and decreased pulsatility may be observed in the spectral waveform distal to the stenosis, and a Doppler bruit may

FIGURE 9.3. Changes in velocity (*white lines*) and associated changes in pressure (*green lines*) through a focal stenosis. The *dashed lines* represent changes through a mild or moderate stenosis; the solid lines represent changes associated with a severe stenosis. V_1 is the stenotic site; V_2 is the poststenotic segment.

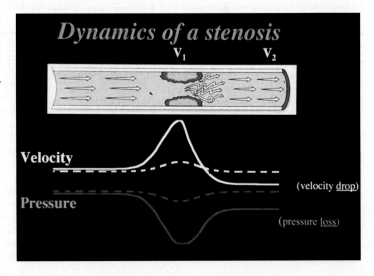

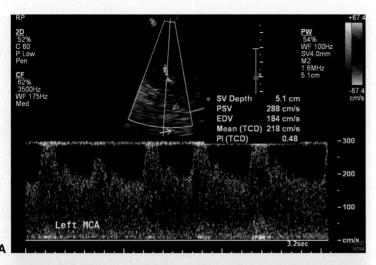

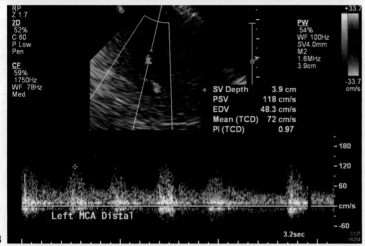

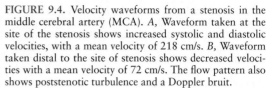

FIGURE 9.4. Velocity waveforms from a stenosis in the middle cerebral artery (MCA). *A*, Waveform taken at the site of the stenosis shows increased systolic and diastolic velocities, with a mean velocity of 218 cm/s. *B*, Waveform taken distal to the site of stenosis shows decreased velocities with a mean velocity of 72 cm/s. The flow pattern also shows poststenotic turbulence and a Doppler bruit.

be present. Since many factors other than the presence of a stenosis influence the velocity of flow in the cerebral arteries (hematocrit, blood volume, blood pressure, cardiac output), absolute velocity thresholds for identifying intracranial arterial stenosis may not be reliable. In general, a focally increased mean velocity of ≥80 cm/s with a decrease of more than 30 cm/s distally is suggestive of a 50% or greater stenosis in the MCA. Higher velocity thresholds, such as ≥100 cm/s or ≥120 cm/s, provide a higher positive predictive value for 50% or greater MCA stenosis.[21-23]

Whenever the previously described normal velocity relationship of MCA > ACA > PCA = BA is disrupted, an abnormality in the basal cerebral arteries should be suspected. Globally high or low flow states may be present. Hyper-dynamic flow is common in younger patients and has been observed with traumatic head injury. Increased velocities in the intracranial arteries can also occur in response to collateral flow and arteriovenous malformations, although in these cases, the velocity increase is typically not focal but is present throughout the involved arterial segments (Fig. 9.5). Diffusely increased velocities occur with vasospasm associated with subarachnoid hemorrhage, and mean velocities of up to 250 cm/s and higher have been observed in that setting. Mean velocity criteria for grading MCA stenosis associated with vasospasm include mild stenosis (>120 cm/s), mild to moderate stenosis (120–150 cm/s), moderate stenosis (150–200 cm/s) and severe stenosis (>200 cm/s).[24]

Step 6. Collateral Flow Patterns

In contrast to a mild or moderate lesion, when a severe extracranial arterial stenosis is present, there are more dramatic hemodynamic consequences. As shown in Figure 9.3, in a severe arterial stenosis the velocity (*solid white line*) shows a marked increase through the stenosis and a drop beyond the stenosis. The corresponding change in pressure (*solid green line*) shows a significant drop through the stenosis, but only a partial recovery beyond the stenosis. In this scenario, a significant pressure gradient develops between the right and left extracranial *inflow* vessels and the intracranial *outflow* vessels of the cerebral circulation. At this critical level, the rerouting of flow will occur very quickly through the collateral pathways. However, the specific path is determined largely by the configuration of the circle of Willis and the status of the communicating arteries (anterior and posterior). Therefore, when a significant extracranial carotid stenosis is present, TCI studies yield invaluable clinical information.

As mentioned previously, differentiating the high velocities associated with collateralization (compensatory flow) from the high velocities associated with a focal stenosis is a potential interpretation pitfall (Figs. 9.4 and 9.5). Keep in mind that the comparatively high flow velocities in collateral channels will be found *throughout all* collateral pathways from the aortic arch branches to the brain. These elevated velocities are due to increased flow volume and show little resemblance to the changes produced by a focal stenosis. The inflow/outflow cerebrovascular map is useful in this context because it enables the user to view the entire network and anticipate in what vessels they may expect increased velocities from compensatory flow.

Alastruey et al[9] developed a computer model of pressure and flow wave propagation in compliant vessels from the left ventricle to the largest arteries that supply the circle of Willis. These authors evaluated the collateral function of a "complete" circle of Willis and its most frequent anatomic variations under normal conditions and after occlusion of an ICA or vertebral artery

CEREBROVASCULAR

FIGURE 9.5. Velocity waveforms from a middle cerebral artery (MCA) with diffusely increased velocities but no focal flow disturbance. *A,* Waveform from the proximal MCA shows increased systolic and diastolic velocities, with a mean velocity of 95 cm/s. *B,* Waveform from the distal MCA shows a similar normal flow pattern with a mean velocity of 79 cm/s.

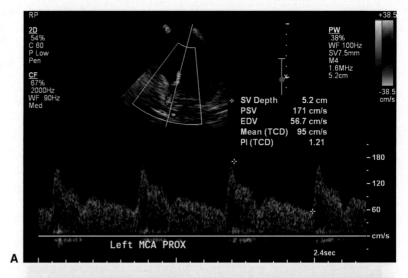

A

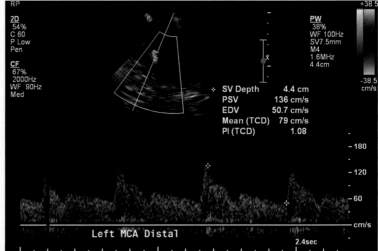

B

(VA). Their research suggests that the system does not require collateral pathways through the communicating arteries to adequately perfuse the brain of normal subjects. They also showed that the ACoA is a more critical collateral pathway than the PCoAs if an ICA is occluded. Occlusions of the VAs proved to be far less critical than occlusions of the ICAs. The worst scenario, in terms of reduction in mean cerebral outflow, is a circle of Willis without the first segment of an ACA combined with an occlusion of the contralateral ICA and a missing PCoA.

Identification of the presence or absence of collateral flow patterns is based on a few basic principles:

- Comparison of TCI flow velocity measurements acquired during the examination with the key relationship model MCA > ACA > PCA. If, for instance, the ACA velocity was greater than the MCA and PCA, this may represent collateral flow through the ACA. If the velocity in the first segment of the PCA (P1) was elevated above the MCA and ACA, this could indicate collateral flow coming through the PCA into the anterior circulation.
- Comparison of findings with the normal flow directions for each artery in the nondiseased state. Because the cerebral arteries (except the MCA) can change their flow direction to shunt collateral flow to an ischemic territory, prior knowledge of the normal flow directions of arteries in the intracranial circulation is essential.
- Understanding of the approximate depth at which each artery should be found, along with its placement in

relation to anatomic landmarks such as the sphenoid wing, petrous ridge, midline (falx), or cerebral peduncles, is critical to accurate vessel identification.
- Knowledge of the main collateral pathways. Being aware that the blood flow will move along the path of least resistance, for example, through a large ACoA rather than through a small PCoA.

There are three major collateral pathways that will be reviewed in the context of a significant stenosis or occlusion of an ICA: intracranial crossover, posterior to anterior, and external to internal. General TCI findings are noted both through a schematic diagram and also in reference to TCI images.

Intracranial Crossover via the ACoA

With intracranial crossover, blood is shunted from the unaffected carotid system to the stenotic side through the ACoA (Fig. 9.6A). This appears to be the first collateral pathway to be recruited because it is generally the path of least resistance, but it is dependent on the presence and diameter of the ACoA. The amount of flow that can pass through the ACoA is directly proportional to the caliber of this vessel. The best identifying feature of intracranial crossover is a 25% higher velocity in the ACA *contralateral* to the ICA lesion compared with the MCA, as shown in Figure 9.6.

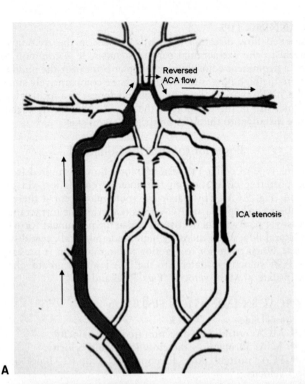

A

FIGURE 9.6. *A*, A stylized map of the arterial network showing the pathway (*in red*) for intracranial crossover from the right to the left hemisphere via the ACoA. Note that the flow direction in the left ACA reverses when this occurs. *B*, Mean velocity in the ACA contralateral to the extracranial carotid stenosis is increased to 113 cm/s (more than 25% higher than the MCA contralateral to the extracranial carotid stenosis). *C*, Mean velocity in the MCA contralateral to the extracranial carotid stenosis is 77 cm/s.

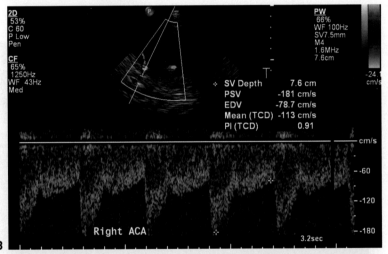

B

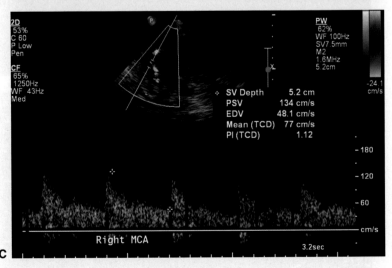

C

TYPICAL EXAMINATION FINDINGS

(Red = flow *toward* the transducer; blue = flow *away* from the transducer.)

Normal Side

- MCA: normal flow direction (red) and velocity.
- ACA: normal flow direction (blue), velocity elevated at least 25% above the adjacent MCA due to compensatory flow (Figs. 9.6 and 9.7).
- PCA: normal flow direction (P1, red; P2, blue as the artery flows toward then bends away from the transducer) and velocity.
- BA: normal flow direction (blue) and velocity.
- Note: There will be compensatory flow noted throughout the CCA and into the ICA, which will elevate velocities throughout this system.

Significant Carotid Stenosis Side

- MCA: normal flow direction (red), velocity will be dependent on the amount of collateral flow being delivered.
- ACA: reversed flow direction (red), turbulence may be present because the flow has just passed through a small collateral channel (ACoA) into the larger channel of the ACA (Fig. 9.7).
- PCA: normal flow direction (P1, red; P2, blue) and velocity.

SCANNING TIPS

Reversed flow direction is usually present in the ACA ipsilateral to the extracranial carotid stenosis. It is common to find a prominent color-flow or Doppler bruit near the midline where the high flow is forced through the comparatively small ACoA. This may act like a stenosis and appear as a focal velocity increase in the position of the ACoA followed by turbulence distally into the ACA on the ispilateral side.

Posterior to Anterior Collateral

In this type of collateral pattern, blood flow is shunted from the posterior circulation to the anterior circulation via the PCoA (Fig. 9.8A). This particular route may occur if there is an absent or hypoplastic ACA, thus rendering the intracranial crossover pathway ineffective. It is also the prominent form of collateral flow when there are high-grade bilateral carotid stenoses. When posterior to anterior collateralization is present, the PCA velocity ipsilateral to the ICA lesion is greater than the ipsilateral MCA velocity (Figs. 9.8B and C).

TYPICAL EXAMINATION FINDINGS

Normal Side

- MCA: norml flow direction (red) and velocity.
- ACA: normal flow direction (blue) and velocity.
- PCA: normal flow direction (P1, red; P2, blue) and velocity.

FIGURE 9.7. *A,* Color-flow image showing normal flow direction (*blue*) in the ACA contralateral to the extracranial carotid stenosis (*arrow*). *B,* Color-flow image showing reversed flow direction (*red*) in the ACA ipsilateral to the extracranial carotid stenosis (*arrow*). In both images MCA flow is in the normal direction (*red*).

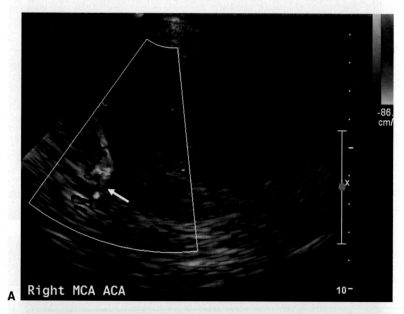

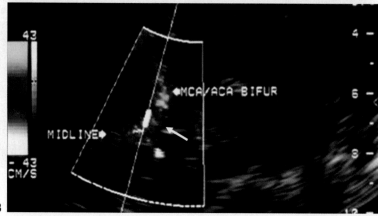

- BA: normal flow direction (blue), velocity will be elevated due to compensatory flow.
- Note: there could be compensatory flow through one or both vertebral arteries, which will elevate the velocities.

Significant Carotid Stenosis Side
- MCA: normal flow direction (red), velocity will be dependent on the amount of collateral flow.
- ACA: normal flow direction (blue) but may have turbulence due to collateral flow coming through the PCoA.
- PCA (P1 segment, red): normal flow direction, velocity elevated and greater than the ipsilateral MCA due to compensatory flow.
- PCA (P2 segment): normal flow direction (blue) and velocity.
- PCoA may be detectable due to the high flow (Fig. 9.8D).

SCANNING TIPS
The flow directions in the MCA (red) and ACA (blue) should be the same for both the right and the left hemispheres. No reversals of flow direction occur in this collateral pattern. There may be turbulence present at the MCA/ACA bifurcation region on the stenotic side. This is generally due to high flow coming through the PCoA into the anterior circulation. A Doppler bruit may be present in the position of the PCoA. The velocity will be elevated in the BA, as will the ipsilateral P1 segment of the PCA and one or both VAs.

External to Internal Collateral

Blood flow can be shunted from the external carotid artery branches into the ophthalmic artery. This produces reversed flow in the ophthalmic artery, which enters the distal ICA just before the level of the PCoA and the MCA/ACA bifurcation. Therefore, normal flow directions remain in the intracranial vessels (Fig. 9.9).

FIGURE 9.8. *A,* A stylized map of the arterial network showing the pathway (*in red*) for posterior to anterior collateral flow via the PCoA. Note that the flow direction in the ACA remains unchanged, and the velocity in the PCoA is elevated. *B* and *C,* The PCA velocity ipsilateral to the extracranial carotid stenosis is greater than the ipsilateral MCA velocity (mean velocities are not shown).

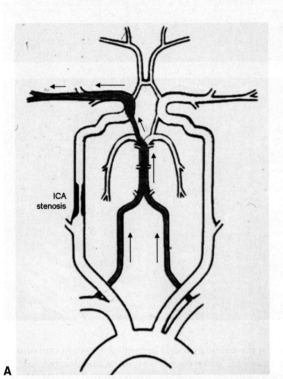

ICA
stenosis

A

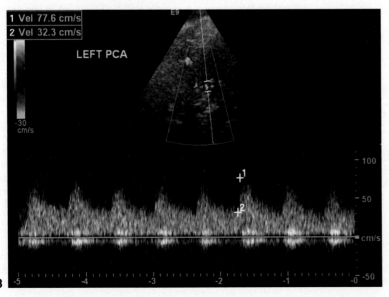

1 Vel 77.6 cm/s
2 Vel 32.3 cm/s

LEFT PCA

B

FIGURE 9.8. (*Continued*) *D*, When there is posterior to anterior collateralization, the PCoA (labeled PCOM) may be seen on color-flow imaging.

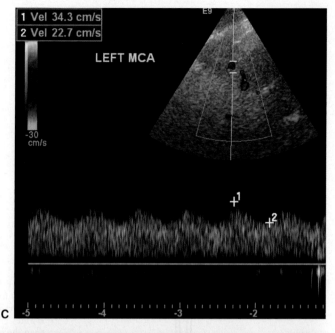

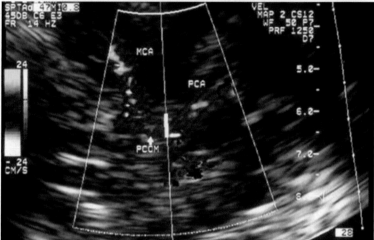

TYPICAL EXAMINATION FINDINGS

Normal Side
- MCA: normal flow direction (red) and velocity.
- ACA: normal flow direction (blue) and velocity.
- PCA: normal flow direction (P1, red; P2, blue) and velocity.

Significant Carotid Stenosis Side
- MCA: normal flow direction (red). Velocity is dependent on adequacy of ophthalmic artery collateral flow.
- ACA: normal flow direction (blue). Velocity is dependent on adequacy of ophthalmic artery collateral flow.
- PCA: normal flow direction (P1, red; P2, blue) and velocity.
- Ophthalmic: reversed flow direction (blue), increased velocity present due to compensatory flow (Fig. 9.10).
- Note: CCA and external carotid artery flow velocities will be elevated due to compensatory flow.

SCANNING TIPS
This is a relatively poor collateral pathway when present in isolation. It rarely delivers adequate flow to the MCA territory, and low flow velocities may be observed in the MCA and ACA. This pathway is used if the ACoA and PCoA are not available.

However, it is sometimes found in conjunction with other functioning collateral patterns such as intracranial crossover or posterior to anterior collaterals. When external to internal collateral flow is present, velocities will be increased in the external carotid artery, particularly the diastolic component.

Combinations of Collateral Flow Patterns

It is possible for more than one of the three basic collateral flow patterns to exist simultaneously in an individual. Usually this occurs when a single collateral pathway is not enough to provide adequate flow, so others are recruited to maintain normal levels of cerebral perfusion (Fig. 9.11). In this situation, the TCI examination can be extremely difficult to perform, and therefore, adherence to a strict scanning protocol is recommended. The findings should be recorded on a map such as the one provided in this chapter. Often, the technologist can piece the puzzle together as he or she is scanning; however, in complex situations, it may not become clear until all of the velocities have been mapped.

SCANNING TIPS
It is important to insonate all vessels in a meticulous manner and to follow a standard routine. For example, begin with the distal MCA and work toward the bifurcation.

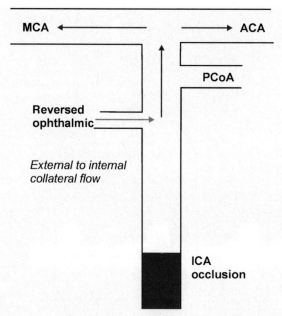

FIGURE 9.9. A schematic showing the entrance of reversed ophthalmic artery flow (*green arrow*) into the distal ICA. The MCA/ACA flow remains in the normal directions with this type of external to internal collateral flow.

Go on to insonate the ACA to the midline only, and follow this by doing the P1 and then P2 segments. Although you may be able to see vessels in the other hemisphere, it is best to change to the opposite temporal window and begin again. Be careful of large sample volumes. Plot velocities and flow directions onto a map. A better idea of the flow patterns should emerge. If things do not make sense, go back and rescan the vessel in question to make sure it was identified properly. Know the depths that the arteries should appear at and check your anatomic landmarks.

Bilateral Carotid Stenosis

Predicting the hemodynamic effects of bilateral extracranial carotid stenosis on the cerebral circulation can be a challenge. The best approach is to first identify the higher-grade ICA stenosis from the carotid duplex scan. Assume that collateral flow will be from the side of the lesser stenosis (higher pressure) to the side of the more severe stenosis (lower pressure) via the path of least resistance. If both stenoses appear similar by duplex, the route of collateral flow may be from the posterior circulation (higher pressure) to the anterior circulation (lower pressure). In this case, there may be collateral flow through both PCoAs. With bilateral carotid stenosis, TCI findings can help to identify the more hemodynamically significant lesion. For instance, if the collateral flow is moving from the left to the right hemisphere, this would indicate that the right side has the more significant extracranial obstruction. A scanning tip is to start the TCI examination on the side of the presumed lesser carotid stenosis, because you are likely to find higher-velocity signals in the MCA/ACA, and therefore, they will be easier to image. It is also technically easier to find an ACA with elevated velocities flowing in the normal direction than an ACA with reversed flow direction.

As noted previously, it is possible that collateral flow will come from more than one pathway simultaneously. TCI has the capability of mapping the collateral flow patterns and also suggesting the adequacy or inadequacy of the resulting flow to the hemispheres. This may be useful for differentiating

ischemic from embolic events. For example, with a hemodynamic stroke, the TCI findings may show low flow velocities in the arteries of interest. However, in an embolic or hemorrhagic stroke, the flow velocities may be within normal limits in the basal cerebral vessels. The adequacy of collateral flow can be assessed by comparing the velocity and pulsatility in the bilateral MCAs. When collateral pathways provide satisfactory flow to both MCAs, the velocities on the two sides will be approximately equivalent with pulsatility indices of greater than 0.50. With poor collaterals, the MCA velocities are often asymmetric and relatively low with pulsatility indices of 0.50 or less (Fig. 9.12).

Step 7. The Transcranial Duplex Imaging Report

The final step in the interpretation of the TCI examination is putting all the information together into a coherent and clinically useful report. Most clinicians are not TCI experts but use the results of the examination as guidance in their management strategy. The formal report should address the clinical questions to be answered. The most important question with carotid stenosis generally concerns flow to the MCA territory and the hemodynamic risk of stroke. Therefore, the report should typically address the following points.

- Compare the MCA flow velocities (stenotic with normal side). If both carotid systems are stenotic and no normal side is present, compare the velocities with known normal values (see Table 9.1) to provide a benchmark.
- Comment on the presence or absence of collateral flow.
- Comment on the pathway(s) used for collateral flow; this could be important for surgical or interventional planning.
- List the useful indices (and be prepared to explain what they mean).
- Comment on other intracranial vessels in terms of flow velocity and direction.

GENERAL SCANNING TECHNIQUE

Preparation

- The status of the extracranial cerebrovascular arteries should be known. The results of a carotid duplex scan should be reviewed whenever available.
- Owing to long examination times of 30 to 60 minutes, the patient should be supine and comfortable. The small size of the cerebral vessels (2 to 4 mm) requires fine motor movement of the hand, and the technologist should be positioned so that the ultrasound controls are nearby.
- The technologist should be familiar with the acoustic windows available on the skull and the course, location, depth, and normal flow directions of the cerebral arteries.

Equipment

- TCI requires a low-frequency (2 to 2.5 MHz), small-footprint (phased array) transducer to penetrate the small acoustic window that is usually (but not always) present as a thin spot in the temporal bone just superior to the zygomatic arch.

FIGURE 9.10. External to internal collateralization via the ophthalmic artery. *A,* Normal ophthalmic artery flow is toward the transducer (out of the orbit) and appears above the zero-flow baseline. *B,* When the ophthalmic artery flow direction is retrograde or reversed due to collateral flow, it appears below the baseline.

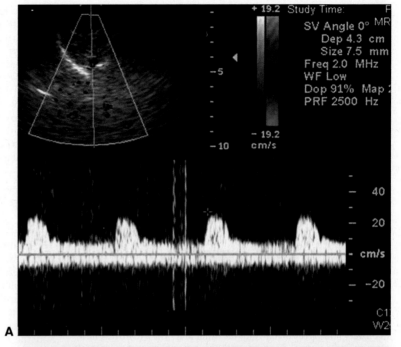

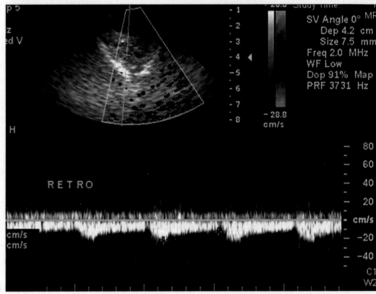

■ All diagnostic information is derived from the spectral waveforms, and the equipment should have the ability to measure PSV and EDV from which mean velocity and indices can be calculated.

Instrument Settings

■ A large sample volume size (5 mm) is used to locate and insonate the cerebral arteries and detect any focal stenoses in the intracranial vessels. Using too small a sample volume will make it difficult to detect a focal high-velocity jet, whereas too large a sample volume will display overlapping velocity profiles from nearby vessels.

■ Sensitivity to low flow can be especially important for locating vessels in abnormal examinations when velocities are very low distal to a severe stenosis or occlusion. In this situation, low pulse repetition frequency (PRF) and wall filter settings and high color frame averaging settings are advised.

■ Never reverse the color-flow direction on the ultrasound display. Determining the flow direction in each artery is critical to the interpretation of collateral flow patterns.

■ Utilize both color and power Doppler. Power mode is useful for finding an artery because it is not angle dependent, and the intracranial arteries are often tortuous. However, once the artery has been located, return to color Doppler as needed to determine flow direction.

Patient/Technologist Positioning

■ The TCI examination can be done from the head of the bed in a manner similar to that preferred by many technologists for a standard carotid/vertebral duplex scan. It is also advantageous to practice scanning from the side of the bed as is required in many portable inpatient or intensive care unit settings.

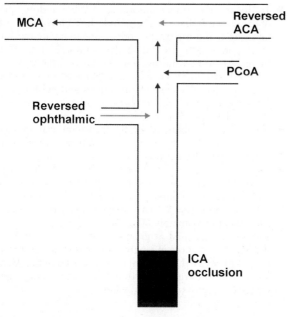

FIGURE 9.11. A schematic showing collateral flow from all three of the major collateral pathways (intracranial crossover, posterior to anterior, and external to internal via the ophthalmic artery) and the flow patterns that should all exist simultaneously.

- The patient is positioned supine for the *transtemporal approach* with the head turned slightly. For the *transorbital approach*, it is recommended that the head be straight up and down. The *transoccipital approach* can be accomplished by rolling the patient on her or his side toward the technologist and asking them to direct their chin slightly downward toward the chest.

Overview

Four steps are taken at each of the examination sites.

1. Locate the acoustic window
   - Studies show that older patients and particularly women tend to have hyperostosis of the temporal bone, and the transtemporal acoustic window may be small and difficult to locate or even absent.[25] With TCI, the transtemporal acoustic window, if present, appears as a sonolucent oval on B-mode image (Fig. 9.13A). If no window is present, the oval will appear "fuzzy" with no discernible bony landmarks (see Fig. 9.13B).
   - Your knowledge of the anatomy and the bony landmarks will direct you into the general location of the artery you wish to insonate.
   - Know the normal flow directions and how these should be color coded as flow toward (red) and away (blue) from the transducer (Fig. 9.14).

FIGURE 9.12. Assessing the adequacy of collateral flow. *A*, MCA waveform showing adequate collateral flow with a mean velocity of 53 cm/s and a normal PI of 1.03. *B*, MCA waveform indicating poor collateral flow with a decreased mean velocity of 32 cm/s and an abnormal PI of 0.47.

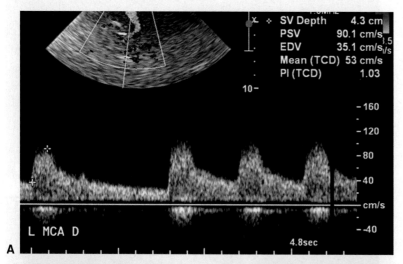

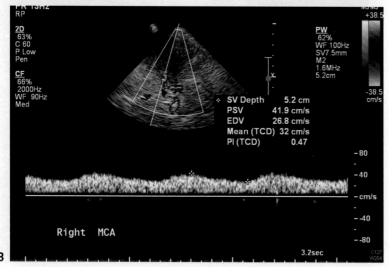

2. Identify the vessel
   - Four criteria are used for vessel identification: depth, flow direction, waveform contour/velocity, and spatial/anatomic position.
3. Insonate each artery at 5-mm intervals, searching for abnormalities.
   - Use digital storage, videotape, or hard-copy prints.
   - Representative PSVs and EDVs are measured for each segment, which can then be used to calculate the mean velocities and indices for interpretation.
   - Locations of spectral abnormalities such as bruits and turbulence should also be recorded.
4. Document normal and abnormal findings

Examination Procedure

The *transtemporal approach* is used to evaluate the MCA, ACA, PCA, and the terminal ICA. The ACoA and PCoA are very small and are not usually seen unless they are functioning as collateral pathways.

- To locate the transtemporal acoustic window, place the transducer flat on the temple just above the zygomatic arch and use the B-mode image to locate the small thin spot usually present in the temporal bone. When there is a good window, one should be able to visualize bony structures such as the sphenoid wing and the petrous ridge. The cerebral peduncles and midline structures such as the falx cerebri can often be appreciated (Figs. 9.13A and 9.14).[26]
- All waveforms obtained via the transtemporal approach should have the same general contour as a normal ICA in a standard extracranial carotid examination.
- The MCA is positively identified by its shallow depth (4 to 6 cm), flow direction toward the transducer (red), and its anatomic course paralleling the lesser wing of the sphenoid bone (Fig 9.14A). Average mean velocity in the MCA is approximately 60 cm/s (Table 9.1).
- The ACA is located at greater depths (6 to 8 cm) than the MCA. It is short in length and located anterior to the proximal MCA. The normal flow direction in the ACA is away from the transducer (blue), and the average mean velocity is approximately 50 cm/s.

FIGURE 9.13. *A,* Example of a good transtemporal acoustic window. Note the clear definition of the sphenoid wing and the petrous ridge. *B,* Example of a poor transtemporal acoustic window. There are no clear bony landmarks present.

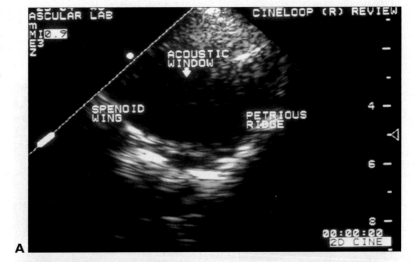

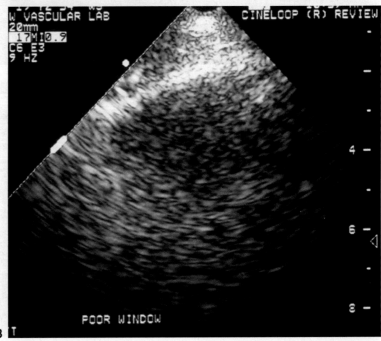

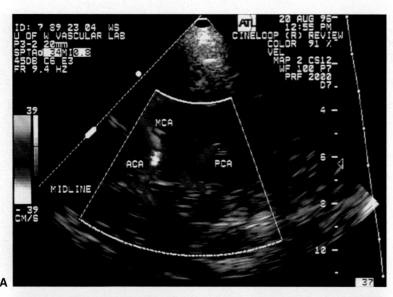

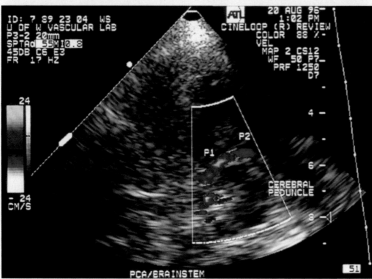

FIGURE 9.14. TCI images taken using a transtemporal acoustic window. *A,* Color-coded image showing normal flow directions in the intracranial arteries (MCA, *red,* ACA, *blue*) with the midline of the brain indicated. Just beyond the midline (in *red*) is the ACA of the opposite hemisphere; although flowing in the normal direction (toward the midline), it is depicted as red because it is viewed from the *contralateral* temporal approach. *B,* Color-coded image showing the PCA P1 segment (in *red*) flowing towards the transducer, and the PCA P2 segment (in *blue*) flowing away from the transducer. The posterior circulation anatomical landmark of the cerebral peduncles is also seen.

- The PCA is also found at deeper depths (6 to 8 cm), but it has a more posterior location and courses around the brainstem with flow direction toward the transducer in the P1 segment (red) and away from transducer in the P2 segment (blue) (Fig. 9.14B). Average PCA mean velocities are approximately 40 cm/s.
- When evaluating hemodynamics via the transtemporal approach, it is essential to remember that MCA mean velocities (~60 cm/s) should always be greater than ACA mean velocities (~50 cm/s), which are greater than PCA mean velocities (~40 cm/s) in a normal patient. Changes in this MCA > ACA > PCA relationship are used to identify collateral pathways.
- The MCA should have three Doppler measurements: proximal (near the bifurcation), mid, and distal. The ACA should have one or two velocity measurements taken. The PCA should have a measurement at the P1 segment and at the P2 segment. If it is possible to take a measurement in the communicating arteries (when there is collateral flow), that should also be documented.

The *transoccipital approach* utilizes the natural opening at the base of the skull, the foramen magnum, to examine the intracranial VAs and the BA.

- Place the probe at the base of the skull with the patient's head tilted forward; the acoustic window is again seen as a somewhat smaller sonolucent oval. The bony structure of the atlas can be used as a B-mode landmark. All waveforms should have the features of normal extracranial VAs. Power Doppler is helpful initially because the vessels can be tortuous and power Doppler is not angle dependent (Fig. 9.15).
- The VAs are found at shallow depths (5 to 8 cm) with normal flow direction away from the probe (blue). The anterior spinal branches are sometimes seen flowing toward the transducer with a higher pulsatility and more resistive waveform, which resembles that seen in a normal external carotid artery.
- The BA can be found at deeper depths (8 to 10 cm) and often appears to be aligned with a dominant VA.
- Document at least one velocity measurement from each of the intracranial VAs and three measurements along the course of the BA.

CEREBROVASCULAR

FIGURE 9.15. Transoccipital approach. The vertebral arteries and basilar artery are identified with power Doppler, which is a helpful imaging technique with small or tortuous arteries. Power Doppler does not provide any information about flow direction.

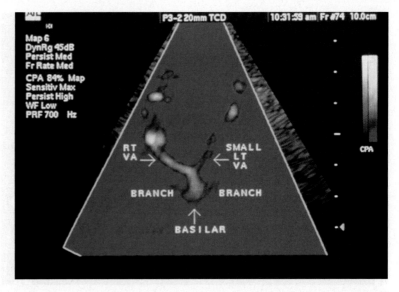

The *transorbital approach* is used to evaluate ophthalmic artery flow direction and the carotid siphon via the optic canal.

- The ophthalmic artery is located at relatively shallow depths (4.5 to 6.0 cm). Ophthalmic artery waveforms should be similar to a normal external carotid artery, and flow direction is normally toward the transducer (Fig. 9.10A).
- The carotid siphon is deeper (6.5 to 7.0 cm) with waveforms that resemble a normal ICA. Flow direction is not meaningful at the carotid siphon because it is possible to locate the paracellar (toward the probe), the genu (dual directional), or the supraclinoid segments of the carotid siphon from this approach. Although this technique has been used for many years throughout the world with no reports of adverse effects, no diagnostic use of ultrasound through the orbit has been granted U.S. Food and Drug Administration approval, and it is prudent to minimize acoustic exposure by decreasing power output/intensity and minimize scanning time whenever possible.

Avoiding Technical Sources of Error

The desired acoustic window should be located and optimized by first using the B-mode image alone without color-flow Doppler. If the technologist spends a few minutes obtaining the best possible B-mode image of the acoustic window and bony landmarks, the positions of the arteries can be more accurately assessed, minimizing errors in vessel identification and ensuring that the best acoustic window is located. Once the acoustic window has been optimized and the color flow is turned on, a whole new set of potential pitfalls arise. One simple error is inverting the color map, which can make directional information confusing. There is generally no need to invert the color map during TCI examinations.

Sensitivity to high or low flow can be a problem, and it is important to make sure that color PRF settings are appropriate. If the PRF is set too high, low flow velocities will not be displayed. If the color PRF is too low, aliasing will make directional information difficult to appreciate. Using a shallow image, depth maximizes frame rate. Although it is sometimes possible to insonate both hemispheres from one transtemporal window, frame rate is a potential source for error, and it is recommended that each hemisphere be evaluated separately

from the ipsilateral window. Using small color-flow boxes also helps to keep the frame rate at manageable levels. Increasing the sample volume size can also lead to errors by making it possible to simultaneously insonate more than one artery at more than one depth.

Incomplete data are another potential source of error. This will occur in difficult studies but can be minimized by strict adherence to protocol. Be sure to document PSV and EDV for each sample depth and to document additional images of any flow disturbances or waveform changes. It will not be possible to insonate all of the basal cerebral vessels in every patient, but mapping the ones that are identified may be enough to obtain a diagnostic study. If a particular vessel is not insonated, describe this in the report noting that it does not indicate that the vessel is occluded, but simply that it is not identified during a difficult imaging examination.

The subject of Doppler angle correction is still an unresolved issue in TCI. On the positive side, it is thought that manually adjusting the Doppler angle should provide more accurate velocity measurements, particularly because the vessels are tortuous and the technologist has very limited options for angle adjustment by manipulating the transducer within the small acoustic windows. On the negative side, only the color-coded Doppler shift is seen in TCI, and the vessel walls are never well visualized. Therefore, it is difficult in repeat examinations to reliably and reproducibly line up the angle cursor with the vessel wall. It is also noteworthy that all current TCI/TCD velocity criteria have been validated without angle correction.

CONCLUSIONS

A TCI examination is most helpful if low CBF is suspected, such as in patients with severe unilateral or bilateral carotid stenoses or multiple lesions in the aortic arch branches. The TCI examination can not only detect the presence of collateral flow pathways but can also infer the adequacy or inadequacy of the resulting flow in the basal cerebral vessels. In addition, TCI has the capability of detecting intracranial arterial stenoses. These lesions are highly variable, being present in 5% to 23% of angiograms done for a stroke.[27-29] The distribution of intracranial arterial stenoses is intracranial ICA 49%, MCA 20%, PCA 11%, vertebrobasilar arteries 11%, and ACA 9%.[28] The TCI/TCD examination has also been proven to detect "embolic signatures," which represent gaseous or particulate emboli passing through the vessels that may be markers of impending TIA or stroke.[29] Examinations for detection of emboli are best performed with nonimaging equipment and specialized probe fixation devices (head gear) for long-term, hands-free monitoring, as described in Chapter 11.

Other important TCI applications are the detection of vasospasm, balloon occlusion testing, CO_2 reactivity testing, autoregulation studies, and intraoperative monitoring (see Chapter 11). Specialized TCI laboratories will often perform these types of studies, because they require additional training and expertise on the part of the technologist and can be extremely time consuming. Therefore, some TCI/TCD applications may not be practical for a routine vascular laboratory setting.

TCI examinations present many challenges to overcome, such as limited insonation windows, small vessels, low velocities, and complex cerebral hemodynamics. However, these examinations can be adequately performed in most vascular laboratories. It is suggested that laboratories use a standardized protocol with anatomic diagrams and a clear worksheet for plotting flow velocities and directions. Experienced technologists are able to build a picture of the hemodynamics in their mind as they scan, but for the less experienced user, mapping velocities onto a picture of the arterial network can be an invaluable learning tool and will facilitate accurate interpretation.

Finally, it should be emphasized that TCI/TCD is an adjunct to carotid duplex imaging and completes the ultrasound examination of the cerebrovascular network (aortic arch to the cerebral circulation). In general, it should be performed only after the extracranial carotid and vertebral studies have been completed and unanswered questions remain.

References

1. Otis SM, Ringelstein EB. The transcranial Doppler examination: Principles and applications of transcranial Doppler sonography. In Tegeler CH, Babikian VL, Gomez CR (eds). *Neurosonology*. St. Louis: Mosby–Year Book, 1996, pp 113-128.
2. Markus H. Doppler embolus detection: Stroke treatment and prevention. In Tegeler CH, Babikian VL, Gomez CR (eds). *Neurosonology*. St. Louis: Mosby–Year Book, 1996, pp 239-251.
3. Lippert H, Pabst R. *Arterial Variations in Man: Classification and Frequency*. Munich: JF Bergmann, 1985.
4. Henderson RD, Eliasziw M, Fox AJ, et al. Angiographically defined collateral circulations and risk of stroke in patients with severe carotid artery stenosis. *Stroke* 2000;31:128-132.
5. Hoksbergen AWJ, Majoie CBL, Hulsmans FJH, et al. Assessment of the collateral function of the circle of Willis: Three-dimensional time-of-flight MR angiography compared with transcranial color-coded duplex sonography. *AJNR Am J Neuroradiol* 2003;24:456-462.
6. Bragoni M, Feldmann E. Transcranial Doppler indices of intracranial hemodynamics. In Tegeler CH, Babikian VL, Gomez CR (eds). *Neurosonology*. St. Louis: Mosby–Year Book, 1996, pp 129-139.
7. Berré J. Pathophysiology of the cerebral circulation. *European Society of Anaesthesiologists Refresher Course*, Vienna, April 1, 2000.
8. Gray H. The arteries. In Pick TP, Howden R (eds). *Gray's Anatomy*, Classic Collector's ed. New York: Crown, 1977, p 507.
9. Alastruey J, Parker KH, Peiró J, et al. Modelling the circle of Willis to assess the effects of anatomical variations and occlusions on cerebral flows. *J Biomech* 2007;40:1794-1805.
10. Aaslid R, Markwalder TM, Nornes H. Noninvasive transcranial Doppler ultrasound recording of flow velocity in basal cerebral arteries. *J Neurosurg* 1982;57:769-774.
11. Hennerici M, Rautenberg W, Schwartz A. Transcranila Doppler ultrasound for the assessment of intracranial arterial flow velocity, part II. *Surg Neurol* 1987;27:523-532.
12. Ringelstein EB, Kahlscheuer B, Niggemeyer E, et al. Transcranial Doppler sonography: Anatomical landmarks and normal velocity values. *Ultrasound Med Biol* 1990;16:745-761.
13. Harders A. Monitoring of hemodynamic changes related to vasospasm in the circle of Willis after aneurysm surgery. In Aaslid R (ed.) *Transcranial Doppler Sonography*. Vienna and New York: Springer-Verlag, 1986.
14. Adams R, Nichols FT, Hess D. Normal values and physiological variables. In Newell DW, Aaslid R (eds). *Transcranial Doppler*. New York: Raven, 1992, pp 41-48.
15. Kety SS. Human cerebral blood flow and oxygen consumption as related to aging. *J Chronic Dis* 1956;3:478-486.
16. Gosling RG, King DH. Arterial assessment by Doppler-shift ultrasound. *Proc Roy Soc Med* 1974;67:447-449.
17. Planiol T, Pourcelot L, Itti R. Radioisotopes, ultrasonics and thermography in the diagnosis of cerebral circulatory disorders. *Rev Electroencephalogr Neurophysiol Clin* 1974;4:221-236.
18. Lindegaard KF. Indices of pulsatility. In Newell DW, Aaslid R (eds). *Transcranial Doppler*. New York: Raven, 1992, pp 68-82.
19. Byrd-Raynor S, Parker K. New transcranial Doppler waveform shape parameters: A repeatability/reproducibility study. *J Vasc Ultrasound* 2007;31:193-205.
20. Byrd-Raynor S, Alastruey J, Hughes A, et al. The relationship between velocity and cerebral resistance during vasomotor reactivity testing: Should we report a different measurement? *J Vasc Ultrasound* 2008;32:67-74.
21. Rorick M, Nichols FT, Adams RJ. Transcranial Doppler correlation with angiography in detection of intracranial stenosis. *Stroke* 1994;25:1931-1934.
22. Felberg RA, Ioannis C, Demchuk AM, et al. Screening for intracranial stenosis with transcranial Doppler: The accuracy of mean flow velocity thresholds. *J Neuroimaging* 2002;12:1-6.
23. Baumgartner RW, Mattle HP, Schroth G. Assessment of ≥50% and <50% intracranial stenosis by transcranial color-coded duplex sonography. *Stroke* 1999;30:87-92.
24. Aaslid R, Huber P, Nornes H. Evaluation of cerebrovascular spasm with transcranial Doppler ultrasound. *J Neurosurg*. 1984;60:37-41.
25. Fujioka K, Douville C. Examination and freehand techniques. In Newell DW, Aaslid R (eds). *Transcranial Doppler*. New York: Raven, 1992, pp 9-31.
26. Byrd S. An overview of transcranial color flow imaging: A technique comparison. *Ultrasound Q* 1998;13:197-210.
27. Hass WK, Fields WS, North RR, et al. Joint study of extracranial arterial occlusion. II. Arteriography, techniques, sites, and complications. *JAMA* 1968;203:961-968.
28. Borozan PG, Schuler JJ, LaRosa MP, et al. The natural history of isolated carotid siphon stenosis. *J Vasc Surg* 1984;1:744-749.
29. Keagy BA, Poole MA, Burnham SJ, et al. Frequency, severity, and physiologic importance of carotid siphon lesions. *J Vasc Surg* 1986;3:511-515.
30. O'Brien E, Bouchier-Hayes D, Fitzgerald D, et al. The arterial organ in cardiovascular disease: ADAPT (arterial disease assessment, prevention, and treatment) clinic. *Lancet* 1998;352:1700-1702.
31. Spencer M. Detection of cerebral arterial emboli. In Tegeler CH, Babikian VL, Gomez CR (eds). *Neurosonology*. St. Louis: Mosby–Year Book, 1996, pp 215-230.

CEREBROVASCULAR

CHAPTER 10 ■ FOLLOW-UP AFTER CAROTID ENDARTERECTOMY AND STENTING

ROBERT M. ZWOLAK AND R. EUGENE ZIERLER

DUPLEX AFTER CAROTID ENDARTERECTOMY
    Ultrasound Findings
    Interpretation of Postoperative Velocity Changes

DUPLEX AFTER CAROTID ARTERY STENTING
    Scanning the Stented Carotid Artery
    Duplex Criteria for In-stent Carotid Restenosis
CONCLUSIONS

Carotid endarterectomy (CEA) and carotid artery stenting (CAS) are procedures performed to prevent atheroembolic stroke. CEA has been a standard therapy since the early 1970s, whereas CAS was added by Medicare in 2005 as a covered treatment modality for symptomatic patients considered to be at high risk for CEA. The decision to cover CAS was made following publication of a randomized trial comparing CAS to CEA in high-risk subgroups.[1] Duplex ultrasound has played a major role in both of these therapies, initially for identifying appropriate treatment candidates and subsequently for following patients after their procedures. This chapter focuses on follow-up after carotid interventions. The general approach to the duplex evaluation of extracranial carotid artery disease is discussed in Chapter 8.

The utilization of CEA increased dramatically from approximately 15,000 cases in 1971 to 107,000 in 1985.[2] However, the total number of CEA cases decreased after that time, purportedly due to uncertainty regarding the specific indications and concerns over operative risk. The randomized clinical trials published in the 1990s compared the results of CEA to the medical management available at that time and helped to clarify the indications for CEA in both symptomatic and asymptomatic patients.[3,4] In the late 1990s, CAS was introduced as a less invasive alternative to CEA, and utilization of CAS increased from 3% of all carotid revascularization procedures in 1998 to 13% in 2008.[5] Even with this increase in CAS, the total number of carotid revascularization procedures decreased over this time period as a result of a larger decrease in the number of CEA operations performed.[6] The outcomes and safety of both CEA and CAS were compared in the Carotid Revascularization Endarterectomy versus Stenting Trial, which was reported in 2010.[7] There was no significant difference between CEA and CAS in the incidence of the primary composite end point of stroke, myocardial infarction, or death in the periprocedural period at 4.5% and 5.2%, respectively. However, there was a difference in the rates of the separate end points, with a lower incidence of stroke in the CEA group and a lower incidence of MI in the CAS group.

Noninvasive evaluation of cerebrovascular disease was the first widespread application of duplex ultrasound scanning.[8,9] As this technique evolved and improved, duplex ultrasound was shown to be sufficiently accurate to serve as the exclusive preoperative testing modality prior to CEA in centers where sonographers and interpreting physicians focused on providing the highest-quality examination possible.[10,11] The safety of CEA has been well established. The largest multicenter prospective trial of CEA in asymptomatic patients in the United States published in 1995 demonstrated a 2.3% incidence of the combined end point of stroke plus death at 30 days.[4] Fifteen years later, the Society for Vascular Surgery Vascular Registry identified a 2.0% incidence of the combined end point of stroke plus death plus myocardial infarction at 30 days in asymptomatic patients.[12] The low morbidity and mortality after CEA is due to a wide range of factors, including careful patient selection, high-quality anesthesia, close attention to technical surgical details, and tightly controlled postoperative care.

Restenosis after CEA and CAS appears to occur infrequently in contemporary series, and duplex ultrasound has been advocated as an appropriate means to detect this complication and help determine the need for reintervention. In the Carotid Revascularization Endarterectomy versus Stenting Trial, restenosis was defined as a diameter reduction of 70% or greater as indicated by a peak systolic velocity (PSV) of 300 cm/s or more.[13] Follow-up by serial duplex scanning for 2 years showed no significant difference between the CEA and CAS groups for a combined end point of restenosis or occlusion with an incidence of 6.3% and 6.0%, respectively. The Kaplan-Meier estimate for the frequency of the combined end point at 4 years was 6.2% for CEA and 6.7% for CAS.

DUPLEX AFTER CAROTID ENDARTERECTOMY

Early reports from authors including Zierler and coworkers,[14] Baker and colleagues,[15] Healy and associates,[16] and others described the use of duplex ultrasound for serial follow-up after CEA, and the range of reported residual or recurrent stenosis varied widely from 4% to 21%. The initial series described by Zierler and coworkers included 76 patients undergoing 89 CEA operations who were followed by duplex scanning for a mean of only 16 months.[14] Duplex findings indicating greater than 50% restenosis (based on velocity criteria for native atherosclerotic lesions) were observed in 32 of the 89 internal carotid arteries; however, some of these early postoperative lesions regressed on serial follow-up, and the

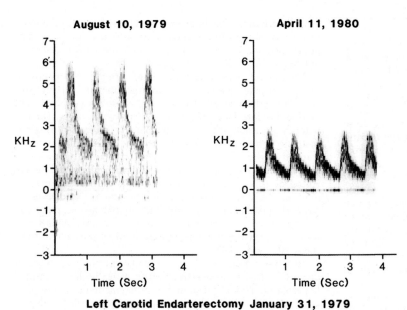

August 10, 1979

April 11, 1980

Left Carotid Endarterectomy January 31, 1979

FIGURE 10.1. Illustration from the 1982 report by Zierler and coworkers showing the Doppler spectral waveforms from an early postoperative stenosis that regressed. *Left,* Examination approximately 6 months after a left carotid endarterectomy shows a flow pattern that is characteristic of a 50% to 79% stenosis with elevated peak systolic frequency. *Right,* A follow-up examination 8 months later (about 14 months postoperatively) is consistent with less than 50% internal carotid artery stenosis. Note that Doppler shift frequencies are shown on the vertical axis because the duplex scanners at the time of this study did not have a velocity scale. (From Zierler RE, Bandyk DF, Thiele BL, et al. Carotid artery stenosis following endarterectomy. *Arch Surg* 1982;117:1408-1415. Reprinted with permission.)

overall incidence of persistent restenosis was 19% (Fig. 10.1). Healy and associates followed 301 patients after CEA, with most of the cases having primary arteriotomy closure without patch angioplasty.[9] By life-table analysis at 7 years, 31% of the patients developed a restenosis of greater than 50%, but 10% of these subsequently regressed. Despite a net restenosis prevalence of 21%, only 3% of patients suffered a stroke during follow-up, and this incidence of postprocedure stroke was no different from that in patients without early restenosis. The authors concluded that a conservative approach could be taken toward restenosis.[16]

Bernstein and coworkers followed 566 patients after CEA and found a 50% or greater restenosis rate at 10 years (life-table analysis) of 14.5% in women and 7.7% in men ($P < 0.003$).[17] Curiously, these authors found early restenosis to be protective—patients with restenosis were statistically less likely to have late symptoms, stroke, or early death than were patients with normal postoperative duplex scans. Mackey and colleagues followed 348 patients after CEA and observed a 16% rate of 50% or greater restenosis at a mean 4-year follow-up.[18] Like Bernstein and coworkers, these authors concluded that the stroke risk related to early restenosis was low. Without performing a formal cost-benefit analysis, this group suggested that routine duplex follow-up after CEA was difficult to justify.

In 1996, Ricotta and DeWeese published a single-center retrospective analysis focusing on progression of contralateral carotid disease in patients undergoing CEA.[19] They reviewed 562 patients who underwent 660 operations over a 13-year period. Approximately 30% of these patients had greater than 50% diameter stenosis in the contralateral carotid artery at initial presentation, and about half of these underwent CEA during early follow-up. For patients with less than 50% contralateral carotid stenosis at presentation, they documented a 10% progression rate to greater than 50% stenosis at 4.5 years mean follow-up. They concluded that patients with minimal contralateral carotid stenosis and a widely patent ipsilateral carotid artery after CEA could be followed using duplex ultrasound at intervals of up to 2 years.

A single-center report by Roth and associates in 1999 assessed the value of duplex scanning during and after CEA.[20] Duplex scans were performed intraoperatively and after operation at 3- to 6-month intervals for a mean follow-up of 27.4 months. Threshold criteria for a 50% to 74% stenosis included PSV greater than 125 cm/s, end-diastolic velocity (EDV) less than 125 cm/s, and an internal carotid artery to common carotid artery (ICA/CCA) PSV ratio greater than 2.5. Threshold criteria to diagnose a 75% to 99% stenosis included PSV greater than 300 cm/s, EDV greater than 125 cm/s, and ICA/CCA PSV ratio greater than 4.0. During follow-up, six arteries (2.7%) developed restenosis greater than 50%, but only one (<1%) developed restenosis greater than 75%, and this latter patient underwent reoperation. Similar to the observations of Ricotta and DeWeese, Roth and associates found a higher rate of progression to severe disease on the side contralateral to the CEA, with 12.7% of patients showing an increase in carotid stenosis by at least one duplex stenosis category during follow-up. Overall, these studies from the 1990s suggested that serial duplex scanning after CEA is more justified for surveillance of contralateral untreated disease than for ipsilateral recurrent stenosis.

These studies form the basis for current duplex follow-up algorithms after CEA. As a related observation, in view of the low morbidity associated with restenosis after CEA documented in these reports, it is noteworthy that a large number of carotid stents have been placed for recurrent stenosis. For instance, 34% of the 480 patients undergoing CAS in the Boston Scientific EPI: A Carotid Stenting Trial for High-Risk Surgical Patients (BEACH) trial of the Boston Scientific WALLSTENT were performed for restenosis after CEA.[21]

The technique of placing a patch for closure of the arteriotomy during CEA (patch angioplasty) likely has a significant impact on the development of restenosis. In a 1987 report, Ouriel and Green found that patch angioplasty was associated with a lower rate of early restenosis.[22] In 1994, Myers and coworkers published a single-center prospective, randomized, controlled trial wherein they were unable to demonstrate superior long-term results with vein patch closure as compared with primary arteriotomy closure during CEA.[23] However, by 2004, Bond and colleagues were able to identify seven randomized, controlled trials involving 1281 operations comparing routine patch closure with primary closure during CEA, and patch angioplasty was associated with a statistically significant reduction in risk for perioperative and late stroke.[24] The strength of these data is such that the National Quality Forum has passed a quality measure supporting patch closure for conventional noneversion CEA.[25]

CEREBROVASCULAR

Ultrasound Findings

Duplex examinations performed on patients in the weeks or months after CEA will most often demonstrate a widely patent endarterectomy site (Fig. 10.2). The proximal initiation point and the distal end point of the endarterectomized segment are usually visible. The location of the proximal "shelf" is determined by surgical technique and the severity of disease in the CCA. The caliber of the lumen and its shape depend on whether primary arteriotomy closure, eversion endarterectomy, or conventional endarterectomy with patch angioplasty closure has been performed. B-mode and color flow imaging typically demonstrate wide patency, although there may be color flow swirling (flow separation) at the CEA site if a patch has been placed (Fig. 10.3). Minor flow disturbances may be seen at the endarterectomy distal end point, but ordinarily, there should be no significantly elevated velocities or extreme flow disturbance. Modest flow disturbances seen early after CEA may disappear on subsequent studies owing to natural vessel remodeling.

The endarterectomy suture line may be visible on B-mode imaging. Sutures appear as small, bright, regularly spaced echoes along the near wall of the vessel, as shown in Figure 10.4. Some surgeons apply stainless steel clips on small arteries and veins during the operation, and these small but highly echogenic objects may cause acoustic shadows that obscure portions of the underlying vessels. Flaps of tissue may be seen in the endarterectomized portion of the artery on intraoperative imaging (Fig. 10.5). Most large flaps that cause

flow disturbances should be treated. The actual natural history of very small flaps in the endarterectomized segment remains poorly defined. Intraoperative assessment of CEA is discussed in Chapter 30.

Ultrasound visualization of a patch after CEA depends on the type of patch material used and the time interval after surgery. Polytetrafluoroethylene (PTFE) is often seen as a bright double-line interface on the near wall of the artery. Dacron patches are thick and also echogenic. If scanned during the first one or two days after surgery, the small amount of air trapped within the PTFE and Dacron material may cause acoustic shadowing and difficulty visualizing the vessel lumen. Autogenous saphenous vein and bovine pericardial patches may not be distinguishable from the native tissue, even in the early postoperative period, but the patched segment can be recognized by a bulging appearance over the endarterectomy site and the possible visualization of adjacent sutures (Figs. 10.3 and 10.4).

Restenosis that occurs in the endarterectomized segment during the first postoperative year is typically due to intimal hyperplasia. This is substantially different tissue than typical atherosclerotic plaque. Lacking any significant calcium deposits, the intimal hyperplastic lesion tends to be echolucent and commonly forms a long uniform narrowing (Fig. 10.6). Peak velocities may be extremely elevated throughout the stenotic segment. Restenosis that occurs 5 to 10 years postoperatively usually represents recurrent atherosclerotic plaque, particularly in an individual whose risk factors have not been successfully treated.

FIGURE 10.2. *A,* One month after carotid endarterectomy (CEA), modest amounts of plaque can be seen on this B-mode image in the common carotid artery proximal to the initiation point of the endarterectomy (*arrow*). *B,* B-mode image of a normal distal internal carotid artery (ICA) end point of a patched CEA 1 month postoperatively (*arrow*). The lumen appears widely patent.

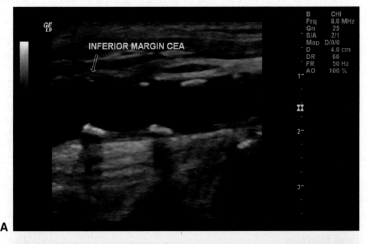

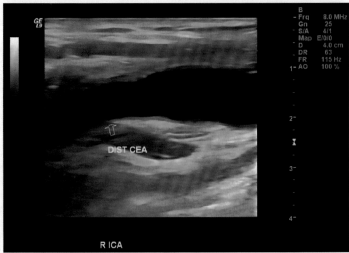

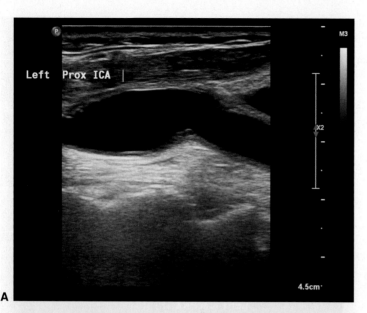

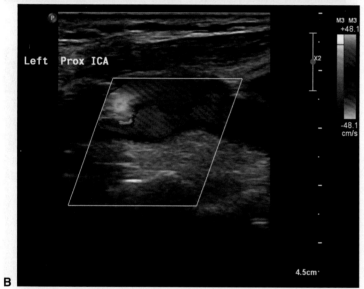

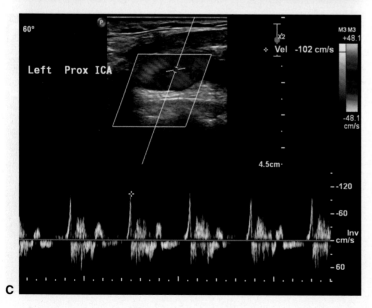

FIGURE 10.3. *A*, B-mode image of a patched internal carotid artery (ICA) 4 months after CEA. The widened lumen is clearly visible. *B*, Color flow image of the same patched ICA showing "swirling" or flow separation. *C*, Doppler spectral waveform from the patched ICA showing periods of forward and reverse flow during the cardiac cycle, characteristic of flow separation.

CEREBROVASCULAR

FIGURE 10.4. B-mode image of a patched internal carotid artery (ICA) showing sutures as bright "dots" on the near wall of the vessel (*arrows*).

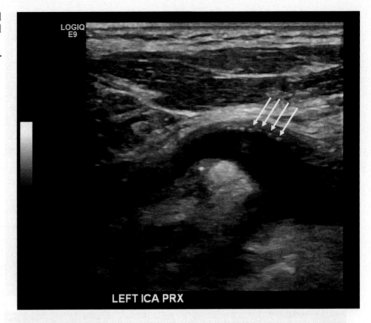

FIGURE 10.5. Intraoperative duplex assessment after carotid endarterectomy. *A*, Longitudinal B-mode image of a flap in the internal carotid artery (*arrow*). *B*, Color flow image of the same flap and a Doppler spectral waveform showing no significant flow disturbance associated with this finding.

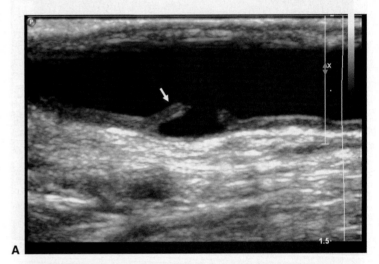

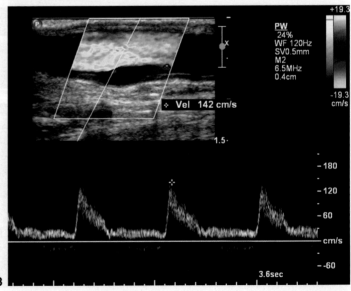

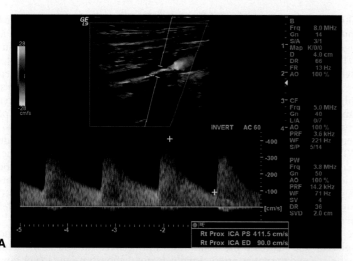

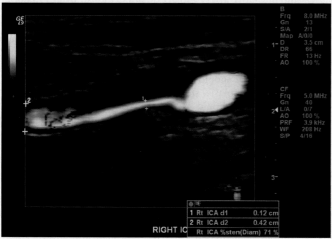

FIGURE 10.6. *A*, The color flow image shows a long segment of stenosis due to intimal hyperplasia in a right internal carotid artery 12 months after endarterectomy (*top*). Elevated peak systolic velocities (411 cm/s) and spectral broadening are apparent in the spectral waveform (*bottom*). *B*, Power Doppler image of the same intimal hyperplastic lesion seen in (*A*). The residual lumen appears to be 1.2 mm in diameter, although little literature support exists to assess the accuracy of this form of measurement.

Interpretation of Postoperative Velocity Changes

Reported experience supports the concept that classifying the severity of restenosis after CEA requires duplex criteria that are different from those for determining the severity of primary or native carotid artery disease. AbuRahma and associates reviewed 200 carotid operations performed between 2003 and 2005 with either PTFE or Dacron patch angioplasty closure, and the patients underwent duplex scans at 6-month intervals postoperatively, with 97% follow-up at a mean of 25 months.[26] Conventional angiography or computed tomography angiography (CTA) were used as the "gold standard," and the authors reported "very good" correlation between these two imaging modalities. These authors found that applying their standard PSV threshold of 140 cm/s to detect a 50% or greater stenosis resulted in a substantial incidence of false positives, meaning that the duplex diagnosis of a 50% or greater restenosis was not confirmed by angiography or CTA. This indicated that the standard PSV threshold for native carotid stenosis was too sensitive and not adequately specific for identification of restenosis after CEA. It was determined that an ICA PSV of greater than 213 cm/s was optimal by receiver operating characteristic (ROC) analysis for diagnosis of 50% or greater restenosis, with a sensitivity of 99% and a specificity of 100%. Similarly, this group's native carotid PSV threshold for 70% or greater stenosis was overly sensitive for restenosis in patched carotid arteries, where the most accurate threshold was found to be a PSV of 274 cm/s or greater, providing 99% sensitivity and 91% specificity for detecting a 70% or

greater restenosis as diagnosed by conventional angiography or CTA. AbuRahma and associates concluded that different carotid duplex velocity criteria should be used to detect restenosis after CEA when a patch closure has been performed.[26]

Although it may be true that intimal hyperplasia causing early restenosis in patched carotid arteries is less compliant and, therefore, results in a higher PSV at the same percentage of stenosis than does native atherosclerotic plaque, the alternative explanation relates to the duplex grading scales used for assessment of native carotid disease. A review of the literature demonstrates a wide range of apparently accurate duplex PSV thresholds for diagnosis of 70% or greater stenosis in native carotid arteries.[27] The consensus conference document published in 2003 identified single-center "most accurate" PSV thresholds ranging from 130 to 325 cm/s.[28] The highest PSV among those was from the vascular laboratory at Oregon Health & Science University.[29] At Dartmouth University, a PSV of 340 cm/s was found to be the most accurate threshold for a 70% or greater stenosis in diseased native carotid arteries. Thus, the issue of variability persists in the search for the most accurate carotid duplex criteria for identifying recurrent stenosis after CEA with patch closure.

DUPLEX AFTER CAROTID ARTERY STENTING

The introduction of CAS into clinical practice again focused attention on the accuracy of duplex scanning for classifying the severity of carotid stenosis. The Centers for Medicare and

Medicaid Services (CMS) approved coverage for CAS in 2005, but major restrictions were also imposed.[30] The CMS National Coverage Determination (NCD) for CAS has been challenged several times, but it remains unchanged. As of March 2015, Medicare coverage for CAS is limited to individuals who suffer lateralizing hemispheric transient ischemic attacks or minor strokes. The beneficiary must also be considered high risk for standard surgical treatment with CEA, for either anatomic or physiologic reasons. Finally, in addition to these two criteria, Medicare CAS coverage is restricted to those patients who have an angiographically proven carotid stenosis of 70% or worse. CMS will also cover CAS when performed in accordance with FDA-approved investigational device exemption (IDE) clinical trials and FDA-approved postapproval studies.

All carotid duplex ultrasound stenosis assessments must be verified by carotid angiography prior to CAS. In its coverage decision memorandum, CMS has written: "The degree of carotid artery stenosis should be measured by duplex Doppler ultrasound or carotid artery angiography and recorded in the patient medical records. If the stenosis is measured by ultrasound prior to the procedure, then the degree of stenosis must be confirmed by angiography at the start of the procedure. If the stenosis is determined to be less than 70% by angiography, then CAS should not proceed." Therefore, in order to avoid subjecting patients to unnecessary carotid angiography, it is increasingly important for all vascular laboratories to review the accuracy of their diagnostic parameters for advanced carotid stenosis.

Scanning the Stented Carotid Artery

Restenosis after CAS appears to be infrequent. Hobson and coworkers[31] followed 114 CAS procedures at 6-month intervals with a median follow-up of almost 2 years and identified 80% or greater diameter reduction in only 4 patients (3.8%). Iyer and colleagues[21] found that 4.7% of CAS procedures in the BEACH trial were associated with a restenosis sufficiently severe to require reintervention. Gurm and associates[32] reported that 2.4% of the CAS procedures in the original Stenting and Angioplasty with Protection in Patients at High Risk for Endarterectomy (SAPPHIRE) trial required target vessel revascularization at 3 years. Thus, like most patients who have undergone CEA, the carotid stent patient's treated carotid artery is typically widely patent (Figs. 10.7 and 10.8). Most commonly, the proximal end of the stent lies in the distal CCA, with the distal end in the ICA and the stent traversing the origin of the external carotid artery. However, some patients receive stents that lie completely in the CCA, whereas a small minority undergo stent placement with a device located entirely in the ICA. Even when the external carotid origin is crossed by the stent, patency of this vessel is usually maintained by flow through the interstices of the stent (Fig. 10.9).

Many of the commonly used carotid stents are tapered (larger proximal diameter and smaller distal diameter) in order to more closely approximate the change in caliber that takes place from the CCA to the ICA (Fig. 10.10). The majority of patients receive only one stent. Stent deployment and apposition of the stent to the arterial wall can be assessed by B-mode imaging (Fig. 10.11). The presence of surrounding plaque, luminal narrowing, or intimal hyperplasia should also be noted. As shown in Figure 10.12, intimal hyperplastic lesions in carotid stents can be echolucent, and not well-visualized on B-mode imaging, making color flow imaging and Doppler spectral waveforms essential for diagnosis.

The proximal transition between the native inflow artery and the stent and the distal transition between the end of the stent and the native artery usually do not demonstrate any major flow abnormalities. However, if increased velocities or other signs of a focal flow disturbance are found, the peak velocities should be recorded and images saved. The Doppler sample volume should be "walked" through the entire length of the stent, sampling velocities throughout. Regions of focal velocity elevation or disordered flow should be noted because these could be signs of intimal hyperplasia, stent deformation, or stent fracture.

An effort should be made to maintain a constant angle of 60 degrees between the Doppler beam and the long axis of the artery (vessel wall) for all velocity measurements in order to minimize variability. If a 60-degree angle cannot be achieved, then a correctly aligned angle of less than 60 degrees is acceptable. A review of experience with duplex scanning in the Carotid Revascularization Endarterectomy versus Stenting Trial showed that angle alignment errors were relatively common, although they resulted in reclassification of stenosis severity in only a small proportion of cases.[33] The ultrasound core laboratory evaluated 1702 pretreatment and 1743 12-month follow-up carotid duplex scans from 111 clinical sites (873 CEA, 870 CAS). There was a high rate of agreement between the site-reported duplex scan results and the results verified by the ultrasound core laboratory. However, based on a threshold PSV for greater than 70% stenosis of greater than 230 cm/s on the pretreatment scans and greater than 300 cm/s on the follow-up scans, the core laboratory review resulted in reclassification of stenosis severity in 75 (4.4%) of the pretreatment scans and 13 (0.75%) of the follow-up scans. The proportion of reclassification at follow-up was greater for CAS (10 scans, 1.2%) than for CEA (3 scans, 0.34%).

FIGURE 10.7. *Top,* B-mode image of a normal carotid stent with the proximal end in the common carotid artery (CCA). *Bottom,* Note the normal "narrow" Doppler spectral waveform with almost no spectral broadening.

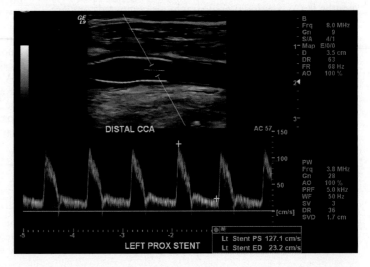

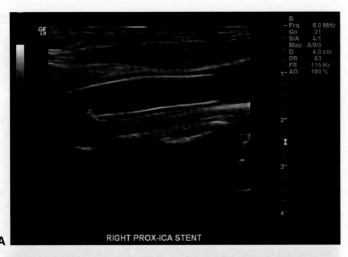

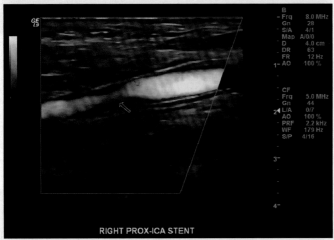

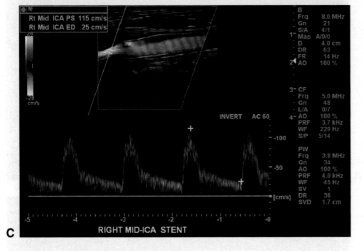

FIGURE 10.8. *A*, Right internal carotid artery (ICA) after stent placement. This chromacolor B-mode image appears to demonstrate a widely patent stent lumen (*arrow*). *B*, Power Doppler image in the same area as (*A*) indicates possible intimal hyperplastic ingrowth, with narrowing of the stented lumen (*arrow*). *C*, Color flow image (*top*) and Doppler spectral waveform (*bottom*) at the same site reveal a peak systolic velocity of 115 cm/s with minimal spectral broadening. Thus, there is no evidence of a hemodynamically significant in-stent restenosis.

It is known that stent fracture may occur in patients who have undergone CAS, with a reported prevalence in the range of 2% to 29% in single-center series.[34,35] In the series from Dartmouth University, multiplanar plain x-ray films were obtained in 100 of the 276 CAS procedures performed between August 2000 and October 2008.[36] Overall, there were 3 stent fractures and 24 deformed stents. All stent fractures occurred in closed-cell stents that had been in place for more than 1 year prior to examination. Neither stent fracture nor deformation was significantly associated with the occurrence of late stroke or reintervention. In some cases of stent fracture, the carotid duplex will be entirely normal, and the fracture can be identified only by plain x-ray. In other cases, a region of flow disturbance will be identified by

duplex ultrasound. The accuracy of duplex scanning for identification of this problem is yet to be determined. Likewise, the clinical significance of stent fracture needs to be further elucidated.

Duplex Criteria for In-stent Carotid Restenosis

Lal and coworkers[37] were among the first to suggest that the currently accepted duplex velocity criteria for native carotid arteries may overestimate the prevalence of restenosis after CAS. Among 90 CAS procedures, only 6 demonstrated in-stent residual stenosis of greater than 20% on completion

FIGURE 10.9. Color flow image and Doppler spectral wave-form from an external carotid artery (ECA), which is being perfused through the interstices of a stent. The stent extended from the mid common carotid artery to the distal internal carotid artery. The ECA appears to be widely patent with no major flow disturbance (peak systolic velocity of 61 cm/s).

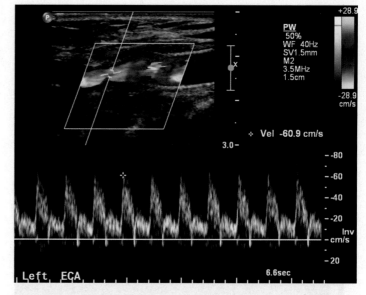

angiography, but immediate postprocedure PSV greater than 130 cm/s was found by duplex in 38 patients. Because a PSV of 130 cm/s or greater corresponded to 50% or greater native carotid stenosis in their laboratory, they concluded that this threshold might be too low for CAS patients, and they suggested that a PSV of less than 150 cm/s corresponded to a normal lumen after CAS.

Stanziale and colleagues[38] from Pittsburgh reviewed 605 patients who had undergone CAS, and among this group, they identified 118 cases in which angiography and duplex were performed within 30 days of each other during follow-up. These investigators also found routine carotid duplex diagnostic criteria to be overly sensitive with low specificity in CAS patients. Based on retrospective analysis of the 118 pairs of studies, they found a PSV of 350 cm/s or greater to have 100% sensitivity and 96% specificity for a 70% or greater restenosis in a stented carotid artery. Likewise, they found a stent/CCA

FIGURE 10.10. A, Color flow imaging of a tapered carotid artery stent in the left carotid bifurcation. B, The mildly elevated peak systolic velocities in this tapered stent (194 cm/s) would not reach the threshold level for diagnosis of a 50% or greater in-stent restenosis based on published recommendations (see Table 10.1).

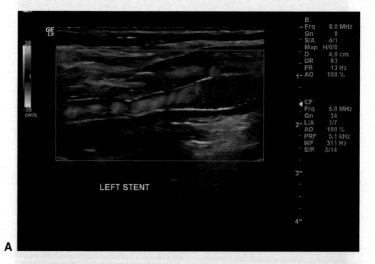

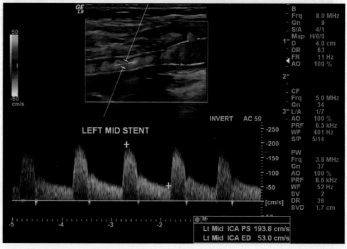

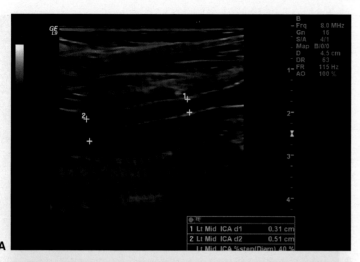

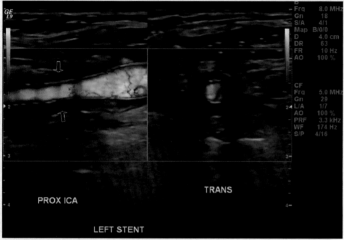

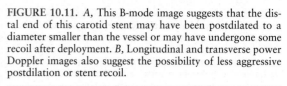

FIGURE 10.11. *A,* This B-mode image suggests that the distal end of this carotid stent may have been postdilated to a diameter smaller than the vessel or may have undergone some recoil after deployment. *B,* Longitudinal and transverse power Doppler images also suggest the possibility of less aggressive postdilation or stent recoil.

PSV ratio of 4.75 or greater to have 100% sensitivity and 95% specificity for 70% or greater restenosis. For a 50% or greater in-stent restenosis, they identified a PSV greater than 225 cm/s and stent/CCA PSV ratio greater than 2.5 as being highly accurate. Although these values require prospective validation, consensus is building that routine native carotid duplex velocity criteria are likely to overestimate the incidence and severity of in-stent restenosis in the CAS patient.

Several additional authors have provided data that support the relative accuracy of the values recommended by Stanziale and colleagues.[38] All of the clinical series are small because restenosis after CAS is a rare event. Nevertheless, Armstrong and associates recommend PSV greater than 300 cm/s, stent/CCA PSV ratio greater than 4, and EDV greater than 125 cm/s as velocity markers of an in-stent carotid restenosis of greater than 75%.[39] Based on 18 carotid arteries with in-stent restenosis greater than 70% by angiography, Zhou and coworkers found a PSV greater than 300 cm/s to have 94% sensitivity and 50% specificity, whereas EDV greater than 90 cm/s had 89% sensitivity and 100% specificity, and stent/CCA PSV ratio greater than 4 demonstrated 94% sensitivity and 75% specificity for a 70% or greater in-stent carotid restenosis.[40]

In a follow-up report, Lal and colleagues reviewed 99 pairs of duplex and CTA measurements, plus 29 pairs of duplex and carotid angiograms, all performed in patients who had undergone CAS.[41] By ROC analysis with acceptable sensitivity and specificity, they recommended a PSV of 220 cm/s or greater and stent/CCA PSV ratio 2.7 or greater for 50% or greater in-stent restenosis and a PSV greater than 340 cm/s and stent/CCA PSV ratio of 4.15 or greater to diagnose 80%

or greater in-stent restenosis. Investigators from laboratories around the country appear to be in relatively closer agreement regarding the duplex diagnosis of in-stent restenosis following CAS than they ever have been on the diagnostic thresholds for native carotid artery disease (Table 10.1).

CONCLUSIONS

Duplex ultrasound is ideally suited for follow-up of patients after CEA and CAS. The incidence of restenosis, occlusion, and neurologic events appears to be low after both of these procedures, and in many cases, the frequency of follow-up testing will be based on the severity of disease in the contralateral untreated internal carotid artery. In the Carotid Revascularization Endarterectomy versus Stenting Trial, the Kaplan-Meier estimate for the frequency of restenosis was 5.8% in both the CEA group (57 of 1105) and CAS group (56 of 1086) at 2 years after revascularization.[13] Further analysis demonstrated that the rates of restenosis were not different in patients with or without neurologic symptoms prior to intervention; however, patients with restenosis were more likely to be women, hypertensive, diabetic, and dyslipidemic. Restenosis was more common in smokers who underwent CEA, but smoking was not associated with restenosis after CAS. Using a similar duplex follow-up protocol, Barros and associates observed a 6.0% frequency of restenosis at 2 years among 96 patients undergoing 100 CAS procedures.[42]

The reported duplex ultrasound velocity thresholds for in-stent restenosis after CAS listed in Table 10.1 indicate that

FIGURE 10.12. *A*, Longitudinal B-mode image of a stent in the common carotid artery (CCA) with some low-level intraluminal echoes suggesting the presence of intimal hyperplasia. *B*, Color flow image of the same CCA clearly showing a narrowed flow channel through the stent. The intimal hyperplastic lesion is echolucent relative to the stent and surrounding tissue. *C*, The presence of an in-stent restenosis is confirmed by a significant focal velocity increase (peak systolic velocity of 485 cm/s).

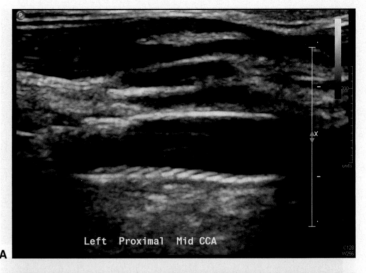

A

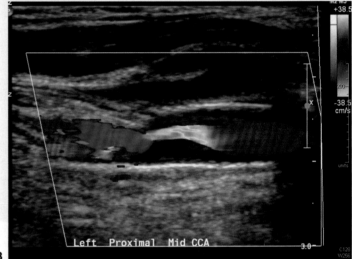

B

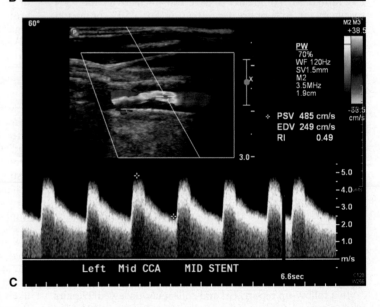

C

the standard velocity criteria for native carotid artery stenosis will overestimate the severity of restenosis after CAS. The velocity threshold used for 70% or greater restenosis in the Carotid Revascularization Endarterectomy versus Stenting Trial was a PSV of 300 cm/s or more.[13] In a unique study of the relationship between the severity of angiographic carotid stenosis and duplex velocity parameters, Beach and colleagues created "scattergrams" based on data from published reports on both native and stented carotid arteries.[27] When a total of 2996 PSV measurements were combined on the same set of axes (Fig. 10.13), it was apparent that PSV increased as angiographic stenosis severity increased, although with significant

RECOMMENDATIONS FOR DUPLEX ULTRASOUND DIAGNOSTIC THRESHOLDS FOR IN-STENT RESTENOSIS AFTER CAROTID ARTERY STENTING*

AUTHORS	DIAMETER REDUCTION BY CONTRAST ANGIOGRAPHY OR CTA			
	50%	70%	75%	80%
PSV Thresholds				
Stanziale et al., 2005[38]	225 cm/s	350 cm/s		
Armstrong et al., 2007[39]			300 cm/s	
Zhou et al., 2008[40]		300 cm/s		
Lal et al., 2008[41]	220 cm/s			340 cm/s
Stent/CCA PSV Ratio Thresholds				
Stanziale et al., 2005[38]	2.5	4.75		
Armstrong et al., 2007[39]			4	
Zhou et al., 2008[40]		4		
Lal et al., 2008[41]	2.7			4.15
EDV Thresholds				
Stanziale et al., 2005[38]				
Armstrong et al., 2007[39]			125 cm/s	
Zhou et al., 2008[40]		90 cm/s		
Lal et al., 2008[41]				

*Based on retrospective comparisons of duplex velocities with carotid angiograms and computed tomography angiography. All series are small due to the low frequency of recurrent stenosis.
CCA, common carotid artery; CTA, computed tomography angiography; EDV, end-diastolic velocity; PSV, peak systolic velocity; stent/CCA PSV ratio, highest PSV in the stented segment/mid-CCA PSV.

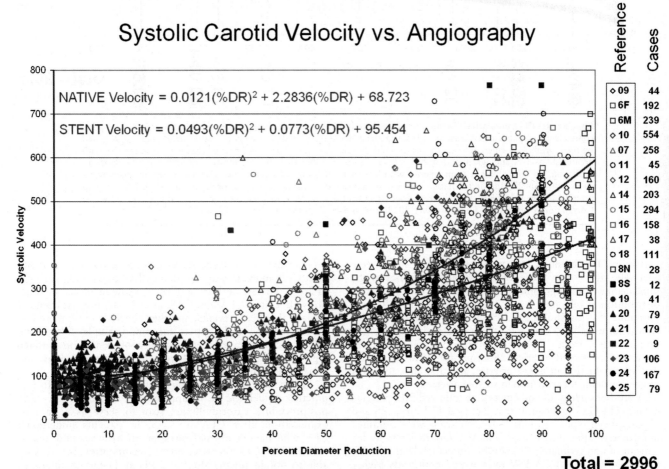

Systolic Carotid Velocity vs. Angiography

NATIVE Velocity = $0.0121(\%DR)^2 + 2.2836(\%DR) + 68.723$

STENT Velocity = $0.0493(\%DR)^2 + 0.0773(\%DR) + 95.454$

Reference	Cases
◇ 09	44
□ 6F	192
□ 6M	239
◇ 10	554
△ 07	258
○ 11	45
◇ 12	160
△ 14	203
○ 15	294
□ 16	158
△ 17	38
○ 18	111
□ 8N	28
■ 8S	12
● 19	41
▲ 20	79
▲ 21	179
■ 22	9
◆ 23	106
● 24	167
◆ 25	79

CEREBROVASCULAR

Total = 2996

FIGURE 10.13. "Scattergram" of peak systolic carotid velocity versus percent diameter reduction by angiography. Compiled results based on 19 publications between 1995 and 2010 including 2996 measurements. Native arteries are represented by *open symbols*; stented arteries are represented by *solid symbols*. Letters after reference numbers indicate separation of cases into males (M) or females (F) and native (N) or stented (S). (From Beach KW, Leotta DF, Zierler RE. Carotid Doppler velocity measurements and anatomic stenosis: Correlation is futile. *Vasc Endovasc Surg* 2012;46:466-474. Reprinted with permission.)

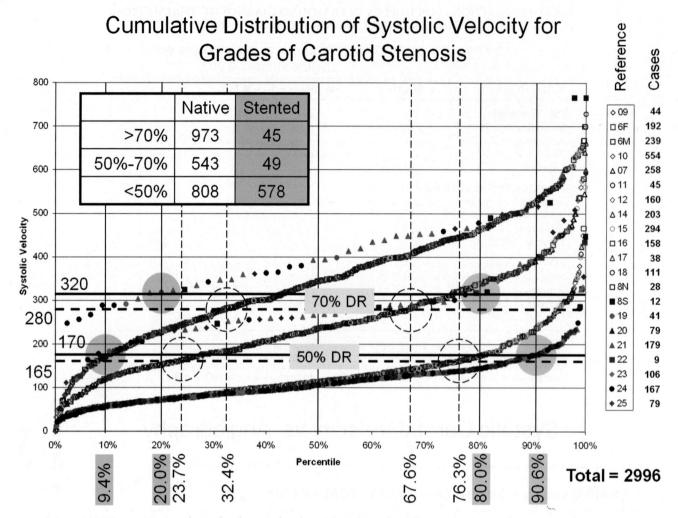

FIGURE 10.14. Cumulative distribution of peak systolic velocity for different stenosis classifications. Compiled results from 19 publications between 1995 and 2010 including 2996 measurements. Native arteries are represented by open symbols; stented arteries are represented by solid symbols. The upper pair of curves is from arteries with greater than 70% angiographic diameter reduction; the middle pair is from arteries with 50% to 70% diameter reduction; the lower pair is from arteries with less than 50% diameter reduction. *Dashed lines* and *open circles* show optimum thresholds for native arteries; *solid lines* and *cyan circles* show optimum thresholds for stented arteries. (From Beach KW, Leotta DF, Zierler RE. Carotid Doppler velocity measurements and anatomic stenosis: Correlation is futile. *Vasc Endovasc Surg* 2012;46:466–474. Reprinted with permission.)

variability. Furthermore, PSV values for carotid stents were generally higher than those for native carotid arteries at the same degree of angiographic stenosis. Based on the cumulative distribution of velocities shown in Figure 10.14, the following optimum PSV thresholds for 50% and 70% carotid stenosis were determined: 165 cm/s for 50% or greater diameter reduction in native arteries, 170 cm/s for 50% or greater diameter reduction in stented arteries, 280 cm/s for 70% or greater diameter reduction in native arteries, and 320 cm/s for 70% or greater diameter reduction in stented arteries.

A study by Hussain and coworkers followed 205 patients having 214 CAS procedures that included 157 open-cell and 57 closed-cell types of stents.[43] Duplex scans were obtained immediately after intervention and at 6-month intervals for a mean of approximately 20 months. Immediately after CAS, both PSV and ICA/CCA PSV ratio were significantly higher for the closed-cell stent group compared to the open-cell stent group, and this difference persisted throughout the follow-up period. The authors concluded that duplex velocity criteria for in-stent restenosis after CAS may need to be modified according to stent type.

A review of evidence relevant to ultrasound surveillance after CEA and CAS was reported by Kallmayer and associates in 2014.[44] These authors confirmed a low incidence of restenosis after both CEA and CAS, as well as a low incidence of ipsilateral ischemic events, and they concluded that there was little evidence-based support for routine duplex ultrasound follow-up. However, the possibility of benefit in selected high-risk subgroups, such as women, diabetics, smokers, and patients with hyperlipidemia, could not be excluded.

In the absence of rigorous clinical evidence or formal practice guidelines, it is appropriate to obtain an early postprocedure carotid duplex scan to serve as a baseline examination after CEA or CAS. In patients undergoing CEA who have a normal intraoperative ultrasound assessment or early postoperative duplex examination, it is reasonable to obtain further duplex scans at 12-month intervals, with more frequent follow-up at 6-month intervals in those patients with ipsilateral carotid abnormalities or significant contralateral carotid disease or those considered to be at high risk for restenosis. Since there has been less reported long-term follow-up after CAS, it is reasonable to obtain duplex scans at 6-month intervals in patients after CAS procedures. If duplex follow-up at 6-month intervals shows widely patent treated arteries for several years after CAS, extending the follow-up interval to 12 months can be considered. Of course, these recommendations are subject to modification as new evidence becomes available.

References

1. Yadav JS, Wholey MH, Kuntz RE, et al. Protected carotid-artery stenting versus endarterectomy in high-risk patients. *N Engl J Med* 2004;351:1493-1501.
2. Pokras R, Dyken ML. Dramatic changes in the performance of endarterectomy for diseases of the extracranial arteries of the head. *Stroke* 1988;19:1289-1290.
3. North American Symptomatic Carotid Endarterectomy Trial Collaborators. Beneficial effect of carotid endarterectomy in symptomatic patients with high-grade carotid stenosis. *N Engl J Med* 1991;15:445-453.
4. Executive Committee for the Asymptomatic Carotid Atherosclerosis Study. Endarterectomy for asymptomatic carotid artery stenosis. *JAMA* 1995;273:1421-1428.
5. Dumont TM, Rughani AI. National trends in carotid artery revascularization surgery. *J Neurosurg* 2012;116:1251-1257.
6. Skerritt MR, Block RC, Pearson TA, et al. Carotid endarterectomy and carotid artery stenting utilization trends over time. *BMC Neurol* 2012;12(17).
7. Brott TG, Hobson RW, Howard G, et al. Stenting versus endarterectomy for treatment of carotid-artery stenosis. *N Engl J Med* 2010;363:11-23.
8. Roederer GO, et al. A simple spectral parameter for accurate classification of severe carotid disease. *Bruit* 1984;8:174-178.
9. Roederer GO, Langlois YE, Jager KA, et al. The natural history of carotid arterial disease in asymptomatic patients with cervical bruits. *Stroke* 1984;15:605-613.
10. Zwolak RM. Expert commentary: Carotid endarterectomy without angiography: Are we ready? *Vasc Surg* 1997;31:1-9.
11. Dawson DL, Zierler RE, Strandness DE, et al. The role of duplex scanning and arteriography before carotid endarterectomy: A prospective study. *J Vasc Surg* 1993;18:673-683.
12. Sidawy AN, Zwolak RM, White RA, et al. Risk-adjusted 30-day outcomes of carotid stenting and endarterectomy: Results from the SVS Vascular Registry. *J Vasc Surg* 2009;49:71-79.
13. Lal BK, Beach KW, Roubin GS, et al. Restenosis after carotid artery stenting and endarterectomy: A secondary analysis if CREST, a randomized controlled trial. *Lancet Neurol* 2012;11:755-763.
14. Zierler RE, Bandyk DF, Thiele BL, et al. Carotid artery stenosis following endarterectomy. *Arch Surg* 1982;117:1408-1415.
15. Baker WH, Hayes AC, Mahler D, et al. Durability of carotid endarterectomy. *Surgery* 1983;94:112-115.
16. Healy DA, Zierler RE, Nicholls SC, et al. Long-term follow-up and clinical outcome of carotid restenosis. *J Vasc Surg* 1989;10:662-668; discussion 668-669.
17. Bernstein EF, Torem S, Dilley RB. Does carotid restenosis predict an increased risk of late symptoms, stroke, or death? *Ann Surg* 1990;212:629-636.
18. Mackey WC, Belkin M, Sindhi R, et al. Routine postendarterectomy duplex surveillance: Does it prevent late stroke? *J Vasc Surg* 1992;16:934-939; discussion 939-940.
19. Ricotta JJ, DeWeese JA. Is routine carotid ultrasound surveillance after carotid endarterectomy worthwhile? *Am J Surg* 1996;172:140-142; discussion 143.
20. Roth SM, Bacj MR, Bandyk DF, et al. A rational algorithm for duplex scan surveillance after carotid endarterectomy. *J Vasc Surg* 1999;30:453-460.
21. Iyer SS, White CJ, Hopkins LN, et al. Carotid artery revascularization in high-surgical-risk patients using the Carotid WALLSTENT and FilterWire EX/EZ: 1-year outcomes in the BEACH Pivotal Group. *J Am Coll Cardiol* 2008;51:427-434.
22. Ouriel K, Green RM. Clinical and technical factors influencing recurrent carotid stenosis and occlusion after endarterectomy. *J Vasc Surg* 1987;5:702-706.
23. Myers SI, Valentine RJ, Chervu A, et al. Saphenous vein patch versus primary closure for carotid endarterectomy: Long-term assessment of a randomized prospective study. *J Vasc Surg* 1994;19:15-22.
24. Bond R, Rerkesem K, Naylor AR, et al. Systematic review of randomized controlled trials of patch angioplasty versus primary closure and different types of patch materials during carotid endarterectomy. *J Vasc Surg* 2004;40:1126-1135.
25. National Quality Forum. Measure #0466 Percentage of patients undergoing conventional (non-eversion) carotid endarterectomy who have patch closure of the arteriotomy; 2008. Available at http://www.qualityforum.org/measures_List.aspx?Keyword=carotid+endarterectomy#
26. AbuRahma AF, Stone P, Deem S, et al. Proposed duplex velocity criteria for carotid restenosis following carotid endarterectomy with patch closure. *J Vasc Surg* 2009;50:286-291.
27. Beach KW, Leotta DF, Zierler RE. Carotid Doppler velocity measurements and anatomic stenosis: Correlation is futile. *Vasc Endovascular Surg* 2012;46:466-474.
28. Grant EG, Benson CB, Moneta GL, et al. Carotid artery stenosis: Grayscale and Doppler US diagnosis—Society of Radiologists in Ultrasound consensus conference. *Radiology* 2003;229:340-346.
29. Moneta GL, Edwards JM, Chitwood RW, et al. Correlation of North American Symptomatic Carotid Endarterectomy Trial (NASCET) angiographic definition of 70% to 99% internal carotid artery stenosis with duplex scanning. *J Vasc Surg* 1993;17:152-159.
30. Phurrough S, et al. Coverage Decision Memorandum for Carotid Artery Stenting. Centers for Medicare and Medicaid Services Coverage and Analysis Group; March 17, 2005. Available at https://www.cms.hhs.gov/mcd/viewdecisionmemo.asp?id=157
31. Hobson RW II, Lal BK, Chukhtoura E, et al. Carotid artery stenting: Analysis of data for 105 patients at high risk. *J Vasc Surg* 2003;37:1234-1239.
32. Gurm HS, Yadav JS, Young N, et al. Long-term results of carotid stenting versus endarterectomy in high-risk patients. *N Engl J Med* 2008;358:1572-1579.
33. Zierler RE, Beach KW, Bergelin RO, et al. Agreement between site-reported and ultrasound core laboratory results for duplex ultrasound velocity measurements in the carotid revascularization endarterectomy versus stenting trial (CREST). *J Vasc Surg* 2014;59:2-7.
34. Varcoe RL, Mah J, Young N, et al. Prevalence of carotid stent fractures in a single-center experience. *J Endovasc Ther* 2008;15:485-489.
35. Ling AJ, Mwipatayi P, Gandhi T, et al. Stenting for carotid artery stenosis: Fractures, proposed etiology and the need for surveillance. *J Vasc Surg* 2008;47:1220-1226; discussion 1226.
36. Chang CK, Huded CP, Powell RJ. Prevalence and clinical significance of stent fracture and deformation following carotid artery stenting (abstract). *J Vasc Surg* 2009;49(5 Suppl):17S.
37. Lal BK, Hobson RW II, Goldstein J, et al. Carotid artery stenting: Is there a need to revise ultrasound velocity criteria? *J Vasc Surg* 2004;39:58-66.
38. Stanziale SF, Wholey MH, Boules TN, et al. Determining in-stent stenosis of carotid arteries by duplex ultrasound criteria. *J Endovasc Ther* 2005;12:346-353.
39. Armstrong PA, Bandyk DF, Johnson BL, et al. Duplex scan surveillance after carotid angioplasty and stenting: A rational definition of stent stenosis. *J Vasc Surg* 2007;46:460-465; discussion 465-466.
40. Zhou W, Felkai DD, Evans M, et al. Ultrasound criteria for severe in-stent restenosis following carotid artery stenting. *J Vasc Surg* 2008;47:74-80.
41. Lal BK, Hobson RW II, Tofighi B, et al. Duplex ultrasound velocity criteria for the stented carotid artery. *J Vasc Surg* 2008;47:63-73.
42. Barros P, Felgueiras H, Pinheiro D, et al. Restenosis after carotid artery stenting using a specific designed ultrasonographic protocol. *J Stroke Cerebrovasc Dis* 2014;23:1416-1420.
43. Hussain HG, Aparajita R, Khan SZ, et al. Closed-cell stents present with higher velocities on duplex ultrasound compared with open-cell stents after carotid intervention: Short and mid-term results. *Ann Vasc Surg* 2011;25:55-63.
44. Kallmayer M, Zieger C, Ahmed AS, et al. Ultrasound surveillance after CAS and CEA: What is the evidence? *J Cardiovasc Surg (Torino)* 2014;55:33-41.

CEREBROVASCULAR

CHAPTER 11 ■ TRANSCRANIAL DOPPLER MONITORING FOR CAROTID REVASCULARIZATION

DEEPAK SHARMA AND K. H. KEVIN LUK

NEUROLOGIC MONITORING DURING CAROTID
ENDARTERECTOMY
TRANSCRANIAL DOPPLER MONITORING FOR CAROTID
ENDARTERECTOMY
   Preoperative Transcranial Doppler

Intraoperative Transcranial Doppler
Postoperative Transcranial Doppler
TRANSCRANIAL DOPPLER MONITORING FOR CAROTID
ARTERY STENTING

Each year, approximately 795,000 people in the United States experience a new or recurrent stroke, and 87% of these strokes are ischemic.[1] The treatment options for atherosclerotic disease of the extracranial carotid artery include carotid revascularization, which may be achieved by open surgical removal of atherosclerotic plaque by carotid endarterectomy (CEA) or endovascular dilation and compression of plaque by carotid artery stenting (CAS). Current guidelines provide a class I recommendation to support CEA and CAS in symptomatic patients with greater than 50% carotid artery stenosis.[2] The guidelines also provide a class IIa recommendation for CEA and a class IIb recommendation for CAS in asymptomatic patients with 70% to 99% stenosis.[2] In 2010, an estimated 100,000 CEAs were performed in the United States.[1] Although the rates of CEA in the Medicare population decreased slightly between 1998 and 2004,[3] the rates of CAS increased dramatically from less than 3% of all carotid revascularization procedures in 1998 to 13% in 2008.[4]

NEUROLOGIC MONITORING DURING CAROTID ENDARTERECTOMY

CEA involves surgical opening of the carotid sheath and exposing the common carotid artery (CCA), internal carotid artery (ICA), and external carotid artery (ECA) followed by removal of the atherosclerotic plaque. In order to maintain a bloodless surgical field and avoid embolization of air and debris to the cerebral circulation, cross-clamping of the carotid branches both distal and proximal to the CCA bifurcation is necessary. The major perioperative neurologic complications of CEA result from[5]:

1. Intraoperative ischemia (due to carotid cross-clamping or due to shunt malfunction if a shunt is used)
2. Intraoperative and postoperative embolism
3. Postoperative carotid thrombosis and
4. Cerebral hyperperfusion

Neuromonitoring during CEA is aimed at early detection of these complications to direct appropriate interventions and minimize neurologic deficits. One option for neuromonitoring is to use regional anesthesia and have an awake, cooperative patient so that cerebral function can be monitored by the patient's executive function and level of consciousness. A decline in neurologic function serves as a surrogate for cerebral ischemia and indicates the need for shunting or other maneuvers. Unfortunately, regional anesthesia is not a viable option for longer and more complex surgeries and for uncooperative patients. When a general anesthetic is used, it is impossible to obtain real-time feedback from the patient and, therefore, additional monitoring is required to detect cerebral ischemia. Since neither technique (general or regional anesthesia) has been shown to be superior to the other,[6] the choice is largely dependent on surgeon preference. Neuromonitoring during CEA may be performed using one or more of the following: electroencephalography (EEG), evoked potentials, cerebral oximetry using near infrared spectroscopy (NIRS), internal carotid stump pressure, and transcranial Doppler (TCD) ultrasonography.[7-9] Each of these techniques has its own advantages and disadvantages, and there are important differences in their sensitivities and specificities for detecting neurologic complications in the setting of CEA.[7-9]

TRANSCRANIAL DOPPLER MONITORING FOR CAROTID ENDARTERECTOMY

No single monitoring technique has been demonstrated to be completely effective in avoiding neurologic complications associated with CEA. However, TCD is the only monitoring method that is able to detect ischemic, hyperemic, and embolic complications, and it can be used for both intraoperative and postoperative monitoring, as well as for preoperative planning.[10] Moreover, it is a continuous, noninvasive, nonradioactive, and nonpharmacologic technique that provides real-time, instantaneous information about changes in cerebral blood flow. Importantly, it is portable and can be performed both in the operating room environment and angiography suite. The report of the Therapeutics and Technology Assessment Subcommittee of the American Academy of Neurology provided a Type B recommendation (Class II to III evidence) to support the use of TCD during CEA to detect hemodynamic and embolic events that may result in perioperative stroke.[11] The applications of TCD monitoring for CEA can be divided into preoperative, intraoperative, and postoperative (Table 11.1).

TABLE 11.1

APPLICATIONS OF TCD MONITORING FOR CEA

Preoperative
- Document presence of adequate temporal acoustic windows
- Evaluation of cerebral collaterals
- Embolus detection
- Assess vasomotor reactivity
- Detection of intracranial arterial stenosis

Intraoperative
- Assessment of cerebral ischemia during carotid clamping and need for a shunt
- Continuous monitoring of shunt function
- Embolus detection
- Evaluation of changes in cerebral flow following clamp release

Postoperative
- Monitoring for hyperperfusion syndrome
- Detection of carotid thrombosis
- Embolus detection

Preoperative Transcranial Doppler

Preoperatively, TCD can be combined with duplex ultrasonography to obtain valuable information for planning CEA. Duplex scanning of the extracranial carotid arteries is discussed in Chapter 8, and the basic principles of TCD are covered in Chapter 9. The TCD assessment prior to CEA includes the following.

a. **Establishing the presence of adequate temporal acoustic windows for insonation of the middle cerebral artery (MCA) during surgery:** In 8% to 10% of the general population, bone density does not allow the ultrasound beam to penetrate the skull, leading to failure of insonation with TCD. Inadequate acoustic windows are more common in women and in older subjects,[12] and the failure rate has been reported to be higher in some series of CEA, most likely due to the relatively older age of the patient population.[8,13]

b. **Evaluating the degree of stenosis and collateralization, including the status of the circle of Willis:** A complete circle of Willis is present in about 30% to 40% of the general population, and the anterior communicating or posterior communicating arteries may be hypoplastic or nonfunctional. The degree of extracranial carotid stenosis and resulting collateralization can be qualitatively assessed by the "reversal of flow" phenomenon seen on TCD. The ophthalmic artery is one of the first branches from the intracranial ICA and forms collateral connections with the internal maxillary branch of the ECA. Flow in the ophthalmic artery is normally directed toward the eye; a reversal in the flow direction of the ophthalmic artery represents ECA to ICA collateralization.[14]

Preoperative TCD is a reliable tool for evaluation of the collateral supply through the circle of Willis in patients with ICA occlusion.[15] A patent anterior communicating artery is indicated on TCD by a reversal of blood flow in the A1-segment of the anterior cerebral artery (ACA) or by a prompt fall in blood velocity in the middle cerebral artery (MCA) after compression of the nonoccluded contralateral carotid artery.[15] Importantly, such carotid compressions must not be performed without first excluding plaques in the carotid system using duplex ultrasonography. In a study evaluating the collateral pathways

through the circle of Willis with TCD and cerebral angiography in 40 patients with ICA occlusion, the sensitivity and specificity of TCD in detecting anterior communicating artery collateral supply were 95% and 100%, respectively.[15] Collateral supply through the basilar artery is usually indicated by (i) a basilar artery blood velocity of more than 70 cm/s; (ii) a marked increase of basilar artery blood velocity after compression of the nonoccluded carotid artery; and (iii) an evident side-to-side asymmetry of the blood velocity in the posterior cerebral arteries with high velocity ipsilateral to the ICA occlusion.[15] For evaluating collateralization via the basilar artery, the sensitivity and specificity of TCD have been reported to be 87% and 95%, respectively.[15]

c. **Preoperative embolus detection:** TCD is also valuable for preoperative detection of cerebral embolization from the carotid lesion and for monitoring therapeutic response using the embolus counts.[16]

d. **Evaluation of hemodynamic significance of carotid stenosis and vasomotor reactivity:** A reversal in the flow direction of the ophthalmic artery represents ECA to ICA collateralization and usually indicates that the lesion in the extracranial carotid artery is long standing and hemodynamically significant.[14] A decrease of mean blood flow velocity more than 70% of the basal value during digital common carotid compression and a critical reduction of vasomotor reactivity (no significant increase of mean blood flow velocity in the MCA during the breath-holding test) also indicate a hemodynamically significant carotid stenosis.[10]

e. **Detecting other intracranial vascular abnormalities:** Preoperative TCD evaluation can also be useful for demonstrating stenosis of the MCA, carotid siphon, and other intracranial arteries.[10]

Although preoperative TCD may provide potentially useful information, some have questioned its utility, arguing that it is not a reliable enough method to modify operative strategy during carotid surgery.[13] However, it is generally agreed that, coupled with arteriography, TCD is a good way to study cerebral hemodynamics.[13]

Intraoperative Transcranial Doppler

Intraoperative monitoring with TCD is aimed at detecting the vascular events leading to cerebral ischemia or hyperemia as they occur, so that appropriate interventions can be made to avoid permanent brain damage.

a. **Probe placement and positioning:** Typically, a 2-MHz pulsed Doppler ultrasound probe is used to insonate the ipsilateral MCA using standard vessel identification criteria. Some surgeons prefer to monitor the MCAs bilaterally. With either approach, it is important to maintain a constant angle of insonation throughout the operation in order to be sure that any observed velocity changes are related to the surgical procedure, because a change in the angle can affect the flow velocity. Hence, it is crucial that a fixation device be used to stabilize the probe position on the patient's head and maintain a constant insonation angle during surgery. Figure 11.1 depicts application of the TCD probe with a head frame for a patient undergoing CEA.

b. **Anesthetic considerations:** Carotid surgery can be performed under regional or general anesthesia. It is important for the person interpreting TCD findings to be aware of the anesthetic technique being used for CEA because this may affect the cerebral blood flow velocities. In general, compared to the awake state, cerebral

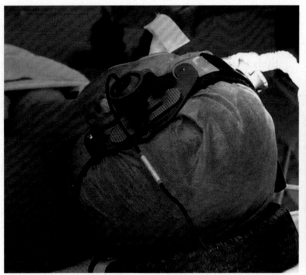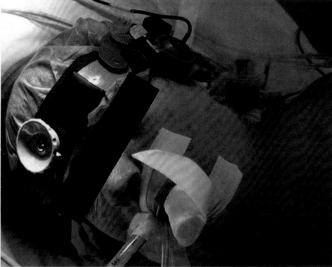

FIGURE 11.1. TCD probe secured over the temporal acoustic window using a commercially available head frame to stabilize the angle of insonation during CEA. The patient is under general anesthesia and intubated.

blood flow velocity decreases with induction of anesthesia, indicating decreased cerebral metabolic activity and flow-metabolism coupling.[17,18] Thereafter, it remains stable unless the anesthetic depth or concentration of the anesthetic agent is changed. Increasing the concentration of volatile anesthetic agent to greater than 1.0 minimum alveolar concentration may increase the MCA velocity if the blood pressure is constant, indicating cerebral vasodilatation.[19] On the other hand, intravenous anesthesia with propofol causes cerebral vasoconstriction and may decrease the MCA velocity.[17]

While there are no data supporting the relative superiority of one anesthetic agent over the other, it is important for the anesthesia provider to ensure that the anesthetic agent and concentration are not changed during crucial periods of the CEA to avoid interference with interpretation of TCD findings. Another physiologic parameter that may affect the interpretation of intraoperative TCD monitoring is the partial pressure of carbon dioxide.[20] Since carbon dioxide is a powerful modulator of cerebrovascular tone, an increase in the partial pressure of carbon dioxide leading to cerebral vasodilatation may cause an increase in the MCA blood flow velocity and vice versa. Therefore, it is important for the anesthesiologist to ensure stable ventilation parameters and avoid inadvertent hypercapnia or hypocapnia during CEA.

c. **Intraoperative monitoring for cerebral ischemia:** Carotid cross-clamping during CEA can cause cerebral ischemia, and the primary goal of neuromonitoring is to determine the need for shunt insertion during the period of cross-clamping to carry blood from the CCA to the ICA and maintain cerebral perfusion. While shunting may prevent cerebral hypoperfusion due to cross-clamping, the routine use of an intraluminal shunt may increase the risk of perioperative stroke due to embolic events.[21,22] Therefore, selective shunting guided by indicators of cerebral hypoperfusion during test clamping is often advocated.[23] It should be acknowledged that there is no definitive evidence that selective shunting is better than routine shunting or nonshunting.[24] However, whenever shunting is planned during CEA, TCD is a useful technique to guide the need for shunt insertion as well as to monitor shunt function.

Most surgeons monitor the MCA ipsilateral to the side of CEA. If insonation of the MCA is started with the patient awake, flow velocity monitoring demonstrates an expected decrease after anesthesia is induced. Thereafter, the velocity remains constant or drifts minimally with no decay over time during prolonged anesthesia.[25] When TCD is used to determine the need for shunting, the immediate "preclamping" mean flow velocity and the relative change (or more specifically, the percent change) following clamping are used. The magnitude of the MCA mean flow velocity decrease following carotid cross-clamping depends on the status of the collateral vessels, and while this decrease may be small in patients with robust collaterals,[21] in others a persistent drop to less than 15% of preclamp values and even complete loss of flow may be seen.[21,26] Approximately 10% of patients exhibit an absolute intolerance to unilateral carotid clamping.[27] Reported studies have indicated various threshold values for the critical decrease in MCA flow velocity that should trigger shunt insertion,[8,9,21,28-31] and consequently, the TCD criteria for shunting vary among centers.

Electroencephalographic findings consistent with cerebral ischemia typically become evident when cerebral blood flow drops below 10 mL/100 g/min,[28,29] which is consistent with an MCA mean flow velocity of 15 cm/s.[28] In general, there appears to be good correlation between the decrease in MCA flow velocity and the frequency of EEG changes after carotid clamping.[26] In the International Transcranial Doppler Collaborators study, cerebral ischemia was considered severe if the MCA mean flow velocity during the first minute after clamping was 0% to 15% of the preclamp value, mild if 16% to 40%, and absent if greater than 40%.[21] These ranges were chosen early in this study and were influenced by ongoing correlative recordings of regional cerebral blood flow (rCBF), EEG, and carotid stump pressure made at some of the 11 participating centers, along with the perioperative rate of severe stroke attributable to intraoperative ischemia.[21] Using the above TCD criteria for cerebral ischemia, it was observed that in patients with persisting ischemia (residual flow velocity 0% to 15%), the rate of severe stroke was very high and shunting was protective against stroke.[21] At the same time, in patients with no ischemia (residual flow velocity >40%), the stroke rate was higher with shunting, although not as high as in the unshunted cases with severe ischemia.[21]

Similarly, Spencer et al[30] using TCD and stump pressure measurements in 97 CEAs observed that a decrease of up to 60% in MCA mean flow velocity after carotid clamping was safe, and a residual mean flow velocity of less than 40% of the preclamp value required shunting.[30] Others have recommended shunting for a drop in MCA mean flow velocity to less than 30% of the preclamping value.[9,31] In a study of 48 patients undergoing CEA with regional anesthesia, a 48% relative reduction in MCA flow velocity after carotid clamping was found to detect clinical neurologic deterioration with 100% sensitivity and 86% specificity.[8]

In summary, most data suggest that a 40% to 50% reduction in the ipsilateral MCA mean flow velocity can be used safely as an indicator for selective shunting during carotid clamping. However, before attributing a decrease in flow velocity to carotid clamping, it should be verified that the angle of insonation, blood pressure, carbon dioxide levels, and anesthetic concentrations are stable. In addition to the flow changes in the ipsilateral MCA, if the contralateral ACA is simultaneously insonated during CEA, the mean flow velocity in the A1 segment of the contralateral ACA can be observed to increase almost instantaneously, within seconds of carotid clamping.[32] The ACA velocity does not change thereafter during clamping, and then typically decreases after the clamp is released.[32] A decrease in pulsatility index (indicating a drop in cerebrovascular resistance), is also observed in the MCA on the side of CEA.[32]

Following shunt insertion, TCD monitoring is helpful in documenting restoration of cerebral perfusion. Published data indicate immediate rebound of MCA flow velocity following shunting to between 50% and 120% of preclamp values.[21,33] Monitoring should be

continued after restoration of flow with a shunt because occasionally a shunt can malfunction due to blockage or kinking. In such situations, TCD can be helpful in early recognition of the problem based on an unexpected decrease in flow velocity.[10,31,34,35] Augmentation of systemic blood pressure is often needed to maintain adequate blood flow through the shunt.[36] Figures 11.2 and 11.3 demonstrate two different scenarios of serial changes in ipsilateral MCA flow velocity during CEA.

d. **Intraoperative and postoperative monitoring for cerebral microemboli:** The principal cause of stroke following CEA is embolism from the operative site.[37,38] Although hemodynamic monitoring by itself cannot reduce perioperative stroke risk, the ability of TCD to detect microemboli is a unique advantage compared to other neuromonitoring techniques for CEA. Studies utilizing TCD have demonstrated that embolization occurs in more than 80% of patients over the course of a CEA.[31,39,40] Intraoperative microembolism may be observed in 5% to 40% of patients during plaque dissection[9,10,39-41] and in about 65% of patients during release of the carotid clamp.[39,41] Microemboli may also be observed with shunting and following wound closure and restoration of blood flow[39-42] and for up to 24 hours postoperatively.[43,44] About 48% of patients have been reported to have one or more emboli detected in the postoperative period, with the majority of these occurring in the first 2 hours.[43]

Monitoring of the MCA using TCD during CEA allows real-time detection of cerebral microemboli. These microemboli can be recognized on TCD as high-intensity transient signals (HITS), and there are potential implications for the number of emboli observed as well as their differentiation into air and particulate types. In general, the majority of emboli observed during the arterial dissection before the arteriotomy and about one-third of those observed immediately after shunt insertion

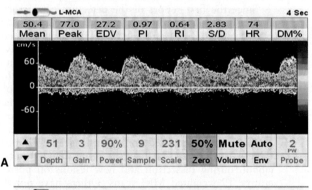

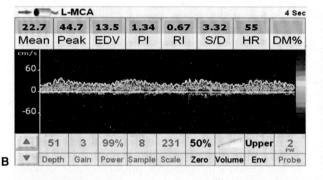

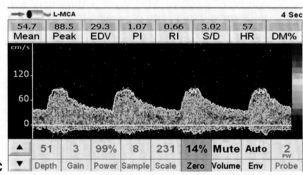

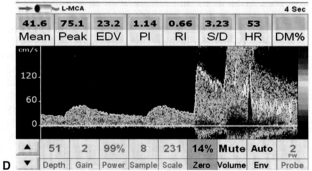

FIGURE 11.2. Serial changes in ipsilateral MCA flow velocity during a CEA. *A,* Preclamp mean flow velocity 50.4 cm/s. *B,* Postclamp mean flow velocity 22.7 cm/s (45% of preclamp value). *C,* Shunt insertion leads to restoration of flow velocity close to the preclamp value (54.7 cm/s), and *D,* Transient hyperemia following completion of the endarterectomy and unclamping of the internal carotid. This patient may not have required a shunt based on the International Transcranial Doppler Collaborators criteria for cerebral ischemia (postclamp flow velocity <40% of preclamp value), but the surgeon elected to shunt.

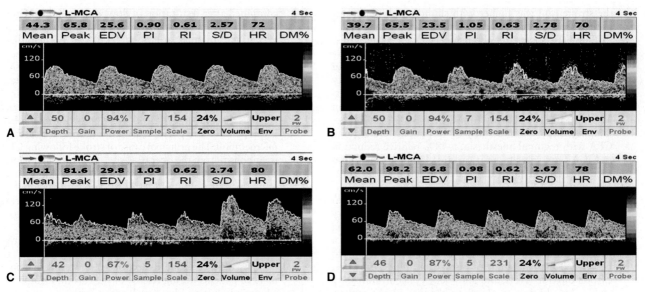

FIGURE 11.3. Serial changes in ipsilateral MCA flow velocity during another CEA. *A*, Preclamp mean flow velocity 44.3 cm/s. *B*, Postclamp mean flow velocity 39.7 cm/s (about 90% of the preclamp value); a shunt was not used. *C*, Unclamping of the internal carotid after endarterectomy is followed by restoration of flow velocity, and *D*, Postoperative mean flow velocity 62 cm/s (140% of the preclamping value). Continued monitoring in the postoperative recovery area for cerebral hyperperfusion syndrome demonstrated no further increase in flow velocity.

are particulate.[41,45] However, the majority of emboli detected in the cerebral circulation after release of the carotid clamp are air, with less than 10% being particulate.[45] It is likely that air emboli, while commonly observed, may have minimal pathologic consequences. Finally, during completion of the operation and closure, particulate emboli are more common. The TCD characteristics of HITS from particulate microemboli are illustrated in Figure 11.4 and include the following[46]:

- Intensity greater than 3 dB above background velocity spectrum
- Duration less than 0.3 seconds
- Unidirectional within the flow velocity spectrum
- Characteristic "chirping," "snapping," or "moaning" sound

It is important to note that HITS on TCD may also be produced as artifacts caused by probe movement, electrical stimuli, or diathermy, and these should be differentiated from microemboli. Bidirectional signatures in the flow velocity waveform are usually artifacts, although air emboli can sometimes produce similar signatures (Fig. 11.5). The major feature of air emboli that makes them grossly distinguishable from particulate emboli is their large dynamic range of around 60 dB compared to the 10 to 15 dB range for particulate emboli (Fig. 11.6). Most commercially available TCD instruments are "overloaded" by signals of such dynamic range, and therefore, air emboli result in signatures that extend outside the normal velocity spectral waveform. This distinction may work for bubbles down to approximately 30 μm in size but not smaller. Although investigators have suggested various techniques, such as the dual

gating method and Wigner spectral analysis, to differentiate between air and particulate emboli,[45] the currently available technology is unable to reliably make this distinction. However, the very high intensity signatures of air emboli, which typically overload the dynamic range of most TCD machines, generally produce some aliasing. On the other hand, the high intensity signals produced by particulate emboli are contained within the velocity waveform and are relatively subtle findings (Fig. 11.4).

Since the first report of the detection of microemboli in the MCA during and in the early postoperative period after CEA,[47] attempts have been made to correlate the number of microemboli detected in a given time period with postoperative neurologic deficits and silent infarction demonstrated on brain imaging. In one of the first attempts to quantify the number of solid microemboli occurring during CEA and determine their clinical significance, Ackerstaff et al[41] noted that microembolism did not result in new morphologic changes in postoperative computed tomography scans, although there was a correlation between more than 10 microemboli during dissection and new lesions on postoperative T2-weighted MRI scans. Others have noted a microembolization rate of greater than 20/hour to be associated with ischemic changes on MRI.[48] In a series of 65 patients where microembolic signals (MES) were detected in 69% of the cases during the first hour postoperatively with counts ranging from 0 to 212/hour, the occurrence of greater than 50 MES/hour in the early postoperative phase was predictive of the development of ipsilateral focal cerebral ischemia.[44] In another study of 81 consecutive patients undergoing CEA with TCD monitoring, Levi et al[49] detected postoperative MES at a

FIGURE 11.4. Microembolic signatures in an MCA velocity waveform indicated by the *black arrows*. Particulate microemboli are typically identified as unidirectional HITS within the flow velocity waveform.

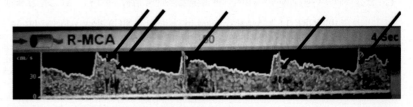

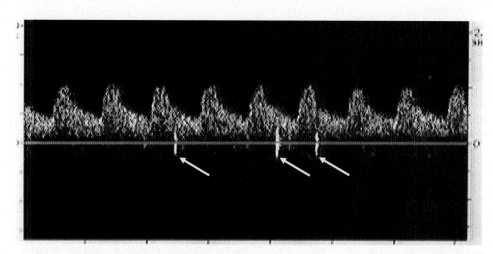

FIGURE 11.5. Signatures consistent with artifacts in a MCA velocity waveform indicated by the *white arrows*. In contrast to true microembolic signatures, these are bidirectional.

rate of more than 50/hour in 8 cases, with 5 of them suffering ischemic neurologic deficits in the territory of the insonated MCA, indicating a strong association between an early postoperative MES count of greater than 50/hour and the development of early cerebral ischemia.

The significance of detecting cerebral microemboli is often questioned because by the time the emboli are detected, they are already in the cerebral circulation. It has been suggested that surgeons could be guided by the documentation of embolic signals to change their operative technique, with the expectation that a decrease in the rate of microembolism would result in a decline in the perioperative stroke rate.[31,41] Moreover, postoperative emboli detection can be used as an indication to intervene with heparin or Dextran to reduce embolization and the consequences thereof.[43,50] In a prospective series of 100 patients who underwent CEA with a 6-hour period of postoperative TCD monitoring, Dextran 40 infusion was started if ≥25 emboli were detected in any 10-minute period.[43] While only five patients developed sustained embolization, in each of these cases, embolization was abolished by Dextran administration, and during the period of this protocol, there was a 0% perioperative morbidity and mortality compared to the same group's previous postoperative thromboembolic stroke rate of 3%.[43]

Other options to decrease cerebral emboli include a combination of clopidogrel or Dextran 40 with dipyridamole/aspirin; however, there has been no difference in the influence of various antiplatelet regimens on embolization detected by TCD following CEA.[51] Subsequent studies have shown that clopidogrel administered the night before surgery, in addition to daily aspirin, significantly reduces postoperative embolization and Dextran utilization.[52] Even when antiplatelet therapy is used preoperatively, TCD monitoring remains useful for determining the need for additional measures such as Dextran 40 in patients who continue to have microemboli during or after CEA.

Postoperative Transcranial Doppler

Successful cerebral revascularization following CEA is usually indicated by the following:

- An increase in ipsilateral MCA and ACA flow velocities compared to preoperative values, which may often exceed the normal values[53]
- Disappearance or a relative reduction of the side-to-side difference in flow velocities[53,54]
- An increase in cerebrovascular reserve capacity[54]
- Normalization of reversed flow or an increase in flow velocity in the ophthalmic artery[55]

Such adaptive changes sometimes take up to 2 weeks to become apparent[54] but may be observed in the immediate postoperative period. As mentioned above, TCD may detect microemboli in the cerebral circulation up to 24 hours after CEA.[41] Other postoperative applications of TCD include the following.

a. **Monitoring for cerebral hyperperfusion syndrome:** A marked increase in cerebral blood flow may occur following CEA in patients undergoing surgery for severe carotid stenosis, most likely due to impairment of cerebral autoregulation. In some patients, such a rebound

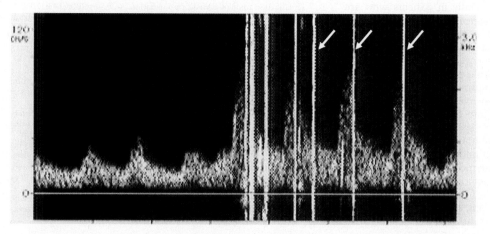

FIGURE 11.6. Multiple microembolic signatures consistent with air emboli in a MCA velocity waveform. These occurred during a CEA immediately following release of the carotid clamp, and some are indicated by the *white arrows*. These display a large dynamic range and extend outside the flow velocity waveform.

increase in blood flow may lead to the "cerebral hyperperfusion syndrome" characterized by ipsilateral headache, hypertension, seizures, and cerebral edema or hemorrhage.[56-58] Risk factors for this syndrome include long-standing hypertension, high-grade carotid stenosis, poor collateral blood flow, contralateral carotid occlusion, impaired cerebral hemodynamic reserve, intraoperative hemodynamic or embolic ischemia, postoperative hypertension, and an ipsilateral increase of $\geq 175\%$ in peak MCA velocity and/or a $\geq 100\%$ increase in pulsatility index.[57,59,60] Intracerebral hemorrhage is reported to occur in 0.4% to 1.8% of patients after CEA and carries a poor prognosis and increased mortality.[56,57,61]

TCD monitoring may be useful to identify such patients as candidates for aggressive pharmacologic measures for blood pressure control. A sustained increase of peak blood flow velocity $\geq 100\%$ or pulsatility index $\geq 100\%$ after declamping should alert the physician about the possible risk of intracerebral hemorrhage.[56,60] However, others have reported low pulsatility with high flow velocity, likely indicating low vascular resistance,[62] and paradoxically, the MCA flow velocity may not be found to be increased if the hemorrhage and neurologic deficit have already occurred.[63] The MCA flow velocity increase is often bilateral, and although the clinical significance of relative flow velocity increases is uncertain, a very high blood flow velocity might be a signal for cerebral hyperperfusion, indicating the need for increased postoperative surveillance and blood pressure control.[64]

b. **Monitoring for thrombosis:** Following successful removal of the carotid atheroma, continued TCD monitoring may be helpful in detecting carotid artery thrombosis. Gaunt and colleagues have reported a decrease in MCA flow velocity and progressively increasing embolization to be indicative of thrombotic occlusion of the carotid artery following CEA and restoration of normal flow.[65] In another example, carotid thrombosis requiring reexploration was diagnosed postoperatively in the setting of progressively increasing embolization, although the flow velocity itself was relatively uncompromised.[66] Hence, TCD monitoring may be useful in differentiating cerebral hyperperfusion syndrome from thrombotic occlusion in a patient with new onset of neurologic deterioration after CEA.

TRANSCRANIAL DOPPLER MONITORING FOR CAROTID ARTERY STENTING

With the advent of endovascular techniques, CAS has become a viable alternative to CEA, especially in patients who are considered to be at high risk for open surgery. The intervention is usually performed under monitored anesthesia care (MAC), such that the patients are conscious and spontaneously breathing, although they may receive some sedation or anxiolysis. Nevertheless, monitoring the cerebral circulation using TCD may provide useful information during and after the procedure. The TCD spectral waveform changes observed during CAS have been classified into four patterns: (1) MES, (2) right-left collateral signals, (3) spectral suppression after balloon inflation, and (4) continuous spectral suppression after balloon removal.[67] The continuous spectral suppression typically appears after stent deployment and balloon dilation and is immediately reversed after removal of the filter device.[67]

The major risk associated with CAS is cerebral embolization of plaque and thrombus causing stroke or asymptomatic brain infarction. Use of embolic protection devices (EPD)

to trap emboli before they reach the brain is now standard practice in CAS. However, emboli smaller than the EPD pores can still reach the brain, and TCD is valuable in detecting these microemboli, which often lead to postintervention ischemic lesions evident on imaging.[68] In a small series, Garami et al[69] demonstrated successful dual probe monitoring with one Doppler probe positioned submandibularly to monitor the ICA and another probe transtemporally to monitor the MCA and ACA during CAS to assess the various EPDs and the techniques of utilization. However, this practice is currently uncommon in routine clinical practice.

Occasionally during CAS, the EPDs may be occluded with fibrin and plaque debris leading to temporary flow impairment.[70] Such decreases in flow may also be detected by TCD. Although originally described after CEA, cerebral hyperperfusion syndrome has also been described after CAS.[71,72] Published data have reported the hyperperfusion syndrome in about 1% of patients following CAS and resulting intracerebral hemorrhage in 0.67% patients.[72] Cerebral hemodynamic monitoring with TCD after CAS may be useful in timely detection of cerebral hyperperfusion.

In summary, CEA and CAS are commonly performed to decrease the risk of stroke in patients with carotid stenosis, and TCD monitoring provides crucial information to the surgeon or interventionalist before, during, and after the procedure. The unique advantages of TCD are the ability to provide continuous, real-time information about cerebral perfusion in a noninvasive manner and the detection of cerebral microemboli. The major limitations of TCD include the absence of adequate acoustic windows in some patients and the need for skilled, experienced personnel. Overall, TCD provides a valuable monitoring technique for carotid revascularization.

References

1. Go AS, Mozaffarian D, Roger VL, et al; American Heart Association Statistics Committee and Stroke Statistics Subcommittee. Executive summary: Heart disease and stroke statistics—2013 update: A report from the American Heart Association. *Circulation* 2013;127(1):143-152.
2. Brott TG, Halperin JL, Abbara S, et al. 2011 ASA/ACCF/AHA/AANN/AANS/ACR/ASNR/CNS/SAIP/SCAI/SIR/SNIS/SVM/SVS Guideline on the Management of Patients with Extracranial Carotid and Vertebral Artery Disease: Executive Summary A Report of the American College of Cardiology Foundation/American Heart Association Task Force on Practice Guidelines, and the American Stroke Association, American Association of Neuroscience Nurses, American Association of Neurological Surgeons, American College of Radiology, American Society of Neuroradiology, Congress of Neurological Surgeons, Society of Atherosclerosis Imaging and Prevention, Society for Cardiovascular Angiography and Interventions, Society of Interventional Radiology, Society of NeuroInterventional Surgery, Society for Vascular Medicine, and Society for Vascular Surgery Developed in Collaboration With the American Academy of Neurology and Society of Cardiovascular Computed Tomography. *J Am Coll Cardiol* 2011;57(8):1002-1044.
3. Goodney PP, Lucas FL, Travis LL, et al. Changes in the use of carotid revascularization among the Medicare population. *Arch Surg* 2008;143:170-173.
4. Dumont TM, Rughani AI. National trends in carotid artery revascularization surgery. *J Neurosurg* 2012;116:1251-1257.
5. Ferguson GG, Eliasziw M, Barr HW, et al. The North American Symptomatic Carotid Endarterectomy Trial: Surgical results in 1415 patients. *Stroke* 1999;30:1751-1758.
6. GALA Trial Collaborative Group, Lewis SC, Warlow CP, Bodenham AR, et al. General anaesthesia versus local anaesthesia for carotid surgery (GALA): A multicentre, randomised controlled trial. *Lancet* 2008;372(9656):2132-2142.
7. Bond R, Rerkasem K, Counsell C, et al. Routine or selective carotid artery shunting for carotid endarterectomy (and different methods of monitoring in selective shunting). *Cochrane Database Syst Rev* 2002;(2):CD000190.
8. Moritz S, Kasprzak P, Arlt M, et al. Accuracy of cerebral monitoring in detecting cerebral ischemia during carotid endarterectomy: A comparison of transcranial Doppler sonography, near-infrared spectroscopy, stump pressure, and somatosensory evoked potentials. *Anesthesiology* 2007;107(4):563-569.
9. Jansen C, Vriens EM, Eikelboom BC, et al. Carotid endarterectomy with transcranial Doppler and electroencephalographic monitoring. A prospective study in 130 operations. *Stroke* 1993;24(5):665-669.

10. Gossetti B, Martinelli O, Guerricchio R, et al. Transcranial Doppler in 178 patients before, during, and after carotid endarterectomy. *J Neuroimaging* 1997;7(4):213-216.

11. Sloan MA, Alexandrov AV, Tegeler CH, et al; Therapeutics and Technology Assessment Subcommittee of the American Academy of Neurology. Assessment: Transcranial Doppler ultrasonography: Report of the Therapeutics and Technology Assessment Subcommittee of the American Academy of Neurology. *Neurology* 2004;62(9):1468-1481.

12. Itoh T, Matsumoto M, Handa N, et al. Rate of successful recording of blood flow signals in the middle cerebral artery using transcranial Doppler sonography. *Stroke* 1993;24:1192-1195.

13. Lagneau P, Baujat B, Anidjar S, et al. Is transcranial Doppler a worthwhile examination for preoperative evaluation of the Circle of Willis? Evaluation of 137 carotid endarterectomies performed under regional anesthesia. *Int Angiol* 1998;17(3):168-170.

14. Tsai CL, Lee JT, Cheng CA, et al. Reversal of ophthalmic artery flow as a predictor of intracranial hemodynamic compromise: Implication for prognosis of severe carotid stenosis. *Eur J Neurol* 2013;20(3):564-570.

15. Müller M, Hermes M, Brückmann H, et al. Transcranial Doppler ultrasound in the evaluation of collateral blood flow in patients with internal carotid artery occlusion: Correlation with cerebral angiography. *AJNR Am J Neuroradiol* 1995;16(1):195-202.

16. van Dellen D, Tiivas CA, Jarvi K, et al. Transcranial Doppler ultrasonography-directed intravenous glycoprotein IIb/IIIa receptor antagonist therapy to control transient cerebral microemboli before and after carotid endarterectomy. *Br J Surg* 2008;95(6):709-713.

17. Ludbrook GL, Visco E, Lam AM. Propofol: Relation between brain concentrations, electroencephalogram, middle cerebral artery blood flow velocity, and cerebral oxygen extraction during induction of anesthesia. *Anesthesiology* 2002;97(6):1363-1370.

18. Thiel A, Zickmann B, Zimmermann R, et al. Transcranial Doppler sonography: Effects of halothane, enflurane and isoflurane on blood flow velocity in the middle cerebral artery. *Br J Anaesth* 1992;68(4):388-393.

19. Bedforth NM, Hardman JG, Nathanson MH. Cerebral hemodynamic response to the introduction of desflurane: A comparison with sevoflurane. *Anesth Analg* 2000;91(1):152-155.

20. Garnham J, Panerai RB, Naylor AR, et al. Cerebrovascular response to dynamic changes in pCO$_2$. *Cerebrovasc Dis* 1999;9(3):146-151.

21. Halsey JH Jr. Risks and benefits of shunting in carotid endarterectomy. The International Transcranial Doppler Collaborators. *Stroke* 1992;23:1583-1587.

22. Cao P, Giordano G, Zannetti S, et al. Transcranial Doppler monitoring during carotid endarterectomy: Is it appropriate for selecting patients in need of a shunt? *J Vasc Surg* 1997;26:973-979.

23. Rerkasem K, Rothwell PM. Routine or selective carotid artery shunting for carotid endarterectomy (and different methods of monitoring in selective shunting). *Cochrane Database Syst Rev* 2009;(4):CD000190.

24. Bond R, Rerkasem K, Rothwell PM. Routine or selective carotid artery shunting for carotid endarterectomy (and different methods of monitoring in selective shunting). *Stroke* 2003;34:824-825.

25. Kuroda Y, Murakami M, Tsuruta J, et al. Blood flow velocity of middle cerebral artery during prolonged anesthesia with halothane, isoflurane, and sevoflurane in humans. *Anesthesiology* 1997;87(3):527-532.

26. Arnold M, Sturzenegger M, Schäffler L, et al. Continuous intraoperative monitoring of middle cerebral artery blood flow velocities and electroencephalography during carotid endarterectomy. A comparison of the two methods to detect cerebral ischemia. *Stroke* 1997;28(7):1345-1350.

27. Sundt TM Jr, Sharbrough FW, Piepgras DG, et al. Correlation of cerebral blood flow and electroencephalographic changes during carotid endarterectomy: With results of surgery and hemodynamics of cerebral ischemia. *Mayo Clin Proc* 1981;56(9):533-543.

28. Halsey JH, McDowell HA, Gelmon S, et al. Blood velocity in the middle cerebral artery and regional cerebral blood flow during carotid endarterectomy. *Stroke* 1989;20(1):53-58.

29. Messick JM Jr, Casement B, Sharbrough FW, et al. Correlation of regional cerebral blood flow (rCBF) with EEG changes during isoflurane anesthesia for carotid endarterectomy: Critical rCBF. *Anesthesiology* 1987;66(3):344-349.

30. Spencer MP, Thomas GI, Moehring MA. Relation between middle cerebral artery blood flow velocity and stump pressure during carotid endarterectomy. *Stroke* 1992;23(10):1439-1445.

31. Spencer MP. Transcranial Doppler monitoring and causes of stroke from carotid endarterectomy. *Stroke* 1997;28(4):685-691.

32. Babikian VL, Schwarze JJ, Cantelmo NL, et al. Collateral flow changes through the anterior communicating artery during carotid endarterectomy. *J Neurol Sci* 1996;138(1-2):53-59.

33. Esses GE, Babikian VL, Cantelmo NL, et al. Hemodynamic considerations during carotid endarterectomy. *J Stroke Cerebrovasc Dis* 1994;4(4):220-223.

34. Naylor AR, Wildsmith JA, McClure J, et al. Transcranial Doppler monitoring during carotid endarterectomy. *Br J Surg* 1991;78(10):1264-1268.

35. Padayachee TS, Bishop CC, Gosling RG, et al. Monitoring cerebral perfusion during carotid endarterectomy. *J Cardiovasc Surg (Torino)* 1990;31(1):112-114.

36. Hayes PD, Vainas T, Hartley S, et al. The Pruitt-Inahara shunt maintains mean middle cerebral artery velocities within 10% of preoperative values during carotid endarterectomy. *J Vasc Surg* 2000;32(2):299-306.

37. Riles TS, Imparato AM, Jacobowitz GR, et al. The cause of perioperative stroke after carotid endarterectomy. *J Vasc Surg* 1994;19(2):206-214.

38. Jacobowitz GR, Rockman CB, Lamparello PJ, et al. Causes of perioperative stroke after carotid endarterectomy: Special considerations in symptomatic patients. *Ann Vasc Surg* 2001;15(1):19-24.

39. Gavrilescu T, Babikian VL, Cantelmo NL, et al. Cerebral microembolism during carotid endarterectomy. *Am J Surg* 1995;170(2):159-164.

40. Gaunt ME, Martin PJ, Smith JL, et al. Clinical relevance of intraoperative embolization detected by transcranial Doppler ultrasonography during carotid endarterectomy: A prospective study of 100 patients. *Br J Surg* 1994;81(10):1435-1439.

41. Ackerstaff RG, Jansen C, Moll FL, et al. The significance of microemboli detection by means of transcranial Doppler ultrasonography monitoring in carotid endarterectomy. *J Vasc Surg* 1995;21(6):963-969.

42. Ackerstaff RG, Moons KG, van de Vlasakker CJ, et al. Association of intraoperative transcranial Doppler monitoring variables with stroke from carotid endarterectomy. *Stroke* 2000;31(8):1817-1823.

43. Lennard N, Smith JL, Dumbille J, et al. Prevention of postoperative thrombotic stroke after carotid endarterectomy: The role of transcranial Doppler ultrasound. *J Vasc Surg* 1997;26:579-584.

44. Levi CR, O'Malley HM, Fell G, et al. Transcranial Doppler detected cerebral microembolism following carotid endarterectomy. High microembolic signal loads predict postoperative cerebral ischaemia. *Brain* 1997;120:621-629.

45. Smith JL, Evans DH, Fan L, et al. Interpretation of embolic phenomena during carotid endarterectomy. *Stroke* 1995;26(12):2281-2284.

46. Basic identification criteria of Doppler microembolic signals. Consensus Committee of the Ninth International Cerebral Hemodynamic Symposium. *Stroke* 1995;26(6):1123.

47. Spencer MP, Thomas GI, Nicholls SC, et al. Detection of middle cerebral artery emboli during carotid endarterectomy using transcranial Doppler ultrasonography. *Stroke* 1990;21:415-423.

48. Cantelmo NL, Babikian VL, Samaraweera RN, et al. Cerebral microembolism and ischemic changes associated with carotid endarterectomy. *J Vasc Surg* 1998;27:1024-1031.

49. Levi CR, Roberts AK, Fell G, et al. Transcranial Doppler microembolus detection in the identification of patients at high risk of perioperative stroke. *Eur J Vasc Endovasc Surg* 1997;14(3):170-176.

50. Levi CR, Bladin CF, Chambers BC, et al. Microembolic watershed infarction complicating carotid endarterectomy. *Cerebrovasc Dis* 1997;7:185-186.

51. de Borst GJ, Hilgevoord AA, de Vries JP, et al. Influence of antiplatelet therapy on cerebral micro-emboli after carotid endarterectomy using postoperative transcranial Doppler monitoring. *Eur J Vasc Endovasc Surg* 2007;34(2):135-142.

52. Sharpe RY, Dennis MJ, Nasim A, et al. Dual antiplatelet therapy prior to carotid endarterectomy reduces post-operative embolisation and thromboembolic events: Post-operative transcranial Doppler monitoring is now unnecessary. *Eur J Vasc Endovasc Surg* 2010;40(2):162-167.

53. Araki CT, Babikian VL, Cantelmo NL, et al. Cerebrovascular hemodynamic changes associated with carotid endarterectomy. *J Vasc Surg* 1991;6:854-860.

54. Barzó P, Vörös E, Bodosi M. Use of transcranial Doppler sonography and acetazolamide test to demonstrate changes in cerebrovascular reserve capacity following carotid endarterectomy. *Eur J Vasc Endovasc Surg* 1996;11(1):83-89.

55. Riiheläinen K, Päivänsalo M, Suramo I. The effect of carotid endarterectomy on ocular blood velocity. *Ophthalmology* 1997;104(4):672-675.

56. Jansen C, Sprengers AM, Moll FL, et al. Prediction of intracerebral haemorrhage after carotid endarterectomy by clinical criteria and intraoperative transcranial Doppler monitoring: Results of 233 operations. *Eur J Vasc Surg* 1994;8(2):220-225.

57. Ouriel K, Shortell CK, Illig KA, et al. Intracerebral hemorrhage after carotid endarterectomy: Incidence, contribution to neurologic morbidity, and predictive factors. *J Vasc Surg* 1999;29(1):82-87.

58. Breen JC, Caplan LR, DeWitt LD, et al. Brain edema after carotid surgery. *Neurology* 1996;46(1):175-181.

59. Piepgras DG, Morgan MK, Sundt TM Jr, et al. Intracerebral hemorrhage after carotid endarterectomy. *J Neurosurg* 1988;68(4):532-536.

60. Russell DA, Gough MJ. Intracerebral haemorrhage following carotid endarterectomy. *Eur J Vasc Endovasc Surg* 2004;28(2):115-123.

61. Schroeder T, Sillesen H, Boesen J, et al. Intracerebral haemorrhage after carotid endarterectomy. *Eur J Vasc Surg* 1987;1(1):51-60.

62. Powers AD, Smith RR. Hyperperfusion syndrome after carotid endarterectomy: Transcranial Doppler evaluation. *Neurosurgery* 1990;26(1):56-59.

63. Karapanayiotides T, Meuli R, Devuyst G, et al. Postcarotid endarterectomy hyperperfusion or reperfusion syndrome. *Stroke* 2005;36(1):21-26.

64. Zachrisson H, Blomstrand C, Holm J, et al. Changes in middle cerebral artery blood flow after carotid endarterectomy as monitored by transcranial Doppler. *J Vasc Surg* 2002;36(2):285-290.

CEREBROVASCULAR

65. Gaunt ME, Ratliff DA, Martin PJ, et al. On-table diagnosis of incipient carotid artery thrombosis during carotid endarterectomy by transcranial Doppler scanning. *J Vasc Surg* 1994;20(1):104-107.

66. Gaunt ME. Diagnosis of early postoperative carotid artery thrombosis determined by transcranial Doppler scanning. *J Vasc Surg* 1994;20(6): 1004-1006.

67. Jeong HS, Song HJ, Lee JH, et al. Interpretation of TCD spectral patterns detected during carotid artery stent interventions. *J Endovasc Ther* 2011;18(4):518-526.

68. Gattuso R, Martinelli O, Alunno A, et al. Carotid stenting and transcranial Doppler monitoring: Indications for carotid stenosis treatment. *Vasc Endovascular Surg* 2010;44(7):535-538.

69. Garami ZF, Bismuth J, Charlton-Ouw KM, et al. Feasibility of simultaneous pre- and postfilter transcranial Doppler monitoring during carotid artery stenting. *J Vasc Surg* 2009;49(2):340-344.

70. Castellan L, Causin F, Danieli D, et al. Carotid stenting with filter protection. Correlation of ACT values with angiographic and histopathologic findings. *J Neuroradiol* 2003;30(2):103-108.

71. Lieb M, Shah U, Hines GL. Cerebral hyperperfusion syndrome after carotid intervention: A review. *Cardiol Rev* 2012;20(2):84-89.

72. Abou-Chebl A, Yadav JS, Reginelli JP, et al. Intracranial hemorrhage and hyperperfusion syndrome following carotid artery stenting: Risk factors, prevention, and treatment. *J Am Coll Cardiol* 2004;43(9): 1596-1601.

SECTION IV ■ AORTOILIAC AND PERIPHERAL ARTERIAL

CHAPTER 12 ■ DUPLEX EVALUATION OF LOWER EXTREMITY ARTERIAL OCCLUSIVE DISEASE

GREGORY L. MONETA AND MOLLY J. ZACCARDI

INSTRUMENTATION
EXAMINATION TECHNIQUE
CLASSIFICATION OF STENOSIS

CLINICAL APPLICATIONS
SUMMARY

Arterial duplex scanning provides detailed anatomic and hemodynamic information from the abdominal aorta to the distal tibial vessels that cannot be obtained by indirect physiologic testing. A prospective comparison of arterial duplex scanning with angiography has established standard criteria for normal and diseased arteries.[1] The sensitivity of duplex scanning for detecting the presence of a hemodynamically significant lesion ($\geq$50% diameter reduction) ranges from 89% at the iliac artery to 68% at the popliteal artery. Overall sensitivities for predicting interruption of patency are 90% for the anterior and posterior tibial arteries and 82% for the peroneal artery. This method is versatile and does not appear to be significantly influenced by the presence of previous operations or multilevel disease.

INSTRUMENTATION

A standard duplex ultrasound system with high-resolution B-mode imaging, pulsed Doppler spectral waveform analysis, and color-flow imaging is adequate for lower extremity arterial scanning. Color-flow imaging facilitates the duplex examination by aiding in the rapid identification of arteries and decreasing the overall time required, particularly in the iliac, popliteal trifurcation, and tibial arteries. Color flow also helps in determining the length of an occlusion and distal sites of reconstitution (Fig. 12.1). However, color flow cannot be used to quantify percent stenosis, and the detailed classification of disease severity is based on analysis of Doppler spectral waveforms.[2]

A variety of transducers is needed for a complete lower extremity arterial duplex examination. Low-frequency (2- or 3-MHz) transducers are best for evaluating the iliac arteries, whereas a higher frequency (5-MHz) transducer is adequate in most patients for the infrainguinal vessels. In general, the highest frequency transducer that provides adequate depth penetration should be used. As for other applications of arterial duplex scanning, Doppler angle correction is important when examining the peripheral arteries. Although 60 degrees is generally regarded as "ideal," angles between 30 and 70 degrees are sufficient to provide clinically accurate information.[3]

EXAMINATION TECHNIQUE

A complete lower extremity arterial duplex examination includes the abdominal aorta; the common and external iliac arteries; the common femoral artery; the profunda femoris artery origin; the proximal, middle, and distal superficial femoral artery; the popliteal artery; and the tibial arteries. Examining patients after a fast of 8 to 12 hours facilitates examination of the intra-abdominal vessels. A complete duplex study in a patient with complicated arterial anatomy may require from 1.0 to 1.5 hours.

The examination begins with the abdominal aorta. With the patient in the supine position, a low-frequency transducer is placed below the xiphoid process and angled cephalad (Fig. 12.2). The proximal abdominal aorta can be seen in long axis with visualization of the origins of the celiac trunk and superior mesenteric artery. This aortic segment is evaluated by both B-mode imaging and pulsed Doppler. The transducer is then angled caudad and moved inferiorly to evaluate the distal abdominal aorta. The aortic bifurcation is visualized by placing the transducer at the level of the umbilicus and using an oblique approach from the patient's left side (Fig. 12.3). It is important to sweep the pulsed Doppler sample volume slowly through the distal aorta and proximal common iliac arteries to detect stenotic lesions. The transducer is placed at the level of the iliac crest to evaluate the middle to distal common iliac and proximal external iliac arteries (Fig. 12.4). This usually requires applying considerable probe pressure. In many cases, the internal iliac artery can also be evaluated from this approach. The internal iliac artery is used as a landmark to separate the common iliac from the external iliac artery.

Next, a higher-frequency transducer is placed in the groin and pointed in a cephalad direction to assess the distal external iliac and common femoral arterial segments (Fig. 12.5). The transducer is moved distally down the leg to identify the origins of the profunda femoris and superficial femoral arteries. The profunda femoris artery is normally evaluated for the first 3 or 4 cm, at which point it begins to descend more deeply into the thigh. Attention then turns back to the superficial femoral artery, which is followed down to the level of the knee. When the superficial femoral artery passes through

FIGURE 12.1. Patient with an embolus to the left common femoral artery. The common femoral artery (CFA) is occluded with absence of color filling (*A*) and a preocclusive "thumping" flow waveform (*B*). More distally the superficial femoral artery (SFA) reconstitutes, as shown by color filling with a low-velocity waveform (*C*).

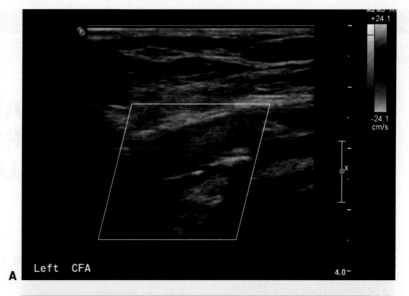

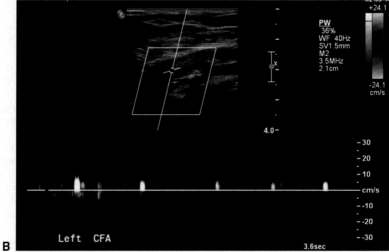

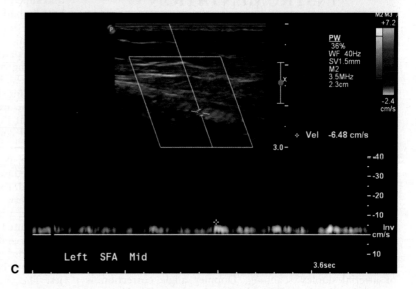

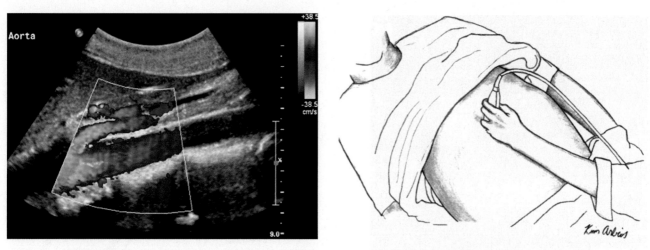

FIGURE 12.2. The transducer is placed just below the xiphoid process and angled cephalad to image the proximal abdominal aorta. The superior mesenteric artery is shown anterior to the aorta in this duplex image.

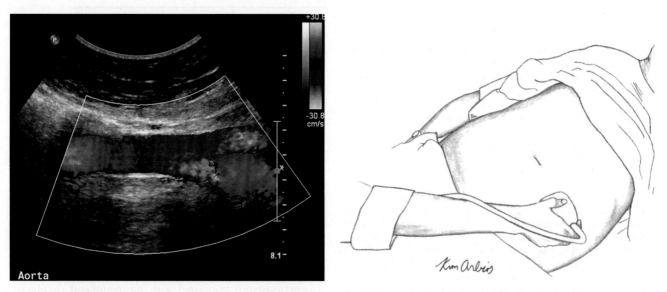

FIGURE 12.3. The transducer is positioned obliquely from the left side at the level of the umbilicus to visualize the distal aorta and proximal common iliac arteries.

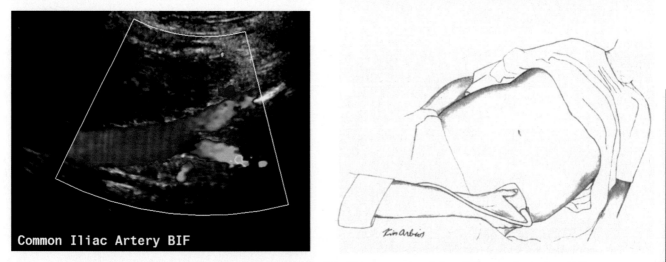

FIGURE 12.4. The transducer is placed at the level of the iliac crest and angled medially to evaluate the middle to distal common iliac artery and the bifurcation (BIF) into the proximal external iliac and internal iliac arteries.

AORTOILIAC AND PERIPHERAL ARTERIAL

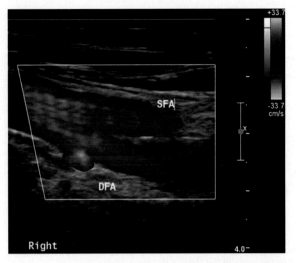 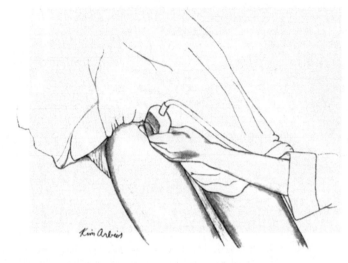

FIGURE 12.5. The transducer is placed in the groin and angled in a cephalad direction to assess the distal external iliac and common femoral arteries. (SFA, superficial femoral artery, DFA, deep femoral artery.)

Hunter's canal, it assumes a deeper position that may make it difficult to assess with the patient supine. At this point, the patient may need to be placed in the prone position to assess the distal superficial femoral and popliteal arteries. As the popliteal artery is scanned in a longitudinal view, the first branch vessel to be encountered is usually the anterior tibial artery.

After the origin of the anterior tibial artery has been identified and interrogated, the technologist places the transducer at the level of the ankle, posterior to the medial malleolus, to visualize the posterior tibial artery (Fig. 12.6). It is possible to follow the posterior tibial artery throughout its entire length up to and including the bifurcation of the tibial-peroneal trunk in the proximal calf. The adjacent paired veins help identify the tibial and peroneal arteries. After scanning the length of the posterior tibial artery, the transducer is placed posterior to the lateral malleolus to assess the distal peroneal artery. Sliding the transducer proximally, the entire length of the peroneal artery is evaluated. Finally, with the transducer

placed anteriorly on the ankle, it is possible to follow the anterior tibial artery up to the level at which it penetrates the interosseous membrane to reach its origin from the popliteal artery.

Velocities should be routinely recorded from specified sites and from any site at which a flow disturbance is identified. Areas of both high velocity (suggestive of a hemodynamically significant stenosis) and low velocity (indicating a more proximal stenosis or occlusion) should be noted. Table 12.1 lists expected blood flow velocities from normal lower extremity arterial segments.

CLASSIFICATION OF STENOSIS

As discussed in Chapter 13, flow waveforms from normal resting lower extremity arteries are triphasic, and end-diastolic flow velocity is near the zero baseline, reflecting the high end-organ resistance associated with the peripheral circulation.

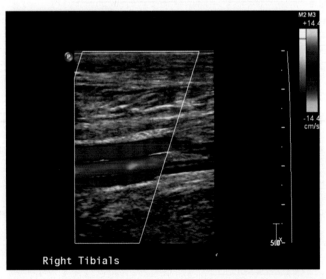 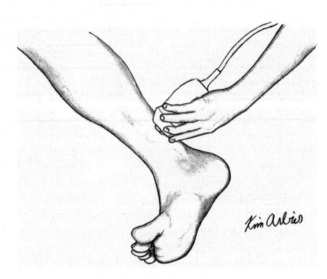

FIGURE 12.6. The transducer is placed at the level of the ankle, posterior to the medial malleolus, to visualize the posterior tibial artery between the adjacent paired veins.

TABLE 12.1

BLOOD FLOW VELOCITIES IN NORMAL LOWER EXTREMITY ARTERIAL SEGMENTS AS MEASURED DURING DUPLEX SCANNING

■ ARTERY	■ PEAK SYSTOLIC VELOCITY (cm/s)
External iliac	119 ± 22
Common femoral	114 ± 25
Superficial femoral	91 ± 14
Popliteal	69 ± 14

This triphasic waveform pattern is maintained throughout the length of the lower extremity, but peak systolic velocity (PSV) decreases from the iliac to the tibial vessels (see Table 12.1). There are no significant differences in velocity measurements among the three tibial/peroneal arteries in normal subjects.

Important changes in the lower extremity flow waveforms that signify occlusive disease include the absence of an end-systolic reverse flow component and focal elevation of the PSV. A 50% reduction in arterial diameter (equivalent to a cross-sectional area reduction of 75%) is associated with a pressure drop across the lesion. The University of Washington criteria for classification of peripheral arterial stenoses by duplex scanning are summarized in Table 12.2 and illustrated in Figure 12.7.

The PSV ratio, obtained by dividing the maximum velocity within a stenosis by the peak velocity in a normal arterial segment just proximal to the stenosis, is also useful for grading stenosis severity. PSV ratios are relatively independent of changes in blood pressure, cardiac output, and vascular compliance. Grading stenoses using the PSV ratio has been found to be highly reproducible.[4,5] Fifty percent or greater stenoses in lower extremity arteries correlate with threshold PSV ratios from 1.4 to 3.0.[1,6-9] A velocity ratio of 2.0 or greater is a reasonable compromise and is used by many vascular laboratories as a threshold for a 50% or greater peripheral arterial stenosis.

CLINICAL APPLICATIONS

Lower extremity duplex scanning can serve as an alternative to arteriography in the preoperative assessment of candidates for arterial intervention. Patients with focal arterial lesions can be identified as most suitable for treatment with endovascular techniques (Fig. 12.8) while patients with more diffuse disease are likely best treated with open surgical reconstruction (Fig. 12.9). In some centers, successful lower extremity revascularization, either by open arterial bypass grafting or with catheter-based techniques, has been reported using only arterial duplex in a high percentage of cases.[10-12] The limiting factor with preoperative arterial duplex is the ability to accurately identify the best site for the distal anastomosis of a bypass graft, especially when the distal anastomotic site is below the knee.[13]

The role of duplex scanning in the surveillance of lower extremity vein grafts has been well documented (Fig. 12.10) and is discussed further in Chapter 17. Repair of graft-threatening stenoses detected by duplex scanning appears to improve secondary graft patency.[14-17] Overall, 20% to 30% of vein grafts will develop a stenosis severe enough to require revision.[18] Approximately 80% of these graft stenoses develop in the first postoperative year; however, graft-threatening lesions can develop at any time. Therefore, surveillance is generally recommended for the life of a graft. A typical protocol for duplex vein graft surveillance is every

Text continues on page 160

TABLE 12.2

UNIVERSITY OF WASHINGTON DUPLEX CRITERIA FOR CLASSIFICATION OF LOWER EXTREMITY ARTERIAL STENOSIS

■ DISEASE SEVERITY	■ SPECTRAL WAVEFORM FEATURES
Normal	Triphasic waveform No spectral broadening
1%-19% Diameter Reduction	Triphasic waveform with minimal spectral broadening PSVs increased <30% relative to the adjacent proximal segment Proximal and distal waveforms remain normal
20%-49% Diameter Reduction	Triphasic waveform usually maintained (although reverse flow component may be diminished) Spectral broadening is prominent, with filling-in of the clear area under the systolic peak PSV is increased from 30% to 100% relative to the adjacent proximal segment Proximal and distal waveforms remain normal
50%-99% Diameter Reduction	Monophasic waveform with loss of the reverse flow component and forward flow throughout the cardiac cycle Extensive spectral broadening PSV is increased > 100% relative to the adjacent proximal segment Distal waveform is monophasic with reduced systolic velocity
Occlusion	No flow detected within the imaged arterial segment Preocclusive "thump" may be heard just proximal to the site of occlusion Distal (collateral) waveforms are monophasic with reduced systolic velocities

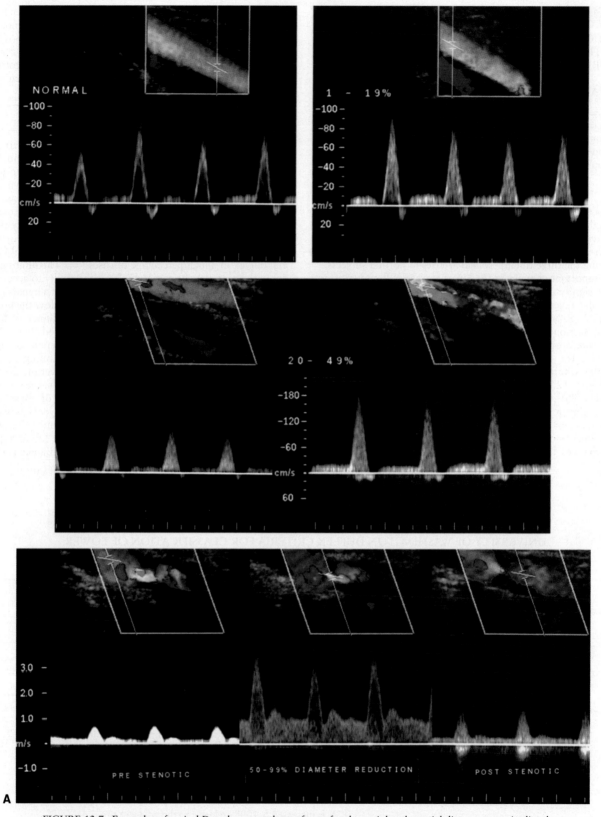

FIGURE 12.7. Examples of typical Doppler spectral waveforms for the peripheral arterial disease categories listed in Table 12.2. (A) Waveforms for normal arteries, 1–19% diameter reduction, 20–49% diameter reduction, and 50–99% diameter reduction.

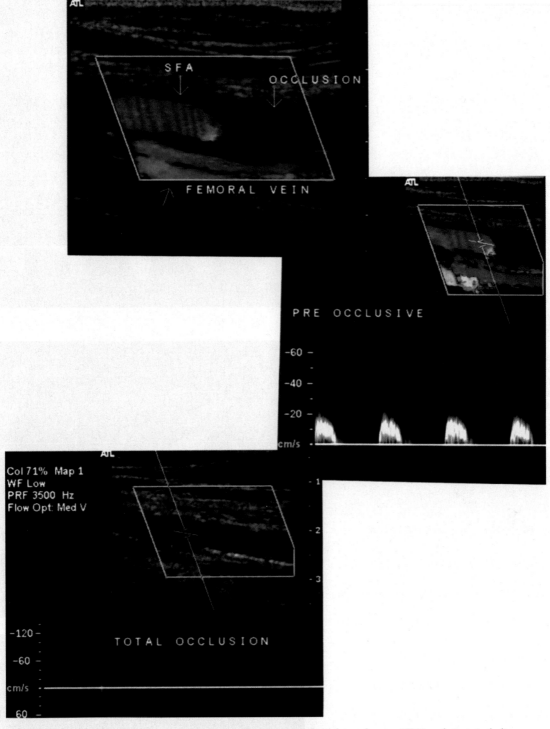

FIGURE 12.7. (*Continued*) (*B*) Findings associated with a superficial femoral artery (SFA) occlusion, including a color-flow image taken just proximal to the site of occlusion, the pre-occlusive waveform, and a B-mode/color-flow image of the occluded segment.

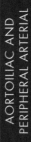

FIGURE 12.7. (*Continued*) (*C*) Distal waveform from an SFA occlusion showing reversed flow direction and monophasic flow in a "re-entry" collateral vessel.

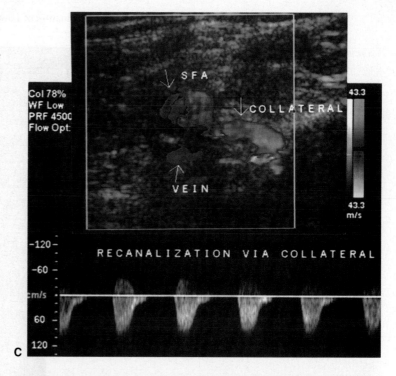

FIGURE 12.8. Duplex examination of the superficial femoral artery (SFA) in a patient with left leg claudication secondary to a high-grade proximal SFA stenosis. Immediately proximal to the stenosis, the waveform is dampened with a relatively low PSV of 28 cm/s (*A*). Within the stenosis, the PSV increases to 356 cm/s (*B*),

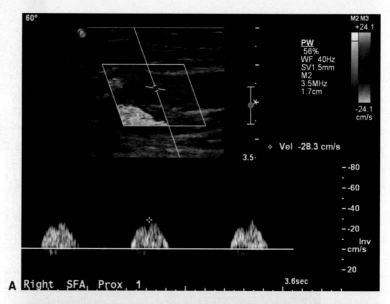

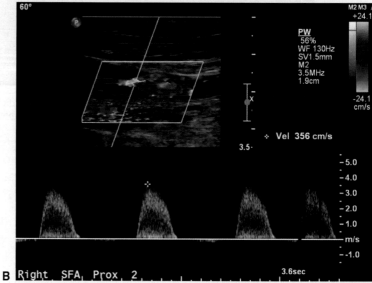

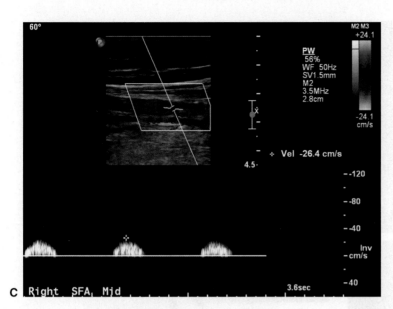

FIGURE 12.8. (*Continued*) while distal to the stenosis, the PSV falls to 26 cm/s (C).

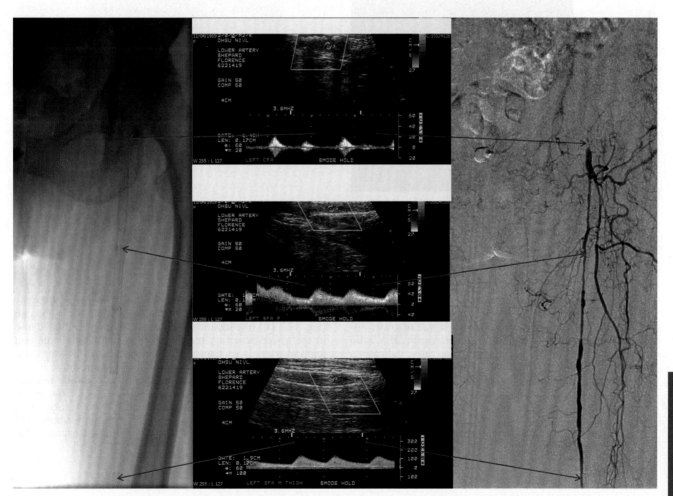

FIGURE 12.9. Arteriogram and duplex images from a patient originally treated with multiple SFA stents for left leg claudication and who now presents with severe ischemic rest pain. The color images show diffuse narrowing of the artery in the previously treated areas with associated dampened and low-velocity waveforms. The common femoral and external iliac arteries are also now occluded.

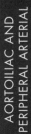

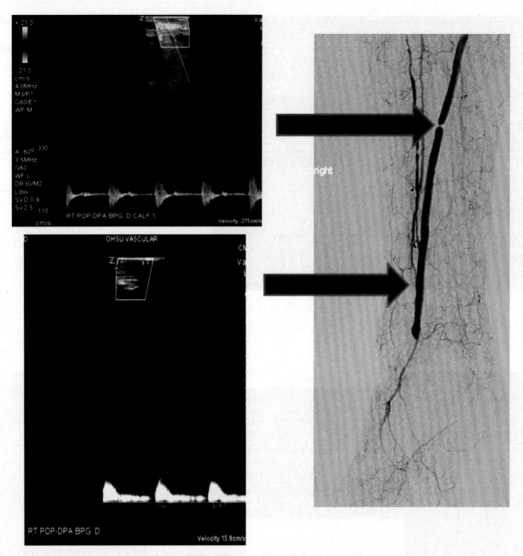

FIGURE 12.10. This arterial duplex examination indicates a high-grade stenosis in the distal segment of a popliteal to dorsalis pedis reversed vein bypass graft. There is an increased flow velocity of 275 cm/s at the site of stenosis and decreased velocity of less than 20 cm/s distally in the graft.

3 months for the first postoperative year and every 6 months thereafter. The examination involves insonation of the proximal inflow arteries, proximal anastomosis, entire graft, distal anastomosis, and the distal outflow arteries. A PSV ratio of 4 or greater, or a PSV of 300 cm/s or greater, indicates a critical graft stenosis, and repair of the lesion by open or catheter-based techniques should be considered.[19] If the PSV ratio is between 2 and 4, the patient should be reevaluated in 3 months.

True peripheral artery aneurysms are relatively infrequently encountered but well recognized. Common femoral and popliteal aneurysms can be easily identified and followed with duplex scanning (Fig. 12.11A). Color flow is particularly useful to document thrombus burden within the aneurysm (Fig. 12.11B). Pseudoaneurysms are also easily evaluated and in the lower extremity most frequently involve the common femoral artery (see Chapter 32). They originate following common femoral artery catheter access, from anastomotic breakdown associated with a prosthetic graft to common femoral artery anastomosis, or from infection (Fig. 12.12). Flow within a pseudoaneurysm secondary to arterial catheterization often demonstrates a "to-and-fro" pattern with flow above and below the baseline as flow within the pseudoaneurysm varies with the cardiac cycle (Fig. 12.13).

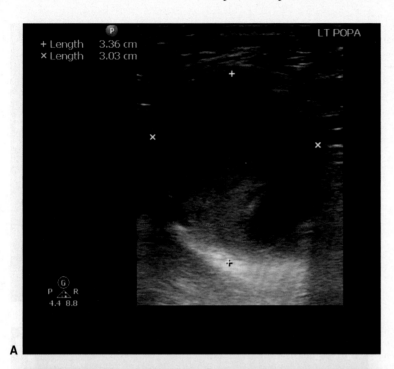

A

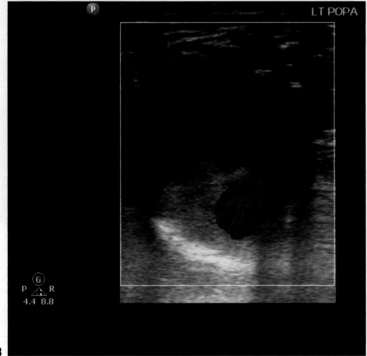

B

FIGURE 12.11. *A*, B-mode image of a 3.36 by 3.03 cm popliteal artery aneurysm. *B*, Color-flow image of the same popliteal artery aneurysm demonstrates a small residual flow channel through the intraluminal thrombus lining the aneurysm. Thrombus within a popliteal artery aneurysm may result in distal embolization or occlusion.

AORTOILIAC AND
PERIPHERAL ARTERIAL

FIGURE 12.12. An infected (mycotic) pseudoaneurysm (>5 cm) of the right common femoral artery secondary to intra-arterial drug injection.

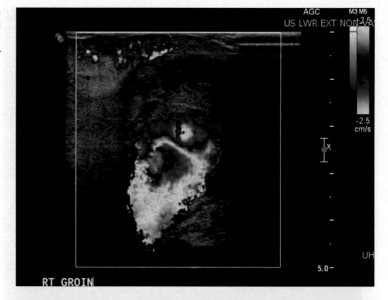

FIGURE 12.13. Color-flow image and velocity waveform from a pseudoaneurysm that resulted from a cardiac catheterization procedure. A "to-and-fro" flow pattern is seen with flow above and below the baseline as flow within the pseudoaneurysm varies with the cardiac cycle.

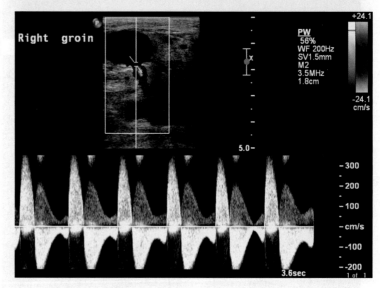

SUMMARY

The noninvasive vascular laboratory provides critically important, objective information to supplement a careful history and physical examination in the evaluation of patients with lower extremity ischemia. Duplex scanning can provide detailed anatomic and hemodynamic information on the status of the lower extremity arteries. When combined with the indirect physiologic tests described in Chapter 13, noninvasive vascular testing establishes the scientific basis for modern therapeutic approaches to the care of patients with arterial occlusive disease.

References

1. Moneta GL, Yeager RA, Antonovic R, et al. Accuracy of lower extremity arterial duplex mapping. *J Vasc Surg* 1992;15:275-284.
2. Jager KA, Ricketts HJ, Strandness DE. Duplex scanning for evaluation of lower limb arterial disease. In Bernstein EF (ed). *Noninvasive Diagnostic Techniques in Vascular Disease.* St. Louis: Mosby, 1985, pp 619-631.
3. Rizzo RJ, Sandager G, Astleford P, et al. Mesenteric flow velocity variations as a function of angle of insonation. *J Vasc Surg* 1990;11:688-694.
4. Whyman MR, Hoskins PR, Leng GC, et al. Accuracy and reproducibility of duplex ultrasound imaging in a phantom model of femoral artery stenosis. *J Vasc Surg* 1993;17:524-530.
5. Leng GC, Whyman MR, Donnan PT, et al. Accuracy and reproducibility of duplex ultrasonography in grading femoropopliteal stenoses. *J Vasc Surg* 1993;17:510-517.
6. Sacks D, Robinson ML, Marinelli DL, et al. Peripheral arterial Doppler ultrasonography: Diagnostic criteria. *J Ultrasound Med* 1992;11:95-103.
7. Jager KA, Phillips DJ, Martin RL, et al. Noninvasive mapping of lower limb arterial lesions. *Ultrasound Med Biol* 1985;11:515-521.
8. Sensier Y, Hartshorne T, Thrush A, et al. A prospective comparison of lower limb colour-coded duplex scanning with arteriography. *Eur J Vasc Endovasc Surg* 1996;11:170-175.
9. de Smet AA, Ermers EJ, Kitslaar PJ. Duplex velocity characteristics of aortoiliac stenoses. *J Vasc Surg* 1996;23:628-636.
10. Elsman BH, Legemate DA, van der Heijden FH, et al. Impact of ultrasonographic duplex scanning on therapeutic decision making in lower-limb arterial disease. *Br J Surg* 1995;82:630-633.
11. Ascher E, Mazzariol F, Hingorani A, et al. The use of duplex ultrasound arterial mapping as an alternative to conventional arteriography for primary and secondary infrapopliteal bypasses. *Am J Surg* 1999;178:162-165.
12. Mazzariol F, Ascher E, Salles-Cunha SX, et al. Values and limitations of duplex ultrasonography as the sole imaging method of preoperative evaluation for popliteal and infrapopliteal bypasses. *Ann Vasc Surg* 1999;13:1-10.
13. Larch E, Minar E, Ahmadi R, et al. Value of color duplex sonography for evaluation of tibioperoneal arteries in patients with femoropopliteal

obstruction: A prospective comparison with anterograde intra-arterial digital subtraction angiography. *J Vasc Surg* 1997;25:629-636.

14. Landry GJ, Moneta GL, Taylor LM Jr, et al. Patency and characteristics of lower extremity vein grafts requiring multiple revisions. *J Vasc Surg* 2000; 32:23-31.

15. Johnson BL, Bandyk DF, Back MR, et al. Intraoperative duplex monitoring of infrainguinal vein bypass procedures. *J Vasc Surg* 2000;31:678-690.

16. Idu MM, Blankenstein JD, de Gier P, et al. Impact of a color-flow duplex surveillance program on infrainguinal vein graft patency: A five-year experience. *J Vasc Surg* 1993;17:42-52; discussion 52-53.

17. Lundell A, Lindblad B, Bergqvist D, et al. Femoropopliteal-crural graft patency is improved by an intensive surveillance program: A prospective randomized study. *J Vasc Surg* 1995;21:26-33; discussion 33-34.

18. Passman MA, Moneta GL, Nehler MR, et al. Do normal early color-flow duplex surveillance examination results of infrainguinal vein grafts preclude the need for late graft revision? *J Vasc Surg* 1995;22:476-481; discussion 482-484.

19. Mills JL Sr, Wixon CL, James DC, et al. The natural history of intermediate and critical vein graft stenosis: Recommendations for continued surveillance or repair. *J Vasc Surg* 2001;33:273-278; discussion 278-280.

CHAPTER 13 ■ INDIRECT PHYSIOLOGIC ASSESSMENT OF LOWER EXTREMITY ARTERIES

GREGORY L. MONETA AND MOLLY J. ZACCARDI

PLETHYSMOGRAPHY	Ankle-Brachial Index
Volume Flow	Segmental Limb Pressures
Pulse Volume Recording	Exercise Testing
Digit Waveforms and Pressure Measurements	Doppler Analog Waveform Analysis
DOPPLER ULTRASOUND	**SUMMARY**

The noninvasive vascular laboratory, in combination with the history and physical examination, plays a critical role in providing objective diagnosis of lower extremity arterial occlusive disease. In many patients, the clinical history and physical examination are all that is necessary to establish a diagnosis of lower extremity intermittent claudication or ischemic rest pain. Almost all such patients will have diminished or absent lower extremity pulses. Palpation of pulses is, however, subjective and poorly reproducible. Therefore, the pulse examination in a patient suspected of having arterial occlusive disease should be supplemented with objective testing in the noninvasive vascular laboratory. Occasionally, a patient will give a history suggesting intermittent claudication yet will have what appear to be normal resting pedal pulses. In this setting, evaluating the response of the ankle systolic pressure to walking exercise is crucial to confirm the diagnosis of intermittent claudication.

Many patients with peripheral arterial disease (PAD) have atypical leg symptoms or are asymptomatic, and these individuals have an increased risk of cardiovascular death similar to that of patients with typical intermittent claudication symptoms. Awareness of these patients has resulted in a renewed interest in screening for the presence of PAD in patients with atypical leg symptoms or atherosclerotic risk factors. Patients with exercise-induced lower extremity or buttock pain should be asked about the location of the pain, its relationship to walking, severity and duration of symptoms, and progression of symptoms over time. Only exercise-induced muscular pain of the calf, thigh, or buttock, relieved within a few minutes of rest and reproduced by additional walking, can be reliably improved by lower extremity arterial revascularization. There are no data on the response of atypical leg symptoms to revascularization in patients with evidence of PAD.

Ischemic rest pain is suspected when a patient complains of pain or numbness in the forefoot, toes, or instep in the resting state. This pain pattern is typically aggravated by elevating the extremity and improved by placing the limb in a dependent position, most likely due to the effect of gravity on hydrostatic pressure and dilatation of collateral vessels. It is also worsened by leg exercise, because patients with ischemic rest pain are clearly at risk for intermittent claudication whenever they walk. Nocturnal leg cramps are generally not manifestations of ischemic rest pain. However, true ischemic rest pain is often worse at night, and some patients seek relief by sleeping in a chair with their legs dependent. As a result, these patients with chronic ischemic rest pain develop profound edema of the symptomatic extremity. This edema is not directly related to arterial insufficiency, but rather to prolonged dependency. Patients with ischemic rest pain will also frequently have thin, atrophic skin on the foot and lower leg, and they exhibit pallor with elevation and rubor with dependency of the foot. Gangrene and ulceration may develop or may be the initial presenting symptoms.

The overall purpose of the vascular laboratory in patients with known or suspected lower extremity PAD is to confirm the presence of arterial insufficiency, provide quantitative and reproducible physiologic data concerning its severity, and document the location and hemodynamic significance of individual arterial lesions. With the exception of determining hemodynamic significance of individual arterial lesions, nonimaging physiologic testing can be used to confirm the presence of arterial disease and provide a very good estimation of disease location.

Lower extremity arterial testing is the one testing area in the vascular laboratory in which nonimaging or indirect physiologic methods are still widely used and provide valuable clinical information. The two categories of nonimaging physiologic testing methods for lower extremity arterial occlusive disease are plethysmography and Doppler ultrasound.

PLETHYSMOGRAPHY

Plethysmography is based on the detection of limb volume changes in response to arterial inflow and venous outflow. In addition to assessing volume flow, this method can be used to measure digit pressures and record pulse volume waveforms. Mercury strain-gauge plethysmography, air plethysmography, and photoplethysmography (PPG) are examples of plethysmographic techniques used clinically.

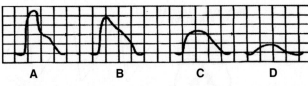

FIGURE 13.1. PVR waveforms. *A,* Normal waveform shows a sharp systolic upstroke, a narrow peak, and a downstroke that bows toward the baseline with a prominent dicrotic notch. *B,* With mild arterial obstruction, the downstroke of the waveform bows away from the baseline with loss of the dicrotic notch. *C,* With moderate arterial obstruction, the amplitude of the waveform is diminished, the upstroke is delayed, and the peak is rounded. *D,* In severe disease, the amplitude of the waveform is even more diminished and the upstroke is more delayed in comparison to moderate disease.

Volume Flow

Calf or foot blood flow can be recorded with a mercury-in-Silastic strain gauge. The electrical resistance of the mercury column depends on the length of the gauge, and when the gauge is wrapped around the limb, small changes in gauge length are proportional to changes in the volume of the extremity. However, there are typically no significant differences in resting calf or foot blood flow between normal subjects and patients with intermittent claudication, even when the symptoms are severe.[1] Hyperemic volume flow is often lower in limbs of patients with arterial occlusive disease, but reactive

hyperemia testing can be quite painful for the patient.[2] Therefore, measurements of volume flow are not very useful in the clinical evaluation of lower extremity ischemia.

Pulse Volume Recording

Air plethysmography can be used to generate pulse volume waveforms, a technique referred to as *pulse volume recording (PVR).*[3] PVR waveforms are obtained with partially inflated air-filled cuffs that detect volume changes sequentially down a limb. The arterial pulse wave causes volume changes in the limb and produces small pressure changes within the cuffs; these changes are displayed as waveforms with the use of appropriate transducers. A normal pulse volume waveform has a sharp systolic upstroke, a narrow peak, and a downstroke that bows toward the baseline and contains a prominent dicrotic notch (Fig. 13.1A). As proximal arterial occlusive disease progresses, the systolic upstroke is delayed, the peak becomes rounded, and the dicrotic notch is lost as the downstroke bows away from the baseline (Fig. 13.1B). With more severe disease, the pulse volume waveform decreases in amplitude and the upstroke and downstroke times become nearly equal (Fig. 13.1C and D). With very severe proximal disease, the pulse volume waveform is absent.[4] Evaluation of pulse volume waveforms is qualitative and based on the shape of the curve, the presence or absence of the dicrotic notch, and the amplitude.[5] Lack of more quantitative data limits the utility of PVR. An example of normal and abnormal lower extremity segmental PVR examinations is shown in Figure 13.2.

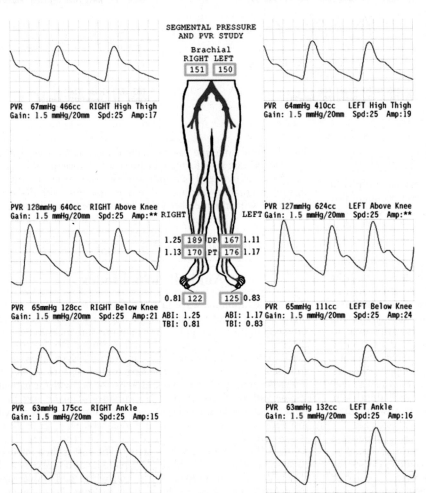

FIGURE 13.2. *A,* Normal lower extremity segmental PVR examination. The pulse volume waveforms at all levels display the normal features shown in Figure 13.1 and described in the text. In addition to the four standard levels (high thigh, above knee, below knee, and ankle), PPG waveforms from the great toes are also shown. The ankle-brachial index (ABI) and toe-brachial index (TBI) are normal bilaterally.

SEGMENTAL PRESSURE AND PVR STUDY

Brachial
RIGHT 151 LEFT 150

PVR 67mmHg 466cc RIGHT High Thigh
Gain: 1.5 mmHg/20mm Spd:25 Amp:17

PVR 64mmHg 410cc LEFT High Thigh
Gain: 1.5 mmHg/20mm Spd:25 Amp:19

PVR 128mmHg 640cc RIGHT Above Knee
Gain: 1.5 mmHg/20mm Spd:25 Amp:**

PVR 127mmHg 624cc LEFT Above Knee
Gain: 1.5 mmHg/20mm Spd:25 Amp:**

RIGHT   LEFT
1.25 189 DP 167 1.11
1.13 170 PT 176 1.17

PVR 65mmHg 128cc RIGHT Below Knee
Gain: 1.5 mmHg/20mm Spd:25 Amp:21

0.81 122   125 0.83

ABI: 1.25   ABI: 1.17
TBI: 0.81   TBI: 0.83

PVR 65mmHg 111cc LEFT Below Knee
Gain: 1.5 mmHg/20mm Spd:25 Amp:24

PVR 63mmHg 175cc RIGHT Ankle
Gain: 1.5 mmHg/20mm Spd:25 Amp:15

PVR 63mmHg 132cc LEFT Ankle
Gain: 1.5 mmHg/20mm Spd:25 Amp:16

PPG RIGHT Great Toe
A Gain: 1 Speed:25 Amp:19

PPG LEFT Great Toe
Gain: 1 Speed:25 Amp:28

FIGURE 13.2. (*Continued*) *B,* Abnormal lower extremity segmental PVR examination. The pulse volume waveforms are abnormal at the right ankle and left below knee, ankle, and toe levels. The right toe pulse volume waveform is borderline. The ABI and TBI are abnormal bilaterally. These findings indicate bilateral disease with more severe involvement on the left.

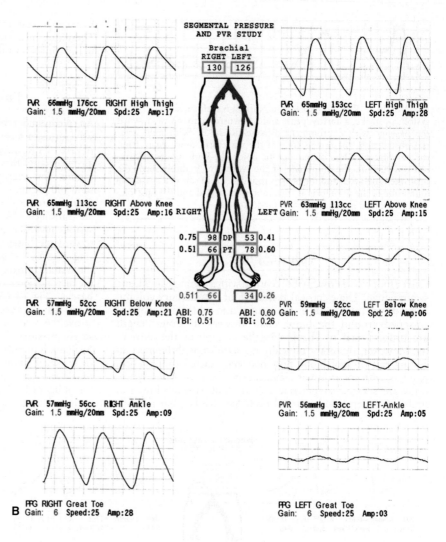

Digit Waveforms and Pressure Measurements

One of the best current applications for plethysmography is in the evaluation of digit blood flow. Air plethysmography, strain-gauge plethysmography, and PPG can all be adapted for this purpose; however, PPG is probably the most widely used technique (Fig. 13.3). It should be noted that the PPG does not record a true volume change and therefore it is not, strictly speaking, a plethysmograph. It consists of an infrared light–emitting diode and a photosensor that detects the light reflected from the tissue. Because red light is attenuated in proportion to the blood content of tissue, the pulse waveform produced by the photosensor has the same features as the true plethysmographic methods. This technique is easily used in combination with pneumatic cuffs to measure digit systolic pressures, as discussed in Chapter 14 for the upper extremity. Digit pressures, as well as comparisons between digit pressures and brachial pressures, are utilized in clinical practice. The toe-to-brachial artery systolic pressure ratio (toe-brachial index or TBI) in normal subjects is greater than 0.70. An absolute digit pressure of less than 50 mm Hg indicates critical ischemia.

PPG-derived digit pressures are particularly useful in patients with highly calcified, noncompressible tibial arteries at the ankle. Digital arteries are less subject to calcification, and in the setting of calcified ankle arteries, toe pressures are a better indicator of the degree of distal ischemia than measurement of ankle pressures. The presence of normal digit PPG waveforms in patients with calcified proximal arteries indicates minimal restriction to blood flow despite the calcific arterial disease. Conversely, an obstructive digit waveform in the presence of normal ankle arterial pulses is frequently an indicator of pedal artery occlusive disease, a situation encountered in many patients with diabetes and those with atheroembolism or connective tissue disorders.

DOPPLER ULTRASOUND

Ankle-Brachial Index

A simple continuous-wave Doppler flow detector can be used along with a set of pneumatic cuffs to measure systolic blood pressures in the lower limb. The site of pressure measurement is determined by cuff placement, and any arterial Doppler signal distal to the cuff can be used. The ratio of ankle systolic pressure to brachial systolic pressure is a very useful measure of overall lower extremity perfusion. This test is performed with the patient supine and after resting for a few minutes to make sure that limb blood flow is at baseline levels. A pneumatic cuff is placed just above the ankle, and the continuous-wave Doppler probe is positioned over the posterior tibial or dorsalis pedis artery distal to the cuff to monitor the flow signal. The cuff is then inflated to suprasystolic levels until the Doppler signal disappears and slowly deflated; the pressure in the cuff when the Doppler signal returns is recorded as the systolic pressure. This sequence is repeated with the other artery at that ankle, and the values compared with the highest brachial artery systolic pressure, also

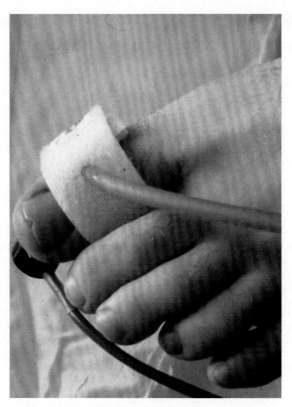

FIGURE 13.3. PPG photosensor and digit cuff attached to the great toe to measure digit pressure.

TABLE 13.2

MODIFIED DEFINITIONS OF NORMAL AND ABNORMAL ABI VALUES

ABI	CLASSIFICATION
>1.40	Noncompressible
1.00-1.40	Normal
0.91-0.99	Borderline
≤0.90	Abnormal

Based on the 2011 ACCF/AHA Focused Update of the Guideline for the Management of Patients With Peripheral Artery Disease. (From Rooke TW, Hirsch AT, Misra S, et al. 2011 ACCF/AHA Focused Update of the Guideline for the Management of Patients With Peripheral Artery Disease (Updating the 2005 Guideline): A Report of the American College of Cardiology Foundation/American Heart Association Task Force on Practice Guidelines. *Circulation* 2011;124:2020-2045.)

obtained with the Doppler. For clinical purposes, the higher ipsilateral dorsalis pedis or posterior tibial artery pressure is divided by the higher brachial artery systolic pressure, yielding the ankle-brachial index (ABI) for that lower extremity. The use of a ratio makes the test relatively independent of day-to-day variations in systemic arterial blood pressure and facilitates serial follow-up and comparisons between patients. As discussed in Chapter 5, a normal ABI is in the range of 1.0 to 1.2, with progressively lower values corresponding to worsening arterial occlusive disease (Table 13.1).[6] A decreased ABI also correlates with an increased risk of cardiovascular death, with the risk increasing as the ABI falls, as discussed in Chapter 26.

The measurement of ABI has several limitations. The brachial systolic pressure used in the calculation is assumed to represent the normal systemic pressure. Although relatively uncommon, significant bilateral subclavian or axillary artery occlusive disease will result in a falsely low systemic pressure measurement and a falsely elevated ABI. Calcified tibial arteries,

which occur most commonly in patients with diabetes or renal failure, may be inadequately or incompletely compressed by the pneumatic cuff. This results in measurement of a falsely elevated ankle pressure and an artificially increased ABI. For this reason, an ABI of 1.4 or greater should be considered abnormal. Such patients have arterial disease and are also at increased risk of cardiovascular death. When the ABI appears to be falsely elevated, qualitative analysis of Doppler-derived analog or plethysmographic waveforms or measurement of digit systolic pressures is a more appropriate indicator of the arterial status of that lower extremity. Other problems with the ABI include confusion with venous signals when the ankle arterial pressure is very low or unmeasurable. A tibial artery can occlude without a change in ABI if the remaining tibial vessels remain patent; high-grade stenosis may also progress to occlusion without a significant change in ABI. Finally, the variability inherent in the measurement should be known. In general, two ABI measurements that are within a range of ±0.15 are not considered to be significantly different.[7] An updated set of guidelines for interpretation of the ABI is shown in Table 13.2.[8]

Segmental Limb Pressures

A series of pneumatic cuffs can be used along the lower extremity to determine the arterial blood pressure at multiple levels. These segmental leg pressures are compared with the higher brachial artery systolic pressure (as for the ABI), with other locations in the ipsilateral leg, and with the corresponding levels in the contralateral extremity. Three or four cuffs may be used on each leg. In the common four-cuff technique, cuffs are placed (1) as far proximal on the thigh as possible (high-thigh), (2) immediately above the knee (above-knee), (3) just below the knee (below-knee), and (4) just proximal to the ankle (ankle). The width of each cuff should be at least 20% greater than the diameter of the limb at the point of application to avoid falsely elevated pressure readings related to using too narrow a cuff.[9] In a large thigh, this may require a single wide cuff. However, use of two thigh cuffs permits an assessment of inflow at or proximal to the common femoral artery with the high-thigh cuff and evaluation for the presence of superficial femoral artery disease with the above-knee cuff. When two thigh cuffs are used, the most proximal thigh cuff is often relatively narrow with respect to the diameter of the thigh, and an artificially elevated high-thigh pressure is then expected—the so-called cuff artifact. The high-thigh index, comparing the proximal thigh pressure with the brachial pressure, is therefore normally about 1.4 with the four-cuff technique and 1.0 to 1.1 with the three-cuff technique.

TABLE 13.1

CORRELATION BETWEEN ABI AND CLINICAL SEVERITY OF ARTERIAL ISCHEMIA[a]

ABI	CLINICAL STATUS
1.11 ± 0.10	Normal
0.59 ± 0.15	Intermittent claudication
0.26 ± 0.13	Ischemic rest pain
0.05 ± 0.08	Impending tissue necrosis

[a]Values are group means from Yao JST. Hemodynamic studies in peripheral arterial disease. *Br J Surg* 1970;57:761-766.
ABI, ankle-brachial index.

AORTOILIAC AND PERIPHERAL ARTERIAL

PRESSURE GRADIENT LOCATION AND CORRESPONDING LOWER EXTREMITY ANATOMIC LOCATION OF OCCLUSIVE DISEASE

■ GRADIENT LOCATION	■ CORRESPONDING ANATOMIC LOCATION	■ NORMAL VERTICAL GRADIENT (mm Hg)
Brachial to high thigh	Aorta, iliac artery, common femoral and superficial femoral arteries	+35 to 46
High thigh to above knee	Superficial femoral artery	−5 to 3
Above knee to below knee	Distal superficial femoral artery, popliteal artery	−12
Below knee to ankle	Trifurcation vessels	−10 to 11
Ankle to toes	Pedal or digital arteries	−10

A continuous-wave Doppler is used to monitor the most prominent arterial flow signal at the ankle, and the examination proceeds from proximal to distal. First, the high-thigh cuff is inflated until the ankle Doppler signal is no longer audible. The cuff is then deflated slowly, and the pressure noted when there is return of the Doppler signal at the ankle is the high-thigh pressure. The above-knee, below-knee, and ankle pressures are similarly determined. If there is no audible arterial Doppler signal at the ankle, the popliteal artery Doppler signal can be used to determine high-thigh and above-knee pressures. Comparison of the pressures measured at each location permits an estimation of the location of occlusive lesions (Table 13.3). An example of a segmental pressure study is shown in Figure 13.4.

There are limitations in the interpretation of segmental limb pressures. In particular, the high-thigh pressure is subject to interpretation difficulties. A diminished high-thigh pressure can reflect an occlusive lesion at or anywhere proximal to the common femoral artery and its proximal branches. Therefore, low high-thigh pressures may reflect a pressure-reducing stenosis in the ipsilateral common or external iliac artery, a common

femoral artery stenosis, tandem pressure-reducing stenoses in the profunda femoris and proximal superficial femoral arteries, or any combination of such lesions. The accuracy of segmental pressures is also affected by mural calcification resulting in artificially elevated pressure measurements, as already described for the tibial arteries at the ankle. Diminished proximal pressures may also mask gradients that exist further down the leg. Segmental pressures do not allow differentiation between short and long segment occlusions or between occluded and patent, but highly stenotic, arteries. These disadvantages are overcome by duplex scanning, as discussed in Chapter 12.

Exercise Testing

Doppler-derived ankle systolic pressures can be combined with treadmill exercise in patients without a contraindication to walking. After determination of resting supine ankle and arm pressures, the patient walks on a treadmill with a predetermined incline at a predetermined speed. The test continues for

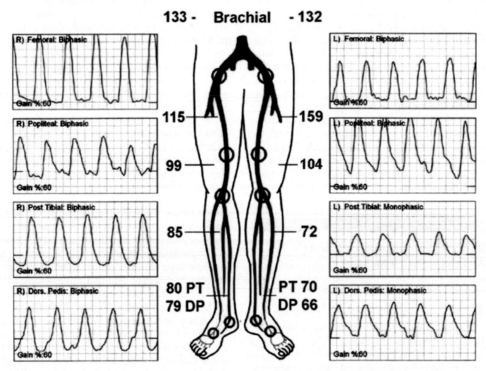

FIGURE 13.4. Abnormal lower extremity segmental pressure study. Based on the observed pressure gradients (see Table 13.3), the right leg has an iliac or common femoral artery lesion, and the left leg has femoropopliteal lesions. Doppler analog waveforms are also shown.

5 minutes or until the patient is forced to stop by any general or localized symptoms. If the patient cannot complete the 5-minute protocol, the type, time to onset, and location of symptoms are recorded. After walking, the patient is immediately placed supine, and the ankle and arm pressures are measured. If the ankle pressure or ABI has dropped from the preexercise baseline, the ankle pressure measurements are repeated at approximately 1-minute intervals until they return to the preexercise level. The magnitude of the drop in ankle pressure and the time required for return to baseline correlate with the severity of arterial occlusive disease in the lower extremity. A worksheet from a treadmill exercise test is shown in Figure 13.5.

In most patients, exercise testing serves only to confirm a diagnosis of intermittent claudication. It is not required in a patient with classic symptoms of claudication, absent peripheral pulses, and a diminished ABI at rest, although it may be helpful to establish the actual limitation in walking ability under controlled conditions. In some cases, exercise testing can document a physiologic response to revascularization or provide an objective assessment of the potential postoperative physiologic benefit.

Exercise testing is particularly useful in the patient with symptoms of claudication who has palpable pedal pulses and a normal or borderline ABI. As discussed in Chapter 5, patients with true intermittent claudication will show a

---

LOWER EXTREMITY ARTERIAL DUPLEX WITH EXERCISE TREADMILL EVALUATION

-PRELIMINARY REPORT-
STUDY WILL BE REVIEWED BY
VASCULAR SURGERY DIVISION

VASCULAR DIAGNOSTIC SERVICE

HISTORY/INDICATION:

62M with pain in the right leg during walking.

Pre-Exercise Ankle Pressures Ankle/Brachial Index (ABI)		
Right		Left
170	Brachial	168
100	Post-Tibial	185
97	Ant-Tibial	185
	Peroneal	
0.59	ABI	1.09

Post-Exercise Ankle Pressures			
RT	Time	LT	ARM
36	1 min	240	225
42	2 min	210	
50	4 min	190	
75	6 min		
85	8 min		
98	10 min		

Exercise Treadmill: Speed __2__ mph Grade __12__ %

Time	Symptoms with Exercise
1:30	Right calf pain first reported
2;10	Worsening right calf pain
2:45	Stopped with severe right calf pain
:	
:	
:	
:	

PRELIMINARY INTERPRETATION DISCUSSED WITH:

☑ PATIENT

☐ MD_____

PRELIMINARY IMPRESSION:
Resting ABI is abnormal on the right at 0.59 and normal on the left at 1.09.
Abnormal treadmill test in the right leg with walking time limited to 2 min 45 sec by right calf pain and a
    decrease in right ankle pressure from 100 to 36 mmHg. Right ankle pressure back to pre-exercise
    baseline at 10 min.
No symptoms noted in left leg and no significant decrease in left ankle pressure.

SIGNATURE: **DATE:**   **TIME:**

PT.NO

NAME

DOB

UW Medicine
Harborview Medical Center – UW Medical Center
University of Washington Physicians
Seattle, Washington
LE ARTERIAL DUPLEX W/ TREADMILL EVAL
VASCULAR EXAMINATIONS

U2145
"U2145"
UH2145 REV AUG 05

PROGRESS — BLUE

FIGURE 13.5. Vascular laboratory worksheet from a treadmill exercise test.

decrease in the postexercise ankle pressure. Exercise testing can also be used to document an ischemic response to exercise in a patient with PAD and other conditions that limit her or his ability to walk. Patients with chronic obstructive pulmonary disease, arthritis, and neurospinal disease are often more limited in their walking ability by these coexisting conditions than by their PAD. If the patients develop lower extremity symptoms during treadmill exercise without a significant drop in ankle pressure, it is highly unlikely that their walking ability would be improved by a revascularization procedure.

The precise end points and techniques of exercise testing are somewhat controversial. Some laboratories exercise patients at low speeds with no inclination of the treadmill, whereas others utilize various inclines and graded increases in treadmill speed. Both initial and absolute claudication distances can be determined. *Initial claudication distance* is the point at which the patient first experiences claudication symptoms; the *absolute claudication distance* is reached when the patient cannot continue walking and the symptoms force him or her to stop. In the vascular laboratory at Oregon Health and Science University, patients are exercised with zero incline at 1.5 mph, and absolute claudication distance is the end point. At the University of Washington, the treadmill is usually set at 2.0 mph with a 12% incline. In either case, the intensity of exercise may have to be modified to accommodate individual patients.

Criteria for a positive treadmill exercise test include a decrease in the ankle pressure of 20 mm Hg or greater or a 20% or greater decrease from the preexercise baseline pressure in the symptomatic extremity, a decrease in the ABI of 0.2 or greater, or failure of the ankle pressure to return to baseline within 3 minutes of completing treadmill walking. Because systemic pressure (and therefore brachial artery pressures) typically increase with exercise, use of the ABI alone to indicate a positive exercise test is incorrect—a decrease in ABI should be accompanied by an absolute pressure drop at the ankle. Failure of the ankle pressure to drop significantly with exercise and failure of the ABI to decrease by 0.2 or more, combined

with a normal resting ABI, substantially rules out arterial insufficiency as the etiology of the patient's exercise-induced symptoms. An exception is the rare patient with buttock claudication that is primarily due to internal iliac artery disease.

Neurogenic claudication may be confused with symptoms of arterial ischemia, as these patients also may present with exercise-induced leg or calf pain. However, careful questioning reveals a pain pattern that differs somewhat from true intermittent claudication. Clinical features that suggest a neurogenic cause for the symptoms include occurrence of the pain with standing, pain relief from leaning forward, worsening of pain with coughing, and a prolonged time for the pain to resolve following exercise. These patients usually have normal ankle pressures at rest that do not decrease with exercise despite onset of symptoms. Failure of the ankle pressures to decrease with exercise in spite of exercise-induced leg symptoms may also be a clue to the presence of other uncommon conditions such as venous claudication and chronic compartment syndromes.

Doppler Analog Waveform Analysis

Continuous-wave Doppler waveforms can be analyzed qualitatively in a manner similar to plethysmographic waveforms; however, the specific characteristics of Doppler flow waveforms are different from those of pulse volume waveforms. As discussed in Chapter 5, normal lower extremity arterial Doppler waveforms are triphasic with a sharp systolic forward flow upstroke, a short reverse flow component in late systole or early diastole, and a smaller phase of forward flow in late diastole (Fig. 13.6A). These normal waveform features are altered with increasing degrees of proximal arterial obstruction. Initially, the reverse flow component disappears (Fig. 13.6B). As the severity of proximal stenosis increases, the rate of rise of the systolic upstroke is decreased, the amplitude of the waveform is

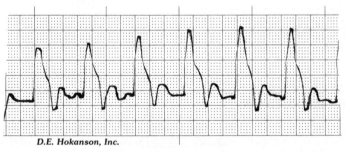

D.E. Hokanson, Inc.

A   **Triphasic (normal)**

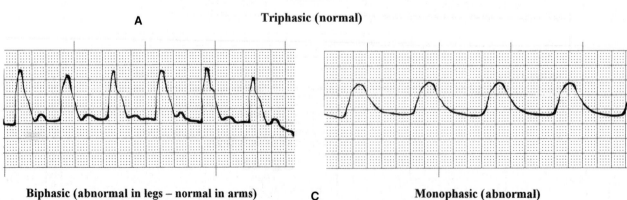

B   **Biphasic (abnormal in legs – normal in arms)**   **C**   **Monophasic (abnormal)**

FIGURE 13.6. Normal and abnormal continuous-wave Doppler analog waveforms. *A*, Triphasic (normal). *B*, Biphasic (abnormal to borderline normal in the lower extremity). *C*, Monophasic (abnormal).

TABLE 13.4

SUMMARY OF MEASUREMENTS AND INDICES FOR PHYSIOLOGIC ASSESSMENT OF LOWER EXTREMITY ARTERIAL OCCLUSIVE DISEASE

■ PARAMETER	■ NORMAL VALUES
Ankle systolic pressure	Exceeds brachial systolic pressure by about 10%
ABI	1.00-1.40[a]
High-thigh systolic pressure	30-40 mm Hg higher than brachial systolic pressure with four-cuff technique
Thigh-brachial index	≥1.2
Segmental pressure gradients	<30 mm Hg between adjacent levels on the same leg or the same levels on the two legs
Toe systolic pressure	70%-90% of brachial systolic pressure
Toe-brachial index	≥0.70
Treadmill exercise test	Walking time 5 min without symptoms or drop in ankle systolic pressure (2 mph, 12% grade)

[a]Based on the 2011 ACCF/AHA Focused Update of the Guideline for the Management of Patients With Peripheral Artery Disease. (From Rooke TW, Hirsch AT, Misra S, et al. 2011 ACCF/AHA Focused Update of the Guideline for the Management of Patients With Peripheral Artery Disease (Updating the 2005 Guideline): A Report of the American College of Cardiology Foundation/American Heart Association Task Force on Practice Guidelines. *Circulation* 2011;124:2020-2045.)

diminished, and diastolic flow increases relative to systolic flow, resulting in a monophasic, dampened waveform (Fig. 13.6C).

Analysis of continuous-wave Doppler analog waveforms is generally used in conjunction with measurement of segmental limb pressures or PVRs. Doppler waveform analysis can also be used to assess iliac artery inflow to the common femoral artery. A monophasic and dampened common femoral artery Doppler waveform indicates hemodynamically significant proximal arterial disease. A summary of measurements and indices for physiologic assessment of lower extremity arterial disease is given in Table 13.4.

SUMMARY

Physiologic testing remains an important component of the noninvasive assessment of lower extremity arterial occlusive disease. In most cases, the ABI is sufficient to establish the presence or absence of hemodynamically significant PAD. Exercise testing is useful to establish the presence or absence of significant PAD in patients where there is discordance between the history and physical examination and the resting ABI. Finally, the combination of segmental pressures or PVR and Doppler waveform analysis can provide a rough estimation of the location of lower extremity hemodynamically significant arterial occlusive lesions. However, in patients under consideration for a therapeutic intervention, imaging studies to more precisely characterize and locate individual arterial lesions should be the next step in the patient's evaluation.

References

1. Yao JST, Needham TN, Gourmos C. A comparative study of strain gauge plethysmography and Doppler ultrasound in the assessment of occlusive arterial disease of the lower extremities. *Surgery* 1972;71:4-9.
2. Yao JST, Flinn WR. Plethysmography. In Kempczinski RF, Yao JST (eds). *Practical Noninvasive Vascular Diagnosis.* Chicago: Year Book Medical, 1987, pp 80-94.
3. Darling RC, Raines JK, Brener BF. Quantitative segmental pulse volume recorder: A clinical tool. *Surgery* 1972;72:873-887.
4. Strandness DE (ed). *Peripheral Arterial Disease: A Physiologic Approach.* Boston: Little, Brown, 1969, pp 112-130.
5. Kempczinski RF. Segmental volume plethysmography: The pulse volume recorder. In Kempczinski RF, Yao JST (eds). *Practical Noninvasive Vascular Diagnosis.* Chicago: Year Book Medical, 1987, pp 140-153.
6. Yao JST. Hemodynamic studies in peripheral arterial disease. *Br J Surg* 1970;57:761-766.
7. Baker JD, Dix DE. Variability of Doppler ankle pressures with arterial occlusive disease: An evaluation of ankle index and brachial-ankle pressure gradient. *Surgery* 1981;89:134-137.
8. Rooke TW, Hirsch AT, Misra S, et al. 2011 ACCF/AHA Focused Update of the Guideline for the Management of Patients with Peripheral Artery Disease (Updating the 2005 Guideline): A Report of the American College of Cardiology Foundation/American Heart Association Task Force on Practice Guidelines. *Circulation* 2011;124:2020-2045.
9. Krikendall WM, Burton AC, Epstein FH, et al. Recommendations for human blood pressure determination by sphygmomanometers: Report of a subcommittee of the Postgraduate Education Committee, American Heart Association. *Circulation* 1967;36:980-988.

AORTOILIAC AND PERIPHERAL ARTERIAL

CHAPTER 14 ■ NONINVASIVE DIAGNOSIS OF UPPER EXTREMITY ARTERIAL DISEASE

GREGORY L. MONETA AND MOLLY ZACCARDI

CLINICAL PRESENTATION	Cold Challenge Testing
PATHOPHYSIOLOGY	Upper Extremity Duplex Scanning
NONINVASIVE DIAGNOSTIC TECHNIQUES	ADDITIONAL TESTING
Segmental Arm Pressures	SUMMARY
Digit Pressures and Plethysmography	

Symptomatic arterial disease of the upper extremity accounts for only about 5% of all cases of extremity ischemia. Unlike the lower extremity, where atherosclerosis is by far the most common pathology, ischemia in the upper extremity may be caused by a variety of local and systemic conditions, and the diagnosis of upper extremity arterial diseases is therefore often complex. A complete history and physical examination, plain x-rays of the neck and shoulder regions, blood tests, and noninvasive and invasive examinations of the upper extremity arteries may all be required.

Surgical intervention is rarely necessary for most etiologies of upper extremity arterial disease. Arteriography is now infrequently required for the diagnosis of upper extremity ischemia, and the anatomic and physiologic information needed for diagnosis can usually be obtained with noninvasive diagnostic testing. Noninvasive vascular laboratory testing for upper extremity arterial disease includes segmental arm pressures, digit pressure measurements and digital plethysmography, and testing for cold-induced vasospasm. Duplex scanning plays somewhat less of a role in the diagnosis of upper extremity ischemia compared to its importance in the evaluation of lower extremity ischemia but is still important in cases amenable to surgical treatment.

CLINICAL PRESENTATION

Raynaud's syndrome is a frequent manifestation of upper extremity arterial disease. Raynaud's syndrome is characterized by episodic attacks of digital artery spasm in response to cold exposure or emotional stimuli. Classic attacks consist of intense pallor of the fingers or distal hand followed by cyanosis and finally rubor upon rewarming. Full recovery requires 15 to 45 minutes after the inciting stimulus is removed (Fig. 14.1). These classic "tricolor" attacks do not occur in all patients. Some patients develop only pallor or cyanosis during the episode, and others complain of cold hands without digit color changes but have abnormal findings on noninvasive testing that are identical to patients with classic digit color changes.

Patients with Raynaud's syndrome are traditionally divided into two groups.[1] The term *Raynaud's disease* is used to describe a benign idiopathic form of intermittent digital ischemia occurring in the absence of known associated diseases. *Raynaud's phenomenon* is used to describe similar symptoms occurring in association with a variety of underlying disease states. It is well recognized that the presence of an underlying disease may not be established at the time a patient presents with Raynaud's syndrome.[2] Therefore, the distinction between Raynaud's disease and Raynaud's phenomenon is somewhat artificial and uncertain. The clinical manifestations of Raynaud's syndrome should be considered as symptoms requiring a diagnosis rather than a diagnosis in itself. In most cases, the diagnosis will be episodic vasospasm without a known associated underlying condition. In cool, damp climates, 6% to 20% of the population, particularly young females, will report symptoms of Raynaud's syndrome.

In about 5% of cases, an underlying condition will be discovered in association with Raynaud's syndrome. The vascular laboratory can play an important role in separating benign episodic vasospasm (Raynaud's disease) from vasospasm associated with serious underlying conditions requiring medical or surgical management (Raynaud's phenomenon).[4,5] With the exception of vasospastic episodes induced by vasopressor medications or ergot, vasospasm alone very rarely results in tissue loss or ulceration. The presence of ulceration or digital gangrene should trigger a workup to confirm the presence of digital artery occlusive disease and an associated condition (Fig. 14.2).

PATHOPHYSIOLOGY

A useful classification scheme for both the diagnosis and the treatment of upper extremity ischemia is to use the physical examination and the vascular laboratory to divide patients into those with large artery disease and those with small artery disease. Patients are then further divided into those with vasospasm alone and those with arterial obstruction (with or without vasospasm) based on vascular laboratory and serologic testing.

Small artery occlusive disease accounts for 90% to 95% of patients presenting with upper extremity ischemia, ulceration, or gangrene (Table 14.1). Small artery occlusive disease may be relatively benign and apparent only as intermittent cold sensitivity of the fingertips. Large artery diseases

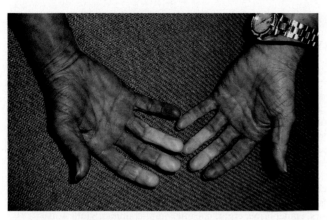

FIGURE 14.1. Raynaud's attack in a 47-year-old woman shows various stages of pallor, cyanosis, and rubor.

NONINVASIVE DIAGNOSTIC TECHNIQUES

Noninvasive vascular laboratory testing of the upper extremity arteries begins with a physical examination. The fingers should be carefully inspected for the presence of ulcers. Hyperkeratotic areas are suggestive of healed ulcers. The hands and fingers should also be examined for telangiectasias, skin thinning, tightening, or sclerodactyly, indicating an associated auto-immune disease. Signs and symptoms of nerve compression syndrome should also be sought. Carpal tunnel syndrome is seen in about 15% of Raynaud's patients.[7] While the physical examination is frequently completely normal in patients with Raynaud's syndrome, a complete pulse examination of all extremities must be performed with attention to the strength and quality of pulses as well as the presence of aneurysms or bruits.

Segmental Arm Pressures

No special patient preparation is required for measurement of segmental arm pressures. Upper extremity segmental pressures are obtained by measuring systolic blood pressure with pneumatic cuffs placed above the elbow, below the elbow, and above the wrist while insonating the radial or ulnar artery at the wrist with a continuous-wave Doppler. Doppler-derived waveforms or plethysmographic waveforms can also be recorded at the different levels. Abnormal waveforms or pressures indicate arterial occlusive disease proximal to the wrist.

A 12-cm-wide blood pressure cuff is usually sufficient for measuring the systolic pressure above the elbow (brachial artery), whereas 10-cm-wide cuffs are used below the elbow and above the wrist (radial and ulnar arteries). However, in general, cuff width should be at least 50% greater than the diameter of the limb in which pressure is being measured. The use of smaller cuffs results in the recording of falsely high pressures. Normally, the gradient between adjacent levels is minimal, and a normal wrist-to-brachial blood pressure ratio is 1.0. If the systolic blood pressure difference between the two arms is more than 15 mm Hg, it is likely that there is a stenosis or occlusion somewhere on the side with the lower pressure. Abnormal Doppler waveforms and decreased pressures at the above-elbow cuff site indicate axillary, subclavian, or brachio-cephalic arterial occlusive disease. Similarly, abnormalities at the below-elbow and above-wrist sites indicate brachial and

generally produce serious upper extremity symptoms by embolization to the digital arteries (Table 14.2). Occlusive disease of the subclavian artery, although very common, is rarely a cause of limb-threatening upper extremity ischemia unless complicated by embolization to the forearm, palmar, or digital arteries.

Patients with purely vasospastic Raynaud's syndrome do not have significant proximal, palmar, or digital artery obstruction and accordingly have normal digit pressures at room temperature. However, a markedly increased force of cold-induced vasospasm causes arterial closure in these patients. Patients with obstructive Raynaud's syndrome have significant occlusive lesions in the arteries between the heart and the distal phalanx of the digit. To experience a Raynaud's attack, the patient must have sufficiently severe arterial obstruction to cause a significant reduction in the resting digit pressure. This requires obstruction of both digital arteries in a single digit. In such patients, a normal vasoconstrictive response to cold is sufficient to overcome the diminished intraluminal distending pressure and cause arterial closure. This theory predicts that all patients with hand arterial obstruction sufficient to cause resting digital hypotension will experience cold-induced Raynaud's attacks.[6] Figure 14.3 schematically demonstrates the relationship between finger pressure and finger temperature for normal individuals and patients with vasospastic or obstructive Raynaud's syndrome.

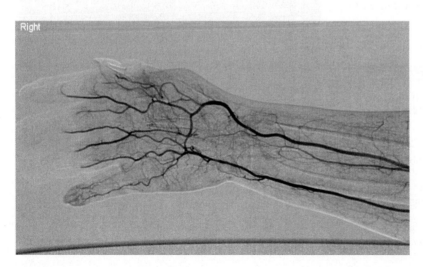

Right

FIGURE 14.2. Arteriogram of digital artery occlusions from a proximal embolic source. Note the lack of filling in the arteries of the index, middle, and ring fingers.

TABLE 14.1

DISEASES ASSOCIATED WITH INTRINSIC DIGITAL ARTERY OCCLUSIONS

■ DISEASE TYPE	■ EXAMPLE
Connective tissue disease	Scleroderma, CREST syndrome, systemic lupus erythematosus, rheumatoid arthritis, Sjögren's syndrome, mixed connective tissue disease, dermatomyositis, small and medium vessel vasculitis
Atherosclerosis and occlusive arterial disease	Atherosclerosis obliterans, atheroembolism, diabetic distal arterial disease, thromboangiitis obliterans (Buerger's disease)
Thromboembolism	Cardiac embolism, arterial embolism, paradoxical embolism
Large vessel vasculitis	Takayasu's arteritis, extracranial temporal arteritis
Dynamic entrapment	Arterial thoracic outlet syndrome
Occupational arterial trauma	Hypothenar hammer syndrome, vibration-induced Raynaud's syndrome
Drug-induced vasospasm	β-Blockers, vasopressors, epinephrine, ergot, cocaine, amphetamines, vinblastine/bleomycin
Infections	Parvovirus, hepatitis B and C antigenemia, sepsis/disseminated intravascular coagulation
Malignancy	Multiple myeloma, leukemia, adenocarcinoma, astrocytoma
Hematologic	Polycythemia vera, thrombocytosis, cold agglutinins, cryoglobulinemia

CREST, calcinosis cutis, Raynaud's phenomenon, esophageal dysfunction, sclerodactyly, telangiectasia.

proximal ulnar/radial arterial occlusive disease, respectively. If the blood pressure difference is more than 15 mm Hg between adjacent levels, or between the radial and ulnar arteries, it is likely due to a stenosis or occlusion (Fig. 14.4).

Digit Pressures and Plethysmography

It is important to measure and record finger temperature before performing digital plethysmography and obtaining finger blood pressures. If the finger temperature is less than 28°C to 30°C, false-positive results may occur secondary to cold-induced vasospasm. Hand or whole-body warming should be performed in patients with low finger temperatures. The technologist should record the finger temperatures to ensure the interpreting physician that the chances of vasospasm have been minimized.

Photoplethysmography (PPG) or strain-gauge plethysmography can be used to measure digit blood pressure[5] and obtain volume pulse waveforms. Alternating current ([AC]-coupled) PPG is preferred because the equipment is easier to use and more durable. An additional advantage of PPG is that it is possible to record the volume pulses from the tips of the digits. This may be useful in documenting obstruction localized to the digital arteries.

TABLE 14.2

CONDITIONS RESULTING IN EMBOLIZATION TO THE UPPER EXTREMITY DIGITAL ARTERIES

■ SOURCE	■ EXAMPLE
Cardiac	Atrial fibrillation, atrial thrombus, valvular disease, myxoma
Trauma	Blunt and penetrating trauma
	Occupational/hypothenar hammer syndrome
Aneurysm	Subclavian artery or more peripheral artery aneurysm (ulnar artery aneurysm)

The PPG photocell is attached to the fingertip pulp with double-sided tape, or a small strain gauge is placed around the fingertip. A 1-inch-(2.5-cm)-wide digital blood pressure cuff is placed around the proximal phalanx (Fig. 14.5). The volume pulse waveforms are recorded using a high sweep speed. This allows the shape of the waveform to be evaluated. Normal waveforms show a rapid upstroke with a time of less than 0.2 second. They may or may not have a prominent dicrotic notch (Fig. 14.6A). An abnormal obstructive waveform will have a prolonged upstroke time and a flattened, rounded peak (Fig. 14.6B). Patients with vasospasm will often have an abnormally shaped waveform termed a *peaked pulse*. These waveforms are thought to represent abnormal elasticity and rebound of the palmar and digital vessels (Fig. 14.6C). The amplitude of the digit volume pulse waveforms is not important. Digit PPG waveforms are not quantitative, and the amplitude depends on the gain setting of the instrument, not blood flow.

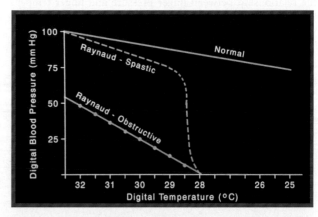

FIGURE 14.3. Finger pressure and temperature in normal individuals and patients with Raynaud's syndrome. The normal response to cold is a linear decline in digital artery pressure. The vasospastic Raynaud's patients have a steeper decline in pressure until a threshold temperature is reached, followed by near-instantaneous occlusion. The obstructive Raynaud's patients have lower normothermic digital artery pressures and a near-normal vasoconstrictive response to cold.

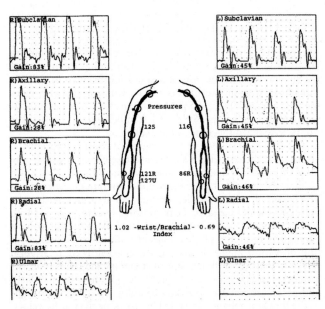

FIGURE 14.4. Segmental arm pressures and Doppler waveforms demonstrate abnormal pressures and waveforms from the radial and ulnar arteries in the left upper extremity. The study indicates arterial occlusive disease distal to the brachial artery in the left upper extremity.

Digit systolic blood pressure is measured by inflating the cuff placed at the base of the finger. The volume pulsations are recorded using a reduced sweep speed while the blood pressure cuff is inflated. When the digit pulsations are obliterated, the cuff is slowly deflated until the pulsations return; the pressure reading at that point is noted and represents the digital artery systolic pressure. Digit systolic blood pressure is normally within 20 to 30 mm Hg of brachial systolic pressure. A ratio of finger systolic pressure to brachial systolic pressure of greater than 0.80 is normal but does not necessarily rule out all digital artery occlusive diseases. It is important to remember that occasional patients with very distal digital artery occlusive lesions have normal finger pressures, because the digit cuff is placed around the proximal phalanx. In addition, occlusive disease in a single digital artery can be missed if the other digital artery in the same finger is normally patent.

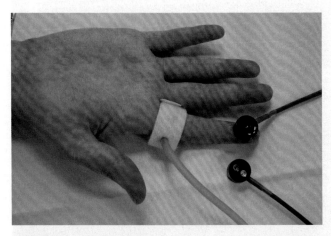

FIGURE 14.5. Application of a finger cuff and a photocell to obtain finger photoplethysmography (PPG) recordings and digit pressures.

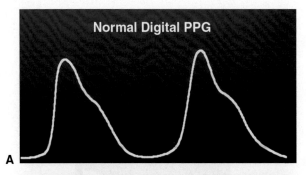

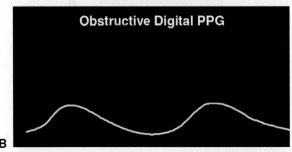

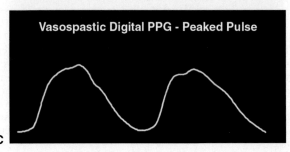

FIGURE 14.6. Volume pulse waveforms. *A,* Normal digit PPG waveform with a rapid upstroke, sharp peak, and typical dicrotic notch on the downslope. *B,* Obstructive digit PPG waveform with a prolonged upstroke and a flattened, rounded peak. *C,* Vasospastic digit PPG waveform with an abnormal peaked pulse. Note that the dicrotic notch is shifted to an earlier point on the waveform and may occur on the distal upstroke.

Cold Challenge Testing

The simplest cold intolerance test is to measure the digit temperature recovery time after immersion of the hand in ice water. Preimmersion digit temperatures must be above 30°C, and hand or body warming may be required before immersion. Using a thermistor probe to measure finger temperatures, the patient's hand is immersed in a container of ice water for 30 to 60 seconds. After the hand is dried, the fingertip pulp temperatures are measured every 5 minutes for 45 minutes, or until the temperature returns to preimmersion levels. Normal individuals will have a recovery time to preimmersion levels of less than 10 minutes. This test is very sensitive for detecting cold-induced vasospasm, but it is nonspecific, and approximately half of the patients with a positive test have no clinical symptoms of cold sensitivity.[8] Cold immersion testing is also uncomfortable and poorly tolerated by patients with significant symptoms of Raynaud's syndrome. Digit pressures often fall to unrecordable levels in such patients.

A better test for cold sensitivity is the digital hypothermic challenge test as described by Nielsen and Lassen[9] (Fig. 14.7).

AORTOILIAC AND PERIPHERAL ARTERIAL

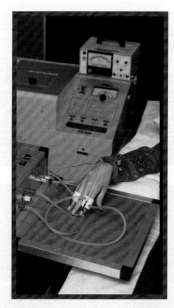

FIGURE 14.7. Device for performance of digital hypothermic challenge or Nielsen's test.

This test involves placing a specially designed finger cuff around the proximal phalanx of the test finger and perfusing the cuff with progressively cooler fluid. The pressure in the test finger is then compared with that of an uncooled reference finger. The Nielsen test is interpreted as positive for abnormal cold-induced vasospasm if the test finger pressure is reduced by more than 17% compared with the reference finger.

Other tests for cold-induced vasospasm include thermal entrainment, digital laser Doppler response to cold, thermography, venous occlusion plethysmography, and digital artery caliber measurement. None of these is widely accepted or employed.[10-12]

Upper Extremity Duplex Scanning

The origins of the brachiocephalic vessels can be difficult to visualize with duplex scanning. For examining the origins of the subclavian arteries, use of a small-footprint 3- or 5-MHz transducer with the sternal notch as a window generally gives the best images (Fig. 14.8). More than 90% of right subclavian artery origins and 50% of left subclavian artery origins can be visualized by color duplex scanning.[13]

Criteria for stenosis at the origins of the brachiocephalic arteries are different than those used elsewhere, because only indirect signs are available when the site of stenosis cannot be directly insonated. If the proximal innominate artery can be visualized, a high-grade stenosis can be implicated when there are focally elevated peak systolic velocities (Fig. 14.9). The presence of a more proximal stenosis is indicated by a dampened, monophasic flow pattern without actual visualization of a focal high-velocity jet. Reversed flow in a vertebral artery is another indirect sign of a significant stenosis in the ipsilateral subclavian artery or the innominate artery. Such additional criteria are necessary to aid in assessing the origins of the brachiocephalic arteries. The use of peak systolic velocities or velocity ratios alone is difficult in this setting and results in higher numbers of both false-positive and false-negative studies.[13]

More distally, the upper extremity arteries are relatively superficial and fairly constant in location. They are best scanned with a higher-frequency 7.5- or 10-MHz transducer. Either a sector or a linear probe may be used, but in either case, a standoff or mound of acoustic gel is helpful to visualize the vessel clearly and assess the flow pattern within it. Color-flow imaging facilitates identification of the vessels (Fig. 14.10) and recognition of tortuosity and other upper extremity arterial features.

The interpretation of duplex findings in the upper extremity beyond the origins of the brachiocephalic arteries is similar to the interpretation of B-mode images and Doppler spectral waveforms gathered in other segments of the arterial system.[14] Normal Doppler waveforms in the upper extremity arteries are usually triphasic. Stenoses will produce focal high-velocity

FIGURE 14.8. Split-screen arterial duplex image of the brachiocephalic artery bifurcation with B-mode (*left*) and color-flow Doppler (*right*) using a sternal notch view. CCA, common carotid artery; SCA, subclavian artery.

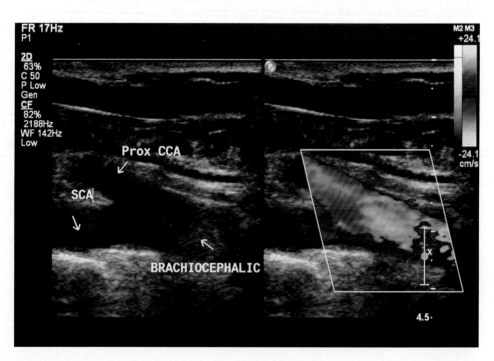

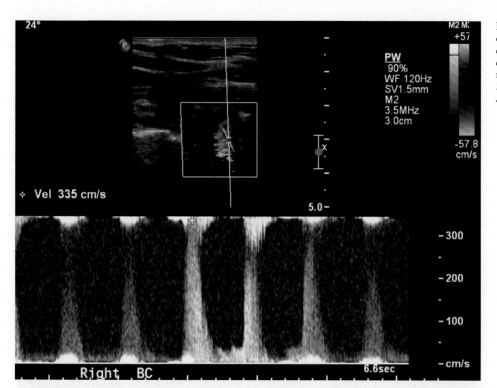

FIGURE 14.9. Arterial duplex image of a high-grade stenosis of the brachiocephalic artery with B-mode and color-flow Doppler using a sternal notch view. Peak systolic velocity is 335 cm/s.

jets, poststenotic turbulence, and dampened distal waveforms (Fig. 14.11). Although there are no specific velocity criteria for classification of stenoses in the upper extremity arteries, some general guidelines are listed in Table 14.3. The diagnosis of arterial occlusion is made by imaging the artery and using the pulsed Doppler to demonstrate no flow within the lumen (Fig. 14.12).

For patients with unilateral upper extremity symptoms who may have a surgically correctable lesion such as a subclavian artery aneurysm (Fig. 14.13) or stenosis, duplex scanning is quite useful.[15] The duplex evaluation of aneurysms is based on the B-mode image appearance, with the most important feature being the size of the enlarged artery and the presence of intraluminal thrombus that may serve as a source of distal emboli. The presence or absence of flow within the aneurysm can be determined using the Doppler component. Duplex scanning may be helpful in patients with suspected embolization to identify proximal

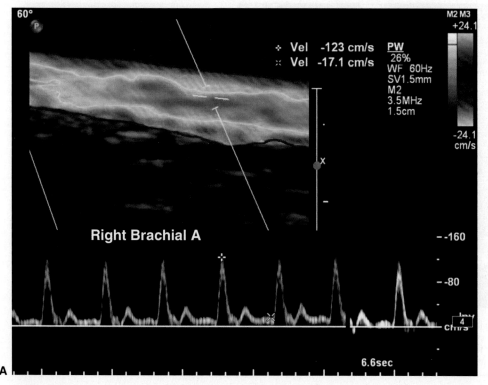

FIGURE 14.10. *A,* Normal brachial artery duplex image shows triphasic spectral waveforms.

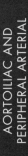

FIGURE 14.10. (*Continued*)
B, Normal radial artery duplex
image shows triphasic spectral
waveforms.

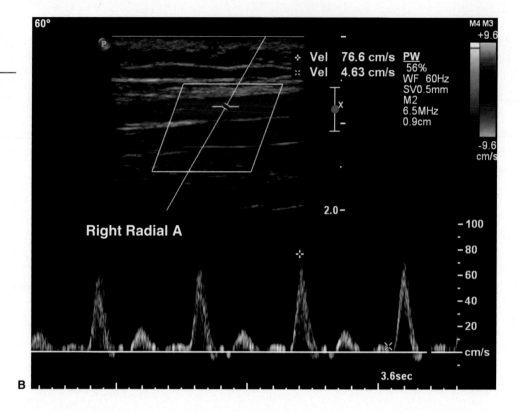

aneurysms. The evaluation should also include echocardiography to look for mural thrombi and valvular lesions. Whereas duplex scanning alone cannot be used to make the diagnosis of Takayasu's arteritis, it can be a helpful adjunct in following the progression or regression of arterial involvement in response to treatment.[16] Upper extremity bypass grafts may also be followed with duplex scanning (Fig. 14.14).

ADDITIONAL TESTING

Tests obtained outside of the vascular laboratory may also be important in the evaluation of patients with upper extremity ischemia. The extent of the evaluation will vary somewhat depending on the history and physical examination and the results of noninvasive vascular testing. Patients with

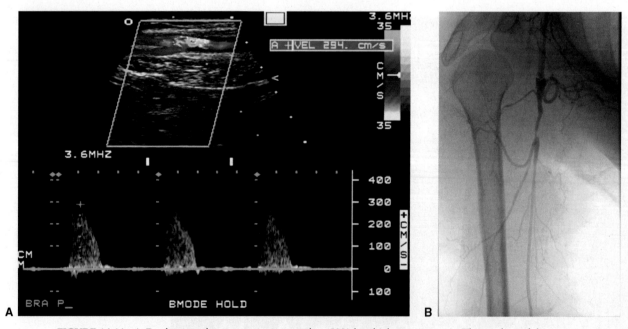

FIGURE 14.11. *A,* Duplex scan demonstrates a greater than 50% brachial artery stenosis. There is loss of the normal triphasic waveform contour, an elevated peak systolic velocity, filling-in of the systolic window, and poststenotic turbulence on the color-flow image. *B,* Arteriogram of the brachial artery from (*A*). The stenotic lesion was likely related to past use of crutches.

TABLE 14.3

GENERAL SPECTRAL WAVEFORM CRITERIA FOR UPPER EXTREMITY ARTERIAL STENOSIS

■ CONDITION	■ CHARACTERISTICS
Normal	Uniform velocity waveforms (no focal changes); biphasic or triphasic flow pattern; clear window beneath the systolic peak
<50% diameter reduction	Focal velocity increase with spectral broadening; persistence of triphasic or biphasic flow pattern
>50% diameter reduction	Focal velocity increase with spectral broadening; loss of triphasic or biphasic flow pattern (monophasic); poststenotic flow (color bruit)
Occlusion	No flow detected

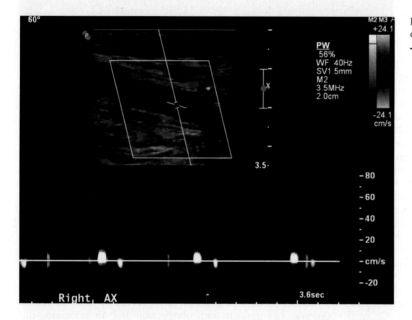

FIGURE 14.12. Duplex image demonstrating occlusion of the right axillary artery secondary to embolism.

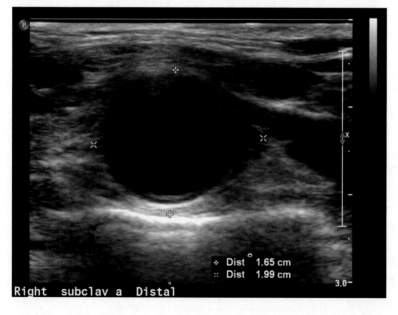

FIGURE 14.13. B-mode image of a right subclavian artery aneurysm.

FIGURE 14.14. Duplex image of the distal anastomosis of a right axillary to radial artery–reversed vein bypass graft.

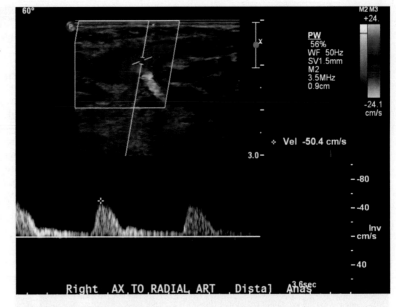

symptoms of upper extremity ischemia with a suspicion for bilateral involvement should have a complete blood count, erythrocyte sedimentation rate, chemistry panel, rheumatoid factor, and antinuclear antibody titer to aid in the diagnosis of any associated autoimmune disease. Hand radiographs may be helpful to evaluate for calcinosis or tuft resorption in patients with a suspected systemic disease. Additional information such as serum protein electrophoresis and antibodies to a variety of nuclear antigens may subsequently be obtained as indicated. Upper extremity nerve conduction tests should be considered if there is any clinical suspicion of carpal tunnel syndrome. Patients with sudden onset of hand ischemia and no evidence of an autoimmune disease should be evaluated for hypercoagulable states. A reasonable, but expensive, hypercoagulable screen consists of prothrombin time/partial thromboplastin time (PT/PTT), antithrombin III, protein C, protein S, lipoprotein (a), and homocysteine levels, as well as screening for antiphospholipid antibodies, anticardiolipin antibodies, hereditary resistance to activated protein C (factor V Leiden), prothrombin gene mutation (G20210A), and dilute Russell's viper venom time (DRVVT). In the minority of cases in which therapeutic intervention is planned, or when the diagnosis cannot be established by noninvasive methods, angiography is still an important diagnostic test in patients with upper extremity arterial disease.

SUMMARY

Upper extremity ischemia is an unusual clinical entity. Evaluation consisting of upper extremity pulse assessment, segmental arm pressures, digit pressures, and digital waveforms will allow the differentiation of large artery disease from small artery disease. Dampened digital waveforms with diminished digit pressures will lead to a diagnosis of occlusive small vessel disease when the proximal arm pressures are normal. Normal digital waveforms and a positive digital hypothermic challenge test will distinguish vasospastic from obstructive disease. Diseases such as scleroderma, Buerger's disease, hypersensitivity angiitis, and hypercoagulable states can also be differentiated and diagnosed with this approach in association with judicious blood testing.

Patients with abnormal arterial pressures in the upper extremity at or proximal to the wrist can be considered to have large artery disease and require further evaluation for correctable lesions. Duplex scanning is proving useful in evaluating patients in whom there is no evidence of a systemic disease process that may be responsible for the obstructive ischemic symptoms. If the diagnosis cannot be established by noninvasive testing, or if therapeutic intervention is planned, angiography still has an important role in the management of upper extremity arterial disease.

Patients with no evidence of large or small artery obstruction and no laboratory abnormalities can be considered to have idiopathic Raynaud's syndrome and have an excellent long-term prognosis with a low probability of developing either a connective tissue disease or ischemic ulcers.[4] Patients with positive serologic tests or other laboratory abnormalities clearly are at increased risk of having or developing an associated disease process, which may or may not require further evaluation and treatment. If these patients have no evidence of obstructive disease, they have an intermediate prognosis along with those patients who have obstruction but no evidence of an associated disease. The patients with obstruction and an associated disease are the group that fare the worst over the long term and are most likely to have or develop digit ulcers and require digit amputation.[4] Approximately one-half of patients who present with digit ulcers will have recurrent ulcers.[3,4]

References

1. Allen E, Brown G. Raynaud's disease: A critical review of minimal requisites for diagnosis. *Am J Med Sci* 1932;83:187-200.
2. Hirschl M, Hirschl K, Lenz M, et al. Transition from primary Raynaud's phenomenon to secondary Raynaud's phenomenon identified by diagnosis of an associated disease: Results of ten years of prospective surveillance. *Arthritis Rheum* 2006;54:1974-1981.
3. Edwards JM. Basic data concerning Raynaud's syndrome. *Ann Vasc Surg* 1994;8:509-513.
4. Landry GJ, Edwards JM, McLafferty RB, et al. Long-term outcome of Raynaud's syndrome in a prospectively analyzed patient cohort. *J Vasc Surg* 1996;23:76-85.
5. McLafferty RB, Edwards JM, Taylor LM Jr, et al. Diagnosis and long-term clinical outcome in patients presenting with hand ischemia. *J Vasc Surg* 1995;22:361-369.
6. Hirai M. Cold sensitivity of the hand in arterial occlusive disease. *Surgery* 1979;85:140-146.
7. Waller DG, Dathan JR. Raynaud's syndrome and carpal tunnel syndrome. *Postgrad Med* 1985;61:161-169.
8. Porter JM, Snider RL, Bardana EJ, et al. The diagnosis and treatment of Raynaud's phenomenon. *Surgery* 1975;77:11-23.
9. Nielsen SL, Lassen NA. Measurement of digital blood pressure after local cooling. *J Appl Physiol Respir Environ Exerc Physiol* 1977;43:907-910.

10. Lutolf O, Chen D, Zehnder T, et al. Influence of local finger cooling on laser Doppler flux and nailfold capillary blood flow velocity in normal subjects and in patients with Raynaud's phenomenon. *Microvasc Res* 1993;46:374-382.

11. Lafferty K, de Trafford JC, Roberts VC, et al. Raynaud's phenomenon and thermal entrainment: An objective test. *Br Med J (Clin Res Ed)* 1983;286:90-92.

12. Singh S, de Trafford JC, Baskerville PA, et al. Digital artery caliber measurement: A new technique of assessing Raynaud's phenomenon. *Eur J Vasc Surg* 1991;5:199-205.

13. Yurdakul M, Tola M, Uslu OS. Color Doppler ultrasonography in occlusive diseases of the brachiocephalic and proximal subclavian arteries. *J Ultrasound Med* 2008;27:1065-1070.

14. Strandness DE. *Duplex Scanning in Vascular Disorders*. New York: Ravens, 1993, pp 159-196.

15. Grosveld WJ, Lawson JA, Eikelboom BC, et al. Clinical and hemodynamic significance of innominate artery lesions evaluated by ultrasonography and digital angiography. *Stroke* 1988;19:958-962.

16. Reed AJ, Fincher RME, Nichols FT. Case report: Takayasu's arteritis in a middle-aged Caucasian woman: Clinical course correlated with duplex ultrasonography and angiography. *Am J Med Sci* 1989;298:324-327.

AORTOILIAC AND
PERIPHERAL ARTERIAL

CHAPTER 15 ■ AORTIC AND PERIPHERAL ANEURYSMS

EUGENE S. LEE, KEVIN LINDHOLM, AND DAVID L. DAWSON

The term "aneurysm" comes from the Greek *aneurysma*, meaning "a widening." Aneurysms are segments of arterial dilatation, usually caused by degenerative changes in the vessel wall. Continued weakening of the vessel wall can lead to aneurysm expansion and vessel rupture. Thrombus can develop in areas of reduced flow velocity within an aneurysm, but the amount of mural thrombus is not an indicator of rupture risk.[1] Major predictors for rupture of an abdominal aortic aneurysm (AAA) are aneurysm diameter, female gender, chronic obstructive pulmonary disease (COPD), higher blood pressure, current tobacco use, cardiac or renal transplant, and critical wall stress.[2] Rapid expansion of an AAA of greater than 0.5 cm within a 6-month interval has been considered a risk factor for rupture and justification for AAA repair. Mural thrombus rarely causes clinically significant problems in aortic aneurysms, but thrombosis and embolism are important causes of complications with peripheral artery aneurysms.[3–6] Aneurysms can also cause complications due to compression of adjacent structures (e.g., nerves[7] or veins[8–10]).

An AAA may be palpable, and aortic palpation is a crucial component of a thorough vascular physical examination. However, the accuracy of detecting an AAA on physical examination is unreliable. Studies have found that the sensitivity of abdominal palpation for determining the presence of an AAA can range from 29% for diameters of 3.0 to 3.9 cm to 76% for large AAAs with diameters over 5.0 cm.[11] Ultrasonography, on the other hand, has a sensitivity and specificity for AAA detection approaching 100%.[2] Hence, the need for vascular sonography in the detection of AAA is crucially important.

Notably, evaluation of the aorta was one of the earliest applications of vascular sonography.[12,13] Because of its safety, low cost, and reliability, ultrasound remains the imaging modality of choice for screening, confirmation of a physical examination finding suggesting the presence of an aneurysm, or follow-up measurements of aneurysms under clinical surveillance.[14,15] Ultrasound imaging is the best noninvasive study for detecting an AAA, though many aneurysms are found incidentally with other imaging studies.

ABDOMINAL AORTIC ANEURYSMS: INDICATIONS AND APPLICATIONS

The infrarenal segment of the abdominal aorta is the most common location for an arterial aneurysm. The presence of an AAA is associated with advancing age, family history of AAA, male sex, and a history of current or past tobacco use.[2] The diagnosis of AAA is made when the aortic diameter is ≥3.0 cm. An AAA is typically asymptomatic until rupture. When rupture does occur, either sudden death ensues or there is immediate onset of excruciating back and abdominal pain. Over 16,000 deaths occur annually from AAA rupture, and this is the 15th leading cause of death in the United States today.

In general, an aortic diameter of ≥5.5 cm is an indication for elective surgical repair.[2] Elective treatment is performed to prevent rupture or thromboembolism.[16] Repair can be done by open surgical replacement of the diseased arterial segment with an interposition graft or by endovascular aortic repair (EVAR). The endovascular approach has become the primary means for AAA treatment for patients with suitable anatomy, which is generally assessed by CT angiography. The lower mortality risk, lower early complication rate, and quicker recovery from EVAR make it preferred over open surgical repair. Further, multiple studies have confirmed the benefit of EVAR over open repair for emergency treatment of ruptured aneurysms. Open repair of a ruptured AAA carries a mortality rate of 42%, compared to emergency EVAR with a mortality rate of 30%.[17] Thus, EVAR has also become the treatment of choice for ruptured AAA if the anatomy permits.

Anatomic Patterns

There are several anatomic patterns of AAAs. The descriptions are clinically relevant, as different techniques for repair are used for different types of aneurysms. The most common type is the *infrarenal* aneurysm, which is located distal to the renal artery origins with a neck of nondilated aorta between the aneurysm and the renal arteries. Infrarenal aneurysms may be repaired with commercially available endografts (See Chapter 16, Fig. 16.5) or by open surgical repair. The aorta may be clamped and sutured distal to the renal arteries with open surgical repair of an infrarenal aneurysm (Fig. 15.1).

Juxtarenal aneurysms have no intervening segment of normal aorta distal to the renal arteries. With this type of aneurysm, endovascular repair is possible with specialized techniques or fenestrated grafts. Commercial fenestrated grafts became available in the in the United States in 2012, with the initial FDA approval for the treatment of AAAs with short infrarenal aortic necks (4 to 15 mm). The proximal segments of these custom-fabricated endografts have holes (fenestrations) so that stents can be placed into the renal arteries, thus providing secure proximal fixation.[18] Endovascular repair also makes use of specialized techniques, including the use of endostapling (where the proximal graft is anchored to a short aortic neck), snorkeling, or the use of endografts that do not rely solely on proximal stent fixation. Open surgical repair is more common for the treatment of juxtarenal aneurysms, but suprarenal or supraceliac aortic clamping is required, increasing the risk of visceral ischemia during the procedure.

Suprarenal aneurysms involve the aorta above the renal arteries, and the renal arteries arise from an aneurysmal segment. Suprarenal aneurysms require concomitant renal or visceral artery reconstruction when open surgical repair is performed. Use of fenestrated or branched endografts for suprarenal aneurysms is an option in some cases, though still experimental in the United States in 2014.

Thoracic aortic aneurysms (TAA) cannot be evaluated by ultrasound due to imaging limitations from the air in the chest (ultrasound is not transmitted through the lungs). Thoracoabdominal aortic aneurysms (TAAA) can involve both the thoracic and abdominal segments of the aorta.[19] Repair of a TAAA requires exposure of the aorta above and below the diaphragm. TAAAs are functionally classified considering the nature of surgical repair required.[20] Suprarenal aortic aneurysms that extend proximally to include the celiac artery origin require aortic clamping and the proximal anastomosis be performed in the chest. This is a Type IV TAAA. Though the thoracic aorta cannot be visualized with ultrasound imaging, the possibility of a TAAA should be considered if the proximal extent of aneurysmal dilatation cannot be defined on an abdominal ultrasound examination. CT or MR angiography is needed for complete evaluation of any TAAA or suprarenal aneurysm.

Pathogenesis

Aneurysms can also be described by their morphology. The most common shape is *fusiform*—widest in the middle and tapering proximally and distally (Fig. 15.2). This descriptor is derived from the Latin *fusus*, meaning "spindle." A more focal dilation is described as a *saccular* aneurysm. A saccular aneurysm resembles a small sac or outpouching. This term is derived from *sacculus*, the Latin word for small pouch or sac.

The most common cause of aortic and iliac artery aneurysms is a chronic degenerative change in the arterial wall leading to a focal arterial dilation. Though patients with aneurysms share risk factors with patients who have atherosclerosis,[21] the term "atherosclerotic aneurysm" is no longer used, as the pathophysiology of AAA is distinct from atherosclerosis. The pathogenesis of an AAA is based on four broad cellular and molecular processes that include proteolytic degradation of the aortic wall, inflammation and immune responses, biomechanical wall stress, and molecular genetics.[22] Multiple factors play a role in localized hemodynamic stress, and genetic predisposition attracts inflammatory cells (monocytes and lymphocytes) to the area of the infrarenal aorta.

Pseudoaneurysms, or "false" aneurysms, are the result of disruption of the arterial wall from injury or infection, or breakdown of an arterial anastomosis, such as the anastomosis of a prosthetic graft to a native artery (Fig. 15.3). Pseudoaneurysms tend to be saccular in appearance. Aneurysms occurring at, or adjacent to, the anastomosis of a graft ("juxta-anastomotic" or "para-anastomotic" aneurysms) are often pseudoaneurysms from disruption of the anastomosis, but they can also represent late aneurysmal degeneration of the remaining native vessel.[23,24] Juxta-anastomotic aneurysms are rare enough that routine, regular surveillance is not recommended after uncomplicated open aortic procedures, at least not for several years after the initial operation.[25] Pseudoaneurysm formation at one or more anastomotic sites can be a late presentation of a prosthetic graft infection.[23,26–31]

Infection is an unusual cause for primary aneurysm formation, although the aorta, peripheral arteries, cerebral arteries, and visceral arteries (in descending order of frequency) can be affected by bacterial arteritis and false aneurysm formation. The most common causal pathogens are *Staphylococcus* and *Streptococcus* species. Imaging features of infected aneurysms include findings of a lobulated vascular mass, an indistinct irregular arterial wall, edema, or a perianeurysmal soft tissue mass. Perianeurysmal gas, aneurysm thrombosis, aneurysmal wall calcification, and disrupted arterial calcification have also been described with infected aneurysms, though these findings are less common.[32]

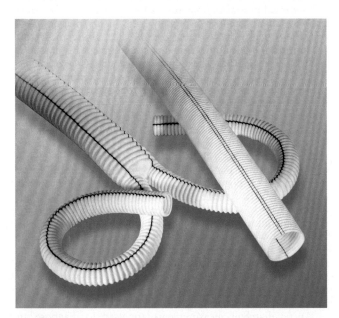

FIGURE 15.1. Prosthetic grafts used for open surgical repair of aneurysms. Grafts may be made of knitted polyester fabric (shown here), woven fabric, or polytetrafluroethylene (ePTFE). (Image provided by MAQUET Medical Systems, USA.)

AORTOILIAC AND PERIPHERAL ARTERIAL

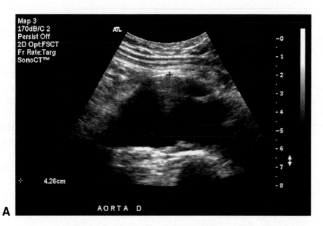 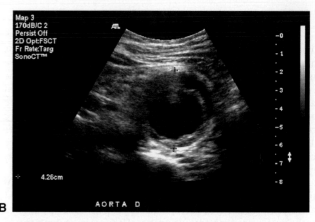

FIGURE 15.2. *A*, Longitudinal B-mode image of a fusiform aneurysm of the infrarenal aorta. The patient's head is to the left of the image. Thrombus is visible in the aortic lumen, and the anterior-posterior (AP) diameter is 4.26 cm. *B*, Transverse B-mode image of the same abdominal aortic aneurysm at the site of maximum diameter (4.26 cm AP).

Threshold for AAA Treatment

Multicenter trials have found that there is no benefit for early surgical repair of small fusiform infrarenal AAAs (the most common type), compared to careful surveillance with serial ultrasound examinations.[33,34] Small aneurysms can be safely observed.[35] Based on a review of published data, the estimated average annual rate of rupture or acute expansion is almost nil for an AAA less than 4.0 cm in diameter.[36] In a meta-analysis of 15,471 patients, small AAAs grew an average of 1.3 to 1.9 mm/year for 3.0 to 3.5 cm AAAs, 2.4 to 3.0 mm/year for 4.0 to 4.5 cm, and 3.6 mm/year for AAAs larger than 5.0 cm. Rupture rates of small aneurysms were found to be very low in this meta-analysis. The growth rates and rupture rates were found to be significantly higher in women than men.[36]

The Society for Vascular Surgery (SVS) guidelines for management of small aneurysms suggest serial ultrasound imaging at intervals that depend on aortic diameter.[2] This strategy appears to be safe for men until the AAA reaches 5.5 cm in diameter, as the expected annual rupture rate is less than the risk of perioperative mortality with surgical repair observed in clinical trials.[16,37–39] Repair is generally recommended if the expansion rate is greater than 0.5 cm in 6 months or if

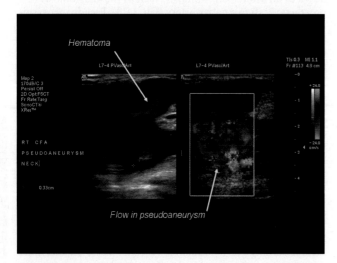

FIGURE 15.3. Pseudoaneurysm (false aneurysm) of the common femoral artery, a complication of arterial catheterization. There is an area of flow within the hematoma overlying the puncture site which communicates with the artery through a narrow "neck."

symptoms develop.[40] Recommendations have been made to consider repair of AAAs at 5.0 cm in diameter for women, as rupture is more common in women with aneurysms, and female gender appears to be a risk factor for adverse outcomes.[41–43]

Because perioperative mortality with EVAR is less than with open repair, it has been suggested that EVAR could be considered at a smaller AAA size threshold. Two recently completed randomized controlled trials evaluated the efficacy of surveillance versus early EVAR for small AAAs. These trials found that mortality and rupture rates for AAAs less than 5.5 cm were low, and no clear advantage was shown with either an early or delayed EVAR strategy. Hence, the authors of both studies concluded that surveillance of small AAAs is safe if careful surveillance is possible.[44–46]

Screening and Ultrasound Diagnosis of AAA

Since AAAs are typically asymptomatic until rupture, screening for AAA is important. This allows AAA treatment in an elective setting. Physical examination is too insensitive to be relied upon for initial diagnosis, especially if the aneurysm is not large or if the patient is heavy,[47] but over 90% of aortic aneurysms are infrarenal in location where ultrasound imaging is practical.

AAA screening has a demonstrated benefit. A large United Kingdom trial, the Multicentre Aneurysm Screening Study (MASS), was a randomized, controlled trial of over 65,000 population-based men 65 to 74 years of age who smoked at least 100 cigarettes in their lifetimes. One-half of the men were invited for AAA screening, while the control group was followed for clinical events but not invited for screening. The results of this multiyear study demonstrated the ability of screening to significantly reduce aneurysm-related deaths as well as reduce all-cause mortality.[48–50] Recognizing the significance of this, Medicare has covered an aortic screening ultrasound (for new Medicare beneficiaries at risk) since 2007. Current recommendations call for a one-time ultrasound screening to be offered to men aged 65 to 75 years who have smoked 100 or more cigarettes in their lifetime or to men and women 50 years of age or older with a family history of AAA.[14] In utilizing these criteria for screening a population at risk for AAA, a prevalence of 5.1% was detected in a contemporary series, which is similar to multiple other studies where the prevalence ranged from 3.9% to 7.2%.[51]

Aortic diameter measurements are used to diagnose an ectatic or aneurysmal aorta, stratify for risk of rupture, and guide the need for long-term follow-up. The normal diameter of the infrarenal aorta is generally less than 2 cm in transverse dimension. The aortic diameter is larger in men, and it increases with body size and age.[52,53] An aneurysm is diagnosed when the abdominal aortic diameter is 1.5 times the normal value or when the aorta is 3 cm or greater in diameter. The aorta is deemed "ectatic" if the aorta measures 2 to 3 cm in diameter (greater than normal aortic size but less than 1.5 times the diameter of the undiseased adjacent aorta). Ultrasound follow-up is recommended for patients with aortic diameters of 2.6 to 2.9 cm at 5-year intervals, 3.0 to 3.4 cm at 3-year intervals, and for those with aortas of 3.5 to 4.4 cm, annual follow-up is recommended. Patients with larger AAAs of 4.5 to 5.4 cm in diameter should be followed at 6-month intervals.[2]

Ultrasonography is recommended for both initial screening and the diagnosis of AAA but is relatively imprecise in measuring aneurysm size. The Intersocietal Accreditation Commission Standards and Guidelines for Vascular Testing state that aneurysms should be measured at the widest point of the aorta from outer wall to outer wall (Fig. 15.4). The outer wall to outer wall measurement was found to have less intraobserver variability and has been suggested as the method for measuring AAA size in the large MASS trial.[54] However, a more recent study has questioned the utility of outer to outer wall measurements and published data that interobserver reliability is greater with the inner wall to inner wall measurement.[55]

Ultrasound imaging may be limited in patients with large body habitus, overlying bowel gas, or those who are unable to cooperate with the examination. In these instances, an abdominal CT scan is more appropriate for making the initial diagnosis of AAA. CT is more reproducible for diameter measurement than ultrasound, and CT is the primary modality for surgical planning. However, in almost all other cases, ultrasound is the preferred modality for initial AAA diagnosis and follow-up.

Given the utility of ultrasonography in screening for AAAs, point-of-care examinations are being used more commonly, especially in underserved and rural areas where primary care clinics are performing AAA screening. The increasing availability of compact, low-cost, ultrasound systems is making point-of-care studies more commonplace, leading experts to believe that ultrasonography will be a basic skill in routine medical practice in the near future (see Chapter 27).[56] The use of contrast-enhanced ultrasonography and 3D ultrasound have found some benefits in follow-up after EVAR, to detect endoleak or to find vascular branches (see Chapter 16), but these advanced applications are not particularly useful in the initial diagnosis of AAA.[57]

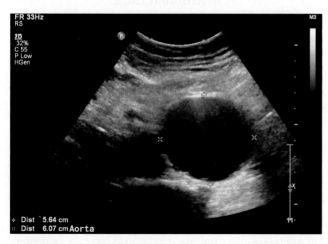

FIGURE 15.4. B-mode image of an abdominal aortic aneurysm in transverse view. The abdominal wall is the most superficial structure at the top of the image, and the vertebral column is deep to the aorta at the bottom of the image. Specular reflections from the deep and superficial walls of the aorta (+) are more distinct than those from the lateral walls (×). Therefore, the lateral resolution of ultrasound is less that the depth resolution, making accurate anterior-posterior (AP) diameter measurements easier to obtain.

Patients presenting with a ruptured AAA need rapid evaluation and treatment. A focused ultrasound study for the presence of an AAA is part of the assessment of an elderly person with hypotension and abdominal pain.[58,59] The diagnosis of AAA can be confirmed in a matter of minutes with a limited examination in the emergency department.[60] If the clinical presentation suggests AAA rupture, there is no need to spend any additional time imaging to confirm the presence of retroperitoneal hematoma or hemoperitoneum, and transfer to the operating room for immediate treatment is indicated. However, a CT scan may be performed first if the patient is stable to guide planning of a possible endovascular repair.

PERIPHERAL ARTERY ANEURYSMS AND PSEUDOANEURYSMS

The utility of ultrasound imaging for the diagnosis and evaluation of peripheral artery aneurysms was established early.[13] The low cost and low risk of ultrasound imaging make it the initial imaging modality of choice for peripheral artery aneurysm evaluations.

Popliteal Artery Aneurysms

The popliteal artery is the most common site for peripheral artery aneurysms, accounting for 70% of all peripheral aneurysms, though the overall incidence is quite low. Arterial diameters are normally larger in men than in women, but normal popliteal artery diameters are typically less than 1.0 cm.[61,62] A popliteal artery is generally considered aneurysmal when the diameter is 1.5 cm, and repair is commonly recommended at 2 cm. Popliteal artery aneurysms occur much more frequently in men, are asymptomatic at the time of diagnosis in one-third, and bilateral in 50% of patients.[63]

Although no controlled trials exist regarding the management of popliteal artery aneurysms, a recent large multicenter registry demonstrated that there is equivalent efficacy between open and endovascular popliteal artery aneurysm repair.[64] The rationale for repair is to prevent thrombosis or embolism, rather than rupture, as thromboembolic complications can lead to acute ischemia and limb loss, and rupture is rare.[65] The reported risk of ischemic complications without surgical repair varies from 8% to 100% (mean 36%), depending on the selection of patients and duration of follow-up.[63]

Elective treatment is recommended for all symptomatic and most large asymptomatic popliteal artery aneurysms. Surgical reconstruction is the standard approach, but endovascular therapy with covered stents appears to be a therapeutic option, at least for some patients. Nonoperative observation with periodic ultrasound surveillance may be considered if the aneurysm measures less than 2.0 cm in diameter and contains no thrombus, or if the patient is at high surgical risk or has limited expected longevity.[66]

Femoral Artery Aneurysms

The common femoral artery (CFA) is the second most frequent site for peripheral artery aneurysms. True aneurysms of the CFA are fusiform and generally do not involve the deep femoral artery, though deep femoral artery aneurysms are seen in rare instances.[67–72] The diameter of the CFA normally increases with age and is related to body size. CFA diameters are larger in males than in females.[73] A CFA aneurysm is diagnosed when there is a focal dilatation of the vessel that is 1.5 to 2 times the diameter of the adjacent nondilated segment.

Symptomatic CFA aneurysms, those larger than 2.5 cm, and those associated with mural thrombus are treated surgically if patients have low operative risk and a reasonable life expectancy.[66,71] However, nonoperative observation may be an option for some asymptomatic CFA aneurysms, as the risk for late complications appears to be less than that of popliteal artery aneurysms.[66] Thorough evaluation for the extent of aneurysmal disease, the presence of concomitant occlusive disease, and the status of inflow and outflow vessels is needed for treatment planning.

Isolated superficial femoral artery (SFA) aneurysms are rare. They are most often found in elderly men and tend to involve the middle third of the artery. The most frequent clinical presentation is localized pain in association with a pulsatile mass. In contrast to popliteal artery aneurysms, SFA aneurysms more frequently present with rupture than with distal ischemia. SFA aneurysm repair is associated with favorable outcomes, with low reported rates of ischemia and limb loss.[74]

The detection of a peripheral artery aneurysm should prompt an evaluation for other aneurysms, including AAA. Finding a peripheral artery aneurysm is a strong predictor for the presence of an AAA, though the converse does not hold. Coexistent AAAs have been reported in 85% of patients with femoral aneurysms[75] and in 62% of those with bilateral popliteal aneurysms,[6] whereas femoral or popliteal aneurysms are present in only 3% to 14% of patients who have AAAs.[76]

Arteriomegaly

Arteriomegaly is the term used to describe diffuse arterial dilation, but this condition is also commonly associated with focal aneurysmal arterial segments.[77–83] There is a risk of thrombosis and embolization with arteriomegaly, as flow is slow through the tortuous, ectatic, irregular vessels. Recognition of arteriomegaly in an arterial segment should prompt a thorough evaluation that includes assessment of the aorta as well as the femoral and popliteal arteries of both extremities. Diffuse enlargement of axial artery segments may also be seen in patients with chronic arteriovenous fistulae or arteriovenous malformations.

Pseudoaneurysm

False aneurysms or pseudoaneurysms of the femoral artery are far more common than true aneurysms in contemporary clinical practice, as the former may be the early or late result iatrogenic complications.

Late degeneration at the site of an arterial anastomosis can lead to pseudoaneurysm formation. This can be a consequence of suture line failure,[84] degradation of graft material,[85] or progressive degeneration of the tissue of the recipient vessel at the suture line.[71,86–93] Anastomotic pseudoaneurysms are usually repaired with surgical revision by replacing the perianastomotic graft segment and reconstructing the arterial anastomosis. Late graft infection should be considered as a potential cause for a graft pseudoaneurysm.[25,27,30,44,94,95] Perigraft fluid, local or systemic signs of inflammation, graft thrombosis, or the presence of multiple or recurrent pseudoaneurysms may suggest the diagnosis of infection. Extra-anatomic reconstruction or use of biologic grafts (autologous vein or arterial allograft) may be needed in such cases.

As discussed in Chapter 32, pseudoaneurysms as a complication of arterial catheterization are pulsatile hematomas that communicate with the artery through the residual defect in the arterial wall. Femoral pseudoaneurysms are well-recognized complications of arterial catheterization, occurring after 0.1% to 0.2% of diagnostic angiograms and after 3.5% to 5.5% of interventional procedures.[66,71,96,97] Puncture-site pseudoaneurysms are associated with longer procedures, use of larger sheaths, systemic anticoagulation, and difficult arterial access. Catheter-related femoral pseudoaneurysms may be difficult to accurately detect with physical examination alone.

Both hematoma and pseudoaneurysm are in the differential diagnosis when ecchymosis and a lump in the groin are present after a femoral artery puncture. Duplex ultrasound, aided by the use of color flow imaging, is used to determine if there is flow outside the vessel, a finding that would confirm the presence of a pseudoaneurysm. In addition, ultrasound imaging can play a role in therapy for postcatheterization pseudoaneurysms, with either ultrasound-guided compression therapy[97–102] or the more favored technique of ultrasound-guided thrombin injection.[103–105]

ULTRASOUND IMAGING OF ANEURYSMS: GENERAL CONSIDERATION

Ultrasound evaluation of an AAA should include abdominal aortic diameter measurement at the suprarenal, pararenal, and infrarenal locations. Common iliac artery diameters and, if indicated, graft anastomotic site diameters should also be included. Diameter measurements are made from a cross-sectional image of the vessel with the scan plane orthogonal to the long vessel axis. Two diameter measurements should be recorded. To avoid confusion about aneurysm size, aneurysm length measurements are generally not reported. A description of aneurysm morphology should be included, such a fusiform, saccular, or pseudoaneurysm.

An ultrasound evaluation of a peripheral artery aneurysm should include the maximum diameter of the artery, flow velocities, and patency of the outflow vessels.[65] An ultrasound evaluation of a femoral pseudoaneurysm should include documenting the size of the pseudoaneurysm (both the active flow cavity and any thrombosed portion), and the flow velocities of the common femoral, superficial femoral, and deep femoral arteries. Also, the concomitant veins are evaluated for the presence of an arteriovenous fistula, venous thrombosis, or compression by the adjacent arterial pseudoaneurysm (see Chapter 32).

SCANNING TECHNIQUE: ABDOMINAL AORTA AND ILIAC ARTERY EVALUATION

Instrumentation

High-quality duplex ultrasound equipment facilitates evaluation of the abdominal aorta and iliac arteries. Transducers with frequencies of 2 to 5 MHz are typically selected for aortic studies to penetrate deep into the abdomen and pelvis. Linear or curved array transducers may be used to evaluate the abdominal aorta, but a low frequency phased array transducer may also be selected for its smaller footprint and good penetration.

Patient Positioning and Examination Preparation

Patients should be instructed to fast for 4 to 6 hours prior to duplex evaluations of the abdomen to reduce obscuring bowel gas and to improve the ease and quality of the study. Ideally, abdominal duplex scans should be scheduled in the morning. For afternoon appointments, a light breakfast may be permitted. Sips of water or small volumes of clear liquids may also be permitted, and all required medications should be taken. Examinations are performed without fasting if the patient needs to eat because of a medical condition or when medications need to be taken with food.

The patient is positioned supine on a gurney or examination table with the abdomen exposed. A small pillow or towel roll under the knees aids patient comfort. Some patients may have difficulty lying flat for various reasons: orthopnea from lung or cardiac conditions, neck and back pain from spinal or joint disease, or other problems. Patients may be more comfortable if the head of the bed is elevated approximately 10 degrees or by using reverse Trendelenburg position.

Imaging the abdominal vasculature can be challenging. Allow at least 60 minutes for an aortic evaluation. This provides sufficient time to attend to setup of the scan room, gather patient information, prepare the patient, perform the examination, record images, and generate the report. The technologist should scan using an ergonomically comfortable position, and the patient should be positioned on the gurney as close as possible to the technologist. This lessens the "reach" required and reduces the stress placed on the technologist's wrist, elbow, shoulder, and back. Positioning the scanned surface below the level of the technologist's waist allows for easier reach to all of the abdomen and better leverage. It is important for the technologist to keep their elbow as straight as possible, as this can lessen joint stress and reduce the likelihood of repetitive strain injuries. For larger patients, it may be necessary to lean into the patient and put more pressure on the abdomen to get the transducer closer to the aorta. A small step stool may be used by shorter technologists to gain the needed height over the patient's abdomen.

Imaging Views and Protocols

The aortic evaluation is begun with transverse imaging, starting at the level of the of the xyphoid process. The visceral segment of the abdominal aorta should be identified at the level of the celiac and superior mesenteric artery origins. The transducer is moved from cephalad to caudal, with transverse imaging of the aorta from the celiac axis to the aortic bifurcation. The umbilicus is the surface anatomy landmark for the approximate location of the aortic bifurcation which is typically at the level of the second lumbar vertebra. Initial examinations should also include imaging of the common iliac, external iliac, and internal iliac arteries, bilaterally.

Transverse diameter measurements should be recorded at multiple levels, including the suprarenal, pararenal, and infrarenal aorta, and at the terminal aorta just proximal to the origins of the common iliac arteries. Two diameter measurements of the aorta are made at each location: the anterior-posterior (AP) and the lateral dimensions. The lateral measurements are usually less accurate due to the lower lateral resolution of B-mode ultrasound compared to its depth resolution (Fig. 15.4).

The suprarenal aorta is generally not parallel to the skin surface. Because of the rigidity of the thoracic cage, the ability to compress with the probe is limited in the upper abdomen, and imaging with optimum alignment of the suprarenal aorta may be difficult. The aorta will appear on the monitor to be rising from a deeper to a more superficial position. Care should be taken to avoid off-axis measurements that overestimate the true diameter. Angle the transducer to obtain true axial diameter measurements. The aorta can also be imaged in a longitudinal (sagittal) plane (See Fig. 15.2A). A single AP measurement is obtained with the longitudinal view.

Color flow Doppler can help to identify the visceral and renal arteries (Fig. 15.5). In the transverse view, the right renal artery will often arise at a 10-o'clock orientation, and the left renal artery will arise at a 4-o'clock position. In many cases, the right renal artery will arise from the aorta more superiorly than the left renal artery. The pararenal aortic diameter can be obtained at either location.

Most AAAs originate below the level of the renal arteries.[16] The infrarenal aorta is the most easily visualized aortic segment, owing to the shallower depth. In the presence of an AAA, the increased diameter makes the aorta easy to recognize. Mural thrombus is often identified (Figs. 15.6 and 15.7). The imaging plane is manipulated to be at right angles to the axis of the aorta to best measure the true diameter (Fig. 15.8). Aneurysmal aortas are often tortuous due to elongation of the aorta, and off-angle imaging will yield a more elliptical cross section. While the minor axis diameter of the elliptical section may be close to the true aortic diameter, the major axis measurement of the elliptical section may result in overestimation of the AAA size. The terminal aorta will often be elliptical in shape, with the lateral measurement greater than the AP measurement.

The relationship of the neck of the AAA to the origin of the renal arteries is clinically important, as this is a major determinant of whether or not the patient is a candidate for endovascular aneurysm repair. If surgical intervention is considered, CT or MR angiography with 3D and multiplanar reconstructions will be performed to provide the additional information needed about the AAA size, length, tortuosity, and its proximity to the renal arteries.

An AAA may extend into the iliac arteries. The common iliac arteries can be easily identified in an axial orientation, just inferior to the umbilicus. Diameters should be obtained in both the proximal and distal common iliac segments. The internal iliac arteries are often difficult to visualize in the axial plane. The common iliac artery bifurcation can be imaged in a longitudinal (oblique sagittal) plane, and a single AP measurement can be obtained (Fig. 15.9). Color flow Doppler can help to identify the common iliac artery bifurcation.

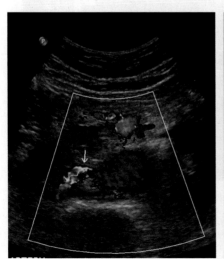 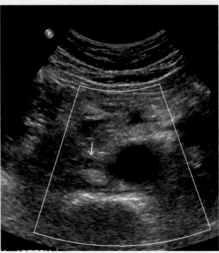

FIGURE 15.5. The use of color Doppler helps to quickly identify renal arteries. Transverse color Doppler image (*left*) and B-mode image alone (*right*) showing a right renal artery (*arrows*).

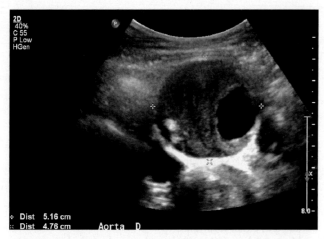

FIGURE 15.6. Extensive mural thrombus in this abdominal aortic aneurysm appears as heterogeneous echoes on the transverse B-mode image, partially filling the aneurysm and surrounding a hypoechoic flow lumen.

FIGURE 15.7. Color Doppler helps distinguish flowing blood from mural thrombus in this transverse image of an abdominal aortic aneurysm. The presence and extent of the mural thrombus generally has little clinical significance.

Pitfalls and Technical Limitations

Obesity and the presence of overlying bowel gas are the most common obstacles to a complete evaluation of the abdominal vasculature. The ultrasound beam is attenuated in the obese patient by the greater distance of the retroperitoneal vessels from the transducer. Increased transmit power may be used in this setting. Applying probe pressure can reduce attenuation and improve image quality, but this may cause patient discomfort. It is a good practice to alert the patient prior to compression maneuvers. A lateral decubitus approach may

also help, though imaging of the suprarenal aorta may still be limited.

The deeper pelvic location of the iliac arteries may make their evaluation difficult with large patients and those with overlying bowel gas. Use of a curved array transducer may be advantageous, as this design offers the ability to scan from different anatomic windows, directing the beam to a desired location by rocking the orientation of the scan head. Most of the course of the common iliac and external iliac arteries can be imaged from a single point in the pelvis, midway between the umbilicus, and the femoral artery in the groin. If bowel gas

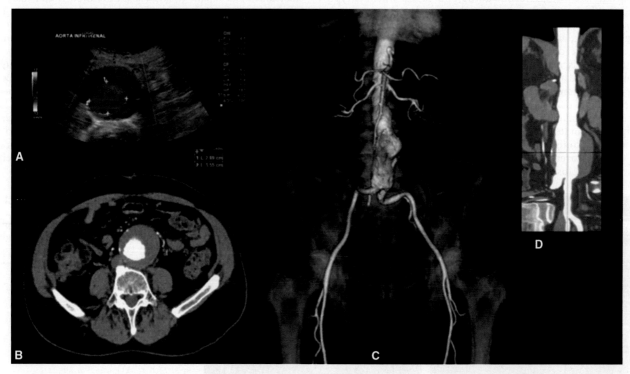

FIGURE 15.8. B-mode and color flow Doppler ultrasound (*A*) are used for abdominal aortic aneurysm screening and surveillance, but axial imaging with CT angiography (*B*) provides a volumetric data set that can be post-processed for 3-D rendering of the aortic flow lumen (*C*) and reformatted in multiple projections. Curved centerline reconstructions (*D*) are used for aortic endograft planning and are essential prior to fenestrated endografts and other complex cases.

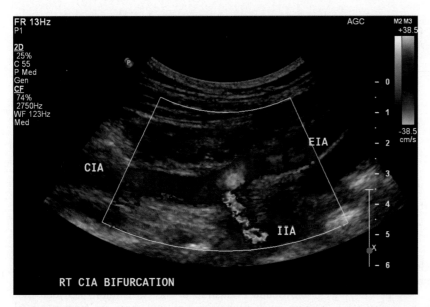

FR 13Hz
P1
2D
25%
C 55
P Med
Gen
CF
74%
2750Hz
WF 123Hz
Med

AGC   M2 M3
                +38.5

EIA   – 0
       .
       – 1
       .
CIA   – 2   –38.5
              cm/s
       – 3
       .
       – 4
IIA   – 5
       X
       – 6

RT CIA BIFURCATION

FIGURE 15.9. Color flow Doppler image of a common iliac artery (CIA) bifurcation (longitudinal view). The internal iliac artery (IIA) can be particularly difficult to identify with B-mode imaging alone. EIA, external iliac artery.

obscures part of the field (as is often the case near the common iliac artery bifurcation), the probe can be moved cranially or caudally along the line of the scan plane and steered superiorly or inferiorly to obtain the needed images.

SCANNING TECHNIQUE: LOWER EXTREMITY PERIPHERAL ARTERY EVALUATION

Instrumentation

For imaging of peripheral artery aneurysms, probe selection is again dictated by depth and geometry of the field to be assessed. Linear array transducers with frequencies of 4 to 10 MHz are typically used. Curved array transducers with lower frequencies, such as those used in the abdomen, can also be selected for situations when the vessel of interest is deeper, such as the femoral artery in the adductor canal or when imaging obese patients.

Patient Positioning and Examination Preparation

Techniques for imaging the extremities for the evaluation of peripheral artery aneurysms are similar to those used for arterial occlusive disease (see Chapter 12). The patient should remove clothing below the waist and don a gown to allow full access to the lower extremity. The patient lies in a relaxed supine position with the knee bent and externally rotated. Some patients with limited range of motion may need to be rotated slightly onto the ipsilateral hip.

Imaging Views and Protocols

Beginning in the inguinal area, the common femoral artery and vein should be identified with the transducer in a transverse orientation. The proximal SFA and profunda femoris artery are also easily identified at this level. The examination continues by

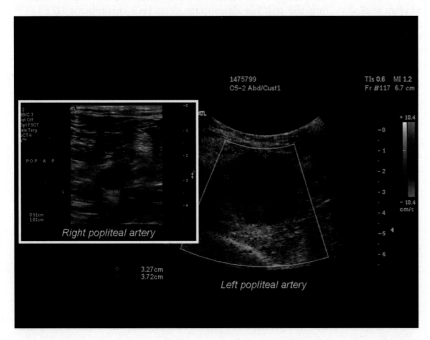

FIGURE 15.10. Transverse views of the left and right (*inset*) popliteal arteries. The left popliteal artery is aneurysmal with the lumen visualized on color Doppler surrounded by mural thrombus.

1475799   TIs 0.6   MI 1.2
C5-2 Abd/Cust1 Fr #117 6.7 cm

POP A P

Right popliteal artery

3.27cm
3.72cm

Left popliteal artery

+ 18.4

– 0
– 1
– 2
– 3
– 18.4
       cm/s
– 4
– 5
– 6

FIGURE 15.11. Combining multiple B-mode images, a feature available on some duplex systems, creates a "panoramic" image of a popliteal artery aneurysm with extensive, irregular mural thrombus.

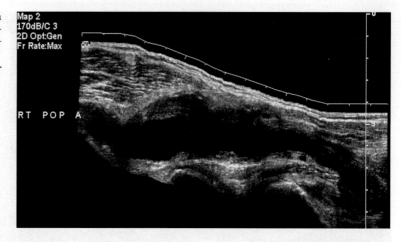

following the course of the SFA through the thigh, sweeping the transducer distally and posteriorly. Areas of abnormal dilatation are readily identified.

As previously mentioned, popliteal artery aneurysms are the most common peripheral artery aneurysms, comprising approximately 80% of all cases.[106] Common clinical presentations include lower extremity ischemia resulting from popliteal aneurysm thrombosis or distal embolization (Figs. 15.10 and 15.11).[107] The popliteal artery is identified behind the knee. When imaging from a posterior approach with the transducer in the popliteal fossa, the artery appears deep to the popliteal vein. The popliteal artery should be evaluated from the level of the adductor canal to the distal segment between the heads of the gastrocnemius muscle. When aneurysmal dilatation of the popliteal artery is focal, it is most commonly seen in the proximal segment. In addition to measuring the maximum transverse dimensions and describing the location and extent of the aneurysm, measurements should be obtained both proximal and distal to any abnormal segment. The presence or absence of mural thrombus should also be noted. Color flow Doppler is helpful for determining arterial patency, as well as for localizing important arterial branches.

Pitfalls and Technical Limitations

Imaging limitations in the lower extremities are most often related to patient comfort or the patient's limited mobility or flexibility. A patient's body habitus can also present limitations; however, this is not as frequent a problem as it is with scanning the aorta

and visceral vessels. Again, the technologist should maintain an ergonomically efficient position during the examination.

Ultrasound evaluation of the extremities often does not require much probe pressure, and there are more potential positions from which to perform the examination. The limb should be close to the technologist, whether the technologist is standing or seated, to allow easy access. The height of the gurney should again be at or just below the level of the technologist's waist. This position allows unobstructed access to the groin and the entire length of the medial thigh.

For some patients, the popliteal fossa is not easily accessible in a supine position due to limited flexure of the hip and knee. In such instances of difficult access, the patient can be positioned prone with either a small pillow or a rolled towel under the feet to bend the knees and reduce the tension of the calf and posterior thigh musculature. The popliteal fossae of both limbs can easily be accessed with the patient in the prone position.

Limitations due to body habitus can usually be solved with correct patient positioning. For very large patients, the pannus can limit access to the groin. By having the patient shift or turn to the side away from the groin being examined, the pannus will shift, improving exposure. The Trendelenburg position may also help.

Peripheral artery aneurysms may compress surrounding structures (Fig. 15.12). Compression of the adjacent deep veins may impair venous return and cause venous stasis, increasing the risk for developing deep vein thrombosis (DVT).[106] Though popliteal artery aneurysms greater than 2.0 cm in diameter may compress and displace the popliteal vein, associated popliteal DVT is relatively rare, perhaps because of

FIGURE 15.12. Color Doppler image of a large common femoral artery aneurysm compressing the common femoral vein (arrow).

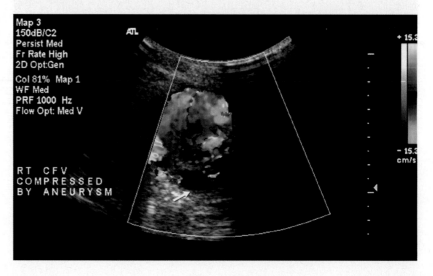

the slow progression of aneurysm growth that allows venous collaterals to develop.[9] Femoral artery aneurysms can compress the adjacent femoral, profunda femoris, and common femoral veins.[108] Care should be taken to identify adjacent deep veins and assess for evidence of extrinsic compression as well as thrombosis.

References

1. Hans SS, Jareunpoon O, Balasubramaniam M, et al. Size and location of thrombus in intact and ruptured abdominal aortic aneurysms. *J Vasc Surg* 2005;41(4):584-588.
2. Chaikof EL, Brewster DC, Dalman RL, et al. SVS practice guidelines for the care of patients with an abdominal aortic aneurysm: executive summary. *J Vasc Surg* 2009;50(4):880-896.
3. Galland RB. History of the management of popliteal artery aneurysms. *Eur J Vasc Endovasc Surg* 2008;35(4):466-472.
4. Galland RB, Magee TR. Management of popliteal aneurysm. *Br J Surg* 2002;89(11):1382-1385.
5. Olcott CT, Holcroft JW, Stoney RJ, et al. Unusual problems of abdominal aortic aneurysms. *Am J Surg* 1978;135(3):426-431.
6. Whitehouse WM Jr, Wakefield TW, Graham LM, et al. Limb-threatening potential of arteriosclerotic popliteal artery aneurysms. *Surgery* 1983;93(5):694-699.
7. Kubacz GJ. Femoral and sciatic compression neuropathy. *Br J Surg* 1971;58(8):580-582.
8. Walsh JJ, Williams LR, Driscoll JL, et al. Vein compression by arterial aneurysms. *J Vasc Surg* 1988;8(4):465-469.
9. Haaverstad R, Fougner R, Myhre HO. Venous haemodynamics and the occurrence of leg oedema in patients with popliteal aneurysm. *Eur J Vasc Endovasc Surg* 1995;9(2):204-210.
10. Cernuda-Morollon E, Ridley AJ. Rho GTPases and leukocyte adhesion receptor expression and function in endothelial cells. *Circ Res* 2006;98(6):757-767.
11. Lederle FA, Simel DL. The rational clinical examination. Does this patient have abdominal aortic aneurysm? *JAMA* 1999;281(1):77-82.
12. Goldberg BB, Ostrum BJ, Isard HJ. Ultrasonic aortography. *JAMA* 1966;198(4):353-358.
13. Holm HH, Kristensen JK, Mortensen T, et al. Ultrasonic diagnosis of arterial aneurysms. *Scand J Thorac Cardiovasc Surg* 1968;2(2):140-146.
14. Fleming C, Whitlock EP, Beil TL, et al. Screening for abdominal aortic aneurysm: a best-evidence systematic review for the U.S. Preventive Services Task Force. *Ann Intern Med* 2005;142(3):203-211.
15. Lederle FA. Ultrasonographic screening for abdominal aortic aneurysms. *Ann Intern Med* 2003;139(6):516-522.
16. Schermerhorn M, Cronentwett J. Abdominal aortic aneurysms. In: Rutherford R (ed.). *Rutherford Vascular Surgery*. 6th ed. Denver: Elsevier Saunders; 2005, pp. 1408-1452.
17. Antoniou GA, Georgiadis GS, Antoniou SA, et al. Endovascular repair for ruptured abdominal aortic aneurysm confers an early survival benefit over open repair. *J Vasc Surg* 2013;58(4):1091-1105.
18. Buck DB, van Herwaarden JA, Schermerhorn ML, et al. Endovascular treatment of abdominal aortic aneurysms. *Nat Rev Cardiol* 2014;11(2):112-123.
19. DeBakey ME, Crawford ES, Garrett HE, et al. Surgical considerations in the treatment of aneurysms of the thoraco-abdominal aorta. *Ann Surg* 1965;162(4):650-662.
20. Crawford ES, Crawford JL, Safi HJ, et al. Thoracoabdominal aortic aneurysms: preoperative and intraoperative factors determining immediate and long-term results of operations in 605 patients. *J Vasc Surg* 1986;3(3):389-404.
21. Singh K, Bonaa KH, Jacobsen BK, et al. Prevalence of and risk factors for abdominal aortic aneurysms in a population-based study: the Tromso Study. *Am J Epidemiol* 2001;154(3):236-244.
22. Ailawadi G, Eliason JL, Upchurch GR Jr. Current concepts in the pathogenesis of abdominal aortic aneurysm. *J Vasc Surg* 2003;38(3):584-588.
23. Curl GR, Faggioli GL, Stella A, et al. Aneurysmal change at or above the proximal anastomosis after infrarenal aortic grafting. *J Vasc Surg* 1992;16(6):855-859; discussion 9-60.
24. Hagino RT, Taylor SM, Fujitani RM, et al. Proximal anastomotic failure following infrarenal aortic reconstruction: late development of true aneurysms, pseudoaneurysms, and occlusive disease. *Ann Vasc Surg* 1993;7(1):8-13.
25. Davidovic L, Vasic D, Maksimovic R, et al. Aortobifemoral grafting: factors influencing long-term results. *Vascular* 2004;12(3):171-178.
26. Edwards MJ, Richardson JD, Klamer TW. Management of aortic prosthetic infections. *Am J Surg* 1988;155(2):327-330.
27. Bandyk DF, Bergamini TM, Kinney EV, et al. In situ replacement of vascular prostheses infected by bacterial biofilms. *J Vasc Surg* 1991;13(5):575-583.
28. McCann RL, Schwartz LB, Georgiade GS. Management of abdominal aortic graft complications. *Ann Surg* 1993;217(6):729-734.
29. Sessa C, Farah I, Voirin L, et al. Infected aneurysms of the infrarenal abdominal aorta: diagnostic criteria and therapeutic strategy. *Ann Vasc Surg* 1997;11(5):453-463.
30. Seeger JM, Back MR, Albright JL, et al. Influence of patient characteristics and treatment options on outcome of patients with prosthetic aortic graft infection. *Ann Vasc Surg* 1999;13(4):413-420.
31. Orton DF, LeVeen RF, Saigh JA, et al. Aortic prosthetic graft infections: radiologic manifestations and implications for management. *Radiographics* 2000;20(4):977-993.
32. Chun KC, Teng KY, Van Spyk EN, et al. Outcomes of an abdominal aortic aneurysm screening program. *J Vasc Surg* 2013;57(2):376-381.
33. Mortality results for randomised controlled trial of early elective surgery or ultrasonographic surveillance for small abdominal aortic aneurysms. The UK Small Aneurysm Trial Participants. *Lancet* 1998;352(9141):1649-1655.
34. Lederle FA, Wilson SE, Johnson GR, et al. Immediate repair compared with surveillance of small abdominal aortic aneurysms. *N Engl J Med* 2002;346(19):1437-1444.
35. Katz DA, Littenberg B, Cronenwett JL. Management of small abdominal aortic aneurysms. Early surgery vs watchful waiting. *JAMA* 1992;268(19):2678-2686.
36. Bown MJ, Sweeting MJ, Brown LC, et al. Surveillance intervals for small abdominal aortic aneurysms: a meta-analysis. *JAMA* 2013;309(8):806-813.
37. Cronenwett JL, Johnston KW. The United Kingdom Small Aneurysm Trial: implications for surgical treatment of abdominal aortic aneurysms. *J Vasc Surg* 1999;29(1):191-194.
38. Greenhalgh RM, Forbes JF, Fowkes FG, et al. Early elective open surgical repair of small abdominal aortic aneurysms is not recommended: results of the UK Small Aneurysm Trial. Steering Committee. *Eur J Vasc Endovasc Surg* 1998;16(6):462-464.
39. Lederle FA. A summary of the contributions of the VA cooperative studies on abdominal aortic aneurysms. *Ann N Y Acad Sci* 2006;1085:29-38.
40. Brewster DC, Cronenwett JL, Hallett JW Jr, et al. Guidelines for the treatment of abdominal aortic aneurysms. Report of a subcommittee of the Joint Council of the American Association for Vascular Surgery and Society for Vascular Surgery. *J Vasc Surg* 2003;37(5):1106-1117.
41. Forbes TL, Lawlor DK, DeRose G, et al. Gender differences in relative dilatation of abdominal aortic aneurysms. *Ann Vasc Surg* 2006;20(5):564-568.
42. McPhee JT, Hill JS, Eslami MH. The impact of gender on presentation, therapy, and mortality of abdominal aortic aneurysm in the United States, 2001–2004. *J Vasc Surg* 2007;45(5):891-899.
43. Sweeting MJ, Thompson SG, Brown LC, et al. Meta-analysis of individual patient data to examine factors affecting growth and rupture of small abdominal aortic aneurysms. *Br J Surg* 2012;99(5):655-665.
44. Cao P. Comparison of surveillance vs Aortic Endografting for Small Aneurysm Repair (CAESAR) trial: study design and progress. *Eur J Vasc Endovasc Surg* 2005;30(3):245-251.
45. Cao P, De Rango P, Verzini F, et al. Comparison of surveillance versus aortic endografting for small aneurysm repair (CAESAR): results from a randomised trial. *Eur J Vasc Endovasc Surg* 2011;41(1):13-25.
46. Ouriel K, Clair DG, Kent KC, et al. Endovascular repair compared with surveillance for patients with small abdominal aortic aneurysms. *J Vasc Surg* 2010;51(5):1081-1087.
47. Fink HA, Lederle FA, Roth CS, et al. The accuracy of physical examination to detect abdominal aortic aneurysm. *Arch Intern Med* 2000;160(6):833-836.
48. Ashton HA, Buxton MJ, Day NE, et al. The Multicentre Aneurysm Screening Study (MASS) into the effect of abdominal aortic aneurysm screening on mortality in men: a randomised controlled trial. *Lancet* 2002;360(9345):1531-1539.
49. Ashton HA, Gao L, Kim LG, et al. Fifteen-year follow-up of a randomized clinical trial of ultrasonographic screening for abdominal aortic aneurysms. *Br J Surg* 2007;94(6):696-701.
50. Thompson SG, Ashton HA, Gao L, et al. Final follow-up of the Multicentre Aneurysm Screening Study (MASS) randomized trial of abdominal aortic aneurysm screening. *Br J Surg* 2012;99(12):1649-1656.
51. Lee ES, Pickett E, Hedayati N, et al. Implementation of an aortic screening program in clinical practice: implications for the Screen For Abdominal Aortic Aneurysms Very Efficiently (SAAAVE) Act. *J Vasc Surg* 2009;49(5):1107-1111.
52. Horejs D, Gilbert PM, Burstein S, et al. Normal aortoiliac diameters by CT. *J Comput Assist Tomogr* 1988;12(4):602-603.
53. Pearce WH, Slaughter MS, LeMaire S, et al. Aortic diameter as a function of age, gender, and body surface area. *Surgery* 1993;114(4):691-697.
54. Thapar A, Cheal D, Hopkins T, et al. Internal or external wall diameter for abdominal aortic aneurysm screening? *Ann R Coll Surg Engl* 2010;92(6):503-505.
55. Hartshorne TC, McCollum CN, Earnshaw JJ, et al. Ultrasound measurement of aortic diameter in a national screening programme. *Eur J Vasc Endovasc Surg* 2011;42(2):195-199.
56. Blois B. Office-based ultrasound screening for abdominal aortic aneurysm. *Can Fam Physician* 2012;58(3):e172-e178.
57. Staub D, Partovi S, Imfeld S, et al. Novel applications of contrast-enhanced ultrasound imaging in vascular medicine. *Vasa* 2013;42(1):17-31.
58. Phelan MP, Emerman CL. Focused aortic ultrasound to evaluate the prevalence of abdominal aortic aneurysm in ED patients with high-risk symptoms. *Am J Emerg Med* 2006;24(2):227-229.

59. Barkin AZ, Rosen CL. Ultrasound detection of abdominal aortic aneurysm. *Emerg Med Clin North Am* 2004;22(3):675-682.
60. Knaut AL, Kendall JL, Patten R, et al. Ultrasonographic measurement of aortic diameter by emergency physicians approximates results obtained by computed tomography. *J Emerg Med* 2005;28(2):119-126.
61. Johnston KW, Rutherford RB, Tilson MD, et al. Suggested standards for reporting on arterial aneurysms. Subcommittee on Reporting Standards for Arterial Aneurysms, Ad Hoc Committee on Reporting Standards, Society for Vascular Surgery and North American Chapter, International Society for Cardiovascular Surgery. *J Vasc Surg* 1991;13(3):452-458.
62. Wolf YG, Kobzantsev Z, Zelmanovich L. Size of normal and aneurysmal popliteal arteries: a duplex ultrasound study. *J Vasc Surg* 2006;43(3):488-492.
63. Dawson I, Sie RB, van Bockel JH. Atherosclerotic popliteal aneurysm. *Br J Surg* 1997;84(3):293-299.
64. Pulli R, Dorigo W, Castelli P, et al. A multicentric experience with open surgical repair and endovascular exclusion of popliteal artery aneurysms. *Eur J Vasc Endovasc Surg* 2013;45(4):357-363.
65. van Bockel EA, Hamand A. Lower extremity aneurysms. In: Rutherford R (ed.). *Rutherford Vascular Surgery*, 6th ed. Denver: Elsevier Saunders, 2005, p. 1534.
66. Hirsch AT, Haskal ZJ, Hertzer NR, et al. ACC/AHA 2005 Practice Guidelines for the management of patients with peripheral arterial disease (lower extremity, renal, mesenteric, and abdominal aortic): a collaborative report from the American Association for Vascular Surgery/Society for Vascular Surgery, Society for Cardiovascular Angiography and Interventions, Society for Vascular Medicine and Biology, Society of Interventional Radiology, and the ACC/AHA Task Force on Practice Guidelines (Writing Committee to Develop Guidelines for the Management of Patients With Peripheral Arterial Disease): endorsed by the American Association of Cardiovascular and Pulmonary Rehabilitation; National Heart, Lung, and Blood Institute; Society for Vascular Nursing; TransAtlantic Inter-Society Consensus; and Vascular Disease Foundation. *Circulation* 2006;113(11):e463-e654.
67. Cutler BS, Darling RC. Surgical management of arteriosclerotic femoral aneurysms. *Surgery* 1973;74(5):764-773.
68. Bergan JJ, Kaupp HA, Trippel OH. Femoral aneurysmectomy. Management of the profunda femoris artery. *Angiology* 1969;20(5):249-255.
69. Furst G, Kuhn FP, Modder U. Color coded duplex sonography in the diagnosis of peripheral vascular disease—applications in the evaluation of peripheral aneurysms, follow-up after arterial graft surgery and deep venous thrombosis. *Acta Radiol* 1991;377:7-14.
70. Levi N, Schroeder TV. Arteriosclerotic femoral artery aneurysms. A short review. *J Cardiovasc Surg* 1997;38(4):335-338.
71. Corriere MA, Guzman RJ. True and false aneurysms of the femoral artery. *Semin Vasc Surg* 2005;18(4):216-223.
72. Harbuzariu C, Duncan AA, Bower TC, et al. Profunda femoris artery aneurysms: association with aneurysmal disease and limb ischemia. *J Vasc Surg* 2008;47(1):31-34; discussion 4-5.
73. Sandgren T, Sonesson B, Ahlgren R, et al. The diameter of the common femoral artery in healthy human: influence of sex, age, and body size. *J Vasc Surg* 1999;29(3):503-510.
74. Leon LR, Jr., Taylor Z, Psalms SB, et al. Degenerative aneurysms of the superficial femoral artery. *Eur J Vasc Endovasc Surg* 2008;35(3):332-340.
75. Graham LM, Zelenock GB, Whitehouse WM, Jr., et al. Clinical significance of arteriosclerotic femoral artery aneurysms. *Arch Surg* 1980;115(4):502-507.
76. Diwan A, Sarkar R, Stanley JC, et al. Incidence of femoral and popliteal artery aneurysms in patients with abdominal aortic aneurysms. *J Vasc Surg* 2000;31(5):863-869.
77. Widmer MK, Blatter S, Schmidli J, et al. Generalized dilating diathesis in patients with popliteal arterial aneurysm. *Vasa* 2008;37(2):157-163.
78. Yamamoto N, Unno N, Mitsuoka H, et al. Clinical relationship between femoral artery aneurysms and arteriomegaly. *Surg Today* 2002;32(11):970-973.
79. Chan O, Thomas ML. The incidence of popliteal aneurysms in patients with arteriomegaly. *Clin Radiol* 1990;41(3):185-189.
80. Hollier LH, Stanson AW, Gloviczki P, et al. Arteriomegaly: classification and morbid implications of diffuse aneurysmal disease. *Surgery* 1983;93(5):700-708.
81. Carlson DH, Gryska P, Seletz J, et al. Arteriomegaly. *Am J Roentgenol Radium Ther Nucl Med* 1975;125(3):553-558.
82. Laureys M, Akkari K, De Wilde JP. Arteriomegaly. *Cardiovasc Intervent Radiol* 2005;28(3):358-359.
83. Thomas ML. Arteriomegaly. *Br J Surg* 1971;58(9):690-694.
84. Moore WS, Hall AD. Late suture failure in the pathogenesis of anastomotic false aneurysms. *Ann Surg* 1970;172(6):1064-1068.
85. Clagett GP, Salander JM, Eddleman WL, et al. Dilation of knitted Dacron aortic prostheses and anastomotic false aneurysms: etiologic considerations. *Surgery* 1983;93(1 Pt 1):9-16.
86. Criado E, Marston WA, Ligush J, et al. Endovascular repair of peripheral aneurysms, pseudoaneurysms, and arteriovenous fistulas. *Ann Vasc Surg* 1997;11(3):256-263.
87. Markovic DM, Davidovic LB, Kostic DM, et al. False anastomotic aneurysms. *Vascular* 2007;15(3):141-148.
88. Sharma NK, Chin KF, Modgill VK. Pseudoaneurysms of the femoral artery: recommendation for a method of repair. *J R Coll Surg Edinb.* 2001;46(4):195-197.
89. Mulder EJ, van Bockel JH, Maas J, et al. Morbidity and mortality of reconstructive surgery of noninfected false aneurysms detected long after aortic prosthetic reconstruction. *Arch Surg* 1998;133(1):45-49.
90. Clarke AM, Poskitt KR, Baird RN, et al. Anastomotic aneurysms of the femoral artery: aetiology and treatment. *Br J Surg* 1989;76(10):1014-1016.
91. Lord JW Jr, Rossi G. Reoperation for femoral anastomotic false aneurysm: a 15-year experience. *Ann Surg* 1988;208(5):670-671.
92. Treiman GS, Weaver FA, Cossman DV, et al. Anastomotic false aneurysms of the abdominal aorta and the iliac arteries. *J Vasc Surg* 1988;8(3):268-273.
93. Youkey JR, Clagett GP, Rich NM, et al. Femoral anastomotic false aneurysms. An 11-year experience analyzed with a case control study. *Ann Surg* 1984;199(6):703-709.
94. Seabrook GR, Schmitt DD, Bandyk DF, et al. Anastomotic femoral pseudoaneurysm: an investigation of occult infection as an etiologic factor. *J Vasc Surg* 1990;11(5):629-634.
95. Ylonen K, Biancari F, Leo E, et al. Predictors of development of anastomotic femoral pseudoaneurysms after aortobifemoral reconstruction for abdominal aortic aneurysm. *Am J Surg* 2004;187(1):83-87.
96. Lumsden A, Peden E, Bush R, et al. In: Rutherford R (ed). *Complications of Endovascular Procedures*, 6th ed. Denver: Elsevier Saunders; 2005.
97. Ahmad F, Turner SA, Torrie P, et al. Iatrogenic femoral artery pseudoaneurysms—a review of current methods of diagnosis and treatment. *Clin Radiol* 2008;63(12):1310-1316.
98. Kang SS, Labropoulos N, Mansour MA, et al. Percutaneous ultrasound guided thrombin injection: a new method for treating postcatheterization femoral pseudoaneurysms. *J Vasc Surg* 1998;27(6):1032-1038.
99. Kumins NH, Landau DS, Montalvo J, et al. Expanded indications for the treatment of postcatheterization femoral pseudoaneurysms with ultrasound-guided compression. *Am J Surg* 1998;176(2):131-136.
100. Feld R, Patton GM, Carabasi RA, et al. Treatment of iatrogenic femoral artery injuries with ultrasound-guided compression. *J Vasc Surg* 1992;16(6):832-840.
101. Hajarizadeh H, LaRosa CR, Cardullo P, et al. Ultrasound-guided compression of iatrogenic femoral pseudoaneurysm failure, recurrence, and long-term results. *J Vasc Surg* 1995;22(4):425-430; discussion 30–3.
102. Hye RJ. Compression therapy for acute iatrogenic femoral pseudoaneurysms. *Semin Vasc Surg* 2000;13(1):58-61.
103. Friedman SG, Pellerito JS, Scher L, et al. Ultrasound-guided thrombin injection is the treatment of choice for femoral pseudoaneurysms. *Arch Surg* 2002;137(4):462-464.
104. Hanson JM, Atri M, Power N. Ultrasound-guided thrombin injection of iatrogenic groin pseudoaneurysm: Doppler features and technical tips. *Br J Radiol* 2008;81(962):154-163.
105. Lonn L, Olmarker A, Geterud K, et al. Prospective randomized study comparing ultrasound-guided thrombin injection to compression in the treatment of femoral pseudoaneurysms. *J Endovasc Ther* 2004;11(5):570-576.
106. Sanjay P, Lewis MH. Deep vein thrombosis and pulmonary embolus associated with a ruptured popliteal aneurysm—a cautionary note. *World J Emerg Surg* 2007;2:34.
107. Parmer SS, Skelly CL, Carpenter JP. Ruptured popliteal artery aneurysm: a case report. *Vasc Endovascular Surg* 2006;40(1):71-74.
108. Dorrucci V, Veraldi GF, Dusi R, et al. True aneurysm of the profunda femoris artery. Case report and literature review. *Minerva Chir* 1998;53(10):847-851.

CHAPTER 16 ■ DUPLEX ASSESSMENT OF AORTIC ENDOGRAFTS

NASIM HEDAYATI, DAVID DEL PIZZO AND DAVID L. DAWSON

Parodi and coworkers[1,2] first reported successful exclusion of an abdominal aortic aneurysm (AAA) by an intraluminal graft in 1991. Since that time, the increased use of endovascular aneurysm repair (EVAR) has led to a decrease in traditional open surgical repair, and currently, nearly 75% of all AAAs are being treated via an endovascular approach.[3–6] Advantages of EVAR include shorter operative time and hospital length of stay, as well as lower perioperative morbidity and mortality compared with those of traditional open AAA repair.[6–9] However, late complications such as aneurysm sac enlargement, endoleaks, stent fracture, endograft migration, and stenosis or occlusion of the iliac graft limbs make lifelong endograft surveillance a necessity.[10]

Surveillance can identify conditions that might represent a risk for aneurysm growth and rupture, such as an endoleak with continued pressurization of the aneurysm sac. Post-EVAR follow-up has traditionally been performed with computed tomography (CT), which has been the "gold standard" for surveillance designed to evaluate aneurysm sac size and detect endoleaks. Follow-up schedules have generally reflected the protocols developed in the clinical trials of EVAR, with postprocedure surveillance CT scans being performed at approximately 1 month, 6 months, 12 months, and annually thereafter.

CT imaging and duplex ultrasonography are the two primary post-EVAR surveillance methods currently being used. Other imaging modalities, such as magnetic resonance angiography (MRA), are rarely used for EVAR surveillance, but the use of duplex ultrasound for the evaluation of abdominal aortic endografts has been gaining wider acceptance. At many institutions, including our own, a duplex ultrasound is performed after the initial post-EVAR CT scan. Subsequent CT imaging is reserved for confirming aneurysm sac enlargement or delineation of an endoleak. An *endoleak* is defined as blood flow outside the lumen of the endograft or in the aneurysm sac, and it is identified in 15% to 32% of all patients who undergo an EVAR.[11–15] An increasing number of studies have compared duplex ultrasound to CT angiography for detecting endoleaks and measuring aneurysm sac diameter. As discussed in this chapter, the efficacy, feasibility, and financial advantages of duplex ultrasonography in comparison with CT angiography for post-EVAR surveillance are well documented.[16–29]

THE ROLE OF SURVEILLANCE AFTER EVAR

One of the most important features of successful aneurysm treatment by EVAR is the absence of an endoleak. Although approximately 50% of all endoleaks will thrombose or resolve spontaneously without intervention,[14] the presence of an endoleak is concerning owing to the possibility of aneurysm sac enlargement and the potential risk for rupture. In addition, endoleak management can greatly increase the overall cost of an EVAR. One estimate of the 5-year postplacement follow-up cost for a patient with an endoleak was $26,739 versus $5706 for a patient without an endoleak.[30] This nearly fivefold increase in cost is associated with the secondary interventional procedures and additional imaging studies.

Classification of Endoleaks

Endoleaks are classified according to the source of the leak, as illustrated in Figures 16.1 and 16.2. A type I endoleak (see Fig. 16.1, *Left*) represents blood flow into the aneurysm sac from the proximal graft attachment site at the infrarenal neck of the aortic aneurysm (type Ia) or the distal attachment site in the iliac arteries (type Ib). Type I endoleaks have been reported in 4% to 7% of all EVARs.[9] If recognized intraoperatively or during postoperative surveillance, type Ia endoleaks can often be treated successfully with balloon angioplasty to better appose the graft to the aortic wall, deploying a proximal aortic cuff, or using a balloon-expandable stent to provide additional proximal fixation and seal. An iliac limb extension can be used to provide a better distal seal for type Ib endoleaks. A persistent type I endoleak not amenable to repair by endovascular techniques may require conversion to open repair.

A type II endoleak results from retrograde flow into the aortic sac from aortic branches such as one or more lumbar arteries, the inferior mesenteric artery, or other collateral vessels (see Fig. 16.1, *Right*). Type II endoleaks are relatively common and have been observed in 27% to 37% of EVAR cases.[11] Some have subcategorized type II endoleaks into type IIa, indicating flow from one branch vessel, and type IIb, representing more than one branch vessel involvement.[11] Others have

FIGURE 16.1. *Left,* Type I endoleaks after endovascular aneurysm repair (EVAR). *Right,* Type II endoleaks.

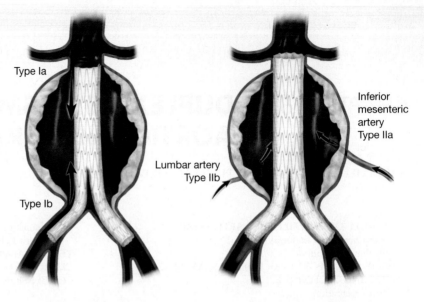

Type I Endoleaks   Type II Endoleaks

described a type IIa endoleak as originating from the inferior mesenteric artery and a type IIb as originating from a lumbar artery. To avoid confusion, it may be better to report the presence of a type II endoleak and specifically describe the branch vessel(s) responsible. Most type II endoleaks can be followed without intervention, because many will resolve spontaneously by thrombosis.[14] Interventions such as coil embolization or vessel ligation are performed when the type II endoleak is associated with evidence of aneurysm sac enlargement or failure of a large aneurysm sac to shrink over time.

A type III endoleak originates from a structural failure of the stent graft, such as a fabric tear or ineffective seal between stent graft components; these occur in less than 3% of cases (see Fig. 16.2, *Left*).[12] Although rare, the presence of a type III endoleak is an indication for intervention by either endovascular revision or open repair because the aneurysm sac is exposed to systemic arterial pressure, and the risk of aneurysm rupture is similar to that with a type I endoleak (or an

unrepaired aneurysm). Type III endoleaks can also be subcategorized into type IIIa, indicating device fabric disruption or holes; type IIIb, separation of modular component devices or junctions; and type IIIc, representing suture holes in the fabric of the graft.[11]

The final endoleak classification is type IV, which is a consequence of graft porosity (see Fig. 16.2, *Right*). Type IV endoleaks have a reported incidence of about 5%[13] but are generally self-limited, resolving quickly as fibrin seals the graft material. Type IV endoleaks are infrequently encountered with the newer generations of endografts that have materials with decreased porosity covering the stents.

The term *endotension* may also be used in conjunction with a post-EVAR evaluation and has been referred to by some as a type V endoleak.[31] Endotension represents pressure in the aneurysm sac or sac enlargement without an identifiable endoleak. Some of these cases are likely associated with endoleaks that are not visualized with the imaging

FIGURE 16.2. *Left,* Type III endoleaks after EVAR. *Right,* Type IV endoleaks.

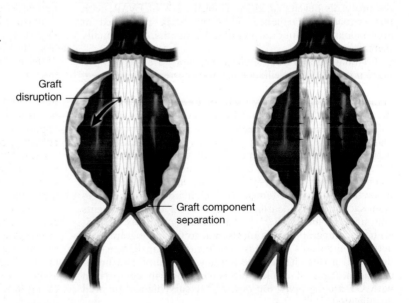

Type III Endoleaks   Type IV Endoleaks

studies performed. Other less likely causes of endotension include a seroma pressurizing the aneurysm sac, pressure transmission from the thrombus around the stent graft, or graft infection.[31]

Imaging Techniques

Although CT angiography is commonly used for post-EVAR surveillance and detection of endoleaks, this approach has a number of disadvantages, including the use of nephrotoxic contrast agents, patient exposure to ionizing radiation, and cost.[17] Furthermore, certain technical factors can limit the accuracy of CT angiography, such as timing of the contrast bolus, the width of image slices, and interobserver variability.[19] Pre- and postcontrast studies, typically with multidetector CT, are needed to distinguish between vessel wall calcification and endoleaks, although newer dual-energy CT systems can better differentiate calcium from contrast. It has been estimated that 33% to 65% of post-EVAR cost is secondary to the necessary radiologic studies, which may include lifelong surveillance with CT imaging.[30,32]

Digital subtraction angiography is usually performed to confirm suspected cases of endoleaks detected by other imaging methods. The feasibility of angiography as a surveillance tool post-EVAR is hindered by its invasiveness, exposure to radiation, and the use of nephrotoxic contrast agents. Furthermore, improper technique or the timing of an angiography contrast injection might result in an endoleak being overlooked.

Duplex Ultrasound

Duplex ultrasound is currently the preferred method for routine diagnosis and surveillance of unrepaired AAAs, as discussed in Chapter 15. In recent years, duplex ultrasonography has also evolved as an effective tool for post-EVAR surveillance. Duplex ultrasound can be used to measure the size of the residual aneurysm sac, detect endoleaks, and evaluate hemodynamic changes or stenosis in the outflow graft limbs and aortic branch vessels. Patency of the renal arteries, which can be compromised by graft fabric impingement, proximal fixation components, or proximal device migration, can be evaluated with duplex ultrasound. With enhanced resolution and better imaging technology, the ability to identify endoleaks with duplex scanning has also improved.[23]

The routine use of post-EVAR duplex ultrasound for surveillance has numerous advantages. Patients with renal insufficiency benefit from avoidance of repeated exposure to nephrotoxic contrast agents with CT imaging. During long-term follow-up, it has been shown that the risk for a decline in renal function is significantly greater after EVAR than after open aneurysm repair in patients with or without preexisting renal insufficiency.[33,34] The ability to eliminate the use of ionizing radiation and its lower cost make abdominal duplex ultrasonography an attractive alternative. A financial analysis of aortic graft surveillance estimated the cost of a CT angiogram at $2779 per study, in comparison to the cost of an abdominal aortic duplex ultrasound at $525 per study.[17] Even with the additional cost of routine abdominal radiographs needed to confirm the position of the stent graft, Bendick and colleagues[17] estimated an average 3-year saving of more than $16,000 per patient followed up with duplex ultrasound rather than CT imaging after EVAR. Other potential benefits include wider availability and portability and the noninvasive nature of the procedure. However, duplex scanning may not be technically satisfactory in every case. Visualization of the aorta and the iliac vessels can be limited by the presence of overlying bowel gas, body habitus, ascites, and vessel tortuosity. Nevertheless, experience has shown that post-EVAR duplex ultrasound is an effective modality for surveillance and evaluation of aneurysm size and the presence of endoleaks.[15–17,20,22–25,35,36]

Duplex ultrasound is an accurate measurement tool for aortic aneurysm size. Aneurysm diameter has been shown to correlate within 5 mm between CT and duplex ultrasound in 70% to 92% of the cases.[16,20,36] Raman and associates[36] performed a retrospective review of 281 patients comparing color-flow duplex ultrasound and CT imaging for post-EVAR surveillance. Routine abdominal radiographs were used to assess the integrity of the stent graft and evaluate for fractures or migration. Minimal variability between the measurements for the minor axis of the aorta was noted between the two diagnostic modalities. Using the abdominal CT scan as the gold standard for post-EVAR evaluation, duplex ultrasonography was demonstrated to have a sensitivity of 42%, a specificity of 96%, a positive predictive value of 54%, and a negative predictive value of 94%. This has been corroborated by Arko and coworkers[19] who examined post-EVAR follow-up CT and ultrasound studies in 201 patients. No significant difference was identified on paired analysis of maximal aortic diameter measurements with either imaging technique. Graft patency was documented to be 99% by both CT scan and duplex ultrasound. Furthermore, in comparison with CT imaging, duplex ultrasonography was shown to have a sensitivity of 81%, a specificity of 95%, a positive predictive value of 94%, and a negative predictive value of 90% for diagnosing an endoleak. The few endoleaks missed by duplex ultrasonography but diagnosed by a CT scan involved small lumbar arteries.

In addition to information regarding aneurysm sac size and endoleaks, iliac limb or outflow graft stenosis after EVAR can be easily diagnosed on duplex ultrasound.[21] Access vessels such as the external iliac arteries are often atherosclerotic with heavy calcification and may need predilation before advancing large sheaths and placing stent grafts. Hemodynamically significant stenosis may require future treatment with balloon angioplasty or stenting. Access vessel complications during EVAR, including dissection, bleeding, false aneurysm, arterial thrombosis, and arterial embolization, were reported in 13% of the patients in the EUROSTAR registry.[37] Subsequent iliac stent graft stenosis has been reported in 5.5% to 9% of cases.[31] Therefore, the evaluation of iliac graft limbs and the native iliac arteries is an essential part of post-EVAR duplex ultrasound surveillance.

Migration of the stent graft, defined as greater than 10-mm displacement, has an incidence of 1.4% during the first year post-EVAR.[31,38] Rarely, graft material may impinge upon the orifices of the renal arteries owing to either a short aneurysm neck or inaccurate deployment of the graft. A compromised renal artery can often be salvaged with stenting during the initial EVAR procedure or during a subsequent angiographic evaluation. It is important for duplex ultrasonography to evaluate the patency and any degree of stenosis in the renal arteries. Although not specifically validated in patients after EVAR, standard interpretation criteria for native renal arteries are usually applied. The duplex criteria for diagnosis of 60% or greater native renal artery stenosis include peak systolic velocity of 200 cm/s or greater and renal-to-aortic velocity ratio (RAR) of 3.5 or greater.[39] There are no standard duplex criteria for stenosis in stented renal arteries, although experience suggests that velocity thresholds for significant stenosis in stented renal arteries are higher than those for native renal arteries (see Chapter 24).

Duplex ultrasound can be used for post-EVAR follow-up and detection of endoleaks with aneurysm sac enlargement. Figure 16.3 shows a patient with a type II endoleak followed up for 2 years. During the EVAR procedure, the patient had a complication with endograft migration requiring stenting of the left renal artery. It was noted on duplex ultrasound that

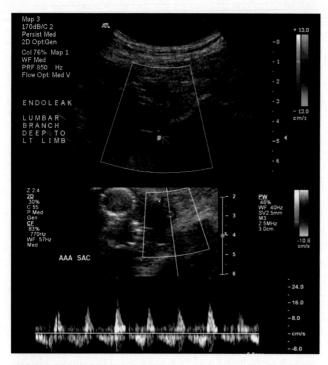

FIGURE 16.3. Duplex ultrasound images of a type II endoleak originating from a lumbar artery. Color flow image (*top*) shows an area of flow outside of the graft limbs (*white arrow*). Pulsed Doppler spectral waveform (*bottom*) shows a "to-and-fro" flow pattern with the sample volume positioned in the aortic aneurysm sac.

despite a small persistent type II endoleak, the aneurysm sac had grown in diameter from 4.9 to 5.6 cm during a 15-month period. An arteriogram revealed an endoleak originating from the iliolumbar artery off the right internal iliac artery, which was then successfully coil embolized (Fig. 16.4).

Aortic intrasac Doppler velocities and flow patterns may also help predict the natural history of endoleaks. Arko and coworkers[19] found that a type II endoleak was more likely to seal spontaneously if it was associated with an intrasac Doppler flow velocity less than 100 cm/s, a small patent inferior mesenteric artery, or fewer paired lumbar arteries. Intrasac velocities less than 100 cm/s correlated well with the likelihood that an endoleak would thrombose without further treatment. Parent and associates[29] observed that type II endoleaks with a "to-and-fro" flow pattern were more likely to resolve spontaneously, while those with a biphasic or monophasic flow pattern tended to persist. A more recent

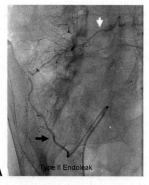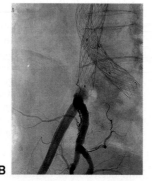

FIGURE 16.4. Type II endoleak. *A*, Angiogram confirms a right iliolumbar branch (*black arrow*) from the right internal iliac artery feeding a lumbar artery (*white arrow*). *B*, Coil embolization of the branch.

study by Beeman and coworkers[15] concluded that intrasac flow velocities in type II endoleaks did not correlate with spontaneous resolution or increases in aneurysm sac size; however, the presence of multiple type II endoleaks and a bidirectional flow pattern were the strongest predictors of an increase in aneurysm sac diameter.

OVERVIEW OF POST-EVAR DUPLEX SCANNING

A general approach to duplex ultrasound for follow-up of aortic endografts can be based on aortic aneurysm sac measurement, stent device patency and integrity, presence of endoleaks, stenosis of outflow graft vessels, and any incidental findings such as renal artery stenosis or thrombus within the graft (Table 16.1). The basic components of the post-EVAR duplex ultrasound examination are aneurysm sac diameter measurement and evaluation for the presence of flow outside the stent graft to identify an endoleak. Determination of the type of endoleak is important, whenever possible, because it may determine the need and urgency for endoleak treatment. This requires fastidious scanning technique by the technologist and the use of multiple views. Measuring the flow velocity in the iliac limbs of the graft and immediately distal to the limbs can provide information about stenosis involving the distal stent graft attachment sites.

Although migration of the stent graft proximally is much less common than migration distally, the renal arteries should be evaluated by duplex ultrasound for any evidence of stenosis secondary to graft material impingement. The common femoral arteries should be evaluated to look for any evidence of access site complications, whether a cutdown or a percutaneous approach was used. Finally, measuring the ankle-brachial indices (ABIs) is important for assessment of arterial perfusion of the lower extremities, and the postoperative ABIs should be compared with preoperative values.

A variety of endografts for infrarenal AAA repair are currently approved for use in the United States (Fig. 16.5). All of these devices consist of graft material supported by self-expanding metal stents. The stent material may be nitinol, stainless steel, or cobalt-chromium alloy. The graft fabric material can be woven polyester or expanded polytetrafluoroethylene (ePTFE). The proximal fixation of the graft can be based on outward radial force of the stent material in the neck of the aneurysm, column strength of the device, or suprarenal stent components. With suprarenal fixation, the device has uncovered metal components above the fabric-covered infrarenal stent that help to secure the graft to the aortic wall above the renal arteries. Suprarenal fixation is intended to provide more secure fixation of the graft to the

TABLE 16.1

COMPONENTS OF POST-EVAR DUPLEX ULTRASOUND

- Measurement of maximum aortic aneurysm sac diameter
- Detection and localization of flow outside the stent graft (endoleaks)
- Assessment of the integrity and patency of the stent graft components
- Detection of thrombus in the aortic stent graft main body or iliac graft limbs
- Measurement of diameters of the common iliac and external iliac arteries
- Evaluation for patency and flow disturbances in the celiac artery, superior mesenteric artery, and renal arteries
- Evaluation of the common femoral arteries for access site complications
- Bilateral ankle-brachial indices

Commercially Available Endografts for AAA

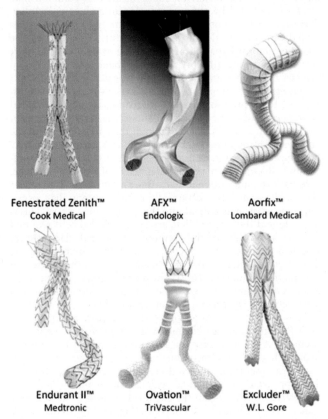

Fenestrated Zenith™
Cook Medical

AFX™
Endologix

Aorfix™
Lombard Medical

Endurant II™
Medtronic

Ovation™
TriVascular

Excluder™
W.L. Gore

FIGURE 16.5. Six commercially available aortic endografts. Images courtesy of Cook Medical, Endologix, Lombard Medical, Medtronic Endovascular, TriVascular, and W.L. Gore and Associates.

aortic wall, improve the seal, and reduce the risk of distal component migration. The use of fenestrated and branched endovascular stent grafts for complex aortic aneurysms has increased in recent years, and a commercially available fenestrated graft system for juxtarenal aneurysms is available in the United States.

Most aortic endografts are bifurcated modular systems with either one or two iliac limbs that "dock" with the aortic main body device. The two iliac limbs of the graft lie in the aortic aneurysm sac, sometimes crossing, and are easily identified on duplex ultrasound. A unibody bifurcated graft is also available that can be seated on the native aortic bifurcation. It is designed to reduce the risk of migration and the need for using multiple stent graft pieces. Newer devices have expanded the indications for EVAR, allowing endovascular treatment of aneurysms with short or angulated aortic necks, or with anatomically challenged access vessels (e.g., tortuous iliac arteries). An important consideration regarding the different stent graft devices available is that endoleak rates may differ based on the type of aortic endovascular graft device.[12]

Although endoleaks are relatively common, their significance and natural history are not completely understood, and many can be followed for months to years without intervention. A persistent endoleak many months postprocedure, or one associated with aneurysm sac enlargement, can be treated by a number of techniques, including transfemoral, transbrachial, or translumbar approaches. One frequently used technique consists of angiography for localization of the endoleak branch vessel and embolization with coils, glue, or other materials. Platinum and stainless steel are commonly used coil materials. Coil embolization may be achieved via access through an internal iliac artery branch connecting to a lumbar

artery or through a branch of the superior mesenteric artery connecting to a branch of the inferior mesenteric artery. Open surgical or laparoscopic ligation of the vessel responsible for a type II endoleak is less frequently performed.

SCANNING TECHNIQUE

Instrumentation

Duplex evaluation of abdominal aortic endografts is one of the most technically challenging and complex examinations performed by vascular technologists. A full-featured ultrasound system with enhanced B-mode, harmonic imaging, high-quality color-flow imaging, high spectral Doppler sensitivity, and other imaging adjuncts better enable the technologist to perform a complete and accurate study. Transducer frequencies ranging from 2 to 5 MHz are used to evaluate the abdominal aorta and visceral vessels. Probe selection depends on the depth of the desired field of view. A low-frequency curved linear array is used to interrogate the abdominal aorta and iliac arteries from an anterior or lateral approach. A small-footprint low-frequency–phased array transducer can be used for intercostal views.

Historically, color flow Doppler imaging has been used as a guide and not as a primary diagnostic tool for arterial examinations. However, color flow Doppler is a requisite part of the abdominal aortic endograft evaluation. Color flow facilitates visualization of flow within the aortic aneurysm sac in the evaluation for endoleaks (see Fig. 16.3). The color flow Doppler pulse repetition frequency (PRF or color scale) should be set low to allow detection of slow flow velocities within the aneurysm sac. A small-sized color box will enable selective positioning within the aneurysm sac and maximize the frame rate. Persistence should be at a medium level. To correctly adjust color gain settings, the technologist should turn the color gain up to the point at which the color "noise" or color speckling is visible on the display and then reduce the color gain to the threshold at which the color "noise" is eliminated. This will ensure that the color gain is set at the highest possible setting without being "overgained."

Patient Preparation and Positioning

Whenever possible, the patient should avoid gas-producing foods for several days before the study and avoid chewing gum or smoking before the examination to minimize intestinal activity and bowel gas. Ideally, the patient should also fast (if not medically contraindicated) for approximately 4 to 6 hours before the examination. Taking medications with a small amount of water is acceptable.

The examination starts with the patient supine and adequately exposed for imaging the abdomen, flanks, and groins. Abdominal aortic endograft evaluations are technically challenging and require numerous views and careful evaluation to detect subtle abnormalities. In general, about 1 to 2 hours should be scheduled for the examination to provide sufficient time to prepare the patient, perform the scan, and generate the preliminary report.

To avoid fatigue and reduce the risk of repetitive stress injury, arrange the imaging system, technologist chair, and patient scanning bed or stretcher for the comfort of both the patient and the technologist. The technologist should be positioned higher than the scanning surface, and the technologist's arm should be supported and moderately flexed and positioned as close to the midline as possible. The technologist may stand during the examination to help apply probe pressure when necessary. If standing, the technologist should attempt to hold the scanning arm as straight and as close as possible, which will allow the technologist to "lean" into the scanning field and apply gentle pressure to displace mobile viscera and position the probe closer to the aorta. The availability of a low-profile step stool may be helpful. The technologist should make the patient aware that pressure may be applied with the ultrasound probe and instruct the patient to report any discomfort. The astute technologist should be aware of the patient's comfort level at all times during the examination. Although probe pressure may be required for best imaging, the technologist can work with the patient to obtain optimal images with the least amount of discomfort.

It may be useful to have the patient turn to the side for right or left lateral decubitus scanning approaches. A lateral scanning approach can help overcome limitations due to depth, vessel tortuosity, and bowel gas. Varying approaches may also improve the patient's comfort level by avoiding continuous probe pressure in the same region throughout the entire examination. It is important to remember that despite proper imaging techniques, image quality may be compromised by bowel gas, body habitus, abdominal wall hernias, presence of ascites, and patient intolerance.[35] Post-EVAR examinations are advanced vascular laboratory studies. Therefore, it is important that the technologist learning to perform these studies be given sufficient time with the expectation that the number of technically limited examinations will decrease as experience is gained.

Examination Protocol

B-Mode Imaging

The examination begins with an anterior approach in a transverse imaging plane. The abdominal aorta should be identified starting at the level of the celiac artery. For difficult evaluations, color flow Doppler can help with branch vessel identification. The hyperechoic walls of most endografts are readily distinguished from the native aortic aneurysm wall (Fig. 16.6). In a transverse view, the endograft is visualized within the abdominal aorta and should be surrounded by thrombus within the aneurysm sac. Most modular bifurcated endograft configurations have the device bifurcation within the abdominal aorta, with two limbs traversing the distal aorta into the iliac arteries. Below the device bifurcation, this results in a "double-barreled" appearance within the abdominal aorta proximal to the native aortic bifurcation (Fig. 16.7). Unibody bifurcated endografts may be seated directly on the aortic bifurcation, and separate iliac limbs will not be visible in the aorta.

Infrequently, an aorto-uni-iliac device may be used to repair an AAA. In these instances, the contralateral common iliac artery is occluded by either disease or an endovascular plug. Perfusion of the contralateral lower extremity is then maintained with a femoral-femoral bypass graft. In these cases, the femoral-femoral bypass graft should be evaluated by duplex surveillance to identify any flow disturbances or increases in velocity that may signify lesions that threaten graft patency.

Measure abdominal aortic diameters at several locations: superior to the proximal extent of the endograft, at the proximal attachment site of the endograft, and at the largest segment of the native aneurysm sac. Also, obtain the circumference of the aneurysm sac, as shown in Figure 16.8. This measurement may be subject to less intertest variability than diameter measurements.[40] Record the maximum diameters of the common iliac, external iliac, and internal iliac arteries. The distal attachment site for the graft limbs is typically in the common iliac artery, but some grafts may extend into the external iliac artery. This is often done if the internal iliac artery is occluded or if required to treat aneurysms of the common or internal iliac arteries. Evaluate the distal attachment sites with measurements of the iliac artery diameter at the most distal aspect of the device and beyond that point (Fig. 16.9). The technologist should describe any unusual endograft appearance, anatomic variations such as tortuosity, and the presence of intragraft echoes.

It is important to interrogate the excluded aneurysm sac with B-mode imaging. Normally, thrombus forms within the excluded AAA and appears as uniform, relatively homogeneous echoes. As the thrombus ages and contracts, the diameter of the aneurysm sac will decrease over time (Fig. 16.10).[41] The appearance of anechoic regions within the thrombus is suggestive of flow within the excluded aneurysm sac and may indicate the presence of an endoleak (Fig. 16.11). To determine the presence of distal endograft migration, measure the distance between the lowest positioned renal artery and the proximal aspect of the endograft device. This may be difficult to do because the renal arteries are rarely visualized while simultaneously imaging the abdominal aorta in a long-axis view.

Doppler Assessment

Evaluate flow patterns throughout the native aorta, endograft main body and graft limbs, outflow vessels, and visceral vessels with the pulsed Doppler and corresponding spectral waveforms. Perform Doppler evaluations using a 60-degree angle of insonation whenever feasible. The Doppler sample volume

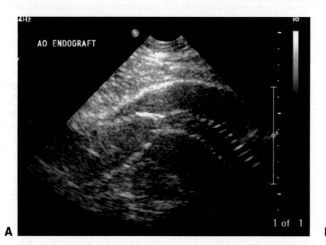
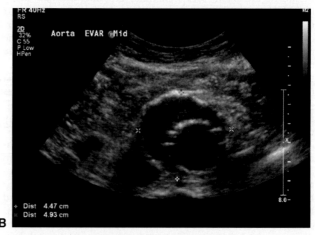

FIGURE 16.6. B-mode images of aortic endografts showing the hyperechoic graft walls within the aneurysm sac. *A*, Longitudinal view with the larger main body of the endograft on the *left* and a smaller iliac limb on the *right*. *B*, Transverse view of the main body of an endograft (*inner ring*) and the aneurysm sac (*outer ring*). Diameter measurements of the aneurysm sac are 4.47 cm × 4.93 cm.

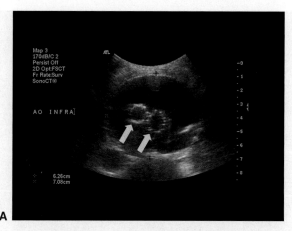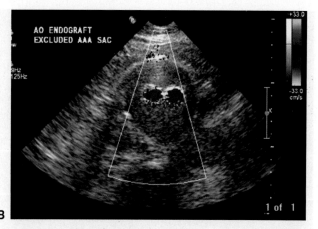

FIGURE 16.7. Endografts typically bifurcate into right and left limbs within the abdominal aorta. *A*, B-mode image of paired graft limbs (*arrows*) in the aneurysm sac. *B*, Color flow image showing flow in the paired graft limbs (*red*), but no flow in the excluded aneurysm sac.

is positioned and swept through the endograft, including the proximal and distal attachment sites. Document any areas of velocity increase, measuring the velocity immediately proximal to, within, and distal to the site of interest.

Although there are no specific validated criteria for the degree of stenosis within an endograft, it has been shown that within peripheral arteries, a velocity ratio of 2.0 or greater is indicative of a narrowing of at least 50% (see Chapter 12).[42] Also, interrogate the origins of the celiac artery, superior mesenteric artery, and the renal arteries. Document peak systolic and end-diastolic velocities as well as flow direction. Finally, evaluate the common iliac, external iliac, and internal iliac arteries beyond the distal attachment sites, as well as the common femoral arteries, with Doppler spectral waveforms for patency, stenosis, and flow characteristics (Figs. 16.12 and 16.13).

Assessing for Endoleak

The principal challenge in post-EVAR imaging is to accurately identify or exclude the presence of an endoleak. The search for endoleaks is technically demanding, because the flow channel associated with an endoleak may be small and the flow velocities may be very low. A careful search is crucial, because a missed endoleak can leave the patient at risk for aneurysm rupture. The

vascular technologist must be diligent and thorough, and scanning should be performed from various approaches, including anterior, oblique, and lateral decubitus views.

Optimized color flow Doppler is needed to identify endoleaks (Figs. 16.14 and 16.15). The technologist should understand the limitations and capabilities of color flow Doppler imaging. Improper color-flow Doppler settings can result in a false-positive test due to color-flow "flash artifact" or color pixels "bleeding" into areas where flow is actually not present. The technologist may also encounter color-flow artifact due to bowel gas, patient movement, and respiratory movement. An endoleak may be missed if the color parameters are not correctly set. It is helpful to decrease the color flow velocity scale (PRF) and to increase color-flow gain and color persistence. Other helpful maneuvers include using a smaller color box size to increase frame rate. Selectively position the color box over the aneurysm sac without involvement of the endograft limbs (see Fig. 16.15). Evaluate the aneurysm sac in its entirety in both transverse and longitudinal planes. Interrogate any areas of color flow visualized within the native aneurysm sac with pulsed Doppler.

When assessing for a type I endoleak, carefully evaluate the proximal and distal endograft attachment sites with both B-mode and color-flow Doppler. Flow signals identified at those sites between the endograft device and the native

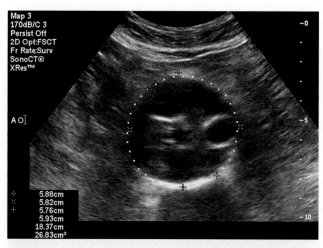

FIGURE 16.8. Diameter and circumference measurements of the abdominal aortic aneurysm are made using electronic elliptical calipers on the B-mode image.

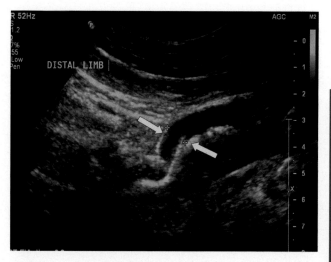

FIGURE 16.9. The diameter of the iliac artery at the distal end of an iliac endograft limb (*blue arrows*) is measured.

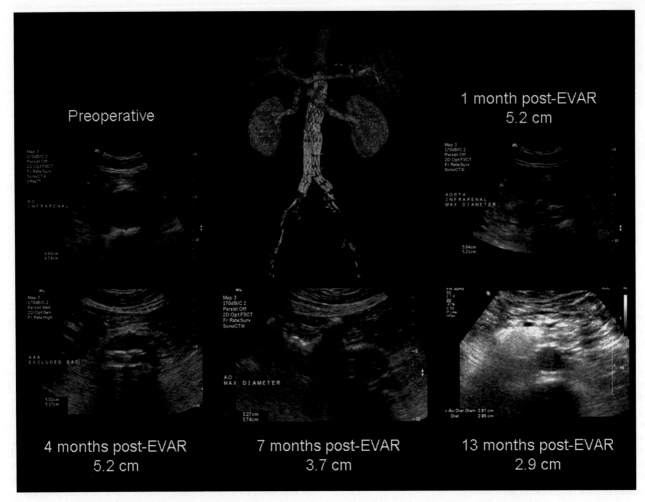

FIGURE 16.10. Serial duplex scans show a decrease in aneurysm sac diameters over 13 months post-EVAR.

arterial wall are indicative of a type I endoleak (Fig. 16.16). B-mode imaging is valuable in these instances to determine whether the device is separated from the native vessel wall as well as to detect any device wall motion at the apposition sites. The typical Doppler flow signal from a type II endoleak will have "to-and-fro" flow characteristics, similar to what is observed in the neck of a peripheral artery pseudoaneurysm (see Chapter 32). Flow appearing to arise from the antero-lateral aspect of the aneurysm wall may be from the inferior mesenteric artery, a type IIa endoleak. Flow arising from the posterolateral aspect of the aorta is more likely from a lumbar artery, a type IIb endoleak (Figs. 16.17 and 16.18).

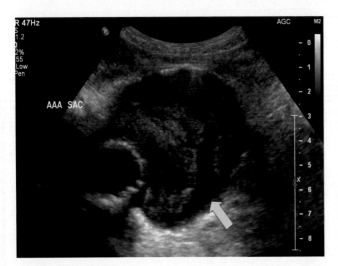

FIGURE 16.11. Hypoechoic areas within the thrombus in the excluded aneurysm sac (*blue arrow*) can be a sign of endoleak.

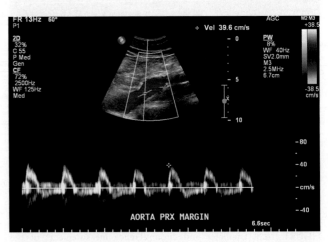

FIGURE 16.12. Velocity measurements are obtained to evaluate for patency and stenosis at the proximal (aortic) end of an endograft.

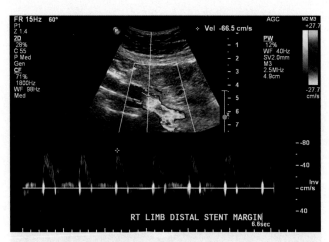

FIGURE 16.13. Peak systolic velocity measurements in the distal limbs of an endograft evaluate for stenosis due to kinking or compression. The native iliac outflow artery should also be assessed.

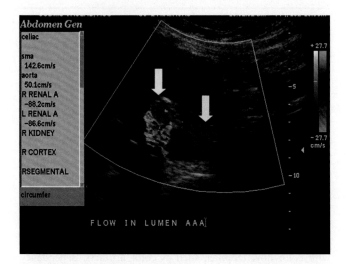

FIGURE 16.14. Color-flow Doppler image demonstrates a low-velocity endoleak (*blue arrow*) adjacent to higher-flow velocities within the endograft (*yellow arrow*).

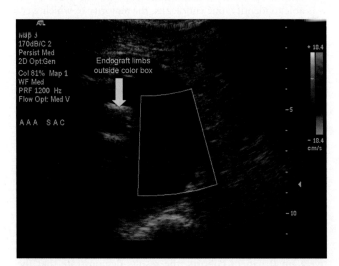

FIGURE 16.15. Selective positioning of the color box can reduce artifacts from high-velocity flow signals in the adjacent endograft lumen.

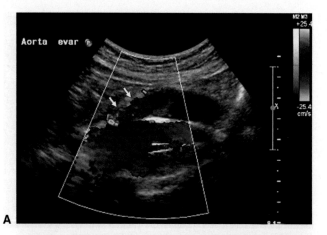

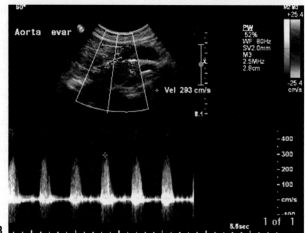

FIGURE 16.16. Type I endoleak at the proximal (aortic) attachment site of an endograft. *A*, Longitudinal color-flow Doppler image shows flow between the native arterial wall and endograft device into the aortic aneurysm sac (*arrows*). *B*, Doppler spectral waveform at the site of this endoleak shows a pulsatile arterial flow pattern.

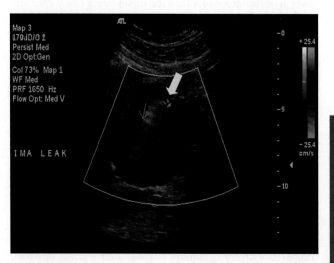

FIGURE 16.17. Retrograde flow within the aneurysm sac arising from the anterior surface of the abdominal aorta. The color flow image shows a type IIa endoleak from a patent inferior mesenteric artery (*blue arrow*).

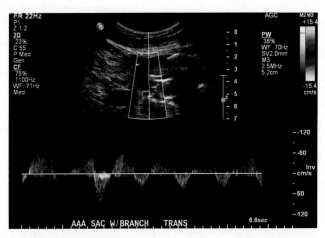

FIGURE 16.18. Color flow image and spectral waveform show the "to-and-fro" Doppler flow signal within a type IIb endoleak from a patent lumbar artery.

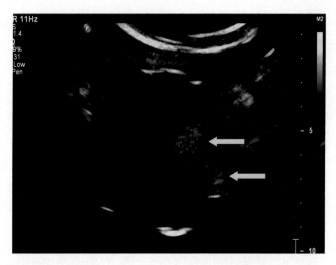

FIGURE 16.19. Contrast-enhanced ultrasound demonstrates flow within the endograft limbs (*blue arrows*). No contrast filling is detected within the aneurysm sac outside the device limbs.

Contrast-Enhanced Ultrasound

Contrast-enhanced ultrasound (CEUS) imaging is currently approved by the U.S. Food and Drug Administration (FDA) for echocardiography, and these contrast agents may also have applications in duplex ultrasonography. CEUS uses stabilized microbubbles to enhance the diagnostic capabilities of current ultrasound technology. The microbubbles have elastic shells that are typically made of sugar matrices, albumin, lipids, or polymers.[43] Contrast agents used with duplex ultrasonography can increase the backscatter of signal intensity, enhancing Doppler analysis. Signal intensity with CEUS is predicted to increase 100 to 1000 times over conventional duplex ultrasound. Because CEUS imaging can detect subtle flow and delineate flow borders without the use of color-flow Doppler, contrast can assist in post-EVAR evaluation. Off-label use of CEUS can be applied selectively in patients with equivocal conventional duplex or CT angiography findings to help identify the presence of an endoleak (Fig. 16.19).

One effective contrast agent is composed of a perflutren gas encapsulated by a lipid- or protein-based microsphere shell that measures 1.1 to 3.3 µm in diameter. The microspheres have lower acoustic impedance than the surrounding blood cells and are therefore highly reflective, enhancing visualization of blood flow with B-mode imaging. Furthermore, the microspheres quickly degrade in the bloodstream and are metabolized in 7 to 10 minutes. The perflutren gas is then exhaled and the outer shell is absorbed. Insonation with ultrasound can induce microsphere rupture; therefore, a low mechanical index of approximately 0.05 is necessary to minimize the transmitted energy. Mechanical index reflects the output power, which in turn corresponds to the local acoustic power.[43]

The contrast agent is activated by rapid shaking. Once activated, the material appears as a white milky substance. Contrast agents can be administered via continuous infusion or a bolus injection. Continuous infusion of 1.3 mL of contrast agent mixed with 50 mL saline, delivered at a rate of 4 mL/min, is generally effective. For bolus infusion, it is recommended to inject 0.5 mL of contrast agent followed by 10-mL normal saline flush. An advantage of the continuous infusion method is that it provides up to 15 minutes of scanning time compared with the 5 minutes possible after a bolus infusion. Another advantage of a longer duration of contrast infusion is that it may allow for delayed filling from small collaterals that are responsible for a type II endoleak.[44]

A vascular laboratory that performs CEUS examinations should have specific protocols for contrast use. The protocols should consider all product labeling and warnings and specify

administering techniques and contraindications for use. The method of contrast administration, imaging techniques, and postinjection patient monitoring should be specified. Assistance of a vascular nurse or other qualified individual is required for administering the contrast agent before the examination and for monitoring the patient during and after the examination. Because of possible side effects, obtain consent from the patient prior to the examination. Common side effects include pain at the injection site, headache, nausea, facial flushing, and a temporary alteration in taste. Cardiovascular and pulmonary side effects might include chest pain and dyspnea. Owing to the lack of any renal or hepatic toxicity, CEUS can be performed in patients with renal or hepatic failure.

CEUS has been shown to be more sensitive than color flow duplex ultrasound for identifying endoleaks.[23,40,44,45] Contrast imaging overcomes some of the inherent challenges associated with color flow Doppler, such as color artifacts, dependency upon angle of insonation, and the poor ability of color flow Doppler to detect very slow flow velocities (Fig. 16.20). Henao and colleagues[41] evaluated the efficacy of CEUS to detect endoleaks in 20 patients. An average volume of 46.8 mL of perflutren (Optison) via continuous infusion was used. CEUS was able to identify nine endoleaks, the majority of which were type II. One of the most important findings in this study was that no endoleaks were discovered on CT imaging that were missed with CEUS. However, three type II endoleaks found on duplex imaging were missed on CT imaging.

In a comparative study of CT imaging with both color flow duplex ultrasound and CEUS, Clevert and associates[18] evaluated endoleaks in 43 patients who had undergone a recent EVAR. The patients underwent all three diagnostic imaging modalities for detection of endoleaks, using the CT scan as the gold standard for surveillance. The sensitivity and specificity of duplex ultrasound were 33.3% and 92.8%, respectively, whereas the sensitivity and specificity of CEUS were 100% and 93%, respectively. The positive and negative predictive values were also significantly higher with CEUS. Furthermore, two false positives noted with CEUS were found to be true positives during follow-up. Napoli and coworkers[44] also established that CEUS has the ability to identify endoleaks missed by other diagnostic modalities. Although these studies may have relatively small patient cohorts, the results demonstrate that the use of ultrasound contrast can significantly improve the sensitivity of duplex scanning for EVAR surveillance and detection of endoleaks. A recent meta-analysis of duplex ultrasound, CEUS, and CT for post-EVAR surveillance demonstrated that

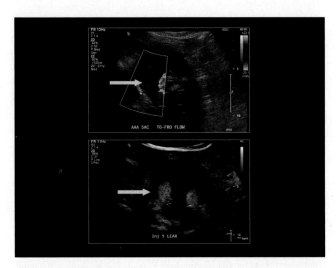

FIGURE 16.20. A type IIb endoleak identified with color flow Doppler (*top*) is well delineated with contrast-enhanced ultrasound (*bottom*). Contrast is clearly visualized within the aneurysm sac.

in comparison to CT, CEUS had a pooled sensitivity of 96% and pooled specificity of 85% for detection of all endoleaks, and for type I and type III endoleaks, the pooled sensitivity and specificity of CEUS were 99% and 100%, respectively.[23]

TECHNICAL PITFALLS AND LIMITATIONS

Duplex evaluations of abdominal aortic endografts are subject to multiple limitations. Patient body habitus and extreme depth can prevent adequate visualization owing to increased ultrasound attenuation. Techniques to overcome depth limitations include ensuring the patient is examined in a fasting state, applying adequate probe pressure, and utilizing multiple scanning approaches. Patient movement or intolerance to probe pressure is another technical difficulty to which the technologist must adapt. Technologist limitations include inexperience and poor body mechanics. The vascular technologist should have a sufficient understanding of the utilization and features of abdominal aortic endografts. The technologist should be cognizant of the limitations of duplex scanning and be able to implement methods to overcome them. Finally, increased technologist experience and training will increase the likelihood of a more complete and diagnostic scan.

It is important that the technologist have the best tools at hand when evaluating abdominal aortic endografts. Modern duplex scanners with advances in B-mode image resolution and penetration are advantageous for visualizing these vessels and devices. Increased color flow Doppler sensitivity is beneficial for identifying endoleaks. Duplex scanners with harmonic imaging features allow the use of ultrasound contrast agents, if desired. Detecting subtle flow disturbances and endoleaks is an integral component of the examination. Current instrumentation and vascular technologists with knowledge and experience are the best means to overcome the pitfalls associated with aortic endograft duplex evaluations.

CLINICAL STUDIES AND GUIDELINES

No large-scale studies have been performed to validate any specific criteria for the post-EVAR evaluation with duplex ultrasonography. However, as discussed in this chapter, the feasibility and efficacy of duplex ultrasonography for post-EVAR

surveillance in comparison with CT imaging has been demonstrated by a number of groups.[15–20,22–25,28] Although some of these studies are small, the correlation between CT imaging and duplex ultrasonography in the detection of endoleaks and other endograft complications supports the incorporation of duplex ultrasonography into the routine follow-up of patients post-EVAR. A meta-analysis that included 25 studies comparing duplex ultrasound to CT for detection of all endoleaks found a pooled sensitivity of 74% and pooled specificity of 94%.[23] There were 13 studies that compared duplex ultrasound and CT for detection of the clinically significant type I and type III endoleaks, and these demonstrated a pooled sensitivity of 83% and pooled specificity of 100%.

The Society for Vascular Surgery (SVS) published guidelines for the care of patients with an AAA in 2009, including recommendations for posttreatment surveillance.[10] While it is generally accepted that the rate of aneurysm-related death is extremely low with all the commercially available endografts, late aneurysm rupture remains a potential risk, and follow-up to detect aneurysm enlargement, endoleak, device migration, and other complications is essential. Protocols for surveillance after EVAR were established by the initial clinical trials and typically consisted of CT scanning at 1, 6, and 12 months following repair and yearly thereafter. Based on the favorable experience with duplex scanning in patients having EVAR, there has been an increasing trend to incorporate duplex ultrasound into post-EVAR surveillance protocols in an attempt to decrease the use of CT imaging. The SVS guidelines recommend CT scanning with contrast at 1 and 12 months during the first year following EVAR. If no endoleak or aneurysm enlargement is detected during that first year, duplex ultrasound (with color flow Doppler) can be considered as a reasonable alternative to CT imaging for continued surveillance. A subsequent increase in aneurysm diameter or detection of an endoleak would prompt a CT scan. The guidelines also point out that the combination of duplex ultrasound and noncontrast CT imaging can be used for post-EVAR surveillance in patients with renal insufficiency.

Implantation of a wireless pressure sensor in the aortic aneurysm sac during placement of an endograft has been used as a method to evaluate the adequacy of aneurysm exclusion with EVAR. The overall sensitivity and specificity of pressure sensors for detecting a type I or type III endoleak compared with angiography were found to be 94% and 80%, respectively,[46] but this technology is no longer commercially available for EVAR.

CONCLUSION

Duplex ultrasound can be used effectively for post-EVAR surveillance. It has the benefits of eliminating the need for nephrotoxic contrast agents, exposure to ionizing radiation, and the high cost associated with CT imaging. In the ongoing effort to improve the quality of care for patients with AAAs, providing efficient, less invasive, and more cost-effective diagnostic studies and procedures becomes increasingly important. Aneurysm sac diameter measurement with duplex ultrasound has been well correlated with CT imaging.[19,20] Furthermore, it has been demonstrated that duplex scanning, particularly with the addition of ultrasound contrast, can provide excellent specificity and sensitivity for detecting endoleaks after EVAR.[18,41,44] In some studies, the relatively low overall sensitivity of duplex ultrasound for the detection of endoleaks compared to CT scanning is offset by the high accuracy for identifying clinically significant type I and type III endoleaks.[10,24]

It is important for any accredited vascular laboratory to have properly trained technologists to improve the quality of the ultrasound studies and be able to identify endoleaks and other potential complications associated with an aortic endograft. For those endografts with no evidence of endoleak or aneurysm enlargement on CT scans during that first year after EVAR, the patient can be safely followed with serial duplex ultrasound examinations. As long as the aneurysm is shrinking or stable in size, continued duplex surveillance is justified; however, CT imaging would be indicated if a new endoleak or an increase in aneurysm sac size were detected. This approach has the potential to decrease the overall cost of an EVAR without jeopardizing quality of care.[10,17] Wider availability of three-dimensional ultrasound imaging systems could also improve the utility of duplex surveillance after EVAR by allowing more accurate assessment of aneurysm sac size and geometry with volumetric measurements.[47]

References

1. Laborde JC, Parodi JC, Clem MF, et al. Intraluminal bypass of abdominal aortic aneurysm: Feasibility study. *Radiology* 1992;184:185-190.
2. Parodi JC, Palmaz JC, Barone HD. Transfemoral intraluminal graft implantation for abdominal aortic aneurysms. *Ann Vasc Surg* 1991;5:491-499.
3. Shah H, Kumar SR, Major K, et al. Technology penetration of endovascular aortic aneurysm repair in southern California. *Ann Vasc Surg* 2006;20:796-802.
4. Berge C, Haug ES, Romundstad PR, et al. Infrarenal abdominal aortic aneurysm repair: Time-trends during a 20-year period. *World J Surg* 2007;31:1682-1686.
5. Hill JS, McPhee JT, Messina LM, et al. Regionalization of abdominal aortic aneurysm repair: Evidence of a shift to high-volume centers in the endovascular era. *J Vasc Surg* 2008;48:29-36.
6. Dua A, Kuy S, Lee CJ, et al. Epidemiology of aortic aneurysm repair in the United States from 2000 to 2010. *J Vasc Surg* 2014;59:1512-1517.
7. Bush RL, Johnson ML, Collins TC, et al. Open versus endovascular abdominal aortic aneurysm repair in VA hospitals. *J Am Coll Surg* 2006;202:577-587.
8. Matsumura JS, Brewster DC, Makaroun MS, et al. A multicenter controlled clinical trial of open versus endovascular treatment of abdominal aortic aneurysm. *J Vasc Surg* 2003;37:262-271.
9. Carpenter JP. Midterm results of the multicenter trial of the powerlink bifurcated system for endovascular aortic aneurysm repair. *J Vasc Surg* 2004;40:849-859.
10. Chaikof EL, Brewster DC, Dalman RL, et al. The care of patients with an abdominal aortic aneurysm: The Society for Vascular Surgery practice guidelines. *J Vasc Surg* 2009;50:2S-49S.
11. Heikkinen MA, Arko FR, Zarins CK. What is the significance of endoleaks and endotension? *Surg Clin North Am* 2004;84:1337-1352, vii.
12. Ouriel K, Clair DG, Greenberg RK, et al. Endovascular repair of abdominal aortic aneurysms: Device-specific outcome. *J Vasc Surg* 2003;37:991-998.
13. AbuRahma AF. Fate of endoleaks detected by CT angiography and missed by color duplex ultrasound in endovascular grafts for abdominal aortic aneurysms. *J Endovasc Ther* 2006;13:490-495.
14. Makaroun M, Zajko A, Sugimoto H, et al. Fate of endoleaks after endoluminal repair of abdominal aortic aneurysms with the EVT device. *Eur J Vasc Endovasc Surg* 1999;18:185-190.
15. Beeman BR, Murtha K, Doerr K, et al. Duplex ultrasound factors predicting persistent type II endoleak and increasing AAA sac diameter after EVAR. *J Vasc Surg* 2010;52:1147-1152.
16. Wolf YG, Johnson BL, Hill BB, et al. Duplex ultrasound scanning versus computed tomographic angiography for postoperative evaluation of endovascular abdominal aortic aneurysm repair. *J Vasc Surg* 2000;32:1142-1148.
17. Bendick PJ, Zelinock GB, Rove PG, et al. Duplex ultrasound imaging with an ultrasound contrast agent: The economic alternative to CT angiography for aortic stent graft surveillance. *Vasc Endovascular Surg* 2003;37:165-170.
18. Clevert DA, Minaifar N, Weckbach S, et al. Color duplex ultrasound and contrast-enhanced ultrasound in comparison to MS-CT in the detection of endoleak following endovascular aneurysm repair. *Clin Hemorheol Microcirc* 2008;39:121-132.
19. Arko FR, Fills KA, Heikkinen MA, et al. Duplex scanning after endovascular aneurysm repair: An alternative to computed tomography. *Semin Vasc Surg* 2004;17:161-165.
20. Badri H, El Haddad M, Ashour H, et al. Duplex ultrasound scanning (DUS) versus computed tomography angiography (CTA) in the follow-up after EVAR. *Angiology* 2010;61:131-136.
21. Blom AS, Troutman D, Beeman B, et al. Duplex imaging to detect limb stenosis or kinking of endovascular device. *J Vasc Surg* 2012;55:1577-1580.
22. Chaer RA, Gushchin A, Rhee R, et al. Duplex ultrasound as the sole long-term surveillance method post-endovascular aneurysm repair: A safe alternative for stable aneurysms. *J Vasc Surg* 2009;49:845-850.
23. Karthikesalingam A, Al-Jundi W, Jackson D, et al. Systematic review and meta-analysis of duplex ultrasonography, contrast-enhanced ultrasonography or computed tomography for surveillance after endovascular aneurysm repair. *Br J Surg* 2012;99:1514-1523.
24. Manning BJ, O'Neill SM, Haider SN, et al. Duplex ultrasound in aneurysm surveillance following endovascular aneurysm repair: A comparison with computed tomography aortography. *J Vasc Surg* 2009;49:60-65.
25. Schmieder GC, Stout CL, Stokes GK, et al. Endoleak after endovascular aneurysm repair: Duplex ultrasound imaging is better than computed tomography at determining the need for intervention. *J Vasc Surg* 2009;50:1012-1018.
26. Beeman BR, Doctor LM, Doerr K, et al. Duplex ultrasound imaging alone is sufficient for midterm endovascular aneurysm repair surveillance: A cost analysis study and prospective comparison with computed tomography scan. *J Vasc Surg* 2009;50:1019-1024.
27. Gray C, Goodman P, Herron CC, et al. Use of colour duplex ultrasound as a first line surveillance tool following EVAR is associated with a reduction in cost without compromising accuracy. *Eur J Vasc Endovasc Surg* 2012;44:145-150.
28. Nagre SB, Taylor SM, Passman MA, et al. Evaluating outcomes of endoleak discrepancies between computed tomography scan and ultrasound imaging after endovascular abdominal aneurysm repair. *Ann Vasc Surg* 2011;25:94-100.
29. Parent FN, Meier GH, Godziachvili V, et al. The incidence and natural history of type I and II endoleak: A 5-year follow-up assessment with color duplex ultrasound. *J Vasc Surg* 2002;35:474-481.
30. Noll RE Jr, Tonnessen B, Munnava K, et al. Long-term postplacement cost after endovascular aneurysm repair. *J Vasc Surg* 2007;46:9-15; discussion 15.
31. Liaw JV, Clark M, Gibbs R, et al. Update: Complications and management of infrarenal EVAR. *Eur J Radiol* 2009;71(3):541-551.
32. Prinssen M, Wixon CL, Buskens E, et al. Surveillance after endovascular aneurysm repair: Diagnostics, complications, and associated costs. *Ann Vasc Surg* 2004;18:421-427.
33. Mills JL Sr, Duong ST, Leon LP Jr, et al. Comparison of the effects of open and endovascular aortic aneurysm repair on long-term renal function using chronic kidney disease staging based on glomerular filtration rate. *J Vasc Surg* 2008;47:1141-1149.
34. Parmer SS, Fairman RM, Karmacharya J, et al. A comparison of renal function between open and endovascular aneurysm repair in patients with baseline chronic renal insufficiency. *J Vasc Surg* 2006;44:706-711.
35. Collins JT, Boros MJ, Combs K. Ultrasound surveillance of endovascular aneurysm repair: A safe modality versus computed tomography. *Ann Vasc Surg* 2007;21:671-675.
36. Raman KG, Missig-Carroll N, Richardson T, et al. Color-flow duplex ultrasound scan versus computed tomographic scan in the surveillance of endovascular aneurysm repair. *J Vasc Surg* 2003;38:645-651.
37. Cuypers P, Buth J, Harris PL, et al. Realistic expectations for patients with stent-graft treatment of abdominal aortic aneurysms. Results of a European multicentre registry. *Eur J Vasc Endovasc Surg* 1999;17:507-516.
38. Criado FJ, Fairman RM, Becker GJ. Talent LPS AAA stent graft: Results of a pivotal clinical trial. *J Vasc Surg* 2003;37:709-715.
39. Soares GM, Murphy TP, Singha MS, et al. Renal artery duplex ultrasonography as a screening and surveillance tool to detect renal artery stenosis: A comparison with current reference standard imaging. *J Ultrasound Med* 2006;25:293-298.
40. Johnson B, Arko FR, Harris EJ, et al. Update: Quantitative duplex ultrasound assessment of aortic aneurysms after endovascular repair. *J Vasc Ultrasound* 2003;27:6.
41. Henao EA, Hodge MD, Felkai DD, et al. Contrast-enhanced duplex surveillance after endovascular abdominal aortic aneurysm repair: Improved efficacy using a continuous infusion technique. *J Vasc Surg* 2006;43:259-264.
42. Kohler TR, Nance DR, Cramer MM, et al. Duplex scanning for diagnosis of aortoiliac and femoropopliteal disease: A prospective study. *Circulation* 1987;76:1074-1080.
43. Correas JM, Bridal JL, Lesavre A, et al. Ultrasound contrast agents: Properties, principles of action, tolerance, and artifacts. *Eur Radiol* 2001; 11:1316-1328.
44. Napoli V, Bargellini I, Sardella SG, et al. Abdominal aortic aneurysm: Contrast-enhanced US for missed endoleaks after endoluminal repair. *Radiology* 2004;233:217-225.
45. Iezzi R, Cotroneo AR, Basilico R, et al. Endoleaks after endovascular repair of abdominal aortic aneurysm: Value of CEUS. *Abdom Imaging* 2010;35:106-114.
46. Ohki T, Ouriel K, Silveira PG, et al. Initial results of wireless pressure sensing for endovascular aneurysm repair: The APEX Trial—Acute Pressure Measurement to Confirm Aneurysm Sac EXclusion. *J Vasc Surg* 2007;45:236-242.
47. Causey MW, Jayaraj A, Leotta DF, et al. Three-dimensional ultrasonography measurements after endovascular aneurysm repair. *Ann Vasc Surg* 2013;27:146-153.

DENNIS F. BANDYK AND KELLEY D. HODGKISS-HARLOW

A vascular laboratory surveillance program based on duplex ultrasound has been recommended as an effective method for improving infrainguinal arterial bypass graft patency.[1–6] Failure of lower extremity autogenous vein and prosthetic arterial bypass grafts is primarily associated with the development of myointimal stenotic lesions that increase the risk of thrombosis by reducing flow. Prospective clinical studies that utilized early duplex testing have established that the majority of stenoses develop within the first year.[5,7,8] Lesions demonstrating velocity spectral features of a high-grade stenosis (peak systolic velocity [PSV] >300 cm/s, end-diastolic velocity >20 cm/s, PSV ratio [Vr] across the stenosis >3.5) or greater than 70% diameter reduction (DR) by confirmatory arteriography are associated with graft failure if not corrected (Fig. 17.1).[2,4,9] The goal of duplex ultrasound surveillance is to identify developing lesions or other abnormalities associated with low graft flow before thrombosis occurs, thereby enabling elective repair and continued graft patency. Revision of the duplex-identified "at-risk" graft significantly improves patency rates compared to surveillance based on clinical symptoms or bypass revision after thrombosis occurs. The 1-year patency following graft revision for duplex-identified stenosis is over 80%, while less than one-third of occluded grafts revised by endovascular or open intervention remain patent.[1,3,5,7]

The concept of duplex ultrasound surveillance with preemptive revision of asymptomatic graft stenosis remains controversial, in part because of the varied threshold criteria for intervention and the success of secondary interventions. Graft occlusion despite duplex surveillance, termed *primary occlusion*, has a reported incidence of 5% and is associated with technical defects related to the bypass graft procedure, such as residual stenosis or low graft flow velocity (GFV), or the lack of adherence to a surveillance protocol, especially failure to undergo early (<1 month) testing.[10] Clinical trials have identified high-risk groups for unheralded graft failure that may benefit from increased surveillance, including women, small-diameter saphenous vein conduits, redo bypasses, and grafts with stenosis on the first or 30-day duplex scan.[5,7]

The progression of myointimal graft stenosis typically occurs without ischemic limb symptoms, especially in the physically inactive patient. Thrombosis of bypasses performed for claudication typically results in the pain-free walking distance returning to prerevascularization levels, but when critical

limb ischemia (CLI) was the indication for bypass grafting, graft thrombosis produces "limb-threatening" ischemia in the majority of patients, with a high likelihood of amputation unless patency can be restored. Compared to elective repair of a duplex-identified graft stenosis, the success of catheter-directed thrombolysis or surgical thrombectomy to restore patency in an occluded graft is associated with reduced long-term patency.[1] A successful infrainguinal graft surveillance program has the outcome features of a low (<5%) incidence of primary graft occlusion, a high (>80%) assisted primary patency rate, reduced need for redo bypass grafting, and, in CLI patients, improved limb salvage.[2,7]

The components of graft surveillance testing include a clinical assessment of the patient for symptoms of limb ischemia, measurement of the ankle-brachial systolic pressure index (ABI), and lower limb duplex ultrasound imaging. The Society for Vascular Surgery (SVS) and American Heart Association (AHA) guidelines for infrainguinal bypass surveillance recommend that testing begin in the immediate postoperative period and be conducted every 6 months thereafter for at least 2 years (level of evidence: A).[10,11] Testing should include duplex imaging along the entire length of the graft with measurement of PSV and calculation of Vr across all lesions. More frequent testing is appropriate if a graft abnormality is identified, using serial duplex imaging to identify progression to greater than 70% DR stenosis. This guideline is contrary to a European multicenter, randomized controlled clinic trial (Vein Graft Surveillance Trial [VGST]), which found no clinical benefit for routine duplex testing after infrainguinal vein bypass based on similar graft patency, amputation rates, and quality-of-life assessments.[12] Limitations of the VGST included recruitment of patients with patent bypasses at 6 weeks or later after operation, resulting in exclusion of early graft failures that account for 10% or more of primary occlusions, and the use of low-threshold duplex interpretation criteria (doubling of PSV, graft PSV <45 cm/s) to identify the "at-risk" bypass graft.

The efficacy of duplex graft surveillance requires appropriate testing methods and interpretation criteria, along with successful and durable repairs of identified stenotic lesions. Duplex testing in the early postoperative period (1 to 4 weeks) will identify a stenosis in approximately one-third of patients, and this finding is predictive of a graft revision for progressive stenosis or thrombosis within 6 months.[1,5,6,12,13] Failure to intervene on grafts with lesions having velocity spectral

FIGURE 17.1. Color-flow duplex image and velocity spectra of a greater than 70% diameter-reducing stenosis in a femoroperoneal saphenous vein bypass based on peak systolic velocity (PSV) at the stenosis of 499 cm/s and end-diastolic velocity of 79 cm/s. Note the tissue bruit in the surrounding perigraft tissue caused by wall vibrations.

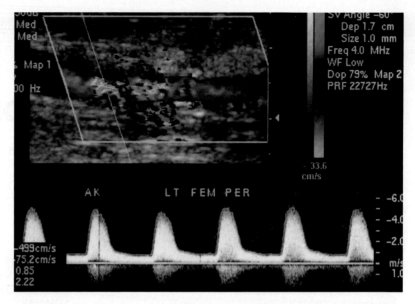

features consistent with greater than 70% stenosis is associated with a high (>80%) thrombosis rate.[1,8] Assessment of graft patency based on the presence of pedal pulses and measurement of ABI is an insensitive technique to detect the "failing" stenotic bypass. Adherence to a duplex surveillance protocol that begins immediately after the procedure, when coupled with timely repair of greater than 70% stenosis and assessment of low PSV (<45 cm/s) grafts, should result in an annual failure rate of less than 3% per year after infrainguinal vein bypass and less than 5% per year after prosthetic bypass grafting.[1,5,12-14] Duplex testing is noninvasive, less expensive, and more accurate than graft imaging using magnetic resonance (MR) or computed tomography (CT) angiographic techniques. Whether graft surveillance imparts a favorable outcome to the patient depends on several factors, including the accuracy of testing in detecting graft-threatening lesions, the success of graft repair, and patient compliance with an ongoing surveillance program to identify new lesions. For patients who require bypass grafting for CLI, postoperative diligence in monitoring functional graft patency is felt to be the cornerstone for long-term limb salvage.

GRAFT SURVEILLANCE METHODOLOGY

Vascular laboratory testing after lower limb bypass grafting is used to verify improvement in limb perfusion and the patient's functional activity. During the patient interview, the vascular technologist should ask about maximum walking distance and any functional limb limitation, the location and character of exercise-induced pain, and recent medical events or hospitalizations. A focused physical examination of the limbs should be performed, including inspection of the foot for signs of ischemia (dependent rubor, ulcer, gangrene), edema, or cyanosis. In patients with recent procedures, nonhealed surgical sites that can interfere with duplex scanning should also be documented. Any unresolved or new symptoms or signs of limb ischemia can be evaluated based on hemodynamic data obtained from physiologic testing and duplex imaging. A review of operative reports for graft type, anastomotic sites, and other concomitant procedures (endarterectomy, angioplasty) on inflow or outflow arteries is extremely useful and helps to minimize examination time. Prior vascular testing results should be available for comparison, so any graft abnormality can be quickly located and assessed for progression or

resolution. It is helpful to include a schematic diagram of the arterial bypass graft in the final report that documents any prior or new graft abnormalities identified by duplex scanning (Fig. 17.2). Finally, a useful quality measure is review of the patient's medications to verify that antiplatelet and statin therapy is prescribed, whenever appropriate.

Arterial Bypass Graft Testing

Lower extremity bypass graft evaluation should include measurement of the resting ABI, toe pressure, and duplex ultrasound imaging of the entire graft including inflow and outflow arteries to the ankle level. Measurement of segmental pressures or pulse volume recordings is not recommended. Linear (5- to 7-MHz) and curved (3- to 5-MHz) array transducers should be available to image both superficial and anatomically tunneled bypass grafts and the aortoiliac segment if necessary. If open wounds are present, transducer or wound covers can be used to scan over these areas. To obtain complete graft imaging, a variety of scanning windows (anterior, medial, lateral, posterior) are necessary, including requiring the patient to rotate the leg from side to side or assume a prone position for imaging grafts to the below-knee popliteal or peroneal artery.

Color Doppler imaging is used to verify graft patency and survey the entire bypass, including anastomotic sites, for aneurysms, stenosis, or lumen defects. Serial duplex velocity spectra are recorded in normal appearing proximal, mid, and distal graft segments to calculate the average peak systolic GFV, as well as at sites of stenosis to classify the DR based on measurement of PSV and the Vr across the stenosis. The technologist imaging and interpretation skills necessary to perform bypass graft surveillance include an ability to differentiate normal versus abnormal color Doppler flow patterns at anastomoses and vein valve sites, an understanding of how graft diameter alters PSV values, recognition of common abnormalities (wound fluid collections, graft mural thrombus), and the ability to identify patent side branches with arteriovenous fistula flow after in situ saphenous vein bypass grafting. Testing should include sufficient image archiving to allow the physician's final interpretation to confirm normal versus abnormal duplex findings, and when a stenosis is identified, determine its severity and impact on graft flow and distal limb or foot perfusion.

Knowledge of the arterial bypass graft type is important to accurate testing because duplex imaging requirements and interpretation criteria may vary. Autogenous vein bypasses

GRAFT TYPE: Date of Surgery:

Indication for Testing:
Current symptoms/walking activity:
Limb ischemia (rest pain, skin lesions, ulcers, gangrene):
Prior testing: Normal:
Graft stenosis:

Atherosclerotic Risk Factors: **Medications:**
Current tobacco use   Antiplatelet
Hypertension   Statin therapy
Diabetes

PHYSIOLOGIC TESTING:

                          ABI:
                          Ankle Pressure:
DUPLEX FINDINGS: **Toe Pressure:**

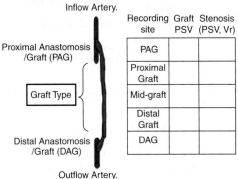

FIGURE 17.2. Essential clinical and test data to be included in the duplex graft surveillance report.

Recording site	Graft PSV	Stenosis (PSV, Vr)
PAG		
Proximal Graft		
Mid-graft		
Distal Graft		
DAG		

Interpretation

Normal:

Abnormal:
   - **stenosis category**
   - **other lesions**
   - **effect on graft flow**

may be constructed using the saphenous (great, small), arm (cephalic, basilic), or femoral veins. The in situ great saphenous vein arterial bypass is located superficially in its normal subcutaneous plane, except near the anastomotic sites. Surgeons attempt to ligate all saphenous vein side branches with an in situ graft, but finding a residual patent branch with arteriovenous flow after operation is not uncommon. When identified, the location of patent side branches and their influence on distal graft flow and limb perfusion pressure (the extent of blood flow "steal" from the bypass graft) should be determined by recording graft velocity proximal and distal to the branch. Endovascular saphenous vein harvest is now commonplace, and these conduits may be used in a reversed or in a nonreversed configuration. The in situ and nonreversed saphenous vein conduits require valve lysis, and this graft technique exposes the vein to possible valvulotome injury or incomplete

valve leaflet incision. It is important to document any residual valve site stenosis along the entire vein bypass length, especially on the first postoperative examination, because these regions of "mild-to-moderate" stenosis defined by a PSV in the 180 to 250 cm/s range are often the precursor of a future critical (>70%) stenosis. At the valve sites in small-caliber (<3 mm diameter) reversed saphenous vein grafts, a functional stenosis (PSV > 180 cm/s, Vr < 2) may be present if the valve leaflets do not lie completely against the vein wall or are sclerotic ("frozen valve").

Prosthetic conduits (Dacron-polyester; polytetrafluoroethylene [PTFE]) are generally easily imaged, with a polyester graft appearing as a corrugated or rippled vessel interface and a PTFE graft appearing as a smooth, double-lined wall conduit (Fig. 17.3). These graft conduits may have external rings to support the graft lumen and prevent compression. The

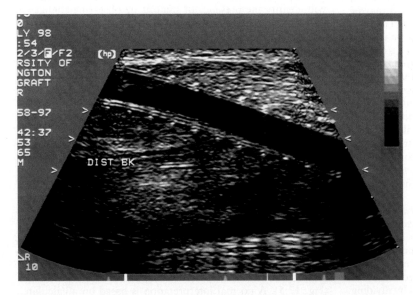

FIGURE 17.3. Longitudinal B-mode image of a ringed polytetrafluoroethylene (PTFE) bypass graft. The graft wall shows the characteristic double line, and the rings are apparent as equally spaced dots along the length of the graft.

FIGURE 17.4. Schematic diagram depicts sites of duplex imaging and calculation of mean or average graft flow velocity (GFV).

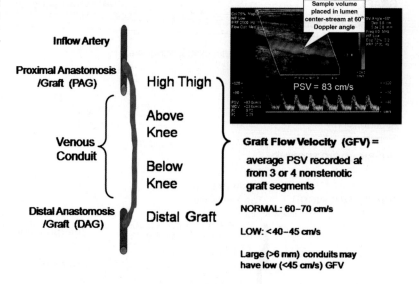

Inflow Artery

Proximal Anastomosis /Graft (PAG)

High Thigh

Above Knee

Venous Conduit

Below Knee

Distal Anastomosis /Graft (DAG)

Distal Graft

Sample volume placed in lumen center-stream at 60° Doppler angle

PSV = 83 cm/s

Graft Flow Velocity (GFV) =

average PSV recorded at from 3 or 4 nonstenotic graft segments

NORMAL: 60–70 cm/s

LOW: <40–45 cm/s

Large (>6 mm) conduits may have low (<45 cm/s) GFV

caliber of prosthetic grafts is typically uniform (6, 7, or 8 mm in diameter), and thus, the PSV should not change significantly (<20 cm/s) along the length of the graft. On transverse imaging, the graft lumen should be circular and mural thrombus should not be visualized.

Duplex Ultrasound Imaging Protocol

Begin the duplex ultrasound evaluation at the inflow artery, which for lower limb bypass grafts is usually the common femoral artery. A more distal graft origin (deep femoral, superficial femoral, popliteal) may have been selected to shorten the vein conduit length. Image the proximal anastomosis graft (PAG) segment for abnormalities (stenosis, aneurysm, mural thrombus) and record inflow velocity spectra to verify the acceleration time (normal <180 ms). Damping of the inflow artery velocity waveform suggests a proximal occlusive lesion and should prompt interrogation of the aortoiliac segment. Color-flow Doppler imaging of anastomotic regions commonly identifies disturbed flow conditions evident by color aliasing and spectral broadening in the pulsed Doppler spectral waveforms. Use real-time B-mode and power Doppler imaging to assess the lumen caliber and presence of mural thrombus. The PSV in the proximal graft segment depends on lumen diameter and propagated flow turbulence produced by the anastomotic configuration and any stenosis, if present; thus, PSV in the proximal graft may be higher or lower than that recorded from the inflow artery.[15]

Perform color-flow mapping of the bypass graft using a longitudinal scan plane, reserving transverse imaging for any sites of graft abnormality. Careful imaging and pulsed Doppler spectral analysis is advised for graft segments showing color-flow turbulence and lumen caliber reduction. Image the entire length of the bypass graft to the extent possible to identify sites of intrinsic or extrinsic stenosis. It is useful to divide the graft into three segments (proximal, middle, and distal) to facilitate study interpretation regarding sites of graft stenosis and communication with the referring physician. Record velocity spectra for measurement of PSV from normal-appearing graft segments (proximal, mid, distal) to determine the mean or average GFV (Fig. 17.4).

When real-time color-flow Doppler imaging locates a stenosis, the pulsed Doppler sample volume is "walked through" the stenotic region to measure PSV proximal to and at the site of maximum flow disturbance. These PSV values recorded proximal to and within the "color-flow jet" are used to calculate a Vr at the stenosis and estimate the DR in three categories (<50%, 50% to 70%, and >70%). Vr is calculated by dividing

the maximum PSV at the site of stenosis (PSV_{max}) by the PSV proximal to the stenosis (PSV_{prox}):

$$Vr = PSV_{max}/PSV_{prox}$$

A PSV_{max} >180 cm/s and Vr >2.0 indicate a greater than 50% DR stenosis. A Vr >3.5 associated with a PSV_{max} >300 cm/s is diagnostic of a greater than 70% DR stenosis (Table 17.1). A stenosis with these severe hemodynamic abnormalities is both pressure and flow reducing, and this has been used as the diagnostic threshold at which to consider graft revision or additional arterial imaging such as angiography. Of note, this degree of graft stenosis has rarely been documented to regress, and it is frequently associated with a concomitant decrease in GFV (>30 cm/s) and ABI (>0.15).[16,17]

The distal anastomosis graft (DAG) segment may terminate in the popliteal artery (above knee, below knee), one of the tibial arteries (posterior, anterior, peroneal), or a pedal artery. Imaging along the course of the bypass conduit is the best way to locate the DAG. Careful duplex interrogation of this graft segment is important because it is the most common site for development of stenosis. Imaging the DAG region may be hampered by its deep location (tibioperoneal trunk, peroneal artery) or the presence of extensive native artery calcification. If duplex imaging is not technically adequate, recording velocity spectra proximal to, within, and distal to the DAG segment will identify the presence of stenosis by observing changes in PSV and spectral waveform pulsatility in the outflow artery. For an end-to-side anastomosis, identify both retrograde and antegrade flow in the native outflow artery distal to the DAG. Scanning technique requires that the technologist sequentially "walk" the pulsed Doppler sample volume through the DAG region, proceeding from the distal graft segment through the outflow artery to identify any focal increases in PSV. The last step in the examination is to record velocity spectra from both the graft outflow artery and other tibial arteries at ankle level to correlate with ABI measurement and detect interval progression of occlusive disease distal to the DAG region.

INTERPRETATION OF GRAFT SURVEILLANCE TESTING

Vascular laboratory testing should allow classification of the graft surveillance study as "normal" (e.g., a patent graft without stenosis or anatomic abnormality) or "abnormal" (e.g., a graft lesion was identified or a low graft flow state was found) (Fig. 17.5). A normal interpretation is based on a calculated

TABLE 17.1

RISK STRATIFICATION FOR GRAFT THROMBOSIS[a]

■ CATEGORY	■ HIGH-VELOCITY CRITERIA PSV (cm/s)	■ VR	■ LOW-VELOCITY CRITERIA GFV (cm/s)	■ ABI CHANGE
I—Highest risk[b] (>70% stenosis with low graft flow)	>300	>3.5	<45, or staccato graft flow	>0.15
II—High risk[b] (>70% stenosis without change or normal graft flow)	>300	>3.5	>45	<0.15
III—Moderate risk[c] (50%-70% stenosis with normal graft flow)	180-300	>2.0	>45	<0.15
IV—Low risk (normal bypass or <50% stenosis with normal graft flow)	<180	<2.0	>45	<0.15

[a]Based on vascular laboratory testing data, including PSV at stenosis, Vr, GFV, and change in ABI.
[b]Forty percent to fifty percent likelihood of stenosis progression or graft thrombosis within 3-6 months.
[c]Twenty percent to thirty percent of early (<3 months) lesions regress, 10% to 20% of lesions remain stable, 40% to 50% progress to >70% stenosis.
ABI, ankle-brachial index; GFV, graft flow velocity; PSV, peak systolic velocity; Vr, PSV ratio.

GFV >45 cm/s, no duplex-detected stenosis, and a normal or unchanged ABI compared with prior testing. Typical values for GFV range from 45 to 100 cm/s (mean, 75 ± 20 cm/s) after successful infrainguinal arterial bypass grafts, with lower or higher values depending on graft diameter and runoff artery status.[1,5,13] Belkin et al.[15] reported that GFV was lower in inframalleolar (pedal) grafts (59 ± 4 cm/s) than in tibial (77 ± 6 cm/s) and popliteal (71 ± 8 cm/s) vein bypasses. Larger-diameter (>6 mm) graft conduits (basilic vein, prosthetic) or bypasses with disadvantaged runoff (pedal bypass, isolated

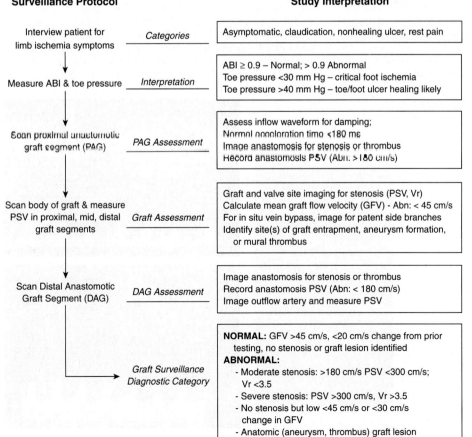

Surveillance Protocol — **Study Interpretation**

Interview patient for limb ischemia symptoms — *Categories* — Asymptomatic, claudication, nonhealing ulcer, rest pain

Measure ABI & toe pressure — *Interpretation* — ABI ≥ 0.9 – Normal; > 0.9 Abnormal / Toe pressure <30 mm Hg – critical foot ischemia / Toe pressure >40 mm Hg – toe/foot ulcer healing likely

Scan proximal anastomotic graft segment (PAG) — *PAG Assessment* — Assess inflow waveform for damping; / Normal acceleration time <180 ms / Image anastomosis for stenosis or thrombus / Record anastomosis PSV (Abn. >180 cm/s)

Scan body of graft & measure PSV in proximal, mid, distal graft segments — *Graft Assessment* — Graft and valve site imaging for stenosis (PSV, Vr) / Calculate mean graft flow velocity (GFV) - Abn: < 45 cm/s / For in situ vein bypass, image for patent side branches / Identify site(s) of graft entrapment, aneurysm formation, or mural thrombus

Scan Distal Anastomotic Graft Segment (DAG) — *DAG Assessment* — Image anastomosis for stenosis or thrombus / Record anastomosis PSV (Abn: < 180 cm/s) / Image outflow artery and measure PSV

Graft Surveillance Diagnostic Category — **NORMAL:** GFV >45 cm/s, <20 cm/s change from prior testing, no stenosis or graft lesion identified / **ABNORMAL:** / - Moderate stenosis: >180 cm/s PSV <300 cm/s; Vr <3.5 / - Severe stenosis: PSV >300 cm/s, Vr >3.5 / - No stenosis but low <45 cm/s or <30 cm/s change in GFV / - Anatomic (aneurysm, thrombus) graft lesion identified

FIGURE 17.5. Graft surveillance testing protocol and study interpretation criteria.

AORTOILIAC AND PERIPHERAL ARTERIAL

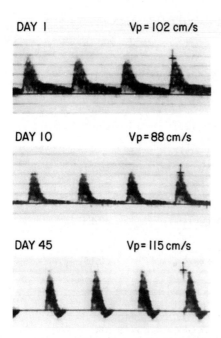

DAY I   Vp = 102 cm/s

DAY 10   Vp = 88 cm/s

DAY 45   Vp = 115 cm/s

FIGURE 17.6. Changes in graft velocity spectra during the early postoperative period with a decrease in flow during diastole indicating an increase in peripheral vascular resistance.

popliteal/tibial artery bypass) may demonstrate a lower GFV in the range of 30 to 50 cm/s. When a low-flow (GFV <40 to 45 cm/s) graft is identified, perform a careful search for a "correctable" lesion. The occlusive lesion may be proximal to (inflow artery), within (graft stenosis), or distal to (outflow artery) the bypass graft. A decrease in GFV of greater than 30 cm/s on serial testing is also an abnormal finding and predicts the development of an occlusive lesion.[5,16,17] Locating the site of abnormality requires complete lower limb arterial mapping, which may be difficult in limbs with anatomically tunneled bypass conduits.

Interpretation of graft surveillance studies during the early postoperative period (1 week to 2 months) requires awareness of changes in graft outflow resistance that occur during this time interval. After successful bypass grafting, the graft velocity spectra evolve from a low-resistance (monophasic waveform) to a higher-resistance (multiphasic waveform) flow pattern, corresponding to the gradual increase in peripheral arterial resistance in skeletal muscle as the revascularization hyperemia abates (Fig. 17.6). These changes in graft outflow resistance are evident as decreases in end-diastolic flow velocity that occur within days in limbs requiring bypass for claudication but may take several weeks in limbs revascularized for CLI. Typically, the GFV does not decrease as this revascularization hyperemia resolves.

When duplex scanning identifies a graft stenosis, the "thrombosis" risk can be classified into one of four categories based on stenosis severity, GFV, and ABI changes (see Table 17.1). A graft at highest risk for thrombosis (category I) has a severe, greater than 70% duplex-detected stenosis, low (<40 to 45 cm/s) GFV, and decreased ABI (Fig. 17.7). Intervention within days to repair the graft stenosis and restore normal graft hemodynamics is recommended, as outlined in Table 17.2.[1,5,13] If "staccato" flow is found on duplex testing (Fig. 17.8), graft flow is minimal and urgent graft revision should be performed; typically, a high-grade, preocclusive stenosis is present downstream from the recording site.

The primary difference between category I and category II "abnormal" bypasses defined in Table 17.1 is the effect of the duplex-detected stenosis on GFV and ABI. When a stenosis with PSV >300 cm/s and Vr >3.5 develops but the GFV remains in the normal range (>45 cm/s) or is decreased less than 30 cm/s from prior studies, the risk for thrombosis is less than that in a "low-flow" bypass. In these cases, an elective revision within 2 to 3 weeks can be recommended to the patient. Often these lesions consist of a focal (<2 cm length) stenosis and are amenable to endovascular repair by balloon angioplasty (cutting, cryoplasty). When duplex testing identifies a category III intermediate graft stenosis (PSV >180 cm/s but <300 cm/s; Vr between 2.0 and 3.4), the risk of thrombosis is low to moderate and depends on the likelihood of disease progression. These lesions are asymptomatic and not associated with a reduction in GFV or ABI.[5] Repeat surveillance at 4 to 6 weeks is sufficient to detect stenosis

FIGURE 17.7. Category I graft stenosis with velocity spectra indicating a greater than 70% stenosis (PSV of 548 cm/s) and a low GFV (18 cm/s). The corresponding arteriographic stenosis is also shown.

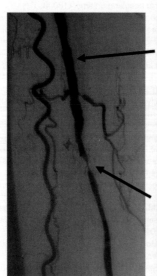

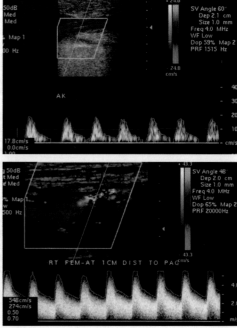

TABLE 17.2

RECOMMENDED MANAGEMENT FOR THE FOUR DUPLEX ULTRASOUND SURVEILLANCE CATEGORIES BASED ON AN ESTIMATED RISK FOR GRAFT OCCLUSION

■ CATEGORY	■ TREATMENT AND SURVEILLANCE RECOMMENDATION
(I) Highest risk	Prompt repair of lesion. Duplex ultrasound assessment of the repair site and bypass 1-2 wk after intervention to exclude residual stenosis and confirm normal graft hemodynamics (GFV >45 cm/s).
(II) High risk	Elective repair of lesion within 2-3 wk. Duplex ultrasound assessment of the repair site and bypass 1-2 wk after intervention to exclude residual stenosis.
(III) Moderate risk	Repeat graft surveillance at 4- to 6-wk intervals with elective repair if stenosis progression to a >70% DR (PSV >300 cm/s; Vr >3.5) is identified.
(IV) Low risk[a]	Surveillance at 6- to 12-mo intervals unless a higher category graft lesion or flow condition develops; exclude complete graft imaging if GFV unchanged and ABI normal (>0.9)

[a]Less than 3% annual incidence of graft failure for arterial bypasses in this duplex surveillance category.
ABI, ankle-brachial index; GFV, graft flow velocity; DR, diameter reduction; PSV, peak systolic velocity; Vr, PSV ratio.

progression or regression, which usually becomes evident within a 3-month interval. Bypasses with the lowest risk for thrombosis (category IV) demonstrate no stenosis or less than 50% stenosis (PSV <180 cm/s; Vr <2.0 within the graft or anastomotic sites; GFV >45 cm/s), and duplex surveillance at 6-month intervals is recommended.[5,16–18]

The likelihood of stenosis development and progression is highest during the first postoperative year and provides the rationale for early serial graft surveillance during this time interval. The rigor or frequency of surveillance can be based on the initial duplex scan results and other characteristics that identify "high-risk" bypasses, such as non–single-segment saphenous vein, vein diameter less than 3 mm, or a redo bypass graft procedure. If the initial postoperative duplex scan identifies an intermediate category III stenosis, the likelihood of graft revision is increased threefold, with a primary patency at 3 years of 28% versus 64% if the duplex scan is normal.[5] Graft surveillance at 3-month intervals for the first postoperative year is recommended for infrainguinal vein bypass grafts with "high-risk" characteristics or sites of mild stenosis (PSV >180 cm/s)

Whether clinical symptoms are present when a greater than 70% graft stenosis is detected depends in large measure on the patient's level of walking activity, as well as their sensitivity to changes in limb perfusion during their daily routine. Many patients treated for CLI or who have a contralateral limb amputation do not walk sufficient distances to develop calf claudication, despite the presence of a category I or II graft stenosis. Most clinicians do not require the presence of symptoms to recommend repair of a progressive high-grade graft stenosis.

The interpretation of graft surveillance studies should address the indication for testing—new symptoms of limb ischemia or asymptomatic protocol surveillance. Graft imaging results, indicating the presence or absence of graft stenosis, an assessment of graft hemodynamics based on GFV, and classification of limb perfusion based on ABI and toe pressure measurements, are integral components of the final interpretation. Some clinicians may elect to confirm the location and severity of a greater than 70% duplex-detected graft stenosis by angiographic imaging and exclude any other graft or native artery abnormalities before proceeding to lesion repair.

LIMITATIONS OF GRAFT SURVEILLANCE

Inability to adequately image the entire bypass graft, incompressible tibial arteries, and poor patient compliance are the major limitations of a graft surveillance program. The vascular technologist must resist the temptation to image only specific sites rather than interrogate the entire graft. Graft abnormalities are often focal when they initially appear and may not produce a significant change in GFV or ABI. If the entire bypass cannot be imaged, notation of this technical limitation should be in the final report. An obese patient with a deeply tunneled graft is a diagnostic challenge; ultrasound imaging will be difficult, and if he or she is not physically active or the ABI measurement is falsely elevated, the clinical signs of a failing graft may escape detection. The diagnostic accuracy of detecting a graft stenosis, and thus the overall efficacy of surveillance, is reduced under these conditions.

Color-flow duplex imaging is a sensitive method for identifying sites of stenosis. Exercise care in recording velocity spectra across the stenotic region using a Doppler angle of 60 degrees or less and positioning the pulsed Doppler sample volume to identify the site of maximum flow disturbance. Superficially located grafts can be compressed by excessive probe pressure, resulting in a false-positive diagnosis of stenosis or overestimation of DR. The findings on duplex scanning should be reproducible and also correlated with limb pressure measurements. A change in ABI and GFV observed on serial testing serves to confirm the duplex scan accuracy when a greater than 70% DR stenosis is found. The absence of an ABI or GFV change should prompt careful imaging of any detected stenosis, because overestimation of lesion severity is possible in that setting. These errors can be minimized by using combined interpretation criteria (PSV and Vr) for grading stenosis severity.

Failure to adequately assess the bypass graft inflow and outflow arteries is another important cause for false-negative surveillance testing. Atherosclerosis disease progression or myointimal stenosis developing at an adjacent angioplasty site can influence the diagnostic accuracy and efficacy of graft surveillance. For example, tibial artery disease progression

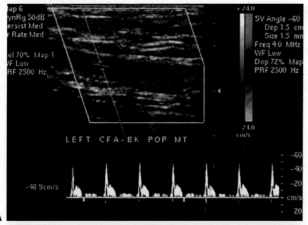

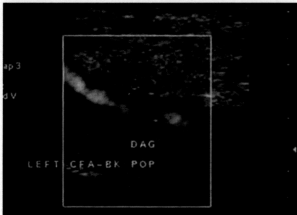

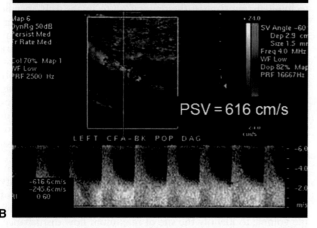

FIGURE 17.8. *A*, Duplex image of a bypass graft with a preocclusive "staccato" velocity pattern indicating minimal flow and high risk for thrombosis. *B*, Two duplex images of the same bypass graft showing a high-grade distal stenosis with a PSV of 616 cm/s.

can be identified on duplex testing by a decrease in GFV to the threshold of a low-velocity, nonstenotic bypass. In some cases, there may not be a viable treatment option by means of angioplasty or a "jump" graft to another leg artery; graft surveillance detected a problem, but graft failure cannot be prevented. Similarly, prosthetic bypasses with low velocity (<45 cm/s) or a monophasic flow pattern are more likely to thrombose than autogenous vein grafts owing to their higher "thrombotic threshold velocity."[13] This contributes to a lower diagnostic accuracy of duplex ultrasound surveillance in predicting prosthetic graft failure—the positive predictive value is less for prosthetic femoropopliteal grafts (57%) than for femorotibial vein grafts (95%).[19] Prosthetic graft failure

is most commonly due to an anastomotic or inflow stenosis, but thrombosis can occur in the absence of a discrete stenosis.[18,19]

IMPLEMENTING A GRAFT SURVEILLANCE PROGRAM

Surveillance after infrainguinal bypass grafting should be considered as part of vascular patient care and is analogous to a routine maintenance program after an automobile purchase. Individualize the frequency of testing according to the patient, the type of arterial bypass, and the results of prior studies. Test all patients within several weeks after bypass grafting to identify residual graft defects and then 3 to 4 months later after graft arterialization or healing has occurred. If the patient is asymptomatic, atherosclerotic risk factors are under control, and initial vascular testing confirms a nonstenotic bypass with normal GFV, subsequent surveillance at 6-month intervals is sufficient. Communication with the patient's primary care physician detailing the rationale for graft surveillance, as well as obtaining a verbal commitment from the patient to adhere to the testing schedule, can improve compliance.

The risk of developing an anatomic lesion decreases with time but remains in the range of 5% to 10% per year in patients requiring vein bypass grafting for CLI.[4,11–17,20] When routine duplex imaging has been included in a graft surveillance program, the incidence of revision for infrainguinal vein graft stenosis ranges from 20% to 40%, with a corresponding primary patency rate of 80% to 60%. Arm vein bypasses, reversed vein conduits, and bypasses with an abnormal early postoperative duplex scan are associated with higher revision rates.[5,11] With aggressive repair of critical stenoses detected by surveillance, assisted primary patency rates should exceed 80% at 4 to 5 years regardless of infrainguinal vein graft type. After prosthetic bypass grafting in the lower limb, the yield of surveillance is less, with a revision rate for stenosis of 10% to 15% and an assisted-primary patency in the range of 50% to 70% at 4 years.[18,19]

In the ambulatory patient with a normal ABI after vein or prosthetic bypass grafting, routine duplex imaging of the entire bypass beyond the first 6 months is not mandatory, as long as the patient is reliable in reporting a decrease in walking distance. The need for detailed graft imaging should be guided by the number of patient-specific risk factors for developing a graft stenosis such as a small-caliber vein, use of arm vein, a redo grafting procedure, infrapopliteal bypass, prior graft revision, and bypass for CLI.[21] If any graft abnormality is identified by duplex scanning, such as focal stenosis with PSV >180 cm/s or aneurysmal dilatation, surveillance at 3-month intervals is recommended during the first postoperative year.[5,11] For bypass grafts with normal duplex testing, an annual evaluation of bypass function is appropriate and reassures the patient and referring physician that atherosclerotic disease progression is not occurring. Certainly, identifying an acquired graft lesion, either high-grade stenosis or aneurysmal degeneration, is valuable for the vascular specialist, because the necessary therapy (endovascular vs. surgical repair) can usually be based on duplex findings alone.

SUMMARY

Vascular laboratory testing is an essential step in the ongoing care of the patient after infrainguinal bypass grafting. Physiologic testing (ABI measurement) and duplex ultrasound imaging testing are necessary to confirm that the arterial bypass has improved perfusion sufficient to relieve CLI or claudication symptoms. Early postoperative duplex imaging is predictive of the subsequent need for bypass graft revision. The natural history of a moderate graft stenosis is relatively benign, and such lesions can be safely followed using serial testing to identify progression. The frequency of testing should be individualized according to the patient, type of arterial bypass, and duplex scan findings. The focus of graft surveillance is on the identification and repair of critical stenoses, as defined by duplex velocity criteria of a PSV >300 cm/s and Vr across the stenosis of greater than 3.5, correlating with greater than 70% DR stenosis. The PSV of prosthetic grafts is an important hemodynamic parameter predictive of patency and if less than 45 cm/s should prompt consideration of oral anticoagulation in addition to antiplatelet therapy. A graft surveillance program should result in a graft failure rate of less than 3% to 5% per year.[5,11]

References

1. Bandyk DF, Schmitt DD, Seabrook GR, et al. Monitoring functional patency of in-situ saphenous vein bypasses: The impact of a surveillance protocol and elective revision. *J Vasc Surg* 1989;9:286-296.
2. Idu MM, Blankstein JD, de Gier P, et al. Impact of a color-flow duplex surveillance program on infrainguinal graft patency: A five-year experience. *J Vasc Surg* 1993;17:42-53.
3. Lundell A, Lindblad B, Berqvist D, et al. Femoropopliteal-crural graft patency is improved by an intensive surveillance program: A prospective randomized study. *J Vasc Surg* 1995;21:26-33.
4. Mofidi R, Kelman J, Bennett S, et al. Significance of the early postoperative duplex result in infrainguinal vein bypass surveillance. *Eur J Vasc Endovasc Surg* 2007;34:327-332.
5. Tinder CN, Chavanpun JP, Bandyk DF, et al. Duplex surveillance after infrainguinal vein bypass may be enhanced by identification of characteristics predictive of graft stenosis development. *J Vasc Surg* 2008;48:613-618.
6. Erickson CA, Towne JB, Seabrook GR, et al. Ongoing vascular laboratory surveillance is essential to maximize long-term in-situ saphenous vein bypass patency. *J Vasc Surg* 2000:32:89-95.
7. Armstrong PA, Bandyk DF, Wilson JS, et al. Optimizing infrainguinal arm vein bypass patency with duplex ultrasound surveillance and endovascular therapy. *J Vasc Surg* 2005;40:724-730.
8. Mills JL, Wixon CL, James DC, et al. The natural history of intermediate and critical vein graft stenosis: Recommendations for continued surveillance or repair. *J Vasc Surg* 2001;33:273-280.
9. Mills JL, Conte MS, Armstrong DG, et al. The Society for Vascular Surgery lower extremity threatened limb classification system: Risk stratification based on wound ischemia, and foot infection (WiFi). *J Vasc Surg* 2014;59:220-234.
10. Oresanya L, Makam AN, Belkin M, et al. Factors associated with primary vein graft occlusion in a multicenter trial with mandated ultrasound surveillance. *J Vasc Surg* 2014;59:996-1022.
11. Anderson JL, Halperin JL, Albert NM, et al. Management of patients with peripheral artery disease ACCF/AHA guideline recommendations: A report of the American College of Cardiology Foundation/American Heart Association task force on practice guidelines. *Circulation* 2013. Published online 2013. http://circ.ahajournals.org/content/early/2013/03/01/CIR.0b013e31828b82aa.citation
12. Davies AH, Hawdon MR, Sydes SG, et al. Is duplex surveillance of value after leg vein bypass grafting? Principle results of the Vein Graft Surveillance Randomized Trial (VGST). *Circulation* 2005;112:1985-1991.
13. Brumberg RS, Back MR, Armstrong PA, et al. The relative importance of graft surveillance and warfarin therapy in infrainguinal prosthetic bypass failure. *J Vasc Surg* 2007;46:1160-1166.
14. Gupta AK, Bandyk DF, Cheanvechai D, et al. Natural history of infrainguinal vein graft stenosis relative to bypass grafting technique. *J Vasc Surg* 1997;25:211-225.
15. Belkin M, Mackey WC, McLaughlin R, et al. The variation in vein graft flow velocity with luminal diameter and outflow level. *J Vasc Surg* 1992;15:991-999.
16. Westerband A, Mills JL, Kistler S, et al. Prospective validation of threshold criteria for intervention in infrainguinal vein grafts undergoing duplex surveillance. *Ann Vasc Surg* 1997;11:44-48.
17. Caps MT, Cantwell-Gab K, Bergelin RO, et al. Vein graft lesions: Time of onset and rate or progression. *J Vasc Surg* 1995;22:466-475.
18. Berceli SA, Hevelone ND, Lipsitz SR, et al. Surgical and endovascular revision of infrainguinal vein bypass grafts: Analysis of midterm outcomes from the Prevent III trial. *J Vasc Surg* 2007;46:1173-1179.
19. Calligaro KD, Doerr K, McAfee-Bennett S, et al. Should duplex ultrasonography be performed for surveillance of femoropopliteal and femorotibial arterial prosthetic bypasses? *Ann Vasc Surg* 2001;15:520-524.
20. Slim H, Tiwari A, Carsten Ritter J, et al. Outcome of infrainguinal bypass grafts using vein conduit with less than 3 millimeters diameter in critical leg ischemia. *J Vasc Surg* 2011;53:421-425.
21. Schanzer A, Hevelone N, Owens CD, et al. Technical factors affecting autogenous vein graft failure: Observations from a large multi-center trial. *J Vasc Surg* 2007;46:1180-1190.

CHAPTER 18 ■ SURVEILLANCE AFTER PERIPHERAL ARTERY ENDOVASCULAR INTERVENTION

DENNIS F. BANDYK AND KELLEY D. HODGKISS-HARLOW

Diagnostic evaluation using duplex ultrasound and limb systolic pressure measurements is integral to quality patient care after open or endovascular intervention for peripheral arterial disease (PAD).[1-4] The rationale for testing is to confirm improvement in limb perfusion and document normal hemodynamics at the treated site. Often, endovascular repair does not restore ankle systolic pressure to normal, that is, ankle-brachial index (ABI) greater than 0.9, due to the presence of multilevel occlusive lesions, especially in the treatment of critical limb ischemia (CLI).[1,3,5-7] Residual stenosis may not be suspected by the interventionist when angiographic monitoring documents a technically successful anatomic end point (<30% angioplasty site stenosis).[8] Duplex ultrasound is recommended as a surrogate for angiography as an anatomic end point to verify stenosis-free patency because it is noninvasive and has a diagnostic accuracy comparable to angiography.[9]

Clinical trials have typically used duplex-acquired peak systolic velocity (PSV) ratios to predict angiographic lumen stenosis, with values of 2.0 to 2.5 corresponding to greater than 50% diameter-reducing (DR) stenosis.[3,9] Clinical device trials that performed early (<1 month) duplex ultrasound testing have demonstrated angioplasty site hemodynamics of a greater than 50% stenosis in 5% to 40% of treated limbs, with a higher incidence after balloon dilation than following stent or stent-graft angioplasty.[5-7] Vascular laboratory testing provides objective hemodynamic data to document whether the improvement in limb perfusion is sufficient for claudication symptoms to abate or ischemic lesions to heal. The relationship between duplex-detected stenosis and clinical outcome, such as recurrent symptoms or angioplasty site thrombosis, is less conclusive.[3,10] At present, immediate (same day) or early (2 to 3 weeks) testing after endovascular intervention is recommended as specific duplex criteria can be used to validate patency and clinical success. Since the PAD patient is prone to occlusive disease through either myointimal hyperplasia (as a response to injury) or atherosclerotic occlusive disease progression, when symptoms of limb ischemia recur, duplex ultrasound is the preferred testing modality to distinguish between angioplasty or stent failure versus progression of atherosclerosis.[3,8-11] The detection of high-grade stenosis within the treated site allows for a preemptive clinical decision to intervene using an endovascular approach before thrombotic failure, thereby extending angioplasty or stent site patency.

THE ROLE OF THE VASCULAR LABORATORY

The goal of testing after lower limb endovascular therapy is to provide objective hemodynamic and anatomic information on the treated arterial segments, classify stenosis severity when present, and provide reliable threshold criteria for reintervention. Duplex ultrasound testing after an open or endovascular intervention can both confirm procedural success and predict the likelihood of failure when a residual stenosis is identified (see Chapter 17).[1,6] Subsequent testing is based on patient symptoms and the presence of clinical risk factors associated with treatment site failure. The application of duplex surveillance to detect and then repair stenotic lesions after arterial intervention has been shown to improve patient outcomes compared with clinical assessment alone after lower limb bypass grafting, endovascular aneurysm repair, and renal/visceral artery angioplasty.[1,5,12,13] After lower limb endovascular intervention, the reported incidence of failure ranges from 20% to 40% within the first year, suggesting that an appropriate surveillance protocol may improve outcomes.[3,12,13] Bui et al.[14] conducted a prospective duplex surveillance study of 94 limbs with femoropopliteal occlusive disease treated by percutaneous transluminal angioplasty. Initial duplex testing was normal in two-thirds of limbs and remained normal in 38 (40%) limbs. New or progressive angioplasty site stenosis occurred in more than one-third of limbs and was associated with a 10% to 20% incidence of arterial thrombosis. Severe (>70%) stenosis was associated with ischemic symptoms in one-half of patients. The sensitivity and specificity of duplex testing to predict occlusion were 88% and 60%, respectively.

The presence of a duplex-detected stenosis after endovascular therapy (atherectomy, transluminal balloon angioplasty, stent angioplasty) is a known risk factor for early (<6 months) procedure failure.[5-7,13,14] This observation has prompted some interventionalists to perform immediate (i.e., intraprocedural) or early (<30 days) duplex scanning to verify that the treated arterial segment has no residual stenosis based on spectral waveform velocity criteria. Early duplex testing indicates that the prevalence of endovascular treatment site stenosis is lowest after stent angioplasty or stent grafting (<5%) and higher after balloon angioplasty (15% to 20%) or atherectomy (25%). An angiogram-monitored angioplasty with less than 20% to 30% residual stenosis does correlate with 30-day patency (i.e., technical success), but does not reliably predict a stenosis-free angioplasty site when evaluated by duplex ultrasound.[3,15-17]

Endovascular intervention has emerged as first-line therapy for symptomatic iliac and femoropopliteal arterial occlusive disease. In 2007, the work group for the Trans-Atlantic Inter-Society Consensus (TASC) updated consensus guidelines (TASC II) for the management of PAD and endorsed endovascular therapy for the treatment of infrainguinal PAD.[11] Most vascular specialists have adopted an "endovascular first" policy for the management of both claudication and CLI. Endovascular intervention for TASC II D lesions can be safely performed with excellent immediate hemodynamic improvement and limb salvage, but restenosis is common, and the success of this clinical approach mandates strict patient follow-up using vascular laboratory testing.[12,13] In the treatment of superficial femoral artery (SFA) occlusive lesions, Schillinger et al.[5] documented that duplex-detected greater than 50% stenosis developed more frequently after balloon angioplasty than after nitinol stenting at both 6 months (45% vs. 25%, $P = 0.06$) and 12 months (63% vs. 37%, $P = 0.01$). Other techniques used to treat native SFA lesions or angioplasty site stenosis, such as cutting or cryoplasty balloon angioplasty, atherectomy, and stent grafting, have a high (>95%) technical success rate, but restenosis and treatment site thrombosis are common and observed in 20% to 50% of limbs by 1 year, depending on TASC lesion severity.[14-18] Duplex criteria for stenosis severity based on PSV correlate with procedural failure.[3] Angioplasty site stenosis with a PSV ratio (Vr) greater than 2.5 was predictive ($P < 0.001$) of recurrent claudication with a sensitivity of 71% and specificity of 72%.[10] Surveillance of stent grafts placed for lower extremity arterial occlusive disease indicated that focal sites of PSV greater than 300 cm/s, Vr greater than 3.0, and, most importantly, a uniformly low PSV less than 50 cm/s throughout the stent graft were predictive of impending thrombosis.[19]

The observed deterioration in primary patency after endovascular intervention is a significant clinical concern, especially in the treatment of CLI, since treatment site thrombosis can result in limb loss. The restoration of secondary patency (after occlusion of a previously treated SFA) is associated with a lower rate of technical success and a risk of distal embolization when mechanical thrombectomy techniques are utilized. It remains a subject of debate as to whether duplex surveillance coupled with reintervention for progressive stenosis is a strategy that will result in improved long-term functional capacity and limb salvage. It is clear that the application of less invasive endovascular therapies for PAD will continue, and further expansion of this technology is expected by both vascular specialists and patients. As device technology and endovascular techniques evolve, improvements in durability are likely. The challenge for the noninvasive vascular laboratory is to provide objective, reliable, anatomic, and hemodynamic information for the complete spectrum of endovascular repairs, assist clinicians in detection of treatment site failure, and provide threshold criteria for intervention when abnormalities are identified.

SURVEILLANCE PROTOCOLS

The essentials of vascular laboratory testing after peripheral endovascular intervention mirror those that apply to bypass graft surveillance and can be summarized as follows:

- Verify the patient's functional activity.
- Document any new or unresolved symptoms or signs of limb ischemia.
- Assess limb perfusion by physiologic testing (limb pressures, duplex velocity spectra).

- Evaluate the treated site using duplex ultrasound for anatomic or flow abnormalities.
- Assign test results to a normal or abnormal diagnostic category.

A proposed testing protocol for angioplasty surveillance is shown in Figure 18.1. The vascular technologist should query the patient for claudication symptoms and examine the limb for signs of ischemia (dependent rubor, ulceration, gangrene, cyanosis). In the patient with claudication, indirect physiologic testing is performed to verify improvement in the ABI to a normal (>0.9) or an improved (increase of >0.2) level, which is predictive that walking distance is likely to be improved. Exercise treadmill testing can be used selectively to document walking ability and ankle pressure response to exercise, as discussed in Chapter 13. In limbs treated for CLI, testing should include measurement of toe systolic pressure, since reliance on ABI alone may not accurately reflect forefoot perfusion due to concomitant plantar arch disease, or the ABI may be falsely elevated in the diabetic patient because of tibial artery calcification and vessel incompressibility. In general, a toe pressure greater than 30 mm Hg is required to relieve rest pain, while a value greater than 40 mm Hg is a reliable predictor of foot wound (ulcer, amputation) healing.

Duplex Testing Protocol

The patient should rest for at least 10 minutes prior to testing to ensure a resting state with pulse and blood pressure at baseline levels. Approximately 30 minutes of examination time should be allotted with testing conducted in a warm (70°F to 74°F) room to minimize vasoconstriction. Duplex scanning is generally performed with the patient supine and the lower limb externally rotated with the knee slightly bent. Prone or lateral decubitus positions can be used to image the popliteal artery, tibioperoneal trunk, and peroneal arteries. A multifrequency 5- to 8-MHz linear array transducer is appropriate for most lower extremity arterial mapping studies and allows the examiner to optimize vessel imaging at varying tissue depths.

The examination begins at the level of the common femoral artery (CFA) to document the presence of normal, multiphasic velocity spectra, indicating that there is no proximal inflow (aortoiliac) occlusive disease (Fig. 18.2). If the CFA velocity waveform is monophasic and has a damped configuration or the acceleration time (i.e., systolic upstroke) is prolonged (>180 ms), duplex imaging of the aortoiliac segment should be performed to characterize the occlusive lesion. Duplex mapping then proceeds from the CFA distally with assessment of the SFA and deep femoral artery origins, imaging the length of the SFA, assessment of the angioplasty or stented site, and recording of ankle-level tibial artery velocity waveforms. Changes in spectral waveform pulsatility from the CFA, to popliteal, to distal tibial arteries are diagnostic of interval development of occlusive disease. When the tibial artery velocity spectral waveforms and ABI are normal, the extent of duplex imaging can be limited to scanning of the treated site to confirm normal (PSV < 180 cm/s) or abnormal hemodynamics. The technologist should provide sufficient duplex images and segmental velocity spectral waveforms for complete study interpretation.

Direct imaging of the endovascular repair includes color flow images and pulsed Doppler spectral waveforms proximal to, throughout, and distal to the treated segment. B-mode imaging (transverse and sagittal scan planes) is used to define vessel and stent diameters as well as to assess the lumen for myointimal stenosis, thrombus, or native artery atherosclerotic

Angioplasty Surveillance Protocol

Test Interpretation

Patient Interview for
Limb Ischemia Symptoms

Categories

Asymptomatic, claudication, nonhealing ulcer, rest pain

Measure ABI & toe pressure

Interpretation

ABI ≥ 0.9 Normal; <0.9—Abnormal
Toe pressure < 30 mm Hg—critical foot ischemia
Toe pressure > 40 mm Hg—toe/foot ulcer healing likely

Scan Angioplasty Site

PTA Assessment

Assess inflow artery waveform for damping;
Normal acceleration time <180 ms
Image angioplasty site for stenosis or thrombus
Record PSV and Vr (Abn:PSV > 180 cm/s, Vr > 2)

Scan tibial arteries
above ankle for calcification
and record segmental
(femoral, popliteal, tibial)
velocity spectra

Limb Assessment

Correlate artery spectra waveform with ABI
Identify waveform damping (PI decrease compared to
PTA site indicating tibial artery occlusive disease

*PTA Surveillance
Diagnostic Category*

NORMAL: PSV < 180 cm/s, no stenosis identified
            ABI > 0.7, ↑ >0.15 from pre-PTA level
ABNORMAL:
  – Moderate stenosis: >180 cm/s PSV < 300 cm/s; Vr < 3.5
  – Severe stenosis: PSV > 300 cm/s, Vr > 3.5
  – No stenosis, but ABI unchanged from pre-PTA level;
     or decreased >0.15 from prior testing.

FIGURE 18.1. Peripheral angioplasty surveillance testing protocol and study interpretation criteria.

---

plaque. Color or power Doppler imaging is used to identify changes in lumen caliber, sites of stenosis, high-velocity flow jets, and turbulent flow. Pulsed Doppler spectral waveforms are recorded using a Doppler angle of 60 degrees or less relative to the vessel or stent wall, and the sample volume is "walked through" the region of stenosis to measure PSV proximal to (PSV_{prox}) and at the site of stenosis (PSV_{max}). These values are used to calculate the velocity ratio (Vr) of the stenosis ($Vr = PSV_{max}/PSV_{prox}$), as illustrated in Figure 18.3. At the site of stenosis, end-diastolic velocity (EDV) should also be measured. The values of PSV_{max}, Vr, and EDV at the stenosis are used to classify stenosis severity. Power Doppler imaging, which is independent of Doppler angle, is useful to demonstrate lumen caliber when low flow velocity conditions are encountered, such as downstream from a high-grade stenosis.

FIGURE 18.2. Schematic diagram depicts sites of duplex scanning, including common femoral artery, angioplasty site, and assessment of distal tibial artery flow. (PTA, percutaneous transluminal angioplasty; PSV, peak systolic velocity.)

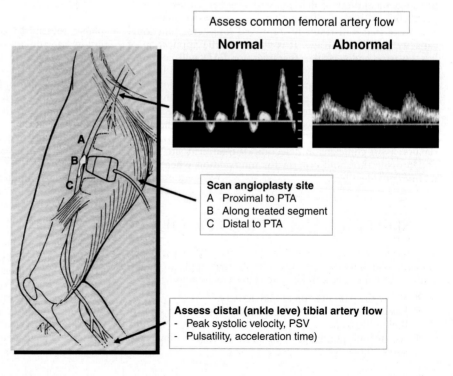

Assess common femoral artery flow

Normal   **Abnormal**

Scan angioplasty site
A Proximal to PTA
B Along treated segment
C Distal to PTA

Assess distal (ankle leve) tibial artery flow
- Peak systolic velocity, PSV
- Pulsatility, acceleration time)

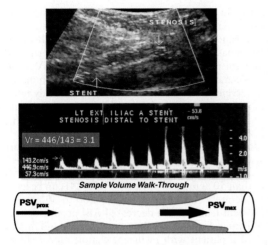

FIGURE 18.3. Color duplex images of a distal external iliac artery stent stenosis (*top*) and velocity spectral waveform (*middle*) show a "walk-through" of the pulsed Doppler sample volume along the stenosis for calculation of the velocity ratio (Vr) based on the recording sites shown in the schematic diagram (*bottom*). (Vr = PSV_{max}/PSV_{prox}; PSV, peak systolic velocity.)

Knowledge of the type of endovascular intervention is important for the vascular technologist to perform accurate duplex surveillance. The artery segment treated (aorta, iliac, CFA, SFA, popliteal, tibial, bypass graft) and the type of intervention performed are important factors to consider in testing and study interpretation. Required scanning and interpretation skills include the ability to discern normal versus abnormal segmental pulsed Doppler spectral waveforms, recognition of stent and stent-graft B-mode ultrasound characteristics, and color flow Doppler patterns within stents and

arterial stenoses. Recording duplex ultrasound findings on a schematic diagram of the lower limb arteries assists in producing a final study interpretation. Prior test results should be available to allow for the diagnosis of stenosis progression. In the majority of patients, duplex scanning can provide sufficient information to identify significant angioplasty or stent site stenosis and aid in a decision to proceed with reintervention.

TEST INTERPRETATION

The recommended duplex velocity spectral waveform criteria for grading angioplasty site and stent stenosis detailed in Figure 18.1 and Table 18.1 are based primarily on threshold PSV and Vr values.[1,8,14-18] The stenosis categories range from normal or less than 50% stenosis to moderate (50% to 70%) stenosis, severe (>70% to 80%) stenosis, or occlusion. Duplex-predicted stenosis severity should be correlated with ABI and toe systolic pressures and with observed changes from prior testing. Test interpretation in limbs treated for CLI indicates whether adequate foot perfusion has been achieved (i.e., toe pressure >30 mm Hg). A normal study interpretation should state that no stenosis was identified at the angioplasty or stent site, and an appropriate increase in ABI has occurred relative to prior or preprocedural testing. A stenotic lesion immediately proximal or distal to the endovascular treatment site should be interpreted as a "new" treatment site abnormality rather than atherosclerotic disease progression.

The velocity criteria recommended for classification of stenosis severity are based on measurements of PSV and Vr. A Vr > 2.0 at the stenotic site is generally regarded as indicating a greater than 50% DR when associated with color Doppler findings of lumen reduction, a focal velocity increase, and turbulent flow. The duplex criteria for grading stenosis shown in Table 18.1 from multiple vascular groups indicate

TABLE 18.1

DUPLEX VELOCITY AND SPECTRAL WAVEFORM CRITERIA FOR GRADING LOWER EXTREMITY ANGIOPLASTY SITE AND STENT STENOSIS

UNIVERSITY OF CALIFORNIA, SAN DIEGO[1]

■ STENOSIS CATEGORY	■ PSV (cm/s)	■ Vr	■ END-DIASTOLIC VELOCITY (cm/s)	■ DISTAL ARTERY WAVEFORM
<50% DR	<180	<2	NA	Normal
>50% DR moderate	180-300	2-3.5	>0	Monophasic
>70% DR severe	>300	>3.5	>45	Damped, monophasic
Occluded			No flow detected	Damped, monophasic

UNIVERSITY OF PITTSBURGH[8]

■ STENOSIS CATEGORY	■ PSV (cm/s)	■ Vr
<50% DR	<190	<1.5
>50% DR	190-275	1.5-3.5
>80% DR	>275	>3.5
Occluded	No flow detected	

PENNSYLVANIA HOSPITAL[20]

■ STENOSIS CATEGORY	■ PSV (cm/s)	■ Vr
Normal, <70% DR	<300	<3.0
Abnormal >70% DR	>300	>3.0

UNIVERSITY OF ARIZONA[14]

■ STENOSIS CATEGORY	■ PSV (cm/s)	■ Vr
Normal	<200	<2.0
Moderate	200-300	2.0-3.0
Severe	>300	>3.0

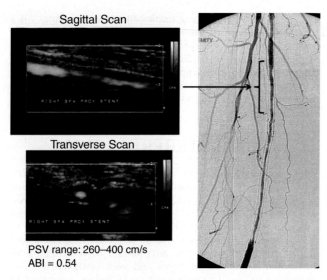

Sagittal Scan

Transverse Scan

PSV range: 260–400 cm/s
ABI = 0.54

FIGURE 18.4. Power Doppler images (sagittal, transverse) and angiogram of a superficial femoral artery stent with diffuse in-stent stenosis. Peak systolic velocity (PSV) ranged from 260 to 400 cm/s within the stent. Measured ankle-brachial index was 0.54.

differences in duplex velocity criteria.[19] At the University of California, San Diego Vascular Laboratory, the same duplex interpretation criteria are used for grading both lower limb arterial bypass graft stenosis and angioplasty site stenosis, including the intervention threshold criteria of PSV > 300 cm/s and Vr > 3.5.[1] Use of the same criteria after open or endovascular intervention improves the reliability of study interpretation among vascular laboratory physicians, the diagnosis of disease progression, and clinical decision-making regarding the surveillance schedule and reintervention.

Endovascular treatment failure may develop in a variety of forms: a focal severe stenosis, diffuse or multiple stenoses, low flow velocity, or thrombotic occlusion. The finding of diffuse greater than 50% in-stent stenosis (Fig. 18.4) can be associated with moderately elevated PSV values (200 to 300 cm/s) along the SFA stent length and a decreased ABI producing recurrent limb ischemia. Figure 18.5 shows angiogram and duplex scan images of a patient with recurrent claudication (ABI = 0.85) after SFA balloon angioplasty. In this case, a focal greater than 70% stenosis was identified by duplex testing; after stent angioplasty of the lesion, the duplex scan images indicate "normal" treatment site patency (ABI = 1.1, PSV = 100 cm/s). An important diagnostic feature of angioplasty failure is the development of a damped, low-velocity spectral waveform at the distal (above ankle) tibial artery recording site.

The incidence of endovascular intervention failure is highest in the first 6 months after the procedure.[5,6] The finding of a residual stenosis in the moderate category (50% to 70% DR) on the initial postprocedure study is a risk factor for failure.[3,6,12,14] In this situation, study interpretation should include a recommendation for repeat testing in 6 to 8 weeks to detect stenosis progression (Fig. 18.6). The ultimate value of surveillance testing is to identify a "failing" endovascular treatment site before thrombosis occurs. In the medically fit patient, the development of a greater than 70% angioplasty or stent site stenosis should be considered as an indication for reintervention. However, in the majority of patients, the initial duplex surveillance study will be normal (<50% DR), and a protocol for follow-up testing in 6 months is appropriate. The patient should also be instructed to return sooner if symptoms of limb ischemia develop.

Angioplasty or stent site failure beyond 6 months is commonly the result of myointimal hyperplasia within the treated region or in the immediately adjacent arterial segment. Stent

substantial agreement on PSV and Vr thresholds for greater than 50% DR. The University of Pittsburgh group reported a positive predictive value of greater than 95% for greater than 50% or greater than 80% in-stent stenosis after femoropopliteal angioplasty for TASC B and C lesions.[8,15] For patients who developed recurrent symptoms and a decrease in ABI of greater than 0.15, the angioplasty site stenosis had a mean PSV of 360 cm/s and Vr of 3.6, exceeding the threshold for severe stenosis in both sets of criteria. The University of Arizona group preferred to report stenosis severity as moderate (PSV 200-300 cm/s, Vr 2.0-3.0 > 2.0) or severe (PSV > 300 cm/s, Vr > 3.0).

In general, PSV values for grading in-stent stenoses are higher than for de novo atherosclerotic stenoses where a value greater than 200 cm/s is a widely accepted threshold for greater than 50% stenosis. Stent angioplasty also changes artery wall compliance and produces abnormal, nonuniform wall shear stress at stent end points, which potentiates the development of myointimal hyperplasia and may account for observed

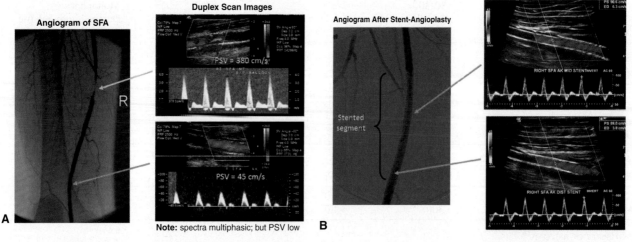

Angiogram of SFA

Duplex Scan Images

PSV = 380 cm/s

PSV = 45 cm/s

Note: spectra multiphasic; but PSV low

Angiogram After Stent-Angioplasty

Stented segment

RIGHT SFA AK MID STENT INVERT

RIGHT SFA AK DIST STENT

A   B

FIGURE 18.5. Angiogram and duplex scan images of a percutaneous transluminal angioplasty (PTA) site restenosis in a superficial femoral artery. A, >70% diameter reduction (DR) stenosis (PSV = 380, Vr = 5, end-diastolic velocity >0) and low popliteal artery PSV of 45 cm/s. B, After reintervention with stent angioplasty, duplex scan demonstrates no stenosis (PSV = 100 cm/s). Ankle-brachial index increased from 0.85 to 1.10. (PSV, peak systemic velocity. SFA, superficial femoral artery.)

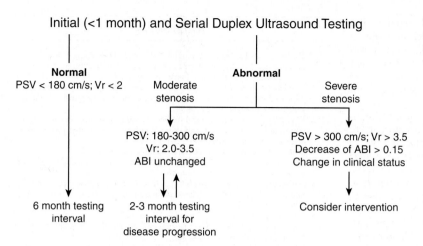

Initial (<1 month) and Serial Duplex Ultrasound Testing

Normal
PSV < 180 cm/s; Vr < 2

Abnormal

Moderate stenosis

Severe stenosis

PSV: 180-300 cm/s
Vr: 2.0-3.5
ABI unchanged

PSV > 300 cm/s; Vr > 3.5
Decrease of ABI > 0.15
Change in clinical status

6 month testing interval

2-3 month testing interval for disease progression

Consider intervention

FIGURE 18.6. A general outpatient surveillance algorithm after infrainguinal endovascular arterial procedures.

fracture is also a known risk factor for stenosis development and thrombosis, but this complication cannot be identified reliably by ultrasound imaging. Stent deformation or kinking can be visualized by careful transverse scanning and should be noted in the final study interpretation. Stent stenosis due to device fracture is typically associated with myointimal hyperplasia, which appears on ultrasound imaging as a homogenous lesion producing lumen narrowing.

APPLICATIONS OF DUPLEX SURVEILLANCE

The success of endovascular therapy should be documented by clinical improvement and treatment site patency, as recommended in the reporting standards published by the American Heart Association.[3] Patency of the treated segment and an increase in ABI of greater than 0.15, in addition to improvement in symptoms or signs of limb ischemia (walking distance, resolution of CLI), are required for a successful procedure. Anatomic failure after endovascular therapy is characterized by a restenosis of greater than 50% DR using duplex criteria (Vr > 2.5) or angiogram measuring techniques; a more strict definition is angioplasty site occlusion or reintervention for stenosis.[19-23] The term *primary patency* denotes a period of uninterrupted patency for the treated target artery segment after endovascular therapy. Any open or percutaneous secondary intervention undertaken to maintain or improve functional patency changes the procedure outcome to *assisted primary patency*. If the angioplasty site is thrombosed and a secondary procedure is performed to restore patency, the outcome status changes to *secondary patency*.

The goal of surveillance is to increase assisted primary patency by timely detection and repair of stenotic lesions. An assisted primary patency of greater than 80% at 3 to 5 years would be an excellent long-term result after an endovascular procedure and compare favorably with open surgical arterial bypass grafting.[1,22-24] Surveillance may begin with an intraprocedural study to assess for technical errors, followed by an outpatient surveillance examination 2 to 4 weeks after the procedure. Ascher et al.[22] published several clinical reports on the treatment of femoropopliteal occlusive disease in which duplex ultrasound was utilized as an alternative to contrast angiography to perform the endovascular procedure and assess the results. This application of duplex-monitored angioplasty showed that a normal angioplasty site immediately after the procedure was associated with early clinical success, and the likelihood of finding a severe stenosis on the initial outpatient study was low (<2%). Documenting normal duplex

ultrasound findings after arterial intervention has predictive value; it confirms the absence of technical error, correlates with early clinical success, and establishes a baseline for subsequent surveillance testing to detect the development of stenosis.

The use of clinical assessment alone, which relies on patient recognition of the symptoms associated with procedure failure, or the use of indirect physiologic testing methods such as the ABI, is not sufficiently sensitive to detect developing myointimal hyperplasia. An abnormal or decreased ABI may indicate an alteration in the circulation, but it does not identify the location of the occlusive lesion or reliably identify angioplasty or stent site stenosis. In addition, ankle pressure measurement and ABI are not reliable in the presence of calcified tibial arteries, as commonly seen in patients with diabetes and end-stage renal disease (see Chapter 13). Duplex surveillance after endovascular revascularization for CLI is superior to physiologic testing. Saarinen et al.[19] found that clinical status or toe pressures alone were inadequate markers of endovascular site failure. Duplex testing was a valuable aid in surveillance and detected significant restenosis or occlusion in one-third of patients.

It is essential to use objective interpretation criteria to grade lesion severity in a surveillance program. This allows for the application of "threshold" criteria for reintervention or a decision to obtain additional arterial imaging. The use of three stenosis categories is sufficient to characterize an arterial repair as "normal" or "abnormal" and further grade any abnormality as one that should be followed for further progression (moderate stenosis) or one that should be considered for repair (severe stenosis, low stent or graft flow velocity).[14,19,23,25] Use of combined PSV and Vr thresholds to identify a severe stenosis (>70% DR) is reliable and associated with a high (>90%) positive predictive value when correlated with angiography.[1,14] Whether duplex testing is used for "screening" or "intervention" decisions depends on the surveillance application. After visceral (mesenteric, renal) artery angioplasty, duplex scanning serves primarily as a screening method to identify stent or angioplasty site stenosis.[26] An abnormal study should prompt additional confirmatory angiographic imaging or pressure gradient measurement to assess lesion severity and clinical significance. Early duplex testing after renal angioplasty and stenting also predicts restenosis and lower postprocedure renal function.[27]

After peripheral artery interventions, duplex testing can be used for patient management decisions, including drug therapy for restenosis, frequency of surveillance, or additional testing to confirm the need for reintervention. The finding of a greater than 70% stenosis on duplex scanning is sufficient anatomic and hemodynamic information, but should be used in conjunction with limb blood pressure measurements or treadmill exercise testing to recommend and proceed with a secondary intervention (endovascular or open surgical repair). Bui et al.[14] recommended caution regarding intervention based on duplex testing alone, since some moderate and severe stenoses were observed to improve on serial examinations. Recurrent limb ischemic symptoms after endovascular therapy were associated with severe angioplasty site stenosis, which, if not treated, progressed to occlusion in 20% of limbs.

A general outpatient surveillance algorithm for infrainguinal endovascular arterial procedures is shown in Figure 18.6. The initial outpatient surveillance examination at 2 to 4 weeks after endovascular therapy should be combined with a vascular surgery clinic visit in order to assess the patient's activity level, document adherence to atherosclerosis risk factor modification, and review relevant drug therapy (antiplatelet agents, statins). If the initial duplex surveillance examination is normal, the interval for follow-up testing is 3 months for patients treated for CLI and 6 months for those treated for claudication. The frequency of testing after iliac artery angioplasty and stenting can be based on the CFA velocity spectral waveform, which when normal, that is, multiphasic, indicates no significant stent stenosis, and a testing interval of 6 to 12 months is recommended.[23,24] If serial clinical follow-up and duplex testing indicate no disease progression, biannual vascular laboratory surveillance is recommended. If duplex surveillance is abnormal, or the patient develops new symptoms, an appointment in vascular surgery clinic is scheduled for a complete physician assessment. Shorter surveillance intervals (i.e., <6 months) may be indicated after treatment of TASC C and D lesions owing to the higher likelihood of endoluminal therapy failure, or if postprocedure scans detected moderate, greater than 50% stenosis.[7,12,25]

In patients treated for single-segment occlusive disease who are asymptomatic and in whom duplex testing remains normal after 2 years, surveillance protocols can be abbreviated to include only ABI and toe systolic pressure measurements, reserving duplex scanning for patients with incompressible tibial arteries, multilevel arterial disease, or those with a change in the indirect physiologic test results.[25,28] However, the use of lower extremity segmental pressure measurements by either the 3 or 4 cuff technique is not recommend after femoropopliteal endovascular interventions.

SUMMARY

Duplex ultrasound surveillance after endovascular intervention using transluminal balloon dilation, stent angioplasty, or stent grafting has been shown to predict treatment site failure, but its routine application remains a decision of the interventionalist. Test interpretation has not been standardized, and the recommended frequency of testing varies among surveillance protocols. Use of duplex velocity criteria predictive of severe, greater than 70% stenosis, may assist in preventing failure of endovascular interventions and concomitantly be associated with improved long-term functional capacity and limb salvage. Some vascular specialists are not convinced that routine duplex surveillance is beneficial or can be used as the sole test prior to reintervention. Our vascular group believes that duplex surveillance is an important adjunct in the clinical follow-up of patients undergoing both open and endovascular lower extremity arterial interventions. Early duplex testing is recommended and when applied correctly is associated with improved outcomes after a variety of open and endovascular arterial procedures. Endovascular therapy is associated with limited functional patency due to the development of myointimal hyperplasia, and in patients with atherosclerotic disease risk factors, a duplex ultrasound surveillance program should be considered as a part of appropriate and necessary medical care.

References

1. Tinder CN, Chavapun JP, Bandyk DF, et al. Duplex surveillance after infrainguinal vein bypass may be enhanced by identification of characteristics predictive of graft stenosis development. J Vasc Surg 2008;48:613-618.
2. Kundell A, Linblad B, Bergqvist D, et al. Femoropopliteal graft patency is improved by an intensive surveillance program: A prospective randomized study. J Vasc Surg 1995;21:26-34.
3. Kinlay S. Outcomes for clinical studies assessing drug and revascularization therapies for claudication and critical limb ischemia in peripheral artery disease. Circulation 2013;127:1241-1250.
4. Scali ST, Beck AW, Nolan BW, et al. Completion duplex ultrasound predicts early graft thrombosis after crural bypass in patients with critical limb ischemia. J Vasc Surg 2011;54:1006-1010.
5. Schillinger M, Sabeti S, Loewe C, et al. Balloon angioplasty versus implantation of nitinol stents in the superficial femoral artery. N Engl J Med 2006;354:1879-1888.
6. Mewissen MW, Kinney EV, Bandyk DF, et al. The role of duplex scanning versus angiography in predicting outcome after balloon angioplasty in the femoropopliteal artery. J Vasc Surg 1992;15:860-866.
7. Humphries MD, Pevec WC, Laird JR, et al. Early duplex scanning after infrainguinal endovascular therapy. J Vasc Surg 2011;53:353-358.
8. Baril DT, Rhee RY, Kim J, et al. Duplex criteria for determination of in-stent stenosis after angioplasty and stent of the superficial femoral artery. J Vasc Surg 2009;49:133-139.
9. Langenberger H, Schillinger M, Plank C, et al. Agreement of duplex ultrasonography vs. computed tomography angiography for evaluation of native and in-stent SFA re-stenosis—findings from a randomized controlled trial. Eur J Radiol 2012;81:2265-2269.
10. Jones DW, Graham A, Connolly PH, et al. Restenosis and symptom recurrence after endovascular therapy for claudication: Does duplex ultrasound correlate with recurrent claudication. Vascular Published online May 2014.
11. Norgren L, Hiatt WR, Dormandy JA, et al. Inter-Society Consensus for the management of peripheral arterial disease (TASC II). J Vasc Surg 2007;45(Suppl):S5-S67.
12. Baril DT, Chaer RA, Rhee RA, et al. Endovascular interventions for TASC II D femoropopliteal lesions. J Vasc Surg 2010;51:627-633.
13. Baril DT, Marone LK. Duplex evaluation following femoropopliteal angioplasty and stenting: Criteria utility of surveillance. Vasc Endovascular Surg 2012;46:353-357.
14. Bui TD, Mills JL Sr, Ihnat DM, et al. The natural history of duplex-detected stenosis after femoropopliteal endovascular therapy suggest questionable utility of routine duplex surveillance. J Vasc Surg 2012;55:246-252.
15. Khan SZ, Khan MA, Bradley B, et al. Utility of duplex ultrasound in detecting and grading de novo femoropopliteal lesions. J Vasc Surg 2011;54:1067-1073.
16. Shrikhandle GV, Graham AR, Aparajita R, et al. Determining criteria for predicting stenosis with ultrasound duplex after endovascular intervention in infrainguinal lesions. Ann Vasc Surg 2011;25:454-460.
17. Kawarada O, Higashimori A, Noguchi M, et al. Duplex criteria for in-stent restenosis of the superficial femoral artery. Catheter Cardiovasc Interv 2013;81:199-205.
18. Kuppler CS, Christie JW, Newton WB, et al. Stent effects on duplex velocity estimates. J Surg Res 2013;183:457-461.
19. Saarinen E, Laukontaus SJ, Alback A, et al. Duplex surveillance after endovascular revascularization for critical limb ischemia. Eur J Vasc Endovasc Surg 2014;47:418-421.
20. Keeling WB, Shames ML, Stone PA, et al. Plaque excision with the Silverhawk catheter: Early results in patients with claudication or critical limb ischemia. J Vasc Surg 2007;45:25-31.
21. Troutman DM, Madden NJ, Dougherty MJ, et al. Duplex ultrasound surveillance of stent-grafts placed for occlusive disease. J Vasc Surg 2014. Published online on September 22, 2014.
22. Ascher E, Marks NA, Hingorani AP, et al. Duplex-guided endovascular treatment for occlusive and stenotic lesions of the femoral-popliteal arterial segment: A comparative study in the first 253 cases. J Vasc Surg 2006;44:1230-1237.
23. Back MR, Novotney M, Roth SM, et al. Utility of duplex surveillance following iliac artery angioplasty and primary stenting. J Endovasc Ther 2001;8:629-637.
24. Al Samaraee A, McCallum I, Cairns T, et al. The results of high-frequency duplex surveillance after iliac arterial stenting in a single center. Vasc Endovascular Surg 2011;45:246-254.
25. Kiguchi MM, Marone LK, Chaer RA, et al. Pattern of femoropopliteal recurrence after routine and selective endoluminal therapy. J Vasc Surg 2013;57:37-43.
26. Hodgkiss-Harlow K. Interpretation of visceral duplex scanning before and after intervention for chronic mesenteric ischemia. Semin Vasc Surg 2013;26:127-132.
27. Christie JW, Conlee TD, Craven TE, et al. Early duplex predicts restenosis after renal artery angioplasty and stenting. J Vasc Surg 2012;56:1373-1380.
28. Hodgkiss-Harlow KD, Bandyk DF. Interpretation of arterial duplex testing of lower extremity arteries and interventions. Semin Vasc Surg 2013;26:95-104.

SECTION V ■ PERIPHERAL VENOUS

CHAPTER 19 ■ ACUTE LOWER EXTREMITY DEEP VEIN THROMBOSIS

DAVID L. DAWSON AND HOLLY M. GRAY

The first reports of the use of Doppler ultrasound for the evaluation of lower extremity venous disease appeared in the late 1960s.[1,2] In 1972, Gene Strandness and his colleague David Sumner published their observations on the use of Doppler ultrasound for the diagnosis of venous thrombosis.[3] A 1982 case report by Steven Talbot, a vascular technologist, is generally regarded as the first publication to describe the use of B-mode imaging for the diagnosis of deep vein thrombosis (DVT).[4,5] Within a few years, ultrasound pioneers recognized the potential for venous duplex scanning.

An area that has been relatively unexplored is the detection of acute venous thrombosis. The veins of the lower extremity from the level of the iliac to the popliteal vessels can be imaged and their blood flow detected. Thus there is little doubt in my mind that duplex scanning can be used for both diagnostic and follow-up purposes for this important aspect of peripheral vascular disease.[6]

—D. Eugene Strandness, Jr. (1985)

The expense, invasive nature, discomfort, and lack of repeatability of ascending venography, coupled with its potential for initiating thrombosis, tarnished the luster of the venography "gold standard."[7,8] Duplex scanning rapidly became the primary imaging modality for the screening, diagnosis, and follow-up of DVT of the lower extremities (Table 19.1).[9,10] Testing for lower extremity DVT is now the most commonly performed study in many vascular laboratories, with applications in numerous clinical settings (Table 19.2).[11] The capability for duplex ultrasound scanning with color flow Doppler is a requisite for any vascular laboratory to be accredited in peripheral venous testing by the Intersocietal Accreditation Commission—Vascular Testing.[12] Clearly, Dr. Strandness' early vision has been realized.

EPIDEMIOLOGY OF VENOUS THROMBOEMBOLISM

DVT and pulmonary embolism (PE), jointly termed "venous thromboembolism" (VTE), represent a major clinical problem. Prevalence estimates suggest that there are over 900,000 VTE cases annually in the United States, with as many as 300,000 PE deaths each year.[13] After heart disease and stroke, VTE is the third most common vascular disease. To put the magnitude of the problem in perspective, it has been pointed out that deaths from PE are five times more common than deaths from breast cancer, motor vehicle accidents, and AIDS combined.[14] Data used by the American College of Chest Physicians (ACCP) for VTE risk estimation have suggested that 31% of hospitalized patients are at risk for VTE, which represents approximately 12 million patients per year.[15]

In addition to the acute risks associated with DVT, many patients subsequently develop symptoms of postthrombotic syndrome (PTS), with pain and limb swelling that can be debilitating (see Chapter 21). These symptoms can develop months or years after the acute episode of thrombosis.[16,17] PTS can substantially impact quality of life. The overall incidence of PTS is estimated to be as high as 30%, although the incidence of symptoms may be higher for some subgroups of DVT patients, in particular those with iliofemoral venous thrombosis.[18]

The significance of VTE as a public health problem prompted the US Surgeon General to issue a "Call to Action to Prevent Deep Vein Thrombosis and Pulmonary Embolism" in 2008.[19] This initiative urged greater understanding of the risk factors and triggering events for developing DVT and PE, better recognition of the symptoms, and implementation of steps to prevent and treat these serious conditions. VTE patient

TABLE 19.1

IMAGING OPTIONS FOR PATIENTS WITH SUSPECTED LOWER EXTREMITY DEEP VEIN THROMBOSIS

■ IMAGING PROCEDURE	■ RATING (Scale: 1 = least appropriate, 9 = most appropriate[a])	■ COMMENTS	■ RELATIVE RADIATION EXPOSURE LEVEL
US lower extremity with Doppler	9		None
MRV lower extremity and pelvis without and with contrast	7	This is the primary modality for pelvic or thigh DVT if US is nondiagnostic.	None
MRV lower extremity and pelvis without contrast	7	This procedure can be performed when contrast is contraindicated.	None
CTV lower extremity and pelvis with contrast	7	This procedure can be performed when MRV is not available or contraindicated.	High
X-ray venography, pelvis	6	This procedure is reserved for inconclusive noninvasive studies or when thrombolysis is planned.	Medium
X-ray venography, lower extremity	4	This procedure is reserved for inconclusive noninvasive studies or when thrombolysis is planned.	Medium

[a]Rating scale: 1, 2, 3 usually not appropriate; 4, 5, 6 may be appropriate; 7, 8, 9 usually appropriate.
Adapted from American College of Radiology ACR Appropriateness Criteria®, 2013.[9]
US, ultrasound; MRV, magnetic resonance venography; CTV, computed tomographic venography; DVT, deep vein thrombosis.

safety measures were developed as a result of the National Consensus Standards for the Prevention and Care of Deep Vein Thrombosis project between the Joint Commission and the National Quality Forum (NQF). Six VTE measures were endorsed by the NQF in May 2008, and these aligned with priorities of the Centers for Medicare and Medicaid Services.[20] Joint Commission Hospital National Patient Safety Goals emphasize the need for appropriate prophylactic measures.[21]

RISK FACTORS

A number of VTE risk factors have been identified, and new factors are currently being investigated. Individuals with an inherited blood clotting disorder or who experience a triggering event such as hospitalization, surgery, or long periods of immobility are more likely to develop DVT or PE. The risk for DVT and PE increases with age, especially after age 50. Women who are pregnant or take hormones (for birth control or menopausal therapy) are at increased risk. Predisposing conditions are summarized in Table 19.3.[41–59] Screening for a hypercoagulable state should be considered for atypical presentations of venous thrombosis,[60] including thrombosis in unusual locations (i.e., mesenteric veins or portal vein), idiopathic venous thrombosis, recurrent venous thrombosis, and superficial venous thrombosis (SVT) in a nonvaricose great saphenous vein.

CLINICAL DIAGNOSIS OF DVT

Anticoagulation for proximal DVT prevents thromboembolic complications in most patients, and it effectively prevents propagation of distal limb thrombi,[61] but anticoagulation is inconvenient and costly and can be associated with serious bleeding complications, so indiscriminant use of anticoagulant therapy is to be avoided. Thus, it is necessary to accurately make the diagnosis of DVT. The clinical diagnosis of DVT is notoriously inaccurate, lacking both sensitivity and specificity.[62] The optimal strategies for clinically assessing DVT risk (pretest probability) consider a combination of demographic and clinical factors. Several risk-scoring algorithms have been developed, including that from Wells et al (Table 19.4).[63] DVT risk estimates based on data from ambulatory and hospitalized populations may differ. Some have suggested that DVT prevalence may be higher in primary care settings than might be expected using the Wells calculations.[64]

D-Dimer

The D-dimer antigen is a marker of fibrin degradation from the action of thrombin, factor XIIIa, and plasmin on thrombus. Fibrin degradation products are created, exposing the D-dimer antigen. D-dimer antigen can exist on fibrin degradation products derived either from soluble fibrin or from fibrin clot that has been degraded by plasmin. D-dimers are unique fibrin degradation products, as they are produced only from the lysis of cross-linked fibrin (factor XIII cross-links the E-element to *two* D-elements).

The D-dimer concentration will be elevated in the presence of DVT, though an elevated D-dimer is nonspecific. In other words, a positive D-dimer result can indicate thrombosis, but it has other potential causes. This means a normal D-dimer measurement can be helpful for the exclusion of acute VTE, but a positive result does not confirm a DVT diagnosis, as D-dimer is a marker of activation of the coagulation system in other settings.[65] The D-dimer level can be high due to liver disease, inflammation, malignancy, trauma, pregnancy, and recent surgery, as well as advanced age. False negatives with D-dimer

TABLE 19.2

AMERICAN COLLEGE OF CARDIOLOGY FOUNDATION (ACCF) APPROPRIATE USE CRITERIA FOR LOWER EXTREMITY VENOUS DUPLEX ULTRASOUND

	APPROPRIATE USE SCORE	LIMB SWELLING	LIMB PAIN (WITHOUT SWELLING)	SHORTNESS OF BREATH	FEVER	KNOWN LOWER EXTREMITY VENOUS THROMBOSIS	SCREENING EXAMINATION FOR LOWER EXTREMITY DVT	POSTENDOVENOUS (GREAT OR SMALL) SAPHENOUS ABLATION	OTHER SYMPTOMS OR SIGNS OF VASCULAR DISEASE
Appropriate	9	Unilateral, acute							
	8	Bilateral, acute	Tender, palpable cord in the lower extremity	Suspected pulmonary embolus		New lower extremity pain or swelling, not on anticoagulation (i.e., contraindication to anticoagulation)		Lower extremity swelling or pain	
	7	Chronic persistent	Nonarticular pain in the lower extremity (e.g., calf or thigh)	Diagnosed pulmonary embolus		Surveillance of calf vein thrombosis for proximal propagation in patient with contraindication to anticoagulation (within 2 wk of diagnosis) New lower extremity pain or swelling while on anticoagulation Surveillance after diagnosis of lower extremity superficial phlebitis—not on anticoagulation, phlebitis location ≤5 cm from deep vein junction		Routine postprocedural follow-up, no lower extremity pain or swelling—within 10 d postprocedure	Physiologic testing positive for venous obstruction Patent foramen ovale with suspected paradoxical embolism for patient without lower extremity pain or swelling obstruction
May Be Appropriate	6	Bilateral, chronic, persistent; no alternative diagnosis identified (e.g., no congestive heart failure or anasarca from hypoalbuminemia)							

(Continued)

TABLE 19.2

AMERICAN COLLEGE OF CARDIOLOGY FOUNDATION (ACCF) APPROPRIATE USE CRITERIA FOR LOWER EXTREMITY VENOUS DUPLEX ULTRASOUND (*Continued*)

APPROPRIATE USE SCORE	LIMB SWELLING	LIMB PAIN (WITHOUT SWELLING)	SHORTNESS OF BREATH	FEVER	KNOWN LOWER EXTREMITY VENOUS THROMBOSIS	SCREENING EXAMINATION FOR LOWER EXTREMITY DVT	POSTENDOVENOUS (GREAT OR SMALL) SAPHENOUS ABLATION	OTHER SYMPTOMS OR SIGNS OF VASCULAR DISEASE
5				Fever of unknown origin (no indwelling lower extremity venous catheter) Fever with indwelling lower extremity venous catheter	Shortness of breath in a patient with known lower extremity DVT before anticipated discontinuation of anticoagulation treatment Surveillance after diagnosis of lower extremity superficial phlebitis—not on anticoagulation, phlebitis location ≥5 cm from deep vein junction			
Rarely Appropriate								
4								
3		Knee pain				After orthopedic surgery, prolonged ICU stay (e.g., >4 d) In those with high risk: acquired, inherited, or hypercoagulable state Positive D-dimer test in a hospital in patient		
2								

Appropriate Care: Median Scores 7 to 9
An appropriate option for management of this patient population due to **benefits generally outweighing risks**; effective option for individual care plans, although not always necessary.

May Be Appropriate Care: Median Scores 4 to 6
At times an appropriate option for management of this patient population due to variable evidence or agreement regarding the benefits/risks ratio, potential benefit based on practice experience in the absence of evidence, and/or variability in the population; effectiveness for individual care must be determined.

Rarely Appropriate Care: Median Scores 1 to 3
Rarely an appropriate option due to the lack of a clear benefit/risk advantage; rarely an effective option for individual care plans; exceptions should have appropriate documentation.

Adapted from: American College of Cardiology Foundation Appropriate Use Criteria Task Force; American College of Radiology; American Institute of Ultrasound in Medicine. ACCF/ACR/AIUM/ASE/IAC/SCAI/SCVS/SIR/SVM/SVS/SVU 2013 appropriate use criteria for peripheral vascular ultrasound and physiological testing. Part II: Testing for venous disease and evaluation of hemodialysis access. *Vasc Med* 2013;18(4):215-231. doi: 10.1177/1358863X13497637. PMID: 23897935.

testing can be encountered if a blood sample is obtained early in the process of thrombus formation, with limited thrombosis (e.g., limited to calf veins), or if testing is delayed for several days. Additionally, use of anticoagulant therapy can interfere with the test. Thus, the principal effectiveness of D-dimer testing is to exclude the diagnosis VTE when its probability is low, based on clinical criteria.[66]

Use of Combined Prediction Rules for DVT Diagnosis

Bayes' theorem is the statistical principle which states that the likelihood of a test yielding a true positive is highest if the test is applied to a population with a high prevalence of the condition that is the subject of the test. The diagnostic accuracy of testing for DVT improves when clinical probability is estimated before diagnostic tests are performd.[67] Due to the poor specificity of D-dimer testing for DVT, this laboratory test should be used as one element of an integrated diagnostic strategy that includes clinical probability assessment and imaging.[68]

In a systematic review of 14 studies involving more than 8,000 outpatients, the value of clinical prediction rules for the diagnosis of DVT, either with or without D-dimer, was evaluated.[69] The studies included all had sufficient information to allow the calculation of the prevalence of DVT for at least one of the three clinical probability estimates (low, moderate, or high) and had patient follow-up for a minimum of 3 months. The prevalence of DVT in the low, moderate, and high clinical probability groups was 5.0%, 17%, and 53%, respectively. The overall prevalence of DVT was 19%. Pooling the studies, the sensitivity and specificity of D-dimer testing in the low-probability group were 88% and 72%; in the moderate-probability group, 90% and 58%; and in the high-probability group, 92% and 45%. The likelihood ratio for a normal result on a highly sensitive D-dimer assay among patients with (1) low clinical suspicion was 0.10, (2) moderate clinical suspicion was 0.05, and (3) high clinical suspicion was 0.07. Thus, it was very uncommon to have a normal D-dimer result in settings where DVT was likely. Patients with low clinical probability on the predictive rules have a prevalence of DVT of less than 5%.

Another review by Fancher et al analyzed 12 studies with more than 5000 outpatients tested with a rapid D-dimer assay after categorization into low, intermediate, or high clinical probability of DVT on the basis of clinical criteria. Using a less sensitive D-dimer assay, the 3-month incidence of VTE was 0.5% among patients with a low clinical probability of DVT and a normal D-dimer concentration. When a highly sensitive D dimer assay was used, the 3-month incidence of VTE was 0.4% among outpatients with low or moderate clinical probability of DVT and a normal D-dimer concentration.[70]

To summarize, in *low-probability* patients with negative D-dimer results, a diagnosis of DVT can be excluded without additional diagnostic testing (e.g., venous duplex scan), but in patients for whom there is a high clinical suspicion for DVT, D-dimer results should not affect clinical decisions.

VASCULAR LABORATORY TESTS FOR DVT

Plethysmography

Plethysmographic techniques are indirect tests that evaluate venous hemodynamics by assessing the changes in limb volume that occur as the venous capacitance vessels fill or empty. These techniques include impedance plethysmography (IPG), air plethysmography (AP),[71] mercury strain gauge plethysmography (SGP),[72,73] photoplethysmography (PPG),[74–76] and foot volumetry. The limb increases in volume when a thigh cuff is inflated to a pressure below arterial but above the venous pressure. Normally, limb volume rapidly returns toward baseline with release of the thigh cuff. In most cases, half of the venous emptying occurs in the first 2 seconds after cuff release.

IPG was an early vascular laboratory standard for diagnosis of DVT associated with hemodynamically significant venous outflow obstruction.[77–80] The impedance plethysmograph measured changes in electrical impedance in an extremity after inflation and release of a proximal venous tourniquet to diagnose the presence of compromised venous outflow.[81–84] A normal IPG test was helpful to rule out the presence of the highest-risk DVT condition, a large proximal DVT.[81]

Plethysmographic techniques do not provide anatomically specific information; they only suggest the diagnosis of DVT. Delayed venous outflow after cuff release indicates a more central obstruction, but the finding is not specific for the location or cause of the outflow obstruction. Plethysmography cannot reliably detect distal (calf vein) or nonocclusive thrombi. Other physiologic or physical abnormalities can produce false-positive tests—including obesity, pregnancy, congestive heart failure, external venous compression, and chronic DVT—but these conditions may also be risk factors for acute DVT. Lack of patient cooperation, arterial occlusive disease, and low-ambient temperatures may also contribute to inadequate venous plethysmography results. Based on these limitations, venous plethysmography is no longer appropriate for the evaluation of suspected acute DVT, although it may have an ancillary role for physiologic evaluations in the vascular laboratory.

Doppler Flow Detection

The use of continuous-wave or pulsed Doppler ultrasound for flow detection was another early technique to assess for venous thrombosis.[85–92] The absence of Doppler-detectable flow in an insonated segment was used as a criterion for the diagnosis of DVT, but the early Doppler ultrasound systems lacked the imaging capability needed to allow the technologist to be certain about which vein was being evaluated, and they did not provide information about anatomic abnormalities.

The early techniques of Doppler flow detection were insensitive to calf vein thrombi and to limited or nonocclusive thrombus. Performance and interpretation of these examinations required highly experienced personnel, as Doppler findings alone were subjective. False-positive examinations resulted from chronic disease interpreted as acute thrombosis or from the interpretation of low amplitude signals as indicative of thrombosis, though this might have been a nonpathologic finding in calf veins, in obese patients, or with excessive Doppler probe pressure impairing venous flow.[93,94] A negative Doppler flow study in a patient with low suspicion for acute DVT was considered sufficient to rule out the diagnosis, but venography was needed when the noninvasive study was equivocal or when the clinical circumstances strongly suggested the diagnosis.[95–97]

Ultrasound Imaging Techniques

First described by Talbot in 1982,[4] B-mode ultrasound imaging for diagnosis of lower extremity venous thrombosis has proved to be practical and widely adopted. DVT is diagnosed by direct visualization of thrombus in the veins. Unlike normal veins that easily collapse with extrinsic compression, thrombosed segments appear dilated and do not collapse with the application of manual (transducer) pressure over the imaged segment.

TABLE 19.3

RISK FACTORS ASSOCIATED WITH VENOUS THROMBOEMBOLISM (VTE)

■ ACQUIRED[22]	■ GENETIC[23–36]	■ HEMATOLOGIC DISEASES[24,37–40]
Age	Activated protein C (APC) resistance/ factor V Leiden mutation	Heparin-induced thrombocytopenia (HIT)
Malignancy		
Surgery (especially orthopedic)	Deficiencies of antithrombin, proteins C and S	Polycythemia rubra vera
Trauma		Essential thrombocytosis
Presence of central venous catheter	Prothrombin 20210A gene variants	Myelodysplasia
Immobilization	Antithrombin deficiency/reduced heparin cofactor II activity	
Oral contraceptive use		
Hormone replacement therapy	Hyperhomocysteinemia	
Tamoxifen, thalidomide, lenalidomide	Dysfibrinogenemia	
Pregnancy and the puerperium	Dysplasminogenemia	
Obesity	Elevated levels of clotting factors XI, IX, VII, VIII, X, and II	
Neurologic and cardiac diseases		
Antiphospholipid antibody syndrome	Elevation in plasminogen activator inhibitor 1	
Inflammatory bowel disease		
Nephrotic syndrome		
Congestive heart failure		

Early validation studies comparing venous ultrasonography to the reference standard of contrast venography identified shortcomings in the use of B-mode imaging as a stand-alone modality, as imaging of deeper structures was limited and some normal venous segments might not collapse with moderate probe pressure (e.g., femoral vein at the level of the adductor hiatus). Venous compressibility can also be limited by obesity, edema, or tenderness. It was soon recognized that duplex scanning, the combination of B-mode imaging *and* Doppler-derived information about the presence and nature of venous flow in the interrogated segments, improved the accuracy of the examination.[98]

Duplex scanning was rapidly adopted for diagnosis of DVT due to its clear advantages over the more cumbersome indirect plethysmographic methods. A review by White et al[99] found the sensitivity of duplex ultrasound for detecting proximal limb thrombi in four well-designed studies (1980–1988) was 92% to 95%, with reported specificity of 97% to 100%. Similar findings were noted in nine other studies that had minor methodologic flaws. It was also recognized that ultrasound imaging could identify a nonthrombotic cause of leg symptoms in 5% to 15% of cases.

Advances in imaging technologies have further improved the accuracy and ease of venous studies for DVT. The addition of color flow Doppler imaging facilitates vessel identification in large limbs and helps with calf vein evaluation. All examination protocols, however, utilize compression as a basic element of the study.

In a clinical practice guideline from the American Thoracic Society, the sensitivity and specificity of various ultrasound techniques for DVT diagnosis were reviewed.[100] In those papers reporting results from appropriately designed prospective studies with venographic correlation, the sensitivity of real-time B-mode (compression) ultrasound for suspected proximal DVT in symptomatic patients was 89% to 100%, with reported specificity ranging from 86% to 100%. Studies of venous duplex scanning reported sensitivities of 88% to 97% and specificities of 80% to 100%. Reports of the accuracy of color flow Doppler ultrasound indicated a sensitivity of 95% to 96% and specificity of 99% to 100%.

Because of its accuracy, low cost, and noninvasive nature, venous duplex scanning is now the diagnostic method of choice for DVT.[101] However, a potentially unwanted effect of the test

TABLE 19.4

WELLS SCORE FOR ESTIMATING PROBABILITY OF DEEP VEIN THROMBOSIS

1 POINT EACH FOR:
Active malignancy
Paralysis, paresis, recent plaster immobilization of lower limb
Recently bedridden for more than 3 d or major surgery in past 4 wk
Localized tenderness along distribution of deep venous system
Entire limb swollen
Calf swelling more than 3 cm compared to asymptomatic leg
Pitting edema
Collateral superficial veins

2 POINTS FOR:
Alternative diagnosis as likely or more likely than that of DVT

PROBABILITY:
High	≥3 points
Intermediate	1–2 points
Low	≤0 points

being so safe, inexpensive, and widely available is its overuse. Providers may tend to request the examination unnecessarily for irrelevant clinical signs and in the absence of any evident DVT risk factors.[102,103]

Point of Care Ultrasound Imaging for DVT

The availability of point of care ultrasound (POCUS) systems in emergency rooms, intensive care units, and other clinical settings can facilitate testing for DVT, but with potential for diagnostic errors.[104] With appropriate training, however, it appears that nonvascular specialist physicians can diagnose femoropopliteal DVT with accuracies approaching those of vascular laboratory professionals.[105] The two-point compression ultrasound examination of the common femoral and popliteal veins as a screening test for acute proximal lower extremity DVT is discussed in Chapter 27. It is anticipated that venous POCUS applications will become increasingly important in clinical practice.

ADVANCED IMAGING MODALITIES

Although venous duplex ultrasonography has become the standard for detection of acute DVT, adjuvant modalities have roles in selected cases.[106]

Magnetic Resonance Imaging

Magnetic resonance venography (MRV) can be used for evaluating the pelvic veins.[107–111] Thrombus is evident either as a venous segment without flow or as a discrete filling defect in the vein lumen with a flow-based approach such as time-of-flight or gradient-focused rapid imaging. MRV is most likely to be useful when venous thrombi are located above the inguinal ligament or when extrinsic compression of the iliac veins mimics the signs and symptoms of DVT, but MRV has also been found useful for femoropopliteal and calf DVT evaluations, with accuracy reported to be greater than 90% in the few series studying this application.[112,113] MRV is contraindicated for patients with pacemakers, and those with claustrophobia do not tolerate the procedure well.

Computed Tomographic Venography

Computed tomography (CT) can also be used to diagnose lower extremity DVT. Similar to MRV, computed tomographic venography (CTV) was originally used for evaluation of the iliac veins.[114,115] There are potential advantages of CTV over iliac vein venography, as CT scanning can identify sources of extrinsic venous compression, as well as diagnose thrombosis. CTV does not, however, yield high-resolution anatomic details of the vein lumen, and CTV may not detect subtle changes from prior episodes of DVT.

CTV obtained in conjunction with CT pulmonary angiography has been evaluated for the diagnosis of DVT in thigh and calf veins.[116–118] Delayed (3-minute) imaging shows good diagnostic performance when compared to contrast venography and ultrasound imaging. This approach offers the potential advantage of screening for both DVT and PE with a single examination, but the accuracy and cost-effectiveness of this approach are not well-established.

DUPLEX SCANNING FOR DVT: ISSUES FOR THE VASCULAR LABORATORY

Bilateral Versus Unilateral Examinations

The noninvasive nature of duplex scanning makes it a suitable test to use for screening or evaluation of asymptomatic limbs. Routinely scanning both extremities, however, appears to be unnecessary in all cases,[119] and unilateral studies are commonly done in many vascular laboratories.[120]

A unilateral approach is justified when a prothrombotic state is not suspected, when there are no systemic symptoms or indications of PE, and when the study is done as a follow-up to assess a limb with known DVT (Fig. 19.1). When outpatients are referred for evaluation of unilateral lower extremity symptoms, it is rare to find unsuspected thrombus in the asymptomatic contralateral limb, unless the patient has risk factors for thrombosis. The incidence of unilateral thrombus in an asymptomatic extremity in an otherwise healthy individual approximates 1%.[121] Outpatients are at risk for clinically silent thrombus in an asymptomatic extremity if they have coagulopathic risk factors such as active malignancy, recent operation or injury, prolonged bed rest, or pregnancy.[122] For

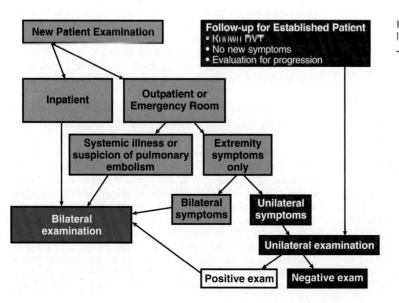

FIGURE 19.1. Algorithm for selecting a unilateral versus bilateral venous duplex examination.

PERIPHERAL VENOUS

these patients, a bilateral study is recommended. Inpatients and patients with bilateral symptoms warrant a bilateral evaluation.[123,124]

Calf Vein Thrombosis

The importance of calf vein thrombosis has been a subject of some controversy. Though isolated calf vein thrombi do not cause clinically relevant PE, these patients are at risk for thrombus progression to involve the femoropopliteal veins. Symptomatic calf vein thrombi are associated with progression or recurrent thrombosis in 15% to 20% percent of patients within 3 months.[125,126] Calf vein thrombosis can be a predictor of thromboembolic risk for which anticoagulation may be indicated.[61] However, routine treatment of all patients with calf DVT does risk overuse of anticoagulation.[127] Factors that appear important in stratifying risk include whether thrombus is confined to the distal limb veins (isolated calf DVT) or also involves the veins of the proximal limb[128–130] and whether the DVT was a first episode of VTE or a second or subsequent episode.[131,132]

In a meta-analysis that included two randomized controlled trials (RCTs) and six cohort studies, PE was significantly less frequent in patients with calf DVT who received anticoagulation compared to those who were not treated, with a trend toward fewer deaths with anticoagulation. When the analysis was limited to RCTs, the benefit of anticoagulation for PE was no longer statistically significant, but the benefit for preventing thrombus progression persisted.[133] Thus, treatment options for patients with calf DVT include either routine anticoagulation or selective anticoagulation if a follow-up duplex scan demonstrates thrombus progression. The ninth edition of the ACCP guidelines recommends serial imaging for 2 weeks, rather than initial anticoagulation, for isolated acute calf vein thrombosis without severe symptoms and when the patient does not have risk factors for thrombus propagation.[134] Patients at increased risk include those who have recently had orthopedic procedures, patients with malignancy, and those who are immobile.[135]

Color flow duplex scanning has been found to be reliable as a method for evaluating calf veins for DVT, but calf veins may be poorly imaged in obese patients or those with chronic edema. Calf vein thrombosis is common in patients who have acute DVT and often occurs as an isolated finding.[136] The peroneal and posterior tibial veins are involved in the majority of cases; thrombi occur much less frequently in the anterior tibial veins.

Calf Muscle Venous Thrombosis

Thrombosis of veins within the gastrocnemius or soleus muscles of the calf either can be an isolated finding or can be found in combination with proximal DVT. Calf muscle venous thrombosis (CMVT) can be associated with localized calf tenderness. In rare cases, there can be propagation and subsequent PE, but isolated CMVT, compared to thrombosis of multiple calf veins, appears to have a lower risk of extension, and if extension is not observed within 2 weeks, it is unlikely to occur.[134,137–139]

Treatment recommendations for isolated CMVT vary. Some studies have shown reduced risk of thrombus progression or PE with anticoagulation therapy, but others showed no benefit.[139] For low-risk patients without active cancer (or other prothrombotic conditions), anticoagulation is not necessary. Patients with transient risk factors, however, should be re-evaluated with duplex scanning 1 week after diagnosis to confirm thrombus resolution or absence of progression.[140]

Diagnosis of Recurrent DVT

Recurrent thromboembolic events after an initial episode of DVT are relatively frequent.[141] Patients with a treated DVT may be referred for repeat studies if they have new symptoms of pain and swelling. Differentiating postthrombotic symptoms from recurrent acute DVT is facilitated if a new baseline is established after a course of anticoagulation has been completed.

The predictive value of sonographic features for establishing the age of a deep vein thrombus is not well-established. The sonographic features that distinguish acute from chronic thrombus need to be considered in the context of the patient's clinical presentation, and it should be emphasized that no imaging feature can be considered reliable in all circumstances. The features of chronic DVT can be confused with acute thrombosis (or "acute-on-chronic DVT"). Understanding the ambiguity of the ultrasound diagnosis can be important, as it is not uncommon for a patient with PTS (including pain and swelling) to be referred to the vascular laboratory to "rule out DVT."

The late appearance of a venous segment can vary significantly after acute DVT. Some segments may remain chronically occluded, or there may be complete or partial recanalization. Thrombus echogenicity can vary, and the appearance of thrombus can be altered by changes in the image-processing settings, and it can be affected by image depth and transducer selection. Incomplete compressibility, a feature of acute non-occlusive DVT, can also be observed with chronic DVT when there is partial recanalization of a previously occluded segment.[142] Veins with acute thrombus typically appear larger than normal veins, and veins with chronic DVT are generally smaller than normal veins, but the ranges of normal and abnormal vein diameters overlap, so size alone cannot be used for the diagnosis of acute versus chronic DVT, except perhaps at "extreme" diameters.[143]

Only when the extent of residual thrombus has been established can the diagnosis of acute-on-chronic thrombosis be made with ultrasound imaging. When a subsequent examination shows thrombosis of previously clear segments, the diagnosis can be made with confidence. On the other hand, visualization of chronic thrombus with no change from prior examinations suggests venous insufficiency from PTS as the cause for recurrent or persistent symptoms. Other features of PTS may include venous reflux (see Chapter 21).

A negative D-dimer test can be used to confirm the absence of new acute thrombosis.[144] For the evaluation of patients with suspected recurrent DVT when a prior ultrasound is not available for comparison, D-dimer testing with a high-sensitivity assay is the recommended first step.[145] As with the initial diagnosis of acute DVT, the finding of an elevated D-dimer is nonspecific, and the abnormal result cannot be taken as an indication that there is recurrent acute thrombosis.

Guiding the Duration of Anticoagulation for DVT

While 3 to 6 months of therapy is a common clinical recommendation for acute DVT, the optimal duration of anticoagulation may differ for individual patients. Anticoagulation continues to reduce the risk of recurrent VTE for as long as it is used, although the absolute risk of recurrent VTE declines over time.[146] While the risk of recurrent VTE is reduced with long-term antithrombotic therapy, this benefit must be weighed against the risk of bleeding, costs, and patient preferences. Patients with an increased risk for bleeding on long-term anticoagulation therapy are those with advanced age, previous bleeding episodes, renal or hepatic impairment, treatment with high-intensity anticoagulation, and concomitant therapy with antiplatelet agents. Because anticoagulation risks persist as treatment benefit declines, the overall efficacy of continued therapy decreases over time.

Clinical prediction rules have been developed to estimate risks of VTE recurrence after a course of anticoagulation for acute DVT, as well as to guide the duration and intensity of continued therapy. The presence of residual thrombus after the completion of a course of anticoagulant therapy was identified as a potential risk factor for recurrent DVT.[22,141,147–149] It has also been identified as a risk factor for other adverse outcomes, including death, suggesting that failure of thrombus resolution may be a marker of vascular dysfunction.[22] In some studies, absence of residual thrombus after treatment was associated with a lower risk for DVT recurrence after discontinuation of anticoagulation.[141,147]

The AESOPUS trial evaluated treatment of DVT, with anticoagulation duration based on the absence or persistence of residual thrombi on ultrasonography.[23] After a 3-month period of anticoagulation, this trial randomized DVT patients to fixed-duration anticoagulation (no further anticoagulation for secondary thrombosis and an extra 3 months for unprovoked thrombosis) or flexible-duration, ultrasound-guided anticoagulation. In the ultrasound-guided treatment group, no further treatment was given if the veins had recanalized, but other patients continued anticoagulation for up to 9 months for secondary DVT and up to 21 months for unprovoked thrombosis. The rate of confirmed recurrent VTE during 33 months of follow-up was 17% in the patients allocated to fixed-duration anticoagulation and 12% for patients allocated to flexible-duration, suggesting that tailoring the duration of anticoagulation on the basis of ultrasound findings might reduce the rate of recurrent VTE in adults with proximal DVT. However, an important limitation of this study was the lack of a comparison group without residual thrombus that was treated with continued anticoagulation.

The PROLONG study evaluated patients with D-dimer testing 1 month after the discontinuation of anticoagulation for an episode of unprovoked proximal DVT. Those with a normal D-dimer level did not resume anticoagulation, while those with an abnormal D-dimer were randomized to either resume anticoagulation or continue without therapy. Patient follow-up averaged 1.4 years. For those with an elevated D-dimer, the adjusted hazard ratio for recurrent VTE was 4.3 for patients who were not anticoagulated compared to those who were.[24] Further analysis of data from this trial suggested that the effect of a persistently elevated D-dimer on recurrent VTE risk was more significant than the persistence of sonographically identified residual thrombosis.[25]

It appears that any component of risk associated with residual venous obstruction (thrombus) as a predictor for recurrent VTE declines over time. In a meta-analysis of ten prospective studies including 2527 patients with a first unprovoked DVT, residual venous obstruction was found in 55% after a median of 6 months. Recurrent VTE occurred in 16% during a median follow-up of 23.3 months. When found 3 months after the acute DVT, residual venous obstruction was associated with increased recurrent VTE risk (hazard ratio 2.2), but there was no significant increase in recurrent VTE risk associated with the finding of residual thrombus after 6 months. This suggests that the presence of persistent chronic thrombus is not an indicator of an ongoing prothrombotic condition.[26] In general, ultrasound findings of residual venous thrombus should not be used as a primary or stand-alone basis for decisions about the duration of anticoagulation for DVT, but they should be considered in the clinical context.

DUPLEX EVALUATION

Instrumentation

Lower extremity deep veins are well-visualized by ultrasound in most patients and generally easy to evaluate for thrombosis. A full-featured, high-resolution duplex scanner enables the technologist to perform a quality examination and to identify subtle segments of abnormalities or thrombosis, even in large patients. Transducer selection depends on the depth of the veins scanned and the approach used. A 5- to 10-MHz linear array transducer is often sufficient for a complete lower extremity venous examination. However, a 3- to 5-MHz curved linear transducer may be necessary when evaluating deeply located vessels such as the inferior vena cava (IVC) and iliac veins or to evaluate obese patients or edematous extremities.

Patient Preparation and Positioning

No special patient preparation is needed before a lower extremity venous duplex examination from the level of the groin to the distal leg, but it is helpful to have the patient fast for 4 to 6 hours if the IVC or iliac veins are to be evaluated to reduce overlying bowel gas that may interfere with imaging. The standard examination is performed with the patient supine and the bed or gurney adjusted to provide moderate reverse Trendelenburg (head up, feet down) positioning. This promotes venous filling in the lower extremities and facilitates ultrasound visualization.

To facilitate a thorough examination of all relevant lower extremity veins (Table 19.5), the extremity being evaluated should be completely exposed to the ankle, and the limb should be externally rotated at the hip and slightly bent at the knee. Positioning the patient as close to the technologist as possible helps the technologist use ergonomically correct body mechanics. However, some patient factors can make patient positioning and scanning difficult, including paraplegia, recent extremity surgery, trauma, or the need to perform the examination in the intensive care unit. Assistance with optimal patient positioning in such cases may facilitate use of scanning positions that reduce stresses on the back, shoulder, and wrist of the technologist.

B-Mode Imaging

Normal Findings

B-mode imaging is used to perform venous compression maneuvers and for direct visualization of intraluminal abnormalities. Vein compression is performed by manual application of enough downward probe pressure to coapt the vein walls without compressing the adjacent artery (Fig. 19.2). A patent, thrombus-free vein will demonstrate complete vein wall coaptation with probe compression along its entire course, with no intraluminal echoes identified (Fig. 19.3). Compressions should be performed in a transverse (cross-sectional) view to make sure that the entire vessel is visualized during the maneuver. If a longitudinal view is used, the probe can slip off the vessel, giving a false impression of complete vein wall compression. Veins should be evaluated for compressibility in segments approximately one probe width apart.

Abnormal Findings

Vein incompressibility reliably indicates the presence of intraluminal thrombus. In the presence of an acute thrombus, the vein will be incompressible and dilated; the vein diameter is usually larger than that of the adjacent artery, and intraluminal echoes are typically anechoic or hypoechoic (Fig. 19.4). Acute thrombus

TABLE 19.5

NOMENCLATURE OF THE DEEP VEINS OF THE LOWER EXTREMITY

Imaging of the locations in **bold text** is required by IAC-Vascular Testing standards for an examination for deep vein thrombosis or obstruction.[150,152,153]

THIGH
Common femoral vein
Saphenofemoral junction
Femoral vein (proximal, mid, and distal thigh)
Deep femoral (profunda femoris) vein
Deep femoral communicating veins (accompanying veins of perforating arteries)
Medial circumflex femoral vein
Lateral circumflex femoral vein
Sciatic vein

KNEE
Popliteal vein
Genicular venous plexus

LEG
Sural veins
Soleal veins
Gastrocnemius veins
Medial gastrocnemius veins
Lateral gastrocnemius veins
Intergemellar vein
Anterior tibial veins
Posterior tibial veins
Fibular or peroneal veins

FOOT
Medial plantar veins
Lateral plantar veins
Deep plantar venous arch
Deep metatarsal veins (plantar and dorsal)
Deep digital veins (plantar and dorsal)
Pedal vein

Adapted from Caggiati A, Bergan JJ. Gloviczki P, et al. Nomenclature of the veins of the lower limbs: an international interdisciplinary consensus statement. *J Vasc Surg* 2002;36(2):416-422; Caggiati A, Bergan JJ, Gloviczki P, et al. Nomenclature of the veins of the lower limb: extensions, refinements, and clinical application. *J Vasc Surg* 2005;41(4):719-724. ICAVL Standards for Accreditation in Noninvasive Vascular Testing. Part II. Vascular Laboratory Operations: Peripheral Venous Testing. 2007; http://www.icavl.org/icavl/pdfs/venous2007.pdf. Accessed June 30, 2009. IAC, Intersocietal Accreditation Commission

may be visualized adherent to the vein wall, or it may demonstrate mobility such as a "free-floating thrombus" or "thrombus tail" (Fig. 19.5). Although the risk of causing thromboembolism is probably small,[27] caution is advised in performing compression maneuvers over a nonoccluding mobile thrombus, as there have been reports of acute embolization of loosely attached thrombi during examinations.[28–30] As previously discussed, it is not possible to reliably determine the age of a venous thrombus by ultrasound; however, some general features that help to distinguish between acute and chronic thrombus are listed in Table 19.6.

Veins may be difficult to completely collapse with probe compression when they are deeply situated or located within relatively incompressible tissues, such as in the pelvis or adductor canal area above the knee. Evaluation with pulsed Doppler or color flow Doppler imaging can confirm the patency of venous segments that do not easily collapse with compression. Outflow obstruction with resulting venous hypertension can make a vein appear dilated, incompressible, and without spontaneous flow. In this unusual circumstance, the segment may be incorrectly reported as occluded.

Color Flow and Pulsed Doppler

Normal Findings

Color flow Doppler and pulsed Doppler spectral waveform analysis are used to evaluate venous flow characteristics. Color flow Doppler is helpful in confirming patency of venous segments that are incompletely evaluated with B-mode imaging (Fig. 19.6). This helps to differentiate between occluding and nonoccluding thrombus and identify anechoic thrombus by visualization of flow around it (Fig. 19.7). The color velocity scale (pulse repetition frequency or PRF) should be at a low setting to detect low-velocity venous flow.

Doppler spectral waveforms should indicate a flow pattern that is spontaneous (present without augmentation) and phasic (varying with the respiratory cycle), as shown in Figure 19.8. By convention, flow waveforms are displayed with normal antegrade venous flow (flow toward the heart) below the baseline. Respiratory phasicity represents the normal variations in lower extremity venous flow that occur in response to changes in abdominal pressure as the diaphragm moves up and down. Venous flow patterns become less phasic and spontaneous with distance from the heart, so these features may not be prominent in the tibial veins. Comparing venous flow waveforms from the left and right sides is helpful in distinguishing normal variation from pathologic findings. Asymmetric flow patterns suggest a unilateral abnormality.

Distal augmentation maneuvers are performed with manual calf compressions while interrogating the common femoral, femoral, and popliteal vein segments. Foot compressions can be used to evaluate the tibial and peroneal veins. A sharp "spike" of antegrade venous flow in response to distal limb compression suggests patency between the level of compression and the site of Doppler interrogation (Fig. 19.9). Blunted or absent augmentation of flow with distal limb compression suggests obstruction below the level being interrogated. Distal augmentation maneuvers are not recommended when an acute deep vein thrombus has already been identified.

The Valsalva maneuver or proximal compression maneuvers may be used to test valvular competency (Fig. 19.10); however, a complete examination for reflux is not required as part of a duplex examination for acute DVT. The evaluation of chronic venous insufficiency is discussed in Chapter 21. Valvular incompetence may be associated with chronic DVT, and it is a feature of the PTS (Figs. 19.11, 19.12, and 19.13).

Abnormal Findings

The absence of color flow within a vein segment while performing distal augmentation maneuvers usually indicates occlusion, most often from thrombus within the vein. Color PRF should be set low and gain should be set high when evaluating a suspected occlusion to minimize the risk of a false-positive finding. Absence of spontaneous and phasic flow patterns may indicate obstruction in the veins cephalad to the level of interrogation. Continuous or high-velocity flow patterns suggest venous stenosis or extrinsic compression. A comparison of the flow characteristics in the common femoral vein on the side of interest to the contralateral common femoral vein is useful for detecting iliac vein thrombus or obstruction.

Scanning Technique and Protocol

Femoropopliteal Segment

The deep veins are evaluated from the level of the inguinal ligament to the distal popliteal fossa with the patient in the supine position. The common femoral, profunda femoris (deep femoral), and femoral veins are best scanned using an

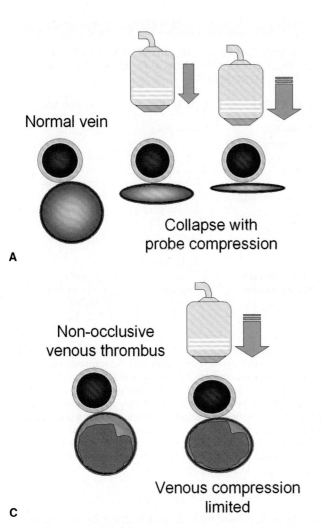

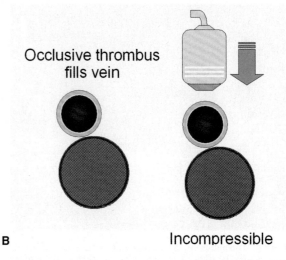

FIGURE 19.2. The presence or absence of thrombus within an imaged vein can be confirmed with probe compression in a transverse view. *A*, Increasing the pressure of the transducer on the examined vein will result in collapse of the normal thin-walled and low-pressure vein. *B*, If the vein is filled with thrombus, it will be incompressible. *C*, Nonocclusive thrombus may allow some but limited compression of the vein.

anterior and medial approach along the thigh. The popliteal vein is visualized with a posterior-medial scanning approach in the popliteal fossa (Fig. 19.14). Probe compressions are obtained at each level, as described previously. Some ultrasound systems allow recording of side-by-side images, a feature that can be used to demonstrate comparable views of the

vein, open and compressed. Alternatively, brief segments of recorded video (cine loops) can be captured to show the vein as it is compressed.

While imaging in a longitudinal view, representative Doppler spectral waveforms are recorded from the common femoral vein, the femoral vein in the proximal thigh, and the

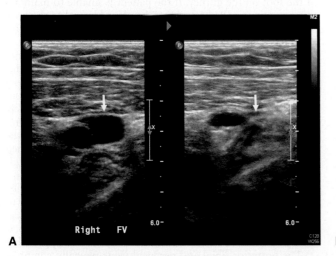

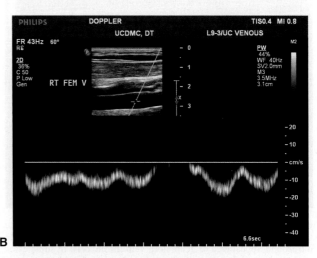

FIGURE 19.3. *A*, Normal femoral vein in transverse view (*arrows*): *Left*, without probe compression; *Right*, with compression and vein walls completely coapted. The adjacent superficial femoral artery is partially compressed. *B*, Normal femoral vein in longitudinal view is seen to have a smooth surface, thin wall, and hypoechoic lumen. A normal, spontaneous, phasic flow pattern is demonstrated.

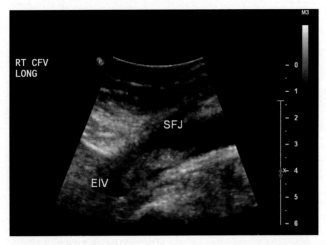

FIGURE 19.4. Thrombus in the common femoral vein (CFV). In some cases, it may be difficult to determine the cephalad extent of iliofemoral thrombus, as iliac veins are deep in the pelvis and may be obscured by bowel gas. (EIV, external iliac vein; SFJ, saphenofemoral junction.)

TABLE 19.6

ULTRASOUND FEATURES THAT MAY HELP TO DISTINGUISH BETWEEN ACUTE AND CHRONIC VENOUS THROMBUS

■ FEATURE	■ ACUTE	■ CHRONIC
Thrombus echogenicity	Hypoechoic	Echogenic
Vein lumen size	Larger, distended	Smaller, irregular
Vein wall	Thin, smooth lumen	Thickened, hyperechoic
Compressibility	Slightly deformable, "spongy" (may not be completely occlusive)	Rigid, incompressible (may be partially recanalized)
Collateral veins	Absent	Present
Valve function	Competent (usually)	Incompetent (reflux)

popliteal vein. The scale or PRF and gain settings are optimized for low flow velocities. Distal augmentation maneuvers are performed while interrogating each of the segments. If the ability to perform calf compressions is limited due to patient discomfort or overlying materials such as a hard cast or splint, the patient can be asked to briskly dorsiflex the foot in order to augment venous flow.

Several conditions may limit this part of the venous duplex examination, possibly leading to false-positive results. The common femoral vein can sometimes be difficult to compress under the inguinal ligament. Using a different probe position or having the patient rotate onto the hip of the side being interrogated helps eliminate this problem. The veins in the adductor canal are deep and may require extreme probe pressure for complete compression. It is helpful to use the opposite hand to apply pressure from the posterior thigh when interrogating the femoral vein, especially where the veins are deep in the distal

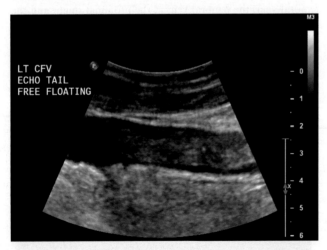

FIGURE 19.5. Homogeneous moderately echoic material filling the lumen of this common femoral vein (CFV) is typical for the B-mode ultrasound appearance of acute deep vein thrombosis. In some cases of thrombosis in large veins, the cephalad end of the thrombus may not be attached to the vein wall ("free floating") and it may be seen to move.

thigh. Also, assuming a more anterior approach in the thigh may yield better visualization and easier compression.

Be aware that the femoral and popliteal veins may be duplicated (Figs. 19.6 and 19.15).[31,32] In this setting, a thorough evaluation of both veins is important, as thrombus can be present in only one of the paired veins.[33–35] In some patients, the profunda femoris vein is the larger, dominant vein in the thigh, and the femoral vein may be small in caliber.[36] Rarely, the profunda femoris vein directly communicates with the popliteal vein in the popliteal fossa.[37]

Calf Veins

Duplex evaluation of the veins in the calf can be more challenging due to their smaller size and variable anatomy. Familiarity with the normal anatomy and examiner patience are required for calf vein evaluation. The limb is slightly flexed at the knee and externally rotated at the hip. The calf muscles should be completely relaxed to allow maximum venous filling. Alternatively, visualization of calf veins may be facilitated by positioning the patient supine with the knee flexed at a 45- to 60-degree angle, pointing the knee upward, with the bottom of the foot on the gurney. If the patient is unable to maintain this position, a rolled towel may be placed lateral to the knee to provide support while the limb is externally rotated. This also helps achieve relaxation of the calf muscles.

The posterior tibial and peroneal veins are evaluated from the ankle to the tibioperoneal trunk vein. These are paired veins that accompany the adjacent artery (Fig. 19.16). The arterial pulsation is a useful landmark for identification of the concomitant veins. Each of the paired veins should be completely evaluated with B-mode imaging using transverse probe compressions. Bony landmarks are also useful in identifying the calf veins. The posterior tibial veins are most easily identified posterior to the medial malleolus. These veins can then be followed proximally to their confluence with the peroneal veins. As a medial scanning approach is most common, the posterior tibial veins appear closer to the transducer (displayed closer to the top of the image), as shown in Figure 19.17. The peroneal veins lie adjacent and posterior to the fibula, appearing superficial to the fibula when scanning from a posterior approach.

The posterior tibial and peroneal veins typically compress easily with probe pressure. Poor patient positioning, obesity, or edema may interfere with effective probe compression of these veins. Manual counter pressure can be applied on the

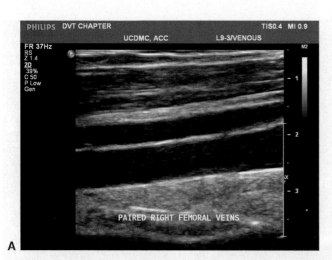

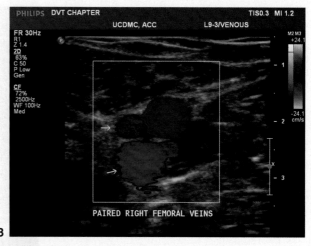

FIGURE 19.6. The deep veins below the knee are paired, but paired veins in the proximal lower limb are a common variant. *A,* Longitudinal B-mode image of paired femoral veins. *B,* Color Doppler imaging in the transverse plane shows the paired femoral veins to be unequal in size, a typical finding when two femoral veins are present.

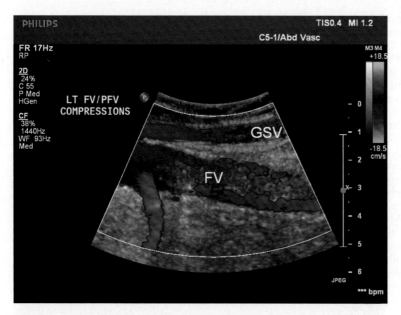

FIGURE 19.7. Acute thrombus may not be tightly attached to the vein wall. Color Doppler demonstrates flow around acute intraluminal thrombus in the femoral vein (FV) with distal thigh compression (augmentation). The great saphenous vein (GSV) is patent.

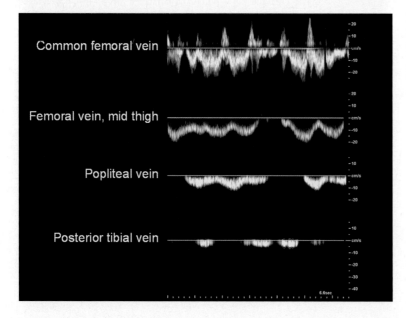

FIGURE 19.8. Normal flow in the lower extremity veins is spontaneous (occurring without calf pump function or augmentation maneuvers) and phasic with respiration. Observed flow patterns are different in various locations, with less spontaneous flow in the small veins of the distal limb.

FIGURE 19.9. Color Doppler image of a normal common femoral vein (CFV). Flow is phasic with respiration. Transient reversal of flow is normally observed in a supine subject, as retrograde flow velocities with respiration may be insufficient for vein valve closure. Augmentation of flow (a brief increase in antegrade flow velocity) can be demonstrated with manual compression of the limb (DST AUGMENT).

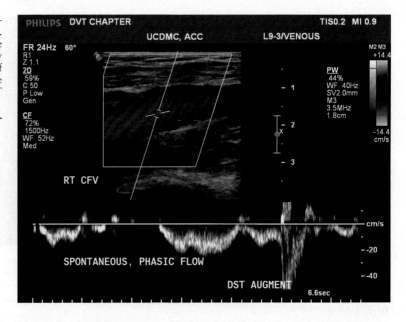

lateral aspect of the calf with the opposite hand while performing probe compression maneuvers in the calf. Scanning of the tibioperoneal trunk is continued cephalad into the popliteal fossa to ensure that the calf vein evaluation overlaps with the evaluation of the popliteal vein. Due to the depth of the tibioperoneal trunk veins, more probe pressure and a slight change in hand and transducer position may be needed for complete coaptation of the vein walls.

Color flow Doppler is especially useful for determining patency of the calf veins and differentiating between occluding and nonoccluding thrombus. Due to the normal lack of spontaneous flow in the calf veins, distal augmentation maneuvers from the foot or calf (distal to the level of insonation) may be needed to confirm calf vein patency with color Doppler. Color flow imaging is particularly helpful when leg swelling or other limitations interfere with B-mode visualization. Thrombosis should be suspected when color flow is absent with distal augmentation, even if thrombus is not directly visualized with B-mode imaging (Figs. 19.18 and 19.19). Occasionally, a posterior tibial vein will appear diminutive or congenitally absent. In these cases, the peroneal veins will be dominant and appear larger than normal.

While the tibial and peroneal veins lie between the muscles, the soleal and gastrocnemius veins are deep veins that lie within the calf muscles. Evaluation of the muscular calf veins may be important, depending on the patient's clinical presentation and symptoms. The soleal veins lie within the soleus muscle of the midleg and drain into the peroneal or posterior tibial veins. These veins are generally small in caliber and may not be routinely visualized; however, they become dilated and more noticeable when thrombosed. The soleal veins can be a common site of thrombus formation in postoperative surgical patients and patients hospitalized with prolonged bed rest.

The gastrocnemius veins are located within the gastrocnemius muscle and drain into the popliteal vein. These veins are most easily identified in the gastrocnemius muscle in the proximal calf or popliteal fossa, superficial to the popliteal vessels. There may be several sets of gastrocnemius veins located in the medial and lateral heads of the muscle (Fig. 19.20). Some of the muscular venous tributaries join before their confluence with the popliteal vein. These veins may be small in diameter but also become dilated and more easily identified when they are thrombosed (Fig. 19.21). Be aware that color Doppler may

FIGURE 19.10. The Valsalva maneuver increases intra-abdominal pressure and causes antegrade flow to cease in the common femoral vein (CFV). With competent valves, only a very brief period (<0.5 seconds) of retrograde flow is seen before valve closure.

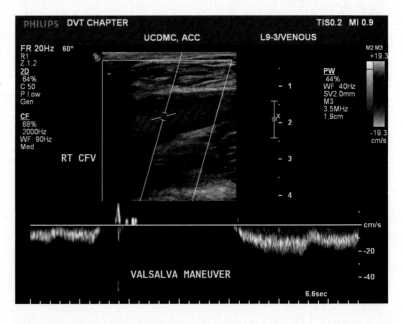

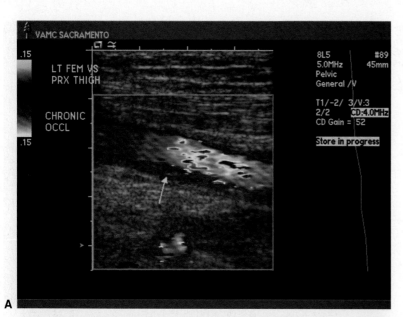

A

FIGURE 19.11. Features associated with chronic postthrombotic changes in deep veins. *A*, Wall thickening in a recanalized segment (*arrow*). *B*, Contracted, thick-walled (sclerotic) incompressible segments (*left*, without compression; *right*, with compression). *C*, Reflux (flow above the baseline) due to loss of valvular competence.

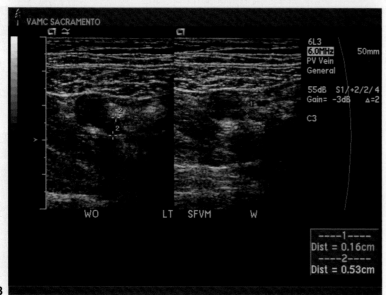

B

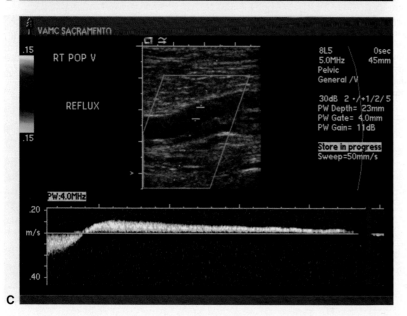

C

FIGURE 19.12. Transverse B-mode image of the common femoral vein (CFV) with chronic thrombus (*arrows*). The vein wall is thickened and the vein is not distended. Hyperechoic chronic thrombus on the deep wall appears heterogeneous.

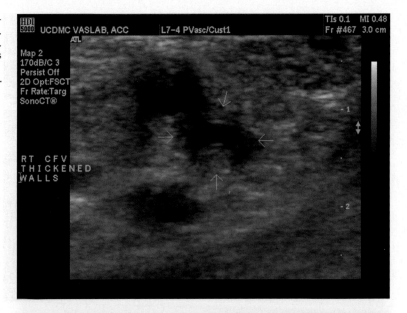

FIGURE 19.13. Chronic occlusion of the external iliac vein, common femoral vein (CFV), and femoral vein (FV). In this example, the profunda femoris vein (PFV) remains patent, but the color Doppler indicates retrograde flow (away from the transducer), consistent with a pattern of chronic collateralization.

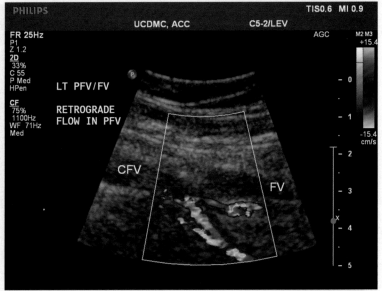

FIGURE 19.14. Acute thrombosis of the popliteal vein (POP), with typical features demonstrated in a transverse B-mode image. The vein is distended and is larger than the adjacent artery (*A*), with homogeneous echoes from the thrombus filling the lumen. Extensive lower extremity venous obstruction in this patient has resulted in edema that is sonographically evident in the soft tissues of the limb.

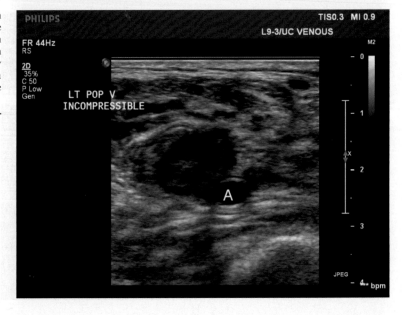

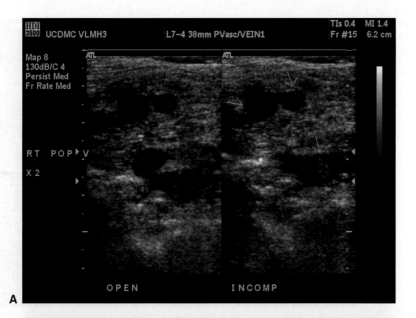

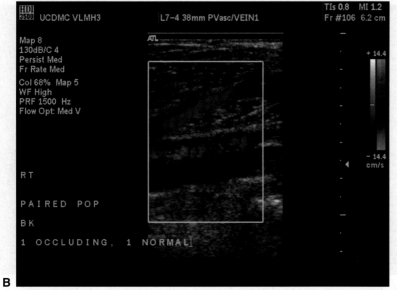

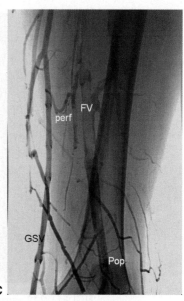

FIGURE 19.15. *A,* Dilated, incompressible muscular veins (gastrocnemius veins) of the calf in a patient with acute, symptomatic deep vein thrombosis (*left,* without compression; *right,* with compression, incompressible veins are indicated by *arrows*). *B,* Thrombus extension is demonstrated into the popliteal vein, where there is no flow detected with color Doppler. In this patient, paired popliteal veins are present, and flow is normal in the smaller of the pair. *C,* Contrast venography demonstrates the filling defect in the popliteal vein (Pop), with extension of thrombus into the femoral vein (FV) in the thigh. The very limited flow of contrast around the femoral vein thrombus produces the characteristic double line or "railroad track sign" of acute thrombosis. The great saphenous vein (GSV) and a major perforating vein (perf) are also demonstrated.

still demonstrate flow with venous thrombosis if acute thrombus is not occlusive or if chronic thrombus has been partially recanalized (Figs. 19.22 and 19.23).

Inferior Vena Cava and Iliac Veins

The IVC and iliac veins, like other intra-abdominal and retroperitoneal vessels, can be difficult to evaluate due to overlying abdominal bowel gas and the decreased resolution of ultrasound when evaluating deeper structures. Whenever possible, the patient should fast for 4 to 6 hours prior to the examination to help reduce bowel gas. The patient should be in a

supine position with the abdomen and pelvis exposed. A low-frequency curved or sector transducer should be used for these deeper vessels. The technologist should utilize correct ergonomic techniques for abdominal scanning.

B-mode imaging and transverse probe compression maneuvers are often not effective when evaluating abdominal or pelvic veins. Therefore, color flow and Doppler spectral waveforms are the primary modalities for this part of the examination. Color scale and gain settings are appropriately adjusted for the increased depth. Flow should be spontaneous and phasic throughout, with greater pulsatility in the IVC due to its proximity to the heart. The absence of detectable flow by

FIGURE 19.16. The posterior tibial veins (PTV) are paired, accompanying the posterior tibial artery. The Doppler spectral waveform shows spontaneous and phasic flow.

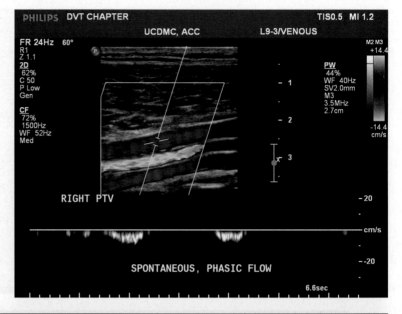

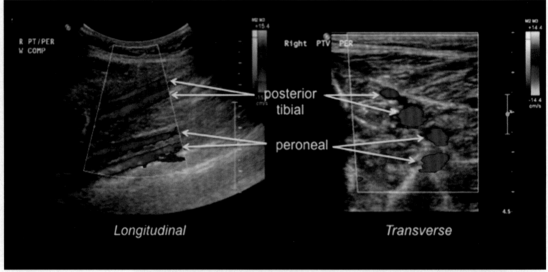

FIGURE 19.17. Imaging of the posterior tibial and peroneal veins: *left*, longitudinal view; *right*, transverse view. Color flow imaging can confirm patency of the posterior tibial and peroneal veins. This finding can help to rule out calf DVT when vein wall coaptation is difficult to visualize with compression maneuvers.

FIGURE 19.18. Peroneal (PER) DVT. *Left*, longitudinal B-mode image shows a thrombus tail (*arrows*). *Right*, transverse color Doppler image shows filling defects in the vein lumen.

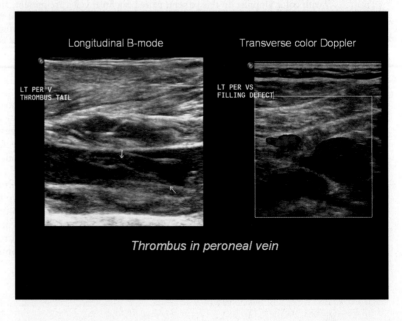

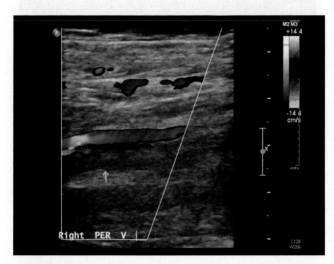

FIGURE 19.19. Peroneal (PER) DVT is recognized by the absence of color filling in one of the paired peroneal veins. The *arrow* indicates the location of intraluminal thrombus.

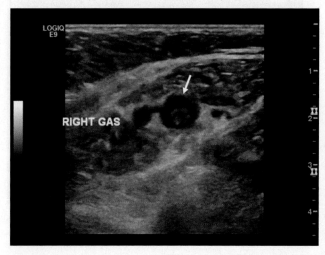

FIGURE 19.21. Acute thrombosis of a muscular calf vein. Thrombus is visualized in a gastrocnemius vein (GAS) in this transverse B-mode image (*arrow*). The vein is dilated with echogenic material in the lumen.

pulsed Doppler and color flow imaging indicates IVC occlusion or thrombosis (Fig. 19.24).

Abnormal flow patterns in lower extremity veins may be an indication of abnormal (central) cardiovascular physiology. Heart failure or tricuspid regurgitation can result in greater flow variation or pulsatility with the cardiac cycle (Fig. 19.25). IVC filters may be imaged and appear as hyperechoic structures within the vein (Figs. 19.26 and 19.27). Imaging prior to planned retrieval of an IVC filter may demonstrate significant thrombosis or emboli within the filter. In these cases, the filter should not be removed without further therapy.

The external iliac and common iliac veins are evaluated with color flow in long axis from the inguinal ligament to the level of the common iliac vein confluence. Augmentations are performed with thigh compressions. Each internal iliac vein is also identified at its confluence

with the external iliac vein. The IVC is evaluated in long axis from the level just below the xiphoid process to the level of the common iliac vein confluence. Transverse evaluation with color flow is also useful in determining complete wall-to-wall color filling.

Complete or partial absence of color flow within the iliac veins or IVC may indicate intraluminal thrombus. Suspicious segments can also be evaluated with B-mode imaging to look for intraluminal thrombus. Absence of spontaneous flow or lack of respiratory phasicity (continuous flow) may indicate a more central venous obstruction (Figs. 19.28 and 19.29). Side-to-side comparison of venous flow characteristics is also important in the external iliac veins as a means to evaluate for common iliac vein obstruction. Flow signals that are continuous with elevated flow velocities may indicate a venous stenosis.

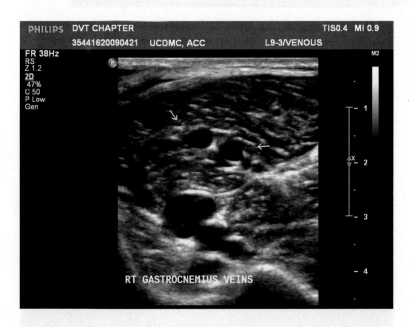

FIGURE 19.20. Transverse imaging of the calf demonstrates the muscular veins. The gastrocnemius veins are prominent here (*arrows*), but they are free of intraluminal echoes that would suggest thrombus. Collapse with probe compression or color Doppler (not shown) confirms patency.

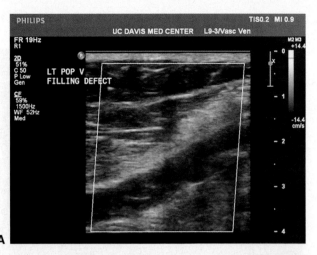
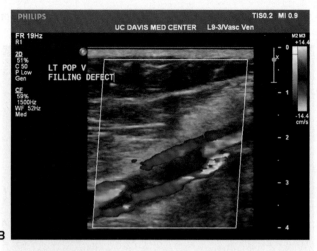

FIGURE 19.22. Flow around an intraluminal venous filling defect can be seen with acute, nonocclusive thrombosis or with partial recanalization of chronic thrombosis. *A,* Longitudinal B-mode image shows mostly hypoechoic thrombus within the lumen of this popliteal (POP) vein. *B,* Color Doppler indicates that there is flow around the nonocclusive thrombus.

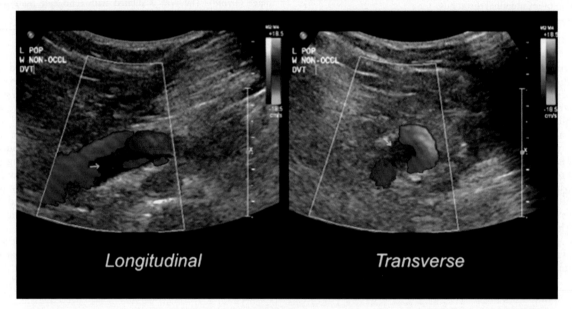

FIGURE 19.23. Nonocclusive thrombus (*arrows*) in a popliteal vein (POP). Color Doppler shows flow around the thrombus (*left,* longitudinal view; *right,* transverse view).

FIGURE 19.24. Thrombosis of the inferior vena cava (IVC), demonstrated in the transverse plane with a low-frequency curved array transducer using color Doppler imaging. The IVC (*green arrow*) is echo-filled with no color flow, while flow is present in the adjacent aorta (Ao). Color Doppler and pulsed Doppler are needed to assess the IVC, as this retroperitoneal vessel may be difficult to manually collapse with probe compression.

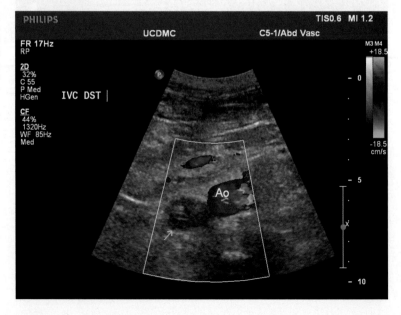

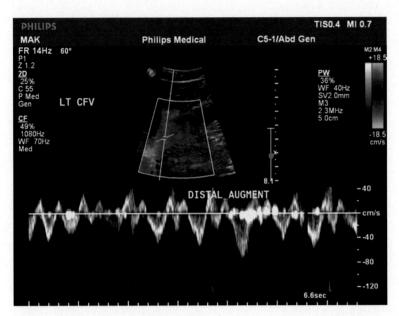

FIGURE 19.25. In the proximal lower extremity deep veins, variation in flow with the cardiac cycle is a sign of volume overload and right heart failure; it may also be seen with tricuspid regurgitation. Increased cardiac pulsatility is evident in this common femoral vein (CFV) flow pattern.

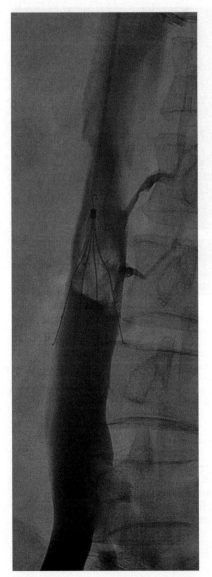

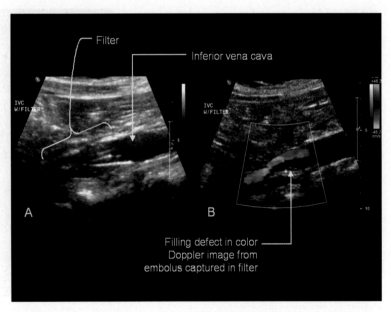

FIGURE 19.26. The inferior vena cava (IVC) can often be directly assessed, although obesity and overlying bowel gas may limit ultrasound imaging in some cases. Duplex scanning may be used to evaluate IVC patency. *A,* The presence of a conical-shaped IVC filter is apparent in this B-mode image. *B,* Color Doppler shows flow only around the periphery of the filter due to the presence of a large captured thromboembolus in the center of the filter.

FIGURE 19.27. A venogram of the inferior vena cava demonstrates a conical filter above the confluence of the iliac veins and below the renal veins. The contrast filling defect seen in the filter is due to the captured embolus (compare to Fig. 19.26).

FIGURE 19.28. Continuous venous flow (loss of normal respiratory phasic variation) is a sign of cephalad (more central) venous obstruction and can be observed with occlusion, nonocclusive thrombosis, chronic narrowing, or extrinsic compression. When seen in one common femoral vein, it indicates an iliac vein obstruction.

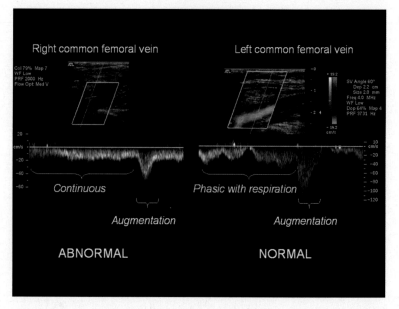

FIGURE 19.29. Common iliac vein occlusion is suggested by the absence of color (*arrow*) in the vein adjacent to the common iliac artery (CIA). This diagnosis is confirmed by the finding of continuous flow in the external iliac vein on pulsed Doppler.

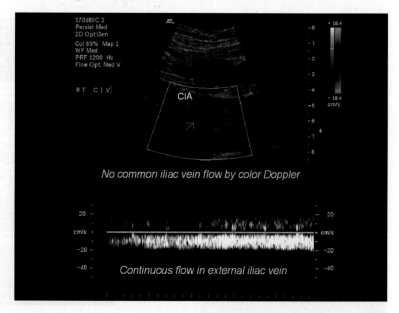

Superficial Veins

Evaluation of the great saphenous vein at the level of the saphenofemoral junction is part of a complete examination of the lower extremity for DVT. A more thorough evaluation of the superficial veins may be appropriate if the patient presents with localized pain, swelling, a palpable cord, or painful superficial varicosities.

The great saphenous and small saphenous veins are evaluated with B-mode imaging and transverse probe compressions. The great saphenous vein can be evaluated from the ankle, anterior to the medial malleolus, to the saphenofemoral junction. The small saphenous vein is located in the posterior calf. It can be followed from the distal calf to the popliteal fossa where it typically drains into the popliteal vein, although the point of confluence with the deep system can be variable. Thrombosis of the superficial veins is easily detectable, as these veins become visibly distended with thrombus (Fig. 19.30).

Pitfalls

While the advantages of duplex scanning as a primary modality for DVT diagnosis are numerous, there are limitations that should be considered (Table 19.7). As previously mentioned, anatomic factors such as obesity, edema, and leg wounds can

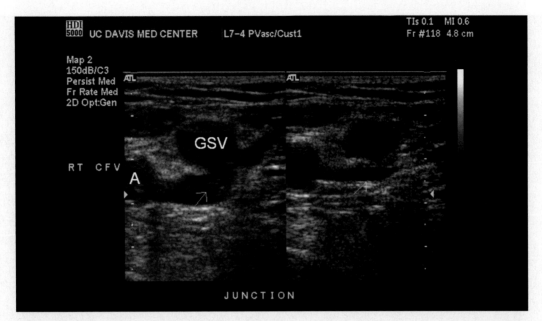

FIGURE 19.30. Superficial venous thrombosis may extend into the deep system. These transverse B-mode images at the level of the saphenofemoral junction show the great saphenous vein (GSV) to be incompressible (*left*, no compression; *right*, with compression). There is minimal change in the appearance of the GSV or the common femoral artery (A) with probe compression. The acute thrombus extends into the common femoral vein (CFV), where it can be visualized (*arrow*).

make the venous scan difficult, but these obstacles can usually be minimized by appropriate patient positioning, use of different transducers, and alternate scanning approaches. When veins cannot be compressed due to depth or surrounding tissues, use of Doppler techniques supplements the imaging findings.

Physiologic abnormalities, such as venous hypertension, can also affect the examination. Several factors can contribute to venous hypertension of the lower extremities, including congestive heart failure, tricuspid valvular insufficiency, and extrinsic compression or thrombosis of the more proximal deep veins. Increased pressure can make collapse of the vein

with probe compression difficult and produce a false-positive examination.

A number of clinical conditions other than DVT can cause lower extremity pain and swelling, including cellulitis, lymphedema, and adenopathy (Fig. 19.31). Patients with a ruptured Baker's cyst,[38–40] gastrocnemius muscle tear or hematoma,[151] or other musculoskeletal problems can present with localized pain and swelling of the posterior calf. It is important to note these incidental findings when they are present. Abnormal venous anatomy (anatomic variations, anomalies, malformations, or venous aneurysms) should be described (Fig. 19.32).

TABLE 19.7

ADVANTAGES AND LIMITATIONS OF DUPLEX SCANNING FOR THE DIAGNOSIS OF ACUTE LOWER EXTREMITY DEEP VEIN THROMBOSIS

■ ADVANTAGES	■ LIMITATIONS
Noninvasive	Operator dependent
Safe	May not distinguish acute from chronic thrombus
Widely available	Not all laboratories have experience with evaluations of calf veins.
Low cost	Limited imaging of pelvic veins and vena cava
Portable	Imaging may be compromised by obesity, marked edema, or recent surgical incisions.
Few contraindications	Casts, splints, or external fixators may limit imaging.
No radiation exposure	
May diagnose other pathology	
Numerous clinical trials to date	

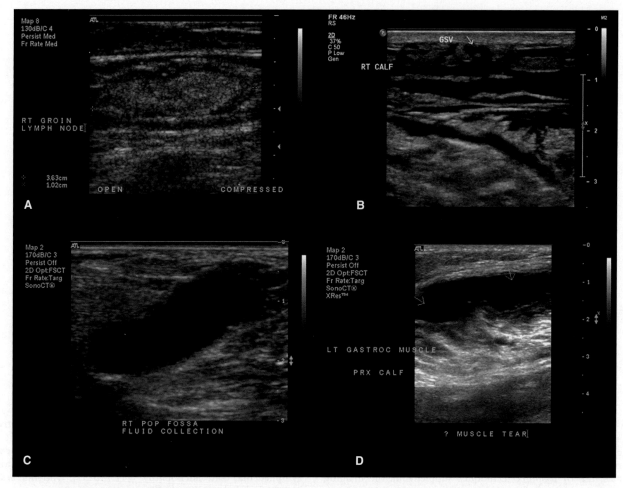

FIGURE 19.31. Vascular technologists and interpreting physicians should be familiar with common non-vascular ultrasound findings encountered in patients referred to the vascular laboratory for evaluation of a swollen, painful limb. *A*, Inguinal lymphadenopathy. *B*, Soft tissue edema in a calf; the great saphenous vein (GSV) is indicated by the *arrow*. *C*, Baker's cyst. *D*, Gastrocnemius muscle tear with hematoma (*arrows*).

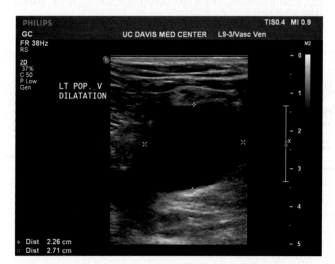

FIGURE 19.32. Transverse B-mode image showing a focal dilatation of a popliteal vein (POP). Aneurysms of deep veins are rare but may predispose to thrombosis and embolization.

References

1. Sigel B, Popky GL, Wagner DK, et al. Comparison of clinical and Doppler ultrasound evaluation of confirmed lower extremity venous disease. *Surgery* 1968;64(1):332-338.
2. Sigel B. A brief history of Doppler ultrasound in the diagnosis of peripheral vascular disease. *Ultrasound Med Biol* 1998;24(2):169-176.
3. Strandness DE, Sumner DS. Ultrasonic velocity detector in the diagnosis of thrombophlebitis. *Arch Surg* 1972;104:180-183.
4. Talbot SR. Use of real-time imaging in identifying deep venous obstruction: A preliminary report. *Bruit* 1982;6:41-42.
5. Talbot SR. B-mode evaluation of peripheral veins. *Semin Ultrasound CT MR* 1988;9(4):295-319.
6. Strandness DE Jr. Echo-Doppler (duplex) ultrasonic scanning. *J Vasc Surg* 1985;2(2):341-344.
7. Albrechtsson U, Olsson CG. Thrombotic side-effects of lower-limb phlebography. *Lancet* 1976;1(7962):723-724.
8. Thomas ML, MacDonald LM. Complications of ascending phlebography of the leg. *Br Med J* 1978;2(6133):317-318.
9. Ho VB, van Geertruyden PH, Yucel EK, et al. ACR Appropriateness Criteria((R)) on suspected lower extremity deep vein thrombosis. *J Am Coll Radiol* 2011;8(6):383-387.
10. Zierler BK. Ultrasonography and diagnosis of venous thromboembolism. *Circulation* 2004;109(12 Suppl 1):I9-I14.
11. American College of Cardiology Foundation Appropriate Use Criteria Task Force, American College of Radiology, American Institute of Ultrasound in Medicine, et al. ACCF/ACR/AIUM/ASE/IAC/SCAI/SCVS/SIR/SVM/SVS/SVU 2013 appropriate use criteria for peripheral vascular ultrasound and physiological testing. Part II: Testing for venous disease and evaluation of hemodialysis access. *Vasc Med* 2013;18(4):215-231.

12. IAC VascularTesting. IAC Standards and Guidelines for Vascular Testing Accreditation. *Section 4B: Peripheral Venous Testing* 2015. http://intersoci-etal.org/vascular/standards/IACVascularTestingStandards2015.pdf.

13. Heit JA, Cohen AT, Anderson FA Jr.; on Behalf of the VTEIAG. Estimated annual number of incident and recurrent, non-fatal and fatal Venous Thromboembolism (VTE) Events in the US (ASH annual meeting abstracts). *Blood* 2005;106(11):910.

14. Wakefield TW, McLafferty RB, Lohr JM, et al. Call to action to prevent venous thromboembolism. *J Vasc Surg* 2009;49(6):1620-1623.

15. Anderson FA Jr., Zayaruzny M, Heit JA, et al. Estimated annual numbers of US acute-care hospital patients at risk for venous thromboembolism. *Am J Hematol* 2007;82(9):777-782.

16. Kahn SR, Shbaklo H, Lamping DL, et al. Determinants of health-related quality of life during the 2 years following deep vein thrombosis. *J Thromb Haemost* 2008;6(7):1105-1112.

17. Hudgens SA, Cella D, Caprini CA, et al. Deep vein thrombosis: Validation of a patient-reported leg symptom index. *Health Qual Life Outcomes* 2003;1:76.

18. Prandoni P, Lensing AW, Prins MR. Long-term outcomes after deep venous thrombosis of the lower extremities. *Vasc Med* 1998;3(1):57-60.

19. SurgeonGeneral.gov. The Surgeon General's call to action to prevent deep vein thrombosis and pulmonary embolism. 2008; http://www.surgeonge-neral.gov/topics/deepvein/calltoaction/call-to-action-on-dvt-2008.pdf.

20. Joint Commission. 2014. http://www.jointcommission.org/venous_throm-boembolism/. Accessed April 26, 2015.

21. Joint Commission. Hospital National Patient Safety Goals. 2015; http://www.jointcommission.org/assets/1/6/2015_NPSG_HAP.pdf. Accessed April 26, 2015.

22. Young L, Ockelford P, Milne D, et al. Post-treatment residual throm-bus increases the risk of recurrent deep vein thrombosis and mortality. *J Thromb Haemost* 2006;4(9):1919-1924.

23. Prandoni P, Prins MH, Lensing AW, et al. Residual thrombosis on ultrasonog-raphy to guide the duration of anticoagulation in patients with deep venous thrombosis: A randomized trial. *Ann Intern Med* 2009;150(9):577-585.

24. Palareti G, Cosmi B, Legnani C, et al. D-dimer testing to determine the dura-tion of anticoagulation therapy. *N Engl J Med* 2006;355(17):1780-1789.

25. Cosmi B, Legnani C, Iorio A, et al. Residual venous obstruction, alone and in combination with D-dimer, as a risk factor for recurrence after antico-agulation withdrawal following a first idiopathic deep vein thrombosis in the prolong study. *Eur J Vasc Endovasc Surg* 2010;39(3):356-365.

26. Donadini MP, Ageno W, Antonucci E, et al. Prognostic significance of residual venous obstruction in patients with treated unprovoked deep vein thrombo-sis: A patient-level meta-analysis. *Thromb Haemost* 2014;111(1):172-179.

27. Baldridge ED, Martin MA, Welling RE. Clinical significance of free-floating venous thrombi. *J Vasc Surg* 1990;11(1):62-67.

28. Schroder WB, Bealer JF. Venous duplex ultrasonography causing acute pulmonary embolism: A brief report. *J Vasc Surg* 1992;15(6):1082-1083.

29. Perlin SJ. Pulmonary embolism during compression US of the lower extremity. *Radiology* 1992;184(1):165-166.

30. Feld R. Pulmonary embolism caused by venous compression ultrasound examination. *J Vasc Surg* 1993;17(2):450.

31. Dona E, Fletcher JP, Hughes TM, et al. Duplicated popliteal and superfi-cial femoral veins: Incidence and potential significance. *Aust N Z J Surg* 2000;70(6):438-440.

32. Gordon AC, Wright I, Pugh ND. Duplication of the superficial femo-ral vein: Recognition with duplex ultrasonography. *Clin Radiol* 1996;51(9):622-624.

33. Quinn KL, Vandeman FN. Thrombosis of a duplicated superficial femoral vein. Potential error in compression ultrasound diagnosis of lower extrem-ity deep venous thrombosis. *J Ultrasound Med* 1990;9(4):235-238.

34. Quinlan DJ, Alikhan R, Gishen P, et al. Variations in lower limb venous anatomy: Implications for US diagnosis of deep vein thrombosis. *Radiology* 2003;228(2):443-448.

35. Screaton NJ, Gillard JH, Berman LH, et al. Duplicated superficial femo-ral veins: A source of error in the sonographic investigation of deep vein thrombosis. *Radiology* 1998;206(2):397-401.

36. Mansour MA. Venous duplex ultrasound of the lower extremity in the diagnosis of deep venous thrombosis. In AbuRahma AF, Bandyk D (eds). Noninvasive Vascular Diagnosis: A Practical Guide to Therapy. 3rd ed. London: Springer-Verlag, 2013,473-481.

37. Jiji PJ, D'Costa S, Prabhu LV, et al. A rare variation of the profunda femoris vein in the popliteal fossa. *Singapore Med J* 2007;48(10):948-949.

38. Volteas SK, Labropoulos N, Leon M, et al. Incidence of ruptured Baker's cyst among patients with symptoms of deep vein thrombosis. *Br J Surg* 1997;84(3):342.

39. Chaudhuri R, Salari R. Baker's cyst simulating deep vein thrombosis. *Clin Radiol* 1990;41(6):400-404.

40. Langsfeld M, Matteson B, Johnson W, et al. Baker's cysts mimicking the symptoms of deep vein thrombosis: Diagnosis with venous duplex scanning. *J Vasc Surg* 1997;25(4):658-662.

41. Armstrong EM, Bellone JM, Hornsby LB, et al. Acquired Thrombophilia. *J Pharm Pract* 2014;27(3):234-242.

42. Henke PK, Schmaier A, Wakefield TW. Vascular thrombosis due to hypercoagulable states. In Rutherford RB (ed). *Vascular Surgery*, 6th ed. Philadelphia: Elsevier Saunders, 2005, pp 568–578.

43. Foy P, Moll S. Thrombophilia: 2009 update. *Curr Treat Options Cardiovasc Med* 2009;11(2):114-128.

44. Martinelli I, Battaglioli T, Tosetto A, et al. Prothrombin A19911G poly-morphism and the risk of venous thromboembolism. *J Thromb Haemost* 2006;4(12):2582-2586.

45. Yilmazer M, Kurtay G, Sonmezer M, et al. Factor V Leiden and prothrom-bin 20210 G-A mutations in controls and in patients with thromboem-bolic events during pregnancy or the puerperium. *Arch Gynecol Obstet* 2003;268(4):304-308.

46. Margaglione M, Brancaccio V, De Lucia D, et al. Inherited throm-bophilic risk factors and venous thromboembolism: Distinct role in peripheral deep venous thrombosis and pulmonary embolism. *Chest* 2000;118(5):1405-1411.

47. McColl MD, Ellison J, Reid F, et al. Prothrombin 20210 G A, MTHFR C677T mutations in women with venous thromboembolism associated with pregnancy. *BJOG* 2000;107(4):565-569.

48. Vargas M, Soto I, Pinto CR, et al. The prothrombin 20210A allele and the factor V Leiden are associated with venous thrombosis but not with early coronary artery disease. *Blood Coagul Fibrinolysis* 1999;10(1):39-41.

49. Bauduer F, Lacombe D. Factor V Leiden, prothrombin 20210A, methy-lenetetrahydrofolate reductase 677T, and population genetics. *Mol Genet Metab* 2005;86(1-2):91-99.

50. Dalen JE. Should patients with venous thromboembolism be screened for thrombophilia? *Am J Med* 2008;121(6):458-463.

51. Franco RF, Middeldorp S, Meinardi JR, et al. Factor XIII Val34Leu and the risk of venous thromboembolism in factor V Leiden carriers. *Br J Haematol* 2000;111(1):118-121.

52. Franco RF, Morelli V, Lourenco D, et al. A second mutation in the methy-lenetetrahydrofolate reductase gene and the risk of venous thrombotic dis-ease. *Br J Haematol* 1999;105(2):556-559.

53. Franco RF, Reitsma PH. Genetic risk factors of venous thrombosis. *Hum Genet* 2001;109(4):369-384.

54. Palareti G, Cosmi B. Predicting the risk of recurrence of venous thrombo-embolism. *Curr Opin Hematol* 2004;11(3):192-197.

55. Rosen SB, Sturk A. Activated protein C resistance—A major risk factor for thrombosis. *Eur J Clin Chem Clin Biochem* 1997;35(7):501-516.

56. Andreotti F, Becker RC. Atherothrombotic disorders: New insights from hematology. *Circulation* 2005;111(14):1855-1863.

57. Nicolaides AN, Breddin HK, Carpenter P, et al. Thrombophilia and venous thromboembolism. International consensus statement Guidelines accord-ing to scientific evidence. *Int Angiol* 2005;24(1):1-26.

58. Mazza JJ. Hypercoagulability and venous thromboembolism: A review. *WMJ* 2004;103(2):41-49.

59. Shantsila E, Lip GY, Chong BH. Heparin-induced thrombocytopenia. A contemporary clinical approach to diagnosis and management. *Chest* 2009;135(6):1651-1664.

60. Johnson CM, Mureebe L, Silver D. Hypercoagulable states: A review. *Vasc Endovascular Surg* 2005;39(2):123-133.

61. Hirsh J, Guyatt G, Albers GW, et al., Physicians ACoC. Antithrombotic and thrombolytic therapy: American College of Chest Physicians Evidence-Based Clinical Practice Guidelines (8th edition). *Chest* 2008;133(6 Suppl):110S-112S.

62. Haeger K. Problems of acute deep venous thrombosis. I. The interpretation of signs and symptoms. *Angiology* 1969;20(4):219-223.

63. Wells PS, Hirsh J, Anderson DR, et al. Accuracy of clinical assessment of deep-vein thrombosis. *Lancet* 1995;345(8961):1326-1330.

64. Oudega R, Hoes AW, Moons KG. The Wells rule does not adequately rule out deep venous thrombosis in primary care patients. *Ann Intern Med* 2005;143(2):100-107.

65. Adam SS, Key NS, Greenberg CS. D-dimer antigen: Current concepts and future prospects. *Blood* 2009;113(13):2878-2887.

66. Wells PS, Anderson DR, Rodger M, et al. Evaluation of D-dimer in the diagnosis of suspected deep-vein thrombosis. *N Engl J Med* 2003;349(13):1227-1235.

67. Palareti G, Cosmi B, Legnani C. Diagnosis of deep vein thrombosis. *Semin Thromb Hemost* 2006;32(7):659-672.

68. Righini M, Perrier A, De Moerloose P, et al. D-Dimer for venous thromboem-bolism diagnosis: 20 years later. *J Thromb Haemost* 2008;6(7):1059-1071.

69. Wells PS, Owen C, Doucette S, et al. Does this patient have deep vein thrombosis? *JAMA* 2006;295(2):199-207.

70. Fancher TL, White RH, Kravitz RL. Combined use of rapid D-dimer test-ing and estimation of clinical probability in the diagnosis of deep vein thrombosis: Systematic review. *BMJ* 2004;329(7470):821.

71. Comerota AJ, Harada RN, Eze AR, et al. Air plethysmography: A clinical review. *Int Angiol* 1995;14(1):45-52.

72. Thomsen TA, Hokanson E, Barnes RW. Automatic quantitation of venous hemodynamics with an electrically calibrated strain gauge plethysmograph. *Med Instrum* 1977;11(4):240-243.

73. Raman ER, Delaruelle J, Vanhuyse VJ, et al. Venous occlusion plethys-mography with mercury-in-rubber strain gauges. *Acta Anaesthesiol Belg* 1980;31(1):5-14.

74. Linhardt GE Jr., Queral LA, Dagher FJ. Noninvasive evaluation of venous insufficiency: photoplethysmography versus strain gauge plethysmography. *Curr Surg* 1982;39(5):319-322.

75. Hirai M, Yoshinaga M, Nakayama R. Assessment of venous insufficiency using photoplethysmography: A comparison to strain gauge plethysmogra-phy. *Angiology* 1985;36(11):795-801.

PERIPHERAL VENOUS

76. van Bemmelen PS, van Ramshorst B, Eikelboom BC. Photoplethysmography reexamined: Lack of correlation with duplex scanning. *Surgery* 1992;112(3):544-548.

77. Wheeler HB. Impedance testing for venous thrombosis. *Arch Surg* 1973;106(6):762-763.

78. Johnston KW, Kakkar VV. Plethysmographic diagnosis of deep vein thrombosis. *Surg Gynecol Obstet* 1974;139(1):41-44.

79. Strandness DE Jr., Sumner DS. Acute venous thrombosis. A case of progress and confusion. *JAMA* 1974;233(1):46-48.

80. Wheeler HB, Anderson FA. Impedance plethysmography. In Kempczinski RF, Yao JST (eds). *Practical Noninvasive Vascular Diagnosis.* Chicago: Year Book Medical Publishers, 1987, pp 407-437.

81. Wheeler HB, Anderson FA Jr., Cardullo PA, et al. Suspected deep vein thrombosis. Management by impedance plethysmography. *Arch Surg* 1982;117(9):1206-1209.

82. Flanigan DP, Goodreau JJ, Burnham SJ, et al. Vascular-laboratory diagnosis of clinically suspected acute deep-vein thrombosis. *Lancet* 1978;2(8085):331-334.

83. Moser KM, Brach BB, Dolan GF. Clinically suspected deep venous thrombosis of the lower extremities. A comparison of venography, impedance plethysmography, and radiolabeled fibrinogen. *JAMA* 1977;237(20):2195-2198.

84. Hume M, Kurlakose TX, Jamieson J, et al. Extent of leg vein thrombosis determined by impedance and 125-I fibrinogen. *Am J Surg* 1975;129(4):455-458.

85. Evans DS, Cockett FB. Diagnosis of deep-vein thrombosis with an ultrasonic Doppler technique. *Br Med J* 1969;2(5660):802-804.

86. Alexander RH, Folse R, Pizzorno J, et al. Thrombophlebitis and thromboembolism: Results of a prospective study. *Ann Surg* 1974;180(6):883-887.

87. Fish P, Kakkar VV, Day TK. Proceedings: The Doppler scan and deep vein thrombosis. *Br J Surg* 1975;62(2):161.

88. Young JR, Evarts CM, Zelch JV. The detection of venous thrombosis. *Clin Orthop Relat Res* 1975(107):123-127.

89. Day TK, Fish PJ, Kakkar VV. Detection of deep vein thrombosis by Doppler angiography. *Br Med J* 1976;1(6010):618-620.

90. Dosick SM, Blakemore WS. The role of Doppler ultrasound in acute deep vein thrombosis. *Am J Surg* 1978;136(2):265-268.

91. Maryniak O, Nicholson CG. Doppler ultrasonography for detection of deep vein thrombosis in lower extremities. *Arch Phys Med Rehabil* 1979;60(6):277-280.

92. Sumner DS, Lambeth A. Reliability of Doppler ultrasound in the diagnosis of acute venous thrombosis both above and below the knee. *Am J Surg* 1979;138(2):205-210.

93. Meadway J, Nicolaides AN, Walker CJ, et al. Value of Doppler ultrasound in diagnosis of clinically suspected deep vein thrombosis. *Br Med J* 1975;4(5996):552-554.

94. Bendick PJ, Glover JL, Holden RW, et al. Pitfalls of the Doppler examination for venous thrombosis. *Am Surg* 1983;49(6):320-323.

95. Russell JC, Becker DR. The noninvasive venous vascular laboratory. A prospective analysis. *Arch Surg* 1983;118(9):1024-1028.

96. Elias A, Le Corff G, Bouvier JL, et al. Value of real time B mode ultrasound imaging in the diagnosis of deep vein thrombosis of the lower limbs. *Int Angiol* 1987;6(2):175-182.

97. Baker WH, Hayes AC. The normal Doppler venous examination. *Angiology* 1983;34(4):283-288.

98. Killewich LA, Bedford GR, Beach KW. Diagnosis of deep venous thrombosis. A prospective study comparing duplex scanning to contrast venography. *Circulation* 1989;79(4):810-814.

99. White RH, McGahan JP, Daschbach MM, et al. Diagnosis of deep-vein thrombosis using duplex ultrasound. *Ann Intern Med* 1989;111(4):297-304.

100. Tapson VF, Carroll BA, Davidson BL, et al. The diagnostic approach to acute venous thromboembolism. Clinical practice guideline. American Thoracic Society. *Am J Respir Crit Care Med* 1999;160(3):1043-1066.

101. Strandness DE Jr. Diagnostic approaches for detecting deep vein thrombosis. *Am J Card Imaging* 1994;8(1):13-17.

102. Seidel AC, Cavalheri G Jr., Miranda F Jr. The role of duplex ultrasonography in the diagnosis of lower-extremity deep vein thrombosis in non-hospitalized patients. *Int Angiol* 2008;27(5):377-384.

103. Fowl RJ, Strothman GB, Blebea J, et al. Inappropriate use of venous duplex scans: An analysis of indications and results. *J Vasc Surg* 1996;23(5):881-885; discussion 885-886.

104. Poley RA, Newbigging J, Sivilotti ML. Estimated effect of an integrated approach to suspected deep venous thrombosis using limited-compression ultrasound. *Acad Emerg Med* 2014;21(9):971-980.

105. Crisp JG, Lovato LM, Jang TB. Compression ultrasonography of the lower extremity with portable vascular ultrasonography can accurately detect deep venous thrombosis in the emergency department. *Ann Emerg Med* 2010;56(6):601-610.

106. Meissner MH, Moneta G, Burnand K, et al. The hemodynamics and diagnosis of venous disease. *J Vasc Surg* 2007;46 (Suppl S):4S-24S.

107. Katsumori T, Kasahara T, Tsuchida Y, et al. MR venography of deep veins: Changes with uterine fibroid embolization. *Cardiovasc Intervent Radiol* 2009;32(2):284-288.

108. Cantwell CP, Cradock A, Bruzzi J, et al. MR venography with true fast imaging with steady-state precession for suspected lower-limb deep vein thrombosis. *J Vasc Interv Radiol* 2006;17(11 Pt 1):1763-1769.

109. Shebel ND, Whalen CC. Diagnosis and management of iliac vein compression syndrome. *J Vasc Nurs* 2005;23(1):10-17; quiz 18-19.

110. Fraser DG, Moody AR, Martel A, et al. Re-evaluation of iliac compression syndrome using magnetic resonance imaging in patients with acute deep venous thromboses. *J Vasc Surg* 2004;40(4):604-611.

111. Spritzer CE, Arata MA, Freed KS. Isolated pelvic deep venous thrombosis: Relative frequency as detected with MR imaging. *Radiology* 2001;219(2):521-525.

112. Fraser DG, Moody AR, Morgan PS, et al. Diagnosis of lower-limb deep venous thrombosis: A prospective blinded study of magnetic resonance direct thrombus imaging. *Ann Intern Med* 2002;136(2):89-98.

113. Totterman S, Francis CW, Foster TH, et al. Diagnosis of femoropopliteal venous thrombosis with MR imaging: A comparison of four MR pulse sequences. *AJR Am J Roentgenol* 1990;154(1):175-178.

114. Zerhouni EA, Barth KH, Siegelman SS. Demonstration of venous thrombosis by computed tomography. *AJR Am J Roentgenol* 1980;134(4):753-758.

115. Andriopoulos A, Wirsing P, Botticher R. Results of iliofemoral venous thrombectomy after acute thrombosis: Report on 165 cases. *J Cardiovasc Surg (Torino)* 1982;23(2):123-124.

116. Loud PA, Katz DS, Klippenstein DL, et al. Combined CT venography and pulmonary angiography in suspected thromboembolic disease: Diagnostic accuracy for deep venous evaluation. *AJR Am J Roentgenol* 2000;174(1):61-65.

117. Ciccotosto C, Goodman LR, Washington L, et al. Indirect CT venography following CT pulmonary angiography: Spectrum of CT findings. *J Thorac Imaging* 2002;17(1):18-27.

118. Cham MD, Yankelevitz DF, Henschke CI. Thromboembolic disease detection at indirect CT venography versus CT pulmonary angiography. *Radiology* 2005;234(2):591-594.

119. Strothman G, Blebea J, Fowl RJ, et al. Contralateral duplex scanning for deep venous thrombosis is unnecessary in patients with symptoms. *J Vasc Surg* 1995;22(5):543-547.

120. Blebea J, Kihara TK, Neumyer MM, et al. A national survey of practice patterns in the noninvasive diagnosis of deep venous thrombosis. *J Vasc Surg* 1999;29(5):799-804, 806.

121. Cronan JJ. Deep venous thrombosis: One leg or both legs? *Radiology* 1996;200(2):323-324.

122. Pennell RC, Mantese VA, Westfall SG. Duplex scan for deep vein thrombosis—Defining who needs an examination of the contralateral asymptomatic leg. *J Vasc Surg* 2008;48(2):413-416.

123. Naidich JB, Torre JR, Pellerito JS, et al. Suspected deep venous thrombosis: Is US of both legs necessary? *Radiology.* 1996;200(2):429-431.

124. Sheiman RG, Weintraub JL, McArdle CR. Bilateral lower extremity US in the patient with bilateral symptoms of deep venous thrombosis: Assessment of need. *Radiology* 1995;196(2):379-381.

125. Lagerstedt CI, Olsson CG, Fagher BO, et al. Need for long-term anticoagulant treatment in symptomatic calf-vein thrombosis. *Lancet* 1985;2(8454):515-518.

126. Masuda EM, Kistner RL, Musikasinthorn C, et al. The controversy of managing calf vein thrombosis. *J Vasc Surg* 2012;55(2):550-561.

127. Righini M, Paris S, Le Gal G, et al. Clinical relevance of distal deep vein thrombosis. Review of literature data. *Thromb Haemost* 2006;95(1):56-64.

128. Hansson PO, Sorbo J, Eriksson H. Recurrent venous thromboembolism after deep vein thrombosis: Incidence and risk factors. *Arch Intern Med* 2000;160(6):769-774.

129. Pinede L, Ninet J, Duhaut P, et al. Comparison of 3 and months of oral anticoagulant therapy after a first episode of proximal deep vein thrombosis or pulmonary embolism and comparison of and 12 weeks of therapy after isolated calf deep vein thrombosis. *Circulation* 2001;103(20):2453-2460.

130. Schulman S, Rhedin AS, Lindmarker P, et al. A comparison of six weeks with six months of oral anticoagulant therapy after a first episode of venous thromboembolism. Duration of Anticoagulation Trial Study Group. *N Engl J Med* 1995;332(25):1661-1665.

131. Ridker PM, Goldhaber SZ, Danielson E, et al. Long-term, low-intensity warfarin therapy for the prevention of recurrent venous thromboembolism. *N Engl J Med* 2003;348(15):1425-1434.

132. Murin S, Romano PS, White RH. Comparison of outcomes after hospitalization for deep venous thrombosis or pulmonary embolism. *Thromb Haemost* 2002;88(3):407-414.

133. De Martino RR, Wallaert JB, Rossi AP, et al. A meta-analysis of anticoagulation for calf deep venous thrombosis. *J Vasc Surg* 2012;56(1):228-237. e221; discussion 236-227.

134. Kearon C, Akl EA, Comerota AJ, et al. Antithrombotic therapy for VTE disease: Antithrombotic Therapy and Prevention of Thrombosis, 9th ed.: American College of Chest Physicians Evidence-Based Clinical Practice Guidelines. *Chest* 2012;141(2 Suppl):e419S-e494S.

135. Singh K, Yakoub D, Giangola P, et al. Early follow-up and treatment recommendations for isolated calf deep venous thrombosis. *J Vasc Surg* 2012;55(1):136-140.

136. Mattos MA, Melendres G, Sumner DS, et al. Prevalence and distribution of calf vein thrombosis in patients with symptomatic deep venous thrombosis: A color-flow duplex study. *J Vasc Surg* 1996;24(5):738-744.

137. Macdonald PS, Kahn SR, Miller N, et al. Short-term natural history of isolated gastrocnemius and soleal vein thrombosis. *J Vasc Surg* 2003;37(3):523-527.

138. Sales CM, Haq F, Bustami R, et al. Management of isolated soleal and gastrocnemius vein thrombosis. *J Vasc Surg* 2010;52(5):1251-1254.

139. Henry JC, Satiani B. Calf muscle venous thrombosis: A review of the clinical implications and therapy. *Vasc Endovascular Surg* 2014;48(5-6):396-401.

140. Schwarz T, Buschmann L, Beyer J, et al. Therapy of isolated calf muscle vein thrombosis: A randomized, controlled study. *J Vasc Surg* 2010;52(5):1246-1250.

141. Prandoni P, Lensing AW, Prins MH, et al. Residual venous thrombosis as a predictive factor of recurrent venous thromboembolism. *Ann Intern Med* 2002;137(12):955-960.

142. Murphy TP, Cronan JJ. Evolution of deep venous thrombosis: A prospective evaluation with US. *Radiology* 1990;177(2):543-548.

143. Hertzberg BS, Kliewer MA, DeLong DM, et al. Sonographic assessment of lower limb vein diameters: Implications for the diagnosis and characterization of deep venous thrombosis. *AJR Am J Roentgenol* 1997;168(5):1253-1257.

144. Cosmi B, Legnani C, Cini M, et al. The role of D-dimer and residual venous obstruction in recurrence of venous thromboembolism after anticoagulation withdrawal in cancer patients. *Haematologica* 2005;90(5):713-715.

145. Bates SM, Jaeschke R, Stevens SM, et al. Diagnosis of DVT: Antithrombotic Therapy and Prevention of Thrombosis, 9th ed: American College of Chest Physicians Evidence-Based Clinical Practice Guidelines. *Chest* 2012;141(2 Suppl):e351S–e418S.

146. Middeldorp S, Prins MH, Hutten BA. Duration of treatment with vitamin K antagonists in symptomatic venous thromboembolism. *Cochrane Database Syst Rev* 2014;8:CD001367.

147. Siragusa S, Malato A, Anastasio R, et al. Residual vein thrombosis to establish duration of anticoagulation after a first episode of deep vein thrombosis: The Duration of Anticoagulation based on Compression UltraSonography (DACUS) study. *Blood* 2008;112(3):511-515.

148. Prandoni P. Risk factors of recurrent venous thromboembolism: The role of residual vein thrombosis. *Pathophysiol Haemost Thromb* 2003;33(5):351-353.

149. Cosmi B, Legnani C, Cini M, et al. D-dimer levels in combination with residual venous obstruction and the risk of recurrence after anticoagulation withdrawal for a first idiopathic deep vein thrombosis. *Thromb Haemost* 2005;94(5):969-974.

150. Caggiati A, Bergan JJ, Gloviczki P, et al. Nomenclature of the veins of the lower limbs: An international interdisciplinary consensus statement. *J Vasc Surg* 2002;36(2):416-422.

151. Liu SH, Chen WS. Medial gastrocnemius hematoma mimicking deep vein thrombosis: Report of a case. *Taiwan Yi Xue Hui Za Zhi* 1989;88(6):624-627.

152. Caggiati A, Bergan JJ, Gloviczki P, et al. Nomenclature of the veins of the lower limb: Extensions, refinements, and clinical application. *J Vasc Surg* 2005;41(4):719-724.

153. ICAVL. Standards for Accreditation in Noninvasive Vascular Testing. Part II. Vascular Laboratory Operations: Peripheral Venous Testing. 2007. http://www.icavl.org/icavl/pdfs/venous2007.pdf. Accessed June 30, 2009.

PERIPHERAL VENOUS

CHAPTER 20 ■ UPPER EXTREMITY VENOUS THROMBOSIS

MICHAEL T. CAPS AND BRIDGET A. MRAZ

In most vascular laboratories, the upper extremity venous duplex examination is performed less frequently than is the lower extremity venous examination. Whereas the basic principles of duplex scanning of the lower extremity venous system also apply to the upper extremity venous system, there are important differences between lower and upper extremity veins with respect to physiology, anatomy, and pathophysiology. An understanding of these differences is a prerequisite for the performance of a proper upper extremity venous duplex evaluation.

There are two major physiologic differences between upper and lower extremity venous flow. First, there is a marked difference in the phasicity of flow related to the respiratory cycle: In the lower extremity veins, flow decreases during inspiration and increases during expiration, whereas in the upper extremity, venous flow has the opposite relationship with respiration. This difference is caused by the interposition of the abdomen between the thorax and the lower extremities. During inspiration, intrathoracic pressure drops, causing an increase in the upper extremity venous pressure gradient and a consequent increase in venous flow from the upper extremities into the chest. However, inspiration is accompanied by descent of the diaphragm with a resulting increase in intra-abdominal pressure. Because veins are collapsible tubes, this increase in intra-abdominal pressure impedes venous outflow from the legs.

A second important physiologic difference between lower and upper extremity venous flow is an often pronounced increase in pulsatility in the upper extremity venous flow pattern, particularly in the more central, axillosubclavian venous segment. This is due to the proximity of the upper extremity veins to the heart. The abdominal venous segments serve as a buffer that dampens out the central venous pressure changes and makes them less detectable in the femoral veins. This increased pulsatility in the upper extremity veins can be particularly marked in patients with elevated right heart pressures due to heart failure, pulmonary hypertension, and tricuspid stenosis or regurgitation. Conversely, pulsatility in these veins may be blunted by the presence of more central venous occlusion.

An important anatomic difference between the upper and lower extremity veins is that a significant portion of the axillosubclavian venous segment lies within the bony thorax or within the thoracic outlet, which can render these veins difficult to image and difficult to compress with the ultrasound probe. As is discussed later in this chapter, these difficulties can often be overcome with the use of small ultrasound probes and color-flow and Doppler spectral waveforms.

A key difference in the pathophysiology of the upper and lower extremity veins is the mechanism by which pathologic conditions in these veins lead to disease states. Deep vein thrombosis (DVT) of the lower extremity is more likely to be associated with clinically significant pulmonary embolism (PE) and limb-threatening venous hypertension (phlegmasia cerulea dolens, venous gangrene) than is upper extremity DVT. Whereas thrombosis of the femoral, popliteal, and calf veins is common and frequently leads to severe symptoms in the lower extremity, analogous thrombosis of the brachial and deep forearm veins (in the absence of axillosubclavian thrombosis) is relatively uncommon and is less often associated with severe clinical symptoms.

Because of their dependent position and longer length, flow in the lower extremity veins is more affected by gravity than is flow in the upper extremity veins. Consequently, venous function in the legs relies more upon the presence of intact and competent venous valves. Although obstruction and incompetence both play important roles in the development of symptoms related to the lower extremity veins, the chronic and often debilitating symptoms of stasis dermatitis and ulceration are more frequently caused by reflux due to venous valvular incompetence. In contrast, these postthrombotic sequelae are less frequently seen in the upper extremity where obstruction (and particularly central venous obstruction) is the predominant pathophysiologic feature.

This chapter describes the technique for performing an upper extremity venous duplex examination for venous thrombosis. In order to provide a clinical context for this application of duplex scanning, the presentation, diagnosis, and treatment of upper extremity venous thrombosis is covered first. This discussion focuses mainly on axillosubclavian venous thrombosis, but jugular, brachial, and forearm DVT, as well as superficial thrombophlebitis of the cephalic and basilic veins, are also mentioned. The related topic of duplex scanning in the evaluation of dialysis access procedures is covered in Chapter 33. Preoperative vein mapping is discussed in Chapter 28.

BRACHIOCEPHALIC VENOUS THROMBOSIS

Etiology

Approximately 5% to 10% of all cases of DVT involve the upper extremity veins.[1-4] Upper extremity DVT is classically divided into two major types: primary and secondary. Thrombosis in both primary and secondary cases of upper extremity DVT usually occurs in the presence of one or more elements of Virchow's triad: endothelial damage, stasis, and hypercoagulability (Fig. 20.1).

First described by Paget and von Schrötter in the late 1800s and subsequently named the "Paget-Schrötter syndrome," a significant fraction of cases of primary upper extremity DVT are caused by compression of the axillo-subclavian venous segment at the thoracic outlet, usually in the vicinity of the first rib. This is commonly referred to as "venous thoracic outlet syndrome." It is hypothesized that thrombosis is preceded by many years of intermittent compression and repetitive trauma to this venous segment, accompanied by the accumulation of scar tissue. In these patients, compression of the subclavian vein can be induced during the performance of upper extremity venography by several provocative body positions, including hyperabduction and external rotation of the shoulder, extension of the neck, and caudal and posterior movement of the shoulder.[5] However, the situation is complicated by the fact that many asymptomatic individuals will also demonstrate these changes on provocative venography. Additionally, a minority of patients with primary upper extremity DVT, many of whom have hypercoagulable states, have no evidence of thoracic outlet compression even with provocative arm and shoulder positioning.

Approximately 75% of upper extremity DVT cases are termed "secondary" DVT, the majority of which are caused by the presence of indwelling medical devices such as central venous catheters and pacemaker wires.[2,6] In addition, the presence of known or occult malignancies, with or without an indwelling catheter, is an important factor in the pathogenesis of secondary upper extremity DVT.[7] In hospital settings, secondary DVT, particularly those cases associated with indwelling catheters and pacemakers, is far more common than is primary upper extremity DVT.

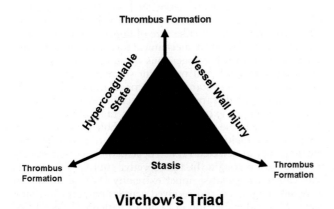

FIGURE 20.1. Virchow's triad of thrombus formation.

Diagnosis

The majority of patients presenting with the Paget-Schrötter syndrome (also called "effort thrombosis") are young, athletic, and often muscular males, although the condition is certainly not limited to this demographic group. The clinical hallmark of the Paget-Schrötter syndrome is ipsilateral upper extremity swelling that typically involves the upper arm, forearm, and hand and is predominantly nonpitting, particularly during the acute phase. Pain is also a frequent symptom, usually described as "tightness" or "heaviness," and is often exacerbated by dependency and partially ameliorated by elevation. Because these patients have venous hypertension in the affected extremity, the veins of the arm and hand are often distended, although this may not be readily apparent because the venous distention is often masked by edema. Although not necessarily present in the acute phase, enlarged venous collaterals are usually visible around the shoulder.

The clinical presentation of patients with catheter-associated upper extremity DVT can be more subtle than the presentation of Paget-Schrötter syndrome.[8] Thrombus associated with indwelling catheters often develops more slowly (allowing more time for the development of venous collaterals) and typically involves a shorter venous segment than primary DVT. Furthermore, the affected patients usually have multiple medical comorbidities (e.g., cancer, heart failure, end-stage renal disease) rendering them far more sedentary than the typical patient with Paget-Schrötter syndrome.

Prior to obtaining objective diagnostic tests, it is possible to stratify patients according to low, intermediate, and high pretest probability for upper extremity DVT in much the same way as has been demonstrated for lower extremity DVT. Constans et al[9] used logistic regression on a derivation sample of 140 patients. These authors developed a clinical scoring system in which a point is added for the presence or absence of swelling, pain, and an indwelling catheter or pacemaker, and a point is subtracted when there is a plausible alternative diagnosis. The scoring system was then tested in a 214 patient validation sample. Among patients with a score of −1 or 0 (low probability), 1 (intermediate probability), and 2 or 3 (high probability), upper extremity DVT was found in 13%, 38%, and 69% of patients, respectively.

Because of its low specificity, a positive D-dimer test cannot be used to diagnose upper extremity DVT. A negative D-dimer result can be used to confidently rule out DVT, particularly among patients with a low pretest probability of upper extremity DVT. However, the clinical usefulness of this approach is limited by the fact that the majority of patients with suspected upper extremity DVT who have cancer or indwelling catheters or pacemakers will also have elevated D-dimer results.[10]

The most commonly employed diagnostic imaging tests are duplex ultrasonography and catheter venography, although magnetic resonance venography (MRV) and computed tomography venography (CTV) may also play important roles depending on local expertise and availability. Although studies of MRV show particularly promising results when performed in centers of excellence, this discussion focuses on duplex scanning because it is far more commonly used in clinical practice, is less costly, and does not involve the use of contrast agents that can pose risks to the patient.

Table 20.1 summarizes the studies in which the accuracy of duplex scanning for the diagnosis of upper extremity DVT has been quantified using catheter contrast venography as the reference or "gold standard."[6,11-16] However, it should be emphasized that venography is not a perfect standard in this setting. When two "blinded" radiologists interpret the same venogram, there is considerable disagreement.[17] In addition, there are cases of nonocclusive upper extremity DVT

TABLE 20.1

SUMMARY OF REPORTED STUDIES IN WHICH THE RESULTS OF DUPLEX SCANNING FOR AXILLARY AND SUBCLAVIAN VENOUS THROMBOSIS WERE VALIDATED USING VENOGRAPHY AS THE "GOLD STANDARD"

■ AUTHORS	■ YEAR	■ NO. OF PATIENTS	■ CATHETER RELATED	■ SENSITIVITY	■ SPECIFICITY
Falk and Smith[13]	1987	14	64%	88%	100%
Knudson et al[15]	1990	20	48%	78%	92%
Haire et al[14]	1991	43	91%	56%	100%
Baxter et al[12]	1991	19	74%	100%	100%
Koksoy et al[16]	1995	94	100%	94%	88%
Prandoni et al[6]	1997	58	14%	100%	93%
Baarslag et al[11]	2002	99	41%	82%	82%
Weighted average		T = 347	62%	86%	90%

diagnosed by duplex scanning in which the venogram is interpreted as being "normal," and venography is clearly inferior to duplex scanning in detecting jugular venous thrombosis. These caveats aside, a well-performed venogram is, in most clinical settings, the final arbiter for the presence or absence of upper extremity DVT.

The accuracy of duplex scanning in diagnosing DVT of the upper extremities has been far less extensively studied than in the lower extremities. The published studies (see Table 20.1) have demonstrated considerable variability in study methodologies, including the proportion of patients with catheter-associated DVT. Taking a weighted average of these studies yields a sensitivity (86%) that is slightly lower than the specificity (90%), but the heterogeneity in reported results is striking, ranging from 56% to 100% for sensitivity and from 82% to 100% for specificity. Some of the variability in results is almost certainly due to the fact that duplex scanning is operator dependent, and this operator dependence is probably more of a factor in the upper extremity venous system owing to the difficulty of imaging underneath the clavicle where most clinically important upper extremity DVT occurs. A list of indications for upper extremity venous duplex scanning is given in Table 20.2.

While upper extremity venous duplex scanning is the most frequently employed imaging test for the diagnosis of DVT in most centers, there is still an important subset of patients who are appropriate for venography. Among patients for whom there is an intermediate or high clinical suspicion of upper extremity DVT, particularly those who would be candidates

for catheter-directed thrombolysis, a strong argument can be made for ignoring a negative duplex scan result or omitting the duplex scan altogether and proceeding directly to venography. Conversely, for patients who are not considered candidates for catheter-directed thrombolysis, the decision to anticoagulate is often based solely on the results of the duplex scan. Among patients who are not considered candidates for thrombolysis and who have had a negative duplex scan, but for whom there is still a high clinical suspicion of upper extremity DVT, venography should be considered and MRV or CTV may also be useful. It should be noted that no studies have examined clinical outcomes resulting from withholding treatment on the basis of a negative duplex scan of the upper extremity veins.

Prognosis

Since the majority of patients with upper extremity DVT are treated with anticoagulation, little is known about the natural history of upper extremity DVT without treatment. Clinically important outcomes include mortality, PE, recurrent thrombosis, and alleviation of acute and chronic ("postthrombotic syndrome") symptoms. In most modern series of upper extremity DVT, mortality rates are substantial owing to the coexistence of cancer, central venous catheters, cardiac disease, pacemakers, and automatic implantable cardiac defibrillators.[3,18-20] The vast majority of these deaths are due to the patient's underlying disease rather than to PE. In contrast, patients with Paget-Schrötter syndrome are typically young and healthy with a markedly better prognosis.

As mentioned previously, PE, and particularly symptomatic PE, is less frequently associated with upper extremity DVT than with lower extremity DVT. Explanations for this difference include the smaller size of upper extremity venous thrombi and variations in mechanical forces and flow dynamics. In studies with heterogeneous combinations of primary and secondary DVT and treatment strategies ranging from no anticoagulation to standard anticoagulation with or without thrombolytic therapy, the incidence of reported PE associated with upper extremity DVT has ranged from 0% to 25%.[4,21-26] Because the majority of emboli associated with DVT of the brachial and cephalic veins are asymptomatic, the frequency of detected PE will depend on how aggressively the diagnosis is sought. In a prospective study of 86 patients with catheter-associated upper extremity DVT, all of whom were anticoagulated and received ventilation-perfusion lung scans, Monreal et al[25] found PE in 13 patients (15%); 11 of these patients were asymptomatic, while 2 had symptomatic and fatal PE.

TABLE 20.2

INDICATIONS FOR UPPER EXTREMITY VENOUS DUPLEX SCANNING

1. Unilateral upper extremity swelling with associated prior event (e.g., shoulder surgery).
2. Presence or history of central venous catheter or PICC line.
3. Screening of central veins prior to placement of central venous catheter, defibrillator, other cardiac device, or heart biopsy.
4. Upper extremity or hand swelling in the presence of a patent dialysis access fistula or graft.
5. Superficial palpable cord.
6. Erythema and tenderness.
7. Facial swelling with prominent chest collaterals (could be a sign of SVC syndrome).

PICC, peripherally inserted central catheter; SVC, superior vena cava.

In a comprehensive literature review of patients with primary upper extremity DVT, Thomas and Zierler[26] found a reported incidence for PE of 12% among those treated without anticoagulation (rest, heat, and elevation of the effected limb) versus 7% for those who were anticoagulated. Although not known with certainty, the rate of PE is most likely similar among patients with primary versus secondary upper extremity DVT. While the data on jugular vein thrombosis are sparse, the available literature suggests a similar risk of PE compared with that of upper extremity DVT.[21,24,27] It is generally believed that isolated DVT occurring distal to the shoulder (i.e., in the brachial or forearm veins), as well as superficial thrombophlebitis involving the cephalic and basilic veins, are both associated with very low risks of PE. However, PE has been reported in both of these subgroups, including one study of 52 patients with isolated brachial vein thrombosis in which the proportion of patients with documented PE was 11.5%.[28]

The risks of recurrent thrombosis and chronic postthrombotic symptoms are also substantially lower following upper extremity DVT compared with lower extremity DVT. The risk of symptomatic upper extremity recurrent thrombosis is 2% to 5% at 12 months and 5% to 15% at 5 years.[3,18,29] The corresponding figures for lower extremity DVT are 5% to 15% at 12 months and 20% to 30% at 5 years.[30,31] As previously mentioned, the risk of long-term postthrombotic symptoms is considerably lower in the arm than in the leg. The proportion of patients suffering long-term postthrombotic symptoms following upper extremity DVT is approximately 15% compared to 30% to 60% following lower extremity DVT.[31-33] Patients who suffer long-term postthrombotic symptoms in the upper extremity are more likely to have residual axillosubclavian vein occlusion and are less likely to have suffered catheter-associated thrombosis.[32]

Treatment

The goals of treatment for patients with upper extremity DVT are to prolong life, alleviate acute symptoms, and minimize the risk of PE, symptomatic recurrent thrombosis, and the postthrombotic syndrome. The treatment of upper extremity DVT may consist of one or more of the following elements: conservative management (rest, heat, elevation, external compression), anticoagulation, central venous catheter removal, thrombolytic therapy, and surgical decompression of the thoracic outlet with or without open or endovascular venous reconstruction.

Because randomized trials of anticoagulant therapy in patients with upper extremity DVT are lacking, recommendations regarding the choice of anticoagulant and duration of therapy for patients with upper extremity DVT are largely extrapolated from data on the treatment of lower extremity DVT. Consensus guidelines from the American College of Chest Physicians provide detailed recommendations for the treatment of upper extremity DVT.[34] Salient points from the most recent 9th edition of this guideline statement are reviewed here.

Unless there are contraindications, patients with acute thrombosis of the subclavian or axillary veins should be anticoagulated.[34] Absolute contraindications to anticoagulation include severe active bleeding, intracranial bleeding, recent brain, eye, or spinal cord surgery, pregnancy, and malignant hypertension. Relative contraindications include recent stroke or major surgery and severe thrombocytopenia. In general, superficial venous thrombophlebitis of the cephalic or basilic veins and isolated DVT involving the brachial or forearm veins do not require anticoagulation. However, there is recent evidence to suggest that patients with superficial venous thrombosis of the lower extremity benefit from treatment with prophylactic dose anticoagulation.[35] Although somewhat controversial, anticoagulation should be considered in patients with extensive and proximal superficial thrombophlebitis or brachial vein thrombosis when there is active cancer and/or indwelling catheters.

Anticoagulant therapy is typically started parenterally in the form of intravenous unfractionated heparin (IVUFH) or subcutaneous low molecular weight heparin (LMWH). Data from several randomized controlled trials and meta-analyses suggest that LMWH is superior to IVUFH with lower mortality and lower risk of recurrent thrombosis and major bleeding.[19,36] Although less compelling, there is evidence to suggest that fondaparinux is also superior to IVUFH for patients with acute DVT and should be considered to have equivalent efficacy and safety compared with LMWH.[34] Because LMWH and fondaparinux have significant renal excretion, they are contraindicated in patients with significant renal impairment (glomerular filtration rate <30 mL/min).

After parenteral therapy is begun, most patients with upper extremity DVT should be treated with a 3-month course of vitamin K antagonists.[34] Selected patients with unprovoked DVT, thrombophilia, or cancer who are at low risk of bleeding complications may benefit from a longer course of therapy. There is evidence from lower extremity DVT trials suggesting that LMWH is superior to vitamin K antagonists for patients with active cancer.[34]

Patients with catheter-associated upper extremity DVT should be anticoagulated similarly. If the catheter is still needed, it should not be removed. If the catheter is no longer needed or is nonfunctional, it should be removed followed by a 3-month course of anticoagulant therapy as outlined above. Anticoagulant prophylaxis for patients with central venous catheters is controversial, but there is no convincing evidence to support it. A meta-analysis of seven trials showed a nonsignificant reduction in the risk of symptomatic thrombosis associated with thromboprophylaxis.[37] This is an area requiring further study.

The use of superior vena cava (SVC) filters is another controversial topic. Major complications such as cardiac tamponade and aortic perforation have been reported in small observational studies.[38] SVC filters should be limited to patients who have a contraindication to anticoagulation and those who have severe symptoms, and they should preferably only be placed in centers with experience using this technique.

Thrombolytic therapy should be limited to patients with severe symptoms, a short (<14 days) duration of symptoms, good functional capacity, and a low risk of bleeding. The majority of patients with secondary upper extremity DVT are not good candidates for thrombolytic therapy for several reasons. First, the symptoms are typically not severe. Second, the patients are often debilitated with significant comorbidities, and the risks of thrombolysis and surgery may be significant. Third, these patients tend to have acceptable results with anticoagulation alone.

In contrast, patients presenting with primary upper extremity DVT are often good candidates for thrombolytic therapy. The rationale for this statement lies in the observation that a significant proportion of patients with primary upper extremity DVT who are treated with anticoagulation alone may have persistent and often severe postthrombotic symptoms in the involved extremity.[39] As previously stated, a significant fraction of patients with primary upper extremity DVT are young and active, and many are athletes. With vigorous exercise, the venous outflow from an upper extremity with a collateralized central venous occlusion often cannot keep up with arterial inflow. These patients have persistent arm swelling and pain exacerbated by extremity exercise. Because these patients are usually quite healthy, there are rarely any contraindications to thrombolytic or surgical therapy. Catheter-directed thrombolytic therapy is performed by embedding a multi–side-holed catheter into the thrombus at the time of venography and infusing a thrombolytic agent, usually tissue-type plasminogen activator (t-PA), typically for 12 to 24 hours. Catheter-directed thrombolysis is often combined with mechanical techniques ("pharmacomechanical thrombolysis") that involve fragmentation and aspiration of the thrombus. These catheter-based approaches are more effective, less damaging to the endothelium, and less morbid than surgical thrombectomy (Fig. 20.2).

Following thrombolysis, the patient will generally fall into one of these four categories based on the appearance of the postlysis venogram.

1. *Complete recanalization with no evidence of residual narrowing with the arm in neutral position or in one of the provocative positions.* This is relatively unusual. These patients should be anticoagulated and worked up for hypercoagulable states and occult malignancy. Thoracic outlet decompression is not indicated.
2. *Complete recanalization with evidence for extrinsic compression, particularly with provocative arm/shoulder positioning.* The treatment of these

patients is somewhat controversial. Some advocate anticoagulation alone for these patients while many surgeons perform immediate or delayed thoracic outlet decompression, usually requiring some combination of first rib removal, scalenotomy, and resection of the costoclavicular ligament done via a supraclavicular, infraclavicular, or transaxillary approach. In addition, some of these patients have cervical ribs that require resection.

3. *Complete or near-complete recanalization with evidence for both extrinsic and intrinsic venous compromise.* The intrinsic compromise is due to residual thrombus, scar tissue, or both. If the intrinsic compromise is severe and does not improve substantially with balloon angioplasty, many advocate thoracic outlet decompression coupled with venous repair involving combinations of endovenectomy, vein patch angioplasty, interposition vein grafting, or jugular vein "turn down." Venous repair usually requires a combined supraclavicular and infraclavicular approach or partial claviculectomy. The use of stents to treat residual stenoses in the axillosubclavian venous segment is generally contraindicated due to high rates of stent fracture, recurrent stenosis, and thrombosis.[40]

4. *Failed thrombolysis with continued axillosubclavian vein occlusion.* These patients should be anticoagulated. Many will experience complete or near-complete

FIGURE 20.2. Case of effort thrombosis. *A*, Initial duplex evaluation shows acute thrombosis of the right subclavian vein with no color Doppler flow. *B*, Initial venogram shows near occlusion of the right subclavian vein (*arrow*).

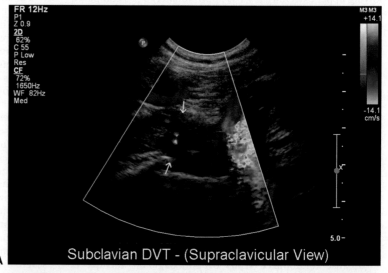

A

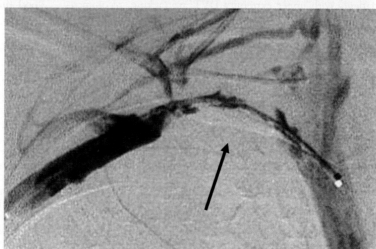

B

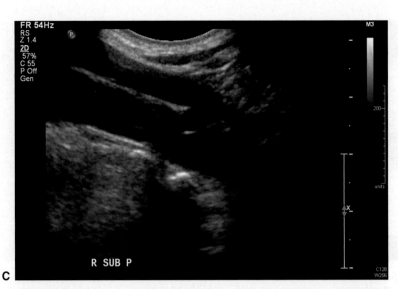

FIGURE 20.2. (*Continued*) *C,* Postthrombolysis B-mode image of the right subclavian vein shows partial residual webbing and a "frozen" valve cusp in the lumen. *D,* Final venogram shows a patent right subclavian vein postthrombolysis.

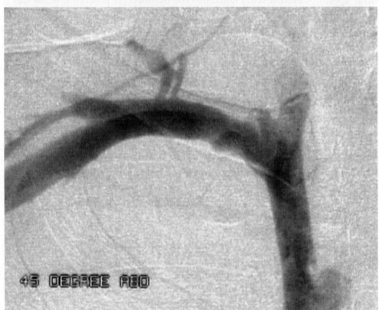

resolution of symptoms. For those with continued severe symptoms and reconstructable venous anatomy, a venous reconstruction with thoracic outlet decompression should be considered.

There are many similarities between upper and lower extremity DVT, as well as some important differences. Many aspects of the diagnosis and treatment of upper extremity DVT require further study including: the role of clinical probability scoring systems, the accuracy of duplex scanning using state-of-the-art equipment and scanning techniques, the role of novel anticoagulants such as the direct thrombin inhibitors and factor Xa antagonists, the optimal duration of anticoagulation as determined by risk stratification on the basis of competing risks of rethrombosis off anticoagulation versus major bleeding risk on anticoagulation, the role of anticoagulation for patients with upper extremity superficial venous thrombophlebitis and brachial and forearm DVT, the role of prophylactic therapy in selected high-risk populations for preventing upper extremity DVT, and optimal criteria for selecting patients for thrombolysis and thoracic outlet decompression.

DUPLEX SCANNING

Instrumentation

A standard duplex ultrasound system is used for the upper extremity venous examination with high-resolution B-mode imaging, color Doppler, and spectral waveform analysis. A midrange-frequency curved transducer (5 to 8 MHz) with a small footprint (as used in neonatal head examinations) is helpful when evaluating the subclavian vein, because access is limited by the clavicle. A high-frequency transducer (10 to 15 MHz) may be helpful for evaluating very superficial veins. Some of the common transducer configurations and their sector image patterns are shown in Figure 20.3.

Venous duplex imaging requires the parameters for color Doppler and Doppler spectral waveforms to be set for optimal detection of low velocity flow. The wall filter should be set at the lowest setting to avoid cutting off low flow velocities. Increasing power and gain maximizes the Doppler flow signal with increasing depth through the tissue. However, overcompensation of the Doppler gain settings produces a mirror image

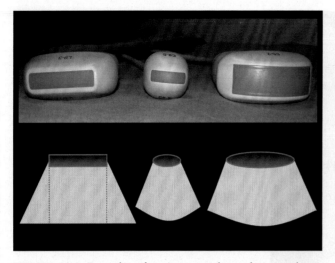

FIGURE 20.3. Examples of various transducer shapes and sector image patterns for scanning of the central and peripheral upper extremity veins.

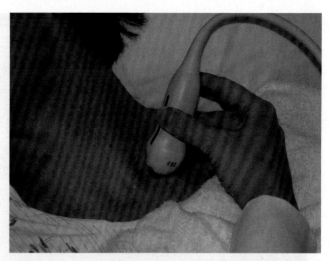

FIGURE 20.4. Patient position for left innominate and proximal subclavian vein evaluation. The transducer is positioned in the supraclavicular fossa.

of flow signals in the spectral display above and below the zero baseline that will be corrected by decreasing the gain. Spectral Doppler and color Doppler settings should be set to optimize peak velocities in the range of 50 to 100 cm/s. The upper extremity venous duplex protocol is summarized in Table 20.3.

Patient Position

For scanning of the central upper extremity veins, it is best for the patient to be supine with the neck turned to the contralateral side and the chin slightly raised, as shown in Figure 20.4. However, if the neck is turned too far to the contralateral side, the sternocleidomastoid muscle will tighten across the neck, making transducer contact difficult and vein wall compression nearly impossible. This is also an uncomfortable position for the patient. If the patient is sitting up, the veins may collapse, making imaging more difficult. Conversely, if the patient's head is

positioned lower than the heart, the veins (particularly the internal jugular vein) may become dilated and difficult to compress.

Deep Venous Anatomy

The internal jugular, innominate or brachiocephalic, and subclavian veins are the central veins that drain the arms and head, as shown in Figure 20.5.

Internal Jugular Veins

The internal jugular vein drains blood from the brain, the face, and the neck. It begins at the jugular foramen at the base of the skull where it is often somewhat dilated, and this dilatation is called the "superior bulb." It also has a common trunk that receives drainage from the anterior branch of the retromandibular vein, the facial vein, and the lingual vein.

TABLE 20.3

UPPER EXTREMITY VENOUS DUPLEX PROTOCOL

	SPECTRAL DOPPLER				COLOR DOPPLER	B-MODE
▪ VESSEL	▪ SPONTANEOUS	▪ PHASIC	▪ PULSATILE	▪ AUGMENT	▪ COMPLETE	▪ VEIN WALLS COMPRESS
Internal jugular vein	✓	✓	✓		✓	✓
Innominate vein	✓	✓	✓		✓	N/A
Subclavian vein	✓	✓	✓		✓	X
Axillary vein	✓	✓	✓	✓	✓	✓
Brachial veins	X	X	X	✓	✓	✓
Radial veins				✓	✓	✓
Ulnar veins				✓	✓	✓
Cephalic vein				✓	X	✓
Basilic vein				✓	X	✓

✓, routine; X, when applicable; N/A, not applicable.

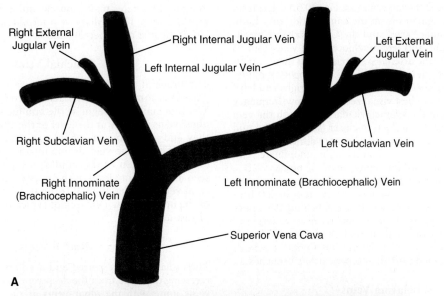

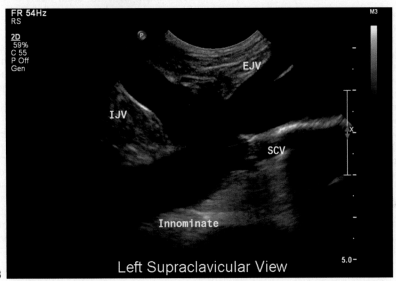

FIGURE 20.5. *A,* The upper extremity central veins. *B,* Corresponding B-mode image of the left upper extremity central veins. EJV, external jugular vein; IJV, internal jugular vein; SCV, subclavian vein.

The internal jugular vein courses vertically down the neck parallel to the internal carotid and common carotid arteries. At the base of the neck, it joins the subclavian vein to form the brachiocephalic (innominate) vein, and just above this confluence is a second dilatation, termed the "inferior bulb." At the base of the neck, the right internal jugular vein is often more lateral than the common carotid artery, and it crosses over the proximal subclavian artery, whereas the left internal jugular vein usually overlaps the common carotid artery. The left internal jugular vein is typically smaller than the right, and each contains a valve about 2.5 cm above the central end of the vessel.

The internal jugular veins are relatively superficial and not protected by bone or cartilage, making them susceptible to injury. There are no valves between the right atrium and the internal jugular vein, so blood can flow back into the internal jugular when the pressure in the right atrium is high. This can be seen externally as a pulsation at the base of the neck with the patient in the supine position, the head of the bed elevated at 45 degrees, and the head turned slightly to the contralateral side. However, unlike the carotid pulse, this jugular venous pulse is not readily palpated. Reasons for jugular venous pressure to be increased include right heart failure, tricuspid stenosis, tricuspid regurgitation, and cardiac tamponade.

Because the internal jugular vein is large, central, and relatively superficial, it is a common site for central line placement, and because it rarely varies in location, it is generally easier to cannulate than other veins. However, there is a risk of missing the vein and puncturing the adjacent carotid artery, especially when venous cannulation is performed without ultrasound guidance, as discussed in Chapter 27. A duplex evaluation of the neck may be requested following an attempted internal jugular vein puncture to evaluate for vascular injury if the patient develops severe swelling or a hematoma. Rarely, a pseudoaneurysm may be found arising from the common carotid or some other artery in the neck.

Brachiocephalic (Innominate) Veins

As previously mentioned, the brachiocephalic veins are also known as the innominate veins. The left and right brachiocephalic veins are formed by the union of the corresponding internal jugular and subclavian veins (see Fig. 20.5A). The term "brachiocephalic" originates from the combination of a Latin term *brachium* meaning "arm" and the Greek *kephale* meaning "head." The right and left brachiocephalic veins join to form the SVC. Unlike the arterial system in which there is typically one innominate artery (on the right), the upper extremity venous system comprises two innominate veins (right and left). The innominate veins are best visualized using a low-frequency transducer scanning in the supraclavicular space with the vein coursing directly away from the transducer (see Figs. 20.4 and 20.5B). The left innominate vein may be more difficult to image because it takes a longer course than the right innominate vein, crossing the midline toward the right side of the heart.

The right brachiocephalic vein passes almost vertically downward in front of the innominate artery, and the left brachiocephalic vein passes from left to right behind the upper part of the sternum. Each of these veins receives a vertebral, deep cervical, deep thyroid, and internal thoracic vein. The left brachiocephalic vein also receives intercostal, thymic, tracheal, esophageal, phrenic, mediastinal, and pericardiac branches.

Subclavian Veins

The subclavian vein is a continuation of the axillary vein and runs from the outer border of the first rib to the medial border of the anterior scalene muscle (Fig. 20.6). The subclavian vein lies anterior and inferior to the subclavian artery as it crosses the first rib; they are separated by the anterior scalene insertion. Anteriorly, the subclavian vein is covered throughout its entire course by the clavicle. Initially, the vein arches upward across the first rib before turning medially, downward, and slightly forward across the insertion of the anterior scalene muscle to enter the thorax where it joins with the internal jugular vein behind the sternoclavicular joint. The thoracic duct drains into the left subclavian vein near its junction with the left internal jugular vein; the right subclavian vein receives the right lymphatic duct.

Axillary Veins

The axillary vein carries blood from the lateral aspect of the thorax, axilla, and upper limb toward the heart, following the course of the corresponding artery. It originates at the lower margin of the teres major muscle and is a continuation of the brachial vein. The axillary vein terminates at the lateral margin of the first rib, where it becomes the subclavian vein.

Brachial Veins

The brachial vein (or veins, because this segment is often paired) accompanies the brachial artery in the upper arm. The brachial veins begin at the confluence of the radial and ulnar veins (usually at the level of the antecubital space), and they end at the border of the teres major muscle (see Fig. 20.6). The basilic vein drains into the brachial vein; however, the location of this confluence is variable and may be seen at nearly any level in the upper arm or axilla. The brachial veins also have small tributaries that drain the muscles of the upper arm which are not typically well seen on duplex ultrasound.

Radial Veins

The radial veins are paired and accompany the radial artery, receiving drainage from the deep veins of the hand. The radial veins unite with the ulnar veins at the antecubital space to form the brachial veins.

Ulnar Veins

The ulnar veins are the paired veins that accompany the ulnar artery in the forearm and drain the ulnar aspect of the forearm and hand. They arise in the hand and join with the radial veins to form the brachial veins.

Superficial Venous Anatomy

The superficial veins in the neck and upper extremities are located superficial to the muscular fascia in the subcutaneous fatty tissue and, in contrast to the deep veins, do not have a corresponding artery. The external jugular vein is the primary superficial venous outflow pathway of the head, whereas the cephalic and basilic veins are the primary superficial venous outflow from the upper extremities.

FIGURE 20.6. The upper extremity veins.

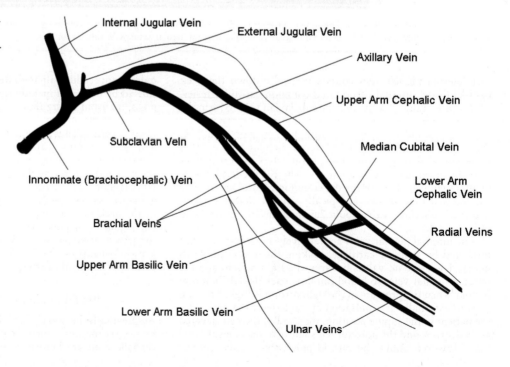

External Jugular Vein

The external jugular vein receives the majority of the venous blood from the scalp and parts of the face. It is formed by the confluence of the posterior division of the posterior facial vein with the posterior auricular vein. It courses down the neck along a line from the angle of the mandible to the middle of the clavicle at the posterior border of the sternocleidomastoid muscle. The external jugular vein crosses the sternocleidomastoid obliquely, perforates the deep fascia, and empties into the subclavian vein lateral to or in front of the anterior scalene muscle. The external jugular vein varies in size and contains a pair of valves—an inferior valve located at the confluence with the subclavian vein and a superior valve about 4 cm above the clavicle. The portion of the external jugular vein between the two valves is often dilated, and is termed the "sinus."

The external jugular vein has a number of tributaries: occipital, posterior external jugular, and near its termination, the transverse cervical, transverse scapular, and anterior jugular veins. Most superiorly, at the parotid gland, it is joined by a large communicating branch from the internal jugular vein. The external jugular vein is not routinely evaluated on duplex scanning, but it may become dilated in the presence of internal jugular or subclavian vein thrombosis, and it is often visualized just superior to the subclavian vein where it may be mistaken for the native subclavian vein (see Fig. 20.5).

Cephalic Vein

The cephalic vein is a superficial vein in the upper extremity that begins on the lateral (radial) side of the wrist and courses up that side of the forearm, communicating with the basilic vein via the median cubital vein at the elbow (see Fig. 20.6). In the upper arm, it is located along the anterolateral surface of the biceps muscle. Superiorly, the cephalic vein passes between the deltoid and the pectoralis major muscles (deltopectoral groove) and through the deltopectoral triangle, where it empties into the axillary vein just beneath the clavicle. Although it usually terminates in the axillary vein, it can also join the external jugular vein. The cephalic vein is often visible through the skin, and its location in the deltopectoral groove is fairly consistent, making identification by ultrasound reliable at that site.

Basilic Vein

The basilic vein is typically the larger of the two main superficial veins in the upper extremity (see Fig. 20.6). It originates on the medial (ulnar) side of the dorsal venous network of the hand, and it travels up that side of the forearm and upper arm. Most of its course is quite superficial. At the antecubital space, the basilic vein typically communicates with the cephalic vein via the median cubital vein. However, the specific anatomy of the superficial veins in the forearm is highly variable from person to person, and there are numerous unnamed superficial veins communicating with the basilic vein. It then runs along the medial margin of the biceps muscle to the middle of the upper arm where it pierces the deep fascia to join with the brachial veins to form the axillary vein. The basilic vein is a common location for a peripherally inserted central catheter (PICC) line to be placed.

Median Cubital Vein

The median cubital vein is a superficial vein in the upper extremity that lies in the antecubital space. It connects the basilic and cephalic veins and is often used for venipuncture. It is separated from the brachial artery by a thickened portion of the deep fascia. There is wide variation in the course of the median cubital vein. Most commonly, the vein forms an H pattern with the cephalic and basilic veins making up the sides. Other forms include an M pattern, in which the vein branches to the cephalic and basilic veins (Fig. 20.7).

Central Venous Lines

A central venous catheter is a line placed through one of the upper extremity central veins, with the tip usually located in the SVC or right atrium. Central venous catheters are utilized to administer medications or total parenteral nutrition (TPN),

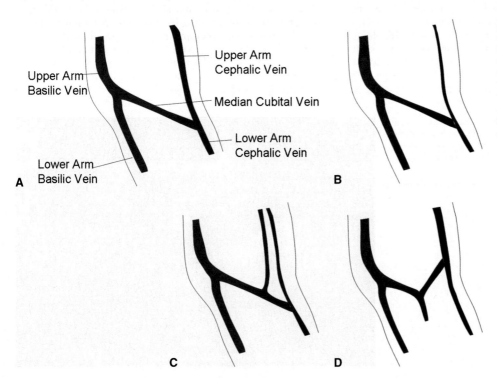

Upper Arm Basilic Vein
Lower Arm Basilic Vein
Upper Arm Cephalic Vein
Median Cubital Vein
Lower Arm Cephalic Vein
A
B
C
D

FIGURE 20.7. Anatomic variations of the superficial veins at the antecubital fossa. A, Most common "H" configuration. B, Dominant upper arm basilic vein with small cephalic vein. C, Dominant basilic vein with two small upper arm cephalic veins. D, Median cubital vein originating from a deep muscular branch.

FIGURE 20.8. B-mode image of a peripherally inserted central catheter (PICC line) in the proximal left subclavian vein. The catheter is seen as two bright parallel lines in the vein lumen (*arrow*).

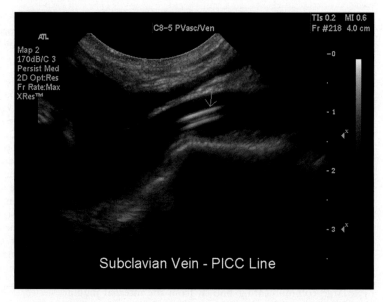

obtain blood samples, perform cardiovascular measurements (central venous pressure), and provide temporary dialysis access. There are several different types of central lines: a PICC, tunneled catheters (Hickman and Groshong), and implanted ports. An understanding of the differences between the types of central venous catheters should improve communication with referring physicians and help direct the upper extremity duplex examination whenever a central line is present.

PICC Lines

A PICC line is inserted into a vein in the arm (peripheral vein) rather than a vein in the neck. PICC lines are usually inserted into the basilic or cephalic vein and advanced until the tip is in the right atrial appendage (Fig. 20.8). A variation is the "midline" catheter which is inserted like a PICC line, but the tip is positioned in the proximal axillary or distal subclavian vein.

Tunneled Catheters

A tunneled catheter is surgically inserted into a vein in the neck or chest and passes through the subcutaneous tissues for a short distance before exiting through the skin. "Tunneling" the catheter under the skin helps keep it in place, allows the patient to move around more easily, and makes it less visible. The external end of the catheter is usually fixed to the skin by a suture or staple and an occlusive dressing. The line is

regularly flushed with saline or heparin to keep it patent and prevent thrombosis. Some lines also contain agents such as antibiotics to reduce the risk of infection.

Two common types of long-term tunneled central venous lines are the Hickman catheter (named for Dr. Robert O. Hickman, a pediatric nephrologist at Seattle Children's Hospital), which uses built-in clamps at the external end to control flow in the line, and the Groshong catheter, which has a valve on the internal tip that opens as fluid is withdrawn or infused and remains closed when not in use. Hickman and Groshong catheters are typically inserted into the internal jugular vein and tunneled under the skin to minimize the risk of infection (Figs. 20.9 and 20.10).

Implanted Ports

An implanted port is similar to a tunneled catheter, but it remains entirely under the skin, and medications are injected through the skin into the catheter. Some implanted ports contain a small reservoir that slowly releases the medication through the catheter into the bloodstream. An implanted port is not visible on the skin and requires very little daily care, so it has less impact on a patient's activities than a PICC line or a tunneled catheter. Ports are used mostly to treat oncology patients, but they have also been adapted for hemodialysis patients (Fig. 20.11).

FIGURE 20.9. B-mode image of an internal jugular vein (IJV) deep vein thrombosis (DVT) associated with a tunneled catheter. The thrombus appears as "softly" echogenic material in the vein lumen that is hypoechoic compared to the surrounding soft tissue.

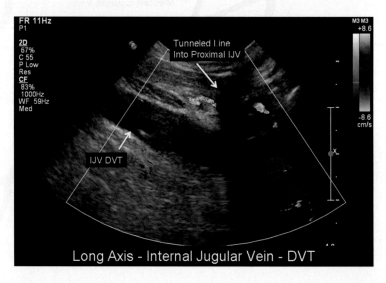

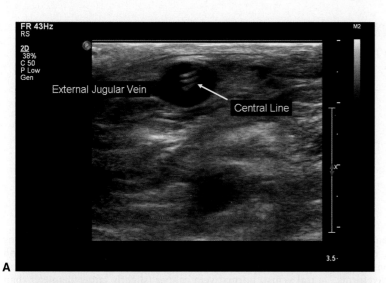

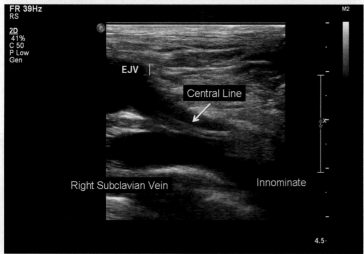

FIGURE 20.10. B-mode images of a right internal jugular vein tunneled line that took a "wrong turn" into the external jugular vein rather than down the innominate vein. *A*, Transverse view shows the line in the external jugular vein. *B*, Long-axis view shows the line in the external jugular vein but not in the innominate vein.

Acute Upper Extremity Deep Vein Thrombosis

The duplex criteria for diagnosis of upper extremity DVT are summarized in Table 20.4. These include B-mode image, color Doppler, and Doppler spectral waveform findings.

B-Mode Image

It has been well documented that vein wall compression by external transducer pressure is the most accurate and direct way to detect venous thrombus. This technique is possible throughout the upper extremity distal to the axilla and in the neck; however, vein wall compressions cannot be performed

FIGURE 20.11. B-mode image of a subclavian deep vein thrombosis (DVT) associated with an implanted port (port-A-Cath).

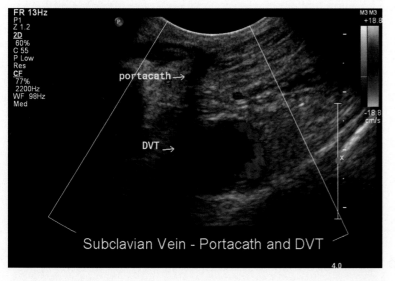

TABLE 20.4

DUPLEX CRITERIA FOR UPPER EXTREMITY DVT

	■ NORMAL	■ ABNORMAL
Spectral Doppler	• Spontaneous • Phasic • Pulsatile • Augmentation with distal compression	• Absent • Continuous • Decreased pulsatility • Diminished augmentation
Color Doppler B-mode	• Complete color filling • Complete vein wall compression	• Incomplete color filling • Incomplete vein wall compression • Intraluminal echoes

for the proximal or central upper extremity veins owing to the location of these vessels posterior to the sternum and clavicle. Therefore, careful collection of B-mode images, demonstration of color Doppler filling, and representative spectral waveforms are crucial for the accurate diagnosis of venous obstruction in the proximal internal jugular, brachiocephalic, and subclavian veins. Selection of the appropriate transducer and careful optimization of the image can help visualize thrombus in these segments. The mid to distal internal jugular vein, axillary and paired brachial, radial, and ulnar veins, and the cephalic and basilic veins can be compressed in their entirety to document the presence or absence of intraluminal thrombus.

Normal deep vein B-mode findings include a hypoechoic or anechoic (echolucent) vessel lumen, normal vein wall motion (due to respiratory phasicity and cardiac pulsatility in the central veins), normal vein caliber (slightly larger diameter than the adjacent artery), and complete vein wall compression with external transducer pressure (Fig. 20.12A). Abnormal B-mode findings with acute DVT include "softly" echogenic material in the lumen of the vein, no detectable vein wall motion (central veins), dilatation of the vein lumen (markedly larger than the adjacent artery), and incompressible vein walls—either fully (occlusive) or partially (nonocclusive)—with external transducer pressure (see Fig. 20.12B).

FIGURE 20.12. *A*, B-mode images of an internal jugular vein with normal vein wall compression (*left*, uncompressed; *right*, compressed). *B*, B-mode images of an internal jugular vein with acute deep vein thrombosis (DVT) and incompressible vein walls (*left*, uncompressed; *right*, compressed). The thrombus appears as "softly" echogenic material in the vein lumen that is hypoechoic compared to the surrounding soft tissue.

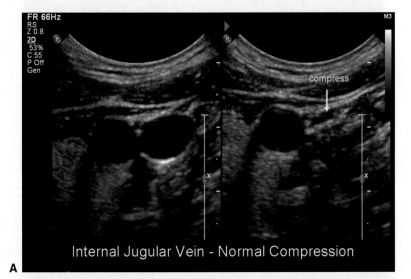

A

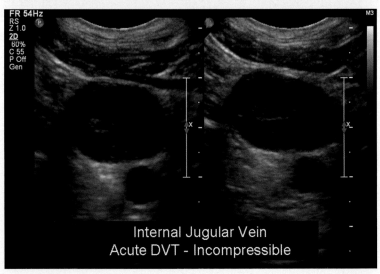

B

Color Doppler

Color Doppler is an invaluable tool in the evaluation of the upper extremity veins. Because the central veins are located between the lungs and the bony structures of the thorax, B-mode image quality is often suboptimal, regardless of transducer selection and system optimization. When properly adjusted, color Doppler will aid in vessel identification and visualization of flow in the vein lumen, sometimes outlining a nonocclusive thrombus. When flow is diminished, the color-scale and gain settings must be adjusted accordingly to detect the decreased velocities. When a major vein is occluded, collateral veins are often visible throughout the region. In some cases, abnormal flow direction in the main veins serves as an indicator of venous collateral pathways.

Normal color Doppler characteristics include spontaneous flow with the most common color mean velocity scale setting of 20 to 30 cm/s (central veins), respiratory phasicity, cardiac pulsatility (most prominent in the central veins and diminishing peripherally), and color filling of the vein lumen (Fig. 20.13A). Abnormal features of acute DVT include absence of color Doppler flow (occlusive) or partial color filling of the lumen (nonocclusive) and spontaneous but continuous color flow (nonocclusive) with loss of respiratory phasicity and cardiac pulsatility (see Fig. 20.13B).

Doppler Spectral Waveforms

Pulsed Doppler spectral waveforms from the upper extremity central venous segments are the most reliable indication of central venous obstruction. Normal spectral waveform characteristics vary from patient to patient, depending on cardiac, respiratory, and positional factors. Therefore, side-to-side comparison of central venous Doppler waveforms is necessary for accurate determination of patency.

Normal Doppler characteristics include spontaneous flow with respiratory phasicity. As previously discussed, venous return from the upper extremities varies with respiration but with a direction opposite to that in the lower extremities. The upper extremity flow pattern also shows cardiac pulsatility (Fig. 20.14A). There is typically a brisk response to distal augmentation in the peripheral veins. With acute DVT, Doppler flow may be absent (occlusive) or there may be minimal Doppler flow (nonocclusive) (see Fig. 20.14B). As for color Doppler, spectral waveforms showing spontaneous and continuous flow with loss of respiratory phasicity indicate

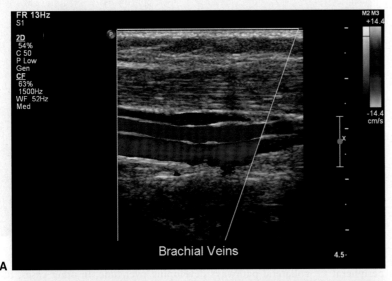

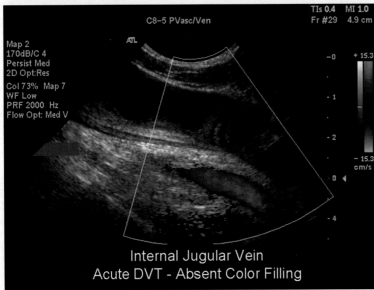

FIGURE 20.13. *A,* Color Doppler image of the paired brachial veins with normal color filling. The brachial artery is shown in *red*; the paired brachial veins are *blue.* *B,* Color Doppler image of acute deep vein thrombosis (DVT) in an internal jugular vein. Note the absence of color filling with echogenic material in the vein lumen. The common carotid artery is shown in *red.*

FIGURE 20.14. *A,* Color Doppler image and spectral waveform of normal pulsatile and phasic flow in an innominate (central) vein. *B,* Color Doppler image and spectral waveform of an acute deep vein thrombosis (DVT) in an internal jugular vein. Note the absence of Doppler flow in the internal jugular vein (see also Fig. 20.13B).

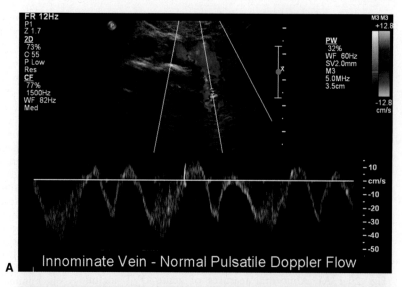

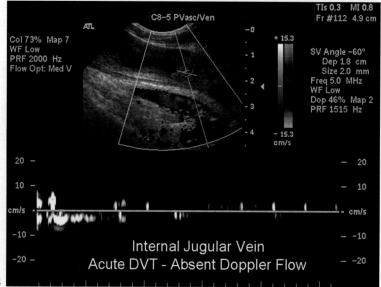

nonocclusive DVT. Distal augmentation from the peripheral veins may be delayed or absent.

Superficial Vein Thrombosis

The cephalic and basilic veins may become acutely thrombosed in association with indwelling catheters such as PICC lines. Figure 20.15 shows a cephalic vein thrombus that extends into the subclavian vein, creating a combined superficial vein thrombosis and DVT. A patent cephalic vein with walls that compress normally is illustrated in Figure 20.16A. An incompressible, thrombosed cephalic vein is shown in Figure 20.16B.

Chronic Upper Extremity Deep Vein Thrombosis

Ultrasound findings in chronic upper extremity DVT are more variable than with acute DVT and range from small, sclerotic veins with prominent collaterals to normal-sized veins with wall thickening or intraluminal scarring or "webbing." Thrombosed veins may contract and remain occluded with

collateral pathways developing over time. In other cases, the veins may recanalize and remain relatively normal in caliber but show chronic thrombotic changes as the walls become thickened and intraluminal webs form.

B-mode findings in chronic DVT include brightly echogenic material in the lumen of the vein, no detectable vein wall motion (central veins), small vein caliber compared with the artery, and nonvisualization of the previously thrombosed vein. Vein walls may be incompressible—either fully (occlusive) or partially (nonocclusive)—with external transducer pressure (Fig. 20.17A). Multiple collateral veins may be visualized in the region of an occlusion (often more pronounced than with lower extremity venous thrombosis), and prominent superficial veins may be visible on the neck, chest wall, and upper extremity.

Color Doppler findings of chronic DVT include partial color filling indicating recanalization (Fig. 20.18; see also Fig. 20.17B and C). Multiple collateral veins may be identified with color Doppler throughout the region of an occlusion. Corresponding Doppler flow characteristics with chronic DVT include minimal flow on spectral waveforms, the presence of reflux flow with respiratory changes (central veins), and reflux Doppler flow following distal augmentation (peripheral veins) (Fig. 20.19; see also Fig. 20.18A).

Text continues on page 268

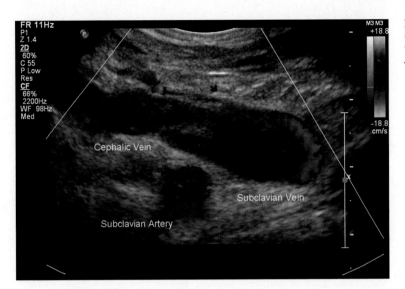

FIGURE 20.15. Color Doppler image of cephalic vein (superficial) thrombosis extending into the subclavian vein, resulting in a DVT.

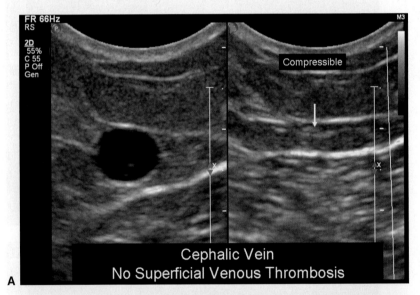

FIGURE 20.16. *A*, B-mode images of a cephalic vein show normal vein wall compression (*left*, uncompressed; *right*, compressed). *B*, B-mode images of a cephalic vein with incomplete vein wall compression, indicating superficial venous thrombosis (*left*, uncompressed; *right*, compressed).

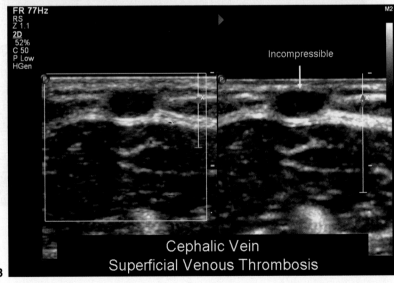

FIGURE 20.17. *A,* Transverse B-mode image of an internal jugular vein with partial compressibility due to chronic deep vein thrombosis (DVT). *B,* Color Doppler image (transverse view) of an internal jugular vein with normal caliber but chronic "webbing" indicative of chronic DVT. *C,* Color Doppler image (longitudinal view) of an internal jugular vein with partially recanalized chronic DVT (*arrows*).

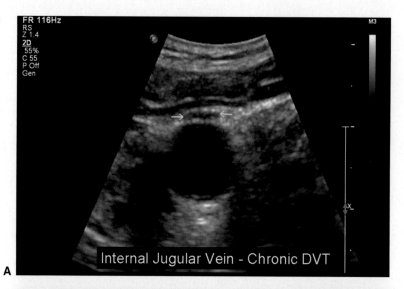

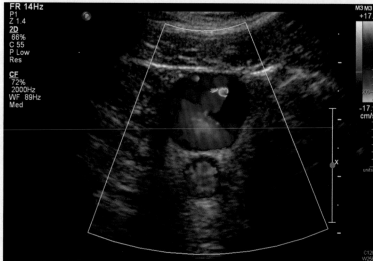

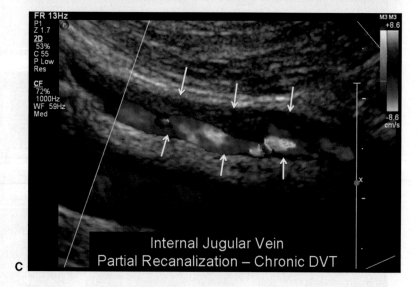

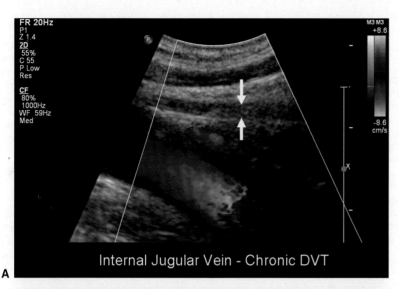

FIGURE 20.18. *A,* B-mode and color Doppler images of a small, contracted internal jugular vein with absent color filling due to chronic deep vein thrombosis (DVT) *(arrows).* The common carotid artery is shown in *red. B,* Color Doppler image of a normal caliber internal jugular vein *(top)* with partial color filling due to chronic webbing from prior DVT. *Bottom,* The common carotid artery is the *color-filled structure.*

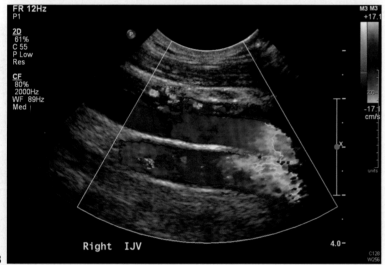

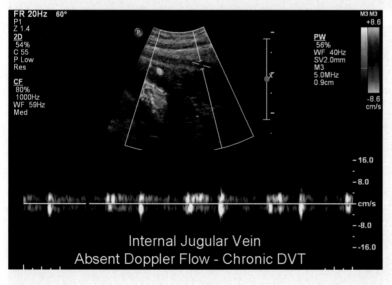

FIGURE 20.19. Color Doppler image and spectral waveform indicate chronic deep vein thrombosis (DVT) of an internal jugular vein (see also Fig. 20.18A).

Collateral Pathways

Innominate Vein Obstruction

Doppler spectral waveforms in the central upper extremity veins are normally pulsatile, unlike those in the lower extremities, which have more prominent respiratory phasicity. This pulsatility is the key to the diagnosis of innominate vein obstruction. Decreased pulsatility in Doppler waveforms from the internal jugular and subclavian veins compared with the contralateral side is a reliable sign of a proximal obstruction in the ipsilateral innominate vein (Fig. 20.20). Chronic occlusion of an innominate vein may result in retrograde flow in the ipsilateral internal jugular vein, causing upper extremity venous outflow from the subclavian vein to course up the internal jugular vein. Innominate vein obstruction may also result in a large collateral vein developing near the jugular-subclavian confluence, carrying flow across the low neck to the contralateral side (Fig. 20.21).

Subclavian Vein Obstruction

Subclavian DVT may rarely result in a collateral vein developing between the subclavian and the axillary veins in the chest that may reverse, carrying flow away from the deep system to superficial chest wall collaterals. These patients have prominent veins that are visible across the chest and shoulder area on the affected side. With subclavian vein obstruction, the external jugular vein will often dilate as a large collateral vein near the clavicle, falsely appearing to be the native subclavian vein (Fig. 20.22).

Superior Vena Cava Syndrome

SVC syndrome results from obstruction of the SVC, leading to venous congestion of the head, neck, and upper extremities. Most cases are associated with cancer or lymphadenopathy compressing the SCV. However, SVC syndrome can also be related to thrombosis or scarring from central venous lines.

FIGURE 20.20. Asymmetrical (normal and abnormal) pulsatility in the subclavian veins from a single patient. *A*, Doppler waveforms from the right subclavian vein show normal pulsatility. *B*, Doppler waveforms from the left subclavian vein show decreased pulsatility with nearly continuous flow, indicating a more proximal venous obstruction.

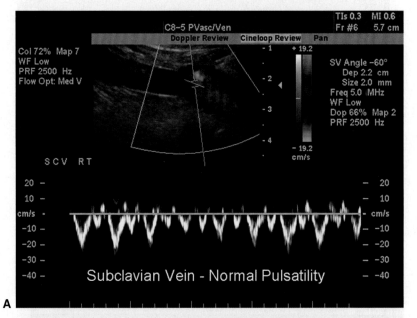

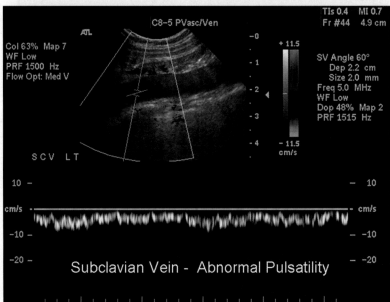

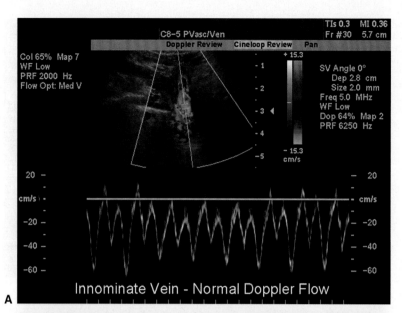

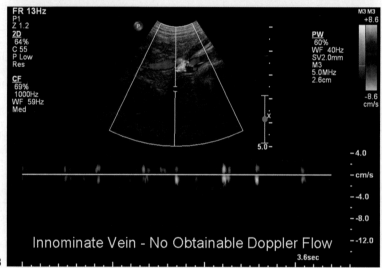

FIGURE 20.21. Asymmetrical innominate vein Doppler waveforms in a single patient. *A,* The right innominate vein shows normal pulsatile central venous flow. *B,* The left innominate vein demonstrates absence of flow with a collateral vein seen coursing medially just superior to the innominate vein.

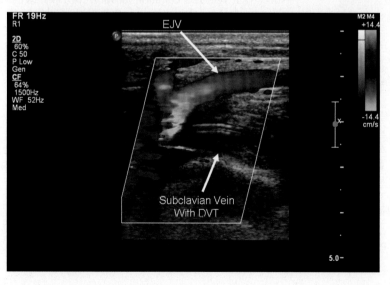

FIGURE 20.22. Color Doppler image of a subclavian deep vein thrombosis (DVT) *(bottom arrow)* secondary to a PICC line, with an enlarged external jugular vein (EJV) *(top arrow)* visualized superior to the subclavian vein.

FIGURE 20.23. Color Doppler image and spectral waveforms show the superior vena cava (SVC) as imaged from just to the right of midline at the suprasternal notch. The confluence of the right and left innominate veins is seen forming the SVC.

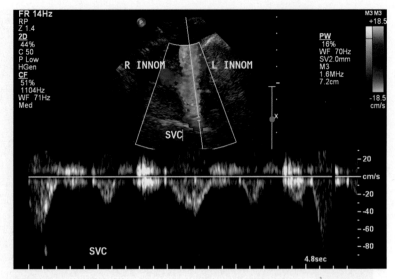

Clinical symptoms may develop over several weeks or longer as increasing venous pressure leads to edema and cyanosis of the head, neck, and arms. Edema may also compromise the function of the larynx or pharynx, resulting in cough and dyspnea. Other common signs include distention of the superficial neck and chest veins.

Venous duplex evaluation of a patient with SVC syndrome can be complicated. Figure 20.23 shows a normal SVC as it is formed by the confluence of the right and left innominate veins. The central veins often show chronic changes with networks of collateral veins (Fig. 20.24). If patent, Doppler flow in the central veins typically displays decreased pulsatility. Although the SVC may not be directly visualized, a carefully performed duplex examination will provide indirect evidence of a "more proximal obstruction," even though the specific level of obstruction may not be identified (Fig. 20.25).

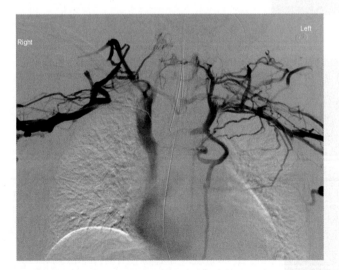

FIGURE 20.24. Venogram of a patient with superior vena cava (SVC) syndrome shows poor filling of the central veins and prominent venous collaterals.

General Limitations and Pitfalls

1. If the B-mode settings are overgained, the image may falsely display intraluminal echoes. However, if the B-mode is undergained, true intraluminal echoes may be masked, especially if they are acute and softly echogenic (hypoechoic).

2. When the color Doppler gain setting is too high, the color Doppler may "overwrite" the B-mode image of a thrombus, particularly when it is acute and softly echogenic (see no. 1, above). Color Doppler filling may appear erroneously partial or limited if the gain settings are too low or when the scale setting is too high.

3. Patient position greatly affects Doppler flow signals and potentially creates false-positive findings for central venous obstruction. Head elevation creates decreased spontaneity and increased pulsatility. If the patient lies slightly to one side or the other, the Doppler flow may be inhibited and appear erroneously continuous.

4. The external jugular vein may be mistaken for the subclavian vein in the supraclavicular view. The proximal subclavian vein is a common location for DVT. When the proximal subclavian vein is thrombosed, the external jugular vein may dilate in the low neck and appear to be the native subclavian vein (see Fig. 20.22).

5. The pleura of the lung may cause a mirror-image artifact, particularly at the level of the proximal subclavian vein in the supraclavicular view (Fig. 20.26).

6. The anatomic variant of a dual brachial vein system is characterized by a high confluence of the radial and ulnar veins. If only one pair of veins is followed in the upper arm, DVT may be missed in the second pair of deep veins.

7. The median nerve can appear as a circular incompressible structure in the upper arm on a transverse image and be mistaken for a DVT. However, unlike a vein with DVT, the nerve has linear striations in a long-axis view. Follow the structure in transverse view to be sure it communicates with another vein (Fig. 20.27).

8. A cold environment (cold room or cold acoustic gel) may cause the veins to vasoconstrict and appear smaller on the B-mode image than in their normal state.

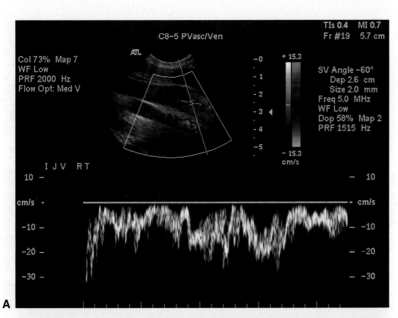

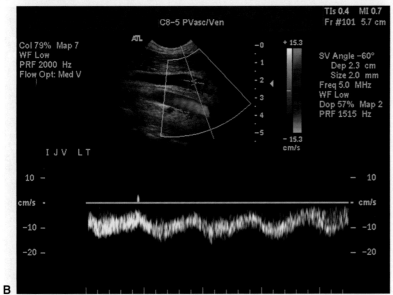

FIGURE 20.25. Decreased phasicity and pulsatility in the right and left internal jugular veins in a patient with superior vena cava (SVC) syndrome. These findings are indirect evidence of a more proximal (central) venous obstruction. A, Spectral waveforms from the right internal jugular vein. B, Spectral waveforms from the left internal jugular vein.

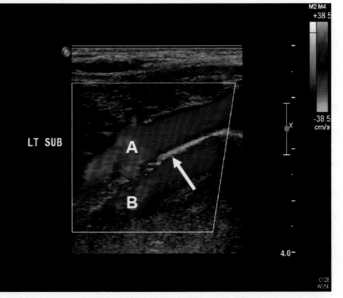

FIGURE 20.26. Color Doppler "mirror image" artifact of the subclavian artery caused by ultrasound reflections from the pleura (arrow). The true location of the subclavian artery is indicated by (A), whereas the artifact appears deep to the pleura (B). This is discussed further in Chapter 7.

FIGURE 20.27. *A,* Transverse B-mode and color Doppler image of a normal size median nerve (*arrows*). *B,* Transverse B-mode and color Doppler image of a large median nerve that may mimic brachial vein thrombosis.

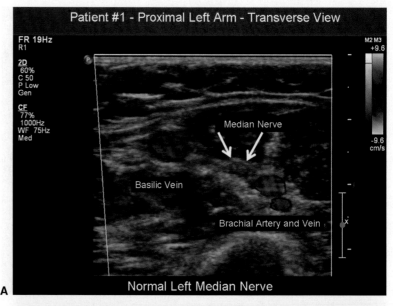

A

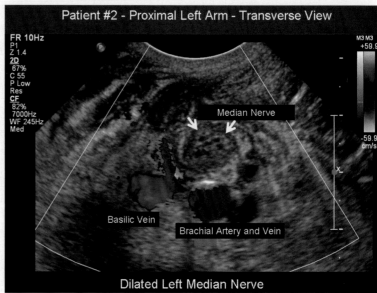

B

References

1. Kucher N, Tapson VF, Goldhaber SZ. Risk factors associated with symptomatic pulmonary embolism in a large cohort of deep vein thrombosis patients. *Thromb Haemost* 2005;93:494-498.
2. Joffe HV, Kucher N, Tapson VF, et al. Upper-extremity deep vein thrombosis: A prospective registry of 592 patients. *Circulation* 2004;110:1605-1611.
3. Munoz FJ, Mismetti P, Poggio R, et al. Clinical outcome of patients with upper-extremity deep vein thrombosis: Results from the RIETE Registry. *Chest* 2008;133:143-148.
4. Spencer FA, Emery C, Lessard D, et al. Upper extremity deep vein thrombosis: A community-based perspective. *Am J Med* 2007;120:678-684.
5. Stevenson IM, Parry EW. Radiological study of the aetiological factors in venous obstruction of the upper limb. *J Cardiovasc Surg (Torino)* 1975;16:580-585.
6. Prandoni P, Polistena P, Bernardi E, et al. Upper-extremity deep vein thrombosis. Risk factors, diagnosis, and complications. *Arch Intern Med* 1997;157:57-62.
7. Girolami A, Prandoni P, Zanon E, et al. Venous thromboses of upper limbs are more frequently associated with occult cancer as compared with those of lower limbs. *Blood Coagul Fibrinolysis* 1999;10:455-457.
8. Lindblad B, Tengborn L, Bergqvist D. Deep vein thrombosis of the axillary-subclavian veins: Epidemiologic data, effects of different types of treatment and late sequelae. *Eur J Vasc Surg* 1988;2:161-165.
9. Constans J, Salmi LR, Sevestre-Pietri MA, et al. A clinical prediction score for upper extremity deep venous thrombosis. *Thromb Haemost* 2008;99:202-207.
10. Merminod T, Pellicciotta S, Bounameaux H. Limited usefulness of D-dimer in suspected deep vein thrombosis of the upper extremities. *Blood Coagul Fibrinolysis* 2006;17:225-226.
11. Baarslag HJ, van Beek EJ, Koopman MM, et al. Prospective study of color duplex ultrasonography compared with contrast venography in patients suspected of having deep venous thrombosis of the upper extremities. *Ann Intern Med* 2002;136:865-872.
12. Baxter GM, Kincaid W, Jeffrey RF, et al. Comparison of colour Doppler ultrasound with venography in the diagnosis of axillary and subclavian vein thrombosis. *Br J Radiol* 1991;64:777-781.
13. Falk RL, Smith DF. Thrombosis of upper extremity thoracic inlet veins: Diagnosis with duplex Doppler sonography. *AJR Am J Roentgenol* 1987;149:677-682.
14. Haire WD, Lynch TG, Lieberman RP, et al. Utility of duplex ultrasound in the diagnosis of asymptomatic catheter-induced subclavian vein thrombosis. *J Ultrasound Med* 1991;10:493-496.
15. Knudson GJ, Wiedmeyer DA, Erickson SJ, et al. Color Doppler sonographic imaging in the assessment of upper-extremity deep venous thrombosis. *AJR Am J Roentgenol* 1990;154:399-403.
16. Koksoy C, Kuzu A, Kutlay J, et al. The diagnostic value of colour Doppler ultrasound in central venous catheter related thrombosis. *Clin Radiol* 1995;50:687-689.
17. Baarslag HJ, van Beek EJ, Tijssen JG, et al. Deep vein thrombosis of the upper extremity: Intra- and interobserver study of digital subtraction venography. *Eur Radiol* 2003;13:251-255.
18. Flinterman LE, Hylckama Vlieg A, Rosendaal FR, et al. Recurrent thrombosis and survival after a first venous thrombosis of the upper extremity. *Circulation* 2008;118:1366-1372.

19. Kucher N. Clinical practice. Deep-vein thrombosis of the upper extremities. *N Engl J Med* 2011;364:861-869.

20. Lee JA, Zierler BK, Zierler RE. The risk factors and clinical outcomes of upper extremity deep vein thrombosis. *Vasc Endovascular Surg* 2012;46:139-144.

21. Ascher E, Salles-Cunha S, Hingorani A. Morbidity and mortality associated with internal jugular vein thromboses. *Vasc Endovascular Surg* 2005;39:335-339.

22. Hingorani A, Ascher E, Hanson J, et al. Upper extremity versus lower extremity deep venous thrombosis. *Am J Surg* 1997;174:214-217.

23. Hingorani A, Ascher E, Lorenson E, et al. Upper extremity deep venous thrombosis and its impact on morbidity and mortality rates in a hospital-based population. *J Vasc Surg* 1997;26:853-860.

24. Major KM, Bulic S, Rowe VL, et al. Internal jugular, subclavian, and axillary deep venous thrombosis and the risk of pulmonary embolism. *Vascular* 2008;16:73-79.

25. Monreal M, Raventos A, Lerma R, et al. Pulmonary embolism in patients with upper extremity DVT associated to venous central lines—a prospective study. *Thromb Haemost* 1994;72:548-550.

26. Thomas IH, Zierler BK. An integrative review of outcomes in patients with acute primary upper extremity deep venous thrombosis following no treatment or treatment with anticoagulation, thrombolysis, or surgical algorithms. *Vasc Endovascular Surg* 2005;39:163-174.

27. Sheikh MA, Topoulos AP, Deitcher SR. Isolated internal jugular vein thrombosis: Risk factors and natural history. *Vasc Med* 2002;7:177-179.

28. Hingorani A, Ascher E, Marks N, et al. Morbidity and mortality associated with brachial vein thrombosis. *Ann Vasc Surg* 2006;20:297-300.

29. Martinelli I, Battaglioli T, Bucciarelli P, et al. Risk factors and recurrence rate of primary deep vein thrombosis of the upper extremities. *Circulation* 2004;110:566-570.

30. Heit JA, Mohr DN, Silverstein MD, et al. Predictors of recurrence after deep vein thrombosis and pulmonary embolism: A population-based cohort study. *Arch Intern Med* 2000;160:761-768.

31. Prandoni P, Lensing AW, Cogo A, et al. The long-term clinical course of acute deep venous thrombosis. *Ann Intern Med* 1996;125:1-7.

32. Elman EE, Kahn SR. The post-thrombotic syndrome after upper extremity deep venous thrombosis in adults: A systematic review. *Thromb Res* 2006;117:609-614.

33. Schulman S, Lindmarker P, Holmstrom M, et al. Post-thrombotic syndrome, recurrence, and death 10 years after the first episode of venous thromboembolism treated with warfarin for 6 weeks or 6 months. *J Thromb Haemost* 2006;4:734-742.

34. Kearon C, Akl EA, Comerota AJ, et al. Antithrombotic therapy for VTE disease: Antithrombotic Therapy and Prevention of Thrombosis, 9th ed: American College of Chest Physicians Evidence-Based Clinical Practice Guidelines. *Chest* 2012;141:e419S-e494S.

35. Decousus H, Prandoni P, Mismetti P, et al. Fondaparinux for the treatment of superficial-vein thrombosis in the legs. *N Engl J Med* 2010;363:1222-1232.

36. van Dongen CJ, van den Belt AG, Prins MH, et al. Fixed dose subcutaneous low molecular weight heparins versus adjusted dose unfractionated heparin for venous thromboembolism. *Cochrane Database Syst Rev* 2004;CD001100.

37. Akl EA, Kamath G, Yosuico V, et al. Thromboprophylaxis for patients with cancer and central venous catheters: A systematic review and a meta-analysis. *Cancer* 2008;112:2483-2492.

38. Owens CA, Bui JT, Knuttinen MG, et al. Pulmonary embolism from upper extremity deep vein thrombosis and the role of superior vena cava filters: A review of the literature. *J Vasc Interv Radiol* 2010;21:779-787.

39. Donayre CE, White GH, Mehringer SM, et al. Pathogenesis determines late morbidity of axillosubclavian vein thrombosis. *Am J Surg* 1986;152:179-184.

40. Urschel HC Jr, Patel AN. Paget-Schroetter syndrome therapy: Failure of intravenous stents. *Ann Thorac Surg* 2003;75:1693-1696.

PERIPHERAL VENOUS

CHAPTER 21 ■ CHRONIC VENOUS DISORDERS

MARK H. MEISSNER AND SARA M. SKJONSBERG

Chronic venous disorders are among the most common afflictions of Western populations affecting 50% to 85% of individuals.[1] It is estimated that as many as 164 of every 1000 people seek medical advice for venous problems.[2] Chronic venous *disorders* include the full spectrum of venous problems, ranging from telangiectasias to venous ulcers, while the term chronic venous *disease* refers to those abnormalities with signs and symptoms warranting further investigation.[1] Chronic venous *insufficiency* specifically refers to advanced manifestations of disease associated with ambulatory venous hypertension including edema, skin changes, and ulceration.

Varicose veins are the most common manifestation of primary chronic venous disease and are defined as dilated, palpable, tortuous veins greater than 3 mm in diameter that do not discolor the overlying skin.[3] In contrast, reticular veins are dilated but nonpalpable blue dermal veins less than 3 mm in diameter and are distinguished from smaller red to purple telangiectasias that are usually less than 1 mm in diameter. The major saphenous trunks are not usually abnormal in patients with telangiectasias and reticular veins but are often incompetent with varicose veins.

Long-standing ambulatory venous hypertension leads to more advanced manifestations of venous disease, including skin changes and ulceration. Hyperpigmentation, most often in a gaiter distribution extending from just below the malleoli to the posterior prominence of the calf muscle, results from the extravasation of red blood cells with subsequent accumulation of hemosiderin within dermal macrophages.[3,4] The subcutaneous tissue later becomes fibrotic and may be associated with cutaneous weeping, scaling, and erythema characteristic of venous eczema. Lipodermatosclerosis refers to the subcutaneous fibrosis and chronic inflammation that result from sustained venous hypertension. Ulceration is the most advanced stage of chronic venous disease.

Chronic venous disorders require a uniform system for describing the clinical manifestations and associated pathologic features, and the CEAP classification has become the international standard.[3,5] As summarized in Table 21.1, the CEAP system includes descriptions of the clinical disease class (C) based upon objective signs; the underlying etiology (E); the anatomic (A) distribution of reflux and obstruction in the superficial, deep, and perforating veins; and the underlying pathophysiology (P). Seven clinical disease categories are recognized including asymptomatic limbs (C_0) and those with telangiectasias (C_1), varicose veins (C_2), edema (C_3), skin changes without ulceration (C_{4a} and C_{4b}), healed ulcers (C_5), and active ulcers (C_6). Etiology is categorized as being congenital (E_c), primary (E_p), or secondary (E_s), while the pathophysiology is defined as being secondary to reflux (P_r), obstruction (P_O), or both (P_{R+O}).

Primary venous disorders are associated either with degenerative changes in the vein wall and valves, resulting in valvular incompetence, or with compressive lesions, most often in the pelvis, leading to venous obstruction. In contrast, secondary venous disorders most often result from a preceding deep venous thrombosis (DVT). When developing after an episode of DVT, manifestations of pain, edema, skin changes, and ulceration are commonly referred to as the postthrombotic syndrome.

Venous claudication, primarily due to iliofemoral venous obstruction, is not included in the CEAP clinical classification and warrants special consideration. Patients with symptoms of venous claudication complain of lower extremity tightness and bursting pain with vigorous exercise.[6] In contrast to arterial claudication, the pain is often less severe and affects the entire limb rather than specific muscle groups; its onset is more gradual and occurs with a higher intensity of activity, and it may require 15 to 20 minutes of rest, frequently with leg elevation, for relief. Associated findings may include swelling of the thigh and calf, cyanosis, and prominence of the superficial veins. Patients may also have other manifestations of chronic venous disease, including varicose veins and ulceration.[7]

It should be clear that the appropriate description and management of chronic venous disorders usually requires more than can be determined from the history and physical examination alone. Precise definition of the underlying etiology, anatomy, and pathophysiology usually requires additional diagnostic studies.

THE DIAGNOSTIC APPROACH TO CHRONIC VENOUS DISORDERS

The manifestations of chronic venous disease may result from either venous reflux or obstruction. Venous reflux is defined as retrograde flow of abnormal duration and may be either axial or segmental.[1] Axial reflux refers to uninterrupted retrograde venous flow from the groin to the calf and may occur through a combination of superficial, deep, and perforator pathways. As discussed below, hemodynamically significant obstruction is difficult to define and is usually based upon anatomic criteria. However, limbs with advanced skin changes and ulceration are more likely to have a combination of reflux and obstruction than either abnormality alone.[8]

The diagnosis of chronic venous disorders has historically relied on a number of clinical tests for venous reflux, such as the Trendelenburg test, supplemented by the findings on continuous wave (CW) Doppler examination.[9,10] Although sensitive,

TABLE 21.1

CLINICAL CLASSIFICATION OF CHRONIC VENOUS DISEASE

Class 0	No visible or palpable signs of venous disease
Class 1	Telangiectasias or reticular veins
Class 2	Varicose veins
Class 3	Edema
Class 4	Skin changes ascribed to venous disease
4a	Pigmentation or eczema
4b	Lipodermatosclerosis or atrophie blanche
Class 5	Skin changes, as defined above, with healed ulceration
Class 6	Skin changes, as defined above, with active ulceration

Adapted from Revision of the CEAP classification for chronic venous disorders: Consensus statement. *J Vasc Surg* 2004;40(6):1248-1252. Ref.[3]

both the clinical tests and CW Doppler have limited specificity, leading to selection of inappropriate procedures in a significant number of limbs [9,11] Not surprisingly, such tests have largely been supplanted by other studies.

Appropriate evaluation of the patient with venous disease depends on the patient's presentation and anticipated treatment plan. Patients with mild symptoms controlled with compression stockings and for whom no intervention is planned do not require an extensive workup. Similarly, it is generally agreed that tests to exclude truncal reflux in patients with telangiectasias are not needed. In contrast, a more precise assessment of the anatomic distribution of venous reflux and obstruction is required in patients in whom the diagnosis is uncertain or for whom intervention is planned. Evaluating the results of an operative procedure requires a more quantitative physiologic test. Unfortunately, most of the diagnostic tests for chronic venous disease display the fundamental dichotomy of providing either anatomic or hemodynamic information. Imaging-based studies such as descending venography, duplex ultrasonography, and intravascular ultrasound (IVUS) can localize reflux and obstruction to specific venous segments and play an important role in planning interventional procedures. However, such studies provide little information regarding the hemodynamic importance of such pathology or improvement following intervention. Physiologic tests, in contrast, provide a global assessment of venous hemodynamics while providing very little anatomic information. Just as the ankle-brachial index and arteriography play complementary roles in evaluating the lower-extremity arterial system, a combination of physiologic and anatomic studies may be necessary to completely characterize the extent of chronic venous disease in an individual patient.

Descending venography and ambulatory venous pressure have historically been the gold standards for the anatomic localization and hemodynamic quantification of reflux. Although descending venography may still have a role in situations such as venous valve reconstruction, it does have several limitations. It provides little information regarding the great and small saphenous veins, may be limited by the presence of competent proximal valves, and can give false-positive results related to hyperbaric contrast streaming past normal valves. Furthermore, the phlebographic grade of reflux is not precisely related to the severity of disease. In contrast, ambulatory venous pressure measurements are physiologic and, to a certain extent, do correlate with the incidence of ulceration.[12,13] However, as the test measures only global hemodynamics, it requires reflux at multiple sites, may be insensitive to isolated segmental reflux, and cannot precisely localize reflux to specific venous segments. The measurement of dorsal foot vein pressures also appears to be relatively insensitive to proximal venous obstruction.[14] Furthermore, since these methods are invasive, they are not easily repeatable and are not appropriate screening tests for patients with chronic venous disease. Accordingly, these tests have largely been supplanted by a number of noninvasive studies that alternatively provide either primarily hemodynamic or anatomic information.

NONINVASIVE PHYSIOLOGIC TESTS FOR VENOUS REFLUX

Photoplethysmography (PPG) and air plethysmography (APG) are the most widely available physiologic tests for chronic venous disease. Both use measurements of venous volume to detect reflux. Photoplethysmography is based on transmission of infrared light into the skin and the measurement of backscattered light by an adjacent photoreceptor. As the patient performs ankle flexion maneuvers in the standing position, the recorded waveform shows a rapid fall from the baseline followed by a gradual return with muscular relaxation. The venous refilling time (VRT) is the time required for return to baseline, and a VRT of ≤20 seconds has often been considered abnormal. Although simple and inexpensive, PPG provides little quantitative information. While a normal VRT excludes significant valvular incompetence and may be useful as a screening test, the specificity of an abnormal result is limited and is poorly correlated with the quantity of reflux and severity of disease.

Air plethysmography measures calf volume changes in response to gravity and exercise as a reflection of reflux. Pressures changes with exercise are measured with a calibrated polyvinyl chloride (PVC) air-filled sleeve that surrounds the calf. After obtaining a baseline recording with the patient supine and the leg elevated to 45 degrees, the patient assumes an upright position (Fig. 21.1). The venous volume (VV) is recorded as the leg fills. The patient is then instructed to plantar flex on both feet to record the ejected volume (EV) followed by 10 tiptoe movements after which the residual volume (RV) is recorded. From this information, it is possible to calculate the venous filling index (VFI = 90% VV/90% venous filling time); the ejection fraction (EF = EV/VV); and the residual volume fraction (RVF = RV/VV). The VFI is an index of global venous reflux, while the EF and RVF reflect calf muscle pump function and ambulatory venous pressure, respectively. The incidence of ulceration increases from 0% with a VFI of less than 5 mL/s to 58% for a VFI greater than 10 mL/s.[15] However, as with other global tests of hemodynamics, APG cannot precisely localize segmental reflux, and the RVF correlates only loosely with the severity of disease. Although the clinical role of APG remains debated, it may have some role in measuring global hemodynamic improvement after venous interventions.

NONINVASIVE VENOUS IMAGING TESTS

Venous duplex ultrasonography has become the most widely used test for the diagnosis of chronic venous disease and indeed has altered its management in many respects. Ultrasound not only permits precise localization of reflux and obstruction, allowing directed venous intervention, but also is used to guide most superficial venous interventions. Both the Society for Vascular Surgery (SVS) and the American Venous Forum (AVF) recommend ultrasound as the first diagnostic test for all patients with suspected chronic venous disease.[16]

FIGURE 21.1. Air plethysmography. A PVC sleeve is placed around the calf and calibrated with air. The venous volume (VV) is measured as the patient stands. The ejection volume (EV) and residual volume (RV) are measured after 1 and 10 toe raises, respectively, and the venous filling index (VFI = 90% VV/90% venous filling time), ejection fraction (EF = EV/VV), and residual volume fraction (RVF = RV/VV) are calculated as indices of reflux volume, calf muscle pump function, and ambulatory venous pressure.

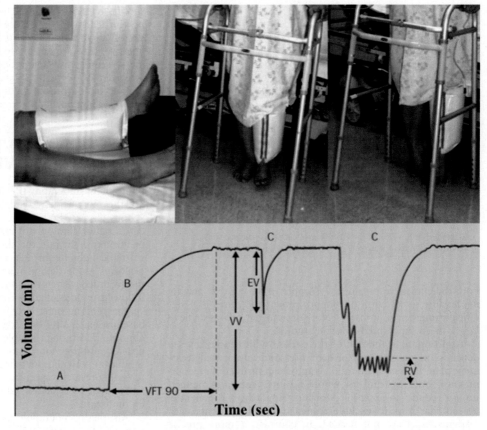

The SVS/AVF guidelines for venous duplex scanning are shown in Table 21.2.

In combining B-mode imaging with pulsed Doppler, duplex scanning is capable of characterizing partial and complete anatomic obstruction as well as valvular incompetence in the deep, superficial, and perforating veins. In evaluating reflux, duplex scanning not only provides the anatomic information lacking from global hemodynamic tests but also avoids the venographic limitations of proximal valve competence and hyperbaric contrast, while permitting valve function to be evaluated under conditions that simulate normal calf muscle pump function.[17] It is the most accurate test for identification of isolated but hemodynamically significant reflux in the distal deep venous segments.[18,19] Although ultrasound is accurate in evaluating chronic infrainguinal venous obstruction, as discussed later in this chapter, it does have some limitations for the diagnosis of iliac vein obstruction.

According to consensus standards, the duplex examination in patients with chronic venous disease should demonstrate the location, competence, and diameters of all saphenous junctions; the extent of saphenous reflux and venous diameters from the groin to the ankle, including the location and

TABLE 21.2

SOCIETY FOR VASCULAR SURGERY/AMERICAN VENOUS FORUM DUPLEX GUIDELINES FOR CHRONIC VENOUS DISEASE

■ GUIDELINE	■ STRENGTH OF RECOMMENDATION[a]	■ LEVEL OF EVIDENCE[b]
We recommend that the history and physical examination in patients with chronic venous disease be complemented by duplex scanning.	1	A
We recommend determination of valvular incompetence in the upright position using Valsalva's maneuver for the common femoral vein and saphenofemoral junction and manual or cuff compression and release for the more distal veins.	1	A
We recommend a threshold value of 1 s for the detection of reflux in the common femoral and popliteal veins and 0.5 s for the great saphenous, small saphenous, tibial, deep femoral, and perforating veins.	1	B
We recommend selective scanning of perforating veins, defining pathologic perforating veins as those with outward flow ≥0.5 s, a diameter ≥3.5 mm, and a location beneath a healed or open ulcer.	1	B

[a]Strength of recommendation: 1, strong; 2, weak.
[b]Level of evidence: A, high quality; B, medium quality; C, low or very low quality.
Adapted from Gloviczki P, Comerota AJ, Dalsing MC et al. The care of patients with varicose veins and associated chronic venous diseases: Clinical practice guidelines of the Society for Vascular Surgery and the American Venous Forum. *J Vasc Surg* 2011;53:2S-48S. Ref.[16]

diameter of any incompetent perforating veins; the source of any superficial varices including nonsaphenous sources; anatomic variants including tortuous venous segments and hypoplastic, atretic, or absent veins; and the state of the deep venous system including any reflux or venous obstruction.[20] Formal training using a standardized protocol has been shown to yield the most precise, reproducible results.[21]

The patient should be examined in a warm environment to avoid venoconstriction that may hinder the detection of reflux. Transducer selection is somewhat dependent on the patient's body habitus and depth of the veins being imaged, but a linear array transducer with a frequency between 7 and 12 MHz is suitable for most infrainguinal deep and superficial veins. The gain and dynamic gain controls should be adjusted to minimize intraluminal echoes while allowing any thrombus to be visualized. A low flow setting should be utilized, generally with a Doppler velocity range of 5 to 10 cm/s and a low wall filter.[20] The spectral display is adjusted to show retrograde flow above the baseline, and the sweep speed should be slowed to demonstrate the longest duration of reflux.

The deep veins of the lower extremity are first imaged in the reverse Trendelenburg position, using standard ultrasound criteria of compressibility, spontaneous flow, augmentation, and respiratory variation to exclude any component of venous obstruction (see Chapter 19).[22] The patient then assumes an upright position with the limb relaxed and slightly bent, weight being borne on the extremity contralateral to that being examined. The transverse B-mode image is used to provide anatomic orientation and determine venous diameters. A longitudinal view is usually used to detect reflux, recording the response of the pulsed Doppler spectral waveform to provocative maneuvers, as discussed below, and measuring the duration of reverse flow. Standard sites for the evaluation of reflux, as well as measurement of venous diameters, include the saphenofemoral junction (terminal and subterminal valves); the great saphenous vein at mid-thigh, knee, and mid-calf; and the saphenopopliteal junction and small saphenous vein at mid-calf.[23] The great saphenous vein is clearly recognized by its position in the saphenous fascial compartment, as opposed to the deep veins beneath the muscular fascia and the tributaries in the epifascial compartment (Fig. 21.2).[23] In evaluating the saphenous veins, attention should be focused on sites of caliber change. Abrupt diameter increases may be associated with entry points of alternative sources of reflux such as the pelvic veins, while decreases are often associated

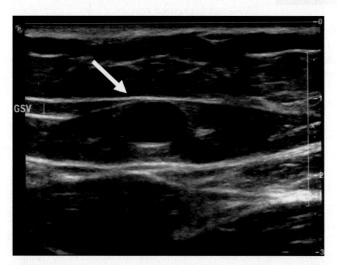

FIGURE 21.2. The great saphenous vein (*arrow*) is enclosed within the saphenous fascia, giving the characteristic saphenous "eye" appearance on a transverse B-mode ultrasound image.

with reflux escape points from the saphenous to the epifascial tributaries.[20] The depth of the saphenous vein from the skin is also an important consideration when endovenous thermal ablation is contemplated (see Chapters 28 and 29). All varicosities should be traced back to their point of origin. A thorough assessment of deep venous reflux is an integral part of the diagnostic evaluation for chronic venous disorders. If associated with overlying varices, skin changes, or ulceration, the perforators in the mid-thigh and calf should also be evaluated for diameter and the presence of bidirectional or outward flow. A visual diagram of the superficial, deep, and perforating veins, their tributaries, and communications should be provided in addition to the text report (Fig. 21.3). As they are a source of significant variability, the report should also detail the time of day the study was performed, the position of the patient, and provocative maneuvers used to elicit reflux.[21]

The ultrasound documentation of reflux is based upon demonstrating reverse flow of abnormal duration in response to provocative maneuvers. As discussed in Chapter 6, the physiologic mechanism of valve closure may be different from the mechanism of valve closure under artificial testing conditions, the latter depending on inducing a transvalvular pressure gradient with a provocative maneuver.[24-26] In the resting, supine position, the lower-extremity valve cusps remain open.[26,27] Valve closure is a passive event initiated by reversal of the resting antegrade transvalvular pressure gradient. As the pressure gradient is reversed, there is a short period of retrograde flow, or reflux, until the gradient becomes sufficient to cause valve closure. Valve closure requires not only the cessation of antegrade flow but also a brief interval of retrograde flow of sufficient velocity to completely coapt the valve cusps. At reverse flow velocities greater than 30 cm/s, normal valve closure occurs within 100 ms and produces a sharp Doppler spectrum with a clear end point (Fig. 21.4A). At velocities less than 30 cm/s, physiologic reflux may occur as reverse flow persists even in the presence of competent valves. The determination of valvular incompetence thus requires that pathologic retrograde flow be demonstrated in response to maneuvers that consistently generate an adequate reverse flow velocity (Fig. 21.4B).

Clinically relevant reflux occurs with calf muscle contraction in the upright position, and valve competence should always be evaluated with the patient standing. The erect position limits the occurrence of physiologic reflux and yields shorter valve closure times in normal subjects.[23,27,28] Detection of reflux in the supine position is unreliable, yielding both false positives, presumably due to failure to generate an adequate reverse flow velocity, and false negatives, possibly due to inadequate reflux volumes.[29] The difference between valve closure times in the supine and upright positions is variable but averages 0.23 second.[21] Methods used to elicit reflux include Valsalva's maneuver, the Parana maneuver, release of distal compression, and standardized pneumatic cuff deflation distal to the venous segment of interest. The ideal method of eliciting reflux would clearly distinguish competent from incompetent venous segments by providing a short duration of reverse flow in normal subjects and a prolonged duration of reflux in symptomatic patients with incompetent valves.

Valsalva's maneuver is most suitable for demonstrating incompetence of the saphenofemoral junction.[30] Sensitivity of Valsalva's maneuver is diminished below proximal competent valves, and it is of little utility below the groin.[18,31,32] The duration of reverse flow across venographically competent valves is also more variable with Valsalva's maneuver.[32] The Parana maneuver, whereby calf muscle contraction is initiated by pushing the patient slightly forward or backward, is widely used outside of the United States and may be helpful in evaluating specific venous segments.[23]

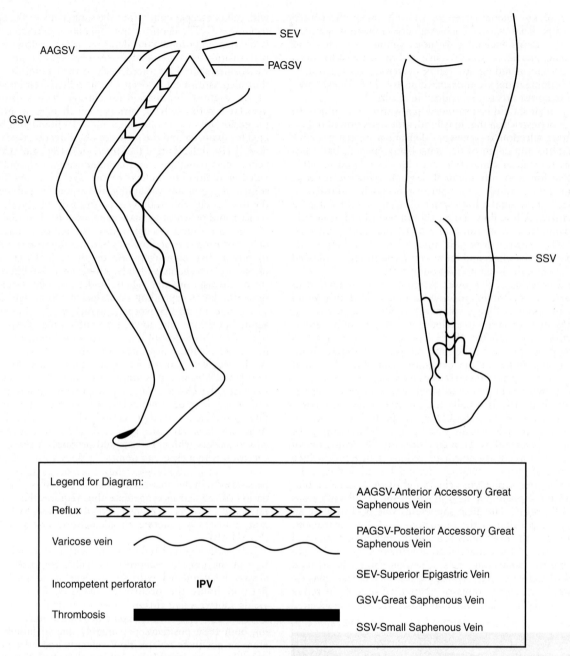

FIGURE 21.3. Visual diagram of refluxing segments and associated varicose tributaries in the great and small saphenous veins. Mapping the sites of reflux provides invaluable assistance in planning interventional procedures.

Proximal compression methods are inferior to release of distal compression, producing variable results with a poor separation between normal and diseased limbs.[27,28] Rapid deflation of a pneumatic cuff distal to the imaged segment in the standing position gives the shortest, most reproducible duration of reverse flow in normal subjects with a sensitivity of 91% and specificity of 100% for the detection of popliteal reflux.[28] Although diligent efforts may produce acceptable results with manual distal compression in the standing position, standing cuff deflation provides a more consistent and standardized approach.[21]

In evaluating reflux using the standing cuff deflation technique, the patient stands with the weight primarily supported by the contralateral limb and the limb being examined slightly bent and relaxed.[17,27,33] A pneumatic cuff is placed distal to the segment of interest and inflation pressure varied according to the hydrostatic pressure at that level. A rapid cuff inflator (Hokanson, Bellevue, WA) is used to provide inflation over approximately 3 seconds and rapid deflation within 0.3 second (Fig. 21.5). The common femoral, proximal femoral, proximal great saphenous, and accessory saphenous veins are evaluated using a 24-cm thigh cuff inflated to 80 mm Hg; the distal femoral, popliteal, and mid-thigh great saphenous veins using a 12-cm calf cuff inflated to 100 mm Hg, and the distal great saphenous and small saphenous veins using a 7-cm foot cuff inflated to 120 mm Hg (Fig 21.6). The spectral waveform display is adjusted to show antegrade flow below the baseline and reverse (reflux) flow above the baseline. Each venous segment is sequentially imaged in a longitudinal plane, and Doppler signals recorded as the cuff is inflated until antegrade flow ceases and then rapidly deflated.

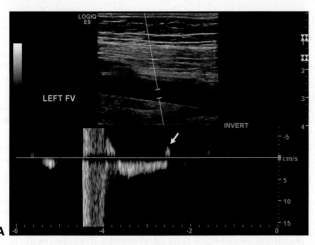
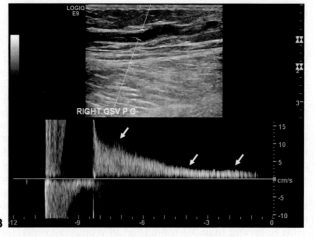

FIGURE 21.4. Ultrasound detection of reflux. The spectral waveform display is adjusted to show retrograde flow, or reflux, above the baseline, and Doppler spectra are recorded during release of distal compression using a pneumatic cuff. *A,* Competent femoral vein segment. There may be a brief (<0.5 second) interval of retrograde flow as the transvalvular pressure gradient causes the cusps to coapt. Valve closure is seen as a sharply demarcated event (*arrow*). *B,* Refluxing great saphenous vein. Valvular incompetence is associated with a prolonged (>0.5 second) duration of retrograde flow displayed above the baseline (*arrows*).

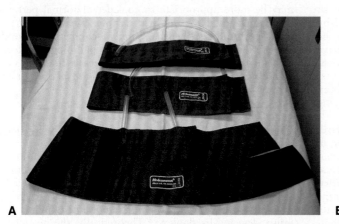
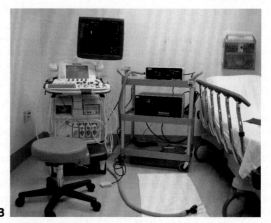

FIGURE 21.5. Standing cuff deflation technique for the detection of reflux. *A,* Pneumatic cuffs (24 cm thigh, 12 cm calf, 7 cm foot) are placed distal to the segment of interest, and inflation pressure varied according to the hydrostatic pressure at that level. *B,* Examination setup for evaluation of reflux using the standing cuff deflation technique. A rapid cuff inflator (Hokanson, Bellevue, WA) is used to provide inflation over approximately 3 seconds and rapid deflation within 0.3 second. A foot pedal is used to facilitate cuff inflation and deflation.

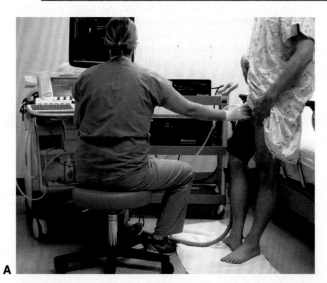
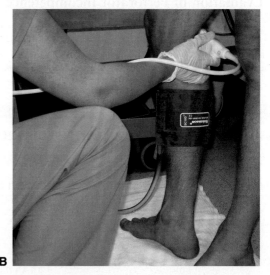

FIGURE 21.6. Standing cuff deflation technique for the detection of reflux. Each venous segment is sequentially imaged in a longitudinal plane, and Doppler spectral waveforms are recorded as the cuff is inflated until antegrade flow ceases and then rapidly deflated. *A,* Evaluation of reflux in the common femoral and great saphenous veins using a 24-cm thigh cuff inflated to 80 mm Hg and rapidly deflated. *B,* Evaluation of reflux in the popliteal vein using a 12-cm calf cuff inflated to 100 mm Hg and rapidly deflated.

Ninety-five percent of normal valves will close within 0.5 second of cuff deflation, a value which provides complete separation between normal volunteers and those with clinical manifestations of chronic venous disease.[27,28] Although a cutoff value of greater than 0.5 second has become the standard definition of lower-extremity reflux, others have noted a shorter duration of reverse flow in normal perforating veins and a longer duration in normal femoropopliteal venous segments. Labropoulos and coworkers found that normal threshold values of ≤0.5 second for the superficial veins and deep calf veins, ≤0.35 second for the perforating veins, and ≤1 second for the femoro-popliteal veins included 96.7%, 97.6%, and 98% of normal veins in each distribution, respectively.[29] Although many vascular laboratories, including our own, use a cutoff value of greater than 0.5 second for all venous segments, the SVS/AVF guidelines endorse the longer greater than 1 second value for the femoral and popliteal veins.[16] However, use of a 1-second cutoff value does tend to yield less reproducible results.[21] Although the duration of retrograde flow can also be measured using color flow Doppler, this may underestimate the duration of reflux in comparison to spectral waveform measurements.[28]

Reflux time measurements are relatively precise with respect to repeatability, although variability is influenced by time of day and patient positioning. Tests performed in the morning and with the patient in the standing position have the lowest variability.[21] Afternoon testing also tends to yield significantly longer reflux times.

The accuracy of standing distal cuff deflation has been compared to reflux determination in the supine position using manual limb compression and Valsalva's maneuvers.[17,31] Considering standing cuff deflation as the reference standard, the supine maneuvers are less sensitive than cuff deflation in identifying reflux at all levels (Table 21.3). Valsalva's maneuver is more sensitive in the proximal segments, while manual compression is more sensitive in the distal segments. When quantified using a multisegment scoring system applied to the entire limb, standing distal cuff deflation provided a sensitivity of 77% and specificity of 85% for the differentiation of clinically mild and severe venous disease in comparison to 61% and 60% for supine duplex and 50% and 41% for descending venography.[17]

Evaluation of Perforator Incompetence

The perforating veins are evaluated in the upright position, scanning along the course of the femoral vein in the mid-thigh and the posterior tibial and posterior accessory (arch) veins in the medial calf. One to five perforating veins are usually traceable as they penetrate the fascia between the superficial and deep venous systems.[34] Perforating veins may occur anywhere along the medial calf, most commonly just below the malleolus and 15 to 19 cm and 30 to 34 cm proximally.[35,36] Unfortunately, although perforating veins may be easily identified with ultrasound, the direction of normal flow and definition of perforating vein reflux remain controversial.[36]

Flow in normal perforating veins is often regarded as unidirectional from the superficial to deep venous system. However, bidirectional flow is commonly observed in both competent and incompetent perforators.[36,37] Incompetent segments are often characterized as having bidirectional flow with outward (reverse) flow occurring during the relaxation phase after distal compression.[35] In general terms, perforator incompetence is defined as outward flow of abnormal duration, with some authorities suggesting that a threshold of 0.35 second may be more appropriate than the 0.5 second used elsewhere in the venous system.[1,29] Perforator incompetence is also related to diameter, with a diameter of greater than 3.9 mm having a 96% specificity, but only 73% specificity for perforator incompetence.[37]

Given the difficulty in defining perforator incompetence, it may be more appropriate to consider abnormal perforators that are clearly associated with venous disease to be "pathologic" perforators rather than simply incompetent perforators. The SVS/AVF guidelines have defined pathologic perforators as being those with an outward flow greater than 0.5 second, a diameter ≥3.5 mm, and a location beneath an open or healed venous ulcer (CEAP class C5–C6).[16]

Quantitative Applications of Duplex Scanning

Although duplex ultrasonography accurately identifies and localizes reflux within the extremity, the relationship of these findings to global venous hemodynamics is less well defined. Abnormal direct venous pressure measurements are present in only 80% of those with common femoral or popliteal venous reflux detected by duplex.[38] Theoretically, the magnitude of duplex detected reflux should correlate with the severity of hemodynamic and clinical derangements, and both anatomic and hemodynamic systems to quantify reflux have been proposed. Anatomic scoring systems, analogous to those used for descending venography, are based upon the axial extent or segmental distribution of reflux and have been more consistent than hemodynamic quantification.[17,33] The quantitative extent of duplex-determined reflux better reflects the clinical severity of disease than standard phlebographic scoring.[17] Quantitative anatomic scores have also been correlated with both invasive and noninvasive indices of reflux.[18]

TABLE 21.3

SENSITIVITY AND SPECIFICITY OF SUPINE MANEUVERS VERSUS STANDING DISTAL CUFF DEFLATION

	VALSALVA		MANUAL COMPRESSION	
■ SEGMENT[a]	■ SENSITIVITY (%)	■ SPECIFICITY (%)	■ SENSITIVITY (%)	■ SPECIFICITY (%)
CFV	75	86	21	98
GSV	67	100	10	100
FV	83	97	50	97
PV	49	98	73	88
PTV	20	99	30	92

[a]CFV, common femoral vein; GSV, great saphenous vein; FV, femoral vein; PV, popliteal vein; PTV, posterior tibial vein.
Adapted from Markel A, Meissner MH, Manzo RA, et al. A comparison of the cuff deflation method with Valsalva's maneuver and limb compression in detecting venous valvular reflux. *Arch Surg* 1994;129:701-705.[31]

Proposed quantitative hemodynamic measures have included valve closure times, maximal reflux velocities, and reflux volume flow. Duplex-derived valve closure times are determined from the duration of reflux on the Doppler spectral waveform, and total valve closure times can be calculated as the sum of segmental closure times in the entire extremity or within the superficial and deep venous systems.[39,40] However, segments included in this calculation have varied between studies, as have the relationship to clinical manifestations and noninvasive measurements of global reflux. Although a relationship between total valve closure times, APG indices of reflux, and the presence of venous ulceration has been noted by some, a poor correlation has been more frequently noted.[39-41] Segmental valve closure times are poorly correlated with reflux volume, since large volumes may reflux over short intervals or small volumes over long intervals.[40] This likely is due to the relationship between the diameter of the refluxing vein and the volume of the capacitor (the varicose vein reservoir) into which the vein refluxes.[29] A small vein refluxing into a large capacitor may show low velocity reflux of long duration, while a large vein refluxing into a small capacitor may demonstrate high-velocity flow of short duration.

Although the clinical importance of maximal reflux velocity remains poorly defined, high-velocity reflux may have relevance in some situations, perhaps reflecting rapid pressure transmission to the microcirculation. For example, a maximal reflux velocity of greater than 10 cm/s in the femoral or popliteal veins has been associated with less clinical and hemodynamic improvement after endovenous ablation.[42] Finally, although not widely utilized, reflux flow volumes calculated from duplex determined reflux velocities and venous cross-sectional areas might also have some utility.[40,43] Peak reflux flows greater than 10 mL/s define a group having a 66% prevalence of skin manifestations in comparison to an absence of skin changes among those with flows less than 10 mL/s.[43]

Unfortunately, the relationship of all quantitative reflux parameters to disease severity remains poorly defined. In comparison to limbs with mild venous disease (CEAP C1–C3), limbs with skin changes and ulceration (C4–C6) have larger saphenous veins, shorter reflux times, higher peak and mean reflux velocities, and higher volume reflux.[44] However, there is significant overlap between groups for all of these measures, and the sensitivity and specificity for the prediction of advanced venous disease is limited. A peak saphenous reflux velocity of greater than 47.8 cm/s appears to be most accurate, although the sensitivity and specificity for advanced venous disease are only 78% and 58%, respectively. This does support the argument that high-velocity, short-duration reflux is worse than low-velocity, long-duration reflux.

TESTS FOR VENOUS OBSTRUCTION

Venous obstruction, particularly of the common iliac veins, also plays an important role in the pathogenesis of chronic venous disorders (see Chapter 25).[8] Unfortunately, the degree at which a venous stenosis becomes significant remains elusive as its hemodynamic importance may be affected by factors such as the length of the stenosis, flow rate, and the number and size of collaterals. Furthermore, the arterial concept of a "critical" stenosis does not apply in the venous circulation.[45] In the arterial circulation, critical stenosis is determined by sharp declines in pressure and flow, while in the venous circulation, the critical parameter is upstream pressure rather

than downstream perfusion. The determinants of a critical venous stenosis are far more complex than in the arterial circulation and include the degree of outflow stenosis, the inflow volume, the Starling (tissue or intra-abdominal) pressure, and right atrial pressure. Unlike in the arterial system, the effects of these components on upstream pressure are not additive but tend to be dominated by the component with the highest pressure. For example, intra-abdominal pressure, representing Starling forces, has a significant influence on the degree of stenosis that increases upstream pressure. Depending on body mass, this varies from less than 1 to greater than 16 mm Hg.[45] At very low Starling pressures, corresponding to low intra-abdominal pressure, stenoses of as little as 10% cause a sharp rise in upstream pressure. In contrast, the degree of stenosis has relatively little effect on upstream pressure at high Starling pressures.

Despite these limitations, a variety of imaging studies, including contrast venography, computed tomographic venography (CTV) and magnetic resonance venography (MRV), duplex ultrasonography, and IVUS have been used to evaluate chronic iliocaval obstruction. Although contrast venography has historically been the gold standard for evaluation of these segments, it requires multiplanar images and frequently underestimates the degree of stenosis. Cross-sectional imaging with CTV or MRV may have some value in screening for iliocaval venous obstruction, although there remain concerns that it may be insufficiently sensitive in comparison to IVUS. Among 78 patients with healed or active ulcers, cross-sectional imaging identified greater than 50% iliocaval venous obstruction in 37%.[46] However, it should also be appreciated that iliac venous compression is a common finding on CTV in patients without venous disease. Among 50 patients undergoing CT scanning for abdominal pain, greater than 50% compression of the left common iliac vein being was identified in 24%.[47]

Venous duplex ultrasound remains the initial test for evaluation of venous obstruction in most patients. Chronic obstruction of the infrainguinal veins is easily recognized using standard ultrasound criteria (see Chapter 19). However, visualization of the iliac veins may be difficult with trans-abdominal ultrasonography, and iliac obstruction is substantially more difficult to identify. Indirect signs such as asymmetry of the common femoral vein Doppler spectral waveforms in comparison to the contralateral side and diminished or absent respiratory variability (Fig. 21.7) are specific for iliac venous obstruction and should be routinely evaluated, but their sensitivity is poor.[16] Direct evaluation of the iliac veins, including planimetric diameter and velocity measurements, is likely more sensitive for the detection of iliac vein stenosis. Early studies have suggested that a peak vein velocity ratio (poststenotic velocity/prestenotic velocity) greater than 2.5 has good correlation with greater than 50% central venous stenosis as determined by pressure measurements.[48]

Because of these limitations, IVUS is regarded as the optimal imaging modality for characterizing stenosis of the iliocaval venous segments (Fig. 21.8).[48] In comparison with IVUS, single plane venography tends to underestimate the degree of stenosis by about 30% with a sensitivity of only 45% for detection of a greater than 70% stenosis.[49] IVUS is also more sensitive than either transabdominal ultrasound or venography in delineating details such as wall thickening, venous webs, and chronic trabeculation (see Chapter 31).[49]

A variety of direct and indirect tests has been proposed to assess the hemodynamic significance of venous obstruction. Most indirect tests rely on plethysmographic techniques (strain gauge, PPG, impedance, and APG) that, although useful in identifying acute proximal obstruction, do not adequately

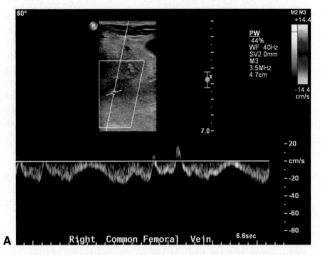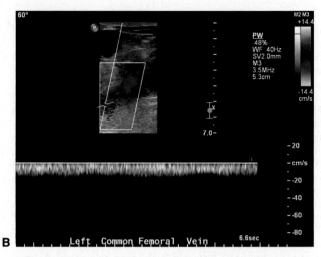

FIGURE 21.7. Doppler spectral waveforms obtained from a common femoral vein in two different patients. *A,* Normal respiratory variability. *B,* Continuous venous flow without respiratory variability is a specific, although insensitive, indirect sign for proximal iliac venous obstruction.

define the significance of chronic lesions. In comparison to limbs with acute venous obstruction, limbs with chronic obstruction have both a higher outflow and venous capacity or "dead space."[50]

Direct tests for deep venous obstruction include a number of pressure measurements. A greater than 2 to 3 mm Hg gradient across a stenosis has often been used to define a greater than 50% stenosis.[48,49] Other measurements have included direct femoral vein pressures, resting arm-foot pressure differentials, and foot pressures after reactive hyperemia.[14,49,51] Unfortunately, none of these measurements are significantly correlated with the degree of stenosis determined by venography

or IVUS.[49] Furthermore, none of these diagnostic tests are able to accurately identify those patients who will clearly benefit from intervention. For the present, treatment must be largely based upon the correlation of the patient's clinical symptoms with the degree of anatomic stenosis determined by IVUS or venography.

SUMMARY

The spectrum of chronic venous disorders extends from cosmetic concerns such as telangiectasias to the severe manifestations of skin changes and ulceration. Such disorders may occur in the absence of an underlying etiology (primary venous disorders) or may follow a previous DVT (secondary venous disorders). Regardless of the underlying etiology, appropriate management depends on precise anatomic localization of any valvular incompetence or venous obstruction, as well as an assessment of the associated hemodynamic significance. Unfortunately, no currently available diagnostic test provides both precise anatomic characterization of the underlying pathology and accurate hemodynamic information. Most symptomatic patients can be effectively managed based upon the anatomic distribution of reflux and obstruction, with the hemodynamic significance of any pathology inferred from the patient's presentation.

With its ability to identify infrainguinal reflux and obstruction, duplex ultrasonography has become the most important diagnostic tool in the management of chronic venous disorders. Examinations for venous reflux are optimally performed in the upright position using a distal compression technique, with retrograde flow of greater than 0.5 second providing an accurate criterion for reflux in most venous segments. The definition of perforator incompetence remains controversial, and it may be more appropriate to define perforators as pathologic rather than simply incompetent. Despite the importance of venous duplex ultrasonography, there remain clinical situations where additional diagnostic information is required. Global hemodynamic information, such as that provided by air plethysmography, is occasionally required for defining the hemodynamic results of an intervention, and intravascular ultrasound is likely the most accurate study for the detection of iliac venous obstruction.

FIGURE 21.8. Intravascular ultrasound of the left common iliac vein. The common iliac vein is flattened and compressed by the overlying right common iliac artery.

References

1. Eklof B, Perrin M, Delis KT, et al. Updated terminology of chronic venous disorders: The VEIN-TERM transatlantic interdisciplinary consensus document. *J Vasc Surg* 2009;49:498-501.
2. Cesarone MR, Belcaro G, Nicolaides AN, et al. "Real" epidemiology of varicose veins and chronic venous diseases: The San Valentino Vascular Screening Project. *Angiology* 2002;53:119-130.
3. Eklof B, Rutherford RB, Bergan JJ, et al. Revision of the CEAP classification for chronic venous disorders: Consensus statement. *J Vasc Surg* 2004;40:1248-1252.
4. Ackerman Z, Seidenbaum M, Loewenthal E, et al. Overload of iron in the skin of patients with varicose ulcers. Possible contributing role of iron accumulation in progression of the disease. *Arch Dermatol* 1988;124:1376-1378.
5. Porter J, Moneta G. Reporting standards in venous disease: An update. *J Vasc Surg* 1995;21:635-645.
6. Killewich LA, Martin R, Cramer M, et al. Pathophysiology of venous claudication. *J Vasc Surg* 1984;1:507-511.
7. Qvarfordt P, Eklog B, Plate G, et al. Intramuscular pressure, blood flow, and skeletal muscle metabolism in patients with venous claudication. *Surgery* 1984;95:191-195.
8. Johnson BF, Manzo RA, Bergelin RO, et al. Relationship between changes in the deep venous system and the development of the postthrombotic syndrome after an acute episode of lower limb deep vein thrombosis: A one- to six-year follow-up. *J Vasc Surg* 1995;21:307-313.
9. Kim J, Richards S, Kent PJ. Clinical examination of varicose veins—A validation study. *Ann R Coll Surg Engl* 2000;82:171-175.
10. Hoare MC, Royle JP. Doppler ultrasound detection of saphenofemoral and saphenopopliteal incompetence and operative venography to ensure precise saphenopopliteal ligation. *Aust N Z J Surg* 1984;54:49-52.
11. Singh S, Lees TA, Donlon M, et al. Improving the preoperative assessment of varicose veins. *Br J Surg* 1997;84:801-802.
12. Nicolaides AN, Hussein MK, Szendro G, et al. The relationship of venous ulceration with ambulatory venous pressure measurements. *J Vasc Surg* 1993;17:414-419.
13. Payne SP, London NJ, Newland CJ, et al. Ambulatory venous pressure: Correlation with skin condition and role in identifying surgically correctible disease. *Eur J Vasc Endovasc Surg* 1996;11:195-200.
14. Kurstjens R, de Wolf M, de Graaf R, et al. Hemodynamic changes in iliofemoral disease. *Phlebology* 2014;29:90-96.
15. Christopoulos D, Nicolaides AN, Szendro G. Venous reflux: Quantification and correlation with the clinical severity of chronic venous disease. *Br J Surg* 1988;75:352-356.
16. Gloviczki P, Comerota AJ, Dalsing MC, et al. The care of patients with varicose veins and associated chronic venous diseases: Clinical practice guidelines of the Society for Vascular Surgery and the American Venous Forum. *J Vasc Surg* 2011;53:2S-48S.
17. Neglen P, Raju S. A comparison between descending phlebography and duplex Doppler investigation in the evaluation of reflux in chronic venous insufficiency: A challenge to phlebography as the "gold standard". *J Vasc Surg* 1992;16:687-693.
18. Baker SR, Burnand KG, Sommerville KM, et al. Comparison of venous reflux assessed by duplex scanning and descending phlebography in chronic venous disease. *Lancet* 1993;341:400-403.
19. Rosfors S, Bygdeman S, Nordstrom E. Assessment of deep venous incompetence: A prospective study comparing duplex scanning with descending phlebography. *Angiology* 1990;41.
20. Coleridge-Smith P, Labropoulos N, Partsch H, et al. Duplex ultrasound investigation of the veins in chronic venous disease of the lower limbs—UIP consensus document. Part I Basic principles. *Eur J Vasc Endovasc Surg* 2006;31:83-92.
21. Lurie F, Comerota A, Eklof B, et al. Multicenter assessment of venous reflux by duplex ultrasound. *J Vasc Surg* 2012;55:437-445.
22. Hamper UM, DeJong MR, Scoutt LM. Ultrasound evaluation of the lower extremity veins. *Radiol Clin North Am* 2007;45:525-547, ix.
23. Zygmunt J. What is new in duplex scanning of the venous system? *Perspect Vasc Surg Endovasc Ther* 2009;21:94-104.
24. Lurie F, Kistner RL, Eklof B. The mechanism of venous valve closure in normal physiologic conditions. *J Vasc Surg* 2002;35:713-717.
25. Lurie F, Kistner RL, Eklof B, et al. Mechanism of venous valve closure and role of the valve in circulation: A new concept. *J Vasc Surg* 2003;38:955-961.
26. van Bemmelen PS, Beach K, Bedford G, et al. The mechanism of venous valve closure. *Arch Surg* 1990;125:617-619.
27. van Bemmelen PS, Bedford G, Beach K, et al. Quantitative segmental evaluation of venous valvular reflux with duplex ultrasound scanning. *J Vasc Surg* 1989;10:425-431.
28. Araki CT, Back TL, Padberg FT, et al. Refinements in the ultrasonic detection of popliteal vein reflux. *J Vasc Surg* 1993;18:742-748.
29. Labropoulos N, Tiongson J, Pryor L, et al. Definition of venous reflux in lower-extremity veins. *J Vasc Surg* 2003;38:793-798.
30. Masuda EM, Kistner RL, Eklof B. Prospective study of duplex scanning for venous reflux: Comparison of valsalva and pneumatic cuff techniques in the reverse trendelenburg and standing positions. *J Vasc Surg* 1994;20:711-720.
31. Markel A, Meissner MH, Manzo RA, et al. A comparison of the cuff deflation method with Valsalva's maneuver and limb compression in detecting venous valvular reflux, *Arch Surg* 1994;129:701-705.
32. Masuda E, Kistner R. Prospective comparison of duplex scanning and descending venography in the assessment of venous insufficiency. *Am J Surg* 1992;164:254-259.
33. Neglen P, Raju S. A rational approach to detection of significant reflux with duplex Doppler scanning and air plethysmography. *J Vasc Surg* 1993;17:590-595.
34. Pierik E, Toonder I, van Urk H, et al. Validation of duplex ultrasonography in detecting competent and incompetent perforating veins in patients with venous ulceration of the lower leg. *J Vasc Surg* 1997;26:49-52.
35. Miller S, Foote A. The ultrasonic detection of incompetent perforating veins. *Br J Surg* 1974;61:653-656.
36. Sarin S, Scurr J, Coleridge SP. Medial calf perforators in venous diseases: The significance of outward flow. *J Vasc Surg* 1992;16:40-46.
37. Labropoulos N, Mansour MA, Kang SS, et al. New insights into perforator vein incompetence. *Eur J Vasc Surg* 1999;18:228-234.
38. Szendro G, Nicolaides AN, Zukowski AJ, et al. Duplex scanning in the assessment of deep venous incompetence. *J Vasc Surg* 1986;4:237-242.
39. Weingarten M, Czeredarczuk M, Scovell S, et al. A correlation of air plethysmography and color-flow-assisted duplex scanning in the quantification of chronic venous insufficiency. *J Vasc Surg* 1996;24:750-754.
40. Rodriguez A, Whitehead M, McLaughlin R, et al, TF OD. Duplex-derived valve closure times fail to correlate with reflux flow volumes in patients with chronic venous insufficiency. *J Vasc Surg* 1996;23:606-610.
41. Iafrati MD, Welch H, O'Donnell TF, et al. Correlation of venous noninvasive tests with the Society for Vascular Surgery/International Society for Cardiovascular Surgery clinical classification for chronic venous insufficiency. *J Vasc Surg* 1994;19:1001-1007.
42. Marston WA, Brabham VW, Mendes R, et al. The importance of deep venous reflux velocity as a determinant of outcome in patients with combined superficial and deep venous reflux treated with endovenous saphenous ablation. *J Vasc Surg* 2008;48:400-405.
43. Vasdekis SN, Clarke GH, Nicolaides AN. Quantification of venous reflux by means of duplex scanning. *J Vasc Surg* 1989;10:670-677.
44. Konoeda H, Yamaki T, Hamahata A, et al. Quantification of superficial venous reflux by duplex ultrasound-role of reflux velocity in the assessment the clinical stage of chronic venous insufficiency. *Ann Vasc Dis* 2014;7:376-382.
45. Raju S, Kirk O, Davis M, et al. Hemodynamics of "critical" venous stenosis. *J Vasc Surg Venous Lymph Disord* 2014;2:52-59.
46. Marston W, Fish D, Unger J, et al. Incidence of and risk factors for iliocaval venous obstruction in patients with active or healed venous leg ulcers. *J Vasc Surg* 2011;53:1303-1308.
47. Kibbe MR, Ujiki M, Goodwin AL, et al. Iliac vein compression in an asymptomatic patient population. *J Vasc Surg* 2004;39:937-943.
48. Labropoulos N, Borge M, Pierce K, et al. Criteria for defining significant central vein stenosis with duplex ultrasound. *J Vasc Surg* 2007;46:101-107.
49. Neglen P, Raju S. Intravascular ultrasound scan evaluation of the obstructed vein. *J Vasc Surg* 2002;35:694-700.
50. Neglen P, Raju S. Detection of outflow obstruction in chronic venous insufficiency. *J Vasc Surg* 1993;17:583-589.
51. Labropoulos N, Volteas N, Leon M, et al. The role of venous outflow obstruction in patients with chronic venous dysfunction. *Arch Surg* 1997;132:46-51.

PERIPHERAL VENOUS

SECTION VI ■ VISCERAL VASCULAR

CHAPTER 22 ■ ULTRASOUND EVALUATION OF THE PORTAL AND HEPATIC VEINS

LESLIE M. SCOUTT, MARGARITA V. REVZIN, HJALTI THORISSON, AND ULRIKE M. HAMPER

VISCERAL VASCULAR

Portal hypertension (PHT) is an extremely common medical problem worldwide. In Western countries, PHT most commonly occurs secondary to underlying liver cirrhosis, either viral or alcohol induced. Morbidity is primarily related to bleeding from gastroesophageal (GE) varices and liver failure. However, these patients are also at increased risk for developing hepatocellular carcinoma (HCC). Although ultrasound cannot directly assess portosystemic pressure gradients, ultrasound remains the most readily accessible, least invasive, and least expensive imaging modality available for screening patients for signs of PHT and HCC. Furthermore, there are no known risks associated with ultrasound examination of the liver. Ultrasound is also an excellent means of evaluating patients for portal vein (PV) thrombosis and Budd-Chiari syndrome (BCS), which may precipitate acute deterioration of liver function in patients with cirrhosis and HCC. In addition, duplex Doppler ultrasound has an important clinical role in monitoring patients following placement of transjugular intrahepatic portosystemic shunts (TIPS), which may serve as an adjunct to medical therapy for the treatment of GE varices or refractory ascites.

PATHOPHYSIOLOGY OF PORTAL HYPERTENSION

PHT is generally defined as an increase in the portosystemic pressure gradient of more than 10 mm Hg. In most cases, the increased portosystemic gradient is largely due to an increase in resistance to portal venous flow or increased peripheral vascular resistance secondary to a combination of morphologic abnormalities as well as circulating vasoconstrictors. The body compensates for the decrease in portal flow by increasing splanchnic blood flow through volume retention, circulating vasodilators, and increased sympathetic tone. Unfortunately, these physiologic adaptations, described as the hyperdynamic circulation, increase congestion in the liver and worsen the portosystemic gradient. The ultimate result of the increased portosystemic gradient is reversal of flow in the PV and the development of portosystemic collaterals. Portosystemic collaterals or varices may arise from dilatation of preexisting portosystemic vascular

channels or from development of new blood vessels (angiogenesis). Splenomegaly and ascites are also common findings in patients with PHT. Hepatic encephalopathy may develop as liver function deteriorates and the liver is no longer able to metabolize the ammonia and manganese absorbed by the blood draining the bowel.

Patients with cirrhosis are at increased risk for developing HCC. The incidence of HCC in patients with cirrhosis is estimated at 3% per year, and patients with cirrhosis due to hepatitis B, hepatitis C, and hemochromatosis seem to have the highest risk for developing HCC. On the other hand, patients with cirrhosis secondary to autoimmune hepatitis, nonalcoholic steatohepatitis, and Wilson's disease are at less risk.[1,2] Hence, patients with cirrhosis are often screened at yearly intervals with ultrasound for HCC and signs of PHT. In addition, if a patient with previously compensated cirrhosis presents with acute decompensation of liver function, workup to exclude HCC or portal/hepatic vein (HV) thrombosis should be considered.[2]

PV pressure is optimally compared to right atrial pressure. A normal gradient is less than 7 mm Hg; a gradient between 7 and 10 mm Hg is consistent with mild PHT; GE varices typically do not form until the portosystemic gradient is greater than 10 to 12 mm Hg. Once the portosystemic gradient exceeds 12 to 15 mm Hg, the risk of variceal bleeding is substantially increased.[3,4] As the morphologic features obstructing portal venous outflow may not be evenly distributed throughout the liver parenchyma, the portosystemic gradient may vary in different hepatic segments.[5]

Many classification systems have been proposed for describing PHT. The most common classification subdivides PHT into prehepatic, intrahepatic, and posthepatic causes (Table 22.1) based on the primary site of increased resistance to portal blood flow. Intrahepatic PHT is often further subdivided into presinusoidal, sinusoidal, and postsinusoidal causes.[6] However, in many cases, increased resistance to flow may occur at more than one site. Hence, there is some overlap within this classification system. Worldwide, the most common cause of PHT is believed to be schistosomiasis.[7] In the United States, alcohol-induced cirrhosis and viral-induced cirrhosis are the most common causes of PHT.[7] Hyperdynamic PHT is the least common type.

TABLE 22.1

CLASSIFICATION OF PORTAL HYPERTENSION

Prehepatic
Portal vein thrombosis
Splenic vein thrombosis

Intrahepatic
Presinusoidal: schistosomiasis, sarcoidosis, primary biliary cirrhosis
Sinusoidal: alcoholic cirrhosis, cryptogenic cirrhosis, postnecrotic cirrhosis, viral hepatitis

Posthepatic
IVC obstruction
Constrictive pericarditis
Right heart failure
Severe tricuspid regurgitation

Hyperdynamic
Arteriovenous fistula
Hereditary hemorrhagic telangiectasia

SCANNING TECHNIQUE AND NORMAL ANATOMY

Duplex ultrasound (DUS) evaluation of the hepatic vasculature is best performed using a 2- to 5-MHz curved array transducer in a fasting (8 to 12 hours) patient. Gray-scale imaging of the liver is initially performed and is optimized by using harmonic imaging, spatial compounding, and multiple acoustic windows. The size, echotexture, and surface contour of the liver should be noted and focal liver lesions excluded. The use of a high-frequency (5 to 10 MHz) linear array transducer may aid in evaluating the liver surface for nodularity suggestive of cirrhosis. The spleen is evaluated for size and focal lesions, and the upper abdomen is screened for ascites and varices.

Oblique imaging, aiming toward the right shoulder, is particularly useful for visualization of the main PV. The porta hepatis is often best visualized in the right decubitus position, as artifact from bowel gas will be eliminated or reduced when the patient turns on the right side, allowing gas in the bowel to rise into the gastric fundus in the left upper quadrant and fluid in the bowel to collect in the gastric antrum and duodenum providing a good acoustic window. When evaluating the hepatic vasculature with pulsed Doppler, spectral waveforms should be obtained from the following vessels: upper abdominal aorta; main, right, and left hepatic arteries; main, right, and left PVs; splenic vein (SV) at the splenic hilum and under the pancreas; superior mesenteric vein (SMV) at the portal confluence; right, middle, and left HVs; and inferior vena cava (IVC). Peak systolic velocity (PSV) is measured in the hepatic arteries as well as in the aorta, and peak velocity is measured in the PVs. Optimally, at least three Doppler spectral waveforms should be obtained in the main PV and main hepatic artery (HA). The highest velocity is recorded.

Machine settings will vary depending upon the vessel examined. When evaluating the PVs, settings should be optimized for the detection of slow flow. The color box should be small; the pulse repetition frequency (PRF) or scale should be set as low as possible before aliasing occurs; the wall filter should be as low as possible until motion artifact occurs; and the gain should be maximized until artifact from noise obscures the image. Spectral Doppler waveforms from the portal and HVs should be obtained during quiet respiration, as deep inspiration will

flatten venous waveforms and decrease PV velocity. However, when evaluating the HA, the PRF and wall filter will need to be increased to avoid aliasing and motion artifact. When measuring PSV with spectral Doppler, the angle of insonation should be 60 degrees or less and the sample volume should encompass the width of the HA. The PRF should be adjusted such that the Doppler waveform is as large as possible before aliasing occurs.

The PV contributes approximately 75% of the blood supply to the liver and is formed by the confluence of the splenic and SMVs. The Doppler spectral waveform from a normal PV demonstrates low-velocity continuous hepatopetal flow. Peak velocity ranges from 10 to 40 cm/s, and normal PV flow demonstrates mild respiratory variation (Fig. 22.1A). During quiet respiration, the PV is normally less than 13 mm in diameter.[8,9] However, diameter and velocity are inversely related. Hence, due to increased intra-abdominal pressure with deep inspiration, PV diameter increases, reaching a maximum of 16 mm, and velocity decreases slightly.[8-11] Occasionally, PV flow may be more pulsatile in the normal patient (see Fig. 22.1B) as cardiac pulsatility is transmitted through the HVs and hepatic sinusoids to the PVs. Contraction of the right atrium at end diastole transmits back pressure to the portal circulation, decreasing forward portal venous flow. Thus, the trough in a pulsatile portal venous waveform corresponds to end diastole.[11] Flow in the SV and SMV is hepatopetal in direction and also demonstrates mild respiratory variation, as well as an increase in diameter on deep inspiration.[10]

In most patients, the celiac artery bifurcates into the common HA and the splenic artery (see Fig. 22.2A). The common HA courses in the hepatoduodenal ligament toward the liver, lying anterior and medial to the PV and inferior to the common bile duct (see Fig. 22.2B). However, in approximately 11% of patients, the right HA arises from the superior mesenteric artery (SMA), and in 4% of patients, the common HA will arise from the SMA. Replaced right or common hepatic arteries course inferior and lateral to the PV. The spectral waveform from the HA demonstrates a sharp systolic upstroke with continuous forward diastolic flow (see Fig. 22.2B). PSV is related to systemic blood pressure and is typically around 100 cm/s, and the resistive index (RI) of the HA normally ranges between 0.55 and 0.7.[11]

The right, middle, and left HVs typically join the IVC near the dome of the liver; however, congenital variations of HV anatomy are common. Normal HV and IVC spectral waveforms are pulsatile, reflecting the variations in right atrial pressure during the cardiac cycle. Flow is primarily directed away from the liver capsule (Fig. 22.3A). The initial S wave is due to filling of the right atrium in early to mid systole. This is followed by the V wave due to overfilling of the right atrium at the end of systole just before the tricuspid valve opens. The subsequent D wave reflects filling of the right atrium in diastole. Lastly, there is a brief reversal of flow heading back toward the liver, the A wave, which corresponds to the right atrial "kick" or contraction at end diastole (see Fig. 22.3B). These changes in HV velocity are extremely sensitive to intra-abdominal pressure. Therefore, if a spectral waveform is obtained in deep inspiration, or if the IVC is compressed by an enlarged liver, ascites, or a large amount of fat in the anterior abdominal wall, the HV and IVC waveforms in may appear artifactually flattened.

ULTRASOUND FINDINGS IN PORTAL HYPERTENSION

Patients with PHT frequently develop splenomegaly (>13 cm in maximal diameter) and ascites (Fig. 22.4). Gamna-Gandy bodies (siderotic nodules containing fibrous tissue, hemosiderin, and calcium salts) may be identified in the spleen

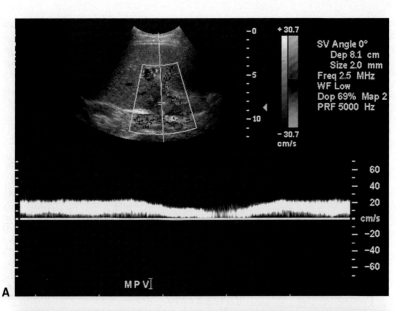

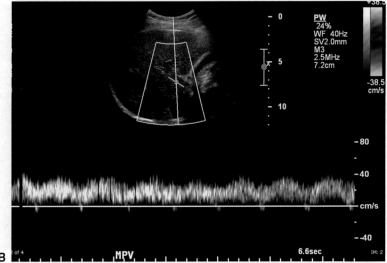

FIGURE 22.1. Normal portal vein. *A*, Spectral waveform from the main portal vein demonstrates flow toward the liver (*red*) with a peak velocity of approximately 25 cm/s. Note the mild respiratory variation. Velocity in the portal vein normally decreases slightly with inspiration. *B*, Spectral waveform from the main portal vein demonstrating mild pulsatility. This can be a normal finding, particularly in thin, athletic patients.

as multiple punctate echogenic foci (Fig. 22.5).[12] In the liver, the stigmata of cirrhosis, namely volume redistribution with a decrease in size of the right lobe and relative increase in size of the caudate lobe and lateral segment of the left lobe, coarse echotexture, surface nodularity, and focal masses may be noted (Fig. 22.6). Any focal mass noted on DUS in a patient with cirrhosis should be presumed to be HCC, irrespective of size and echogenicity, until proven otherwise (see Fig. 22.6E and F). Although regenerative nodules are the most common cause of focal liver lesions in patients with cirrhosis, they are uncommonly visualized on ultrasound examination. While cirrhosis is the most common cause of PHT in the United States, it should be remembered that cirrhosis can be present in the absence of PHT, and PHT can occur without cirrhosis.

Ultrasound findings of PHT progress as the portosystemic gradient increases. Initially, the diameter of the PV increases: greater than 13 mm in quiet respiration and greater than 16 mm in deep inspiration (Fig. 22.7A). This change in PV diameter has been reported to have a very high specificity (near 100%) though a low sensitivity (~45% to 50%) for PHT.[13,14] In addition, the PV, SV, and SMV will not increase in diameter with deep inspiration in patients with PHT. A less than 20% increase in the diameter of the SV and SMV following deep inspiration has been reported to have a sensitivity of 81% and specificity of 100% for the diagnosis of PHT.[10-14] On spectral Doppler

interrogation, loss of respiratory variation occurs in the PV, and the waveform will flatten. As PV diameter increases, velocity decreases (see Fig. 22.7B). Eventually, bidirectional flow (above and below the baseline) will be observed (see Fig. 22.7C), and ultimately flow in the PV will reverse, becoming hepatofugal (see Fig. 22.7D).[15-18] As flow in the PV decreases, flow in the HA typically increases, and the HA becomes dilated and tortuous with a so-called corkscrew appearance (Fig. 22.8). Waveforms in the HVs may also flatten (Fig. 22.9).[19]

However, none of these progressive findings in the PV, HA, or HVs directly correlate with specific measurements of the portosystemic gradient, and not all of the above findings are specific for PHT. The most common pitfall in DUS evaluation of the PV is poor visibility due to increased depth secondary to a large liver or ascites. In some patients, flow in the PV may be of such low velocity and volume that it cannot be detected by pulsed Doppler despite optimization of imaging parameters, thereby mimicking PV thrombosis. Dilatation of the PV is a nonspecific finding and can be seen with congestive heart failure, although in patients with heart failure the waveform in the PV is typically pulsatile, and dilatation of the IVC and HVs is common with prominence of the A wave. Furthermore, the absence of the findings described above cannot be used to exclude the possibility of PHT. Therefore, Doppler ultrasound cannot be used to assess the severity or progression of PHT.

FIGURE 22.2. Normal hepatic artery. *A,* Transverse color Doppler image demonstrating the celiac artery (*arrow*) arising anteriorly from the aorta (A). The celiac artery branches in a T-shape configuration into the hepatic artery (HA), which courses to the right, and the splenic artery (SA), which courses to the left. *B,* Spectral Doppler waveform from the main hepatic artery demonstrates a sharp systolic upstroke with continuous forward diastolic flow. In the porta hepatis, the main hepatic artery is found anterior to the main portal vein.

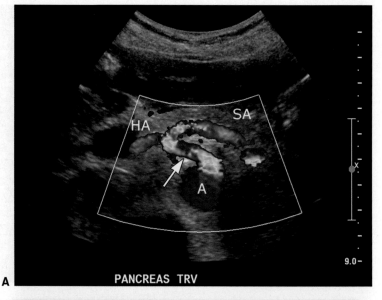

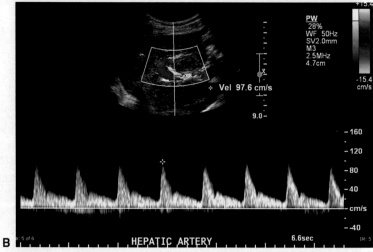

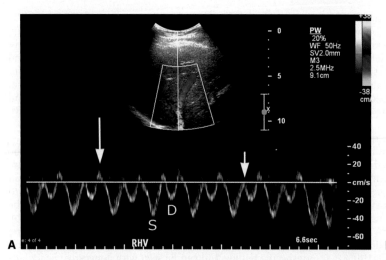

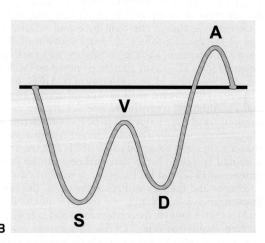

FIGURE 22.3. Normal hepatic vein. *A,* The Doppler waveform from a normal HV is pulsatile, reflecting pressure changes in the right heart. Flow is hepatofugal or directed away from the liver (*blue*). The initial S wave occurs during filling of the right atrium (S). The V trough (*short arrow*) reflects overfilling of the right atrium before the tricuspid valve opens. Subsequent hepatofugal flow as the right atrium fills in diastole creates the D wave. Last, flow is pushed back toward the liver (hepatopetal) as the right atrium contracts causing the A wave (*long arrow*), a short reversal of flow above the baseline. *B,* Schematic representation of the effect of transmitted right heart pressure on the hepatic venous waveform. S, V, D, and A as described above for 22.3*A.*

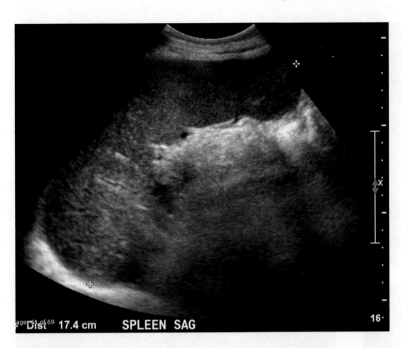

FIGURE 22.4. Splenomegaly. The spleen in this patient with cirrhosis measures 17.4 cm in maximum sagittal dimension. The spleen should normally measure less than 13 cm in an adult. Splenomegaly is a nonspecific finding. In addition to cirrhosis, other causes of splenomegaly include myeloproliferative disorders and infection.

VISCERAL VASCULAR

The most specific finding of PHT is the visualization of portosystemic shunts or varices, although occasionally collateral vessels may develop secondary to mesenteric or SV thrombosis. Varices may develop secondary to reversal of flow in existing veins or recanalization of embryonic channels. Up to 65% to 90% of varices can be visualized on DUS, provided one looks systematically throughout the abdomen and retroperitoneum (Fig. 22.10).[15,20-22]

Identification of GE varices is critical, as rupture of GE varices may result in death if bleeding cannot be controlled. It is estimated that 30% to 40% of patients with Child-Pugh class A compensated cirrhosis have GE varices, and up to 60% to 65% of patients with Child-Pugh classes B and C.[23,24] Hence, the incidence of varices appears to be related to the severity of the liver disease. Additionally, the risk of bleeding from GE varices is directly related to the portosystemic pressure gradient. Once the portosystemic gradient exceeds 12 to 15 mm Hg, the risk of variceal bleeding is substantially increased.[3,4] Endoscopic screening is the most sensitive way of identifying GE varices, and some groups recommend that patients with established cirrhosis be routinely screened with endoscopy.[25,26] However, such screening is invasive and costly. On ultrasound, GE varices are most easily found by locating the echogenic diaphragm near the aorta in a sagittal plane and imaging with color Doppler (Fig. 22.11). Alternatively, one may follow the coronary vein cephalad toward the GE junction from the portal confluence. The coronary vein runs craniocaudally in a plane parallel to the SMV or aorta and joins the SV from above, usually just medial and superior to the confluence of the SV with the SMV. The coronary vein is considered abnormal if flow is heading toward the head or if the diameter is greater than 4 mm. The risk of bleeding from GE varices increases if the coronary vein is greater than 7 mm in diameter.[15,27]

The paraumbilical vein runs in the ligamentum teres between the medial and lateral segments of the left lobe of the liver (Fig. 22.12). It extends from the left PV toward the capsule of the liver, continues anteriorly and superficially coursing under the anterior abdominal wall, and drains into the inferior epigastric veins. Blood returns to the systemic circulation via the external iliac vein. A paraumbilical vein is considered abnormal

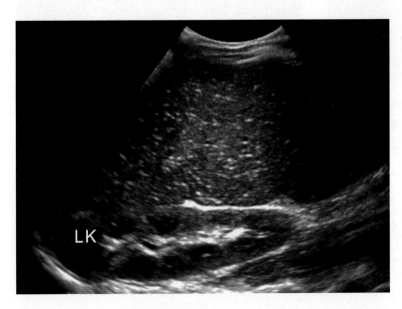

FIGURE 22.5. Gamna-Gandy bodies. Note multiple tiny punctate echogenic foci that represent the siderotic nodules found in the spleen in patients with cirrhosis. Gamna-Gandy bodies are visualized more commonly on magnetic resonance imaging than on ultrasound. LK, left kidney.

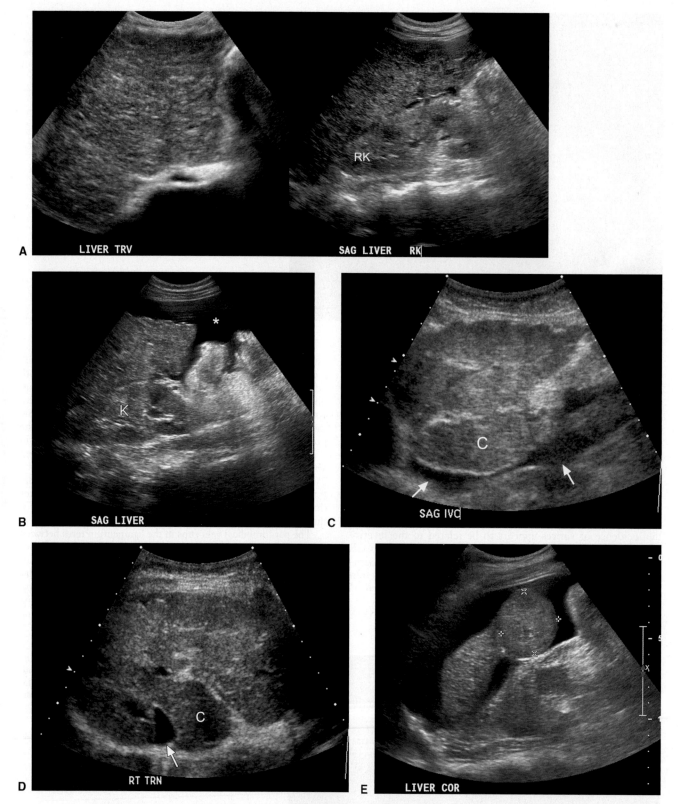

FIGURE 22.6. Ultrasound findings in cirrhosis. *A*, Gray-scale images of the liver from two patients with cirrhosis demonstrating coarse echotexture of the liver parenchyma. The coarseness or graininess of the parenchymal echotexture in the patient on the right is so pronounced with scattered ill-defined areas of decreased echogenicity that it is difficult to exclude underlying focal masses. RK, right kidney. *B*, Note the nodular surface of the liver. Nodularity of the liver surface is often best appreciated in patients with ascites (*) and by using a high-frequency linear array transducer. K, right kidney. Sagittal (*C*) and transverse (*D*) views of the liver demonstrating an enlarged caudate lobe (C). *Arrows* indicate the IVC. *E*, Note coarsened echotexture of the liver, ascites, and exophytic liver mass (calipers). This HCC was relatively isoechoic to the liver parenchyma.

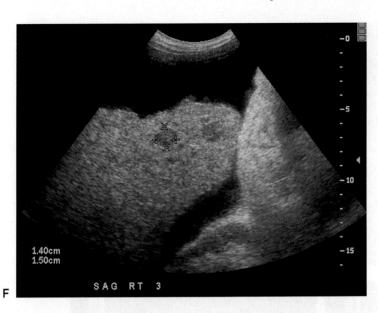

FIGURE 22.6. (*Continued*) F, Note two small hypoechoic nodules (calipers), biopsy-proven HCCs. The liver is coarse in echotexture, the liver surface is nodular, and ascites is present in this patient with long-standing cirrhosis.

if it is greater than 3 mm in diameter or if flow extends beyond the liver capsule. A patent vein in the ligamentum teres less than 2 mm in diameter can be seen in some normal patients and can even demonstrate low-velocity (<5 cm/s) flow away from the liver capsule.[28-30] If a patient with PHT develops a patent paraumbilical vein, flow often remains hepatopetal in the main PV despite elevation of the portosystemic gradient. However, a patent paraumbilical vein does not significantly decompress the liver or reduce the portosystemic gradient. Hence, patients with patent paraumbilical veins remain at risk for developing GE varices.

Short gastric or left gastric varices are found below the left lobe of the liver (Fig. 22.13). In patients with spontaneous splenorenal shunts, a direct communication, often "U-shaped," will be observed between the splenic and left renal veins (Fig. 22.14). The left renal vein is typically dilated and flow will be reversed in the main PV. Spontaneous portocaval shunts are less common, but if large are associated with focal dilatation of the IVC at the level of the shunt as well as hepatic encephalopathy, since a large amount of blood draining from the bowel will be shunted into the systemic circulation without detoxification by the liver. Surgical shunts appear similar to spontaneous shunts on DUS examination. Although these are the most readily ultrasound-detected variceal patterns, varices can occur virtually anywhere in the retroperitoneum or abdomen (Figs. 22.15 and 22.16).

It is estimated that approximately one-third of patients with GE varices will present with significant variceal bleeding.[24,31,32] Risk factors for hemorrhage include large varices, a portosystemic gradient greater than 12 to 15 mm Hg, a coronary vein greater than 7 mm in diameter, ascites, acute alcohol binge, and exercise.[3,4,15,33] Medical management of significant bleeding from GE varices includes endoscopic sclerotherapy, variceal band ligation, vasoconstrictors (vasopressin, nitroglycerin, somatostatin, and octreotide), and balloon tamponade. Bleeding is controlled by a combination of endoscopic and pharmacologic treatment in up to 80% to 90% of cases.[24,32,34-36] However, approximately 70% of patients will rebleed,[35-37] and the mortality rate in such patients is extremely high (30% to 40%) despite aggressive medical management including prophylactic treatment with β-blockers.[35-38]

For patients with persistent uncontrolled bleeding from GE varices or recurrent bleeding following medical management, the next step is placement of a TIPS. The role of TIPS placement in managing patients with cirrhosis has evolved over the past few decades, and currently, TIPS placement is preferred over creation of a surgical shunt as it avoids general anesthesia and major abdominal surgery. In addition, TIPS placement does not alter the extrahepatic vascular anatomy, allowing a patient to remain on the liver transplantation list for definitive treatment of liver disease. The most common current indications for TIPS placement are secondary prevention of variceal bleeding, variceal bleeding refractory to medical and endoscopic therapy, and ascites refractory to medical management.[39] Less frequent but also commonly accepted indications for TIPS placement include hepatorenal syndrome, BCS, hepatic venoocclusive disease, and hepatic hydrothorax.[39] Generally accepted absolute contraindications to TIPS placement include severe right heart failure (as shunting of significant blood volume into the IVC through the TIPS may produce volume overload and precipitate cardiac decompensation), severe tricuspid regurgitation (TR), severe pulmonary hypertension (mean pulmonary pressure >45 mm Hg), and uncontrolled sepsis.[39] Other often accepted contraindications to TIPS placement include preexisting severe hepatic encephalopathy (as creation of a TIPS may worsen the encephalopathy), inadequate liver reserve (as TIPS placement may result in fulminant liver failure on the basis of ischemia in such patients), sepsis, and multiple hepatic cysts (due to lack of adequate surrounding liver parenchyma that is necessary to keep the TIPS stable in location).[39] Relative contraindications, while dependent upon the aggressiveness of the interventionist and the expected length of patient survival, include HCC (especially in the right lobe or central in location), biliary obstruction (due to risk of bile leak), and moderate pulmonary hypertension.[39] The presence of PV thrombosis makes TIPS placement difficult although not impossible.[40]

Most centers report close to a 90% technical success rate for TIPS placement,[41-43] with bleeding controlled in up to 90% of patients[43-46] and an approximately 2% mortality rate.[47] The complication rate ranges in most series from approximately 10% to 16%.[45,46] Factors that increase post-TIPS mortality include Childs-Pugh class C, emergent placement for acute uncontrolled variceal hemorrhage, serum bilirubin greater than 3 mg/dL, alanine aminotransferase levels greater than 100 IU/L, and pre-TIPS encephalopathy.[48] More recently, the Model for End-Stage Liver Disease (MELD) score, which is based on serum creatinine, INR, and bilirubin levels, has become a widely used standard to predict 3-month post-TIPS mortality. A score greater than 18 is associated with significantly increased mortality.[49-51] Causes of acute morbidity include hemorrhage from transcapsular puncture, which may occur in up to 33% of cases,[39] stent migration,

Text continues on page 296

VISCERAL VASCULAR

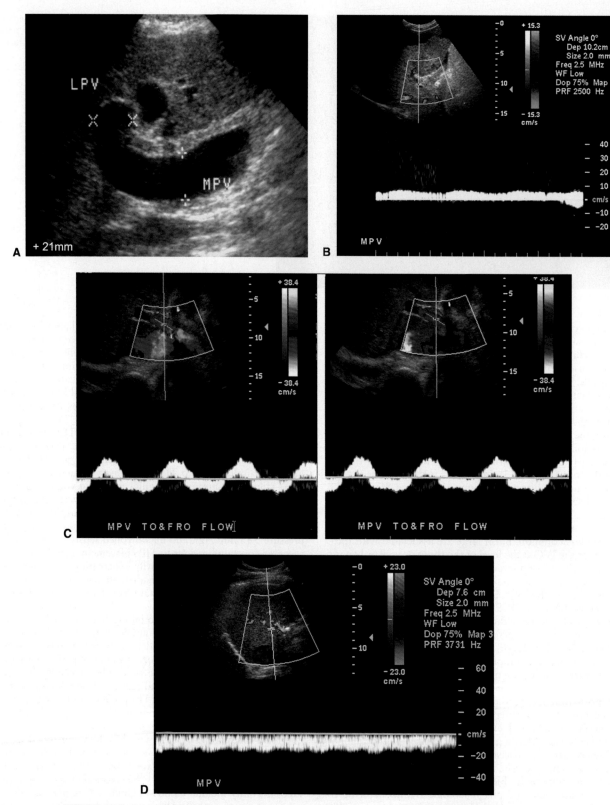

FIGURE 22.7. Portal Hypertension: Doppler findings in the portal vein. *A,* Enlargement of the portal vein. The PV (calipers) is 21 mm in diameter in this patient with PHT. The normal portal vein measures less than 13 mm during quiet respiration. Color Doppler interrogation revealed no evidence of thrombus. MPV, main portal vein, LPV, left portal vein. *B,* Spectral Doppler waveform from the portal vein demonstrating decreased velocity (<10 cm/s). Flow remains hepatopetal, heading toward the liver. *C,* Spectral waveform from the portal vein demonstrating "to-and-fro" flow, above and below the baseline. Depending on when the color image is frozen, flow may be red/hepatopetal (*left image*) or blue/hepatofugal (*right image*). *D,* Spectral Doppler waveform demonstrating reversed flow in the main portal vein (*blue*). Flow is in the opposite direction (*red*) in the hepatic artery, which lies anterior to the main portal vein. Reversed flow in the portal vein usually indicates relatively severe PHT and is a late finding.

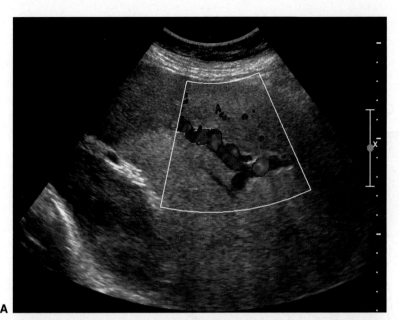

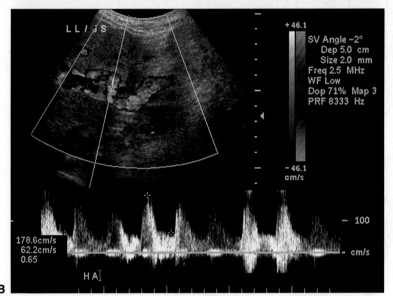

FIGURE 22.8. Portal hypertension: Doppler findings in the hepatic artery. *A*, Color Doppler image demonstrating a tortuous, redundant hepatic artery (*red*), the so-called corkscrew hepatic artery. Flow is reversed (*blue*) in the portal vein, also consistent with PHT. *B*, In another patient with long-standing PHT, the main hepatic artery is markedly dilated and tortuous. PSV is elevated at 178.6 cm/s.

VISCERAL VASCULAR

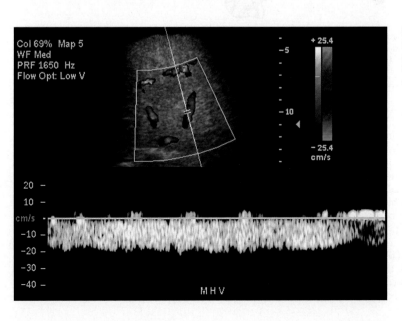

FIGURE 22.9. Portal hypertension: Doppler findings in the HVs. Spectral Doppler waveform from the middle HV demonstrates a flat, even waveform with loss of the normally transmitted cardiac pulsatility.

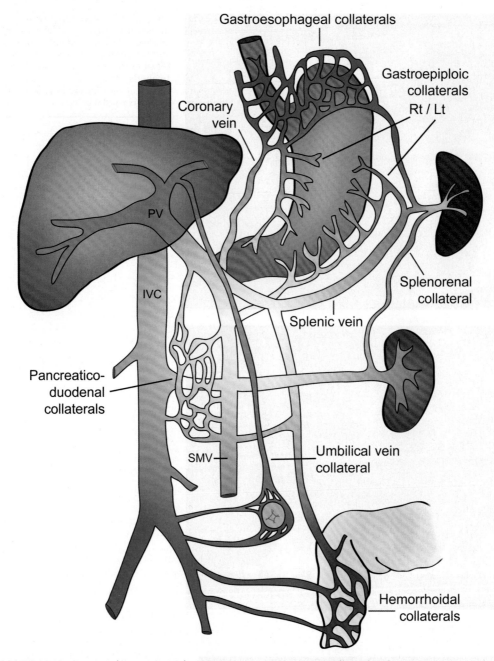

FIGURE 22.10. Diagram demonstrating the most common portosystemic collateral pathways in patients with cirrhosis. (Modified after image 32-4, p 591 in Zweibel WJ. Ultrasound Assessment of the Hepatic. In Zweibel WJ, Pellerito JS (eds). *Introduction to Vascular Ultrasonography*. Philadelphia: Elsevier/Saunders, 2005, pp 585-609 [used with permission from the publisher].)

cardiopulmonary failure (due to volume overload), infection, and hepatic encephalopathy. Hepatic encephalopathy is most likely caused by shunting of ammonia and other potentially toxic metabolites directly into the systemic circulation without being detoxified by the liver. The larger the TIPS diameter, the more blood is shunted through the liver and the higher the risk of hepatic encephalopathy. Shunt reduction or occlusion may be required if the patient does not respond to protein restriction, lactulose, and vancomycin therapy.

Recurrent variceal bleeding following successful TIPS placement is usually due to TIPS malfunction from stenosis, thrombosis, or stent retraction. Stenoses within a TIPS usually occur at the hepatic end. Causes of early TIPS stenoses have been postulated

to include biliary-TIPS fistulae due to thrombogenic and inflammatory factors in the bile, kinking, or other technical factors.[52] Later TIPS stenoses or thromboses are most commonly caused by pseudointimal hyperplasia and turbulent blood flow, which may cause endothelial damage resulting in an outflow stenosis in the draining HV.[52] TIPS stenoses and thromboses are relatively common when "bare" stents are used. Primary patency rates for bare stents are reported to be in the range of 25% to 78% at 1 year[39,43,45,53,54] and as low as 13% at 5 years.[53] If stenoses in bare stents are corrected, the assisted patency rate is higher, close to 85% at 1 year[41,45] and 36% at 5 years.[53]

The recent introduction of the partially covered Viatorr polytetrafluoroethylene (PTFE) stent graft for TIPS creation

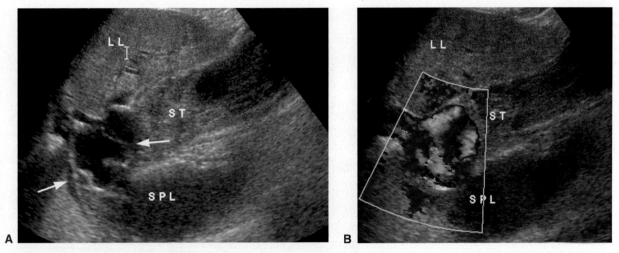

FIGURE 22.11. Gastroesophageal varices. Gray-scale (*A*) and color Doppler (*B*) images demonstrating dilated serpiginous vessels (*arrows*) underneath the diaphragm above the stomach. LL, left lobe of the liver, SPL, spleen, ST, stomach.

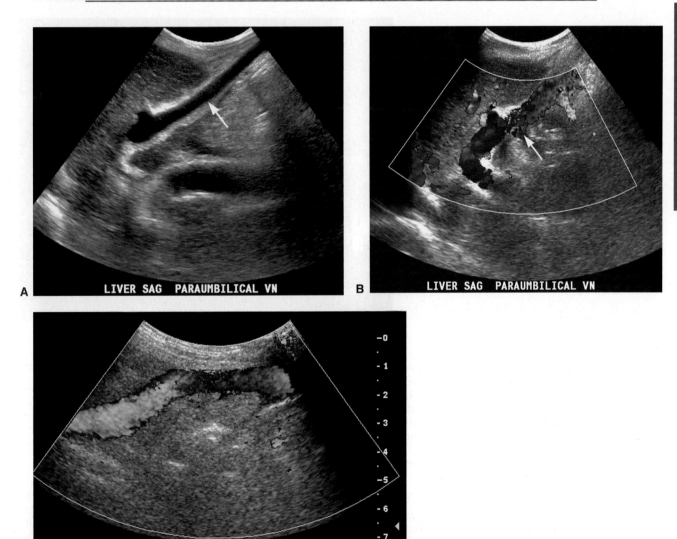

FIGURE 22.12. Patent paraumbilical vein. Gray-scale (*A*) and color (*B*) Doppler images demonstrating an enlarged patent paraumbilical vein (*arrow*). This collateral arises from the umbilical segment of the left portal vein and runs within the echogenic falciform ligament directing flow toward the liver capsule (*red*). After exiting the liver, this collateral travels inferiorly into the pelvis running under the anterior abdominal wall (*C*).

VISCERAL VASCULAR

FIGURE 22.13. Short Gastric Varices. Gray-scale (*A*) and duplex (*B*) images demonstrating massively dilated veins underneath the left lobe of the liver (L). Such varices usually originate from the short gastric veins.

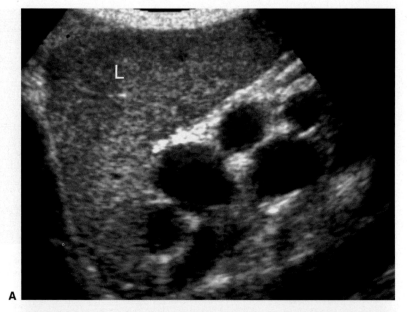

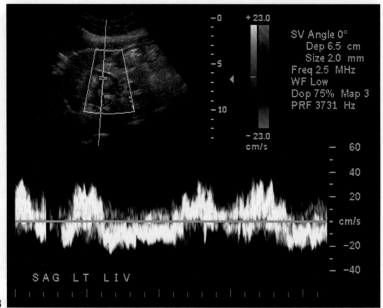

has significantly improved primary patency, with a reported 6-month patency rate of up to 90% and a 24-month patency rate of up to 75%.[55-57] The Viatorr stent graft has a 2-cm segment of bare metal stent that is placed in the PV and a variable length of PTFE-covered stent extending to the HV-IVC confluence. Use of the partially covered Viatorr stent graft has now become standard of care for TIPS creation. However, even with the partially covered stent graft, identifying an underlying stenosis in a TIPS before it becomes symptomatic is of the utmost clinical importance, as reintervention and revision may prevent TIPS failure. Since most TIPS stenoses are found in asymptomatic patients, surveillance is still often recommended.[58] DUS is the least invasive and least expensive method for screening patients for TIPS stenoses. A baseline examination followed by DUS at 6 months, 12 months, and then annually is considered a reasonable surveillance schedule.[40] However, because the primary patency rate of PTFE-covered stents is so high, it remains controversial whether or not long-term surveillance with DUS is necessary.[59]

Duplex Follow-up of TIPS Procedures

The DUS imaging protocol for patients with TIPS should include evaluation for recurrent varices or ascites, since recurrence suggests that the TIPS is not working effectively and is likely to be stenosed or occluded. Direct interrogation of the shunt typically requires a 2.5-MHz curved array transducer, as the TIPS is usually placed deep in the right lobe of the liver. Doppler interrogation requires numerous acoustic windows and velocity scales. Higher scales are required for interrogation of the TIPS than for the intrahepatic veins because velocities are typically substantially higher within a normally functioning TIPS. PV and shunt velocity will decrease with deep inspiration, so velocity should be measured at the end of gentle respiration. Velocities should be obtained from the main PV 2 to 3 cm proximal to the TIPS, in the proximal, mid, and distal shunt, and in the IVC or draining vein. Direction of flow should be noted in the main and intrahepatic portal, splenic, and hepatic veins.

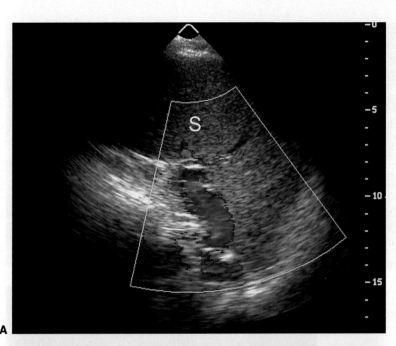

A

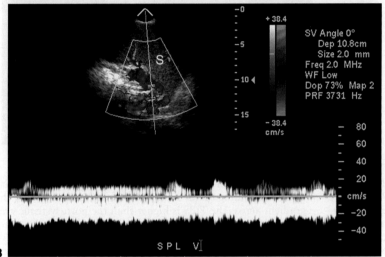

B

FIGURE 22.14. Spontaneous splenorenal shunt. Color Doppler (*A*) and duplex (*B*) images demonstrating an enlarged SV coursing inferiorly from the splenic hilum. This large varix makes a "U" turn to join the left renal vein. S, spleen.

The stent walls are very echogenic and should be smooth and parallel. When covered stents are first placed, air embedded in the covering fabric typically causes dense shadowing along the entire length of the stent, preventing Doppler interrogation and mimicking thrombosis (Fig. 22.17).[40,60] This air is gradually absorbed, and the shadowing disappears within 2 to 3 days, allowing ultrasound evaluation. Color should fill the lumen of the stent and extend to the echogenic walls (Fig. 22.18A). Spectral Doppler findings in patients with TIPS are variable and likely depend on the cause and severity of PHT, the diameter and type of stent graft used, and the residual portosystemic gradient following TIPS placement. In general, flow velocity is high in the shunt, ranging from 100 to 200 cm/s, and there is little change over the length of the shunt in a given patient (see Figs. 22.18B-D). Increased flow velocity (>40 cm/s) will be observed in the main PV (see Fig. 22.18E), and flow in the HA is also typically increased (>130 cm/s).[45,46,61-65] Optimally, the gradient across the shunt following TIPS placement will be less than the residual gradient in the liver parenchyma and, therefore, flow will be directed toward the shunt (hepatofugal) in the right and left intrahepatic PVs (see Fig. 22.18F).[40] However, depending upon technical success

and the effect of reduced hepatic congestion on the residual portosystemic gradient in the liver parenchyma, in some patients, the residual parenchymal gradient may not be higher than the gradient across the TIPS in all segments of the liver. In such patients, flow may not reverse in all of the intrahepatic PVs. For this reason, a baseline examination of the intrahepatic PVs is extremely important to assess the direction of flow.

Reappearance of varices, refractory ascites, and pleural effusion are associated with TIPS occlusion or stenosis. Lack of detectable flow on color and pulsed Doppler interrogation, in combination with intraluminal echoes, is highly accurate in diagnosis of TIPS thrombosis or occlusion (Fig. 22.19), although occasionally it may be difficult to demonstrate flow within a TIPS if it is located too deep in the abdomen.[45,46,60-65] Reported DUS diagnostic criteria for TIPS stenoses vary from institution to institution, likely in part related to differences in patient population and the type and diameter of TIPS shunt, as well as angiographic and DUS technique.[40] Velocity less than 30 cm/s in the main PV, velocity less than 50 to 60 cm/s within the TIPS shunt, a focal increase in velocity of greater than 200 to 250 cm/s in the TIPS, and a focal increase or decrease in velocity of greater than 50 cm/s over time (from one study

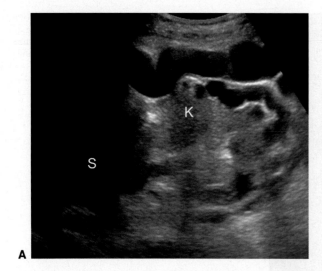

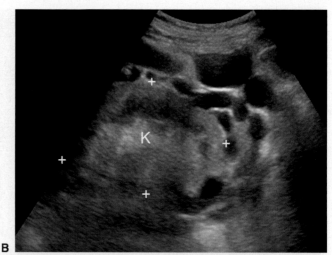

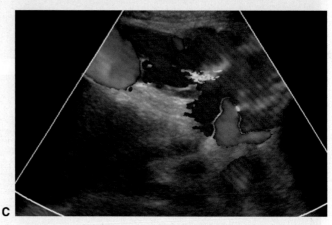

FIGURE 22.15. Retroperitoneal varices. Gray-scale (*A*) and (*B*) and color Doppler (*C*) images demonstrating large collateral vessels lateral to the spleen and left kidney. S, spleen. K, left kidney.

to the next) or spatially along the length of the TIPS are the velocity criteria most often used to diagnose TIPS stenoses (Figs. 22.20 and 22.21).[45,46,61-65] In addition, a focal narrowing on color or power Doppler imaging with color aliasing or intraluminal thrombus may be noted (see Fig. 22.20A). A change in direction of flow from hepatofugal to hepatopetal in the left or right PVs (see Fig. 22.20D), or from hepatopetal to hepatofugal in the main PV, has been reported as a relatively late finding of TIPS malfunction and indicative that the gradient across the TIPS is higher than the portosystemic gradient in the liver parenchyma.[40,63] No single Doppler criterion has been reported to have adequate sensitivity or positive predictive value for the diagnosis of TIPS stenosis; however, sensitivity increases when multiple criteria are used.[65]

FIGURE 22.16. Varices. *A,* Sagittal gray-scale image demonstrating large collaterals (*arrow*) below the left lobe of the liver (L) anterior to the celiac axis and superior mesenteric arteries. A, aorta.

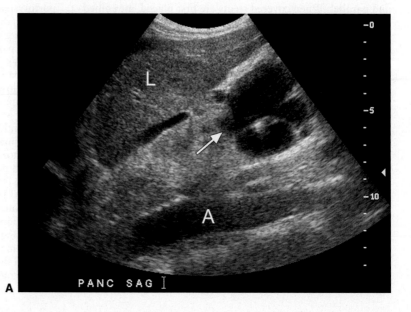

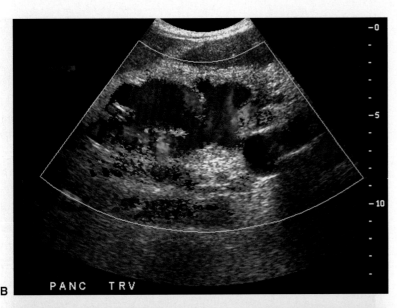

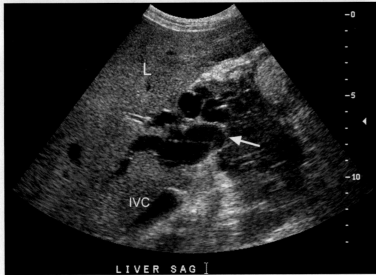

FIGURE 22.16. *(Continued) B,* Transverse color Doppler image demonstrating these large midline varices. *C,* This patient also had periportal varices *(arrow).* Varices involving multiple collateral pathways are common in an individual patient. IVC, inferior vena cava. L, liver.

False-positive diagnoses of TIPS stenosis and thrombosis have been reported. Since a TIPS is curvilinear in configuration, multiple imaging planes and angles are required for evaluation. If the TIPS is imaged out of a midline longitudinal plane, partial voluming of the back wall may suggest a TIPS stenosis.[60] Occasionally, the depth is too great to document flow on color Doppler imaging. In addition, flow may not be apparent on color Doppler imaging if part of the TIPS is imaged in a plane perpendicular to the ultrasound beam.[60] If the color scale is set too high, incomplete color saturation will occur, mimicking the appearance of intraluminal thrombus. On some machines, paradoxically, if the scale and PRF are set too low, high-velocity normal flow may not be detected.[40]

Despite these pitfalls and variations in diagnostic criteria, ultrasound remains the most readily available, inexpensive, and noninvasive surveillance modality for TIPS stenoses. However, specific Doppler criteria for TIPS stenoses must be tailored to each individual patient. Both the sonographer and physician must recognize that sensitivity and specificity are inversely related in this setting. Thus, clinical correlation and patient history are critically important to determine when to intervene, and increases in sensitivity of Doppler criteria must be balanced by the tolerance of both patient and clinician for referral to either short interval ultrasound follow-up or angiography. Recently,

several studies have reported that the use of intravenous ultrasound contrast agents increases the sensitivity of the Doppler examination for the diagnosis of TIPS dysfunction.[66,67]

PORTAL VEIN THROMBOSIS

Patients with acute portal vein thrombosis (PVT) may be completely asymptomatic or present with abdominal pain and abnormal liver function tests. Patients with chronic PVT most often present with signs and symptoms of PHT (varices, esophageal hemorrhage, splenomegaly), jaundice, or abnormal liver function tests. However, patients with presinusoidal PHT from causes such as PVT rarely develop significant ascites unless there is associated sinusoidal PHT (cirrhosis), in contrast to patients with postsinusoidal PHT, for example, from BCS, who often develop massive ascites.[6] PVT is one of the common causes of acute deterioration of liver function tests in cirrhotic patients. In children, the most common cause of PVT is omphalitis. In adults, 25% of patients with PVT have cirrhosis.[6] Other causes include hypercoagulable states (deficiencies of antithrombin, protein C or protein S, antiphospholipid antibody syndrome, and polycythemia vera), neoplasia (especially hepatocellular and pancreatic carcinoma), oral contraceptive use, pancreatitis,

Text continues on page 306

FIGURE 22.17. Covered polytetrafluoroethylene (PTFE) transjugular intrahepatic portosystemic shunt (TIPS): Early postplacement ultrasound appearance—pitfall mimicking stenosis/occlusion. *A,* Sagittal gray-scale image obtained 6 hours postplacement demonstrates the curvilinear, echogenic near wall *(arrows).* The lumen and back wall are obscured by shadowing from air in the fabric of the covered stent. *B,* Color Doppler image demonstrates a thin rim of color in the TIPS lumen just under the near wall. *C,* Spectral Doppler waveform reveals very low-velocity flow of 12.3 cm/s. Initially, this was interpreted as a near TIPS occlusion or high-grade stenosis. However, when a PTFE-covered TIPS is evaluated with Doppler early postplacement (<72 hours), air within the wall of the stent commonly obscures visualization of the lumen. Follow-up ultrasound 3 days later demonstrated that the TIPS was widely patent.

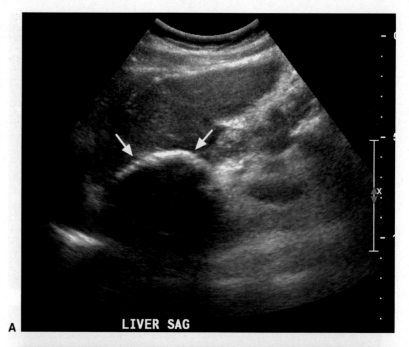

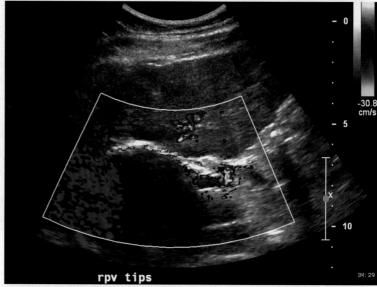

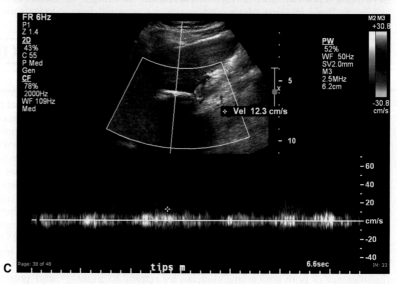

FIGURE 22.18. Normal TIPS: Duplex Doppler Appearance. *A,* Color Doppler interrogation demonstrates that color flow fills the lumen of the TIPS, extending all the way to the stent wall, which is extremely echogenic and striated in appearance. Spectral Doppler interrogation demonstrates normal peak velocity in the proximal (*B*), mid (*C*), and distal (*D*) segments of the TIPS. (*Continued*)

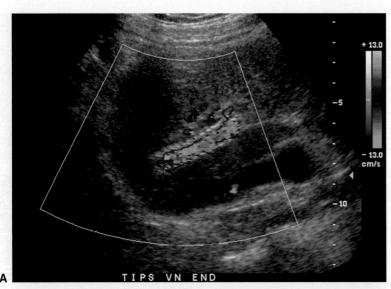

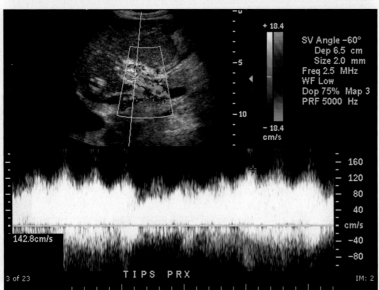

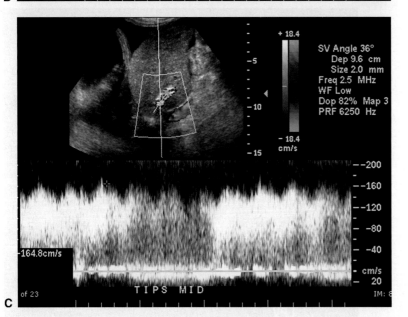

FIGURE 22.18. (*Continued*) (Velocity in a normal TIPS should range between 100 and 200 cm/s depending upon diameter of the stent and portosystemic gradient. Velocity should not vary appreciably (>50 cm/s) along the length of the TIPS. *E*, Peak velocity in the main portal vein is 104 cm/s with flow heading toward the liver (*red*). Normal velocity in the main portal vein should be greater than 40 cm/s in a patient s/p TIPS placement. *F*, In a patient with a normally functioning TIPS, flow in the intrahepatic portal veins will be reversed and opposite in direction from the hepatic arteries. Flow in the intrahepatic portal veins should be directed toward the TIPS if the gradient across the TIPS is less than the gradient in the liver parenchyma. Note that flow in the hepatic artery is color coded red while flow in the left portal vein is color coded blue, indicating reversed flow. The spectral Doppler waveform demonstrates flow in the hepatic artery above the baseline and flow in the left portal vein below the baseline.

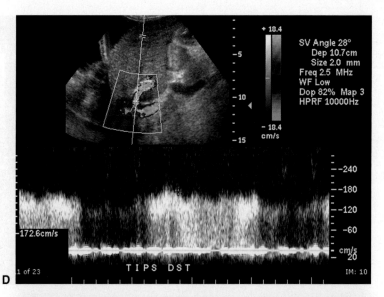

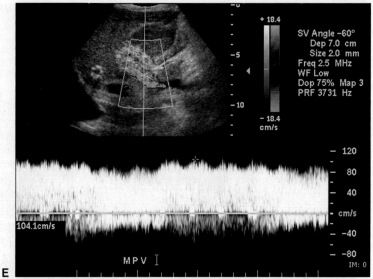

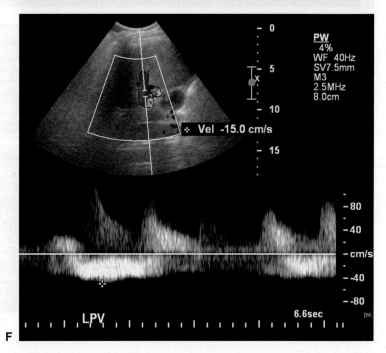

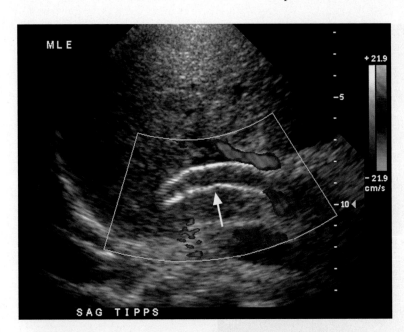

FIGURE 22.19. TIPS occlusion. Color Doppler image reveals no flow in the lumen of the TIPS (*arrow*). Note intraluminal echoes consistent with thrombus.

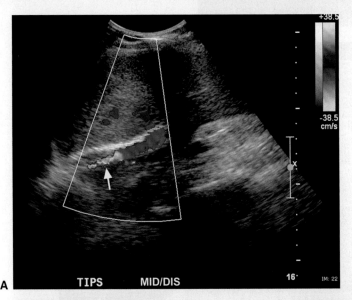

FIGURE 22.20. TIPS stenosis. *A,* Color Doppler image demonstrating color aliasing and narrowing of the lumen (*arrow*) at the hepatic (distal) end of the TIPS. *B,* Spectral waveform obtained in the proximal TIPS reveals markedly reduced flow with velocity of 44.3 cm/s. (*Continued*)

VISCERAL VASCULAR

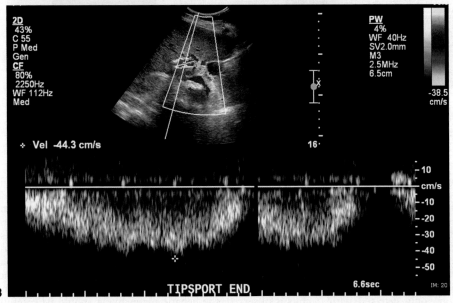

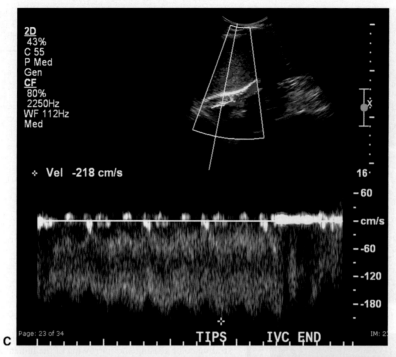

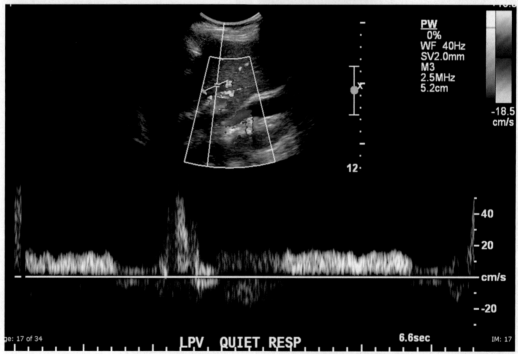

FIGURE 22.20. *(Continued) C*, Peak velocity at the site of the stenosis is markedly elevated at 218 cm/s. *D*, Flow in the left portal vein is now hepatopetal, directed away from the TIPS and in the same direction as the hepatic artery.

inflammatory bowel disease (including appendicitis and diverticulitis), sepsis, collagen vascular diseases, myeloproliferative syndromes, postoperative states, and trauma. However, in many cases, the cause is unknown or idiopathic.[6,15]

Ultrasound findings in patients with acute PVT include distension of the PV and absence of flow on color, power, and spectral Doppler imaging (Fig. 22.22).[68,69] In patients with nonocclusive thrombus, color Doppler imaging will outline the echogenic thrombus within the PV.[68] Acute thrombus may be completely anechoic and, therefore, only detected with color Doppler imaging. Subacute or chronic thrombus will demonstrate internal echoes. Typically, chronic thrombus is more echogenic than is subacute thrombus. PVT may extend into the splenic, superior mesenteric, or intrahepatic portal veins (Figs. 22.22 and 22.23). The intrahepatic PVs may also thrombose and dilate, mimicking the appearance of a tumor. The presence of arterial flow signals within the thrombus can be used to distinguish malignant tumor thrombus from bland, avascular thrombus (Fig. 22.24). If arterialization of thrombus is observed, the hepatic parenchyma should be carefully

Text continues on page 310

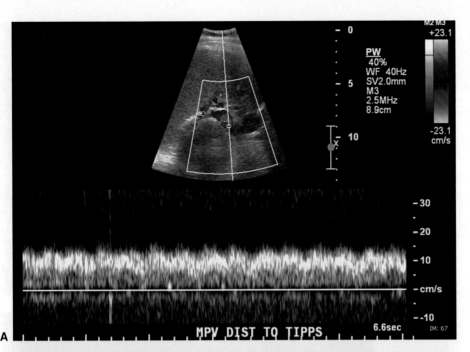

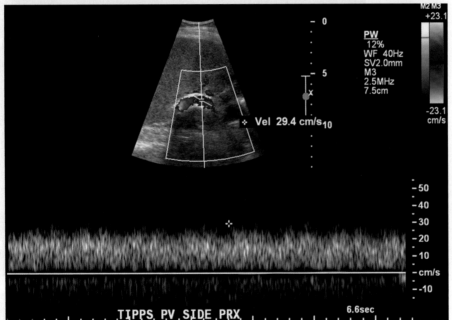

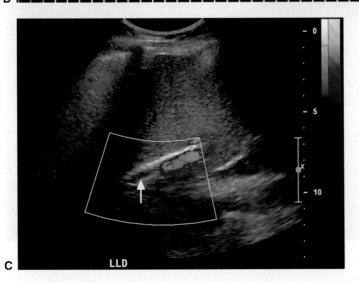

FIGURE 22.21. TIPS occlusion. *A,* Spectral waveform from the main portal vein proximal to the TIPS reveals decreased flow (<18 cm/s), suspicious for TIPS malfunction. *B,* Flow in the proximal TIPS is markedly reduced at 29 cm/s. *C,* Power Doppler image reveals no evidence of flow (*arrow*) in the distal TIPS, consistent with occlusion.

VISCERAL VASCULAR

FIGURE 22.22. Portal vein thrombosis. Gray-scale (*A*) and color-flow (*B*) images of the main portal vein (*arrow*) reveals intraluminal echoes and no evidence of flow, consistent with thrombus. *C*, The thrombus extends into the portal confluence (C) and SV (*long arrow*). A, aorta. IVC, inferior vena cava. *Short arrow*, right renal artery.

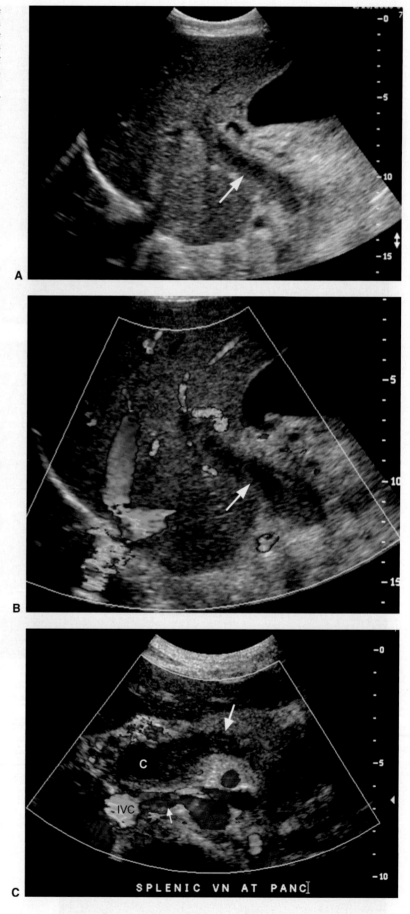

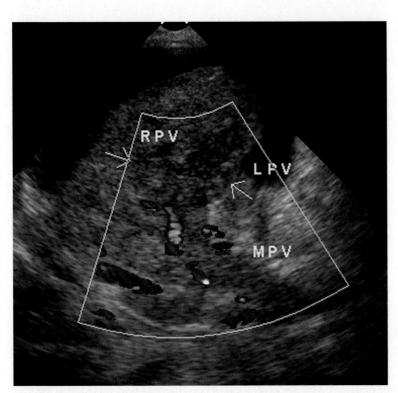

FIGURE 22.23. Intrahepatic portal vein thrombosis. Note absence of color flow and presence of intraluminal echoes consistent with thrombus in the main portal vein (MPV), right portal vein (RPV), and left portal vein (LPV). When the intrahepatic portal veins are distended with tumor, as in this patient, the ultrasound appearance can mimic the presence of a focal liver mass.

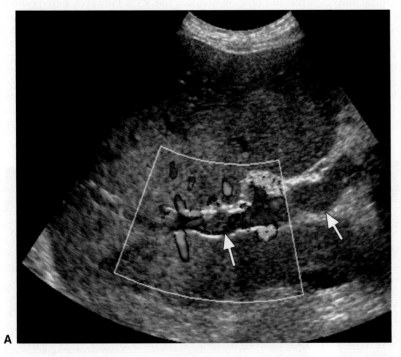

FIGURE 22.24. Malignant portal vein thrombosis. A, Color Doppler image demonstrates nonocclusive thrombus (*arrows*) in the main portal vein. Some peripheral color flow is seen. (*Continued*)

VISCERAL VASCULAR

FIGURE 22.24. (*Continued*) *B*, Spectral Doppler waveform reveals arterial signal within the thrombus. Arterial flow would not be expected in bland thrombus and indicates invasion of the portal vein by tumor.

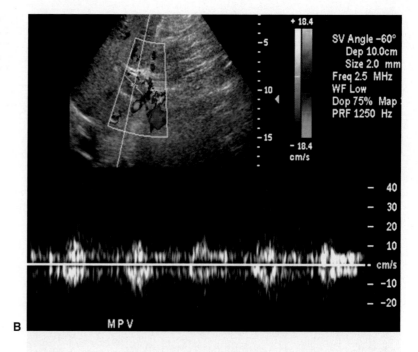

evaluated for focal lesions consistent with HCC or metastatic disease. In long-standing PVT, the thrombus will become more echogenic, and the PV will decrease in caliber due to fibrosis. In some patients, the PV will not be visualized.[18] Cavernous transformation of the PV, the development of periportal and perigallbladder portosytemic collaterals within the hepatoduodenal ligament and lesser omentum, may occur as early as 6 to 20 days after the development of PVT. On color Doppler, a tangle or cluster of irregular vessels will be noted in the porta hepatis or gallbladder wall (Fig. 22.25).[70,71] Intrahepatic collaterals or recanalization of the PV may also be noted.[70]

Color Doppler has been reported to have a sensitivity of 89%, a specificity of 92%, an accuracy of 92%, and a negative predicative value of 98% for the diagnosis of PVT.[69]

In patients with clinical concern for PVT, a DUS examination with demonstration of portal venous flow on color or spectral Doppler is adequate to exclude PVT, and no further workup is necessary,[69] although rarely color "bleeding" will overwrite and obscure nonocclusive PVT. However, false-positive diagnoses of PVT are more common, as it may be difficult on Doppler ultrasound to differentiate PVT from slow flow. To improve accuracy, machine settings should be adjusted to maximize sensitivity for slow flow. A small color box, low wall filter, and the highest gain and lowest scale possible without image degradation due to motion artifact and color aliasing, respectively, should be used in order to maximize sensitivity to slow flow (Fig. 22.26). The incident color Doppler angle should be kept at less than 90 degrees. A color Doppler finding

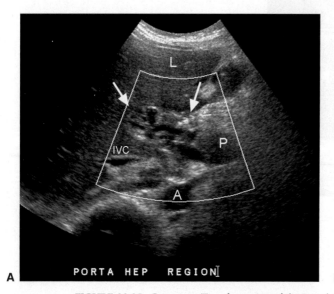

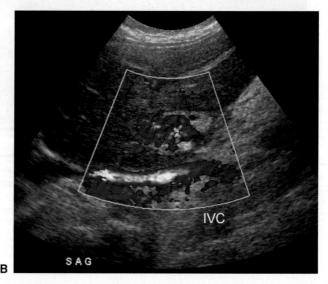

FIGURE 22.25. Cavernous Transformation of the Portal Vein. *A*, Gray-scale image demonstrating numerous tangled, serpiginous anechoic tubular structures in the porta hepatis (*arrows*). A, aorta. IVC, inferior vena cava. L, liver. P, pancreas. *B*, Color Doppler image reveals that these structures are vessels. The main portal vein could not be identified. Cavernous transformation can occur as early 1 week following PVT. As these small vessels do not adequately decompress the portosystemic gradient in the liver, esophageal and other varices are frequently associated.

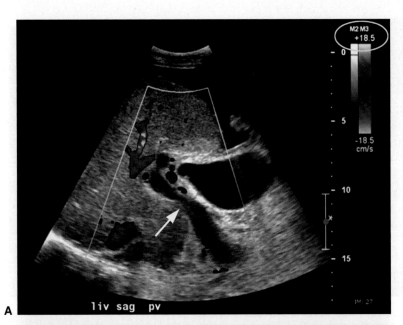

FIGURE 22.26. False-positive diagnosis of PVT. *A*, Initial color Doppler image reveals no flow in the main portal vein (*arrow*), suggestive of PVT. No intraluminal echoes are seen. However, acute PVT may appear anechoic on ultrasound. Note the color scale (*yellow circle*). *B*, When the color scale (*yellow circle*) is lowered from 18.5 to 7.7 in, flow fills the lumen of the portal vein.

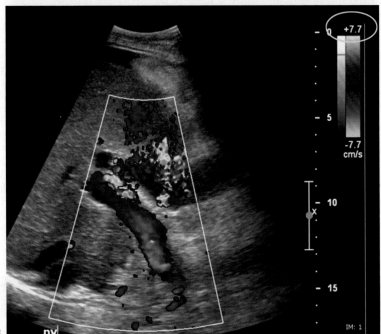

VISCERAL VASCULAR

of no flow suggesting occlusive thrombus should be confirmed with power and spectral Doppler imaging, since these Doppler modes are more sensitive than color Doppler for the detection of low-velocity flow. If no flow is seen on color Doppler interrogation and the PV is distended with echogenic thrombus, or if color Doppler outlines nonocclusive thrombus, confirmatory studies are not necessary; however, CT or MR imaging may be helpful for documentation of the extent of thrombus or to evaluate for underlying malignancy. In addition, referral for further evaluation with CT or MR should be considered if it is not possible to differentiate nondetectable slow flow from thrombus on DUS examination.

BUDD-CHIARI SYNDROME

BCS can be caused by venous outflow obstruction at the level of the hepatic venules, large HVs, or IVC. BCS is classified as primary when the venous outflow obstruction is due to an intrinsic

venous problem (thrombus, stenosis, or webs) and secondary if it is related to extrinsic compression.[72] If untreated, BCS will result in increased hepatic sinusoidal pressure and PHT. Venous stasis and hypoxia in the hepatic parenchyma result in centrilobular necrosis, fibrosis, nodular regenerative hyperplasia, and eventually cirrhosis.[73] The presenting symptoms are variable depending upon the exact site of occlusion. Patients may present with a fulminant, acute, subacute, or chronic course.[73] The subacute form is most common, and these patients present with ascites, abdominal pain, hepatomegaly, jaundice, abnormal liver function tests, and hypertrophy of the caudate lobe. Lower extremity swelling is common if the IVC is thrombosed. The most common predisposing risk factors are myeloproliferative disorders (especially polycythemia vera), hypercoagulable states, and malignancy (especially hepatocellular, adrenal, and renal cell carcinomas). Other risk factors include oral contraceptives, pregnancy, malnutrition, collagen vascular diseases (especially Behcet's disease), paroxysmal nocturnal hemoglobinuria, IVC webs, and infections. Webs and stenoses within

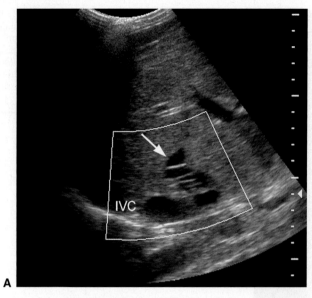

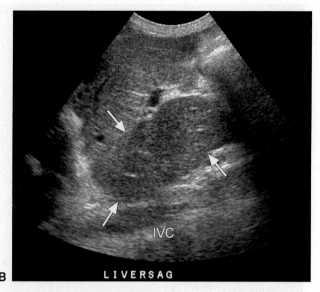

FIGURE 22.27. Budd-Chiari syndrome. *A*, Gray-scale image of a dilated middle HV (*arrow*) reveals numerous echogenic intraluminal linear structures, consistent with webs. *B*, Transverse image of the liver reveals marked hypertrophy of the caudate lobe (*arrows*), a frequent finding in BCS. IVC, inferior vena cava.

the IVC are a much more common cause of BCS in Southeast Asia in comparison to the United States.[74] No identifiable cause is found in 10% to 20% of patients.[73,75,76]

Ultrasound is considered as the primary diagnostic imaging modality for patients with suspected BCS. Findings include hepatomegaly with hypertrophy of the caudate lobe, ascites, and findings of PHT (Fig. 22.27). Although BCS is much less common than PVT, as many as 25% of patients with BCS may have associated PVT.[11,75] Doppler interrogation will reveal absence of flow with echogenic intraluminal thrombus in or nonvisualization of the HVs or IVC (Figs. 22.28 and 22.29) If thrombus is acute, the HVs may be distended. Veins may also dilate proximal to a stenosis. A dampened monophasic Doppler waveform in the peripheral HVs suggests more central obstruction (see Fig. 22.29), although a dampened

hepatic venous waveform pattern may be observed in patients following deep inspiration or secondary to extrinsic compression of the IVC.[19] Intrahepatic collaterals, especially subcapsular in location (Fig. 22.30), have been described as relatively specific findings in BCS but may also be seen in patients with PHT or cirrhosis.[74,77,78] DUS has been estimated to have a sensitivity and specificity of at least 85% for the diagnosis of BCS.[79] Inability to visualize the HVs has been reported to be suggestive of BCS,[74,77] but this is a nonspecific finding also seen in cirrhosis and extensive fatty infiltration of the liver. Narrowing of the IVC or HVs may be noted in association with high-velocity flow and color aliasing at the site of stenosis (Fig. 22.31).[74] Association of HV or IVC thrombus with an adrenal, renal, or liver mass should raise concern for tumor thrombus. The presence of arterial flow within the thrombus will confirm this diagnosis.[11]

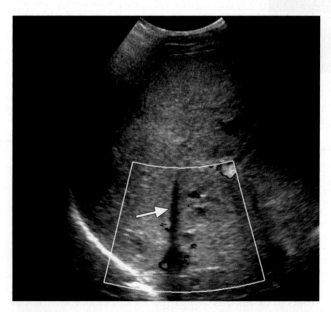

FIGURE 22.28. Budd-Chiari syndrome. Color Doppler image reveals no flow in the middle HV (*arrow*), consistent with thrombosis.

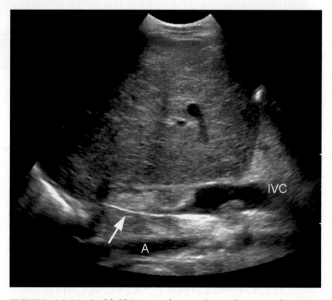

FIGURE 22.29. Budd-Chiari syndrome. Sagittal gray-scale image showing echogenic thrombus (*arrow*) in the inferior vena cava (IVC) adjacent to the liver. A, aorta.

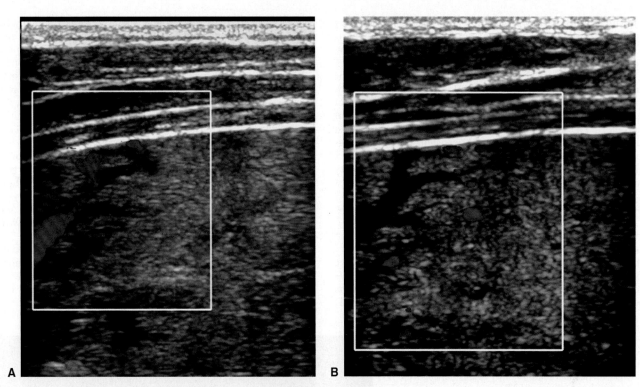

FIGURE 22.30. Budd-Chiari syndrome. *A* and *B,* Color Doppler images demonstrating dilated subcapsular and pericapsular branching vessels. Collateral vessels in this location are most commonly due to BCS or arteriovenous malformations and are less commonly seen in patients with PHT.

HEPATIC VENOOCCLUSIVE DISEASE

Hepatic venoocclusive disease (VOD) occurs most commonly in patients following hematopoietic stem cell transplantation. In one series, VOD occurred in 54% of patients following blood or bone marrow transplantation.[80] Preexisting liver disease increases the risk of developing VOD, and VOD is also more common in women.[81] Other risk factors include mismatched donor bone marrow, prior radiation therapy to the abdomen, and therapy with acyclovir or vancomycin.[81,82] More rarely, VOD occurs as a sequela of chemotherapy, alkaloid toxin ingestion, high-dose radiation therapy, or liver transplantation.[81] Patients typically present with hepatomegaly, tenderness of the liver, right upper quadrant pain, swelling, weight gain, ascites, jaundice, and abnormal liver function tests. Symptoms most often begin 3 to 6 days following transplantation.[82] Patients with severe disease may develop renal or cardiopulmonary failure and mental status changes.[81]

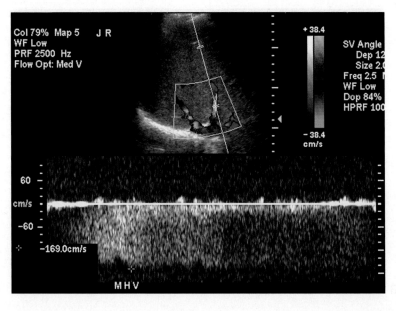

FIGURE 22.31. Hepatic vein stenosis. This color Doppler image demonstrates narrowing with color aliasing in the right and middle (Doppler sample gate) HVs, consistent with stenosis. The spectral waveform demonstrates increased velocity of 169 cm/s in the middle HV.

Hepatic venous outflow obstruction in VOD occurs secondary to nonthrombotic fibrous occlusion in the terminal hepatic venules and hepatic sinusoids, which is thought to be precipitated by injury to the venous endothelium.

Most patients are diagnosed clinically by elevation of the total bilirubin level to more than 2 mg/dL, hepatomegaly, right upper quadrant pain, or a greater than 2% body weight gain.[81-83] However, these clinical signs and symptoms are not specific.[84] The differential diagnosis includes graft versus host disease, sepsis, cardiac failure, and persistent tumor. Findings on Doppler ultrasound include elevated HA resistive index (RI > 0.75) and reversal of flow in the PV.[85-87] The sensitivity and specificity of these ultrasound findings are not known.

MISCELLANEOUS CONDITIONS

In patients with congestive heart failure, TR, or pulmonary hypertension, the HVs and IVC become dilated and the A wave becomes more pronounced (Fig. 22.32A). In addition, the PVs may demonstrate pulsatile flow (Fig. 22.32B).[88,89] In patients with TR, the S wave will typically not be as deep as the D wave. If the TR is severe enough, the S wave may actually be above the baseline and the S wave may merge with the A and V waves resulting in a single large retrograde "A-S-V" complex or reversed S wave.[11] In patients with TR, the V wave becomes abnormally tall[11]; however, in patients with competent tricuspid valves and severe right-sided heart failure, the A and V waves also became abnormally tall, but the S wave will remain deeper than the D wave.[11] These are nonspecific findings, as pulsatile portal venous flow may also be observed in thin, young patients or in patients with arteriovenous malformations.

Arteriovenous malformations may occur in the liver secondary to trauma, Rendu-Osler-Weber syndrome, and cirrhosis. Shunts may be arterioportal, portovenous, or arteriovenous; DUS findings depend on the exact nature of the shunt but typically include dilated or tangled vessels, direct visualization of a shunt, color aliasing, and high-velocity/low-resistance flow in the feeding vessel and draining vein (Fig. 22.33).[90]

Pseudoaneurysms in the liver are rare, occurring most commonly following trauma and less frequently due to infection. Color Doppler will demonstrate "yin-yang" swirling flow in the aneurysm and "to-and-fro" flow above and below the baseline in the neck (Fig. 22.34).

FIGURE 22.32. Congestive heart failure. *A,* Spectral waveform demonstrates a prominent A wave *(arrow)* in the middle HV. *B,* Spectral waveform from the portal vein reveals marked pulsatility in this patient with congestive heart failure and TR.

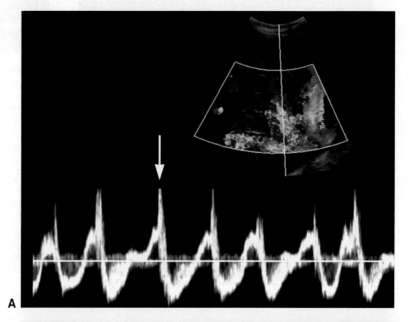

A

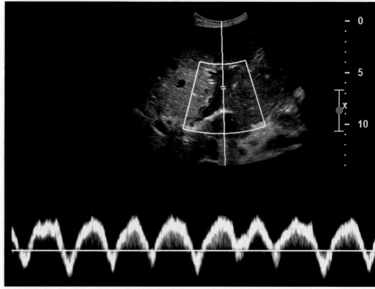

B

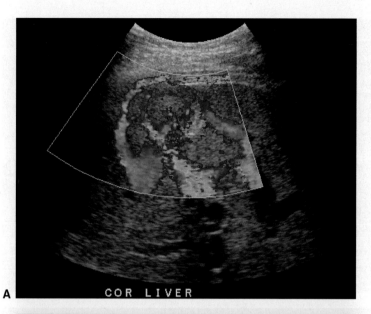

A   COR LIVER

FIGURE 22.33. Arteriovenous malformation. *A*, Color Doppler image reveals a group of dilated tangled subcapsular vessels in a patient with hereditary telangiectasia and right upper quadrant pain. Spectral Doppler reveals a low-resistance waveform with increased diastolic flow in the hepatic artery (*B*) and pulsatile flow in the draining vein (*C*) consistent with an arteriovenous malformation.

VISCERAL VASCULAR

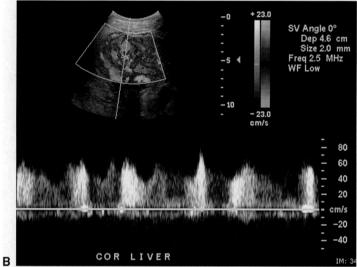

B   COR LIVER

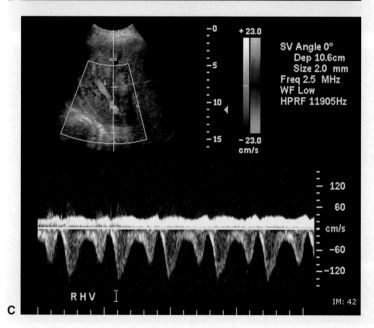

C

FIGURE 22.34. Hepatic artery pseudoaneurysm. *A*, Gray-scale image from a patient with pancreatitis presenting with abdominal pain demonstrates a cystic structure (calipers) underneath the left lobe of the liver (*L*). *B*, Color Doppler image shows flow within the cystic structure with a "yin-yang" appearance (*arrows*). Findings are consistent with a pseudoaneurysm. A, aorta. *, portal confluence. *C*, Duplex Doppler image demonstrates that the pseudoaneurysm arises from the hepatic artery (*arrow*). Spectral waveform demonstrates the classic finding of "to-and-fro" flow in the neck of the pseudoaneurysm (sample gate) with flow heading toward the pseudoaneurysm during systole and flowing away during diastole. *, portal vein.

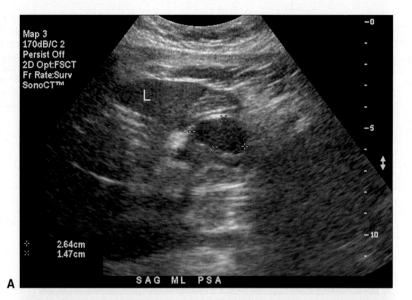

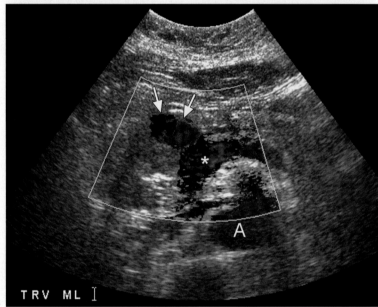

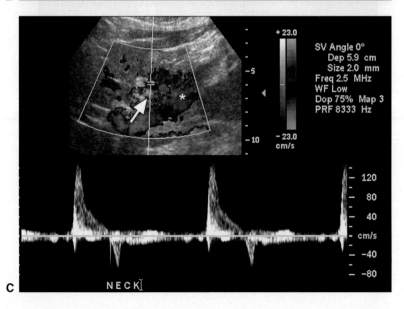

HEPATIC TRANSPLANTATION

Hepatic transplantation is now accepted as the treatment of choice for most patients with end-stage liver disease as well as early-stage hepatic malignancies. Despite recent advances in medical therapy, there is no known cure for viral hepatitis or alcoholic liver disease, which are the most common causes of cirrhosis and end-stage liver disease in the United States. On the other hand, advances in surgical technique, postoperative immunosuppression protocols, and organ distribution via the United Network for Organ Sharing (UNOS) have resulted in significant improvement in patient mortality and morbidity following hepatic transplantation. As of January 2013, the Organ Procurement and Transplantation Network (OPTN) reported that the 1-year survival rate (YSR) in the United States was 86.3% for a deceased donor graft and 90.1% for a living donor graft, and the 5 YSR was 72.0% for a deceased donor graft and 77.7% for a living donor graft.[91] Survival rates are lowest for repeat transplants, recipients over age 65 years, and donors under age 5 years or over age 50 years. Patients transplanted due to hepatic malignancy, acute hepatic necrosis, or noncholestatic cirrhosis also have lower survival rates. The MELD score, which is based on serum creatinine, total serum bilirubin, and INR, is a relatively accurate predictor of the severity of liver disease as well as patient mortality and is also used to prioritize patients on the liver transplant waiting list.

Primary nonfunction of the graft is the most common cause of graft loss, followed by biliary and vascular complications; however, biliary and vascular complications are interrelated as the HA provides the sole blood supply to the biliary tree in the transplanted liver. Postoperative bleeding and infection are also significant causes of mortality and morbidity. Due to diagnostic accuracy, portability, noninvasive nature, and relatively low cost, DUS is generally considered to be the imaging modality of choice for suspected vascular complications, biliary tract abnormalities, and perihepatic collections in the transplant recipient. However, DUS has no role in establishing the diagnosis of rejection, which generally requires liver biopsy.

Over 6,000 liver transplants are performed yearly in the United States. The most common indications for liver transplantation are listed in Table 22.2. Note that the eligibility of patients with HCC is determined by the Milan criteria: single HCC < 5 cm in diameter or fewer than three HCCs each less than 3 cm in diameter.[92] Commonly accepted contraindications for liver transplantation are listed in Table 22.3.[93] However, considerable controversy exists regarding differentiation between absolute and relative contraindications, and practice may vary from institution to institution. As of January 2013, there were 16,551 patients on the liver transplant waiting list.

Surgical Considerations

Most liver transplants are performed by orthotopic transplantation of a whole liver deceased donor graft. However, due to the relative shortage of donors, patients may also receive a split liver deceased donor allograft or a living donor segmental or lobar (partial) transplant. The exact configuration of the HA, PV, IVC/HVs, and biliary anastomoses depends upon the type of graft and the presence of congenital anomalies or preexisting disease in either the donor or recipient vessels or biliary tree.

In patients undergoing an orthotopic liver transplant, the donor liver is placed in the same anatomic location and orientation as the resected native liver. The hepatic arterial anastomosis is most commonly constructed using an end-to-end anastomosis of the recipient HA at the bifurcation or origin of the gastroduodenal artery with either the donor celiac axis or common HA. The PV anastomosis is most commonly created by a direct end-to-end anastomosis between the donor and recipient main PVs. Conventionally, the donor IVC is placed as an interposition graft between the suprahepatic and infrahepatic recipient IVC after the recipient intrahepatic IVC is resected and explanted with the diseased liver, requiring both a suprahepatic and infrahepatic end-to-end anastomosis (Fig. 22.35). However, currently, a "piggy-back" approach is

---

TABLE 22.2

INDICATIONS FOR HEPATIC TRANSPLANTATION

Cirrhosis (End-Stage Liver Disease)
  Viral hepatitis
  Alcoholic liver disease
  Autoimmune hepatitis
Acute Hepatic Necrosis
  Tylenol overdose
Nonalcoholic Fatty Liver Disease (NAFLD) and
  Nonalcoholic Steatohepatitis (NASH)
Primary Biliary Cirrhosis
Primary Sclerosing Cholangitis
Hepatic Tumors
  HCC (Milan criteria apply: single HCC <5 cm in diameter
    or up to three HCCs each <3 cm in diameter)
  Neuroendocrine tumors
  Cholangiocarcinoma
Metabolic and Genetic Disorders
  Hemochromatosis
  Wilson's disease
  α-1 Antitrypsin deficiency
  Glycogen storage diseases

TABLE 22.3

CONTRAINDICATIONS FOR HEPATIC TRANSPLANTATION

Absolute
  Extrahepatic malignancy not in remission
  HCC >5 cm in diameter or more than three tumors >3 cm
    in diameter (Milan criteria)
  Uncontrolled systemic infection
  Active substance or alcohol abuse
  Severe cardiopulmonary disease
  Multisystem failure (beyond liver failure)
  Noncompliance

Relative
  Older age
  Cholangiocarcinoma
  Portal vein thrombosis
  Active/refractory infection (including HIV)
  Previous malignancy
  Psychiatric disorder
  Advanced chronic renal failure

Factors That Increase Risk
  Chronic HBV
  Severe abdominal atherosclerosis
  Massive ascites
  Severe malnutrition
  Prior biliary tract surgery
  Prior transjugular portosystemic shunt (TIPS)
  Surgery involving portal vein

FIGURE 22.35. Diagram demonstrating the most common vascular and biliary anastomoses in a whole liver deceased donor orthotopic hepatic transplant with an interposition IVC graft.

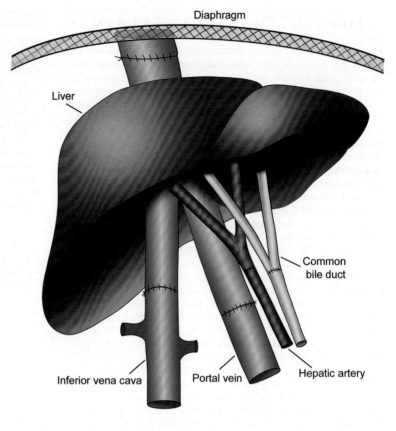

often performed whereby the suprahepatic donor IVC (or HV in the case of a partial liver transplant) is sutured end-to-side with the recipient hepatic venous confluence. Drainage from the caudate veins generally keeps the donor IVC patent, which is tied off distally (Figs. 22.36 and 22.37). Advantages of the "piggy-back" technique include decreased retroperitoneal dissection, less blood loss, and shorter operating time, as well as the need to create only one IVC anastomosis. In addition, intraoperative venous bypass is not required, as caval flow is not interrupted in the recipient during surgery. The gallbladder is routinely removed, and biliary drainage is typically achieved by creation of an end-to-end anastomosis between the donor common bile duct and the recipient common

hepatic or common bile duct. Choledochojejunostomies are typically only constructed if the recipient or donor common bile duct is diseased.

Duplex Ultrasound Evaluation

While protocols vary from institution to institution, in many centers, screening of the transplanted liver with DUS is performed daily for the first 3 days postoperatively and subsequently at 1, 6, and 12 months posttransplantation. A successful DUS examination requires the use of numerous acoustic windows, especially in the immediate postoperative

FIGURE 22.36. Diagram of a "piggy-back" inferior vena cava (IVC) anastomosis.

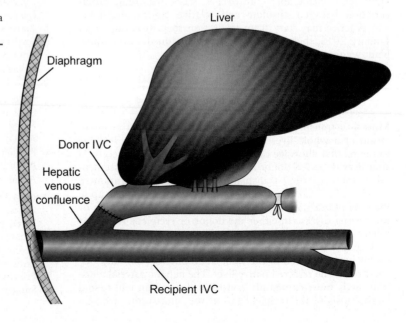

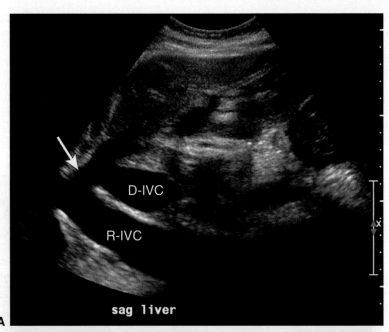

A

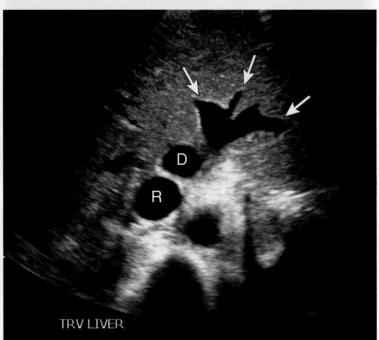

B

FIGURE 22.37. Normal postoperative anatomy of a "piggy-back" IVC anastomosis. *A,* Sagittal gray-scale image demonstrating the anastomosis of the suprahepatic donor inferior vena cava (D-IVC) with the recipient hepatic venous confluence (*arrow*). The recipient inferior vena cava (R-IVC) is left in situ, thus avoiding extensive retroperitoneal Dissection. *B,* Transverse gray-scale image demonstrates the donor (D) IVC above the recipient IVC (R) in cross section below the right, middle, and left HVs (*arrows*). The aorta is to the left of the recipient IVC.

VISCERAL VASCULAR

period when ultrasound access is more difficult due to overlying bandages and immobility of the patient. A curved array 2- to 5-MHz transducer is generally used to obtain gray-scale and color images as well as spectral Doppler waveforms of the main, right, and left HAs and PVs, the right, middle, and left HVs, IVC, and aorta. The RI, PSV, and acceleration time (AT—the time interval between the onset of systole and the first systolic peak) should be measured in the main, right, and left HAs. Every attempt should be made to visualize all vascular anastomoses. In addition, gray-scale evaluation of the liver parenchyma, biliary tree, and perihepatic spaces should be performed.

The normal HA waveform demonstrates a sharp systolic upstroke with an AT of less than 0.08 seconds and continuous forward diastolic flow with an RI between 0.5 and 0.8 (Fig. 22.38A). PSV in the HA is typically less than 200 cm/s, although difficulty in obtaining a correct Doppler angle in a tortuous vessel may result in a false elevation of PSV.[94-96] However, decreased diastolic flow resulting in elevation of the RI >0.8 is commonly observed in the immediate postoperative period (Fig. 22.39). Although this finding was initially considered suspicious for impending hepatic artery thrombosis (HAT), it is now considered a normal postoperative finding, likely due to increased peripheral vascular resistance or decreased vessel compliance due to some combination of congestive heart failure and volume overload resulting in hepatic congestion, reperfusion edema, and vasospasm. The RI typically normalizes by the end of the first postoperative week.[96-102] Imaging after administration of intravenous ultrasound contrast agents or nifedipine (a vasodilator)[103-106] can be useful to distinguish between HAT or hepatic artery stenosis (HAS) and absent or decreased diastolic flow merely due to poor visualization of vessels.

The normal PV waveform is monophasic with hepatopetal flow and mild respiratory variation (Fig. 22.38B). Mismatch in diameter between the donor and recipient PV is particularly common in pediatric transplant recipients and such a "step-off" should not be misconstrued as PV stenosis. The IVC and HVs should have a triphasic, pulsatile waveform reflecting transmitted cardiac pulsatility with predominately hepatofugal flow except during the A wave, which corresponds to right atrial contraction (Fig. 22.38C). While a monophasic hepatic venous waveform is considered a nonspecific abnormal finding, deep inspiration and external compression of the IVC or liver due to overlying adipose tissue, large volume ascites, or a large liver

transplanted into a small space may also cause a monophasic hepatic venous waveform. On the other hand, accentuated pulsatility in the IVC, HVs, and even in the PVs (Fig. 22.40) is noted relatively commonly in the immediate postoperative period due to right heart failure, often exacerbated by volume overload or TR.

HAT is the most common vascular complication following liver transplantation and usually occurs within the first 6 weeks. The reported incidence ranges from 3% to 12% in adults[94,107-112] but is much higher in children, likely

FIGURE 22.38. Normal postoperative spectral Doppler waveforms following hepatic transplantation. *A,* Spectral Doppler waveform from the main hepatic artery in the porta hepatis above the portal vein demonstrating a sharp systolic upstroke with continuous forward diastolic flow. The RI is 0.65. *B,* Spectral Doppler waveform from the main portal vein demonstrating monophasic hepatopetal flow with slight respiratory variation. Velocity decreases slightly during inspiration.

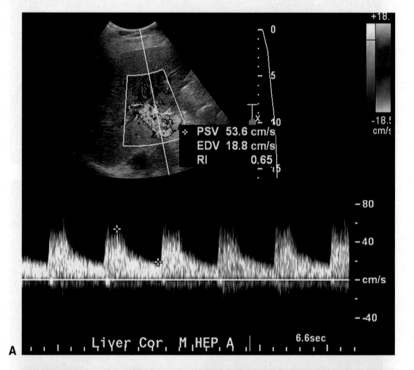

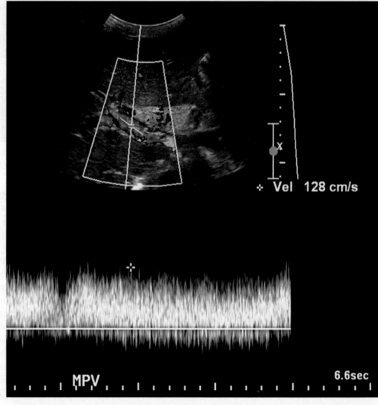

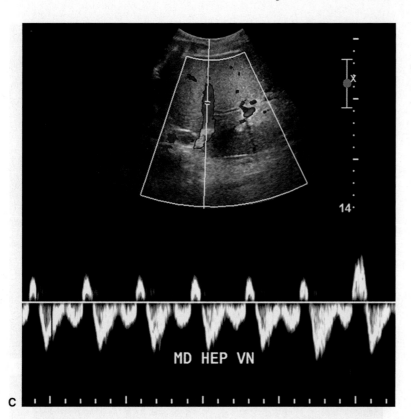

FIGURE 22.38. (*Continued*) C, Normal waveform from the middle HV has a pulsatile pattern reflecting right heart pressure with flow primarily directed away from the liver capsule (hepatofugal). Waveforms in the IVC as well as the right, middle, and left HVs should appear similar.

secondary to the smaller size of the vessels. Most patients present with fulminant hepatic failure due to hepatic necrosis, liver infarction, or biliary complications such as biliary necrosis, bile leaks, bilomas, or biliary strictures, as the HA provides the sole blood supply to the biliary tree in the transplanted liver. Abscess formation, bacteremia, and sepsis are common sequelae of HAT. Risk factors include vessel diameter mismatch between the donor and recipient HA, small size of one or both HAs, complex arterial reconstructions (especially interposition grafts), prolonged donor liver ischemic time,

retransplantation, hypercoagulable states, and extensive blood loss during surgery.[109-115] If thrombectomy or thrombolysis is not successful, most patients require emergency retransplantation. The mortality rate is estimated at slightly over 31%.[110,112,113]

The diagnosis of HAT is made on DUS by documenting absence of flow in the main and intraparenchymal HAs using color, power, and spectral Doppler (Fig. 22.41). The reported accuracy of DUS in the diagnosis of HAT is close to 92%.[116] False-positive diagnoses may occur when flow is not

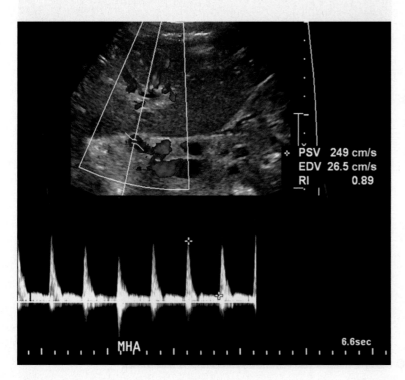

FIGURE 22.39. High-resistance postoperative hepatic artery (HA) waveform. One day post-op, the PSV in the HA is elevated, and diastolic flow is significantly reduced resulting in an elevated RI of 0.89. While this type of waveform was initially considered worrisome for impending HAT, it is relatively common in the immediate postoperative period, most likely due to a combination of vasospasm and increased peripheral vascular resistance secondary to hepatic parenchymal edema. One week later, diastolic flow had normalized.

FIGURE 22.40. Congestive heart failure. Note increased pulsatility of the waveforms in both the middle HV (*A*) and main portal vein (*B*). Waveforms were similar in the IVC, left and right HVs, and left and right PVs. This patient has right-sided congestive heart failure as well as pulmonary hypertension. Note reversal of diastolic flow in the main HA (*C*) due to increased peripheral vascular resistance secondary to hepatic congestion. Waveforms in all vessels normalized following diuretic therapy.

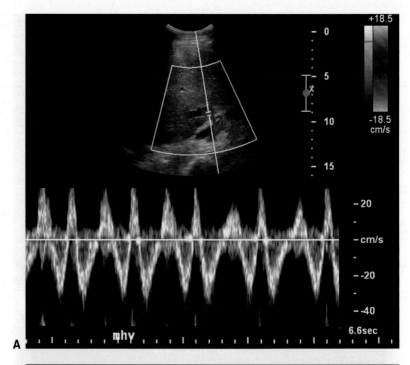

A

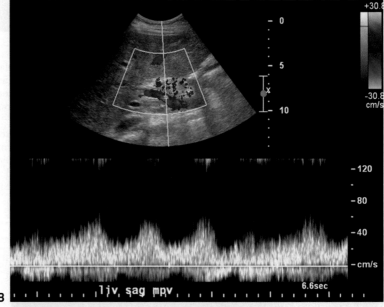

B

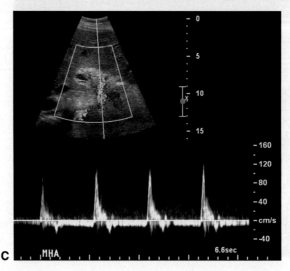

C

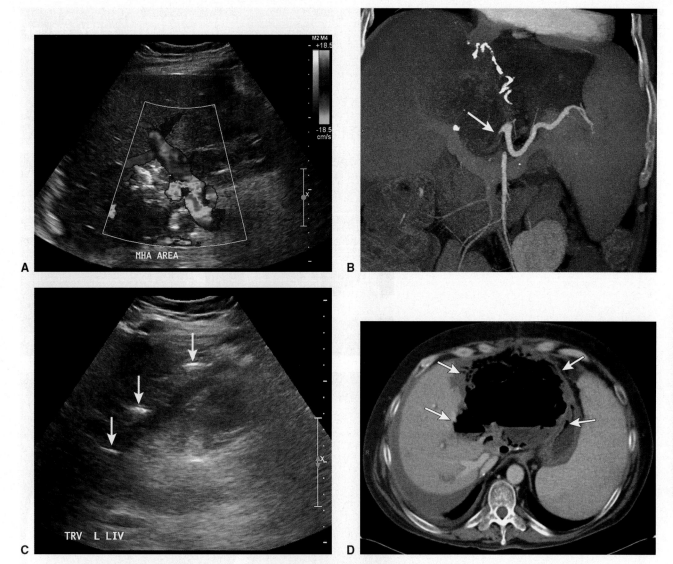

FIGURE 22.41. Hepatic artery thrombosis (HAT). *A,* Color Doppler image of the porta hepatis demonstrates flow in the main portal vein, but no flow in the area of the main hepatic artery (MHA). *B,* Coronal volume rendered contrast-enhanced CT image demonstrating an abrupt cut off of the MHA (*arrow*) consistent with HAT. *C,* Gray-scale image of the left hepatic lobe demonstrates linear echogenic areas (*arrows*) with distal shadowing consistent with gas in the liver parenchyma. *D,* The presence of air within a large abscess (*arrows*) in the left lobe of the liver is confirmed on follow-up axial contrast-enhanced CT image. Infarction with subsequent superinfection and abscess formation is a known sequela of HAT. (This figure was published in Reid SA, Scoutt LM, Hamper UM. *Ultrasound Clinics: Vascular Ultrasound. Vascular Complications of Liver Transplants: Evaluation with Duplex Doppler Ultrasound,* Vol 6. Elsevier, 2011, pp 519. Copyright Elsevier, Philadelphia, PA 2011. Reprinted with permission from the publisher.)

visualized secondary to poor technique, compression of the HAs due to severe hepatic edema, vasospasm, HAS, and low flow states. Imaging with contrast-enhanced ultrasound or following the administration of nifedipine can reduce false-positive examinations and should be considered rather than more invasive imaging if HA flow cannot be documented and the clinical scenario is not concerning for HAT, particularly in the immediate postoperative state when visualization of the HA is most difficult.[103-106] Rarely, a false-negative examination may occur due to visualization of intraparenchymal arterial flow derived from the development of collateral arterial flow in some patients with HAT.

HAS is estimated to occur in 2% to 11% of liver transplant recipients and most commonly occurs at the anastomotic site, although stenoses may occur anywhere along the length of the HA.[109,117,118] Predisposing risk factors include rejection,

injury from surgical clamps or perfusion catheters, complex arterial reconstructions, and small arteries.[119] Similar to HAT, HAS can cause biliary ischemia and necrosis (Fig. 22.42). Patients may present with a wide range of symptoms. While some patients are completely asymptomatic, others present with bile leaks, strictures, liver abscess or infarction, and even hepatic dysfunction and graft loss. Angioplasty with stent placement is the preferred treatment option but may not be durable, and occasionally, surgical revision and even retransplantation must be performed.

Doppler criteria for the diagnosis of HAS are somewhat controversial. A PSV > 200 cm/s in the HA has been reported to have a positive predictive value of 95% (Fig. 22.43).[119] Focal narrowing and color aliasing may be observed in the main HA. The presence of a tardus parvus waveform (Fig. 22.43) in the intraparenchymal HA with an AT > 80 ms

FIGURE 22.42. Hepatic artery stenosis (HAS). *A*, Spectral Doppler waveform demonstrating increased PSV of 289 cm/sec in the main HA suggestive of HAS. Mild intrahepatic biliary ductal dilation was also noted (not shown). *B*, Image from ERCP demonstrates a stricture (*arrow*) at the common bile duct anastomoses that required stent placement.

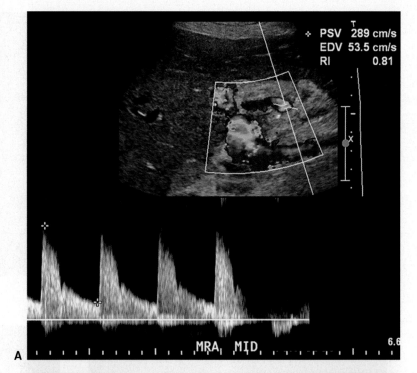

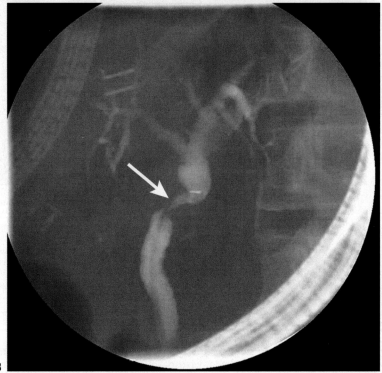

and RI < 0.5 has been reported to have a sensitivity of 73% for HAS and should raise concern even in the absence of a documented increase in PSV, as visualization of the HA anastomosis may be obscured by overlying bowel gas.[119,120] However, a more recent study reported that the finding of a tardus parvus waveform alone has a much lower positive predictive value,[121] as a similar waveform pattern may be observed in patients with HAT and collateral flow, aortic or celiac artery stenosis, or even reperfusion injury. These authors recommended combining this finding with a PSV of less than 48 cm/s in the HAs, which yielded a positive predictive value of 88% and sensitivity of 69%.[121] It should

be cautioned that a similar waveform pattern is commonly noted in the first 48 hours posttransplantation, likely due to peripheral vasodilatation secondary to reperfusion injury. Thus, a tardus parvus waveform in the intraparenchymal HA is much more concerning for HA stenosis more than 48 hours posttransplantation.

PVT is a relatively rare complication following liver transplantation with a reported incidence of only 1% to 3%.[108,109,122,123] Patients may present with findings of PHT or liver failure. Risk factors include vessel injury, complex venous anastomoses or reconstructions, hypercoagulable states, hypovolemia, vessel size mismatch, history of PVT, prior surgery

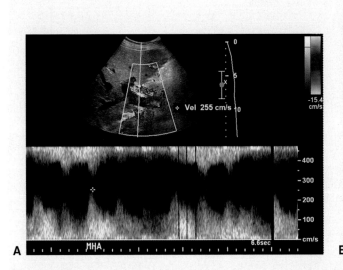
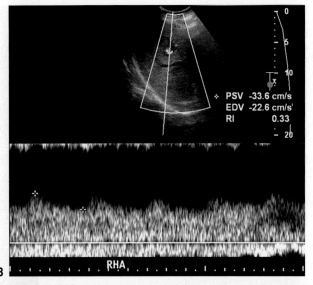
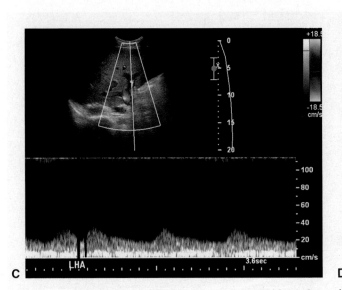
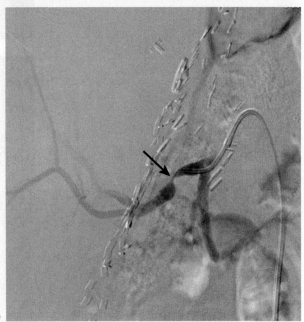

VISCERAL VASCULAR

FIGURE 22.43. Hepatic artery stenosis (HAS). *A,* Spectral Doppler waveform from the main HA demonstrating elevated PSV of 255 cm/s. Spectral Doppler waveforms from the right (*B*) and left (*C*) intrahepatic HAs show a pronounced tardus parvus waveform pattern with a significant delay in systolic acceleration and relatively increased diastolic flow resulting in a decreased RI of 0.33. Tight stenosis (*arrow*) at the HA anastomosis was confirmed on angiography (*D*).

involving the PV, and prior TIPS placement.[123,124] The diagnosis of PVT is made on DUS by demonstrating absence of flow in cases of occlusive PVT or a color void in cases of nonocclusive PVT on color or power Doppler imaging. Findings should be confirmed with spectral Doppler interrogation.[94] Intraluminal echogenic thrombus may be seen on gray-scale imaging (Fig. 22.44). However, acute thrombus may be anechoic and, therefore, not visible on gray-scale imaging alone. In cases of chronic PVT, the PV may not be visualized (Fig. 22.45). DUS has been reported as being both sensitive and specific for the diagnosis of PVT.[19,20,28] Treatment options include thrombolysis, thrombectomy, stent placement, or surgical revision with placement of an interposition graft or TIPS.

Portal vein stenosis (PVS) typically occurs at the anastomosis, and the clinical presentation is quite variable. Patients with mild PVS may be asymptomatic, but once the PV diameter is reduced by over 80%, patients commonly present with symptoms of PHT.[123] Care must be taken not to misinterpret diameter mismatch between the donor and recipient PV as true PVS. Thus, long segment narrowing of the PV is more concerning for PVS. In addition, comparison with immediate postoperative imaging may be helpful. Color Doppler interrogation will demonstrate narrowing and focal color aliasing. Suggested DUS criteria for the diagnosis of PVT include: diameter less than 2.5 to 5 mm, peak velocity greater than 125 cm/s, or PV velocity ratio pre- and poststenosis greater than 2.5 or 3:1 (Fig. 22.46).[125,126] If treatment is necessary, angioplasty with stent placement is generally tried prior to resorting to surgical reconstruction.

Thrombosis or stenosis of the HVs or IVC is extremely uncommon following liver transplantation, occurring in well under 2% of transplant recipients.[95,107,109] While often

FIGURE 22.44. Portal vein thrombosis (PVT). *A,*-Gray-scale longitudinal image of the main portal vein (*arrow*) demonstrates intraluminal echoes consistent with thrombus. *B,* Power Doppler image confirms that there is no blood flow in the main portal vein, consistent with PVT. Flow is present in the IVC posteriorly. (This figure was published in Reid SA, Scoutt LM, Hamper UM. *Ultrasound Clinics: Vascular Ultrasound. Vascular Complications of Liver Transplants: Evaluation with Duplex Doppler Ultrasound,* Vol 6. Elsevier, 2011, pp 523, Copyright Elsevier, Philadelphia, PA 2011. Reprinted with permission from the publisher.)

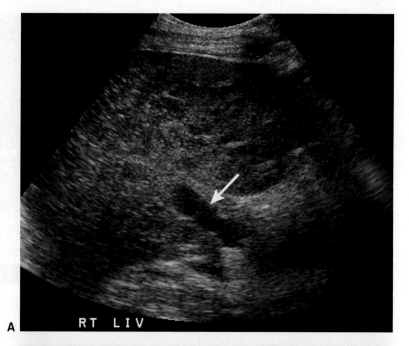

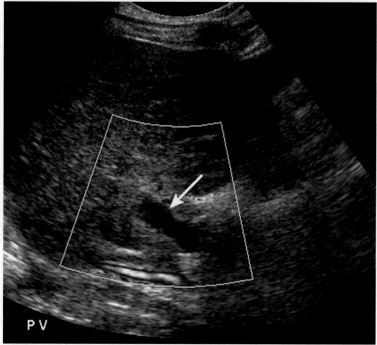

asymptomatic, patients may present with abdominal pain, hepatomegaly, ascites, or peripheral edema. IVC stenoses most often occur at the anastomotic sites.[123] Risk factors include vessel injury, hypercoagulable states, kinking of the vessels, or external compression.[125-127] Fibrosis, chronic thrombosis, or intimal hyperplasia may lead to delayed development of thrombosis or stenosis of the IVC. Intraluminal echoes or vessel narrowing may be noted on gray-scale or color Doppler (Figs. 22.47 and 22.48). A color void will be noted on color or power Doppler interrogation in patients with venous thrombosis. In cases of HV or IVC stenosis, focal color aliasing with an increase in velocity by a factor of 3 to 4 will be noted, along with dampening or flattening of the more peripheral HV waveforms (Fig. 22.49).[94,95] A pulsatility index less than 0.45 has been reported to be 95% specific

for the diagnosis of significant HV or outflow IVC stenosis, while a pulsatility index of greater than 0.75 is considered normal.[125,127] Monophasic waveforms in the HVs may indicate more cephalad stenosis, but this is a nonspecific finding and may be seen in normal patients or when there is extrinsic compression of the IVC.[127,128]

Although extremely uncommon, HA pseudoaneurysms (PSAs) are potentially serious vascular complications due to the risk of rupture and hemorrhage. Extrahepatic PSAs arise at the HA anastomosis and may be associated with infection or poor surgical technique. Intrahepatic PSAs are most commonly iatrogenic secondary to liver biopsy, transhepatic cholangiography, or drainage catheters but also may be mycotic secondary to bacteremia. Risk factors include Roux-en-Y hepaticojejunostomy, pancreatitis, sepsis, and technically difficult arterial

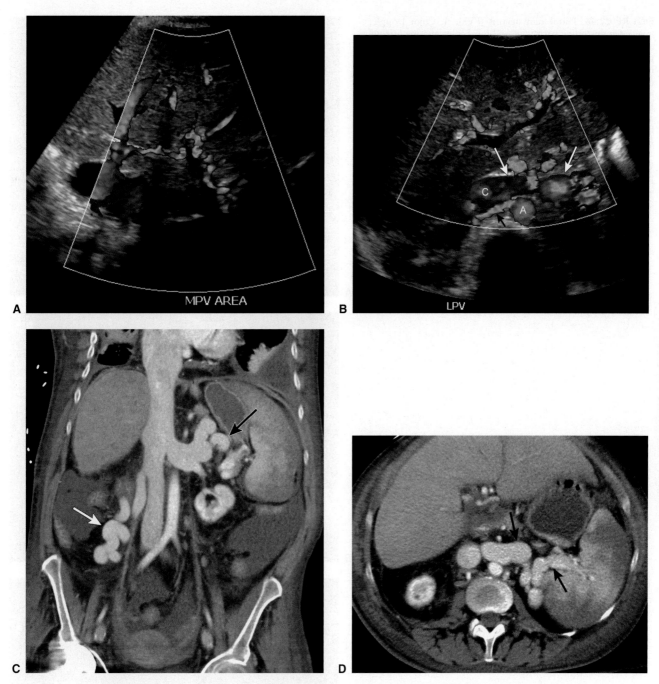

VISCERAL VASCULAR

FIGURE 22.45. Chronic portal vein thrombosis. *A,* Color Doppler image of the porta hepatis reveals a dilated, tortuous main HA; however, the main portal vein is not seen. *B,* Transverse color Doppler image in the mid-abdomen demonstrates a massively enlarged left renal vein (*white arrows*) consistent with a large patent splenorenal shunt. C, inferior vena cava. A, aorta. Black *arrow,* right renal artery. Coronal (*C*) and transverse (*D*) images from a contrast-enhanced CT demonstrating spontaneous splenorenal shunt (*black arrows*) and additional varices in the right retroperitoneum (*white arrow*). (Courtesy of Dr. Jonathan Kirsch, Yale University School of Medicine.)

reconstructions.[129] Gray-scale imaging will demonstrate a cystic area, typically anechoic, adjacent to the HA; however, the diagnosis is made by the demonstration of swirling blood flow in a "yin-yang" pattern within the pseudoaneurysm on color Doppler imaging (Fig. 22.50), as well as "to-and-fro" flow above and below the baseline in the neck of the PSA on spectral Doppler interrogation. A thrombosed hepatic artery PSA may be difficult to differentiate from a parenchymal hematoma. Intrahepatic hepatic artery PSAs are most commonly treated either by exclusion with a covered stent or embolization. Surgical revision is generally required for extrahepatic PSAs.

HA to PV fistulae are rare complications following liver biopsy. Most are small and resolve spontaneously. Characteristic ultrasound findings are the presence of a focal color bruit in the surrounding soft tissues, high PSV and end-diastolic velocity isolated to the feeding artery, and pulsatile flow with increased velocity in the draining vein.

FIGURE 22.46. Portal vein stenosis (PVS). *A,* Color Doppler image demonstrating narrowing and focal color aliasing (*arrow*) of the main portal vein (MPV). Spectral waveform from the MPV proximal to the stenosis (*B*) demonstrates a velocity of 30 cm/s in comparison to 166 cm/s obtained at the site of the stenosis (*C*). The velocity ratio is 5.5, which is suggestive of a hemodynamically significant stenosis. While the clinical significance of PVS is uncertain, stenting could be considered in the setting of abnormal liver function tests and no other explanation. (This figure was published in Mathur M, Ginat DT, Rubens D, et al. Evaluation of Organ Transplants. In *Introduction to Vascular Ultrasonography*, 6th ed, Chapter 34. Elsevier, 2012, pp 607, Copyright Elsevier, 2012. Reprinted with permission from the publisher.)

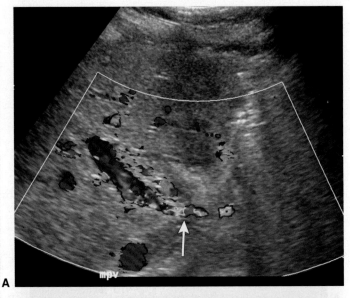

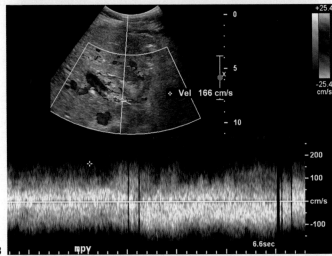

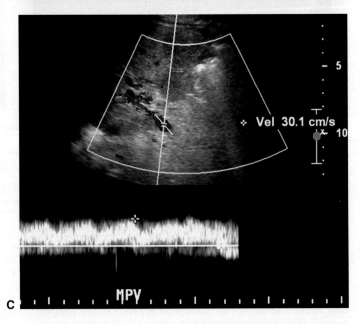

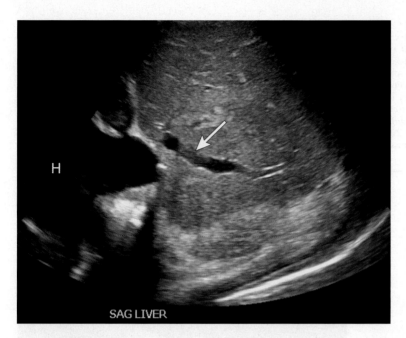

FIGURE 22.47. Hepatic vein thrombosis. Note intramural echoes (*arrow*) in one of the HVs on this sagittal gray-scale image of the liver. H, heart.

Nonvascular Ultrasound Findings

Ultrasound examination can also have an important role in the evaluation of nonvascular complications following liver transplantation. In the immediate postoperative period, most patients will be found to have perihepatic hemorrhage (Fig. 22.51) or ascites, as well as right-sided pleural effusions. Biliary complications including stricture, necrosis, or leakage resulting in biliary ductal dilation, bilomas (Fig. 22.52), or abscess formation (Fig. 22.53) are relatively common and are often associated with HA abnormalities (HAT or HAS) or complex biliary reconstructions. While such focal collections are often well marginated and anechoic, internal echoes may be present, and the observation of echogenic speckles with ring-down artifact is strongly suggestive of air and superinfection. HAT or HAS may also lead to infarction of the hepatic parenchyma. Hepatic infarcts are often wedge-shaped and peripheral with indistinct margins on ultrasound examination and may appear either hypoechoic

or echogenic depending upon time course and whether or not hemorrhage or superinfection has occurred (Fig. 22.54). The presence of solid hepatic masses, irrespective of echogenicity (Fig. 22.55), should raise concern for malignancy, either recurrent tumor or posttransplant lymphoproliferative disorder (Fig. 22.56).

Conclusion

The DUS examination following liver transplantation plays an important role in screening patients for vascular complications, which can threaten graft and patient survival unless accurately diagnosed and treated. Such complications are more common in patients receiving partial liver transplants, in patients requiring complex vascular reconstructions, and in patients undergoing retransplantation. The examination is difficult to perform, especially in the immediate postsurgical setting. A clear understanding of the surgical approach and type of transplantation will facilitate the examination.

Text continues on page 336

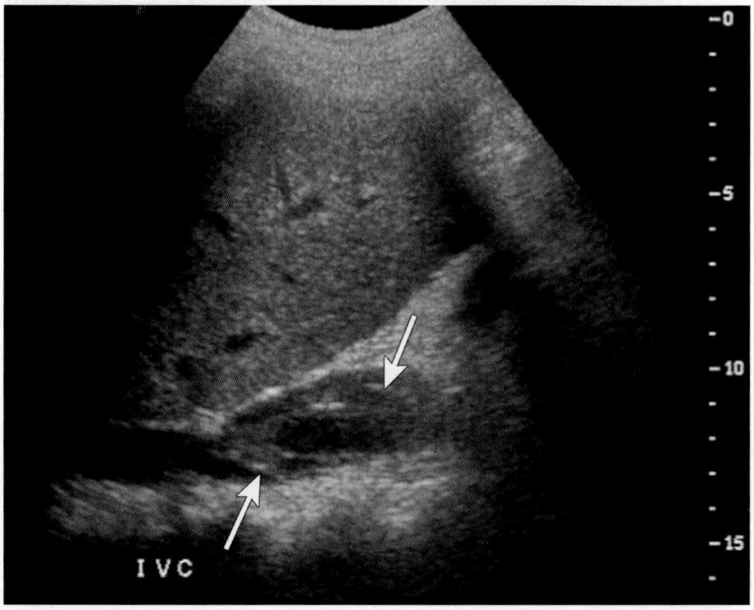

FIGURE 22.48. Inferior vena cava (IVC) thrombosis. Intraluminal echoes (*arrows*) in the intrahepatic IVC on this sagittal gray-scale image are consistent with nonocclusive IVC thrombus. (This figure was published in Reid SA, Scoutt LM, Hamper UM. *Ultrasound Clinics: Vascular Ultrasound. Vascular Complications of Liver Transplants: Evaluation with Duplex Doppler Ultrasound*, Vol 6. Elsevier, 2011, pp 527, Copyright Elsevier, Philadelphia, PA 2011. Reprinted with permission from the publisher.)

VISCERAL VASCULAR

FIGURE 22.49. Stenosis of inferior vena cava (IVC). *A,* Color Doppler sagittal image of the IVC demonstrating focal color aliasing and narrowing of the lumen (*arrow*), consistent with stenosis. *B,* Spectral Doppler waveforms demonstrate markedly increased velocity (309 cm/s) at the site of the stenosis and a flat, nonpulsatile waveform (*C*) in the proximal middle hepatic vein (MHV). (This figure was published in Reid SA, Scoutt LM, Hamper UM. *Ultrasound Clinics: Vascular Ultrasound. Vascular Complications of Liver Transplants: Evaluation with Duplex Doppler Ultrasound*, Vol 6. Elsevier, Philadelphia, PA 2011, pp 526. Copyright Elsevier, 2011. Reprinted with permission from the publisher.)

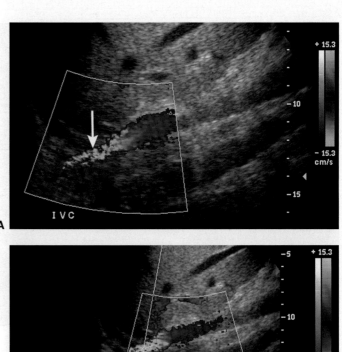

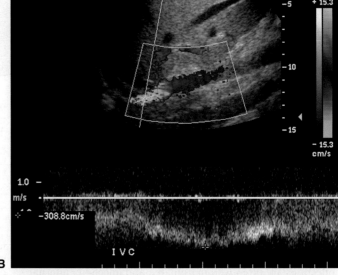

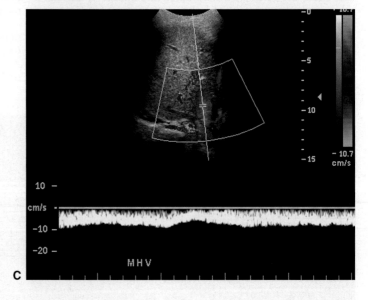

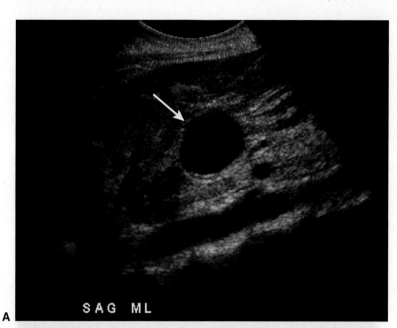

A

SAG ML

FIGURE 22.50. Hepatic artery pseudoaneurysm (PSA). *A,* Gray-scale image of a native liver demonstrates an anechoic cyst-like area (*arrow*) near the porta hepatis. *B,* Color flow with a "yin-yang" swirling pattern is documented on color-flow imaging. In a transplanted liver, intraparenchymal PSAs most commonly arise secondary to iatrogenic trauma or infection. (This figure was published in Reid SA, Scoutt LM, Hamper UM. *Ultrasound Clinics: Vascular Ultrasound. Vascular Complications of Liver Transplants: Evaluation with Duplex Doppler Ultrasound,* Vol 6. Elsevier, 2011, pp 522, Copyright Elsevier, Philadelphia, PA 2011. Reprinted with permission from the publisher.)

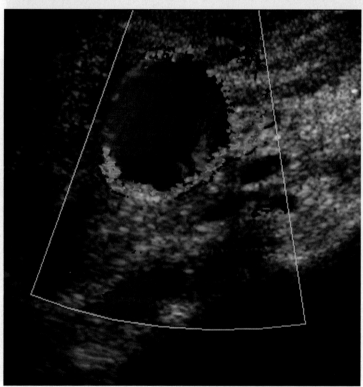

B

VISCERAL VASCULAR

FIGURE 22.51. Postoperative perihepatic hematoma. *A,* Gray-scale coronal image demonstrating a large complex collection (*arrows*) under the inferior margin of the left lobe of the liver. The patient did well with supportive therapy despite initial hematocrit drop. Follow-up examination (*B*) demonstrates that the post-op hematoma (*arrow*) has decreased in size and become more uniformly anechoic, consistent with evolution of a postoperative seroma.

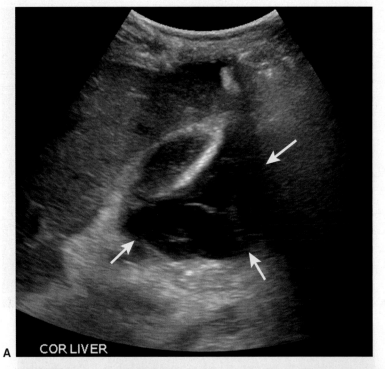

A   COR LIVER

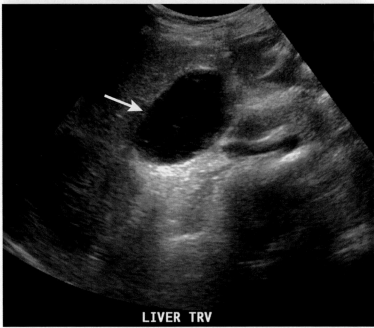

B   LIVER TRV

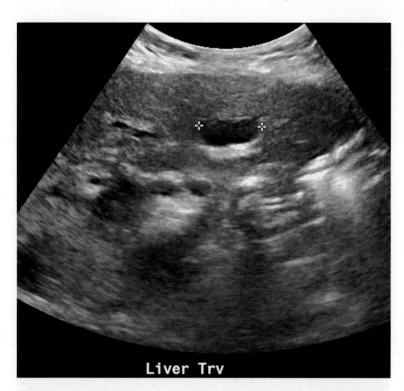

FIGURE 22.52. Biloma. Transverse gray-scale image of the left lobe of the liver demonstrating an anechoic lesion adjacent to the portal triads (*calipers*). This patient had biliary necrosis with numerous small bile leaks, which resulted in the development of several small intraparenchymal bilomas. Findings were confirmed on MRI and aspiration.

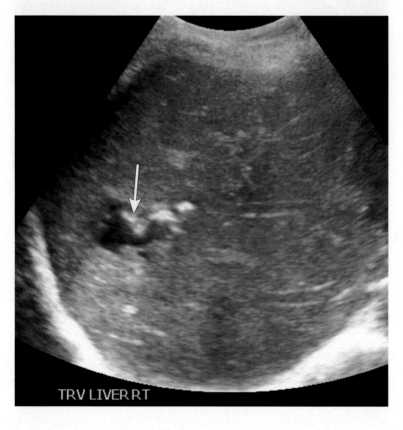

FIGURE 22.53. Abscess. This patient had a tight stricture at the common bile duct anastomosis and developed a bile leak with formation of a biloma, which became superinfected. Note complex fluid collection with increased through transmission in the right lobe of the liver on this gray-scale image. Punctate echogenic foci (*arrow*) represent air in the abscess.

VISCERAL VASCULAR

FIGURE 22.54. Infarct. *A,* Gray-scale image demonstrates a peripheral, irregular hypoechoic focus in the left lobe of the liver, suspicious for hepatic parenchymal infarct (*arrows*). *B,* Axial contrast-enhanced CT image demonstrates two classic wedge-shaped areas of infarction (*arrows*). (This figure was published in Reid SA, Scoutt LM, Hamper UM. Ultrasound Clinics: Vascular Ultrasound, Vascular Complications of Liver Transplants: Evaluation with Duplex Doppler Ultrasound, Vol 6. Elsevier, Philadelphia, PA 2011, pp 520, Copyright Elsevier, 2011. Reprinted with permission from the publisher.)

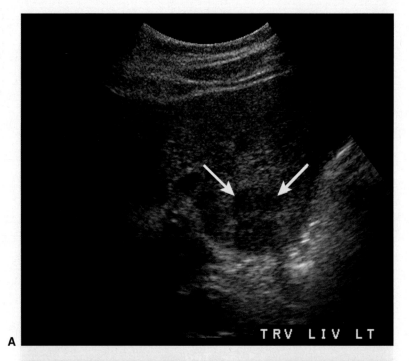

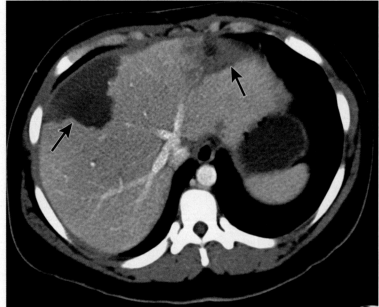

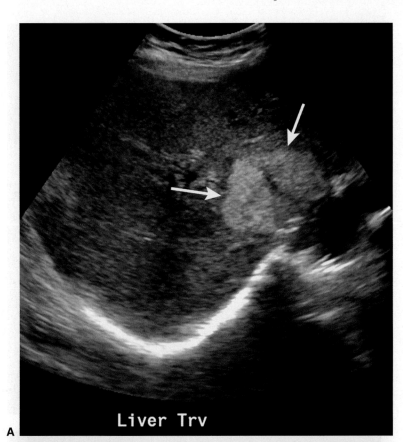

FIGURE 22.55. Focal liver lesion. *A*, Gray-scale image demonstrates a new echogenic well marginated solid liver lesion (*arrows*) in a patient 2 years post liver transplantation. *B*, Color Doppler image demonstrates a vessel running through the lesion and no mass effect on surrounding blood vessels, consistent with focal fatty infiltration. The diagnosis was confirmed on MRI. This is an unusual occurrence and atypical location for fatty infiltration. All new solid lesions should be carefully evaluated to exclude malignancy irrespective of echogenicity. Hypoechoic lesions are particularly worrisome for posttransplant lymphoproliferative disorder, metastases, and HCC.

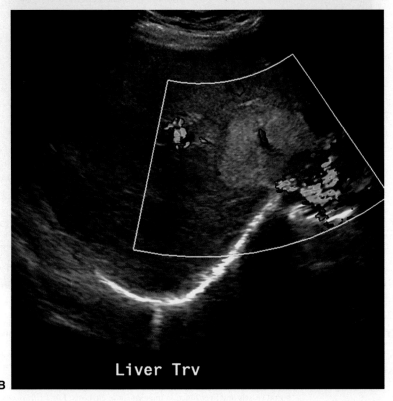

FIGURE 22.56. Posttransplant lymphoproliferative disorder. *A*, Coronal gray-scale image of the liver reveals two small hypoechoic solid masses (*arrows*) that correspond to FDG-avid lesions (*yellow*) on PET CT (*B*), consistent with posttransplant lymphoproliferative disorder. (Courtesy of Dr. Jonathan Kirsch, Yale University School of Medicine.)

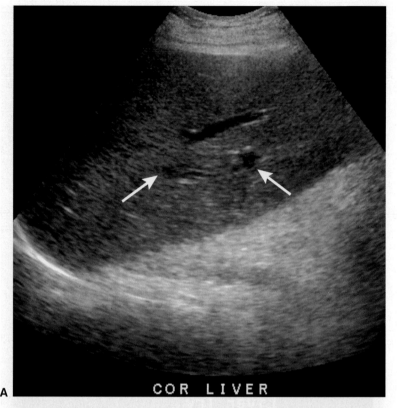

A

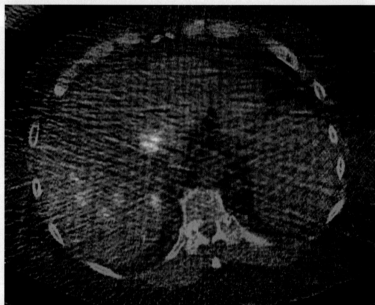

B

ACKNOWLEDGMENTS

The authors wish to acknowledge the contributions of Lisa M. Hribko for her administrative support and Geri Mancini for her illustrations and photography.

References

1. Colombo M, deFranchis R, Del Ninno E, et al. Hepatocellular carcinoma in Italian patients with cirrhosis. *N Engl J Med* 1991;325:675.
2. Goldberg E, Chopra S. Overview of the complications, prognosis and management of cirrhosis. In Bonis PAL, Runyon BS (eds). *Cirrhosis*. Waltham: UpToDate, 2008. Available at www.uptodate.com
3. Nevens F, Bustami R, Scheys I, et al. Variceal pressure is a factor predicting the risk of a first variceal bleeding: A prospective cohort study in cirrhotic patients. *Hepatology* 1998;27:15.
4. Schafer EA. Portal hypertension. In Beers MH, Porter RS, Jones TV, et al (eds). *The Merck Manual of Diagnosis and Therapy*, 18th ed. Whitehouse: Merck Research Laboratories, 2006.
5. Tarantino L, Giorgio A, de Stefano G, et al. Reversed flow in intrahepatic portal vessels and liver function impairment in cirrhosis. *Eur J Ultrasound* 1997;6:171-177.
6. Sanyal AJ. Extraportal vein obstruction (portal vein thrombosis). In Chopra S, Bonis PAL (eds). *Cirrhosis*, 2008. Available at www.update.com
7. Shearman DJC, Finlayson NDC. Portal hypertension. In Meyer HS, Eldredge JD (eds). *Diseases of the Gastrointestinal Tract and Liver*, 2nd ed. New York: Churchill Livingstone, 1989, pp 2013-2040.
8. Weinreb J, Kumari S, Phillips G, et al. Portal vein measurements by real-time sonography. *AJR Am J Roentgenol* 1982;139:497-499.
9. Rahim N, Adam EJ. Ultrasound demonstration of variations in normal portal vein diameter with posture. *Br J Radiol* 1985;58:313-314.

10. Zoli M, Dondi C, Marchesini G, et al. Splanchnic vein measurements in patients with liver cirrhosis: A case-control study. *J Ultrasound Med* 1985;4:641-646.

11. McNaughton DA, Abu-Yousef MM. Doppler US of the liver made simple. *Radiographics* 2011;31:161-188.

12. Bhatt S, Simon R, Dogra VS. Gamna-Gandy bodies: Sonographic features with histopathologic correlation. *J Ultrasound Med* 2006;25:1625-1629.

13. Bolondi L, Gamrolfi L, Arienti V, et al. Ultrasonography in the diagnosis of portal hypertension: Diminished response of portal vessels to respiration. *Radiology* 1982;142:167-172.

14. Bolondi L, Mazziotti A, Arienti V, et al. Ultrasound sonographic study of portal venous system in portal hypertension and after portosystemic shunt operations. *Surgery* 1984;95:261-269.

15. Zwiebel WJ. Ultrasound assessment of the hepatic vasculature. In Zwiebel WJ, Pellerito JS (eds). *Introduction to Vascular Ultrasonography.* Philadelphia: Elsevier/Saunders, 2005, pp 585-609.

16. Ralls PW. Color Doppler sonography of the hepatic artery and portal venous system. *AJR Am J Roentgenol* 1990;155:517-524.

17. Tchelepi H, Ralls P, Radin R, et al. Sonography of diffuse liver disease. *J Ultrasound Med* 2002;21:1023-1032.

18. Wachsberg RH, Bahramipour P, Sofocleous CT, et al. Hepatofugal flow in the portal venous system: Pathophysiology, imaging findings, and diagnostic pitfalls. *Radiographics* 2002;22:123-140.

19. Ohta M, Hashizume M, Tomikawa M, et al. Analysis of hepatic vein waveform by Doppler ultrasonography in 100 patients with portal hypertension. *Am J Gastroenterol* 1994;89:170-175.

20. Dokmeci AK, Kimura K, Matsutani S, et al. Collateral veins in portal hypertension: Demonstration by sonography. *AJR Am J Roentgenol* 1981;137:1173-1177.

21. Subramanyam BR, Balthazar EJ, Madamba MR, et al. Sonography of porto-systemic collaterals in portal hypertension. *Radiology* 1983;146:161-166.

22. Juttner H-U, Jenney JM, Ralls PW, et al. Ultrasound demonstration of portosystemic collaterals in cirrhosis and portal hypertension. *Radiology* 1982;142:459-463.

23. Garcia-Tsao G. Current management of the complications of cirrhosis and portal hypertension: Variceal hemorrhage, ascites, and spontaneous bacterial peritonitis. *Gastroenterology* 2001;120:726-748.

24. D'Amico G, Pagliaro L, Bosch J. The treatment of portal hypertension: A meta-analytic review. *Hepatology* 1995;22:332-354.

25. de Franchis R. Evolving consensus in portal hypertension: Report of the Baveno IV Consensus Workshop on Methodology of Diagnosis and Therapy in Portal Hypertension. *J Hepatol* 2005;43:167-176.

26. Grace ND, Groszman RJ, Garcia-Tsao G, et al. Portal hypertension and variceal bleeding: An AASLD single topic symposium. *Hepatology* 1998;28:868-880.

27. Lafortune M, Marleau D, Breton D, et al. Portal venous system measurements in portal hypertension. *Radiology* 1984;151:27-30.

28. Saddekni S, Hutchinson DE, Cooperberg PL. The sonographically patent umbilical vein in portal hypertension. *Radiology* 1982;145:411-443.

29. Aagaard J, Jenson LI, Sorenson TIW, et al. Recanalized umbilical vein in portal hypertension. *AJR Am J Roentgenol* 1982;139:1107-1109.

30. Lafortune M, Constantin A, Breton G, et al. The recanalized umbilical vein in portal hypertension: A myth. *AJR Am J Roentgenol* 1985;144:549-553.

31. Roberts LR, Kamath PS. Pathophysiology and treatment of variceal hemorrhage. *Mayo Clin Proc* 1996;71:973-983.

32. Pagliaro L, D'Amico G, Sorensen TI, et al. Prevention of first bleeding in cirrhosis: A meta-analysis of randomized trials of non-surgical treatment. *Ann Intern Med* 1992;117:59-70.

33. Garcia-Tsao G. Portal hypertension. *Opin Gastroenterol* 2002;18:351-359.

34. Sanyal AJ. Role of transjugular intrahepatic portosystemic shunts in the treatment of variceal bleeding. In Chopra S, Bonis PAL (eds). *Cirrhosis*, 2008. Available at www.uptodate.com

35. Graham DY, Smith JL. The course of patients after variceal hemorrhage. *Gastroenterology* 1981;80:800.

36. Burroughs AK. The natural history of varices. *J Hepatol* 1993;17:S10.

37. Grace ND. Diagnosis and treatment of gastrointestinal bleeding secondary to portal hypertension. *Am J Gastroenterol* 1997;92:1081-1091.

38. Sanyal AJ, Freedman AM, Leuketic VA, et al. Transjugular intrahepatic portosystemic shunts for patients with active variceal hemorrhage unresponsive to sclerotherapy. *Gastroenterology* 1996;111:138-146.

39. Fidelman N, Kwan SW, LaBerge JM, et al. The transjugular intrahepatic portosystemic shunt: an update. *AJR Am J Roentgenol* 2012;199:746-755.

40. Middleton WD, Teefey SA, Darcy MD. Doppler evaluation of transjugular intrahepatic portosystemic shunts. *Ultrasound Q* 2003;19:56-70.

41. Darcy M. Minimally invasive therapy for portal hypertension. *Probl Gen Surg* 1999;16:28-43.

42. Coldwell DM, Ring EJ, Rees CR, et al. Multicenter investigation of the role of TIPS shunt in management of portal hypertension. *Radiology* 1995;196:335-340.

43. Ong JP, Sands M, Younossi ZM. Transjugular intrahepatic portosystemic shunts (TIPS): A decade later. *J Clin Gastroenterol* 2000;30:14-28.

44. Brown RS Jr, Lake JR. Transjugular intrahepatic portosystemic shunt as a form of treatment for portal hypertension: Indications and contraindications. *Adv Intern Med* 1997;42:485-504.

45. Kerlan RK Jr, LaBerge JM, Gordon RL, et al. Transjugular intrahepatic portosystemic shunts: Current status. *AJR Am J Roentgenol* 1995;164:1059-1066.

46. Rossle M, Siegerstetter V, Huber M, et al. The first decade of the transjugular intrahepatic portosystemic shunt (TIPS): State of the art. *Liver* 1998;18:73-89.

47. Freedman AM, Sanyal AJ, Tisnado J, et al. Complications of transjugular intrahepatic portosystemic shunt: A comprehensive review. *Radiographics* 1993;13:1185-1210.

48. Chalasani N, Clark WS, Martin LG, et al. Determinants of mortality in patients with advanced cirrhosis after transjugular intrahepatic portosystemic shunting. *Gastroenterology* 2000;118:138-144.

49. Ferral H, Vasan R, Speeg KV, et al. Evaluation of a model to predict poor survival in patients undergoing elective TIPS procedures. *J Vasc Interv Radiol* 2002;13:1103-1108.

50. Schepke M, Roth F, Flimmers R, et al. Comparison of MELD, Child-Pugh, and Emory model for the prediction of survival in patients undergoing transjugular intrahepatic portosystemic shunting. *Am J Gastroenterol* 2003;98:1167-1174.

51. Kamath PS, Wiesner RH, Malinchoc M, et al. A model to predict survival in patients with end stage liver disease. *Hepatology* 2001;33:464-470.

52. Cura M, Cura A, Suri R, et al. Causes of TIPS dysfunction. *AJR Am J Roentgenol* 2008;191:1751-1757.

53. Zhuang ZW, Teng GJ, Jeffrey RF, et al. Long-term results and quality of life in patients treated with transjugular intrahepatic portosystemic shunts. *AJR Am J Roentgenol* 2002;179:1597-1603.

54. Sterling KM, Darcy MD. Stenosis of transjugular intrahepatic portosystemic shunts: Presentation and management. *AJR Am J Roentgenol* 1997;168:239-244.

55. Vignali C, Bargellini I, Grosso M, et al. TIPS with expanded polytetrafluoroethylene-covered stent: Result of an Italian multicenter study. *AJR Am J Roentgenol* 2005;185:472-480.

56. Bureau C, Pagan JC, Layrargues GP, et al. Patency of stents covered with polytetrafluoroethylene in patients treated by transjugular intrahepatic portosystemic shunts: Long-term results of a randomized multicenter study. *Liver Int* 2007;27:742-747.

57. Rossi P, Salvatori FM, Fanelli F, et al. Polytetrafluoroethylene covered nitinoil stent-graft for transjugular intrahepatic portosystemic shunt creation: 3-year experience. *Radiology* 2004;231:820-830.

58. Dacry M. Evaluation and management of transjugular intrahepatic portosystemic shunts. *AJR Am J Roentgenol* 2012;199:730-736.

59. Carr CE, Tuite CM, Soulen MC, et al. Role of ultrasound surveillance of transjugular intrahepatic portosystemic shunts in the covered stent era. *J Vasc Interv Radiol* 2006;17:1297-1305.

60. Wachsberg RH. Doppler ultrasound evaluation of transjugular intrahepatic portosystemic shunt function: Pitfalls and artifacts. *Ultrasound Q* 2003;19:139-148.

61. Feldstein VA, Patel MD, LaBerge JM. TIPS shunts: Accuracy of Doppler US in determination of patency and detection of stenoses. *Radiology* 1996;201:141-147.

62. Foshager MC, Ferral H, Nazarian GK, et al. Duplex sonography after TIPS shunt: Normal hemodynamic findings and efficacy in predicting shunt patency and stenosis. *AJR Am J Roentgenol* 1995;165:1-7.

63. Kanterman RY, Darcy MD, Middleton WD, et al. Doppler sonographic findings associated with TIPS shunt malfunction. *AJR Am J Roentgenol* 1997;168:467-472.

64. Chong WK, Malisch TA, MAzer MJ, et al. TIPS shunt: Ultrasound assessment with maximum flow velocity. *Radiology* 1993;189:789-793.

65. Zizka J, Elias P, Krajina A, et al. Value of Doppler sonography in revealing transjugular intrahepatic portosystemic shunt malfunction: A 5 year experience in 216 patients. *AJR Am J Roentgenol* 2000;175:141-148.

66. Uggowitzer MM, Kugler C, Machan L, et al. Value of echo-enhanced Doppler sonography in evaluation of transjugular intrahepatic portosystemic shunts. *AJR Am J Roentgenol* 1998;170:1041-1046.

67. Zfurst G, Malms J, Heyer T, et al. Transjugular intrahepatic portosystemic shunts: Improved evaluation with echo-enhanced color Doppler sonography, power Doppler sonography, and spectral duplex sonography. *AJR Am J Roentgenol* 1998;170:1047-1054.

68. Tessler FN, Gehring BJ, Gomes AS, et al. Diagnosis of portal vein thrombosis: Value of color Doppler imaging. *AJR Am J Roentgenol* 1991;157:293-296.

69. Gansbeke FV, Avni EF, Delcour C, et al. Sonographic features of portal vein thrombosis. *AJR Am J Roentgenol* 1985;144:749-752.

70. De Gaetano AM, Lafortune M, Patriquin H, et al. Cavernous transformation of the portal vein: Patterns of intrahepatic and splanchnic collateral circulation detected with Doppler sonography. *AJR Am J Roentgenol* 1995;165:1151-1155.

71. Weltin G, Taylor KJW, Carter AR, et al. Duplex Doppler: Identification of cavernous transformation of the portal vein. *AJR Am J Roentgenol* 1985;144:999-1001.

72. Ferral H, Behrens G, Lopera J. Budd-Chiari Syndrome. *AJR Am J Roentgenol* 2012;199:737-745.

73. Menon NKV, Shah V, Kamath P. The Budd-Chiari syndrome. *N Engl J Med* 2004;350:578-585.

74. Chaubal N, Dighe M, Hanchate V, et al. Sonography in Budd-Chiari syndrome. *J Ultrasound Med* 2006;25:373-379.

VISCERAL VASCULAR

75. Valla DC. The diagnosis and management of the Budd-Chiari syndrome: Consensus and controversies. *Hepatology* 2003;38:793-803.
76. Hauser SC. Etiology of Budd-Chiari syndrome. In Chopra S, Bonis PAL (eds). Waltham: UpToDate, 2007. Available at www.uptodate.com
77. Bargallo X, Gilabert R, Nicolau C, et al. Sonography in Budd-Chiari syndrome. *AJR Am J Roentgenol* 2006;187:W33-W42.
78. Brancatelli G, Vilgrain V, Federle M, et al. Budd-Chiari syndrome: Spectrum of imaging findings. *AJR Am J Roentgenol* 2007;188:503.
79. Bolondi L, Gaiani S, Li Bassi S, et al. Diagnosis of the Budd-Chiari syndrome by pulsed Doppler ultrasound. *Gastroenterology* 1991;100:1324-1331.
80. Carreras E, Bertz H, Arcese W, et al. Incidence and outcome of hepatic veno-occlusive disease after blood or marrow transplantation: A prospective cohort study of the European Group for Blood and Marrow Transplantation. *Blood* 1998;92:3599.
81. Negrin RS, Bonis PAL. Pathogenesis and clinical features of hepatic–veno-occlusive disease following hematopoetic cell translation. In Chao NJ, Lardaw SA (eds). Waltham: UpToDate, 2006. Available at www.uptodate.com
82. McDonald GB, Sharma P, Matthews DE, et al. Veno-occlusive disease of the liver after bone marrow transplantation: Diagnosis, incidence and predisposing factors. *Hepatology* 1984;4:116.
83. McDonald GB, Hinds MS, Fisher LD. Veno-occlusive disease of the liver and multiorgan failure after bone marrow transplantation: A cohort study of 355 patients. *Ann Intern Med* 1993;118:255.
84. Carreras E, Granena A, Navasa M, et al. On the reliability of clinical criteria for the diagnosis of hepatic veno-occlusive disease. *Ann Hematol* 1993;66:77.
85. Herbetko J, Grigg AP, Buckley AR, et al. Veno-occlusive liver disease after bone marrow transplantation: Findings at duplex sonography. *AJR Am J Roentgenol* 1992;158:1001.
86. Teefey S, Brink JA, Borson RA, et al. Diagnosis of veno-occlusive disease of the liver after bone marrow transplantation: Value of duplex sonography. *AJR Am J Roentgenol* 1995;164:1397.
87. Sharafuddin MJ, Foshager MC, Steinbuch M, et al. Sonographic findings in bone marrow transplant patients with symptomatic hepatic veno-occlusive disease. *J Ultrasound Med* 1997;16:575.
88. Duerinckx AJ, Grant EG, Perrella RR, et al. The pulsatile portal vein in cases of congestive heart failure: Correlation of duplex Doppler findings with right atrial pressures. *Radiology* 1990;176:655-658.
89. Abu-Yousef MM, Milam SG, Farner RM. Pulsatile portal vein flow: A sign of tricuspid regurgitation on duplex Doppler sonography. *AJR Am J Roentgenol* 1990;155:785-788.
90. Bodner G, Siegfried P, Karner M, et al. Nontumorous vascular malformations in the liver. *J Ultrasound Med* 2002;21:187-197
91. Organ Procurement and Transplantation Network. http://optn.transplant. hrsa.gov/latestData/viewDataReports.asp (Accessed in 2013)
92. Mazzaferro V, Regalia E, Doci R, et al. Liver transplantation for the treatment of small hepatocellular carcinomas in patients with cirrhosis. *N Engl J Med* 1996;334:693-699.
93. O'Leary JG, Lepe R, Davis GL. Indications for liver transplantation. *Gastroenterology* 2008;134:1764-1776.
94. Crossin JD, Muradali D, Wilson SR. US of liver transplants: Normal and abnormal. *Radiographics* 2003;23:1093-1114.
95. Singh AK, Nachiappan AC, Verma HA, et al. Postoperative imaging in liver transplantation: What radiologists should know. *Radiographics* 2010;30:339-351.
96. Brody MB, Rodgers SK, Horrow MM. Spectrum of normal or near normal sonographic findings after orthotopic liver transplantation. *Ultrasound Q* 2008;24:257-265.
97. Propeck PA, Scanlan KA. Reversed or absent hepatic arterial diastolic flow in the liver transplants shown by duplex sonography: A poor predictor of subsequent hepatic artery thrombosis. *AJR Am J Roentgenol* 1992;152:1199-1201.
98. Hedegard WG, Wade C, Bhatt, S. Hepatic arterial waveforms on early post-transplant Doppler ultrasound. *Ultrasound Q* 2011;27:49-54.
99. Garcia-Criado A, Gilabert R, Salmeron JM, et al. Significance of and contributing factors for a high resistive index on Doppler sonography of the hepatic artery immediately after surgery: Prognostic implications for liver transplant recipients. *AJR Am J Roentgenol* 2003;181:831-838.
100. Garcia-Criado A, Gilabert R, Berzigotti A, et al. Doppler ultrasound findings in the hepatic artery shortly after liver transplantation. *AJR Am J Roentgenol* 2009;193:128-135.
101. Chen W, Facciuto ME, Rocca JP, et al. Doppler ultrasonographic findings of hepatic arterial vasospasm early after liver transplantation. *J Ultrasound Med* 2006;25:631-638.
102. Sanyal R, Lall CG, Lamba R, et al. Orthotopic liver transplantation: Reversible Doppler US findings in the immediate post-operative period. *Radiographics* 2012;32:199-211.
103. Hom BK, Shrestha R, Palmer, et al. Prospective evaluation of vascular complications after liver transplantation: Comparison of conventional and microbubble contrast-enhanced US. *Radiology* 2006;241:267-274.
104. Berry JD, Sidhu PS. Microbubble contrast enhanced ultrasound in liver transplantation. *Eur Radiol* 2004;14(Suppl 8):P96-P103.
105. Hom BK, Shrestha R, Palmer SL et al. Prospective evaluation of vascular complications after liver transplantation: Comparison of conventional and microbubble contrast-enhanced US. *Radiology* 2006;241:267-274.
106. Sidhu PS, Shaw AS, Ellis SM, et al. Microbubble ultrasound contrast in the assessment of hepatic artery patency following liver transplantation: Role in reducing frequency of hepatic artery angiography. *Eur Radiol* 2004;14:21-20.
107. Caiado AH, Blasbalg R, Marcelino AS, et al. Complications of liver transplantation: Multimodality imaging approach. *Radiographics* 2007;27:1401-1417.
108. Quiroga S, Sebastia C, Pallisa E, et al. Complications of orthotopic liver transplantation: Spectrum of findings with helical CT. *Radiographics* 2001;21:1085-1110.
109. Wozney P, Zajko AB, Bron KM, et al. Vascular complications after liver transplantation: A 5 year experience. *AJR Am J Roentgenol* 1986;147:657-663.
110. Strange BJ, Glanemann M, Nuessler NC, et al. Hepatic artery thrombosis after adult liver transplantation. *Liver Transplant* 2003;9:612-620.
111. Duffy JP, Hong JC, Famer DG, et al. Vascular complications of orthotopic liver transplantation: Experience in more than 4,200 patients. *J Am Coll Surg* 2009;208:896-905.
112. Bekker J, Ploem S, de Jong KP. Early hepatic artery thrombosis after liver transplantation: A systemic review of the incidence, outcomes and risk factors. *Am J Transplant* 2009;9:746-757.
113. Bhattacharjya S, Gunson BK, Mirza DF, et al. Delayed hepatic artery thrombosis in adult orthotopic liver transplantation—a 12-year experience. *Transplantation* 2001;71(11):1592-1596.
114. Langnas AN, Marujo W, Stratta RJ, et al. Vascular complications after orthotopic liver transplantation. *Am J Surg* 1991;161:76-82.
115. Berrocal T, Parron M, Alvarez-Luque A, et al. Pediatric liver transplantation: A pictorial essay of early and late complications. *Radiographics* 2006;26:1187-1209.
116. Flint EW, Sumkin JH, Zajko AB, et al. Duplex sonography of hepatic artery thrombosis after liver transplantation. *AJR Am J Roentgenol* 1998;151:481-483.
117. Sanchez-Bueno F, Robles R, Acosta F, et al. Hepatic artery complications after liver transplantation. *Clin Transplant* 1994;8:399-404.
118. Abbasoglu O, Levy MF, Vodapally MS, et al. Hepatic artery stenosis after liver transplantation-incidence, presentation, treatment, and long term outcome. *Transplantation* 1997;63:250-255.
119. Dodd GD, Memel D, Zajko A, et al. Hepatic artery stenosis and thrombosis in transplant recipients: Doppler diagnosis with resistive index and systolic acceleration time. *Radiology* 1994;192:657-661.
120. Friedwald SM, Molmenti E, DeJong MR, et al. Vascular and nonvascular complications of liver transplants: Sonographic evaluation and correlation with other imaging modalities and findings at surgery and pathology. *Ultrasound Q* 2003;19:71-85.
121. Park YS, Kim KW, Lee J, et al. Hepatic arterial stenosis assessed with Doppler US after liver transplantation: Frequent false-positive diagnoses with tardus parvus waveform and value of adding optimal peak systolic velocity cutoff. *Radiology* 2011;260:884-900.
122. Uzochukwu LN, Bluth EI, Smetherman DH. Early poster-operative hepatic sonography as a predictor of vascular and biliary complications in adult orthotopic liver transplant patients. *AJR Am J Roentgenol* 2005;185:1558-1570.
123. Settmacher U, Nussler NC, Glanemann M, et al. Venous complications after orthotopic liver transplantation. *Clin Transplant* 2000; 14: 235-241.
124. Kyoden Y, Tamura S, Sugawara Y, et al. Portal vein complications after adult-to-adult living donor liver transplantation. *Transplant Int* 2008;21:1136-1144.
125. Chong WK, Beland JC, Weeks SM. Sonographic evaluation of venous obstruction in liver transplants. *AJR Am J Roentgenol* 2007;188:515-521.
126. Huang TL, Cheng YF, Chen TY, et al. Doppler ultrasound evaluation of postoperative portal vein stenosis in adult living donor liver transplantation. *Transplant Proc* 2010;42:879-881.
127. Ko EY, Kim TK, Kim PN. Hepatic vein stenosis after living donor liver transplantation: Evaluation with Doppler US. *Radiology* 2003;229:806-810.
128. Rossi AR, Pozniak MA, Zarvan NP. Upper inferior vena caval anastomotic stenosis in liver transplant recipients: Doppler US diagnosis. *Radiology* 1993;187:387-389.
129. Marshall MM, Muiesan P, Srinivasan P, et al. Hepatic pseudoaneurysms following liver transplantation: Incidence, presenting figures and management. *Clin Radiol* 2001;56:579-587.

CHAPTER 23 ■ MESENTERIC ARTERIES

AARON C. BAKER

Evaluation of the mesenteric arteries is an important duplex application because it allows the noninvasive vascular laboratory to diagnose chronic mesenteric ischemia, a life-threatening disorder. Mesenteric duplex scanning can help prevent severe morbidity and mortality in these patients who often go undiagnosed for prolonged periods of time. The diagnosis of chronic mesenteric ischemia is difficult because the natural history is not well understood and the symptoms are often nonspecific. Prior to the validation of duplex ultrasound for evaluating the mesenteric arteries, the only way to confirm mesenteric artery stenosis in a patient with the clinical suspicion for chronic mesenteric ischemia was contrast arteriography. Nicholls et al from the University of Washington were among the first to report the use of ultrasound for the diagnosis of mesenteric artery disease in 1986.[1] These investigators described the hemodynamic characteristics of normal and abnormal mesenteric arteries based on Doppler velocity waveforms. In 1991, two large retrospective studies identified duplex flow velocities that allowed accurate identification of severe mesenteric artery stenosis.[2,3] Since then, the mesenteric duplex examination has been widely adopted, and several prospective studies have established the accuracy of the velocity thresholds.[4,5] Like renal duplex scanning (see Chapter 24), the mesenteric duplex examination entails a substantial learning curve for both the sonographer and the interpreting physician. However, when mastered, this is a valuable and rewarding study.

The goals of intervention for chronic mesenteric ischemia are to alleviate symptoms, restore normal body weight, and prevent bowel infarction. The number of mesenteric revascularizations has increased substantially over the last decade, largely because of improved diagnosis and the decreased morbidity associated with endovascular therapy. In most centers, mesenteric angioplasty and stenting is the first choice of treatment over open surgical revascularization in patients with chronic mesenteric ischemia who have suitable lesions.[6–8] While there are no prospective randomized comparisons between the two therapeutic approaches, retrospective reviews show decreased 30-day mortality, decreased perioperative morbidity, and shorter length of stay and convalescence time with endovascular revascularization compared to open surgery. However, open mesenteric bypass offers better patency, lower rates of reintervention, and improved freedom from recurrent symptoms.[6,8–18]

INDICATIONS FOR MESENTERIC ARTERY SCANNING

Mesenteric duplex scanning is an excellent screening test for patients with symptoms of chronic mesenteric ischemia. The most common cause of chronic mesenteric ischemia is atherosclerotic disease, and the majority of patients will have a history of smoking, hypertension, and hyperlipidemia; however, nonatherosclerotic conditions including vasculitis, dissection, fibromuscular dysplasia, radiation arteritis, mesenteric venous occlusion, drug-induced arteriopathy, and midaortic syndrome can present with a similar clinical picture. Classic signs and symptoms include abdominal pain, weight loss, and "food fear." Typically, the pain is mid abdominal and dull or crampy, and it begins within 30 minutes after meals and can last for as long as six hours. Some patients learn to avoid certain foods or complain of nausea, vomiting, or a change in bowel habits, all without postprandial onset.

Although it may be argued that patients with the textbook presentation of postprandial pain, weight loss, and "food fear" should proceed directly to diagnostic angiography, duplex scanning is an appropriate starting point for patients with less classic presentations. Most patients with symptomatic chronic mesenteric ischemia are found to have severe stenosis or occlusion in multiple mesenteric arteries. The role of duplex scanning in the evaluation of suspected acute mesenteric ischemia is much more limited because those patients are usually critically ill and are difficult to examine with ultrasound.

Mesenteric duplex scanning is being used for follow-up after endovascular interventions, including superior mesenteric artery (SMA) and celiac artery stents.[19–22] Given that these stents are prone to restenosis, duplex scanning is an ideal surveillance method. While a few retrospective studies have shown that the velocity thresholds used to diagnose native mesenteric artery stenosis overestimate the severity of stenosis in stented mesenteric arteries, there are currently no standard duplex criteria for the detection of mesenteric in-stent restenosis.[19–21]

Duplex ultrasound has also been used in diagnosing median arcuate ligament syndrome. While the pathophysiology and clinical significance of median arcuate ligament syndrome are controversial, mesenteric duplex can be a useful adjunct in determining the presence of this condition. An elevated peak systolic velocity (PSV) in the celiac artery during expiration, which normalizes with deep inspiration, is typically found; however, this respiratory variation can be a normal physiologic finding in healthy, asymptomatic patients.[23] There are currently no duplex ultrasound findings that have been validated for the diagnosis of median arcuate compression of the visceral arteries. Ultimately, the diagnosis and decision to intervene are made in combination with the clinical history, physical examination, and additional imaging studies. Finally, duplex scanning may be used for the evaluation of portal, mesenteric, and hepatic venous disorders (see Chapter 22).

VISCERAL VASCULAR

DUPLEX TECHNIQUE

It is important to perform the mesenteric duplex examination after the patient has fasted overnight, or for at least 4 hours prior to the examination, because the SMA velocity waveform changes from a low-flow, high-resistance pattern to a high-flow, low-resistance pattern after eating. Velocity thresholds for identifying significant stenosis of the celiac artery and SMA have been established for patients in the fasting state, so application of these standard criteria requires that the examination be performed in fasting patients. Typically, the patient should be instructed not to eat or drink anything starting at midnight and schedule the duplex scan early the next day to minimize abdominal gas. Regular medications can be taken with a few sips of water. Diabetic patients are instructed to consult with their primary care provider to alter insulin or other medications appropriately, and all patients are asked to refrain from smoking or chewing gum on the morning of the examination.

The mesenteric duplex examination is performed with the patient supine. A slight reverse Trendelenburg (feet down) position or head elevation may be helpful. Alternatively, a lateral decubitus position may be used in patients with large abdominal girth or when bowel gas interference is encountered with the patient supine. Low-frequency transducers are required, with the exact frequency range determined by the body habitus of the patient.

The scan head is initially placed just below the xiphoid process and slightly to the left of the midline for identification of the most proximal abdominal aorta. B-mode is used initially, scanning transversely through the length of the abdominal aorta for determining maximum size and presence of plaque to the level of the bifurcation. The aorta, celiac artery, common hepatic artery, and SMA should be interrogated thoroughly by pulsed Doppler, and spectral waveforms should be recorded from these vessels. This will require a combination of sagittal and transverse views. The Doppler sample volume should be "walked" from the aorta into the origins of the celiac artery and the SMA to identify the highest PSV and end-diastolic velocity (EDV). Attempts should be made to identify and assess the inferior mesenteric artery (IMA), particularly if significant occlusive disease is found in the celiac artery or SMA.

The celiac artery arises from the anterior aspect of the aorta 1 to 2 cm below the diaphragm and is usually best imaged in a transverse plane, showing its origin and bifurcation into the common hepatic artery (going toward the liver on the patient's right) and the splenic artery (going toward the spleen on the patient's left). This view is often referred to as the "seagull sign" and allows for accurate flow velocity measurements at the origin of the celiac artery utilizing a relatively small or zero degree Doppler angle (Fig. 23.1). The normal Doppler waveform from the celiac artery has a low-resistance pattern with antegrade flow continuing throughout systole and diastole. This Doppler waveform morphology occurs because the celiac artery supplies two low-resistance solid organs—the liver and spleen (Fig. 23.2).

Careful attention to Doppler angle correction for velocity measurements is necessary because these vessels may be tortuous. Close attention should also be given to the Doppler pulse repetition frequency (PRF) and the orientation of the color-scale bar. The colors on the top half of the scale are assigned to flow coming toward the scan head, and the colors on the bottom half represent flow away from the scan head. Flow direction becomes especially important when the celiac artery is occluded or severely stenotic. In this situation, low pressure in the celiac artery induces SMA collaterals to divert blood toward the liver and spleen through the gastroduodenal artery (GDA). The GDA backfills the common hepatic artery such that retrograde flow in the common hepatic artery crosses the celiac artery origin to perfuse the splenic artery (Fig. 23.3). The finding of retrograde flow direction in the common hepatic artery is always associated with severe celiac artery stenosis or occlusion. Additionally, poststenotic turbulence in the splenic and hepatic arteries can be indirect signs of a celiac artery stenosis.

The SMA typically originates from the anterior surface of the aorta 1 to 2 cm below the celiac artery. It is best visualized in a sagittal plane as it courses parallel to the aorta with the left renal vein running between the SMA and aorta. The normal fasting SMA Doppler spectral waveform is triphasic (high resistance) with a brief phase of reversed flow followed by little or no flow in the second half of the cardiac cycle, similar to the pattern found in the major upper and lower extremity arteries (Fig. 23.4). The SMA should be scanned as far distally as possible, obtaining Doppler spectral waveforms from the proximal, middle, and distal segments.

The IMA is most easily identified in a transverse view by locating the aortic bifurcation and then scanning proximally up the distal abdominal aorta for 1 to 2 cm. The IMA usually originates from the aorta slightly to the left of the anterior midline (i.e., the 1 or 2 o'clock position on a transverse image) (Fig. 23.5). Normal Doppler spectral waveforms from the IMA resemble those from the fasting SMA with a high-resistance pattern.

FIGURE 23.1. Color flow image in transverse view of the origin of the celiac artery from the aorta. The "seagull sign" is formed by the celiac artery bifurcation into the common hepatic and splenic arteries. The blue color in the splenic artery is caused by flow away from the transducer relative to the ultrasound scan lines.

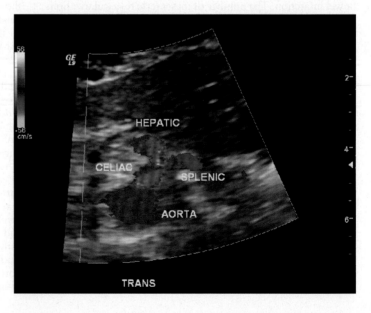

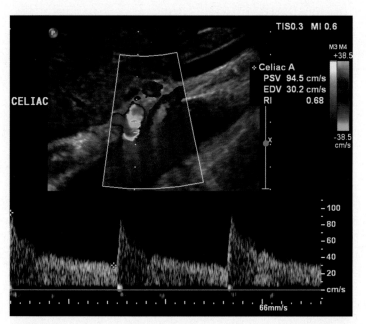

FIGURE 23.2. Color flow image and Doppler spectral waveform from a normal celiac artery. The flow pattern is typical of a low-resistance vascular bed, with forward flow throughout the cardiac cycle. Peak systolic velocity (PSV) is 94 cm/s and end-diastolic velocity (EDV) is 30 cm/s.

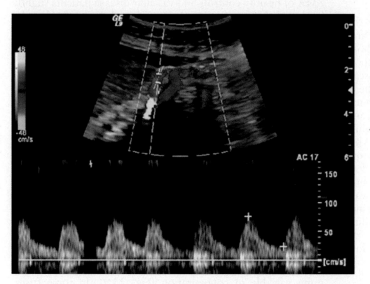

FIGURE 23.3. Color flow image and Doppler spectral waveform illustrating the importance of color scale and pulse repetition frequency (PRF). The pulsed Doppler sample volume is positioned in the common hepatic artery, and both the spectral waveform and the color flow image (*red*) indicate flow toward the scan head. This represents retrograde collateral flow in the common hepatic artery, crossing the celiac bifurcation and providing antegrade flow in the splenic artery away from the scan head (*blue*).

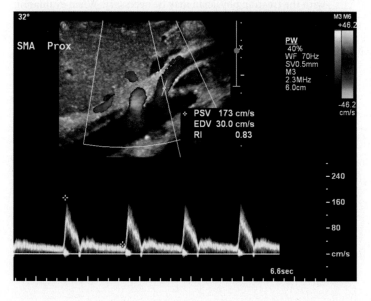

FIGURE 23.4. Color flow image and Doppler spectral waveform from a normal superior mesenteric artery (SMA) showing a high-resistance triphasic flow pattern in a fasting patient. The color flow image shows the origin and proximal segment of the SMA in sagittal view. Note placement of the angle cursor for Doppler angle correction along the curve near the vessel origin. Peak systolic velocity (PSV) is 173 cm/s and end-diastolic velocity (EDV) is 30 cm/s.

FIGURE 23.5. Transverse color flow image of a normal inferior mesenteric artery (IMA) originating from the distal aorta slightly to the left of the anterior midline at about the 1 o'clock position. The spectral waveform shows a high-resistance (triphasic) flow pattern with a peak systolic velocity of 223 cm/s.

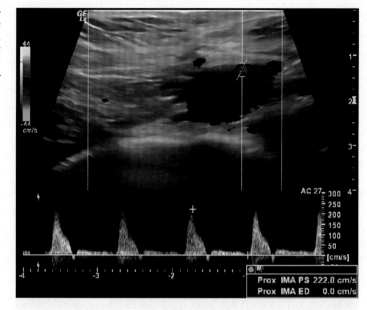

Scanning Tips

Attempts should be made to visualize the origins of both the celiac artery and the SMA in the same duplex image to confirm correct identification of these vessels, particularly when both arteries have elevated velocities and abnormal Doppler spectral waveforms (Fig. 23.6). This may require rotating the scan head slightly or moving laterally and angling the scan head back toward the midline. As with the renal duplex examination, there is movement of these arteries with respiration, and asking the patient to suspend breathing momentarily while recording Doppler waveforms can be very helpful. It is possible for the Doppler sample volume to inadvertently slip from one artery to the other, and keeping these vessels as still as possible helps avoid errors. If there is air in the epigastrium, light pressure with the scan head can push it out of the way. When midline scars from abdominal surgery cause shadowing, moving the scan head laterally and angling toward the midline may help with visualization.

Measurement of both fasting and postprandial blood flow velocities is not necessary to identify hemodynamically significant SMA stenosis, and a postprandial evaluation adds little information to the fasting duplex examination.[24,25] Comparison of fasting and postprandial duplex ultrasound

velocities with angiographic stenosis measurements in the SMA of healthy controls and vascular disease patients slightly increased the specificity and positive predictive value but did not improve overall accuracy.[24] However, it has been shown that PSV and EDV increase following a meal in the SMA but not in the celiac artery, reaching a maximum around 45 minutes after eating, with the EDV showing the largest proportional increase (Fig. 23.7).[25] Ingestion of water alone does not result in an increase in the SMA velocity parameters.

When scanning patients with possible median arcuate ligament compression syndrome, representative Doppler spectral waveforms should be obtained from the celiac artery and SMA during deep inspiration and compared with waveforms obtained during complete expiration and normal respiration (Fig. 23.8). Transient compression of the celiac artery origin by the median arcuate ligament of the diaphragm is apparent during expiration but resolves with descent of the diaphragm during inspiration.

For mesenteric bypass grafts and stented mesenteric arteries, it is important to know the locations of the proximal and distal anastomoses or the sites of stent placement before attempting to perform the scan, as these reconstructions are quite variable in configuration (Fig. 23.9). In some cases, review of the procedure based on operative notes or discussion with the treating physician may be necessary. When evaluating

FIGURE 23.6. Color flow image showing the origins of both the celiac artery and the superior mesenteric artery (SMA) from the aorta in a sagittal view.

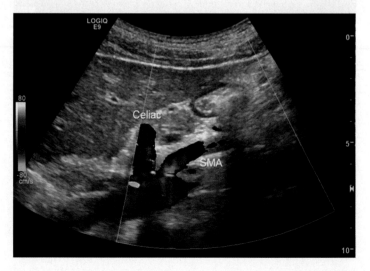

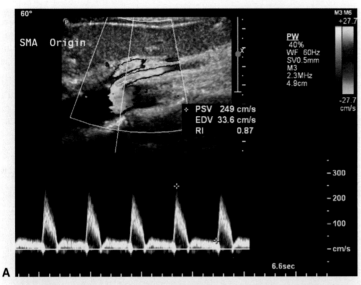

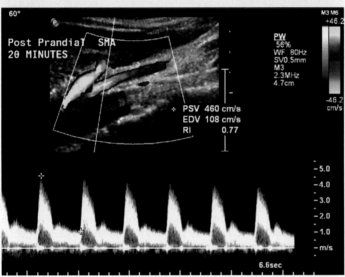

FIGURE 23.7. Fasting and postprandial flow velocities in a normal superior mesenteric artery (SMA). *A*, Color flow image and Doppler spectral waveform in the fasting state with peak systolic velocity (PSV) of 249 cm/s and end-diastolic velocity (EDV) of 34 cm/s. *B*, Repeat evaluation 20 minutes after eating shows PSV of 460 cm/s and EDV of 108 cm/s.

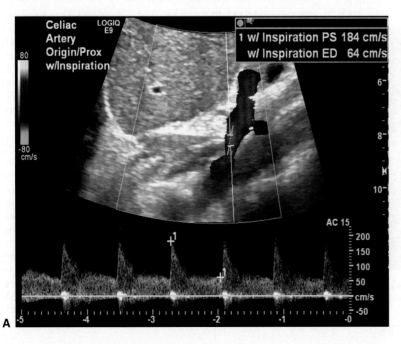

FIGURE 23.8. Color flow images and Doppler spectral waveforms from the celiac artery during inspiration (*A*) and expiration (*B*) illustrate the findings with median arcuate ligament compression. Note the change in peak systolic velocity (PSV) from 184 (inspiration) to 258 cm/s (expiration) and end-diastolic velocity (EDV) from 64 (inspiration) to 138 cm/s (expiration). These changes are due to compression of the celiac artery by the median arcuate ligament during expiration that resolves with inspiration. The color flow images also show some "straightening" of the proximal celiac artery during inspiration. (*Continued*)

FIGURE 23.8. (*Continued*)

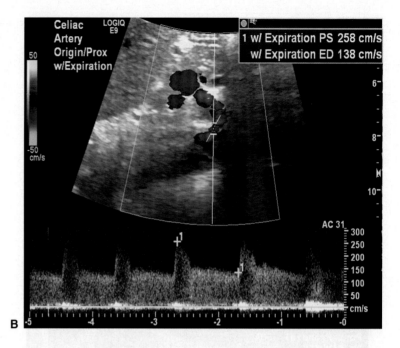

bypassed or stented mesenteric arteries, representative B-mode images and Doppler spectral waveforms with velocity measurements should be recorded at the proximal, mid, and distal sites. The inflow and outflow arteries must be included along with Doppler spectral waveforms throughout the stent or graft. The Doppler sample volume should be "walked" through the proximal anastomosis, the body of the graft, the distal anastomosis, and into the outflow artery (Figs. 23.10 to 23.12).

Anatomic Considerations

Anomalous mesenteric artery anatomy has been reported in approximately 20% of the general population, and this can increase the complexity of a mesenteric duplex examination substantially. Awareness of the possible anomalies facilitates recognition of unusual ultrasound findings. A right hepatic artery originating from the SMA rather than the common

hepatic (replaced right hepatic artery) is the most common anomaly, with a prevalence of approximately 17%. This finding should be suspected when a low-resistance flow pattern (flow throughout diastole) is found in an otherwise normal proximal SMA. Occasionally, a replaced right hepatic artery may be identified by duplex arising from the SMA and arching back toward the liver. Other important mesenteric artery anomalies include the common hepatic artery originating from the SMA (2% to 3%), the common hepatic artery originating from the aorta (1% to 2%), and a common origin of the celiac artery and SMA (celiacomesenteric artery) from the aorta (<1%). The IMA is the smallest of the mesenteric arteries and typically becomes relevant only in advanced cases of chronic mesenteric ischemia when it provides collateral flow into the SMA territory through a meandering mesenteric artery.

CRITERIA FOR INTERPRETATION

The normal SMA Doppler spectral waveform has a sharp systolic upstroke with a narrow band of frequencies or velocities (clear systolic window). As noted previously, the normal SMA flow pattern reflects a high-resistance outflow bed in the fasting state. This typically includes a brief reverse flow phase at the end of systole and little or no forward flow at the end of each cardiac cycle. The PSV in the normal SMA is usually less than 125 cm/s. Diagnostic velocity data focusing on PSV criteria were determined retrospectively and then tested prospectively, as reported by Moneta et al.[3,4] In their validation study, these authors found excellent accuracy for diagnosis of a 70% or greater angiographic stenosis in the SMA by using a threshold PSV of 275 cm/s or higher, with 92% sensitivity and 96% specificity. In parallel studies, the Dartmouth group focused on EDV for diagnosis of a 50% or greater angiographic SMA stenosis. These values were also established by retrospective analysis then tested prospectively.[2,5] An EDV of 45 cm/s or greater in the SMA resulted in 90% sensitivity and 91% specificity.[5]

Doppler waveforms recorded from the normal celiac artery also demonstrate a sharp systolic upstroke and PSV less than 125 cm/s, but with a low-resistance flow pattern characterized by forward flow throughout the cardiac cycle. The PSV criterion reported by Moneta et al for 70% or greater angiographic celiac artery stenosis is 200 cm/s or higher, a lower

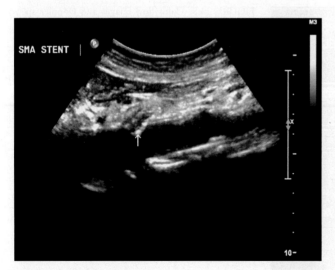

FIGURE 23.9. B-mode image of a stent in the superior mesenteric artery (SMA). In this sagittal plane view, the proximal end of the stent is protruding slightly into the adjacent aorta (*arrow*).

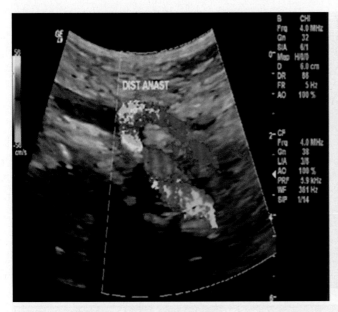
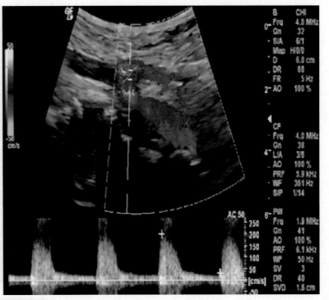

FIGURE 23.10. Duplex images of a retrograde external iliac artery to superior mesenteric artery (SMA) bypass graft. *Left*, color flow image shows a patent bypass graft with the distal anastomosis to the SMA. *Right*, Doppler spectral waveform at the distal anastomosis shows a high-resistance flow pattern.

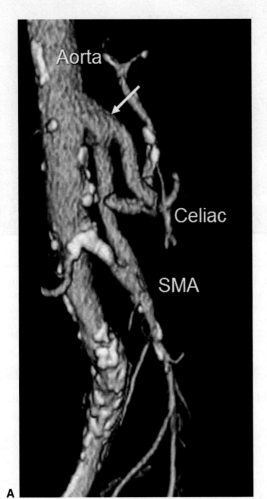

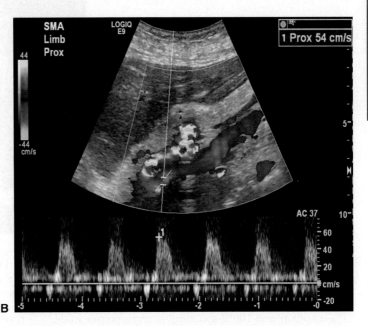

FIGURE 23.11. *A*, 3D rendering from a CT angiogram showing an antegrade bypass graft from the supraceliac aorta to the celiac artery and superior mesenteric artery (SMA). The main body of the bifurcated graft is indicated by the *arrow*. *B*, Duplex image of the bypass graft with the pulsed Doppler sample volume positioned in the SMA limb and a peak systolic velocity of 54 cm/s.

FIGURE 23.12. *A,* B-mode image of the celiac limb of the antegrade aorta to celiac and superior mesenteric artery bypass graft (BPG) shown in Figure 23.11. *B,* Color flow image and Doppler spectral waveform of the celiac limb showing a low-resistance flow pattern with a peak systolic velocity of 87 cm/s.

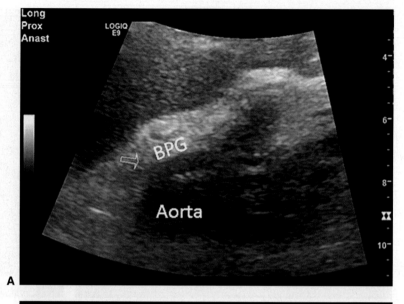

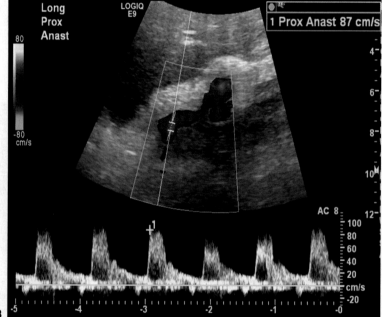

threshold than that determined for the SMA.[4] When tested prospectively, this threshold demonstrated a sensitivity of 87% and a specificity of 80%. The Dartmouth criterion for celiac artery stenosis is an EDV of 55 cm/s or greater, with 93% sensitivity and 100% specificity in a prospective study.[5] These criteria are summarized in Table 23.1.

Doppler evaluation of the IMA has received little attention in the duplex literature, but AbuRahma et al reported a greater than 50% angiographic stenosis of the IMA with a peak systolic velocity of greater than 250 cm/s.[26] This retrospective review showed a sensitivity of 90%, specificity of 96%, and overall accuracy of 95% for the 250 cm/s threshold. An IMA

TABLE 23.1

SUMMARY OF VELOCITY THRESHOLDS FOR DIAGNOSIS OF CELIAC ARTERY AND SUPERIOR MESENTERIC ARTERY STENOSIS BY DUPLEX SCANNING

■ AUTHOR	■ ARTERY	■ % STENOSIS	■ PSV (cm/s)	■ EDV (cm/s)	■ SENSITIVITY (%)	■ SPECIFICITY (%)
Moneta[3,4]	Celiac	≥70	≥200		87	80
	SMA	≥70	≥275		92	96
Zwolak[2,5]	Celiac	≥50		≥55	93	100
	SMA	≥50		≥45	90	91

EDV, end-diastolic velocity; PSV, peak systolic velocity; SMA, superior mesenteric artery.

PSV to aortic PSV ratio of >4.0 had an overall accuracy of 93%. No prospective validation of duplex criteria for the IMA has been reported to date.

Interpretation Tips

Elevated velocities may be observed in a normal mesenteric artery when compensatory flow through collaterals occurs in response to a critical stenosis or occlusion of a companion visceral artery. This is particularly common in the mesenteric circulation due to the abundant collateral pathways that often develop when there is occlusive disease in the celiac artery, SMA, or IMA. Van Petersen et al confirmed this finding in a retrospective review of 228 patients with chronic mesenteric ischemia.[27] Overall, the presence of a celiac artery stenosis and visceral collaterals resulted in a significantly higher PSV in a normal SMA without stenosis, and vice versa with a SMA stenosis and normal celiac artery. Thus, stenosis in one mesenteric artery and the resulting collateral flow may lead to overestimation of stenosis in another mesenteric artery.

To differentiate a velocity elevation related to a stenosis from compensatory flow in a widely patent artery, sequential Doppler velocity measurements are helpful. A stenosis typically produces a focal flow disturbance with a high-velocity jet and poststenotic spectral broadening. Compensatory flow usually demonstrates minimal spectral broadening and diffusely elevated velocities throughout the imaged artery.

DUPLEX OF STENTED VISCERAL ARTERIES

A few retrospective studies have provided evidence that the duplex velocity criteria for stenosis in a native SMA will overestimate the severity of stenosis after the vessel has undergone stent placement. However, these retrospective studies have been unable to establish definite criteria for determining mesenteric in-stent restenosis. Mitchell et al from the Oregon Health and Science University followed 35 patients who underwent SMA stent placement for presumed mesenteric ischemia.[20] Angiographic SMA stenosis of 70% or more was documented

in 91% of these patients at the time of treatment. Poststent residual stenosis was less than 30% by completion angiography in all patients, and for the 22 patients who underwent SMA pressure gradient measurements pre- and poststent, there was a significant reduction in the gradient. Despite confirmation of improvement by these anatomic and physiologic measures, early poststent duplex scanning in 13 patients revealed SMA PSV ranging from 279 cm/s to 416 cm/s, with a mean posttreatment SMA PSV of 336 cm/s (Fig. 23.13).

Additional studies have been performed by Baker et al and AbuRahma et al.[19,21] Both of these reports confirmed that the PSV in a successfully stented SMA often remains higher than the native SMA 70% stenosis threshold of 275 cm/s. Baker et al evaluated 24 patients who underwent 31 SMA stenting procedures for chronic mesenteric ischemia with a mean follow-up period of 14 months.[19] In patients who did not undergo reintervention, the PSV of the stented SMA did not significantly change in comparison to a baseline poststenting PSV. In patients who did require a reintervention for in-stent restenosis, the PSV either doubled from the initial poststenting baseline PSV or approached 500 cm/s. AbuRahma et al retrospectively reviewed 43 patients with 62 stents (32 SMA and 30 celiac artery) who had postintervention duplex scans and angiograms confirming in-stent restenosis.[21] A receiver operating characteristic (ROC) analysis was then used to determine optimal duplex velocity criteria for detecting ≥50% and ≥70% in-stent restenosis. The optimal PSV for ≥50% celiac artery restenosis was 274 cm/s (sensitivity 96%, specificity 86%, accuracy 93%) versus 240 cm/s for ≥50% native celiac artery stenosis. The PSV for ≥70% celiac artery restenosis was 363 cm/s (sensitivity 88%, specificity 92%, accuracy 90%) versus 320 cm/s for ≥70% native celiac artery stenosis. When evaluating stents in the SMA, the optimal PSV for detecting ≥50% SMA restenosis was 325 cm/s (sensitivity 89%, specificity 100%, accuracy 91%) versus 295 cm/s for ≥50% native SMA stenosis. The threshold for detecting ≥70% SMA restenosis was 412 cm/s (sensitivity 100%, specificity 100%, accuracy 97%) versus 400 cm/s for native SMA stenosis.

Until duplex ultrasound criteria for stented mesenteric arteries are standardized, an early postintervention duplex ultrasound should be obtained to serve as a baseline for comparison with future surveillance examinations. These serial scans will facilitate the detection of progressively increasing velocities and allow for detection of developing in-stent restenosis.

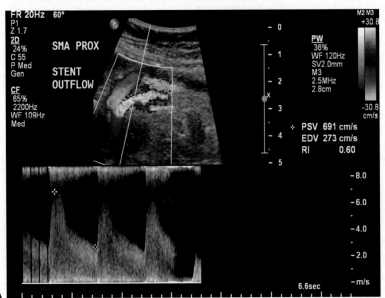

A

FIGURE 23.13. Duplex images of superior mesenteric artery (SMA) stents. *A,* This color flow image and Doppler spectral waveform show a markedly elevated in-stent peak systolic velocity (PSV) of 691 cm/s, consistent with an in-stent restenosis. (*Continued*)

FIGURE 23.13. (*Continued*) *B,* This stented SMA has a PSV of 343 cm/s without any significant restenosis. Note that this in-stent PSV is higher than the native SMA velocity threshold for greater than 70% stenosis.

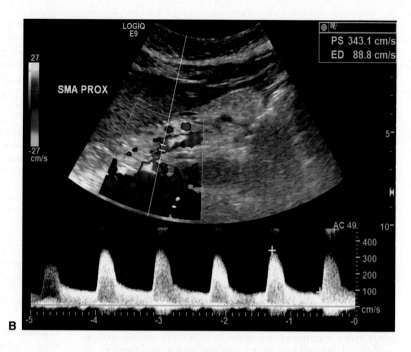

ACKNOWLEDGMENT

This chapter is based in part on Chapter 22 from the 4th edition by Robert M. Zwolak and Anne Musson.

References

1. Nicholls SC, Kohler TR, Martin RL, et al. Use of hemodynamic parameters in the diagnosis of mesenteric insufficiency. *J Vasc Surg* 1986;3:507-510.
2. Bowersox JC, Zwolak RM, Walsh DB, et al. Duplex ultrasonography in the diagnosis of celiac and mesenteric artery occlusive disease. *J Vasc Surg* 1991;14:780-786; discussion 6-8.
3. Moneta GL, Yeager RA, Dalman R, et al. Duplex ultrasound criteria for diagnosis of splanchnic artery stenosis or occlusion. *J Vasc Surg* 1991;14:511-518; discussion 8-20.
4. Moneta GL, Lee RW, Yeager RA, et al. Mesenteric duplex scanning: A blinded prospective study. *J Vasc Surg* 1993;17:79-84; discussion 5-6.
5. Zwolak RM, Fillinger MF, Walsh DB, et al. Mesenteric and celiac duplex scanning: A validation study. *J Vasc Surg* 1998;27:1078-1087; discussion 88.
6. Oderich GS, Bower TC, Sullivan TM, et al. Open versus endovascular revascularization for chronic mesenteric ischemia: Risk-stratified outcomes. *J Vasc Surg* 2009;49:1472-1479.e3.
7. Oderich GS, Gloviczki P, Bower TC. Open surgical treatment for chronic mesenteric ischemia in the endovascular era: When it is necessary and what is the preferred technique? *Semin Vasc Surg* 2010;23:36-46.
8. Schermerhorn ML, Giles KA, Hamdan AD, et al. Mesenteric revascularization: Management and outcomes in the United States, 1988–2006. *J Vasc Surg* 2009;50:341-348.e1.
9. van Petersen AS, Kolkman JJ, Beuk RJ, et al. Open or percutaneous revascularization for chronic splanchnic syndrome. *J Vasc Surg* 2010;51:1309-1316.
10. Aburahma AF, Campbell JE, Stone PA, et al. Perioperative and late clinical outcomes of percutaneous transluminal stentings of the celiac and superior mesenteric arteries over the past decade. *J Vasc Surg* 2013;57:1052-1061.
11. Tallarita T, Oderich GS, Gloviczki P, et al. Patient survival after open and endovascular mesenteric revascularization for chronic mesenteric ischemia. *J Vasc Surg* 2013;57:747-755; discussion 54-55.
12. Tallarita T, Oderich GS, Macedo TA, et al. Reinterventions for stent restenosis in patients treated for atherosclerotic mesenteric artery disease. *J Vasc Surg* 2011;54:1422-1429.e1.
13. Atkins MD, Kwolek CJ, LaMuraglia GM, et al. Surgical revascularization versus endovascular therapy for chronic mesenteric ischemia: A comparative experience. *J Vasc Surg* 2007;45:1162-1171.
14. Kasirajan K, O'Hara PJ, Gray BH, et al. Chronic mesenteric ischemia: Open surgery versus percutaneous angioplasty and stenting. *J Vasc Surg* 2001;33:63-71.
15. Oderich GS, Malgor RD, Ricotta JJ II. Open and endovascular revascularization for chronic mesenteric ischemia: Tabular review of the literature. *Ann Vasc Surg* 2009;23:700-712.
16. Rawat N, Gibbons CP. Surgical or endovascular treatment for chronic mesenteric ischemia: A multicenter study. *Ann Vasc Surg* 2010;24:935-945.
17. Sivamurthy N, Rhodes JM, Lee D, et al. Endovascular versus open mesenteric revascularization: Immediate benefits do not equate with short-term functional outcomes. *J Am Coll Surg* 2006;202:859-867.
18. Pecoraro F, Rancic Z, Lachat M, et al. Chronic mesenteric ischemia: Critical review and guidelines for management. *Ann Vasc Surg* 2013;27:113-122.
19. Baker AC, Chew V, Li CS, et al. Application of duplex ultrasound imaging in determining in-stent stenosis during surveillance after mesenteric artery revascularization. *J Vasc Surg* 2012;56:1364-1371; discussion 71.
20. Mitchell EL, Chang EY, Landry GJ, et al. Duplex criteria for native superior mesenteric artery stenosis overestimate stenosis in stented superior mesenteric arteries. *J Vasc Surg* 2009;50:335-340.
21. Aburahma AF, Mousa AY, Stone PA, et al. Duplex velocity criteria for native celiac/superior mesenteric artery stenosis vs in-stent stenosis. *J Vasc Surg* 2012;55:730-738.
22. AbuRahma AF, Stone PA, Srivastava M, et al. Mesenteric/celiac duplex ultrasound interpretation criteria revisited. *J Vasc Surg* 2012;55:428-436 e6; discussion 35-36.
23. Gruber H, Loizides A, Peer S, et al. Ultrasound of the median arcuate ligament syndrome: A new approach to diagnosis. *Med Ultrason* 2012;14:5-9.
24. Gentile AT, Moneta GL, Lee RW, et al. Usefulness of fasting and postprandial duplex ultrasound examinations for predicting high-grade superior mesenteric artery stenosis. *Am J Surg* 1995;169:476-479.
25. Moneta GL, Taylor DC, Helton WS, et al. Duplex ultrasound measurement of post-prandial intestinal blood flow: Effect of meal composition. *Gastroenterology* 1988;95:1294-1301.
26. AbuRahma AF, Scott Dean L. Duplex ultrasound interpretation criteria for inferior mesenteric arteries. *Vascular* 2012;20:145-149.
27. van Petersen AS, Kolkman JJ, Meerwaldt R, et al. Mesenteric stenosis, collaterals, and compensatory blood flow. *J Vasc Surg* 2014;60:111-119, 9 e1-e2.

CHAPTER 24 ■ RENAL DUPLEX SCANNING

R. EUGENE ZIERLER AND KARI A. CAMPBELL

VISCERAL VASCULAR

Like the other major branches of the aorta, the renal arteries can develop both occlusive and aneurysmal disease. The processes responsible for renal artery pathology include atherosclerosis, fibromuscular dysplasia (FMD), thromboembolism, dissection, and arteritis. The principal lesions associated with renal artery stenosis are atherosclerosis and FMD. Atherosclerosis is by far the most common cause of renovascular disease, accounting for approximately 90% of cases. These lesions are typically located at the origins or in the proximal segments of the renal arteries and are found in patients older than 50 years with significant aortoiliac or lower extremity atherosclerotic occlusive disease (Fig. 24.1). In a study of 395 patients undergoing routine arteriography for peripheral arterial disease, a renal artery stenosis of more than 50% diameter reduction was found in 38% with abdominal aortic aneurysms, 33% with aortoiliac occlusive disease, and 39% with lower extremity occlusive disease.[1] FMD is usually found in patients younger than age 40 and affects the middle or distal segments of the renal arteries with a characteristic "string-of-beads" appearance (Fig. 24.2).

Occlusive disease of the renal arteries may result in hypertension or ischemic nephropathy. Hypertension affects about 50 million individuals in the United States, and the proportion with a renovascular etiology is in the range of 1% to 6%.[2,3] However, the prevalence of renovascular hypertension in patients with severe hypertension (diastolic blood pressure >105 mm Hg) may be as high as 30% to 40%.[4] Ischemic nephropathy can be defined as a progressive decline in renal function secondary to global renal ischemia. It has been estimated that 60,000 to 120,000 patients in the United States have azotemia on this basis, and ischemic nephropathy may account for 5% to 15% of the patients who develop end-stage renal disease each year and require renal replacement therapy.[5,6]

Because many patients are found to have unilateral or bilateral renal artery stenosis without severe hypertension or renal insufficiency, it is clear that not all renal artery lesions are physiologically or clinically significant. Therefore, diagnostic tests must address both the anatomy and the physiology of renovascular disease.

DIAGNOSTIC EVALUATION FOR RENOVASCULAR DISEASE

The purpose of diagnostic testing in patients with suspected renal artery stenosis is to identify those individuals most likely to benefit from renal artery interventions for management of hypertension or renal insufficiency. Severe hypertension occurring in children or young adults is particularly likely to be renovascular in origin, although the etiology in these cases would be nonatherosclerotic. Other general features that suggest the presence of renovascular hypertension rather than essential hypertension are sudden onset of hypertension, an abdominal bruit, resistance to standard antihypertensive therapy with multiple medications, an atrophic kidney or size discrepancy between the two kidneys, flash pulmonary edema, and acute azotemia during treatment with angiotensin-converting enzyme inhibitors or angiotensin receptor blockers. Although these features can be used to increase the positive yield of screening tests, they do not have sufficient discriminative value to exclude patients from further diagnostic evaluation. Therefore, the principal criterion for renal artery disease screening remains the severity of hypertension, particularly the diastolic component.

Establishing a diagnosis of renovascular hypertension or ischemic nephropathy is especially complicated because these conditions involve physiologic as well as anatomic abnormalities. Historically, a variety of screening tests have been used for this purpose. Peripheral plasma renin assays, rapid-sequence intravenous pyelography, and isotope renography have all been tried, but they lack sufficient sensitivity to serve as reliable screening tests.[7] Captopril renal scintigraphy is based on the pathophysiology of renovascular hypertension, and it has been advocated as a screening test.[8] Contrast arteriography remains the "gold standard" for the anatomic diagnosis of renal artery disease, but it is unsuitable for use as a screening test owing to its high cost and invasive nature. The potential nephrotoxicity of radiographic contrast is another factor that has limited the use of arteriography in patients with renal artery disease and renal insufficiency.

FIGURE 24.1. Arteriogram of atherosclerotic renal artery stenosis. The lesions are located in the proximal right and left renal artery segments and are associated with significant aortic involvement. There is poststenotic dilatation distal to the left renal artery lesion.

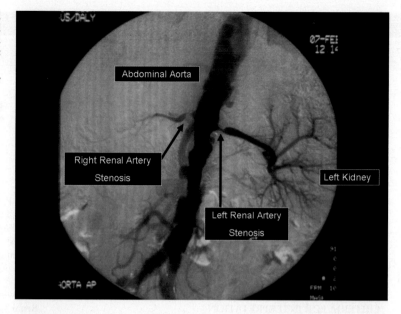

FIGURE 24.2. *A,* Arteriogram of renal artery fibromuscular dysplasia (FMD). The "string-of-beads" lesion involves the middle and distal segments of the renal artery. *B,* B-mode image of FMD in a distal renal artery.

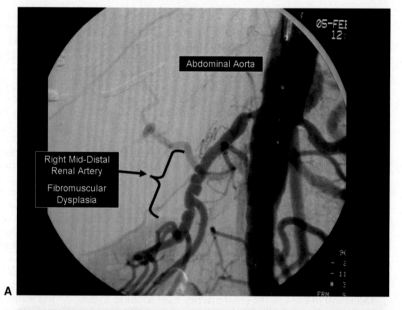

A

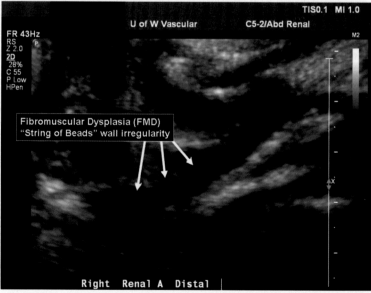

B

Computed tomography angiography (CTA) and magnetic resonance angiography (MRA) are also being used to image the renal arteries. Although sensitivities and specificities of greater than 90% have been reported for detection of main renal artery stenosis by CTA, this approach may not be suitable for many patients because it requires relatively large volumes of iodinated contrast.[9,10] Calcification in atherosclerotic plaques interferes with arterial imaging by CTA, and accessory renal arteries may not be reliably identified.[11] MRA does not require injection of iodinated contrast and can produce images that appear similar to those of standard arteriograms. Gadolinium is a noniodinated contrast agent that improves the quality of MRA images and enhances the ability to identify accessory renal arteries. Excellent sensitivities and specificities have been reported for imaging of main renal artery stenoses by MRA, but the resolution in the smaller distal renal artery branches may not be optimal.[12,13] The main disadvantage of MRA is that it may overestimate the severity of stenosis and produce false-positive results. As with all magnetic resonance studies, the test cannot be performed on patients with pacemakers or other metal devices. It is now recognized that there is an association between nephrogenic systemic fibrosis (NSF) and the use of gadolinium-based contrast agents in patients with renal insufficiency, with reported prevalences of up to 18%.[14,15] Therefore, these contrast agents should be avoided in patients with abnormal renal function, particularly those with severe renal insufficiency and patients requiring hemodialysis.

When a hemodynamically significant renal artery stenosis is found, functional studies may be indicated to determine whether the lesion is truly responsible for the clinical findings. This can be accomplished by either renal vein renin determinations or split renal function studies. However, both of these methods are complex and invasive. The most commonly used approach is to measure the renin concentration in blood sampled from each renal vein to detect unilateral renin hypersecretion. The test is considered positive if there is a ratio of at least 1.5 to 1.0 when the stenotic and nonstenotic sides are compared. Split renal function studies are infrequently used and require cystoscopy with ureteral catheterization to measure urine flow and urinary concentration from each kidney. Unfortunately, these functional studies have numerous sources for error, and the results are not uniformly reliable, particularly in the presence of bilateral renal artery disease or renal artery stenosis involving a solitary kidney.[5]

Duplex ultrasound scanning was developed in the 1970s as a direct noninvasive method for evaluating the extracranial carotid arteries. Subsequent advances in ultrasound technology, particularly the availability of improved B-mode imaging systems, color-flow Doppler imaging, and lower-frequency ultrasound transducers, have extended the applications of duplex scanning to the more complex and deeply located vessels of the abdomen. Duplex scanning is currently the only method available in the noninvasive vascular laboratory for evaluating the renal arteries.

DUPLEX SCANNING TECHNIQUE

The principal challenge in renal duplex scanning is to locate the arteries and obtain satisfactory pulsed Doppler spectral waveforms using a favorable angle of insonation. Renal arteries are especially difficult to examine because of their small size, deep location, and variable anatomy. The effects of respiratory motion and overlying bowel gas can also limit the success of renal duplex scanning. Whereas some renal duplex examinations can be performed in 30 to 45 minutes, evaluating the entire renovascular system can be time consuming, and it is preferable to allow up to 1 hour for a routine renal duplex scan.

The general principles of renal duplex scanning are identical to those for other arterial sites that supply low-resistance vascular beds. The renal arteries are visualized by B-mode and color-flow imaging, the pulsed Doppler sample volume is placed within the vessels, and spectral waveform analysis is used to characterize the flow patterns and classify the severity of disease. A localized flow disturbance with a high-velocity jet indicates the presence of a high-grade stenosis. In addition to the renal artery evaluation, the renal veins and renal parenchyma are also evaluated as described in the following sections.

Equipment

Ultrasound evaluation of the aorta, renal arteries, renal veins, and kidneys requires a low-frequency, 2.5- to 3.0-MHz phased array or curved linear transducer to obtain adequate depth penetration. Color-flow imaging is extremely helpful when performing abdominal vascular duplex examinations, in order to help define anatomic relationships and identify blood vessels. In addition, it can be beneficial to have a stretcher that has a reverse Trendelenburg (feet-down) position, which will sometimes drop the bowel out of the scan plane and improve visualization of the deeper structures.

Patient Preparation

The main barrier to a successful abdominal duplex examination is bowel gas, so the focus of patient preparation is on efforts to minimize this problem. To maximize patient comfort and for optimal technical results, renal artery duplex examinations should be scheduled in the morning, preferably before 10:00 AM. Whenever possible, have the patient fast for about 8 hours before the examination. If the study is scheduled as a first appointment in the morning, a low-residue diet on the day before the study and fasting after midnight are usually adequate. Smoking and gum chewing should be discouraged on the morning of the examination. Some laboratories employ additional methods such as a full bowel preparation (laxatives and enemas) or use of over-the-counter medicines containing simethicone. However, the effectiveness of these measures compared with fasting alone has not been proved.

Because the majority of patients take oral medications, they should be instructed to take these medications with small sips of water as directed. If food is recommended with the medication, or if the patient is diabetic, she or he should eat low-residue food in small amounts. About 5% of examinations will be incomplete because of bowel gas, depth of vessels, respiratory motion, or lack of patient cooperation. If the patient is not well prepared as outlined previously, a repeat scan after optimal preparation should be considered.

Examination Protocol

The renal duplex examination is always bilateral, unless a limited study is specifically requested. Some indications for a unilateral or limited renal duplex scan are known absence of a kidney (congenital or surgical), previously documented occlusion of a renal artery, and follow-up of a unilateral renal artery intervention. Position the patient on the examining table in the supine position with his or her arms resting comfortably at his or her side. The position of the technologist is equally important and somewhat unique for the renal duplex examination. Abdominal vascular scanning requires a significant amount of pressure with the transducer, and using proper ergonomic technique will reduce distractions due to shoulder, arm, wrist, and hand discomfort (Figs. 24.3 and 24.4). If visualization is poor owing to abdominal gas, firm downward pressure on the transducer into the abdomen will often disperse the gas and bring the vasculature closer to the transducer for enhanced

FIGURE 24.3. An ergonomically *incorrect* position for a technologist performing a renal artery duplex evaluation. The scanning arm is elevated at the shoulder and positioned away from the body.

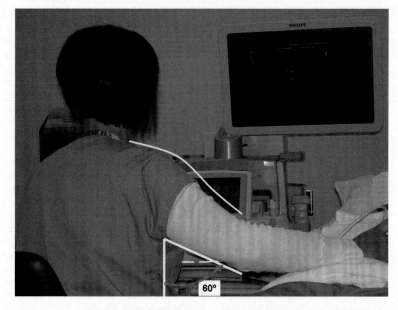

image quality. However, it is important to be aware of the amount of pressure applied and the patient's comfort level.

When patient respirations are rapid or deep, excessive motion of the kidney and renal artery may occur. If the patient is able to cooperate and is not in respiratory distress, instruct her or him to take in a deep breath and either hold it or let it out part way and then hold it. This causes the kidney to move inferiorly for better visualization and provides a short time interval for recording more optimal images and spectral waveforms.

Abdominal Aorta and Branches

Starting in the midline, place the transducer in the subxiphoid position and visualize the proximal abdominal aorta and inferior vena cava (IVC) in the transverse plane. If bowel gas prevents imaging of the abdominal aorta from the midline, slide the transducer laterally to either side and angle back toward the midline to obtain better visualization. The spine lies immediately posterior to the aorta, providing a highly reflective echo interface and anatomic landmark (Fig. 24.5). When the transverse colon obscures visualization of the proximal abdominal aorta, slide the transducer superiorly onto the

xiphoid process, increase the image depth, and use gentle pressure with the transducer. Often the proximal abdominal aorta and the celiac and superior mesenteric artery (SMA) origins can be visualized using this approach.

Obtain diameter measurements of the proximal abdominal aorta at the level of the celiac and SMA origins. Continue scanning the aorta inferiorly until the bifurcation into the common iliac arteries is identified, measuring the aorta at the mid- (infrarenal) segment and again at the distal segment just above the iliac artery origins. Keep in mind that the aorta tapers, becoming smaller in diameter distally. If there is evidence of occlusive or aneurysmal disease in the abdominal aorta, evaluate it at this time. Perform Doppler evaluation of the aorta with the vessel in a longitudinal view, moving the pulsed Doppler sample volume along the length of the vessel. Use a small (1.5- to 2.0-mm) sample volume size and a 60-degree angle of insonation. Record a Doppler spectral waveform at the level of proximal (suprarenal), mid- (infrarenal), and distal (just superior to the bifurcation) abdominal aorta. Evaluate any areas of suspected abnormality with pulsed Doppler and document with spectral waveforms as appropriate. It is important to obtain a Doppler peak systolic velocity (PSV) in the abdominal

FIGURE 24.4. An ergonomically *correct* position for performing a renal artery duplex evaluation. The scanning arm is relaxed at the shoulder and held closer to the body (see Fig. 24.3).

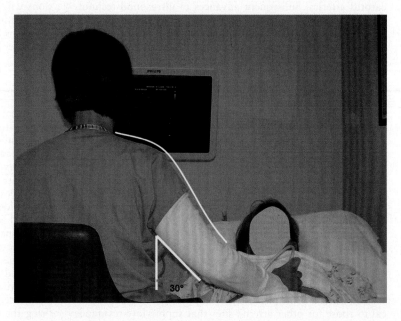

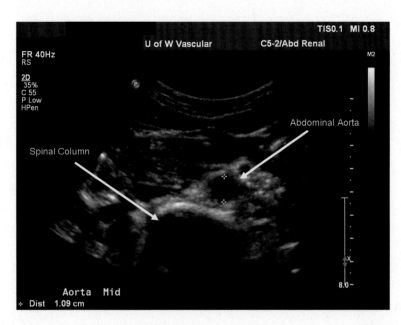

FIGURE 24.5. B-mode image of the abdominal aorta in transverse orientation. The spine is visualized posterior to the aorta providing a highly reflective echo interface (at about 5.0 cm depth) with acoustic shadowing.

aorta at the level of the SMA origin for use in calculating the renal-to-aortic ratio (RAR). Aortic PSVs are typically in the range of 80 to 100 cm/s at this level, although higher velocities are often observed in young normal individuals. The spectral waveform in the suprarenal aorta usually shows forward flow throughout diastole (low-resistance pattern); below the level of the renal arteries, a reverse flow component is present and there is less flow in diastole (high-resistance pattern). These changes in the aortic flow pattern are related to the normal low vascular resistance of the kidneys (Fig. 24.6).

After the abdominal aorta has been evaluated, return the transducer to the subxiphoid position with a transverse orientation and scan inferiorly until the first major branch of the abdominal aorta is identified. This will be the celiac artery originating from the anterior surface of the aorta just below the diaphragm. The SMA is the second major branch of the abdominal aorta and is located anteriorly about 1.0 to 2.0 cm below the celiac artery. A longitudinal view of the upper abdominal aorta often shows the origins of the celiac artery and SMA (Fig. 24.7A). A transverse view of the celiac artery is shown in Figure 24.7B. When viewed in a transverse plane, the SMA is a small round structure anterior to the abdominal aorta. At approximately the level of the renal artery origins, the SMA is separated from the aorta by the left renal vein, as shown in Figure 24.8.

The inferior mesenteric artery (IMA) is the third and last anterior unpaired branch of the abdominal aorta and originates between the level of the renal arteries and the aortic bifurcation. The IMA is smaller than the celiac artery and SMA and runs inferiorly from the aorta and to the patient's left. Whereas it is not necessary to scan the mesenteric arteries in detail during a renal duplex examination unless there is a specific indication, the celiac artery and SMA are relatively constant in location and provide helpful anatomic landmarks for finding the origins of the renal arteries. If a color Doppler bruit or aliasing is noted in the mesenteric arteries, it may be clinically useful to evaluate these vessels.

Renal Arteries and Veins

The renal arteries usually arise from the aorta just distal to the level of the SMA, although their location is variable. The right renal artery tends to originate from the lateral aspect of the aorta at about the 10-o'clock position in a transverse view, and it runs posterior to the IVC (retrocaval) toward the right

kidney. The left renal artery arises from the lateral or posterolateral aspect of the aorta (the 3- or 4-o'clock position). These relationships are illustrated in Figure 24.9.

Both renal arteries lie posterior to their companion renal veins. Once they have been located with B-mode and color-flow imaging, evaluate the renal arteries throughout their length using a small (2.0-mm) pulsed Doppler sample volume. Sweeping the sample volume from the abdominal aorta directly into the renal artery is valuable, because atherosclerotic renal artery lesions are typically continuous with aortic plaque and involve the renal artery ostium (Fig. 24.10). Spectral waveforms are obtained at the origin and the proximal, middle, and distal portions of the right and left renal arteries (Fig. 24.11). Give special attention to any focal abnormalities such as high-velocity jets or aneurysmal changes. Figure 24.12 demonstrates the unusual appearance of a renal artery aneurysm. It is important to document the highest flow velocity in each renal artery, along with any flow disturbance distally (Fig. 24.13). The distal renal artery may be difficult to visualize with the patient in a supine position, and a lateral decubitus or lateral posterior oblique position may provide better ultrasound access. It is helpful to roll the patient onto his or her side when using the flank approach. An example of insonating the origin of the renal artery from a flank approach is shown in Figure 24.14. After evaluating the main renal arteries, attempt to locate and evaluate accessory renal arteries, which are present in up to 17% of kidneys (Fig. 24.15).[16] A relatively common location for an accessory renal artery is arising from the right lateral aspect of the aorta around the level of the IMA and running anterior to the IVC to the inferior pole of the right kidney.

The duplex technique for evaluation of renal artery stents does not differ significantly from that for native renal arteries (Fig. 24.16). Interrogation of stents ideally involves documentation of Doppler flow velocity and waveform contour present, at the proximal end of the stent, midstent, at the distal end of the stent, and poststent. However, as these stents are small in caliber and usually very short, this is not always feasible. Sweep the Doppler sample volume through the stent to identify any focal velocity increase. When present, attempt to identify the specific location of stenosis (e.g., at the distal end of the stent), as demonstrated in Figure 24.17. As previously mentioned, atherosclerotic renal artery stenosis is predominantly continuous with aortic plaque that involves the renal artery ostium. For this reason, renal artery stents are

Text continues on page 361

VISCERAL VASCULAR

FIGURE 24.6. *A*, Duplex image demonstrates low-resistance spectral waveform contour in the abdominal aorta proximal to the renal artery origins. The Doppler sample volume is located at the level of the celiac and superior mesenteric artery origins. Forward flow is present throughout the cardiac cycle (*arrow*).) *B*, High-resistance spectral waveform in the abdominal aorta distal to the renal artery origins. The Doppler sample volume is in the midabdominal aorta, distal to the level of the left renal artery origin. The flow pattern is triphasic with a reverse-flow component and a final brief forward-flow phase (*arrow*).

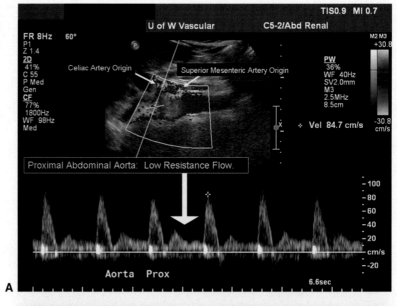

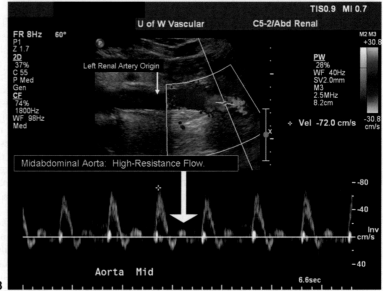

FIGURE 24.7. *A*, Longitudinal B-mode image of the proximal abdominal aorta shows the origins of the celiac and superior mesenteric arteries.

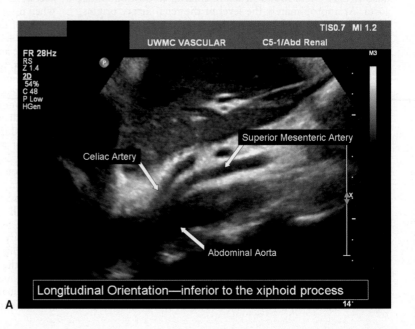

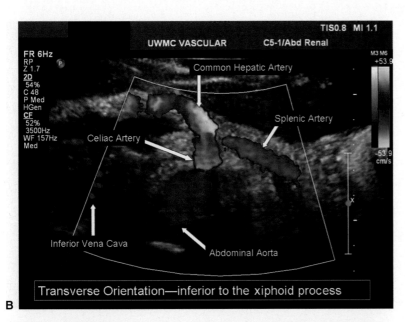

B

FIGURE 24.7. (*Continued*) *B*, Transverse duplex image of the abdominal aorta and the celiac artery, including the common hepatic and splenic artery branches.

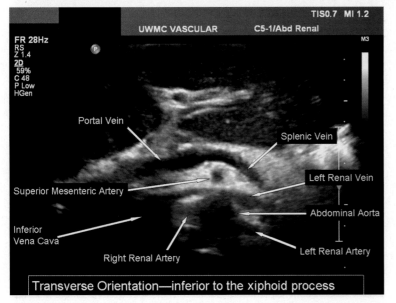

FIGURE 24.8. Transverse B-mode image of the structures at the level of the renal arteries. The left renal vein is seen running between the superior mesenteric artery and the aorta.

VISCERAL VASCULAR

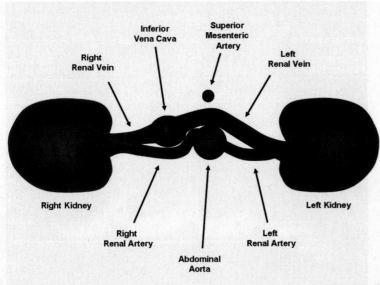

A

FIGURE 24.9. *A*, Cross-sectional diagram shows the typical relationships of the renal artery origins to the aorta, inferior vena cava, and renal veins. (*Continued*)

FIGURE 24.9. (*Continued*) *B*, Corresponding transverse color-flow image of the abdominal aorta (AO), with the origins of the right (RT) and left (LT) renal arteries.

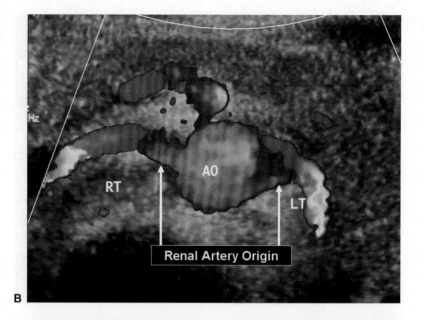

FIGURE 24.10. Spectral waveforms from the abdominal aorta and right renal artery. The sample volume is shown in the abdominal aorta on the color-flow image. In the spectral display, the sample volume is slowly moved from the aorta (AO) into the origin of the right renal artery (RRA), demonstrating no stenosis at this site.

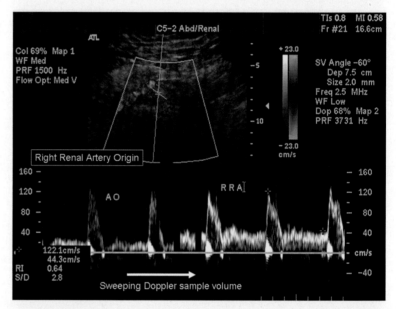

FIGURE 24.11. *A*, Normal spectral waveform from the proximal segment of the left renal artery. The peak systolic velocity (PSV) is 110 cm/s.

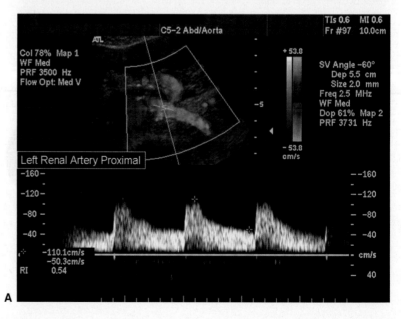

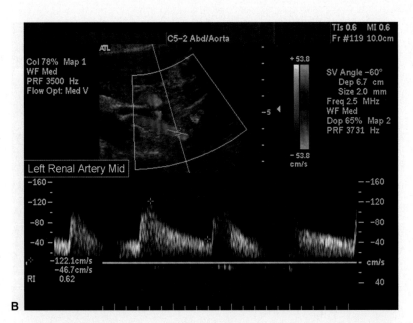

B

FIGURE 24.11. (*Continued*) *B*, Normal spectral waveform from the midsegment of the left renal artery. The PSV is 122 cm/s.

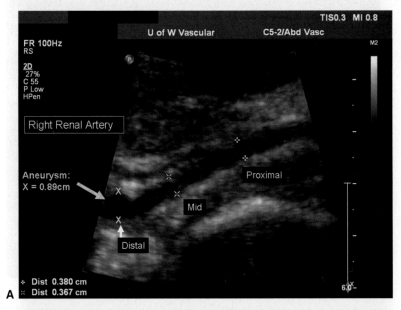

A

FIGURE 24.12. *A*, B-mode image of an aneurysm in the distal segment of the right renal artery. The proximal and midrenal arteries measure 0.37 to 0.38 cm in diameter; the distal renal artery measures 0.89 cm in diameter. *B*, Color-flow image of the same distal renal artery aneurysm.

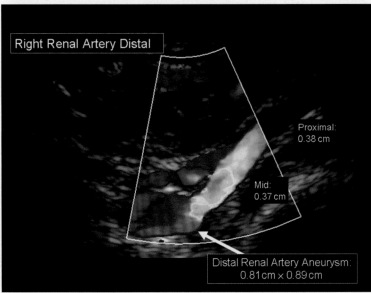

B

FIGURE 24.13. *A*, Abnormal spectral waveform from the proximal right renal artery. The PSV is 428 cm/s, and there is a visible Doppler bruit indicative of a hemodynamically significant stenosis. *B*, Spectral waveform from the distal right renal artery. Poststenotic turbulence is present with a PSV of 99 cm/s.

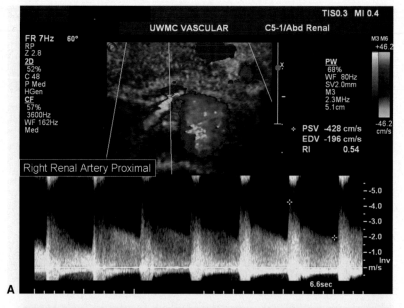

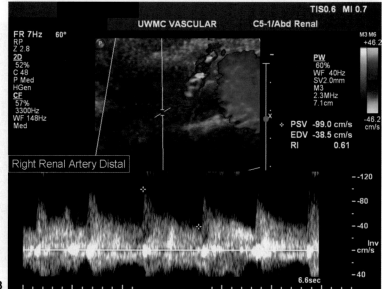

FIGURE 24.14. This right renal artery is being insonated from the flank approach. The kidney is near the top of the image, and the abdominal aorta is near the bottom. The spectral waveform is taken from the right renal artery origin using a 0-degree Doppler angle, resulting in a PSV of 79 cm/s.

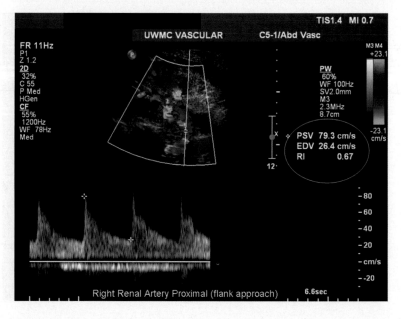

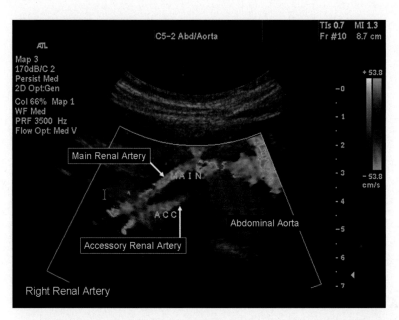

FIGURE 24.15. Color-flow image of an accessory renal artery. The abdominal aorta is shown in transverse orientation with the right main renal artery at the 10-o'clock position and an accessory renal artery arising at the 9-o'clock position.

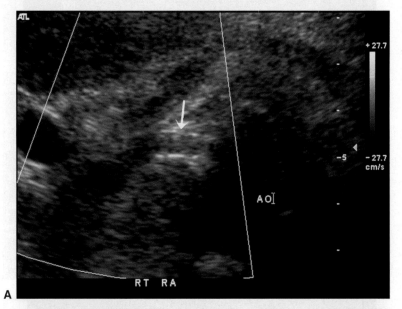

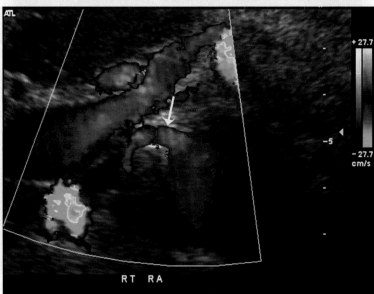

FIGURE 24.16. *A,* Transverse B-mode image of a right renal artery stent (*arrow*). The stent extends into the lumen of the adjacent aorta (AO). *B,* Color-flow image of the same right renal artery stent (*arrow*) running deep to the left renal vein and IVC.

VISCERAL VASCULAR

FIGURE 24.17. *A*, Color-flow image of a stenosis in a left renal artery stent (*arrows*). *B*, Spectral waveforms obtained by sweeping the pulsed Doppler sample volume from the aorta into the left renal artery stent with an increase in the PSV to 286 cm/s in the proximal stent segment. *C*, Spectral waveform taken at the distal end of the left renal artery stent with a PSV of 682 cm/s (maximum for the scale shown). This focal velocity increase indicates a stenosis at this site.

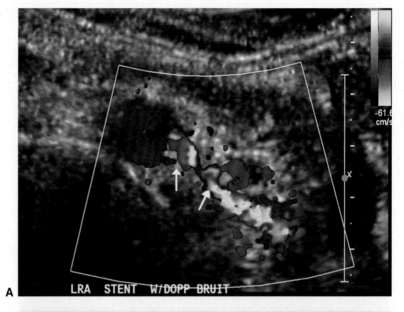

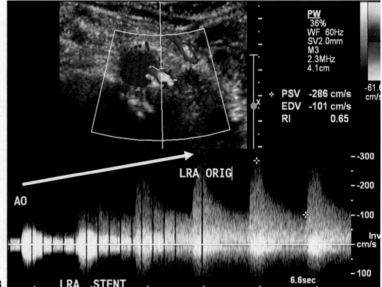

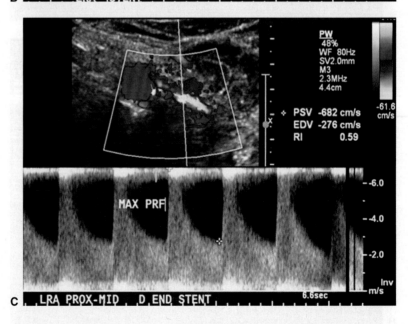

intentionally placed extending into the lumen of the aorta, rather than flush with the aortic wall. Where applicable, visualize the stent with B-mode imaging, noting any stent defects or areas of poor apposition to the artery wall.

Renal artery bypass grafts are relatively uncommon compared to stents. The usual proximal anastomotic site is the infrarenal aorta, but these grafts may originate from the hepatic artery on the right or the splenic artery on the left, as well as the iliac arteries or suprarenal aorta. Ideally, renal bypass grafts should be visualized in their entirety, including the anastomotic segments, with 60-degree Doppler angles; however, in the abdomen this is not always possible. Identify the inflow artery to the bypass graft, documenting flow velocity and waveform contour to look for hemodynamically significant inflow obstruction. Sweep the Doppler sample volume through the inflow anastomosis of the graft, documenting a representative flow velocity. Obtain a midgraft Doppler flow velocity, sampling throughout the graft if possible. Sweep the Doppler sample volume through the outflow anastomosis, again documenting a representative flow velocity. Finally, evaluate Doppler velocity and waveform contour through the outflow segments of the main renal artery. When the graft cannot be evaluated in its entirety due to overlying abdominal gas, even the documentation of a midgraft Doppler flow velocity and waveform contour can be useful in verifying graft patency.

Although it is not necessary to scan the renal veins in detail during a routine renal duplex evaluation, document patency of the right and left renal veins (Fig. 24.18). The right renal vein is shorter than the left renal vein and is best imaged with the transducer placed in the right lateral abdomen over the right kidney and angled medially. The left renal vein is best imaged with the transducer placed in the midline of the abdomen in a transverse orientation just inferior to the origin of the SMA where it courses between the SMA and the aorta to enter the left lateral aspect of the IVC. The renal veins typically have a pulsatile flow pattern near their entry into the IVC owing to transmitted pulsations from the right atrium. However, closer to the renal hilum, the renal vein flow pattern is more phasic with respiration. The presence of pulsatile flow throughout the bilateral renal veins into the hilar branches is usually due to increased central venous pressure and is found in patients with congestive heart failure, cardiomyopathy, or pulmonary edema (Fig. 24.19).

Renal vein thrombosis may occur in association with renal carcinoma, nephrotic syndrome, trauma, or compression secondary to an extrinsic tumor. The renal vein will be dilated proximal to an occlusion, and thrombus may be visualized in the vessel lumen. In the acute phase, the thrombus appears isoechoic to the surrounding blood, no venous flow is identified by Doppler, and the affected kidney is enlarged with a loss of the normal renal architecture. In long-standing cases of renal vein occlusion, the thrombus appears more echogenic, and there may be abnormal, continuous venous flow present in the recanalized lumen.

In some patients, it is possible to insonate a renal artery in its entirety from the flank, particularly when the patient is lying on his or her side. This approach often allows the entire renal artery to be imaged in one view from the aorta to the hilum of the kidney, as shown in Figure 24.14. In addition, individual segmental branches of the renal artery can often be differentiated from the distal main renal artery segment (Fig. 24.20).

Renal Hilum and Parenchyma

A renal duplex evaluation should include the vessels in the hilum of the kidney and the renal parenchyma. By definition, the hilum is the part of an organ where the blood vessels enter and leave. The distal main renal artery divides into segmental branches that enter the renal parenchyma and subsequently divide into interlobar, arcuate, and interlobular arteries. The renal sinus contains the segmental vessels and the collecting system (calyces and pelvis of the ureter) embedded in fatty tissue and appears as a relatively echogenic (bright) central area in the kidney on B-mode imaging (Fig. 24.21).

The hilar or segmental branches are typically evaluated with the kidney in longitudinal or transverse view using either the liver (on the right) or the spleen (on the left) as an acoustic window. Because the hilar vessels are small and numerous, it is not practical to evaluate them individually, so a large (10.0-mm) sample volume is used at a 0-degree angle to acquire a Doppler signal that includes multiple vessels. Doppler spectral waveforms taken at the hilar level are similar to those from the distal renal artery; however, the velocities are usually lower. Hilar spectral waveforms are easier to obtain than waveforms from the main renal artery but, as is discussed later, they have less diagnostic value.

Parenchymal arteries that can be evaluated during a renal duplex examination are the interlobar and arcuate arteries (Fig. 24.22). Perform the parenchymal Doppler evaluation

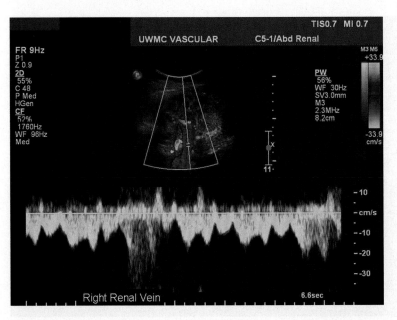

FIGURE 24.18. Duplex image of the right renal vein at the hilum of the kidney taken from the flank approach. The spectral waveform shows a normal phasic and pulsatile renal vein flow pattern.

FIGURE 24.19. Spectral waveform from the right renal vein in a patient with congestive heart failure shows a strongly pulsatile flow pattern secondary to increased central venous pressure.

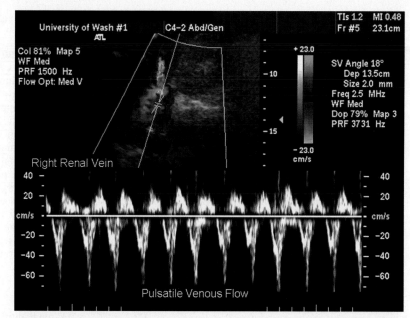

FIGURE 24.20. Color-flow image of a distal left renal artery with extraparenchymal segmental branches.

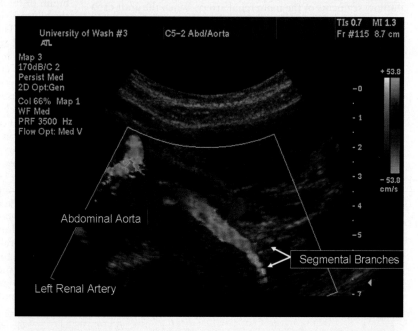

FIGURE 24.21. B-mode image of a kidney in longitudinal orientation. Renal length is 10.5 cm.

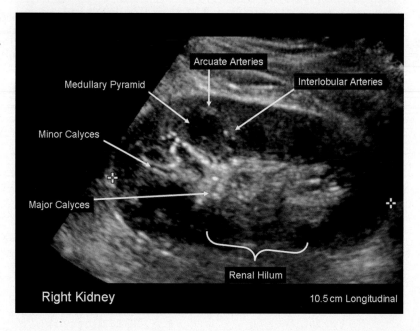

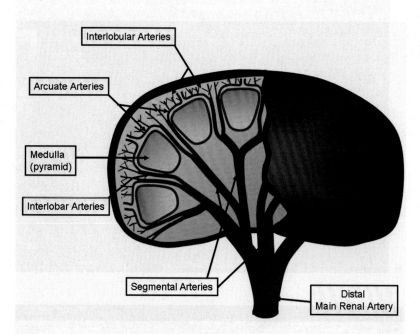

FIGURE 24.22. Anatomy of the extra- and intraparenchymal renal arteries.

using a small (1.5- to 2.0-mm) sample volume size and a 0-degree angle. Color-flow or power Doppler imaging facilitates visualization of these arteries. Use a low wall filter setting when obtaining Doppler waveforms within the renal parenchyma, as a high wall filter prevents detection of low diastolic flow velocities. Identify interlobar arteries between the calyces of the collecting system, and obtain Doppler spectral waveforms from the upper and lower poles of the kidneys. Peak systolic flow velocities in the interlobar arteries are normally in the range of 30 to 40 cm/s, slightly lower than those in the hilum (Fig. 24.23A). Obtain Doppler spectral waveforms from the upper and lower pole arcuate arteries, which are identified at the junction of the renal parenchymal cortex and medulla (the corticomedullary junction). Doppler flow velocities continue to decrease peripherally into the renal parenchyma, and arcuate artery PSVs are in the range of 20 to 30 cm/s (Fig. 24.23B). In the presence of severe renal parenchymal disease, arterial flow may be highly resistive or absent.

Two distinct areas of the kidney parenchyma can be differentiated on B-mode ultrasound surrounding the renal sinus: the medulla and the cortex. The medulla is immediately adjacent to the renal sinus and contains the hypoechoic pyramids. The diuretic status of the patient affects the ultrasound appearance of the medulla; when there is an increase in diuresis, the pyramids become more prominent and are easier to visualize. The cortex is the most peripheral portion of the renal parenchyma and is located between the medulla and the renal capsule. The normal echogenicity of the adult renal cortex is comparable with that of the liver or spleen at the same depth. The corticomedullary junction is recognized by the relatively echogenic arcuate arteries, which appear as bright dots or lines as they arch over the tops of the pyramids (Fig. 24.24). Identification of the corticomedullary junction is an important step in the measurement of cortical thickness. It is a normal finding for the kidney cortex and outer capsule to have a "scalloped" appearance (Fig. 24.25).

Measurements of kidney size have diagnostic value and should be included in the routine renal duplex evaluation. The kidneys are located in the retroperitoneum under the costal margin, with the right kidney slightly lower than the left.

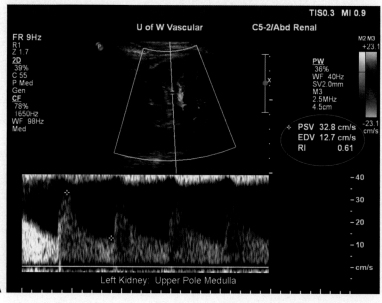

FIGURE 24.23. A, Normal low-resistance Doppler flow pattern obtained in the upper pole medulla of the kidney (interlobar arteries): PSV = 33 cm/s; end-diastolic velocity (EDV) = 13 cm/s; resistance index (RRI) = 0.61 (end-diastolic ratio [EDR] = 0.39). (Continued)

FIGURE 24.23. *(Continued) B,* Normal low-resistance flow obtained in the upper pole cortex of the kidney (arcuate arteries): PSV = 25 cm/s; EDV = 11 cm/s; RRI = 0.58 [EDR = 0.42].

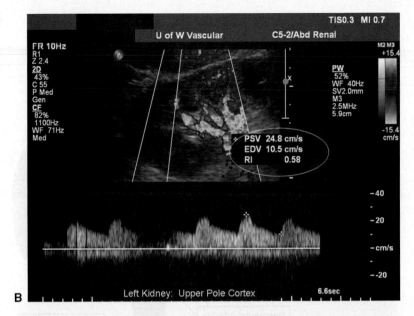

FIGURE 24.24. B-mode image shows the arcuate arteries, which mark the internal border of the cortex. The cortical thickness measurement is 0.74 cm.

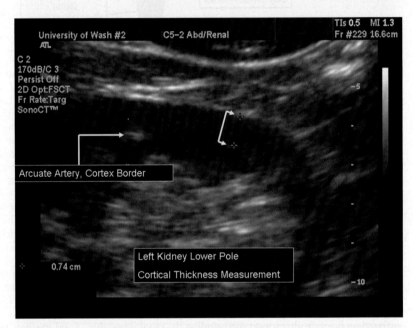

FIGURE 24.25. B-mode image of a kidney with an irregularly shaped cortex, appearing "scalloped."

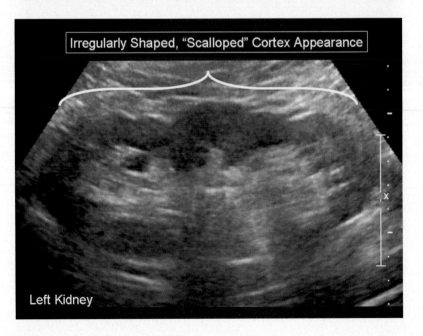

A thin, fibrous capsule, perirenal fat, and Gerota's capsule surround each kidney. During inspiration, the kidneys may move downward by as much as 2.5 cm; therefore, asking the patient to take a deep breath may improve the visualization of the kidneys. The normal adult kidney is about 10.0 to 12.0 cm long and 4.5 to 6.0 cm wide, with men having slightly larger kidneys than women. Kidney size tends to be symmetrical within an individual, so a difference in length of more than about 2.0 cm between sides is significant.

The right kidney is best imaged using the liver as an acoustic window with the patient in either a supine or a left lateral decubitus position, scanning through the anterior axillary line, intercostally or subcostally. The left kidney is best imaged using the spleen as an acoustic window with the patient in a right lateral decubitus position, scanning through the posterior axillary line in an intercostal space. When the left upper pole cannot be identified because of rib or bowel gas interference, a fluid-filled stomach can be used as an acoustic window. Alternatively, as mentioned previously, simply having the patient take a deep breath in and hold it will cause the kidney to be displaced from beneath the ribs and become more accessible to ultrasound imaging.

The optimal view for length measurement displays the kidney longitudinally as shown in Figure 24.26, with both poles clearly visualized. Obtain three separate pole-to-pole kidney length measurements using the renal capsule as a landmark. Average these three measurements and report them as one length measurement for that kidney. Some vascular laboratory protocols may include renal width measurements as part of the routine evaluation. To measure renal width, rotate the transducer, so the kidney appears in a transverse view and obtain three kidney width measurements using the renal artery and renal vein as landmarks. The three kidney width measurements are also averaged. In addition to kidney length and width, cortical thickness reflects the status of the renal parenchyma. Measurements are made from the corticomedullary junction (arcuate arteries) to the renal capsule, as illustrated in Figure 24.24. Take cortical thickness measurements from the upper and lower poles of the kidneys, and average these two and report them as one measurement. Normal cortical thickness is in the range of 1.0 to 1.5 cm when this approach is used.

Incidental Findings

Unsuspected pathology not directly related to the renal vasculature, or "incidental" findings, is relatively common in renal duplex scanning. Although the vascular sonographer, as well as some interpreting physicians, may not have expertise in nonvascular imaging, it is still important to report these findings so that their significance can be established by other appropriate diagnostic tests.

Simple renal cysts are a frequent ultrasound finding, increasing in prevalence with age, and they have been observed in up to 50% of individuals older than 55 years.[17,18] Single cysts are most common, but they can be multiple and located anywhere in the kidney. The characteristic features of a renal cyst on ultrasound are a smooth, clearly demarcated cyst wall, round or slightly oval shape, absence of internal echoes, and acoustic enhancement beyond the cyst (compared with the brightness of echoes from the adjacent renal parenchyma). This typical appearance is shown in Figure 24.27. Some renal cysts may contain septations or loculations. Polycystic kidneys are often bilateral, and the presence of multiple cysts makes measurement of kidney size difficult. Figure 24.28 illustrates the appearance of a polycystic kidney. Parapelvic cysts are located in the renal sinus or hilum. Although they may compress the renal pelvis, they have no direct communication with the collecting system. Parapelvic cysts develop from lymphatic or other nonparenchymal tissues and are less common than simple cysts. The characteristic ultrasound feature of parapelvic cysts is their hilar location, making them difficult to distinguish from hydronephrosis.

Solid renal masses are also readily detected by ultrasound. These lesions are characterized by internal echoes that produce a different echogenicity than normal renal parenchyma and do not result in acoustic enhancement beyond the mass (Fig. 24.29). Renal cell carcinoma is the most common malignant tumor of the kidney and may produce a bulge or distortion in the normal kidney shape. Thrombosis of a renal vein secondary to tumor extension can also occur with renal cell carcinoma. Benign renal tumors include lipomas, leiomyomas, and hemangiomas. Whereas flow is often detected in solid renal masses by pulsed or color-flow Doppler, no hemodynamic features reliably differentiate between benign and malignant tumors.

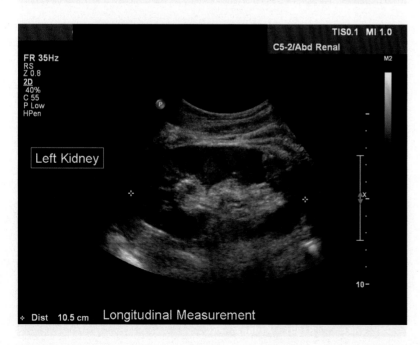

FIGURE 24.26. B-mode image of a left kidney in longitudinal orientation with a caliper length measurement of 10.5 cm. The image should be "horizontal" across the screen when the length measurement is taken.

FIGURE 24.27. B-mode image of a right kidney with a cyst in the lower pole. The tissues are brighter deep to the cyst owing to acoustic enhancement. This cyst measures approximately 4.8 × 3.6 cm.

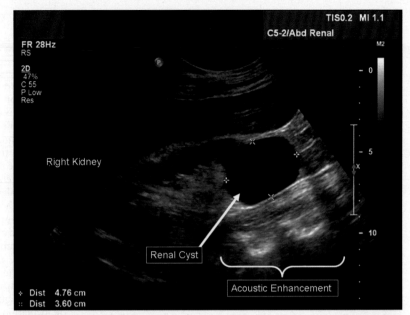

FIGURE 24.28. B-mode image of a polycystic kidney. Multiple small cysts are visible throughout the renal parenchyma.

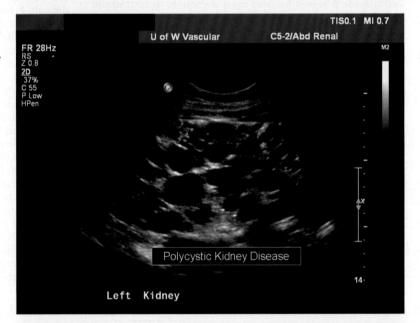

FIGURE 24.29. B-mode image of a kidney with renal cell carcinoma. A solid echogenic mass is visible in the upper pole with characteristics that clearly differ from the surrounding tissues. The mass measures 3.25 × 3.49 cm.

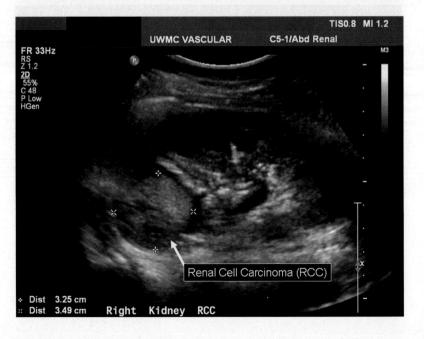

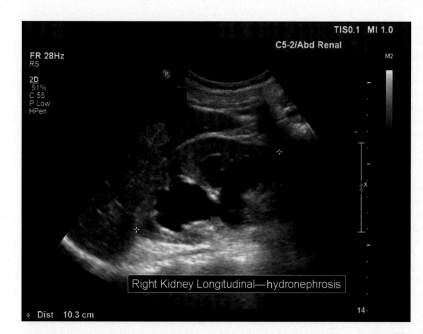

FIGURE 24.30. B-mode image of a right kidney with hydronephrosis. The calyces are markedly dilated throughout the kidney.

Hydronephrosis represents dilatation of the renal pelvis and calyces due to obstruction of urine outflow. The increased pressure in the collecting system is transmitted back into the renal parenchyma and causes compression of the vasculature and renal atrophy. The key ultrasound finding in hydronephrosis is a splaying or separation of the normally dense central echoes in the renal sinus (Fig. 24.30). This feature becomes more prominent as hydronephrosis progresses. In severe hydronephrosis, a large echolucent sac is seen, along with thinning of the renal parenchyma. If hydronephrosis is suspected, it is important to have the patient void and repeat the scan to avoid a false-positive diagnosis resulting from a full bladder. Kidney stones may also be identified on ultrasound as reflective structures in the renal collecting system associated with acoustic shadowing. The presence of hydronephrosis generally makes visualization of stones easier.

Scanning of Kidney Transplants

Kidney transplantation has become a standard treatment for end-stage renal disease. Tissue transplanted from one human to another is referred to as an *allograft*, so a transplanted kidney is a renal allograft. A transplant procedure involves placement of the kidney in the iliac fossa of the recipient on the side contralateral to the original location of the kidney in the donor. The renal allograft is located extraperitoneally in a relatively superficial location. A recipient's native kidneys are usually left in place unless removal is required to treat infection or some other renal condition. The renal artery of the allograft is anastomosed to the common iliac, internal iliac, or external iliac artery of the recipient, most often in an end-to-side fashion. If the artery is short, a vein interposition graft may be necessary. The renal vein is anastomosed end to side to the common or external iliac vein. Because the vascular anatomy is quite variable, it is helpful to obtain an operative report for reference during duplex scanning. The allograft ureter is passed through an oblique tunnel in the bladder wall, which functions as a valve to prevent reflux of urine into the transplanted kidney. Renal allografts are subject to numerous early and late complications, including acute tubular necrosis (ATN), acute or chronic rejection, infection, ureteral obstruction, extrarenal fluid collections, and vascular stenosis or thrombosis.

The superficial location of the renal allograft allows excellent ultrasound visualization, without the limitations imposed by transabdominal scanning for native kidneys. Because the renal allograft is rotated before placement, the hilar structures are medial to the renal parenchyma, with the renal pelvis and ureter anterior, the renal vein posterior, and the renal artery lying between these two structures. Scan the patient in a supine position with a full, but not distended, urinary bladder. Images can be obtained by scanning along the surgical incision and angling the transducer toward the allograft. The general techniques described previously for scanning native kidneys can be applied to renal allografts. A normal transplanted kidney should have B-mode and Doppler characteristics that are similar to those of native kidneys. It is helpful to obtain a duplex evaluation in the early posttransplant period to establish a baseline for subsequent follow-up. The renal allograft normally hypertrophies during the first 2 to 4 weeks after transplantation; in adults, the volume of the kidney typically increases 30% or more.

Rejection of a renal allograft has been associated with a variety of ultrasound findings.[19] These include a sudden increase in kidney size (more rapid than the expected posttransplant hypertrophy), enlargement of the medullary pyramids, increased echogenicity of the renal cortex, and decreased echogenicity of the renal sinus. Some of these signs are seen only in cases of severe rejection, and a normal duplex scan does not rule out early or mild rejection. Parenchymal Doppler waveforms often indicate abnormally high vascular resistance, a flow pattern characterized by sharp narrow systolic peaks, flow reversal in early diastole, and minimal or absent diastolic flow. The most common cause of acute posttransplant renal failure is ATN, but no ultrasound findings are unique to this condition.

Mild hydronephrosis in a renal allograft is commonly seen during the first few weeks after transplantation and may persist. However, this is not clinically significant if urine output and renal function are satisfactory and the degree of dilatation does not progress. Severe or progressive posttransplant hydronephrosis can be associated with serious urologic abnormalities and generally requires correction. Fluid collections are common after renal transplantation.[20] A small amount of serous fluid adjacent to the allograft and in the area of surgical dissection is expected in the immediate postoperative period, but this should resolve and not increase in volume over time. Large or expanding fluid collections are likely to be abnormal whenever they appear and require further evaluation. The differential diagnosis for abnormal fluid collections after renal transplantation includes seroma, hematoma, abscess, urine (urinoma), and lymphocele.

VISCERAL VASCULAR

The general approach to scanning the arteries and veins of a renal allograft is similar to that for native renal vessels, taking into account the variations in vascular anatomy described previously. It is usually possible to evaluate the allograft vessels completely from their anastomoses to the kidney. Vascular complications that may be encountered include stenosis, occlusion, arteriovenous fistula, and pseudoaneurysm. Arterial stenoses are the most common vascular complications in transplanted kidneys, with a prevalence of about 10%.[20] These lesions result from intimal hyperplasia at the anastomosis, rejection, or stenosis of the proximal native iliac artery. Stenosis of a renal allograft artery may present clinically with new onset of hypertension. A focal stenosis is identified by a high-velocity jet and poststenotic turbulence. If no arterial Doppler signals can be obtained from the imaged artery, occlusion is likely. Segmental infarction is documented by the absence of arterial flow signals within one portion of the kidney when signals are detected elsewhere.

Renal vein thrombosis is uncommon and occurs primarily in the early posttransplant period. Ultrasound findings in this condition include enlargement of the kidney secondary to congestion, hypoechoic regions in the renal parenchyma due to hemorrhage, and a high-resistance flow pattern in the allograft renal artery. Flow is absent in the renal vein, which is typically distended with thrombus visualized in the lumen. Arteriovenous fistulas in the parenchyma of a renal allograft are the result of trauma from biopsies.[21] These may be asymptomatic incidental findings or associated with hypertension, and they produce a characteristic high-flow color bruit on color-flow imaging (Fig. 24.31). Pseudoaneurysms in the parenchyma of renal allografts are also usually related to biopsies. Their appearance is similar to that of renal cysts on B-mode imaging, but color-flow imaging shows blood flow in the cavity. Pseudoaneurysms can also involve the allograft vessel anastomoses but are very uncommon.

CRITERIA FOR INTERPRETATION

Renal Arteries

The classification of renal artery disease by duplex scanning is based on spectral waveforms from the renal artery and adjacent abdominal aorta. The triphasic flow pattern seen in the distal abdominal aorta and iliac and lower extremity arteries is a result of the relatively high vascular resistance in the normal peripheral circulation. In contrast, the normal kidney offers a low vascular resistance, and the renal artery velocity waveform shows forward flow throughout the cardiac cycle (Fig. 24.32). As in other arterial segments, hemodynamically significant renal artery narrowing results in a focal elevation of the PSV. Normal renal arteries typically show PSV values of less than 180 cm/s.[22] Because the PSV associated with a renal artery stenosis increases relative to aortic PSV, the ratio of PSVs in the renal artery and aorta can be used as an index of renal artery stenosis severity. This is referred to as the *renal-to-aortic ratio* or RAR (Fig. 24.33). Like the ankle-brachial pressure index, this type of diagnostic ratio compares the arterial site of interest with a presumed normal "reference" site, which in the RAR is the perirenal aorta. Consequently, if the aortic PSV is abnormal, the RAR will be invalid. Because aortic PSV is normally between about 40 and 100 cm/s, the RAR should not be used when aortic PSV values are outside this range.

The duplex scanning criteria developed at the University of Washington for classification of disease in the main renal arteries are given in Table 24.1.[22,23] Four categories are defined based on the highest PSV in the renal artery and the RAR: normal, less than 60% diameter reduction, 60% or greater diameter reduction, and occlusion. The threshold of 60% diameter reduction for a significant renal artery stenosis was based on work in experimental models that showed a pressure gradient across lesions of that severity.[24] In those cases with an aortic PSV outside the normal range, the highest PSV in the main renal artery can be used to classify the severity of stenosis, as outlined later. Renal artery occlusion is present when the artery is visualized, but no flow signal can be detected by pulsed or color-flow Doppler. Very low parenchymal velocities or absent parenchymal flow signals will also be found with renal artery occlusion. In cases of chronic renal artery occlusion, the kidney will usually be atrophic (<8 cm in length). It is generally recognized that duplex scanning does not reliably detect all accessory renal arteries; however, isolated stenosis in an accessory renal artery is rare, and the majority of these lesions are associated with main renal artery disease.[16] There are no specific velocity criteria for stenoses in accessory renal arteries, but when there is a focal jet near the origin with a PSV of 200 cm/s or more, suspect a significant stenosis.

FIGURE 24.31. Duplex image of an arteriovenous fistula in a transplanted kidney. Increased velocities and a color bruit are present.

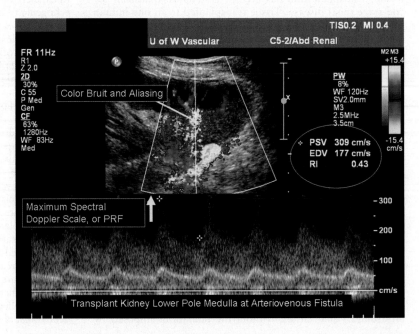

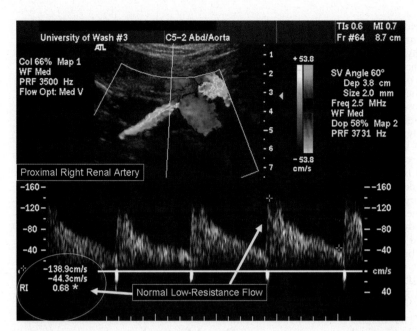

FIGURE 24.32. Normal spectral waveform from a proximal right renal artery with low-resistance characteristics (forward flow throughout the cardiac cycle).

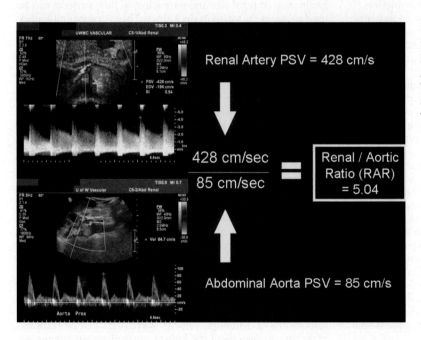

FIGURE 24.33. Calculation of the renal-to-aortic ratio (RAR). The spectral waveform from the proximal renal artery (*top*) has a PSV of 428 cm/s, and the PSV from the abdominal aorta at the level of the celiac/SMA origins (*bottom*) has a PSV of 85 cm/s. The RAR is 5.04, which is consistent with 60% or greater stenosis (see Table 24.1).

TABLE 24.1

CRITERIA FOR CLASSIFICATION OF NATIVE RENAL ARTERY DISEASE BY DUPLEX SCANNING

RENAL ARTERY DIAMETER REDUCTION	RENAL ARTERY PSV	RAR
Normal	<180 cm/s	<3.5
<60%	≥180 cm/s	<3.5
≥60%	≥180 cm/s	≥3.5
Occlusion (100%)	No signal	No signal

PSV, peak systolic velocity; RAR, renal-to-aortic ratio (ratio of highest PSV in the renal artery to the PSV in the adjacent abdominal aorta).

The criteria in Table 24.1 were validated by Hoffman and coworkers in a series of 41 patients with 74 renal arteries evaluated by both duplex scanning and arteriography.[22] A renal artery PSV of 180 cm/s or greater discriminated between normal and diseased renal arteries with a sensitivity of 95% and specificity of 90%. Based on 60% diameter reduction as the threshold for a hemodynamically significant stenosis, an RAR of 3.5 or greater identified renal artery stenosis with a sensitivity of 92% and specificity of 62%. This relatively low specificity was due to a large number of "borderline" lesions that had RAR values greater than 3.5 but were interpreted as being in the range of 50% to 60% diameter reduction by arteriography. It is noteworthy that several of these borderline renal artery stenoses were treated by angioplasty or surgery with a successful clinical outcome, suggesting that the stenoses were hemodynamically significant, as predicted by the duplex scan. Occluded renal arteries were correctly identified by duplex scanning in 10 of 11 cases; however, accessory or branch renal artery stenoses were not reliably detected.

Other groups have used similar methods and criteria to validate renal duplex scanning, with reported sensitivities and specificities in the range of 91% to 98%.[25-27] Hansen and colleagues found that a focal renal artery PSV of 200 cm/s or greater in combination with a "turbulent" distal velocity waveform correlated highly with an arteriographic renal artery stenosis of 60% or greater diameter reduction.[25] Among 122 kidneys with single renal arteries in 74 patients, duplex scanning correctly identified 67 of 68 arteries that were normal or had less than 60% stenosis and 35 of 39 arteries with 60% to 99% stenosis. All 15 renal artery occlusions were correctly identified. This resulted in a sensitivity of 93%, a specificity of 98%, a positive predictive value of 98%, a negative predictive value of 94%, and an overall accuracy of 96%. However, among the 14 patients who had 20 kidneys with multiple renal arteries, the sensitivity of duplex scanning decreased to 67%, with a corresponding negative predictive value of 79%.

A variety of duplex ultrasound criteria and diagnostic thresholds have been described for renal artery stenosis. Some groups recommend using the RAR whenever it is valid, whereas others prefer to rely on the renal artery PSV alone. Excellent sensitivities and specificities have been reported for RAR thresholds from 2.5 to 3.5 and renal artery PSV thresholds in the range of 170 to 200 cm/s.[28-30] Based on this cumulative experience, it is important for every laboratory to validate its own diagnostic criteria by comparison with other imaging methods to make sure the laboratories are obtaining accurate studies. Finally, it should be emphasized that the criteria summarized previously have been developed and validated primarily for atherosclerotic lesions in the main renal arteries, and they may not apply as well to FMD and other types of renal artery lesions.

Hilar Parameters

The rationale for renal hilar duplex scanning is that velocity waveforms obtained distal to a hemodynamically significant renal artery stenosis should be dampened and display a more gradual systolic upstroke. Because pulsed Doppler signals are relatively quick and easy to obtain from the renal hilum using a flank approach, it has been suggested that a hilar duplex scan could serve as a rapid screening test for renal artery stenosis. Renal hilar waveform parameters include the acceleration time (AT), acceleration index (AI), and the early systolic peak (ESP) and tardus/parvus pattern (TPP). The AT is the time interval from the onset of systolic flow to the initial peak in milliseconds (Fig. 24.34A), and AI is the slope of the initial systolic acceleration of the waveform (Fig. 24.34B). An AT of more than 100 ms and an AI of less than 300 cm/s^2 are generally considered abnormal. The ESP is defined as the peak of the acceleration phase of the velocity waveform, which is normally followed by a short deceleration phase and a second acceleration phase before the true systolic peak (Fig. 24.34C). Absence of the ESP is considered abnormal; however, distinguishing between the initial or compliance peak and the true systolic peak can be difficult because of variations in the normal hilar waveform. The TPP refers to an abnormally prolonged early systolic acceleration and low rounded peak in the hilar waveform, features that are qualitatively related to the AT and AI (Fig. 24.34D).

Although the reported specificity of the hilar parameters is typically greater than 90%, the sensitivity is more variable, with a range of 32% to 93%.[31-33] Therefore, whereas the renal hilar scan appears to be reliable when it is positive, false-negative results are relatively common, and the low sensitivity makes it unsuitable for use as a primary screening test. In addition, the limited hilar duplex scan cannot distinguish between renal artery stenosis and occlusion, localize the site of a stenosis, or identify less than 60% stenosis.

Renal Parenchyma

Evaluation of renal size and parenchymal flow patterns can be used to assess the status of the kidney. The average adult kidney length as measured by ultrasound is approximately 11.0 cm, with measurements running about 5.0 mm longer in men than in women.[34] A kidney length of more than 7.0 or 8.0 cm has been advocated as a parameter favoring revascularization in patients with renal artery stenosis. In contrast, decreasing kidney size has received little attention as a parameter for clinical follow-up and is rarely considered as an indication for intervention. Based on a variability study using normal subjects, a single examiner, and the same duplex scanner, a difference of more than 1.0 cm can be considered as a significant change in kidney length between examinations.[35] Cortical thickness measurements have not been as widely used or reported as kidney length. In one ultrasound study of 194 adults without known renal disease, the mean cortical thickness was 1.6 cm.[36]

Doppler spectral waveforms obtained from the renal parenchyma reflect not only the adequacy of renal artery inflow but also the parenchymal vascular resistance and compliance.[37] Two parameters that have been used to quantify renal parenchymal resistance are the end-diastolic ratio (EDR) and the renal resistive index (RRI). The EDR is defined as (end-diastolic velocity/peak systolic velocity), while the RRI is the inverse of the EDR [(peak systolic velocity − end-diastolic velocity)/PSV]. Although velocity waveforms can be recorded from various regions of the kidney, cortical measurements are easier to obtain and appear to be less variable. Normal cortical EDR values are in the range of 0.30 to 0.47, and values less than 0.30 in patients with atherosclerotic renal artery disease have been associated with progressive renal parenchymal disease and diminished potential for reversibility of hypertension or renal insufficiency.[38] The RRI has been more widely used in the clinical setting, with the upper limit of the normal range being 0.70 or 0.80.[39] RRI is a nonspecific indicator of renal parenchymal disease and has been shown to correlate with age, coronary heart disease, increased blood pressure, estimated glomerular filtration rate, and diabetic nephropathy.[40-42] Abnormal RRI values have also been associated with clinical failure of renal artery interventions.[43] An association between RRI and renal allograft rejection has been observed in some studies; however, the use of RRI to assess the status of renal allografts remains controversial.[44,45] An example of normal and abnormal renal parenchymal waveforms is given in Figure 24.35.

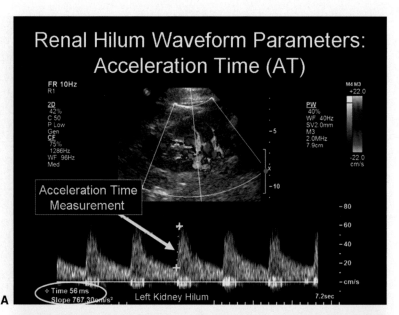

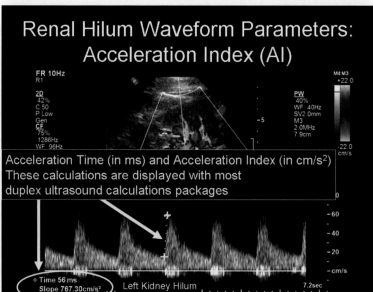

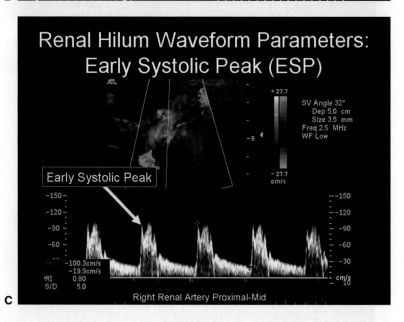

FIGURE 24.34. Duplex images demonstrate renal hilar waveform parameters. *A,* Acceleration time (AT) measurement of 56 ms. *B,* Acceleration index (AI) measurement is indicated as the slope of the systolic portion of the waveform (767.30 cm/s^2). *C, Arrow* demonstrates the early systolic peak (ESP). The presence of an ESP indicates normal arterial waveform contour. (*Continued*)

FIGURE 24.34. (*Continued*) *D*, Tardus/parvus pattern (TPP) is characterized by decreased pulsatility, delayed acceleration time, a rounded systolic peak, and low flow velocity.

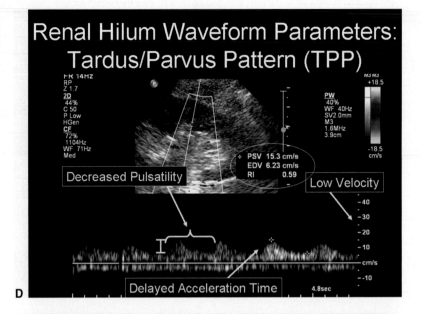

FIGURE 24.35. *A*, Spectral waveform from the cortex of a kidney with normal renovascular resistance (PSV = 24 cm/s; EDV = 10 cm/s; RRI = 0.56; EDR = 0.44). *B*, Spectral waveform from the medulla of a kidney with abnormally increased renovascular resistance (PSV = 27 cm/s; EDV = 4 cm/s; RRI = 0.86; EDR = 0.14).

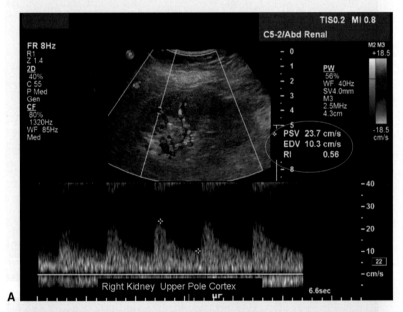

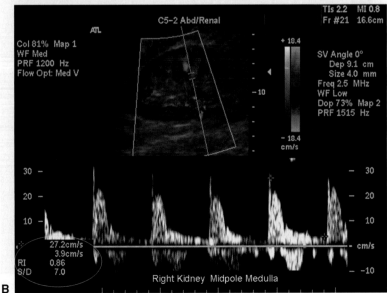

Renal Allograft Vessels

As discussed previously, stenosis of a transplant renal artery is documented following the same general principles that apply to native renal arteries. Stenotic lesions are particularly likely to occur at the anastomotic site or in the native iliac arteries where vascular clamps have been placed. A focal velocity increase with a PSV of 200 cm/s or more with poststenotic turbulence is highly specific for an allograft artery stenosis.[21,46] The RAR does not apply to allografts, because the transplant renal artery does not originate from the aorta; however, a renal-to-iliac artery ratio (RIR) has been described that uses the ratio of PSVs in the allograft renal artery and proximal iliac artery. An RIR of 2.5 to 3.0 or greater is consistent with a significant stenosis in the allograft renal artery.[46]

CLINICAL APPLICATIONS

Current applications of renal duplex scanning include screening of patients with hypertension or renal failure, predicting the outcome of renal artery interventions, intraoperative assessment of renal artery reconstructions, follow-up after renal artery interventions, evaluation of renal transplants, and natural history studies.

Screening

Ideally, a screening test for renal artery disease should be able to detect and classify lesions in all segments of the main renal arteries as well as accessory renal arteries. As previously discussed, renal duplex scanning is reliable for assessing the main renal arteries, but it does not consistently identify accessory renal arteries or lesions in the segmental branches. When renovascular hypertension is suspected, it is important to assess the status of the main renal arteries and any accessory or polar arteries. Although hypertension can result from a stenosis isolated to an accessory renal artery, this situation is extremely uncommon, with a prevalence of only 1.5%.[16] Therefore, failure to detect a hemodynamically significant stenosis in an accessory renal artery may occasionally result in a false-negative screening test, and additional imaging studies should be considered when a duplex scan shows normal main renal arteries and there is a strong clinical suspicion for renovascular hypertension. Unlike renovascular hypertension, ischemic nephropathy results from "total" renal ischemia, so there must be hemodynamically significant lesions in both main renal arteries (or in a single main renal artery in patients with a solitary kidney) for this condition to be present. Consequently, if one or both main renal arteries are shown to be widely patent, ischemic nephropathy can be ruled out.

Labropoulos and associates determined the prevalence of renal artery stenosis among 324 consecutive patients referred to a hospital-based vascular laboratory for renal duplex scanning.[47] This group included 169 females and 155 males, with a mean age of about 63 years. The indication for testing was hypertension in 78% of these patients, and the primary criteria for a significant renal artery stenosis were a renal artery PSV of greater than 200 cm/s and an RAR greater than 2.5. The RRI was also measured, and a value of 0.80 or more identified patients with severe parenchymal disease. Duplex scanning identified unilateral renal artery stenosis in 14% and bilateral renal artery stenosis in 7% of the patients, with 2% found to have renal artery occlusions. The highest prevalence of renal artery stenosis (55%) occurred in hypertensive patients taking three or more antihypertensive drugs. An abnormal RRI was found in 120 patients (37%). Incidental findings were present in 24% of the patients and included abdominal aortic aneurysms; aortic or mesenteric artery stenoses; renal artery aneurysms; and renal cysts, stones, and cancer. These unsuspected abnormalities altered management in 26% of the patients with incidental findings. This experience indicates that there is a relatively high prevalence of renal artery stenosis among patients referred to a vascular laboratory for screening. The high prevalence of clinically significant incidental findings increases the overall diagnostic value of renal duplex scanning in this setting.

Predicting Clinical Outcome of Interventions

Parenchymal flow patterns have been used to predict the clinical response to renal artery interventions. Elevated renal parenchymal resistance, which is associated with low EDR or high RRI values, occurs in kidneys with severe parenchymal disease, and this may be a factor in failures of renal artery interventions.[38,43,48] In a review of 23 patients undergoing 31 renal revascularizations, Cohn and coworkers found that the mean preintervention EDR was significantly higher in those patients who had a favorable blood pressure response or improvement in renal function.[48] A preintervention EDR of less than 0.30 correlated with a poor clinical outcome. Radermacher and colleagues reported similar results using the RRI in a cohort of 138 hypertensive patients with unilateral or bilateral renal artery stenosis who had 131 technically successful interventions.[43] Among the 35 patients with an RRI of 0.80 or more, 34 showed no significant decrease in blood pressure, and renal function deteriorated in 28. However, 90 of 96 patients with an RRI less than 0.80 showed a decrease in blood pressure of 10% or more. These authors concluded that an RRI value of 0.80 or greater identifies a group of patients who are unlikely to respond to renal revascularization. Yuksei and associates reviewed 73 consecutive patients undergoing percutaneous interventions for atherosclerotic renal artery stenosis who were followed for a mean period of approximately 12 months and found that a preintervention RRI of 0.75 or less was associated with significantly better clinical outcomes compared to patients with higher RRI values.[49] These outcomes included serum creatinine levels, estimated glomerular filtration rate, systolic and diastolic blood pressure, and need for antihypertensive medications.

Intraoperative Assessment

Assessment of the technical result is an essential step in arterial reconstructive surgery that facilitates immediate correction of any problems that could lead to vessel occlusion, thromboembolic complications, or graft thrombosis (see Chapter 30). Simple observation and palpation of arteries or bypass grafts are not adequate because these methods are subjective and may not detect significant abnormalities. Operative arteriography is a more objective method for intraoperative assessment; however, it does not provide any physiologic information on blood flow patterns in the visualized vessels. It also requires arterial puncture and injection of contrast material. The need for less invasive and more physiologic approaches has led to the use of ultrasound for intraoperative assessment, and duplex scanning is ideally suited for this purpose.

The general approach to intraoperative duplex scanning is based on the same principles as the preoperative and postoperative evaluations. A small linear array probe with a transmitting frequency of 7 to 10 MHz is typically used. The

VISCERAL VASCULAR

probe and cable are covered with a sterile plastic sleeve filled with acoustic gel, and a small amount of saline or blood is used to couple the probe to the vessel or skin surface. Both B-mode images and Doppler spectral waveforms are recorded from anastomotic sites, from endarterectomy end points, and along vein conduits. Inflow and outflow vessels adjacent to the arterial reconstruction can also be assessed. When Okuhn and associates performed intraoperative duplex scans on 61 patients having renal or visceral artery reconstructions, the mean scanning time was about 8 minutes per patient.[50] Among the 96 reconstructed arteries, 65 (68%) were normal, 27 (28%) had minor defects, and 4 (4%) had major defects. The major defects (3 occlusions and 1 floating thrombus) were repaired. An example of images from an intraoperative assessment of an aortorenal bypass graft is shown in Figure 24.36.

Follow-up after Interventions

The options for renal revascularization include percutaneous transluminal angioplasty (PTA) with or without stenting and a variety of open surgical procedures. Most patients with atherosclerotic renal artery disease have comorbidities that increase their risk for open surgery, so a percutaneous approach is the initial procedure of choice. Stenting is required in the majority of cases, because PTA alone is not effective for these typically orificial and proximal stenoses. Duplex ultrasound provides a practical noninvasive method for assessing the results of renal artery interventions. In 1989, Taylor and coworkers reported on 16 renal artery stenoses of 60% or greater diameter reduction that were followed after interventions.[51] Six arteries in five patients were treated by PTA, and surgical bypass was performed on 10 arteries in seven patients. The PTA group was

FIGURE 24.36. Intraoperative assessment of an aortorenal bypass graft. *A,* B-mode image of the aortic anastomosis. *B,* Color-flow image of the aortic anastomosis.

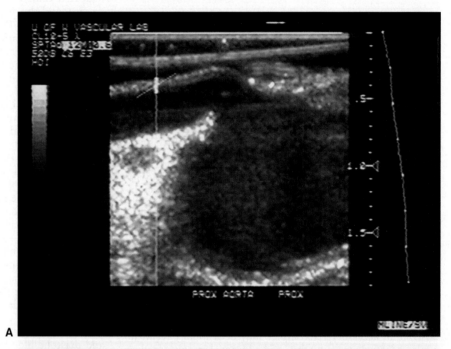

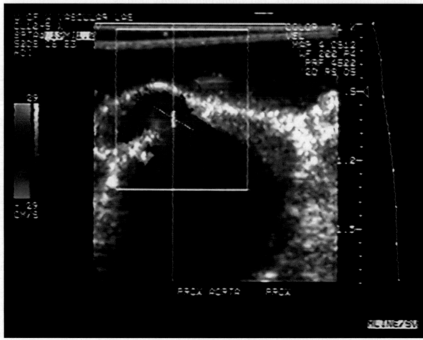

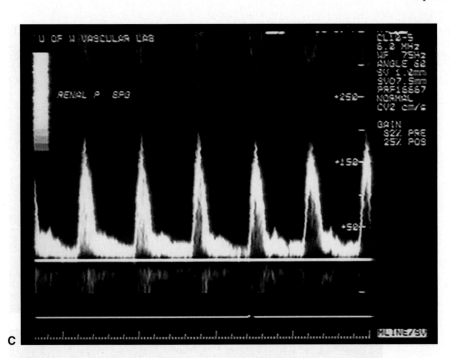

C

VISCERAL VASCULAR

FIGURE 24.36. (*Continued*) C, Spectral waveform taken from the bypass graft shows normal inflow with a relatively high-resistance flow pattern.

followed for a mean of 6.5 months. Duplex scanning documented relief of renal artery stenosis in two patients whose hypertension improved after PTA and persistent stenosis in three patients whose hypertension did not improve. Follow-up of the surgical bypass group for a mean of 9 months showed eight patent and two occluded grafts. In another follow-up study of 51 renal artery interventions in 36 patients, including 8 PTAs, the diagnostic accuracy of duplex scanning was 86%, with a sensitivity of 80% and a specificity of 87%.[52] A larger study of 61 renal artery interventions (44 surgical repairs, 17 PTAs) indicated that duplex scanning had an overall accuracy of 92%, a sensitivity of 69%, and a specificity of 98%.[53] The duplex scan results were adversely affected by the presence of branch renal artery disease, and a separate analysis of the 50 interventions for main renal artery lesions yielded an accuracy of 96%, a sensitivity of 89%, and a specificity of 98%.

The duplex evaluation of aortorenal bypass grafts is similar to that for native renal arteries, except that bypass grafts are typically larger and usually originate from the infrarenal aorta, making them easier to scan (Fig. 24.37). The presence of a stent does not limit ultrasound interrogation of the vessel

(Figs. 24.16, 24.17, and 24.38). Reported experience suggests that velocity thresholds for significant stenosis in stented renal arteries are higher than those listed in Table 24.1 for native renal arteries.[54-57] Mohabbat and colleagues reported on 518 renal arteries in 287 patients who were treated with stents or stent-grafts at the time of endovascular aortic aneurysm repair and followed for a mean of 25 months.[54] The optimal criteria for a significant (60% to 99%) in-stent stenosis were a PSV of more than 280 cm/s and an RAR of more than 4.5. Fleming and associates reviewed 30 patients who had both angiography and duplex scanning following 66 renal artery stenting procedures.[56] These authors found that the best velocity threshold for a 60% or greater in-stent stenosis was a PSV of 250 cm/s. Chi and coworkers compared 67 patients with suspected restenosis after renal artery stenting and 55 patients without renal artery stents who also underwent duplex scanning and angiography.[57] The velocity thresholds of 395 cm/s for PSV and of 5.1 for RAR were most predictive of a 70% or greater in-stent stenosis. Finally, del Conde and colleagues reported on a series of 132 stented renal arteries that were evaluated by both duplex scanning and angiography, including 88 with 0

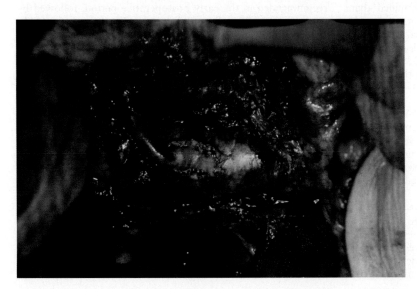

FIGURE 24.37. Operative photograph of a left aortorenal vein graft originating from the infrarenal aorta. The patient's head is to the left. Both the aortic and the renal anastomoses are visible.

FIGURE 24.38. Duplex evaluation of a right renal artery after percutaneous transluminal angioplasty (PTA) and stenting. *A*, Color-flow image of flow through the stent. *B*, The pulsed Doppler sample volume is positioned at the distal end of the stent, and the spectral waveform shows a PSV of 99 cm/s.

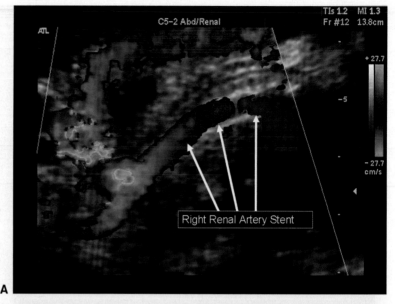

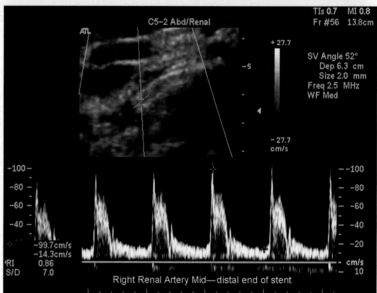

to 59% stenosis and 44 with 60% to 99% stenosis.[55] Using receiver-operator characteristics curves, they determined that both PSV and RAR were very good discriminators, although PSV was a single better predictor of in-stent renal artery stenosis. A PSV of less than 241 cm/s was accurate for excluding 60% to 99% stenosis, while a PSV of greater than 295 was accurate for predicting 60% to 99% stenosis; PSVs in the range of 241 to 295 cm/s were indeterminate. An RAR of 4.4 or greater was optimal for predicting 60% to 99% stenosis.

The incidence of restenosis after renal artery PTA and stenting is in the range of 10% to 21% within 3 to 40 months.[58,59] Although the ideal timing of postintervention surveillance has not been established, frequent follow-up during the first 12 to 24 months appears justified. Clinical indications for duplex follow-up include recurrent hypertension and deteriorating renal function.

Renal Transplant Evaluation

The duplex evaluation of renal allografts has been discussed in previous sections. While duplex scanning can detect a variety of abnormalities following renal transplantation, the focus in most cases is on vascular complications. A baseline scan is recommended in the early postoperative period, followed by scans at about 2 weeks and 3 months. The frequency of subsequent follow-up is determined by the clinical course of the patient.

Natural History Studies

The goal of natural history studies is to provide data on the course of a disease either without specific treatment or with "usual" medical management. This information can serve as a basis for comparison with new treatment options, particularly in patients with asymptomatic or minimally symptomatic disease where the indications for intervention are uncertain. A prospective study on the natural history of atherosclerotic renal artery stenosis was initiated in the vascular research laboratory at the University of Washington in 1990.[60] The study population included patients with renal artery disease who did not require immediate intervention. All renal arteries were classified by duplex scanning according to the criteria listed in Table 24.1. Eligible patients had at least one abnormal renal artery with a

TABLE 24.2

ANALYSIS OF BASELINE RISK FACTORS FOR RENAL ARTERY DISEASE PROGRESSION

■ RISK FACTOR	■ RR	■ 95% CI	■ P VALUE
Systolic blood pressure ≥160 mm Hg	2.1	(1.2, 3.5)	0.006
Diabetes mellitus	2.0	(1.2, 3.3)	0.009
≥60% Ipsilateral renal artery stenosis	1.9	(1.2, 3.0)	0.004
≥60% Contralateral renal artery stenosis	1.7	(1.0, 2.8)	0.04

95% CI, 95% confidence interval; RR, relative risk.

PSV of 180 cm/s or greater or an RAR of 3.5 or greater. Disease progression in a renal artery was defined as (1) an increase in renal artery PSV of 100 cm/s or greater relative to prior examinations (hemodynamic); (2) an increase in renal artery stenosis severity to a 60% or greater diameter reduction (anatomic); or (3) occlusion of a previously patent renal artery.

Caps and associates reported on 170 patients (85 males, 85 females; mean age, 68 years) who were followed for a mean of 33 months.[60] The baseline status of the 295 eligible renal arteries was normal in 56, less than 60% stenosis in 96, and 60% or greater stenosis in 143. Hemodynamic disease progression was detected in 91 of the 295 renal arteries (31%), and the 3-year cumulative incidence was 18%, 28%, and 49% for renal arteries initially classified as normal, less than 60% stenosis, and 60% or greater stenosis, respectively. Based on the duplex criteria, the 3-year cumulative incidence of anatomic renal artery disease progression was 13% from normal to 60% or greater stenosis and 56% from less than 60% to 60% or greater stenosis. Only 9 of the 295 renal arteries progressed to occlusion during the follow-up period, and all of these either had 60% or greater stenosis at the baseline examination or progressed to 60% or greater stenosis before occlusion.

Analysis of baseline risk factors indicated that the following four were independently associated with hemodynamic renal artery disease progression: increased systolic blood pressure, diabetes mellitus, presence of a high-grade ipsilateral renal artery stenosis, and a high-grade contralateral renal artery stenosis (Table 24.2). Systolic hypertension showed the strongest association, with a 2.1-fold increase in risk of progression for a value of 160 mmHg or greater. Renal arteries exposed to all four of the baseline risk factors listed in Table 24.2 would have a predicted 2-year cumulative incidence of disease progression of 65%; however, if none of these factors was present, the cumulative incidence would be only 7%.

Changes in renal size were also documented in 122 patients with a total of 204 eligible kidneys over a mean follow-up interval of 33 months.[35] Renal atrophy was defined as a decrease in kidney length of 1 cm or greater during follow-up compared with the baseline length measurement. A decrease in kidney length of 1 cm or greater was observed in 33 (16%) of the 204 kidneys. The cumulative incidence of renal atrophy at 2 years was 6% for kidneys with normal renal arteries, 12% for kidneys having less than 60% stenosis, and 21% for kidneys having 60% or greater stenosis at baseline. Three baseline factors were strongly associated with renal atrophy: systolic hypertension, severity of renal artery stenosis, and diminished renal cortical blood flow velocity.

Natural history studies of atherosclerotic renal artery stenosis have defined the clinical risk factors for disease progression and renal atrophy. These results suggest that early renal revascularization could be beneficial for selected patients with severe renal artery stenoses in terms of improved blood pressure control and preservation of renal function. However, specific clinical recommendations will depend on the results of randomized clinical trials.

References

1. Olin JW, Melia M, Young JR, et al. Prevalence of atherosclerotic renal artery stenosis in patients with atherosclerosis elsewhere. Am J Med 1990;88:46N-51N.
2. Chobanian AV, Bakris GL, Black HR, et al. The Seventh Report of the Joint National Committee on Prevention, Detection, Evaluation, and Treatment, of High Blood Pressure (The JNC 7 Report). JAMA 2003;289:2560-2572.
3. Simon N, Franklin SS, Bleifer KH, et al. Clinical characteristics of renovascular hypertension. JAMA 1972;220:1209-1218.
4. Dean RH. Screening and diagnosis of renal vascular hypertension. In Novick A (ed). Renovascular Disease. Philadelphia: WB Saunders, 1998, pp 225-233.
5. Jacobson HR. Ischemic renal disease: An overlooked clinical entity. Kidney Int 1988;34:729-743.
6. Rimmer JM, Gennari J. Atherosclerotic renovascular disease and progressive renal failure. Ann Intern Med 1993;118:712-719.
7. Grim CE, Luft FC, Weinberger MH. Sensitivity and specificity of screening tests for renal vascular hypertension. Ann Intern Med 1979;91:617-622.
8. Meier GH, Sumpio B, Black HR, et al. Captopril renal scintigraphy: An advance in the detection and treatment of renovascular hypertension. J Vasc Surg 1990;11:770-777.
9. Olbricht CJ, Prokop M, Chavin A, et al. Minimally invasive diagnosis of renal artery stenosis by spiral computed tomography angiography. Kidney Int 1995;48:1332-1337.
10. Beregi JP, Elkohen M, Deklunder G, et al. Helical CT angiography compared with arteriography in the detection of renal artery stenosis. AJR Am J Roentgenol 1996;167:495-501.
11. Elkohen M, Beregi JP, Deklunder G, et al. A prospective study of helical computed tomography angiography versus angiography for the detection of renal artery stenoses in hypertensive patients. J Hypertens 1996;14:525-528.
12. Kent KC, Edelman RR, Kim D, et al. Magnetic resonance imaging: A reliable test for the evaluation of proximal atherosclerotic renal artery stenosis. J Vasc Surg 1991;13:311-317.
13. Gedroyc WMW, Neerhut P, Negus R, et al. Magnetic resonance angiography of renal artery stenosis. Clin Radiol 1995;50:436-439.
14. Sadowski EA, Bennett LK, Chan MR, et al. Nephrogenic systemic fibrosis: Risk factors and incidence estimation. Radiology 2007;243:148-157.
15. Thomsen HS. Contrast media safety—an update. Eur J Radiol 2011;80:77-82.
16. Bude RO, Forauer AR, Caoili EM, et al. Is it necessary to study accessory arteries when screening the renal arteries for renovascular hypertension? Radiology 2003;226:411-416.
17. Pollack HM, Banner MP, Arger PH, et al. The accuracy of gray-scale renal ultrasonography in differentiating cystic neoplasms from benign cysts. Radiology 1982;143:741-745.
18. Bartholomew TH, Slovis TL, Kroovand RL, et al. The sonographic evaluation and management of simple cysts in children. J Urol 1980;123:732-736.
19. Hricak H, Cruz C, Eyler WR, et al. Acute post-transplantation renal failure: Differential diagnosis by ultrasound. Radiology 1981;139:441-449.
20. Coyne SS, Walsh JW, Tisnado WH, et al. Surgically correctable renal transplant complications: An integrated clinical and radiologic approach. AJR Am J Roentgenol 1981;136:1113-1119.
21. Dodd GD, Tublin ME, Shah A, et al. Imaging of vascular complications associated with renal transplants. AJR Am J Roentgenol 1991;157:449-459.
22. Hoffman U, Edwards JM, Carter S, et al. Role of duplex scanning for the detection of atherosclerotic renal artery disease. Kidney Int 1991;39:1232-1239.
23. Kohler TR, Zierler RE, Martin RL, et al. Noninvasive diagnosis of renal artery stenosis by ultrasonic duplex scanning. J Vasc Surg 1986;4:450-456.
24. Norris CS, Pfeiffer JS, Rittgers SE, et al. Noninvasive evaluation of renal artery stenosis and renovascular resistance. J Vasc Surg 1984;1:192-201.

25. Hansen KJ, Tribble RW, Reavis S, et al. Renal duplex sonography: Evaluation of clinical utility. *J Vasc Surg* 1990;12:227-236.

26. Olin JW, Piedmonte MR, Young JR, et al. The utility of duplex ultrasound scanning of the renal arteries for diagnosing significant renal artery stenosis. *Ann Intern Med* 1995;122:833-838.

27. Nchimi A, Biquet JF, Brisnois D, et al. Duplex ultrasound as a first-line screening test for patients suspected of renal artery stenosis: Prospective evaluation in high-risk group. *Eur Radiol* 2003;13:1413-1419.

28. Soares GM, Murphy TP, Singha MS, et al. Renal artery duplex ultrasonography as a screening tool to detect renal artery stenosis. *J Ultrasound Med* 2006;25:293-298.

29. Stauub D, Canevascini R, Huegli RW, et al. Best duplex-sonographic criteria for assessment of renal artery stenosis—correlation with intra-arterial pressure gradient. *Ultraschall Med* 2007;28:45-51.

30. Li J, Jiang Y, Zhang S, et al. Evaluation of renal artery stenosis with hemodynamic parameters of Doppler sonography. *J Vasc Surg* 2008;48: 323-328.

31. Motew SJ, Cherr GS, Craven TE, et al. Renal duplex sonography: Main renal artery versus hilar analysis. *J Vasc Surg* 2000;32:462-471.

32. Stavros TA, Parker SH, Yakes WF, et al. Segmental stenosis of the renal artery: Pattern recognition of tardus and parvus abnormalities with duplex sonography. *Radiology* 1992;184:487-492.

33. Kliewer MA, Tupler RH, Carroll BA, et al. Renal artery stenosis: Analysis of Doppler waveform parameters and tardus-parvus pattern. *Radiology* 1993;189:779-787.

34. Emamian SA, Nielsen MB, Pederson JF, et al. Kidney dimensions at sonography: Correlation with age, sex, and habitus in 665 adult volunteers. *AJR Am J Roentgenol* 1993;160:83-86.

35. Caps MT, Zierler RE, Polissar NL, et al. The risk of atrophy in kidneys with atherosclerotic renal artery stenosis. *Kidney Int* 1998;53:735-742.

36. Bucholz NP, Abbas F, Biyabani SR, et al. Ultrasonographic renal size in individuals without known renal disease. *J Pak Med Assoc* 2000;50: 12-16.

37. Bude RO, Rubin JM. Relationship between the resistive index and vascular compliance and resistance. *Radiology* 1999;211:411-417. Frauchiger B, Zierler RE, Bergelin RO, et al. Prognostic significance of intrarenal resistance indices in patients with renal artery interventions: A preliminary study with duplex ultrasound. *Cardiovasc Surg* 1996;4:324-330.

38. Riehl J, Schmitt H, Bongartz D, et al. Renal artery stenosis: Evaluation with colour duplex ultrasonography. *Nephrol Dial Transplant* 1997; 12:1608-1614.

39. Galesic K, Brkljacic B, Sabljar-Matovinovic M, et al. Renal vascular resistance in essential hypertension: Duplex-Doppler ultrasonographic evaluation. *Angiology* 2000;51:667-675.

40. Gaurav K, Yalavarthy U, Chamberlain N, et al. Correlation between renal resistive index and estimated glomerular filtration rate in patients with hypertension. *J Vasc Ultrasound* 2008;32:82-84.

41. Ohta Y, Fujii K, Arima H, et al. Increased renal resistive index in atherosclerosis and hypertensive nephropathy assessed by Doppler sonography. *J Hypertens* 2005;23:1905-1911.

42. Radermacher J, Chiavan A, Bleck B, et al. Use of Doppler ultrasonography to predict the outcome of therapy for renal artery stenosis. *N Engl J Med* 2001;344:410-417.

43. Don S, Kopecky KK, Filo RS, et al. Doppler US of renal allografts: Causes of elevated resistive index. *Radiology* 1989;171:709-712.

44. Naesens M, Heylen L, Lerut E, et al. Intrarenal resistive index after renal transplantation. *N Engl J Med* 2013;369:1797-1806.

45. De Morais RH, Muglia VF, Mamere AE, et al. Duplex Doppler sonography of transplant renal artery stenosis. *J Clin Ultrasound* 2003;31:135-141.

46. Labropoulos N, Ayuste B, Leon LR, et al. Renovascular disease among patients referred for renal duplex ultrasonography. *J Vasc Surg* 2007;46: 731-737.

47. Cohn EJ, Benjamin ME, Sandager GP, et al. Can intrarenal duplex waveform analysis predict successful renal artery revascularization? *J Vasc Surg* 1998;28:471-480.

48. Yuksei UC, Anabtawi AGM, Cam A, et al. Predictive value of renal resistive index in percutaneous renal interventions for atherosclerotic renal artery stenosis. *J Invasive Cardiol* 2012;24:504-509.

49. Okuhn SP, Reilly LM, Bennett JB, et al. Intraoperative assessment of renal and visceral artery reconstruction: The role of duplex scanning and spectral analysis. *J Vasc Surg* 1987;5:137-147.

50. Taylor DC, Moneta GL, Strandness DE Jr. Follow-up of renal artery stenosis by duplex ultrasound. *J Vasc Surg* 1989;9:410-415.

51. Eidt JF, Fry RE, Clagett P, et al. Postoperative follow-up of renal artery reconstruction with duplex ultrasound. *J Vasc Surg* 1988;8:667-673.

52. Hudspeth DA, Hansen KJ, Reavis SW, et al. Renal duplex sonography after treatment of renovascular disease. *J Vasc Surg* 1993;18:381-390.

53. Mohabbat W, Greenberg RK, Mastracci T, et al. Revised duplex criteria and outcomes for renal stents and stent grafts following endovascular repair of juxtarenal and thoracoabdominal aneurysms. *J Vasc Surg* 2009;49:827-837.

54. del Conde I, Galin ID, Trost B, et al. Renal artery duplex ultrasound criteria for the detection of significant in-stent restenosis. *Catheter Cardiovasc Interv* 2014;83:612-618.

55. Fleming SH, Davis RP, Craven TE, et al. Accuracy of duplex sonography scans after renal artery stenting. *J Vasc Surg* 2010;62:953-958.

56. Chi YW, White CJ, Thornton S, et al. Ultrasound velocity criteria for renal in-stent restenosis. *J Vasc Surg* 2009;50:119-123.

57. Blum U, Krumme B, Flugel P, et al. Treatment of ostial renal-artery stenosis with vascular endoprostheses after unsuccessful balloon angioplasty. *N Engl J Med* 1997;336:459-465.

58. Balk E, Raman G, Chung M, et al. Effectiveness of management strategies for renal artery stenosis: A systematic review. *Ann Intern Med* 2006; 145:901-912.

59. Caps MT, Perissinotto C, Zierler RE, et al. A prospective study of atherosclerotic disease progression in the renal artery. *Circulation* 1998;98: 2866-2872.

CHAPTER 25 ■ PELVIC CONGESTION SYNDROME

DEREK P. NATHAN AND MARK H. MEISSNER

Pelvic congestion syndrome was first described by Taylor in 1949.[1] He, as well as others, demonstrated that pelvic varicosities and venous congestion were consistently found in women with what was then known as the pelvic pain syndrome.[2] Reflux and obstruction affecting the pelvic veins may present in a variety of ways including chronic pelvic pain; varicose veins affecting the legs, vulva, perineum, or gluteal cleft; or with symptoms of flank pain and hematuria associated with the nutcracker syndrome.

Chronic pelvic pain is defined as pain below the umbilicus that lasts for 6 months or longer. It affects 15% of women 18 to 50 years of age in the United States and may be associated with significant disability and distress.[3] Fifteen percent of women with chronic pelvic pain report time lost from employment, and 45% report decreased work productivity. Despite the significant clinical and socioeconomic impact, a definitive diagnosis is made in fewer than 40% of women with chronic pelvic pain. Although a variety of disorders, including endometriosis, uterine leiomyoma, and pelvic inflammatory disease, may be associated with chronic pelvic pain, pelvic congestion syndrome is the second leading cause of chronic pelvic pain and accounts for as many as 31% of cases.[4] The modern diagnosis of pelvic congestion syndrome is based upon correlation of the patient's clinical presentation with diagnostic imaging findings demonstrating reflux and/or obstruction in the pelvic venous system.

CLINICAL PRESENTATION

Pelvic venous disorders primarily affect premenopausal, multiparous women and may be associated with a variety of clinical presentations. Among 42 women with pelvic varices, the mean onset of symptoms was after the second pregnancy at a mean age of 31.9 years. Symptoms were related to vulvar varices in 74%, lower extremity varices in 43%, and chronic pelvic pain in 26%.[5]

Beard et al[6] compared the clinical features of women with chronic pelvic pain due to pelvic congestion to those of women with pain due to other pelvic pathologies. Women with symptomatic pelvic congestion were younger and more often multiparous. Pain associated with pelvic congestion is often described as dull and aching with occasional sharp exacerbations. It is improved in the supine position but worsened in positions that increase pelvic blood flow, such as standing or sitting, as well as during menstruation.[4,7] Such patients may also report dyspareunia, dysmenorrhea, and dysuria, and they

have higher rates of anxiety and depression than do women with chronic pelvic pain from other causes.[4] Symptoms usually improve or resolve with menopause.[6]

Pelvic venous disorders may also be associated with varicose veins, with or without pelvic pain. Atypically distributed varices, specifically those localized below the gluteal crease, on or below the perineum in the medial thigh, or on the vulva, should raise the suspicion of pelvic venous reflux. However, more typically distributed varices may also arise from communications between the deep and superficial external pudendal tributaries of the great saphenous vein and the internal iliac veins. Importantly, depending on demographics, one-quarter to one-third of recurrent varicose veins in women arise from a pelvic source.[8]

Aortomesenteric compression of the left renal vein (the nutcracker syndrome) may be associated with left flank pain and hematuria as well as pelvic congestion symptoms in women and a left-sided varicocele in men.[9] The nutcracker syndrome has a bimodal age distribution, with one peak in adolescents and young adults and a second peak in women in their third to fourth decades.

ANATOMY AND PATHOPHYSIOLOGY

The diagnosis and management of pelvic venous disorders requires a thorough understanding of the complicated venous anatomy. The venous drainage of the pelvis occurs through the ovarian veins, tributaries of the internal iliac veins, and the femoral veins. These three systems have multiple interconnections, including frequent drainage across the pelvis.[10] The ovarian veins drain the venous territories of the parametrium, cervix, mesosalpinx, and pampiniform plexus, which may also drain through the internal iliac veins as a collateral pathway. These plexuses form the ovarian vein, which may have two to three trunks before classically forming a single vein at the level of the fourth lumbar vertebra. Although variations occur, the right ovarian vein usually drains directly into the inferior vena cava, while the left ovarian vein drains into the left renal vein. Together with the left adrenal, ascending lumbar, hemiazygous, peri-ureteric, and capsular veins, the left ovarian vein may be the primary drainage of the left kidney in cases of aortomesenteric compression of the left renal vein. The normal ovarian vein has a diameter of approximately 3 mm, although this increases with pregnancy, and it usually has two or three valves.

379

The internal iliac vein is formed by the union of the obturator, branches of the internal pudendal, and gluteal veins, which originate in the thigh, perineum, and buttock, respectively. The internal iliac vein may have multiple collaterals, both across the pelvis and through the internal pudendal and obturator tributaries to the ovarian and femoral veins. Four pelvic escape points have been described as connections between internal iliac tributaries and the lower extremity veins: the inguinal (I) point arising from the round ligament vein, the perineal (P) point arising from the pudendal veins, the obturator (O) point carrying reflux from the obturator vein, and the gluteal (G) points arising from the superior and inferior gluteal veins.[11]

As with other venous disorders, pelvic venous syndromes may result from either reflux or obstruction. Both the ovarian veins and the internal iliac tributaries contain valves that can become incompetent, leading to pelvic venous reflux. Ovarian vein reflux may be demonstrated in up to 47% of women. Pregnancy is associated with as much as a 60-fold increase in pelvic blood flow as well as hormonally mediated ovarian and uterine vein dilation.[7,12,13] Ovarian vein dilation ultimately leads to valvular incompetence and retrograde flow or reflux. The high capacitance of the pelvic venous system is facilitated by the pelvic veins' lack of a supporting sheath of fascia as in the veins of the lower and upper extremities. The central role of hormonally mediated changes in the pelvic venous circulation in pelvic congestion syndrome is demonstrated by the significant improvement in symptoms with pharmacologic ovarian suppression.[4] The role of pelvic vein dilatation is similarly demonstrated by the observation that dihydroergotamine, a vasoconstrictive agent that increases venous tone and reduces venous capacitance, is effective in reducing venographic venous diameters, increasing contrast clearance, and decreasing venous congestion in women with chronic pelvic pain.[14]

Pelvic congestion syndrome may also result from venous obstruction, usually related to compression of the common iliac veins, resulting in internal iliac venous reflux, or compression of the left renal vein, resulting in left ovarian venous reflux. May-Thurner syndrome, which most commonly arises from compression of the left common iliac vein by the right common iliac artery, and the nutcracker syndrome, which most commonly represents compression of the left renal vein by the superior mesenteric artery, are the most common compression syndromes in the abdomen. Less commonly, a retroaortic left renal vein may be compressed between the aorta and vertebral column (posterior nutcracker syndrome). Although most commonly associated with deep venous thrombosis, iliac vein compression may occasionally lead to varices associated with internal iliac venous reflux.[13] As discussed above, the left ovarian vein may also function as a refluxing collateral pathway draining the kidney in cases of symptomatic aortomesenteric compression of the left renal vein.

DIAGNOSTIC CONSIDERATIONS

The diagnosis of pelvic congestion syndrome can be difficult, and it is common for women to consult multiple physicians prior to obtaining a definitive diagnosis. The differential diagnosis is quite broad, including endometriosis, pelvic adhesions, atypical menstrual pain, pelvic inflammatory disease, leiomyoma, urologic disorders, pelvic congestion syndrome, and irritable bowel syndrome. Furthermore, a high prevalence of psychiatric disorders among women with pelvic congestion syndrome, such as depression and anxiety, may obfuscate the diagnosis.[4] As described above, the anatomy and

pathophysiology are quite complex, with both reflux and obstruction in multiple interconnected venous beds. Finally, the availability and quality of the imaging studies used to establish the diagnosis may vary widely between institutions.

Selective left renal, bilateral ovarian, and bilateral internal iliac venography is often considered the gold standard for the diagnosis of pelvic congestion syndrome (Fig. 25.1). Either a common femoral vein or right internal jugular vein approach may be utilized for catheter access, although due to the acute angulation of its confluence with the inferior vena cava, selective catheterization of the right ovarian vein may be difficult from the groin. Based on transuterine pelvic venography, Beard et al[2] described the venographic criteria for pelvic congestion as (1) an ovarian vein diameter ≥6 mm, (2) contrast retention within the pelvic veins of greater than 20 seconds, and (3) congestion of the pelvic venous plexus and/or opacification of the ipsilateral (or contralateral) internal iliac vein. Each variable is assigned a value of 1 to 3 depending on the degree of abnormality with a score greater than 5 being diagnostic of pelvic congestion syndrome. Venographic filling of vulvovaginal and thigh varicosities is also diagnostic of a pelvic source of reflux (Fig. 25.2).

The invasive nature of venography has led to the investigation of noninvasive imaging modalities for diagnosis of pelvic congestion syndrome. Both computed tomographic (CT) and magnetic resonance (MR) venography can be used to document compression of the left renal and iliac veins, to measure ovarian vein diameters, and to identify pelvic varices. CT- and MR-based criteria for pelvic congestion syndrome include an ovarian vein diameter greater than 8 mm and more than four tortuous parauterine veins measuring greater than 4 mm in diameter (Fig. 25.3).[15] Unfortunately, standard cross-sectional imaging gives no physiologic information regarding the hemodynamic significance of reflux or

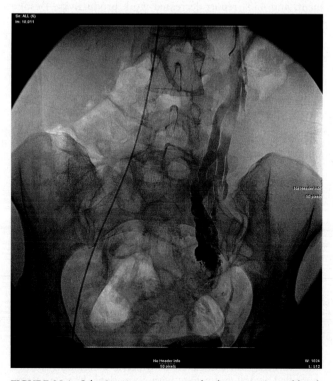

FIGURE 25.1. Selective contrast venography demonstrating a dilated, refluxing left ovarian vein communicating with extensive pelvic varicosities.

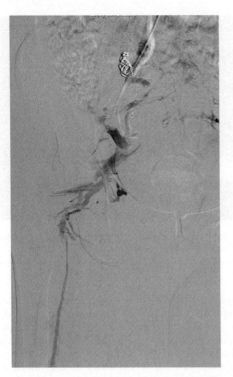

FIGURE 25.2. Balloon occlusion contrast venography demonstrating communication between internal iliac venous tributaries and the great saphenous vein.

obstruction, and the quality of studies varies widely between institutions.

Ultrasound provides a noninvasive means for identifying women who might benefit from diagnostic and therapeutic pelvic venography. Moreover, ultrasound can identify other conditions, such as leiomyoma or endometriosis, which are important in the diagnostic workup of the patient. Both transabdominal and transvaginal ultrasound have been widely used, sometimes in combination, for the evaluation of pelvic congestion syndrome.

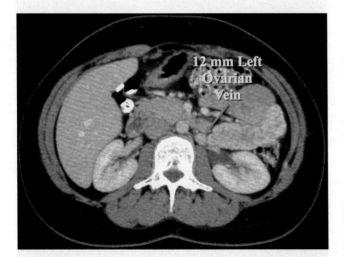

FIGURE 25.3. Computed tomographic (CT) venogram demonstrating dilation of the left ovarian vein to 12 mm in diameter (arrow). Note the position of the ovarian vein immediately above the psoas muscle.

ULTRASOUND TECHNIQUE

The ultrasound evaluation of pelvic congestion syndrome is performed in the fasting patient in both steep reverse Trendelenburg and standing positions. A low-frequency curved array abdominal transducer (2 to 4 MHz) is generally preferred. Setting the Doppler pulse repetition frequency high enough to prevent aliasing but low enough to detect slow venous velocities should optimize evaluation of venous flow.

The inferior vena cava and common iliac veins are initially assessed in a steep reverse Trendelenburg position. The left common iliac vein is specifically examined for evidence of compression by the right common iliac artery that may lead to reflux in the internal iliac veins (Fig. 25.4). The diameters of the internal iliac veins are measured and reflux is identified by asking the patient to perform a Valsalva maneuver, which also accentuates venous filling and improves visualization of pelvic varicosities. The normal pelvic plexus should appear as one or two straight venous structures less than 5 mm in diameter.[16] Reflux in dilated parauterine veins is identified during the Valsalva maneuver and their diameters are measured. The external iliac and common femoral veins are also interrogated for evidence of reflux, obstruction, or prominent venous collaterals.

The right and left ovarian veins are identified above the psoas muscle in the retroperitoneum at about the level of the fourth lumbar vertebra. The right ovarian vein is typically more difficult to identify than the left.[10,16] These veins are then followed to their confluence with the inferior vena cava and left renal vein, respectively (Fig. 25.5). Alternatively, the left ovarian vein can be initially identified in the left upper abdomen in a transverse plane as it joins the left renal vein.[16] Moving the transducer into a longitudinal plane demonstrates the tubular left ovarian vein as it joins the left renal vein at a right angle. The right ovarian vein can be similarly identified centrally in the abdomen at its confluence with the inferior vena cava. Vein diameters are measured along the course of both ovarian veins. Retrograde flow during a Valsalva maneuver is evaluated with both color-flow (Fig. 25.6) and spectral Doppler waveforms (Fig. 25.7).

The left renal vein should also be evaluated for evidence of aortomesenteric compression (nutcracker syndrome). The aorta and superior mesenteric artery are visualized, and the angle between the aorta and proximal superior mesenteric artery is determined in a longitudinal view (Fig. 25.8).

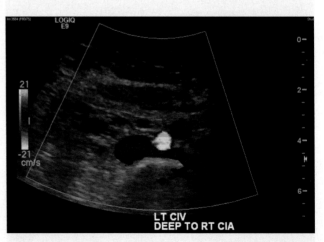

FIGURE 25.4. Cross-sectional color-flow duplex image demonstrating crossing of the left common iliac vein (blue) beneath the right common iliac artery (color aliased—yellow, orange, and blue).

VISCERAL VASCULAR

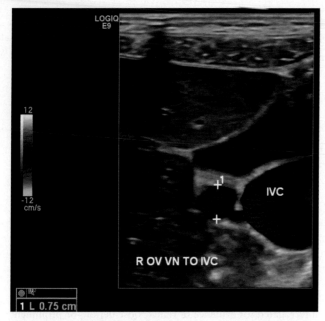

FIGURE 25.5. Color-flow duplex image demonstrating a dilated right ovarian vein at its confluence with the inferior vena cava (IVC). The right ovarian vein measures 0.75 cm in diameter. The ovarian vein is located immediately above the psoas muscle.

Cross-sectional views of the aorta and superior mesenteric artery, with the left renal vein crossing between them, are then obtained in order to measure both diameters and velocities in the left renal vein on the caval side of the aorta, at the aorto-mesenteric angle, and on the renal side of the aorta (Fig. 25.9). Diagnostic accuracy is improved if the examination is then repeated with the patient standing, focusing on the evaluation of the internal iliac veins, ovarian veins, and left renal vein.

Finally, if the patient presents with lower extremity varicosities, the specific pelvic escape points should be evaluated as a source.[11] This should include imaging of the inguinal (I) point at the superficial origin of the inguinal canal and the perineal

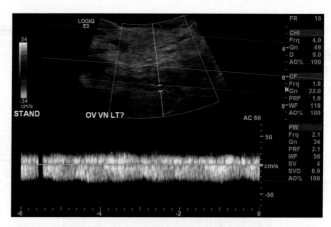

FIGURE 25.7. Doppler spectral waveform showing prolonged reflux in the left ovarian vein in response to a Valsalva maneuver.

(P) point located at the perineal membrane. The obturator (O) point communicating with the common femoral vein and the superior and inferior gluteal (G) points at the midportion of the buttocks and infragluteal fold should similarly be assessed.

Although transvaginal ultrasound is outside the technical scope of most vascular laboratories, it does allow enhanced visualization of the pelvic venous plexus and associated anatomy.[17] The transvaginal ultrasound examination for pelvic congestion syndrome is performed initially in the supine position and then repeated in a steep reverse Trendelenburg position to accentuate venous filling. A higher-frequency transducer is used than for transabdominal ultrasonography, such as a 5- to 9-MHz intracavitary probe. Performed in this manner, the transvaginal ultrasound examination is particularly helpful for evaluating the pelvic venous plexus and associated reflux, the volume of the uterus, and the presence of crossing veins in the uterine myometrium.[16,18] It can also be helpful

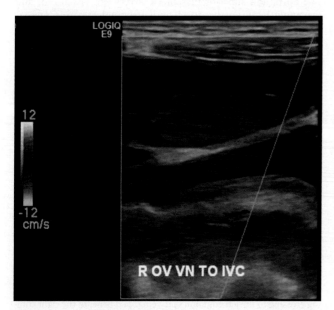

FIGURE 25.6. Color-flow duplex image demonstrating retrograde flow (reflux) in the right ovarian vein in response to a Valsalva maneuver.

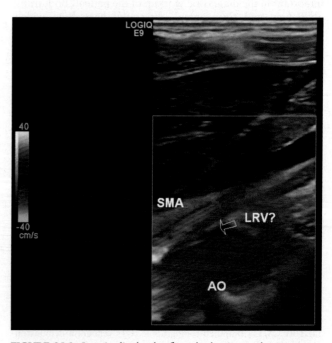

FIGURE 25.8. Longitudinal color-flow duplex image demonstrating compression of the left renal vein (LRV) within the angle formed by the superior mesenteric artery (SMA) anteriorly and the aorta (AO) posteriorly.

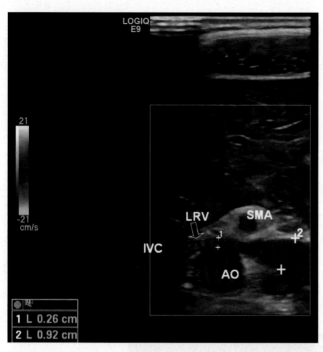

FIGURE 25.9. Cross-sectional image of the left renal vein (LRV) as it passes between the aorta (AO) and superior mesenteric artery (SMA). Velocities and diameters of the left renal vein are measured on the caval (0.26 cm diameter) and renal (0.92 cm diameter) sides of the aorta to determine the respective ratios.

for identifying other pelvic pathologies as a cause of pelvic pain. Unfortunately, it provides little information outside of the pelvis and usually must be supplemented with transabdominal ultrasound to clearly define all sources of reflux and obstruction.[10]

DIAGNOSTIC CRITERIA

As discussed above, the diagnosis of pelvic congestion syndrome depends upon demonstrating complex patterns of reflux and obstruction in the ovarian and internal iliac veins as well as the femoral vein tributaries. Reflux is inferred both from an evaluation of venous diameters and demonstration of retrograde flow during the Valsalva maneuver. Park et al[16] found the mean diameter of the left ovarian vein to be 0.79 cm in women with pelvic congestion syndrome as compared to 0.49 cm in women with other pelvic pathologies. Most vascular laboratories consider an ovarian vein diameter of ≥6 mm to be suggestive of ovarian vein incompetence.[10,16] In comparison to CT or contrast venography, duplex ultrasound has a sensitivity of 100% and specificity of 57% for the detection left ovarian vein dilation. This is somewhat reduced for the right ovarian vein, where the corresponding sensitivity and specificity are 67% and 90%, repectively.[10]

The direction of flow in the left ovarian vein can be visualized in two-thirds of patients with pelvic congestion syndrome and in almost half of the patients with other pelvic pathologies.[16] Retrograde flow in the left ovarian vein was found in 100% of the patients with pelvic congestion syndrome, but in only 25% of the patients who did not have pelvic congestion syndrome. Unlike the lower extremity veins, there are no validated criteria for the duration of retrograde flow that constitutes pathologic reflux in the ovarian or pelvic veins. However, when present, such retrograde flow is usually prolonged and often more than 2 seconds.[10]

Examination of the pelvis in patients with pelvic congestion syndrome should demonstrate dilated, tortuous veins greater than 5 mm in diameter around the ovary and uterus.[16] Dilated myometrial arcuate veins may also be seen crossing the uterus. A Valsalva maneuver should produce a corresponding change in the color-flow image or spectral waveform. Among 32 patients with pelvic congestion syndrome reported by Park et al,[16] pelvic varices were present in 100%, while changes in the Doppler waveform with Valsalva were variable with reversal of flow direction in only 27%.

Similar criteria have been developed for the diagnosis of pelvic congestion syndrome based upon transvaginal ultrasound.[16] Dilated, tortuous parauterine veins greater than 5 mm in diameter can reliably distinguish pelvic congestion syndrome from other pelvic pathologies.[16,19] Reflux is demonstrated by changes in the spectral waveform and color-flow direction with a Valsalva maneuver (Fig. 25.10). Other findings may include an increase in uterine volume and polycystic ovaries as indicators of other estrogen-dependent processes. Among those patients reported by Park et al,[16] varices were identified in all patients with pelvic congestion syndrome in comparison to only 17% of women with chronic pelvic pain due to other pathologies. The mean diameter of the largest left pelvic vein was 0.68 cm in the pelvic congestion group and 0.42 cm in the control group, while the corresponding diameters of the largest right pelvic vein were 0.64 and 0.35 cm, respectively.

Venous obstruction, most commonly from compression of the left common iliac vein or left renal vein, as a contributing factor to pelvic congestion symptoms can also be inferred from ultrasound. Absent or reduced respiratory phasicity in the common femoral vein flow pattern, particularly in comparison to the contralateral side, is suggestive of more proximal iliac vein obstruction (Fig. 25.11). However, normal respiratory flow variability does not exclude subtle degrees of partial obstruction that may be of clinical importance.[11] Others have found a poststenotic to prestenotic velocity ratio of >2.5 to have a sensitivity of 90% for the detection of a >50% venous stenosis in comparison to invasive pressure measurements.[20]

Criteria for diagnosis of the nutcracker syndrome are based on venous diameters and velocities. Examination in the upright position significantly improves diagnostic accuracy. As described above, the left renal vein anterior-posterior diameter is measured at the aortomesenteric angle and near the left renal hilum (Fig. 25.9). A diameter ratio of greater than 5.0 has been reported to have a sensitivity of 69% and specificity

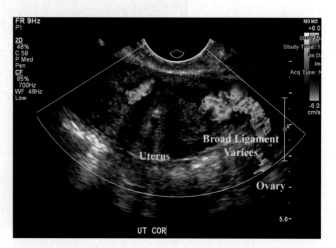

FIGURE 25.10. Transvaginal ultrasound image showing dilated parauterine varices. Reflux, as demonstrated by aliasing of the color-flow image, is seen with a Valsalva maneuver.

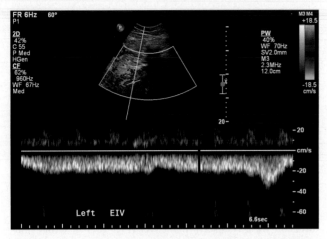

FIGURE 25.11. Continuous venous flow in the absence of respiratory phasicity suggests an obstruction proximal to this patent left external iliac vein (EIV).

of 89% for venographically confirmed nutcracker syndrome. Similarly, the peak velocity is measured at the aortomesenteric angle and near the left renal hilum (Fig. 25.12A and B). A peak velocity ratio of greater than 5 has a sensitivity and specificity of 80% and 94%, respectively.[21] Other potentially important ultrasound findings include the presence of collateral veins on color-flow imaging[22] and the absence of respiratory flow variation in the hilar portion of the vein.[23]

TREATMENT

The treatment of pelvic congestion syndrome is critically dependent on accurate diagnosis of the underlying pathology with options that include medical, endovascular, and surgical approaches. Although ovarian suppression with goserelin, a luteinizing hormone releasing hormone agonist, or medroxyprogesterone provides symptomatic improvement, it is associated with significant undesirable side effects and is not appropriate for long-term management.[4]

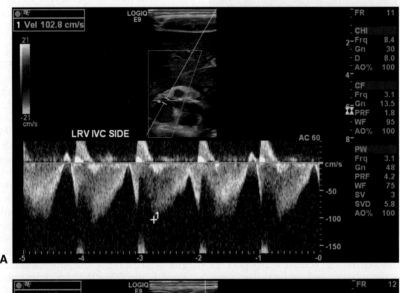

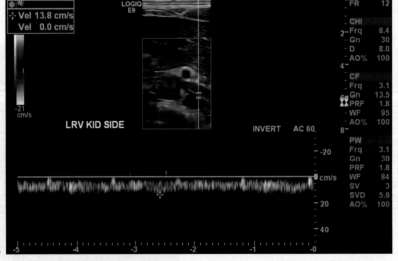

FIGURE 25.12. Nutcracker syndrome. Peak left renal vein velocities are measured (A) at the point of compression beneath the superior mesenteric artery and (B) in the proximal renal vein (kidney side). A velocity ratio greater than 5 is suggestive of aortomesenteric compression (nutcracker syndrome). In this case, the velocity ratio is 102.8/13.8 = 7.45.

VISCERAL VASCULAR

Surgical options for the management of pelvic reflux include hysterectomy and bilateral salpingo-oophorectomy, a morbid procedure with significant reproductive implications, and open or laparoscopic division of the ovarian veins.[24,25] However, such surgical options have largely been replaced by endovascular treatment with sclerotherapy of the pelvic venous plexus and coil embolization of refluxing ovarian and internal iliac veins.[26] Chung and Huh[27] randomized 106 women with chronic pelvic pain unresponsive to medical treatment to ovarian vein embolization; laparoscopic hysterectomy, bilateral salpingo-oophorectomy, and hormone replacement; or laparoscopic hysterectomy and unilateral oophorectomy. Mean pain scores were significantly improved among those undergoing ovarian vein embolization or bilateral oophorectomy, but not among those undergoing unilateral oophorectomy. Pain reduction at 12 months was greatest in those undergoing embolotherapy.

Case reports describe successful treatment of symptomatic internal iliac vein reflux due to compression of the common iliac vein with iliac vein stenting. Although a variety of procedures for management of the nutcracker syndrome have been suggested, the greatest experience has been with left renal vein transposition and endovascular stenting.[28-30] Both procedures appear to provide good relief of flank pain and hematuria, although adjunctive endovascular treatment of associated pelvic varies or varicocele may be required. Surgical morbidity and a small but not insignificant risk of stent migration represent competing risks of the two procedures.

SUMMARY

Reflux and obstruction of the pelvic veins can present in a variety of ways, including classical symptoms of pelvic congestion; vulvar, perineal, gluteal, or more typically distributed great saphenous varicosities; or pelvic symptoms in association with flank pain and hematuria characteristic of the nutcracker syndrome. Appropriate treatment depends on identifying often complex patterns of reflux and obstruction in the interconnected ovarian, internal iliac, and femoral venous systems. Both transabdominal and transvaginal ultrasound play an important role in this regard. The diagnosis of ovarian vein reflux depends on demonstrating retrograde flow in veins larger than 6 mm in diameter, while identification of internal iliac vein reflux similarly depends on showing reflux in response to a provocative Valsalva maneuver. Obstruction associated with compression of the common iliac veins or left renal vein can also cause reflux in the pelvic veins, and diagnosis is based on demonstrating a diameter reduction in these veins with elevated velocity ratios. Although definitive diagnosis and treatment usually rely on contrast venography, ultrasound plays a critical role in identifying patterns of venous disease in symptomatic patients and guiding interventional treatment.

References

1. Taylor HC Jr. Vascular congestion and hyperemia; their effect on function and structure in the female reproductive organs; etiology and therapy. *Am J Obstet Gynecol* 1949;57:654-668.
2. Beard RW, Highman JH, Pearce S, et al. Diagnosis of pelvic varicosities in women with chronic pelvic pain. *Lancet* 1984;2:946-949.
3. Mathias SD, Kuppermann M, Liberman RF, et al. Chronic pelvic pain: Prevalence, health-related quality of life, and economic correlates. *Obstet Gynecol* 1996;87:321-327.
4. Soysal ME, Soysal S, Vicdan K, et al. A randomized controlled trial of goserelin and medroxyprogesterone acetate in the treatment of pelvic congestion. *Hum Reprod* 2001;16:931-939.
5. Sculetus AH, Villavicencio JL, Gillespie DL, et al. The pelvic venous syndromes: Analysis of our experience with 57 patients. *J Vasc Surg* 2002;36:881-888.
6. Beard RW, Reginald PW, Wadsworth J. Clinical features of women with chronic lower abdominal pain and pelvic congestion. *Br J Obstet Gynaecol* 1988;95:153-161.
7. Alimi YS, Hartung O. Iliocaval venous obstruction: Surgical treatment. In: Cronenwett JL, Johnson KW (eds). *Rutherford's Vascular Surgery*, 7th ed. Philadelphia: Saunders, 2010, pp. 919-945.
8. Whitely AM, Taylor DC, Dos Santos SJ, et al. Pelvic venous reflux is a major contributory cause of recurrent varicose veins in more than a quarter of women. *J Vasc Surg: Venous and Lym Dis* 2014; In press.
9. Garland BT, Meissner MH. Renal vein entrapment: The nutcracker syndrome. In: Stanley JC, Veith F, Wakefield TW (eds). *Current Therapy in Vascular Surgery*, 5th ed. Philadelphia: Elsevier Saunders, 2014, pp. 932-935.
10. Malgor RD, Adrahtas D, Spentzouris G, et al. The role of duplex ultrasound in the workup of pelvic congestion syndrome. *J Vasc Surg* 2014;2:34-38.
11. Zygmunt J, Pichot O, Daulplaise T. Venous anatomy. In: Kabnick LS, Sadick N (eds). *Venous Ultrasound*. Boca Raton: CRC Press, 2013, pp. 11-29.
12. Hodgkinson CP. Physiology of the ovarian veins during pregnancy. *Obstet Gynecol* 1953;1:26-37.
13. Rastogi N, Kabutey NK, Kim D. Incapacitating pelvic congestion syndrome in a patient with a history of May-Thurner syndrome and left ovarian vein embolization. *Ann Vasc Surg* 2012;26:732.e7-11.
14. Reginald PW, Beard RW, Kooner JS, et al. Intravenous dihydroergotamine to relieve pelvic congestion with pain in young women. *Lancet* 1987;2:351-353.
15. Coakley FV, Varghese SL, Hricak H. CT and MRI of pelvic varices in women. *J Comput Assist Tomogr* 1999;23:429-434.
16. Park SJ, Lim JW, Ko YT, et al. Diagnosis of pelvic congestion syndrome using transabdominal and transvaginal sonography. *AJR Am J Roentgenol* 2004;182:683-688.
17. Phillips D, Deipolyi AR, Hesketh RL, et al. Pelvic congestion syndrome: Etiology of pain, diagnosis, and clinical management. *J Vasc Interv Radiol* 2014;25:725-733.
18. Durham JD, Machan L. Pelvic congestion syndrome. *Semin Intervent Radiol* 2013;30:372-380.
19. Giacchetto C, Cotroneo GB, Marincolo F, et al. Ovarian varicocele: Ultrasonic and phlebographic evaluation. *J Clin Ultrasound* 1990;18:551-555.
20. Labropoulos N, Borge M, Pierce K, et al. Criteria for defining significant central vein stenosis with duplex ultrasound. *J Vasc Surg* 2007;46:101-107.
21. Kim SH, Cho SW, Kim HD, et al. Nutcracker syndrome: Diagnosis with Doppler US. *Radiology* 1996;198:93-97.
22. Takebayashi S, Ueki T, Ikeda N, et al. Diagnosis of the nutcracker syndrome with color Doppler sonography: Correlation with flow patterns on retrograde left renal venography. *AJR Am J Roentgenol* 1999;172:39-43.
23. Hartung O, Grisoli D, Boufi M, et al. Endovascular treatment of pelvic vein congestion caused by nutcracker syndrome: Lessons learned from the first five cases. *J Vasc Surg* 2005;42:275-280.
24. Beard RW, Kennedy RG, Gangar KF, et al. Bilateral oophorectomy and hysterectomy in the treatment of intractable pelvic pain associated with pelvic congestion. *Br J Obstet Gynaecol* 1991;98:988-992.
25. Gargiulo T, Mais V, Brokaj L, et al. Bilateral laparoscopic transperitoneal ligation of ovarian veins for treatment of pelvic congestion syndrome. *J Am Assoc Gynecol Laparosc* 2003;10:501-504.
26. Venbrux AC, Lambert DL. Embolization of the ovarian veins as a treatment for patients with chronic pelvic pain caused by pelvic venous incompetence (pelvic congestion syndrome). *Curr Opin Obstet Gynecol* 1999;11:395-399.
27. Chung MH, Huh CY. Comparison of treatments for pelvic congestion syndrome. *Tohoku J Exp Med* 2003;201:131-138.
28. Chen S, Zhang H, Shi H, et al. Endovascular stenting for treatment of Nutcracker syndrome: Report of 61 cases with long-term followup. *J Urol* 2011;186:570-575.
29. Reed NR, Kalra M, Bower TC, et al. Left renal vein transposition for nutcracker syndrome. *J Vasc Surg* 2009;49:386–393; discussion 93-94.
30. Wang X, Zhang Y, Li C, et al. Results of endovascular treatment for patients with nutcracker syndrome. *J Vasc Surg* 2012;56:142-148.

SECTION VII ▪ PREOPERATIVE PLANNING, INTRAOPERATIVE ASSESSMENT AND PROCEDURAL GUIDANCE

CHAPTER 26 ■ CARDIOVASCULAR RISK ASSESSMENT IN THE VASCULAR LABORATORY

THAIS COUTINHO AND IFTIKHAR J. KULLO

Cardiovascular (CV) disease remains the leading cause of death in the United States, with an overall rate of death attributable to CV diseases of 236 per 100,000 per year.[1] An estimated 635,000 Americans have a first myocardial infarction (MI) or coronary artery disease–related death, and 610,000 Americans suffer a new stroke each year.[1] These statistics highlight the need for better risk stratification schemes in order to identify those at greatest CV risk and to implement lifestyle and pharmacologic interventions aimed at preventing CV events. Coupled with standard clinical evaluation, newer noninvasive techniques allow earlier and more accurate risk assessment and targeted interventions. This chapter focuses on four noninvasive techniques that can be used in the vascular laboratory for CV risk assessment: ankle-brachial index (ABI), carotid intima-media thickness (CIMT), tonometry for measurement of arterial stiffness, and assessment of endothelial function with brachial artery reactivity.

ANKLE-BRACHIAL INDEX

As discussed in Chapter 13, the ABI is a simple and inexpensive test that can be performed in the vascular laboratory to objectively document the presence and severity of peripheral arterial disease (PAD).[2] Compared to invasive lower extremity angiography, the ABI has high sensitivity (79% to 95%) and specificity (95% to 96%) to detect hemodynamically significant (>50% stenosis) arterial narrowings[3,4] and thus is used as a first-line test for detecting PAD.

A low ABI is indicative of PAD, even in the absence of symptoms, and identifies individuals at higher risk of mortality and CV events who require greater attention toward risk factor management and preventive measures.[5,6] Patients with PAD have a 20% to 60% higher risk of MI, a 40% greater risk of stroke, and a two- to sixfold increase in coronary heart disease death than the general population.[7-9] To help identify these individuals at higher risk of CV events, the American College of Cardiology Foundation/American Heart Association Practice Guidelines for Patients with Peripheral Arterial Disease[10]

recommend obtaining an ABI in patients with suspected PAD, even when they are asymptomatic (Table 26.1).

Patient Preparation, Technique, and Protocol

The patient should be resting supine for 5 to 10 minutes prior to commencing the examination. The ABI is obtained by comparing the blood pressure (BP) in the lower extremities (ankles) with the BP in the upper extremities (brachial arteries). In healthy individuals, pulse wave reflection and peripheral BP augmentation cause the ankle systolic BP to be 10 to 15 mm Hg higher, on average, than the brachial artery systolic pressure. Therefore, the normal ABI is greater than 1.00. Lower ABIs

TABLE 26.1

INDICATIONS FOR MEASURING THE RESTING ANKLE-BRACHIAL INDEX

Symptomatic patients:
Leg symptoms with exertion (suggestive of claudication)
Ischemic rest pain in the lower extremities

Asymptomatic patients:
Age ≥ 65 y
Age ≥ 50 y with a history of diabetes or smoking
Nonhealing lower extremity wounds
Abnormal lower extremity pulse examination

Adapted from the 2011 ACCF/AHA Focused Update of the Guidelines for the Management of Patients with Peripheral Arterial Disease (Rooke TW, et al. 2011 ACCF/AHA focused update of the guideline for the management of patients with peripheral artery disease (updating the 2005 guideline): A report of the American College of Cardiology Foundation/American Heart Association Task Force on Practice Guidelines: Developed in collaboration with the Society for Cardiovascular Angiography and Interventions, Society of Interventional Radiology, Society for Vascular Medicine, and Society for Vascular Surgery. *Catheter Cardiovasc Interv* 2012;79(4):501-531.)

indicate the presence of lower extremity atherosclerotic plaques causing a drop in lower extremity pressures, and thus the ABI varies inversely with PAD severity.

The first step in the examination is to sequentially obtain the systolic BP from both brachial arteries using a stethoscope and calibrated sphygmomanometer. If the brachial BPs differ by more than 10 mm Hg, bilateral brachial BPs should be obtained *simultaneously* by two examiners. If the brachial BP difference persists on simultaneous measurements, this may indicate the presence of subclavian or axillary artery occlusive disease and should be reported. The *higher* of the two brachial BPs should be used as the denominator for the ABI calculations.

Following documentation of the brachial BP, the examiners should turn their attention to recording of the ankle systolic BPs (Fig. 26.1). For optimal lower extremity pressure measurement, BP cuffs should be appropriately sized for the patient's

lower calf (immediately above the ankles); the width of the cuff should be at least 20% greater than the diameter of the limb. A 5- to 10-MHz handheld Doppler should be used, and a clear arterial pulse signal should be heard. The cuff is then inflated to at least 20 mm Hg above the point where the Doppler sounds disappear and then slowly deflated until the Doppler sounds reappear. The BP at which the Doppler signal of the arterial pulse reappears is the systolic BP for that vessel. For each leg, systolic BPs should be documented for both the dorsalis pedis and posterior tibial arteries, and the *higher* BP of the two pedal arteries should be used in the numerator for ABI calculation. For example, in a patient with a right brachial systolic BP of 100 mm Hg, a left brachial systolic BP of 90 mm Hg, a right dorsalis pedis systolic BP of 70 mm Hg, and a right posterior tibial systolic BP of 80 mm Hg, the right lower extremity ABI is calculated as 80 mm Hg/100 mm Hg = 0.80. ABI values should be reported to the second decimal.

Postexercise Ankle-Brachial Index

In a subset of patients with PAD, the resting ABI may be normal. In other patients who have atypical leg symptoms, differentiation of true claudication from pseudoclaudication is warranted. In these cases, measurement of ABI postexercise is helpful. Indications for postexercise ABI are outlined in Table 26.2. From a risk assessment standpoint, obtaining a postexercise ABI is recommended in asymptomatic patients with suspected PAD (see Table 26.1) who have a normal or borderline normal resting ABI (0.91 to 1.40). The resting ABI may fail to document PAD in some patients with mild to moderate disease. In such cases, obtaining postexercise ABIs increases the sensitivity of the test.

Assessment of postexercise ABIs should follow the measurement of resting baseline ABIs. Exercise is performed using a motorized treadmill, and protocols used are less strenuous than are those implemented for assessment of coronary artery disease. Different exercise protocols have been reported.[11,12] In the Mayo Clinic vascular laboratory, patients walk on a treadmill at a steady speed of 2 mph at a 10% grade for 5 minutes or until development of limiting symptoms, whichever comes first. If patients cannot walk at 2 mph, alternative protocols using steady lower speeds (1 or 1.5 mph) are used. Patients should be instructed to walk until maximally tolerated symptoms. Additional information that can be obtained from the exercise test includes: total walking time and distance, time and distance walked before development of leg symptoms (initial claudication distance), laterality of symptoms and muscle groups involved, and presence of nonclaudicatory symptoms such as angina, dyspnea, palpitations, joint pain, or generalized fatigue. Concomitant electrocardiogram (ECG) monitoring allows identification of cardiac arrhythmias or myocardial ischemia. If significant arrhythmias or marked signs of myocardial ischemia (i.e., ST-segment depression >2 mm in ≥2 contiguous leads) occur, the test should be interrupted regardless of leg symptoms.

If measurement of postexercise ABI is indicated but patients are unable to walk on the treadmill (e.g., due to balance problems), up to 50 standing plantar flexions can be performed instead,[13] and the ABI should be repeated immediately following exercise as described above.

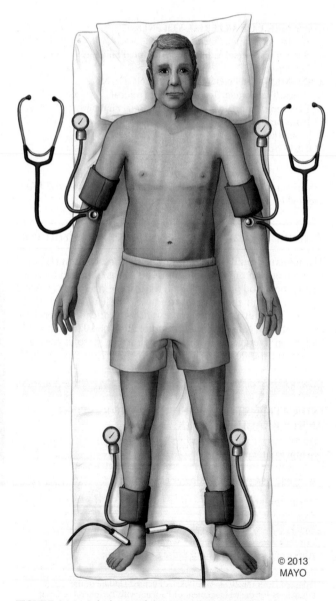

© 2013
MAYO

FIGURE 26.1. Calculation of the ABI. While the patient lies supine, a brachial BP is obtained sequentially in the right and left upper extremities. The higher of the two brachial BPs should be used for ankle-brachial index (ABI) calculation. With cuffs applied to the ankles, a 5- to 10-MHz handheld Doppler is used to measure systolic BP at the dorsalis pedis (DP) and posterior tibial (PT) arteries in both lower extremities. For each leg, the higher of the DP and PT pressures is used for ABI calculation.

Reporting, Normal Values, and Abnormal Findings

ABIs should be reported according to the recommendations from the 2011 ACCF/AHA Focused Update of the Guidelines for the Management of Patients with Peripheral Arterial

TABLE 26.2

INDICATIONS FOR MEASURING THE POSTEXERCISE ANKLE-BRACHIAL INDEX

■ INDICATION	■ RECOMMENDATION
Patients with symptoms of intermittent claudication who have a normal resting ABI (0.91-1.40)	Class I
Patients with atypical leg symptoms, to differentiate true intermittent claudication from nonarterial claudication ("pseudoclaudication")	Class I
Patients with claudication who are to undergo exercise training, with the goal of determining functional capacity, assessing nonvascular exercise limitations, and demonstrating the safety of exercise	Class I
Asymptomatic patients with suspected PAD (age ≥65 y; age ≥50 y with a history of diabetes or smoking; presence of nonhealing lower extremity wounds or abnormal lower extremity pulse examination) who have a normal resting ABI (0.91-1.40)	Class IIa

Adapted from the 2011 ACCF/AHA Focused Update of the Guidelines for the Management of Patients with Peripheral Arterial Disease (Rooke TW, et al. 2011 ACCF/AHA focused update of the guideline for the management of patients with peripheral artery disease (updating the 2005 guideline): A report of the American College of Cardiology Foundation/American Heart Association Task Force on Practice Guidelines: Developed in collaboration with the Society for Cardiovascular Angiography and Interventions, Society of Interventional Radiology, Society for Vascular Medicine, and Society for Vascular Surgery. *Catheter Cardiovasc Interv* 2012;79(4):501-531.)

Disease,[10] as outlined in Table 26.3. A special comment should be made about patients with ABI values >1.40. In patients with stiff, calcified leg arteries that cannot be compressed by the ankle BP cuff (such as seen in the elderly, diabetics, or those with chronic renal insufficiency), pedal systolic BPs will be very high (>240 mm Hg), causing the ABI to exceed 1.40. In such patients with poorly compressible arteries, the risk of death is high, even higher than that observed among patients with documented PAD (ABI ≤ 0.90) (Fig. 26.2).[14]

In addition, gender and race differences in ABI have been previously demonstrated and should be recognized, especially when reporting "borderline abnormal" ABI values. The ABI is lower in African Americans than in non-Hispanic white individuals[15-17] and in women than in men.[17] Applying a single cut-off value for normality in large population studies may lead to overestimation of the prevalence of PAD in women and in African-Americans.

TABLE 26.3

INTERPRETATION OF THE ANKLE-BRACHIAL INDEX

■ ABI VALUE	■ INTERPRETATION
At Rest	
1.00-1.40	Normal
0.91-0.99	Borderline
≤0.90	Abnormal
• *0.81-0.90*	• *Mild disease*
• *0.51-0.80*	• *Moderate disease*
• *≤0.50*	• *Severe disease*
>1.40	Poorly compressible
Postexercise	
0.91-1.40	Normal
0.50-0.90	Mild disease
0.20-0.49	Moderate disease
<0.20	Severe disease

ABI, ankle-brachial index.
Adapted from the 2011 ACCF/AHA Focused Update of the Guideline for the Management of Patients with Peripheral Arterial Disease (Rooke TW, et al. 2011 ACCF/AHA focused update of the guideline for the management of patients with peripheral artery disease (updating the 2005 guideline): A report of the American College of Cardiology Foundation/American Heart Association Task Force on Practice Guidelines: Developed in collaboration with the Society for Cardiovascular Angiography and Interventions, Society of Interventional Radiology, Society for Vascular Medicine, and Society for Vascular Surgery. *Catheter Cardiovasc Interv* 2012;79(4):501-531.)

CAROTID INTIMA-MEDIA THICKNESS

Historically, arterial disease has been evaluated by the presence of atherosclerotic plaques and luminal narrowing. However, such an approach only allows identification of patients with established disease in whom lifestyle and pharmacologic measures are less likely to prevent development of CV events. The mechanisms leading to thickening of the arterial wall are not fully understood, but increased CIMT is thought to represent arterial aging and may be related to intimal or medial hypertrophy or a combination of both, as an adaptive response to changes in flow, wall tension, or lumen diameter.[18] Since atherosclerosis is a complex process that begins in the arterial wall, the process leading to intimal thickening is thought to be similar, although not identical, to that underlying atherosclerosis.[19] This is the basis for the assessment of CIMT, which is an ultrasound-based, sensitive, well-validated, and reproducible technique that can be used for the purpose of CV risk assessment and stratification.

Greater CIMT is associated with CV risk factors[20] and has been shown to be independently associated with a higher risk of adverse CV events. In the Atherosclerosis Risk in Communities (ARIC) study, patients with extreme CIMT values (>1 mm) had a much higher (unadjusted) risk of stroke (hazard ratios of 8.5 in women and 3.6 in men)[21] and MI (hazard ratios of 5.1 in women and 1.9 in men)[22] after 6 to 9 years when compared to those with CIMT <0.6 mm. Similar associations of CIMT with MI and stroke were also observed in the Cardiovascular Health Study[23] and in the Rotterdam Study.[24] Based on these findings, CIMT can be performed to refine risk stratification in asymptomatic patients with intermediate risk of CV events.[25] Indications for measuring CIMT are outlined in Table 26.4. Of note, assessment of CIMT is not of value in patients with established atherosclerotic disease or if the results would not be expected to change clinical management. In addition, there is great interest in assessing CIMT for measuring atherosclerosis progression or regression, but at this time, serial studies of CIMT to monitor disease in clinical practice are not recommended.

PREOPERATIVE PLANNING, INTRAOPERATIVE ASSESSMENT AND PROCEDURAL GUIDANCE

FIGURE 26.2. Risk of mortality based on the ankle-brachial index (ABI) in patients referred for noninvasive lower extremity evaluation. Among patients referred for lower extremity evaluation, those with peripheral arterial disease (PAD; ABI < 0.9) had a higher risk of mortality than those with a normal ABI. In addition, patients with poorly compressible arteries (PCA; ABI > 1.40) had the highest risk of mortality. (Adapted with permission from Arain FA, et al. Survival in patients with poorly compressible leg arteries. *J Am Coll Cardiol* 2012;59(4):400-417.)

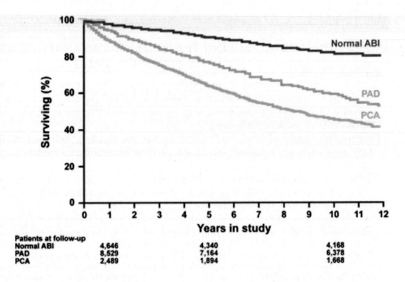

Patient Preparation, Technique, and Protocol

The patient should be lying supine on the examination table with the head slightly tilted toward the opposite side of the carotid artery being examined, while the sonographer is positioned at the head as shown in Figure 26.3. The study should be performed at a standard depth of 4 cm (or higher for patients with thicker necks) using a state-of-the-art ultrasound machine that possesses a linear array transducer with a minimal fundamental frequency of 7 MHz and capable of storing digital images. B-mode imaging is used, and zoom functions should be avoided in order to optimize image resolution.[26]

The first step in the examination is to screen the carotid arteries for the presence of atherosclerotic plaques, defined as areas of wall thickening measuring at least 1.5 mm, or ≥50% thicker than the surrounding walls.[26] The sonographer should then image in the longitudinal plane that visualizes the common carotid artery (CCA) and carotid bulb bifurcating into internal and external carotid arteries, which is considered standard for CIMT assessment (Fig. 26.4). Transducer tilt and pressure as well as image focus and gain should be optimized so that "double lines" are seen in the near and far walls of the CCA (Fig. 26.5). This region should be imaged at three angles (anterior, posterior, and lateral) as indicated in Figure 26.6. A cine loop and three optimized R-wave gated still images of the longitudinal CCA should be obtained from each of these three imaging angles.

The intima-media portion of the vessel wall starts at the luminal edge of the artery and ends at the boundary between the media and the adventitia. The image that most clearly depicts the interface between blood and the intima-media portion of the vessel wall ("double line") should be chosen for analysis, and CIMT should be measured in the far wall of the distal 1 cm of the CCA using a leading edge-to-leading edge technique (Fig. 26.5). Three separate measurements of CIMT should be obtained (one from each imaging angle) and averaged to obtain a final value for each CCA. Although CIMT can be measured manually, use of semi-automated border detection software can improve reproducibility and reduce error and reading time.[27]

TABLE 26.4

INDICATIONS FOR MEASURING CAROTID INTIMA-MEDIA THICKNESS

Asymptomatic adults with intermediate risk of cardiovascular events based on the Framingham Risk Score[a]
Family history of premature cardiovascular disease in a first-degree relative (men <55 y old, women <65 y old)[b]
Adults ≤ 60 y old with severe abnormalities in a single risk factor (e.g., genetic dyslipidemia) who otherwise would not be candidates for pharmacotherapy[b]
Women younger than 60 y with at least two CVD risk factors[b]

[a]Recommendation by the ACCF/AHA guideline for assessment of cardiovascular risk in asymptomatic adults (Greenland, P, et al. 2010 ACCF/AHA guideline for assessment of cardiovascular risk in asymptomatic adults: a report of the American College of Cardiology Foundation/American Heart Association Task Force on Practice Guidelines. *Circulation* 2010;122(25):e584-e636.)
[b]Recommendation by the Consensus Statement from the American Society of Echocardiography Carotid Intima-Media Thickness Task Force (Stein JH, et al. Use of carotid ultrasound to identify subclinical vascular disease and evaluate cardiovascular disease risk: a consensus statement from the American Society of Echocardiography Carotid Intima-Media Thickness Task Force. *Am Soc Echocardiogr* 2008;21(2):93-111; quiz 189-190.)

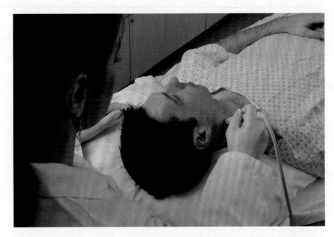

FIGURE 26.3. Proper scanning position for CIMT assessment. Patients lie supine on the examination table with their heads slightly tilted toward the opposite side of the carotid artery being examined while the sonographer is positioned at the head of the bed.

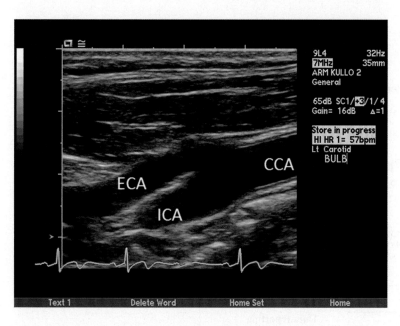

FIGURE 26.4. "Standard" longitudinal plane for CIMT assessment. Sonographers should identify the longitudinal plane that visualizes the common carotid artery (CCA) and carotid bulb bifurcating into internal (ICA) and external (ECA) carotid arteries.

Reporting, Normal Values, and Abnormal Findings

A template for reporting CIMT studies has been recommended by the Consensus Statement from the American Society of Echocardiography Carotid Intima-Media Thickness Task Force[28] and is depicted in Table 26.5. The report should include patient information, indication, standard statements, description of plaques and acoustic shadowing (if present), mean CIMT for each carotid artery, interpretation of the patient's CV risk based on the CIMT values, and relevant incidental findings.

CIMT increases with age, even in the absence of atherosclerosis, and by age 90, CIMT is usually threefold greater than at age 20.[29] In addition, CIMT varies based on race as well as between men and women. Thus, CIMT results need to be interpreted within the context of age, gender, and race. The age-specific CIMT percentiles recommended by the Consensus Statement from the American Society of Echocardiography Carotid Intima-Media Thickness Task Force are listed in Table 26.6.[28] The CIMT values presented here were derived from the Multi-Ethnic Study of Atherosclerosis (MESA), but values obtained from other cohort studies can also be found in the Consensus Statement.

Each patient's CIMT values should be interpreted and reported in terms of CV risk: CIMT values ≤25th percentile represent low CV risk, values between the 25th and 75th percentiles are indicative of average CV risk, and CIMT values ≥75th percentile are associated with high CV risk.

Limitations

Reliable measurement of CIMT requires extensive training and expertise. Technical issues such as body habitus or acoustic shadowing may preclude optimal visualization of the intima-media layer and lead to inaccurate CIMT measurements. There are also multiple protocols for CIMT assessment with different levels of complexity, different measurement sites and angles, and different methods of reporting. Strictly speaking, CIMT values can only be compared if they are obtained using the exact same protocol. The use of a semiautomated edge detection software/algorithm may potentially overestimate CIMT if the computer selects the

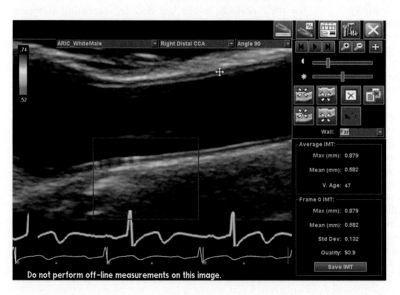

FIGURE 26.5. Carotid intima-media thickness measurement. Images should be optimized so that "double lines" are seen in the near and far walls of the CCA. Border detection software is preferred to achieve accurate measurements of CIMT.

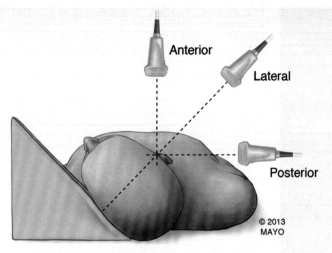

FIGURE 26.6. Angles for imaging the CCA for CIMT assessment. Each carotid artery should be imaged at three angles: anterior, posterior, and lateral.

wrong pixels for measurement. On the other hand, manual measurement of CIMT is subject to greater interobserver variability.[30]

ASSESSMENT OF ARTERIAL STIFFNESS

The aorta is an elastic reservoir that interacts directly with the heart and the end organs, and as such, its role in the human body extends beyond delivery of blood to the peripheral tissues. In individuals with compliant aortas, ventricular-arterial coupling is optimized, thereby maximizing ejection of blood from the left ventricle, while minimizing swings in BP. In addition, by buffering the ample pulsatile load generated by the left ventricle, the elastic aorta protects end organs from the deleterious effects of high pulsatility.[31] The arterial flow pulse is composed not only of forward waves but also reflected pressure waves. With each cardiac cycle, a forward pressure wave is generated by the interaction of the left ventricle with the aorta and is propagated in the arterial wall along the arterial tree. At areas of impedance mismatch (such as branching points and arterioles), part of the pressure wave is reflected back toward the heart. In the setting of preserved aortic elasticity, the velocity of pulse transmission along the compliant arterial wall is low, and the timing and amplitude of reflected waves occur in such a way as to allow mild augmentation of the diastolic pressure at the level of the aortic root, thereby enhancing coronary artery perfusion. Thus, an elastic aorta maximizes the efficiency of the cardiovascular system and protects the end organs from excess pulsatility.

With aging, there is progressive stiffening of the aorta[32] due to fatigue and fragmentation of elastic fibers and increased collagen deposition in the arterial wall. Aortic stiffening is further exacerbated in the presence of CV risk factors, especially hypertension, diabetes, and renal insufficiency.[33] As the aorta stiffens, afterload (particularly pulsatile load) increases, leading to an imbalance in ventricular-arterial coupling.[34] One consequence of this is an increased risk of heart failure, particularly heart failure with preserved ejection fraction.[35,36] In addition, a stiffer aorta leads to greater variations in pressure during cardiac ejection, increasing pulse pressure and promoting the delivery of highly pulsatile energy to the end organs. This can be particularly deleterious in organs with high blood

TABLE 26.5

REPORTING OF CAROTID INTIMA-MEDIA THICKNESS STUDIES FOR CARDIOVASCULAR RISK ASSESSMENT

Patient information
- Name, date of birth, medical record/identification number
- Sex
- Race/ethnicity
- Ordering health care provider
- Indication

Statements
- This is a screening carotid ultrasound study for CVD risk assessment.
- This study is not a replacement for a clinically indicated carotid duplex ultrasound.
- This study measures the thickness of the walls of the carotid arteries and identifies the presence of carotid plaques.
- Percentile values do not represent percent stenosis.
- Summary of scanning protocol (i.e., right and left CCA)

Data reporting
- Describe carotid plaques (presence/absence, carotid segment, near or far wall)
- Presence of acoustic shadowing (optional)
- Mean CIMT values for each side
- Percentile range for each CIMT value, relative to the patient's age, sex, and race/ethnicity
- Other clinically relevant findings (i.e., possible obstructive carotid artery disease, thyroid abnormalities, lymphadenopathy)
- Interpretation
- Level of CVD risk and relative risk associated with patient's CIMT

Adapted from the Consensus Statement from the American Society of Echocardiography.
Carotid Intima-Media Thickness Task Force Endorsed by the Society for Vascular Medicine (Stein JH, et al. Use of carotid ultrasound to identify subclinical vascular disease and evaluate cardiovascular disease risk: a consensus statement from the American Society of Echocardiography Carotid Intima-Media Thickness Task Force. *Am Soc Echocardiogr* 2008;21(2):93-111; quiz 189-190.)

flow and low impedance, such as the brain and the kidneys. As such, increased arterial stiffness has been shown to be associated with target-organ damage.[30,37,38]

For these reasons, in the last decade, increasing attention has been given to the function and elastic properties of the aorta. Greater arterial stiffness is a predictor of adverse CV events,[39,40] total and CV mortality,[41,42] and is also associated with the incidence of heart failure,[43] atrial fibrillation,[44] cerebral small vessel disease,[45] and cognitive decline.[46,47] Furthermore, measuring arterial stiffness is useful in helping to more accurately classify CV risk.[48,49] The European Societies of Cardiology and Hypertension currently recommend measuring arterial stiffness in all hypertensives, where the technique is available, in order to better assess risk of CV diseases and end-organ damage.[50]

Arterial stiffness can be measured in the peripheral and central (aorta) arteries, but since the aorta is the most compliant artery in the human body, its assessment is the most robust for risk assessment purposes. The carotid-femoral pulse wave velocity (cfPWV), also called aortic pulse wave velocity, can be measured by several techniques, but arterial tonometry is considered the gold standard for noninvasive measurement of aortic stiffness.[51] This measurement requires relatively little technical expertise, is reproducible, and has the

TABLE 26.6

COMMON CAROTID ARTERY CIMT VALUES (in mm) ACCORDING TO AGE, SEX, RACE, AND PERCENTILES

RIGHT COMMON CAROTID ARTERY—MEAN OF FAR WALL MEASUREMENTS (in mm)

	WHITE MALES				WHITE FEMALES				BLACK MALES				BLACK FEMALES			
Age (years)	45-54	55-64	65-74	75-84	45-54	55-64	65-74	75-84	45-54	55-64	65-74	75-84	45-54	55-64	65-74	75-84
25th percentile	0.52	0.57	0.65	0.72	0.51	0.55	0.65	0.72	0.58	0.61	0.71	0.74	0.55	0.60	0.65	0.71
50th percentile	0.62	0.68	0.77	0.83	0.58	0.65	0.75	0.83	0.67	0.74	0.85	0.85	0.64	0.71	0.76	0.83
75th percentile	0.71	0.81	0.92	0.97	0.67	0.76	0.87	0.93	0.80	0.92	0.99	1.02	0.74	0.81	0.92	0.96

	CHINESE MALES				CHINESE FEMALES				HISPANIC MALES				HISPANIC FEMALES			
Age (years)	45-54	55-64	65-74	75-84	45-54	55-64	65-74	75-84	45-54	55-64	65-74	75-84	45-54	55-64	65-74	75-84
25th percentile	0.54	0.56	0.62	0.66	0.55	0.54	0.59	0.67	0.53	0.60	0.65	0.71	0.51	0.57	0.65	0.63
50th percentile	0.64	0.70	0.73	0.79	0.60	0.63	0.71	0.77	0.62	0.67	0.78	0.81	0.58	0.69	0.76	0.78
75th percentile	0.73	0.83	0.92	0.98	0.70	0.77	0.84	0.96	0.73	0.82	0.90	0.92	0.67	0.77	0.87	0.92

LEFT COMMON CAROTID ARTERY—MEAN OF FAR WALL MEASUREMENTS (in mm)

	WHITE MALES				WHITE FEMALES				BLACK MALES				BLACK FEMALES			
Age (years)	45-54	55-64	65-74	75-84	45-54	55-64	65-74	75-84	45-54	55-64	65-74	75-84	45-54	55-64	65-74	75-84
25th percentile	0.54	0.57	0.67	0.71	0.50	0.55	0.63	0.70	0.56	0.63	0.69	0.72	0.54	0.59	0.63	0.68
50th percentile	0.63	0.69	0.81	0.85	0.58	0.64	0.73	0.80	0.69	0.75	0.82	0.85	0.63	0.67	0.76	0.78
75th percentile	0.78	0.82	0.95	1.00	0.67	0.75	0.85	0.94	0.81	0.92	0.99	1.02	0.73	0.80	0.90	0.91

	CHINESE MALES				CHINESE FEMALES				HISPANIC MALES				HISPANIC FEMALES			
Age (years)	45-54	55-64	65-74	75-84	45-54	55-64	65-74	75-84	45-54	55-64	65-74	75-84	45-54	55-64	65-74	75-84
25th percentile	0.55	0.57	0.62	0.69	0.49	0.52	0.58	0.64	0.55	0.61	0.68	0.72	0.51	0.58	0.62	0.68
50th percentile	0.63	0.70	0.72	0.84	0.58	0.63	0.71	0.76	0.64	0.72	0.80	0.86	0.58	0.68	0.72	0.77
75th percentile	0.73	0.84	0.86	0.97	0.67	0.72	0.87	0.94	0.75	0.85	0.98	0.97	0.68	0.79	0.86	0.91

Values obtained from the Consensus Statement from the American Society of Echocardiography Carotid Intima-Media Thickness Task Force Endorsed by the Society for Vascular Medicine (Stein JH, et al. Use of carotid ultrasound to identify subclinical vascular disease and evaluate cardiovascular disease risk: a consensus statement from the American Society of Echocardiography Carotid Intima-Media Thickness Task Force. *Am Soc Echocardiogr* 2008;21(2):93-111; quiz 189-190.)

PREOPERATIVE PLANNING, INTRAOPERATIVE ASSESSMENT AND PROCEDURAL GUIDANCE

largest amount of evidence for predicting CV events.[41] This parameter assesses the velocity of transmission of the pressure wave along the aortic wall, based on the principle that pulse wave velocity (PWV) varies directly with the stiffness of the arterial wall:

$$PWV = \sqrt{(Yh/2\rho r)}$$

where Y is Young's modulus (a measure of stiffness of an elastic material), h is wall thickness, ρ is blood viscosity, and r is arterial radius. The carotid and femoral arteries are used for measuring aortic PWV since these are superficial, easily accessible, and the distance between them comprises most of the length of the aorta.

Arterial tonometry also allows systolic pulse contour analysis (SPCA), which yields several central arterial hemodynamic parameters, such as the central systolic, diastolic, and pulse pressure and the aortic augmentation index. The central pulse pressure (CPP) is a global measure of arterial stiffness and has been shown to be a better predictor of CV events than brachial pulse pressure,[52,53] highlighting the incremental benefit of assessing central hemodynamics instead of relying on brachial BP alone. In a recent meta-analysis, each 10 mm Hg increase in CPP led to a 14% increase in the risk of CV events.[42] The augmentation index (AIx) is a measure of peripheral wave reflections and has also been shown to predict adverse CV events and mortality[42]; however, its prognostic value in community-based cohorts remains poorly defined.

Patient Preparation, Technique, and Protocol

Arterial stiffness can be measured using a variety of techniques including arterial tonometry, carotid ultrasound, aortic magnetic resonance imaging, and finger photoplethysmography.[51] This discussion will focus on arterial tonometry, a relatively simple, noninvasive technique that can be performed in the office or in the vascular laboratory.

Several preparatory steps help to ensure accurate data. The patient should be instructed to refrain from smoking, eating, or drinking beverages containing caffeine for a minimum of 3 hours, and from drinking alcoholic beverages for at least 10 hours prior to the study. Patients should rest supine for at least 10 minutes before commencing the examination, which is also performed in the supine position. Patients should not speak or sleep during the study. In cases of repeated measurements on the same patient, studies should be performed at the time of the day. ECG leads should be applied to the chest and connected to the arterial tonometry system, since all measurements are signal-averaged based on the ECG. Brachial BP should be measured three times, at 2-minute intervals, using a stethoscope and calibrated sphygmomanometer; the mean of the three BPs is entered into the system and used for calibration of the arterial pressure waveforms. The measurement of cfPWV is performed by arterial tonometry, utilizing one of several commercially available systems.

The examiner should record the distances between the carotid artery sampling site and the sternal notch, and between the sternal notch and the femoral artery sampling site using body surface calipers. Measurement tapes should be avoided since they may overestimate the sternal notch-femoral artery distance in patients with large abdominal girth. The distance from the carotid location to the sternal notch is then subtracted from the distance between the sternal notch and the femoral location, and this final distance is used to estimate aortic length for the cfPWV calculation. Next, the examiner should sequentially obtain carotid and femoral artery pressure tracings using a high-fidelity applanation tonometer, avoiding delays between measurements at the two sites (Fig. 26.7). Such tracings are obtained by identifying the carotid and femoral artery pulses, then pressing the tonometer against these sites, causing gentle flattening of the artery and allowing recording of the arterial pressure waveform. Excessive pressure can lead to loss of the features of the contour of the pressure waveform and should be avoided. Pressure and tilt of the tonometer should be optimized until clear arterial tonometry waveforms are consistently obtained. For carotid tonometry, if respiratory motion interferes with the quality of the pressure signal, patients should be asked to hold their breath for a few seconds until a steady, high-quality signal is obtained. When obtained properly, pressure waveforms from arterial tonometry are virtually identical to those obtained with intra-arterial catheters. Examples of high-quality carotid and femoral artery tonometry pressure tracings are depicted in Figure 26.8. Once the carotid and femoral pressure tracings are recorded, the system utilizes the R-wave of the ECG signal as the fiducial point to estimate the time delay between the carotid and femoral artery waveforms. The cfPWV (in m/s) is then calculated as:

$$PWV = D/t$$

where D is the distance between the carotid and femoral sampling sites (in meters) and t is the time delay between carotid and femoral artery waveforms (in seconds).

For SPCA, an aortic pressure waveform is derived, which can be obtained using: (1) a carotid pressure waveform as a surrogate for central aortic pressure (given its proximity to the aorta) or (2) a radial artery pressure waveform using a validated transfer function (Fig. 26.7).[54,55] Once the aortic pressure waveform is obtained, several hemodynamic parameters can be calculated (Fig. 26.9). The CPP is calculated as the difference between central systolic and diastolic BP, represented by the peak and trough of the arterial waveform. The systolic portion of the aortic waveform has two peaks: The first peak (P1) represents the forward pressure wave, and the second peak (P2) represents the contribution of the reflected pressure wave to the central systolic BP. Thus, the augmented pressure (AP) is calculated as P2-P1, and the AIx as the ratio AP/CPP. The time of arrival of the reflected waveform (Tr), in milliseconds, can also be calculated as the time delay between the onset of P1 and the onset of P2.

Other important central hemodynamic parameters, such as the aortic characteristic impedance, total arterial compliance, proximal aortic compliance, the global reflection coefficient, and the amplitude of the forward and reflected pressure waves, can also be obtained by integrating arterial tonometry with echocardiography.[36,56] However, given the lack of prognostic data associated with these measures, these are currently only measured in the research setting.

Reporting, Normal Values, and Abnormal Findings

Several previous studies have suggested reference values for arterial stiffness parameters; however, results vary based on the population studied (general population, normotensives, hypertensives, young or elderly). The reader is referred to the Expert Consensus Statement on Arterial Stiffness for a summary of previously reported normal values for different arterial stiffness measures.[51]

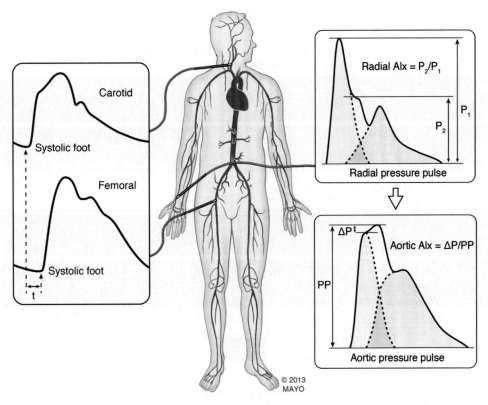

FIGURE 26.7. Carotid-femoral pulse wave velocity measurement and derivation of central pressure waveform from radial artery tonometry. *LEFT:* The distances from the suprasternal notch to the carotid pulse (SSN-C) and to the femoral pulse (SSN-F) are measured in meters with calipers, and aortic length (L) is estimated as (SSN-F) – (SSN-C). Arterial tonometry waveforms are obtained with ECG gating at the carotid and femoral arteries, and the time delay from onset of the carotid waveform to onset of the femoral waveform (t) is documented in seconds. Carotid-femoral pulse wave velocity is calculated as: cfPWV = D/t in m/s. *RIGHT:* An aortic pressure waveform can be derived from a radial artery pressure waveform using a validated transfer function.

Limitations

The presence of atrial dysrhythmias, such as atrial fibrillation or frequent ectopy, may preclude accurate measurements of central hemodynamics by arterial tonometry and results should be interpreted with caution in that setting. Despite being considered the gold standard measure of aortic stiffness, the cfPWV does not accurately reflect the stiffness of the proximal ascending aorta, given the parallel blood flow transmission to the carotid arteries and aortic arch. Also, calculation of cfPWV relies on skin surface measurements to estimate the length of the aorta, which may be inaccurate, especially in patients with tortuous aortas. A limitation of the AIx in the prediction of CV risk is that, starting at about age 60, the AIx tends to plateau and even slightly decline due to predominant stiffening of the aorta and a decrease in the impedance mismatch between the aorta and distal arteries.[56] Consequently, AIx may not accurately predict CV risk in elderly patients.

ASSESSMENT OF ENDOTHELIAL FUNCTION

The vascular endothelium is a biochemically active paracrine organ that, in the healthy state, balances the production of vasodilatory, antimitogenic, and antithrombotic substances. A hallmark of endothelial dysfunction is reduced nitric oxide

bioavailability. Nitric oxide is not only a potent vasodilator, but it also inhibits platelet adhesion and aggregation, leukocyte adhesion and migration, and smooth muscle cell proliferation,[57] processes that are implicated in atherogenesis. Thus, endothelial dysfunction is considered the first stage in the atherosclerotic process and has been shown to precede morphologic arterial changes.[58] For this reason, there is intense interest in noninvasively assessing endothelial function for CV risk assessment, with the intent of identifying individuals at early stages of the atherosclerotic cascade.

Initial methods of assessing endothelial function were invasive and involved infusing acetylcholine in a coronary arterial bed followed by assessment of change in blood flow.[59] Subsequently, noninvasive techniques utilizing peripheral arterial beds have been used, since endothelial dysfunction is thought to be a systemic process. The two main methods used for endothelial function assessment are brachial artery reactivity testing (BART) and EndoPAT (peripheral arterial tonometry). Since BART is the most widely used noninvasive technique for assessing endothelial function and yields the greatest amount of prognostic data, it will be the focus of this discussion.

BART involves evaluation of vasodilation of the forearm arteries in response to ischemic hyperemic flow. Several parameters can be obtained from BART, including baseline forearm blood flow, reactive hyperemic flow, and flow-mediated dilation (FMD). This technique is based on the principle that, in a person with healthy endothelium, forearm arteries and arterioles will dilate in response to a marked increase in forearm

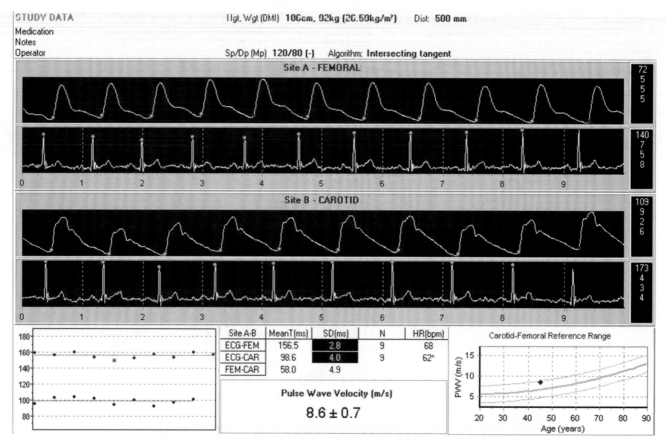

FIGURE 26.8. High-quality femoral and carotid artery pressure tracings obtained with an applanation tonometer.

blood flow during reactive hyperemia. This increase in reactive hyperemic flow itself is thought to be nitric oxide dependent[60,61] and to reflect the endothelial function of the microvasculature. In addition, the increase in shear stress at the endothelial surface caused by hyperemic blood flow leads to dilation of the brachial artery, mainly due to nitric oxide, prostacyclin, and other endothelial vasodilators.[61] This increase in diameter of the brachial artery during hyperemia is called FMD and is thought to represent the endothelial function of larger conduit arteries. Peripheral endothelial function assessed by BART correlates modestly with coronary endothelial function.[62]

Previous studies have investigated the association of BART with CV events. BART is associated with adverse CV events in patients with PAD,[63] in healthy postmenopausal women,[64] in patients being evaluated for chest pain,[65] and in community-dwelling subjects without known vascular disease.[66-68] The prognostic value of BART has also been confirmed in large epidemiologic studies. In the MESA study, low FMD (less than the median of 4.2% in women and 3.6% in men) independently predicted CV events, and using FMD in combination with the Framingham Risk Score classified a subject's risk better than each strategy alone.[69] Similarly, in elderly subjects from the Cardiovascular Health Study, those with normal FMD had higher event-free survival than those with low FMD, independent of conventional risk factors.[70] However, the incremental risk information was small, and at present, the utility of BART for CV risk assessment in the vascular laboratory is unclear.

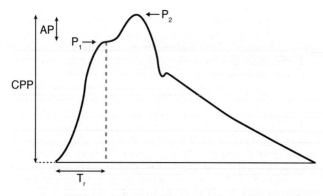

FIGURE 26.9. Central (aortic) pressure waveform. Several hemodynamic parameters can be obtained from the central pressure waveform. The difference between central systolic and diastolic BPs is the central pulse pressure (CPP). The difference between the second systolic peak (P2) and the first systolic peak (P1) is the augmented pressure (AP). The ratio AP/CPP is the augmentation index (AIx). The time from the foot of the pressure wave to the arrival of the reflected wave is the reflected wave arrival time (Tr).

Patient Preparation, Technique, and Protocol

Several steps should be followed prior to BART, since caffeine, tobacco, alcohol, certain foods, and vasoactive drugs may temporarily alter endothelial function. Beginning 8 to 12 hours before the study patients should be instructed to fast and refrain from exercising, smoking, or consuming caffeinated beverages, vitamin C, or high-fat foods. Brachial BP should be measured before commencing the study. Then, a BP cuff is placed at the forearm, below the antecubital fossa, in preparation for BART.

BART should be performed in a quiet, dark room with controlled temperature and the patient lying in the supine position.

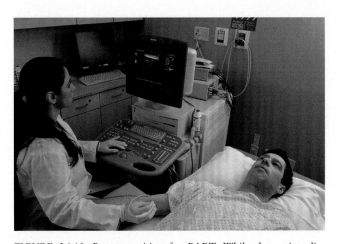

FIGURE 26.10. Proper position for BART. While the patient lies supine, the right arm (or left, if scanning is done from the left side) should be extended and rest comfortably on a support board in order to expose the brachial artery.

The right arm (or left, if scanning is done from the left side) should be extended and rest comfortably on a support board in order to expose the brachial artery (Fig. 26.10). ECG leads should be applied to the chest and connected to the ultrasound machine. The study should be performed using ultrasound systems equipped with vascular software and a high-frequency vascular transducer (broadband linear array transducer with a minimal frequency of 7 MHz).

The brachial artery is imaged in the antecubital fossa at baseline, longitudinally in gray-scale 2D mode (Fig. 26.11), and a segment showing a distinct blood/vessel wall interface and clear visualization of the intima should be chosen for examination. Transducer pressure and tilt, and image depth and gain, should be adjusted to optimize image quality. During image acquisition, the sonographer should note surrounding anatomic landmarks, such as veins and fascial planes, in order to maintain a steady image during the examination. Where available, a probe-holding device can be used to ensure a constant image location. The second step is to utilize pulsed-wave Doppler to estimate resting brachial blood flow (Fig. 26.12). The angle of insonation should be kept at less than 60 degrees.

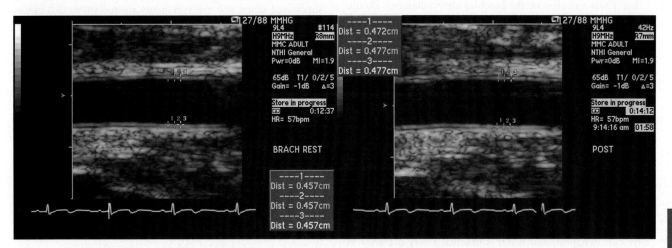

FIGURE 26.11. Longitudinal 2D image of the brachial artery at baseline and during hyperemia. *Left,* Brachial artery diameter at baseline. *Right,* Brachial artery diameter after cuff release (hyperemia). The average of three measurements is obtained both at baseline and during hyperemia. In this example, the average brachial artery diameter was 0.46 cm at baseline and 0.48 cm during hyperemia. The flow-mediated dilation (FMD) was 4%.

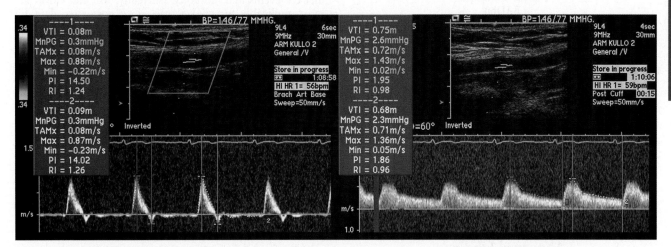

FIGURE 26.12. Baseline and hyperemic brachial artery flow. *Left,* Pulsed-wave Doppler of the brachial artery is obtained to estimate baseline brachial artery flow. *Right,* Pulsed-wave Doppler of the brachial artery is obtained immediately after cuff release to estimated hyperemic brachial artery flow. Note that, in this example, the brachial artery velocity-time integral (VTI) increased nearly eightfold during hyperemia.

The third step is to induce ischemia by inflating a BP cuff on the forearm to at least 50 mm Hg above systolic BP for 5 minutes. Of note, the brachial artery should be imaged continuously, starting at 30 seconds before cuff inflation and ending at 2 minutes after cuff deflation. Brachial artery pulsed-wave Doppler is then repeated immediately upon cuff release and no longer than 15 seconds after cuff deflation to estimate reactive hyperemic flow (Fig. 26.12).

An optional fourth step consists of administering nitroglycerin to assess endothelium-independent vasodilation. Patients should be allowed to rest for 10 minutes after cuff deflation. The longitudinal image of the brachial artery should be obtained again to reestablish a baseline brachial artery diameter. Then, a sublingual 0.4-mg tablet or spray of nitroglycerin is administered to the patient, as an exogenous nitric oxide donor, to assess endothelium-independent vascular smooth muscle function. Contraindications to nitroglycerin administration include significant bradycardia, hypotension, or use of phosphodiesterase type 5 inhibitors within the preceding 24 hours. The brachial artery should be imaged continuously for 5 minutes, as peak vasodilation is expected to occur 3 to 4 minutes after nitroglycerin administration.

For FMD calculation, the brachial artery diameter should be recorded before cuff inflation and 60 seconds after cuff deflation and measured again before and 3 to 4 minutes after nitroglycerin administration utilizing the extra-arterial anatomic landmarks to ensure that the measurement site is the same before and after. The boundaries for brachial artery diameter measurement consist of the lumen-intima interfaces on the near and far walls, and this can be done either manually using electronic calipers or automatically with the use of edge detection software. Brachial artery diameter should always be measured at the same part of the cardiac cycle, preferably during diastole (using the ECG for points of reference). FMD (endothelium-dependent vasodilation) is calculated as:

$$\frac{(BADh - BADr)}{BADr}$$

where BADh is brachial artery diameter during hyperemia (after cuff deflation) and BADr is brachial artery diameter at resting baseline. Similarly, brachial artery diameter should be measured before and after nitroglycerin administration, and the endothelium-independent vasodilation is calculated as:

$$\frac{(BADan - BADbn)}{BADbn}$$

where BADan is brachial artery diameter after nitroglycerin and BADbn is brachial artery diameter before nitroglycerin. To estimate reactive hyperemia flow, the velocity-time integral obtained by pulsed-wave Doppler before cuff inflation and in the first 15 seconds after cuff deflation is recorded. At least three cardiac cycles should be measured, and their average is used for analysis. Reactive hyperemia flow is expressed as:

$$\frac{(BAFh - BAFb)}{BAFb}$$

where BAFh is the brachial artery flow during hyperemia and BAFb is baseline brachial artery flow.

Reporting, Normal Values, and Abnormal Findings

FMD and reactive hyperemic flow are generally reported as a percent of the baseline brachial artery diameter and flow, respectively. Currently, normative data for brachial FMD and

hyperemic flow are lacking. Among healthy individuals, different studies reported mean FMD to be as high as 19.2%.[71]

Peripheral Arterial Tonometry (Endopat)

Peripheral arterial tonometry (EndoPAT) is another noninvasive tool for endothelial function assessment. With the use of plethysmography, it detects pressure changes in the finger tips caused by the arterial pulse, translating them into a peripheral arterial tone (PAT). Endothelium-mediated changes in vascular tone after occlusion of the brachial artery reflect a downstream hyperemic response that correlates with endothelial function. Simultaneous measurements on the contralateral arm are used to control for non–endothelium-dependent changes in vascular tone.[72]

Limitations

BART requires extensive training due to the precise site, sequence, and timing of the images obtained. One hundred supervised scans and measurements are recommended before independent scanning, and 100 yearly scans are recommended to maintain competency.[73] In addition, since FMD is calculated based on diameter changes that are fractions of a millimeter, BART is subject to inter- and intraobserver variability, which is likely related to issues such as different locations of measurements and different durations of cuff occlusion.[73] In addition, factors such as mental or physical stress, a recent meal, medications, vitamins, exogenous hormones, the menstrual cycle, and time of day can potentially affect BART results. Since there are no current reference values for FMD or hyperemic flow, the clinical applicability of this technique is limited, and its main use remains in the scientific arena.

CONCLUSIONS

Prevention and early detection should be at the forefront of clinical care and global health policies in order to limit the devastating clinical and socioeconomic consequences of adverse CV events. Several noninvasive techniques, such as ABI, CIMT, arterial stiffness assessment, and BART, have been shown to correlate with CV risk factors and also to predict CV events and mortality. Currently, ABI and CIMT are most applicable for clinical use, since normative data for these techniques are available. However, arterial stiffness assessment is also a useful risk assessment tool with robust prognostic data, and its clinical utility will be enhanced by publication of reference values based on large community-based cohorts. Assessment of endothelial dysfunction by BART remains primarily a research tool, as its clinical utility is not fully defined.

References

1. Go AS, et al. Heart disease and stroke statistics—2013 update: A report from the American Heart Association. *Circulation* 2013;127(1):e6-e245.
2. Meijer WT, et al. Peripheral arterial disease in the elderly: The Rotterdam Study. *Arterioscler Thromb Vasc Biol* 1998;18(2):185-192.
3. Carter SA. Clinical measurement of systolic pressures in limbs with arterial occlusive disease. *JAMA* 1969;207(10):1869-1874.
4. Lijmer JG, et al. ROC analysis of noninvasive tests for peripheral arterial disease. *Ultrasound Med Biol* 1996;22(4):391-398.
5. Hooi JD, et al. Risk factors and cardiovascular diseases associated with asymptomatic peripheral arterial occlusive disease. The Limburg PAOD Study. Peripheral Arterial Occlusive Disease. *Scand J Prim Health Care* 1998;16(3):177-182.

6. Hooi JD, et al. Incidence of and risk factors for asymptomatic peripheral arterial occlusive disease: A longitudinal study. *Am J Epidemiol* 2001;153(7):666-672.

7. Leng GC, et al. Incidence, natural history and cardiovascular events in symptomatic and asymptomatic peripheral arterial disease in the general population. *Int J Epidemiol* 1996;25(6):1172-1181.

8. Kornitzer M, et al. Ankle/arm pressure index in asymptomatic middle-aged males: An independent predictor of ten-year coronary heart disease mortality. *Angiology* 1995;46(3):211-219.

9. Criqui MH, et al. Mortality over a period of 10 years in patients with peripheral arterial disease. *N Engl J Med* 1992;326(6):381-386.

10. Rooke TW, et al. 2011 ACCF/AHA focused update of the guideline for the management of patients with peripheral artery disease (updating the 2005 guideline): A report of the American College of Cardiology Foundation/American Heart Association Task Force on Practice Guidelines: Developed in collaboration with the Society for Cardiovascular Angiography and Interventions, Society of Interventional Radiology, Society for Vascular Medicine, and Society for Vascular Surgery. *Catheter Cardiovasc Interv* 2012;79(4):501-531.

11. Gardner AW, et al. Progressive vs single-stage treadmill tests for evaluation of claudication. *Med Sci Sports Exerc* 1991;23(4):402-408.

12. Nagle FJ, Balke B, Naughton JP. Gradational step tests for assessing work capacity. *J Appl Physiol* 1965;20(4):745-748.

13. McPhail IR, et al. Intermittent claudication: An objective office-based assessment. *J Am Coll Cardiol* 2001;37(5):1381-1385.

14. Arain FA, et al. Survival in patients with poorly compressible leg arteries. *J Am Coll Cardiol* 2012;59(4):400-407.

15. Kullo IJ, et al. Ethnic differences in peripheral arterial disease in the NHLBI Genetic Epidemiology Network of Arteriopathy (GENOA) study. *Vasc Med* 2003;8(4):237-242.

16. Singh S, Bailey KR, Kullo IJ. Ethnic differences in ankle brachial index are present in middle-aged individuals without peripheral arterial disease. *Int J Cardiol* 2013;162(3):228-233.

17. Aboyans V, et al. Intrinsic contribution of gender and ethnicity to normal ankle-brachial index values: The Multi-Ethnic Study of Atherosclerosis (MESA). *J Vasc Surg* 2007;45(2):319-327.

18. Bots ML, Hofman A, Grobbee DE. Increased common carotid intima-media thickness. Adaptive response or a reflection of atherosclerosis? Findings from the Rotterdam Study. *Stroke* 1997;28(12):2442-2447.

19. Pignoli P, et al. Intimal plus medial thickness of the arterial wall: a direct measurement with ultrasound imaging. *Circulation* 1986;74(6):1399-1406.

20. Salonen R, Salonen JT. Determinants of carotid intima-media thickness: A population-based ultrasonography study in eastern Finnish men. *J Intern Med* 1991;229(3):225-231.

21. Chambless LE, et al. Carotid wall thickness is predictive of incident clinical stroke: The Atherosclerosis Risk in Communities (ARIC) study. *Am J Epidemiol* 2000;151(5):478-487.

22. Chambless LE, et al. Association of coronary heart disease incidence with carotid arterial wall thickness and major risk factors: The Atherosclerosis Risk in Communities (ARIC) study, 1987–1993. *Am J Epidemiol* 1997;146(6):483-494.

23. O'Leary DH, et al. Carotid-artery intima and media thickness as a risk factor for myocardial infarction and stroke in older adults. Cardiovascular Health Study Collaborative Research Group. *N Engl J Med* 1999;340(1):14-22.

24. Bots ML, et al. Common carotid intima-media thickness and risk of stroke and myocardial infarction: the Rotterdam Study. *Circulation* 1997;96(5):1432-1437.

25. Greenland P, et al. 2010 ACCF/AHA guideline for assessment of cardiovascular risk in asymptomatic adults: a report of the American College of Cardiology Foundation/American Heart Association Task Force on Practice Guidelines. *Circulation* 2010;122(25):e584-e636.

26. Touboul PJ, et al. Mannheim intima-media thickness consensus. *Cerebrovasc Dis* 2004;18(4):346-349.

27. Wendelhag I, et al. A new automated computerized analyzing system simplifies readings and reduces the variability in ultrasound measurement of intima-media thickness. *Stroke* 1997;28(11):2195-2200.

28. Stein JH, et al. Use of carotid ultrasound to identify subclinical vascular disease and evaluate cardiovascular disease risk: a consensus statement from the American Society of Echocardiography Carotid Intima-Media Thickness Task Force. Endorsed by the Society for Vascular Medicine. *J Am Soc Echocardiogr* 2008;21(2):93-111; quiz 189-190.

29. Nagai Y, et al. Increased carotid artery intimal-medial thickness in asymptomatic older subjects with exercise-induced myocardial ischemia. *Circulation* 1998;98(15):1504-1509.

30. Bots ML, et al. Reproducibility of carotid vessel wall thickness measurements. The Rotterdam Study. *J Clin Epidemiol* 1994;47(8):921-930.

31. Mitchell GF. Effects of central arterial aging on the structure and function of the peripheral vasculature: Implications for end-organ damage. *J Appl Physiol* 2008;105(5):1652-1660.

32. Izzo JL Jr, Mitchell GF. Aging and arterial structure-function relations. *Adv Cardiol* 2007;44:19-34.

33. Mitchell GF. Arterial stiffness and wave reflection in hypertension: pathophysiologic and therapeutic implications. *Curr Hypertens Rep* 2004;6(6):436-441.

34. Chantler PD, Lakatta EG. Arterial-ventricular coupling with aging and disease. *Front Physiol* 2012;3:90.

35. Borlaug BA, et al. Global cardiovascular reserve dysfunction in heart failure with preserved ejection fraction. *J Am Coll Cardiol* 2010;56(11):845-854.

36. Coutinho T, et al. Sex differences in arterial stiffness and ventricular-arterial interactions. *J Am Coll Cardiol* 2013;61(1):96-103.

37. Safar ME, et al. Pulse pressure, arterial stiffness, and end-organ damage. *Curr Hypertens Rep* 2012;14(4):339-344.

38. Coutinho T, Turner ST, Kullo IJ. Aortic pulse wave velocity is associated with measures of subclinical target organ damage. *JACC Cardiovasc Imaging* 2011;4(7):754-761.

39. Mitchell GF, et al. Arterial stiffness and cardiovascular events: The Framingham Heart Study. *Circulation* 2010;121(4):505-511.

40. Mattace-Raso FU, et al. Arterial stiffness and risk of coronary heart disease and stroke: the Rotterdam Study. *Circulation* 2006;113(5):657-663.

41. Vlachopoulos C, Aznaouridis K, Stefanadis C. Prediction of cardiovascular events and all-cause mortality with arterial stiffness: A systematic review and meta-analysis. *J Am Coll Cardiol* 2010;55(13):1318-1327.

42. Vlachopoulos C, et al. Prediction of cardiovascular events and all-cause mortality with central haemodynamics: a systematic review and meta-analysis. *Eur Heart J* 2010;31(15):1865-1871.

43. Chae CU, et al. Increased pulse pressure and risk of heart failure in the elderly. *JAMA* 1999;281(7):634-639.

44. Mitchell GF, et al. Pulse pressure and risk of new-onset atrial fibrillation. *JAMA*; 2007:297(7):709-715.

45. Poels MM, et al. Arterial stiffness and cerebral small vessel disease: the Rotterdam Scan study. *Stroke* 2012;43(10):2637-2642.

46. Scuteri A, et al. Arterial stiffness as an independent predictor of longitudinal changes in cognitive function in the older individual. *J Hypertens* 2007;25(5):1035-1040.

47. Hazzouri AZ, et al. Pulse wave velocity and cognitive decline in elders: The Health, Aging, and Body Composition study. *Stroke* 2013;44(2):388-393.

48. Muiesan ML, et al. Pulse wave velocity and cardiovascular risk stratification in a general population: the Vobarno study. *J Hypertens* 28(9):1935-1943.

49. Ben-Schlomo Y, et al. Aortic pulse wave velocity improves cardiovascular event prediction: an individual participant meta-analysis of prospective observational data from 17,635 subjects. *J Am Coll Cardiol* 2014;63(7):636-646.

50. Mancia G, et al. 2007 Guidelines for the management of arterial hypertension: The Task Force for the Management of Arterial Hypertension of the European Society of Hypertension (ESH) and of the European Society of Cardiology (ESC). *Eur Heart J* 2007;28(12):1462-1536.

51. Laurent S, et al. Expert consensus document on arterial stiffness: Methodological issues and clinical applications. *Eur Heart J* 2006;27(21):2588-2605.

52. Pini R, et al. Central but not brachial blood pressure predicts cardiovascular events in an unselected geriatric population: The ICARe Dicomano Study. *J Am Coll Cardiol* 2008;51(25):2432-2439.

53. Roman MJ, et al. Central pressure more strongly relates to vascular disease and outcome than does brachial pressure: The Strong Heart study. *Hypertension* 2007;50(1):197-203.

54. Chen CH, et al. Estimation of central aortic pressure waveform by mathematical transformation of radial tonometry pressure. Validation of generalized transfer function. *Circulation* 1997;95(7):1827-1836.

55. Gallagher D, Adji A, O'Rourke MF. Validation of the transfer function technique for generating central from peripheral upper limb pressure waveform. *Am J Hypertens* 2004;17(11 Pt 1):1059-1067.

56. Mitchell GF, et al. Hemodynamic correlates of blood pressure across the adult age spectrum: Noninvasive evaluation in the Framingham Heart study. *Circulation* 2010;122(14):1379-1386.

57. Cannon RO III. Role of nitric oxide in cardiovascular disease: Focus on the endothelium. *Clin Chem* 1998;44(8 Pt 2):1809-1819.

58. Juonala M, et al. Interrelations between brachial endothelial function and carotid intima-media thickness in young adults: The cardiovascular risk in young Finns study. *Circulation* 2004;110(18):2918-2923.

59. Ludmer PL, et al. Paradoxical vasoconstriction induced by acetylcholine in atherosclerotic coronary arteries. *N Engl J Med* 1986;315(17):1046-1051.

60. Meredith IT, et al. Postischemic vasodilation in human forearm is dependent on endothelium-derived nitric oxide. *Am J Physiol* 1996;270(4 Pt 2):H1435-H1440.

61. Loscalzo J, Vita JA. Ischemia, hyperemia, exercise, and nitric oxide. Complex physiology and complex molecular adaptations. *Circulation* 1994;90(5):2556-2559.

62. Anderson TJ, et al. Close relation of endothelial function in the human coronary and peripheral circulations. *J Am Coll Cardiol* 1995;26(5):1235-1241.

63. Huang AL, et al. Predictive value of reactive hyperemia for cardiovascular events in patients with peripheral arterial disease undergoing vascular surgery. *Arterioscler Thromb Vasc Biol* 2007;27(10):2113-2119.

64. Rossi R, et al. Flow-mediated vasodilation and the risk of developing hypertension in healthy postmenopausal women. *J Am Coll Cardiol* 2004;44(8):1636-1640.

65. Neunteufl T, et al. Late prognostic value of flow-mediated dilation in the brachial artery of patients with chest pain. *Am J Cardiol* 2000;86(2):207-210.

PREOPERATIVE PLANNING, INTRAOPERATIVE ASSESSMENT AND PROCEDURAL GUIDANCE

66. Anderson TJ, et al. Microvascular function predicts cardiovascular events in primary prevention: Long-term results from the Firefighters and Their Endothelium (FATE) study. *Circulation* 2011;123(2):163-169.

67. Shechter M, et al. Long-term association of brachial artery flow-mediated vasodilation and cardiovascular events in middle-aged subjects with no apparent heart disease. *Int J Cardiol* 2009;134(1):52-58.

68. Hirsch L, et al. The impact of early compared to late morning hours on brachial endothelial function and long-term cardiovascular events in healthy subjects with no apparent coronary heart disease. *Int J Cardiol* 2011;151(3):342-347.

69. Yeboah J, et al. Predictive value of brachial flow-mediated dilation for incident cardiovascular events in a population-based study: The multi-ethnic study of atherosclerosis. *Circulation* 2009;120(6):502-509.

70. Yeboah J, et al. Brachial flow-mediated dilation predicts incident cardiovascular events in older adults: the Cardiovascular Health Study. *Circulation* 2007;115(18):2390-2397.

71. Bots ML, et al. Assessment of flow-mediated vasodilatation (FMD) of the brachial artery: Effects of technical aspects of the FMD measurement on the FMD response. *Eur Heart J* 2005;26(4):363-368.

72. Kuvin JT, et al. Assessment of peripheral vascular endothelial function with finger arterial pulse wave amplitude. *Am Heart J* 2003;146(1):168-174.

73. Corretti MC, et al. Guidelines for the ultrasound assessment of endothelial-dependent flow-mediated vasodilation of the brachial artery: A report of the International Brachial Artery Reactivity Task Force. *J Am Coll Cardiol* 2002;39(2):257-265.

CHAPTER 27 ■ VASCULAR APPLICATIONS IN POINT OF CARE ULTRASOUND

R. EUGENE ZIERLER

The use of ultrasound for medical diagnosis began in the late 1940s and early 1950s based on experience with SONAR (sound navigation and ranging) and metal flaw detection devices. These military and industrial applications of ultrasound paved the way for research on ultrasound as a noninvasive tool for characterizing biologic tissues. However, commercial ultrasound equipment did not become available until the 1960s, and those early devices were limited to A-mode (amplitude mode) displays that produced a one-dimensional tissue image and continuous-wave (CW) Doppler for detection of blood flow.[1,2] Two-dimensional gray-scale imaging was introduced in the 1970s, initially with static imaging systems and later with real-time ultrasound displays. The combination of a real-time B-mode imaging system with a pulsed Doppler and spectral waveform analyzer—the "duplex" scanner— was first described in 1974.[3] Color Doppler capabilities were added to ultrasound systems in the 1980s, and three-dimensional gray-scale imaging was developed in the 1990s. Medical ultrasound now has applications in numerous specialties, including radiology, cardiology, obstetrics, neurology, and vascular surgery.

While technical advances in ultrasound led to better diagnostic capabilities and a wider range of clinical applications, the instrumentation was complex and required specialized training and expertise to operate. This gave rise to the profession of diagnostic medical sonography as a distinct allied health specialty. Some of the regulatory issues relevant to vascular ultrasound, specifically credentialing and accreditation, are discussed in Chapter 3. Over the last two decades, ultrasound systems have become smaller, lower in cost, and easier to use, prompting physicians, nurses, and other health care providers to start using them in offices, clinics, and hospitals, that is, at the "point of care." However, these "nontraditional" users of medical ultrasound are not replacing or duplicating the role of dedicated ultrasound professionals; instead, they rely on ultrasound as a tool for use during a patient encounter, much like they would use a stethoscope. In this setting, the goal is to acquire additional information that can be used immediately to guide diagnosis and treatment.

The differences between traditional diagnostic ultrasound and point of care ultrasound are summarized in Table 27.1 and are important to emphasize. A traditional diagnostic ultrasound examination is performed on a patient by a sonographer in an ultrasound facility at the request of a health care provider, and the "product" of that examination is a report of the ultrasound findings interpreted by a qualified physician. In contrast, point of care ultrasound is performed by a health care provider during a patient encounter to address a specific clinical question or for procedural guidance, and a formal report or interpretation is not absolutely necessary (although it may be required for billing purposes or clinical documentation). The current scope of point of care ultrasound includes the FAST (focused assessment with sonography for trauma) examination, pulmonary ultrasonography, focused cardiac echocardiography, screening for abdominal aortic aneurysms, and procedural guidance (arterial and venous access, thoracentesis, paracentesis, arthrocentesis, and regional anesthesia).[4-8]

Although point of care ultrasound examinations can be performed with the standard, full-featured ultrasound systems used by ultrasound professionals (Fig. 27.1), these relatively expensive and complicated instruments are not typically available to health care providers in the clinical setting. Fortunately, there are now a variety of smaller, less expensive, and easier to use ultrasound instruments that are well suited for point of care applications (Fig. 27.2), and some of these systems have features that approach those of the larger systems.

Most vascular applications of point of care ultrasound are abbreviated or simplified versions of the complete diagnostic tests discussed elsewhere in this book. To be most effective, each application should be used to answer a specific clinical question, and the interpretation criteria should be clearly defined—preferably as a dichotomous choice (yes/no, present/ absent, positive/negative). This chapter reviews some aspects that are unique or especially relevant to the use of ultrasound by a health care provider to facilitate clinical decision making or a therapeutic intervention in a patient with vascular disease.

EVALUATION OF SUSPECTED LOWER EXTREMITY ISCHEMIA

The concept of using ultrasound at the point of care is not really new in vascular surgery. In 1967, Strandness et al[2] published a paper titled *Ultrasonic Flow Detection—A Useful Technic in the Evaluation of Peripheral Vascular*

TABLE 27.1

FEATURES OF TRADITIONAL DIAGNOSTIC ULTRASOUND VS. POINT OF CARE ULTRASOUND

	■ DIAGNOSTIC ULTRASOUND	■ POINT OF CARE ULTRASOUND
Requested by:	Health care provider	No formal order or request
Performed by:	Diagnostic medical sonographer or physician specializing in sonography	Health care provider
Typical purpose	Definitive diagnosis, screening	Immediate diagnosis, screening, or procedural guidance
Instrumentation	Full-featured ultrasound system (expensive)	Small, limited feature ultrasound system (inexpensive)
Typical setting	Dedicated ultrasound facility	Clinic, medical office, or bedside
Interpretation by:	Physician specializing in sonography	Health care provider
Formal report	Routinely provided to requesting health care provider	Not required

Disease in which they described their initial experience with a commercially available Doppler device. Their approach was simply to listen to the audible flow signals and learn to recognize the sounds associated with various arterial and venous abnormalities. When used in this fashion, the Doppler assessment was an extension of the physical examination. In their own words, "Since the clinician uses the instrument as he would a stethoscope, the major requirements for success are experience and normal auditory acuity." Although this seems primitive by modern standards, these authors were able to accurately assess acute and chronic arterial occlusions, detect flow alterations produced by arteriovenous fistulas, evaluate extremity veins for thrombosis, and monitor the results of arterial reconstructions. In the summary of this paper, they state, "When used in a similar manner to a stethoscope, the examiner may learn to recognize normal arterial velocity signals and those that result from narrowing or occlusion of the arteries. With stenoses the frequency of the signal over the narrowed segment is higher than that observed in the pre-stenotic segment. With arterial occlusion, both acute and chronic, the velocity signal is absent from the involved area." Although

written almost 50 years ago, this description can still be applied at the point of care today.

Doppler Evaluation of Peripheral Arterial Pulses

A simple CW Doppler device can be used to assess peripheral arterial pulses during the physical examination (Fig. 27.3). As discussed in Chapter 7, CW Doppler signals do not allow for depth resolution and are not ideal for spectral waveform analysis; however, they can provide information on flow direction and produce signals that are suitable for audible interpretation. Experienced examiners can readily differentiate between the normal multiphasic peripheral arterial flow signal and the dampened, monophasic flow signal that is heard distal to a severe stenosis or occlusion. As described by Strandness and colleagues in 1967, a focal, high-pitched arterial signal represents the high-velocity jet within a stenosis.[2] These qualitative findings can be used to establish the presence or absence of peripheral arterial disease and determine its approximate location and severity.

FIGURE 27.1. Examples of full-featured ultrasound systems. *A*, GE Logiq 9, photo courtesy of GE Healthcare. *B*, Philips iU22, photo courtesy of Philips Healthcare.

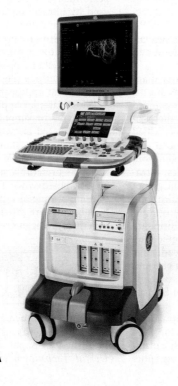

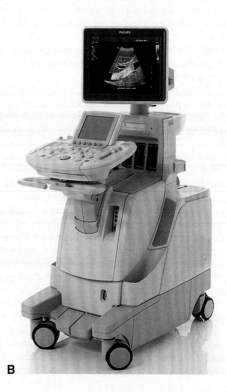

A   B

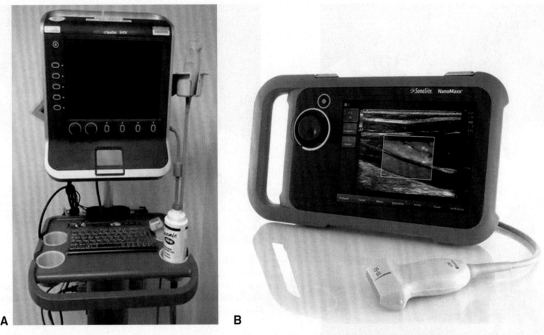

FIGURE 27.2. Examples of compact point of care ultrasound systems. *A*, SonoSite S-Series, photo courtesy of Amy Morris, MD. *B*, SonoSite NanoMaxx, photo courtesy of SonoSite, Inc.

Ankle-Brachial Indices (without Doppler waveforms)

The measurement of systolic ankle pressures and calculation of the ankle-brachial indices is a simple quantitative method for assessing the status of the lower extremity arterial circulation (see Chapter 13). Although tibial artery flow waveforms are routinely recorded with the ankle pressures in a formal vascular laboratory examination, this step is not necessary at the point of care. Measurement of ankle and brachial systolic pressures and audible interpretation of the CW Doppler signals from the distal tibial arteries will provide a valuable physiologic assessment of the overall severity of lower extremity arterial occlusive disease. Figure 27.4 shows Dr. Strandness performing an ankle pressure measurement in the 1970s.

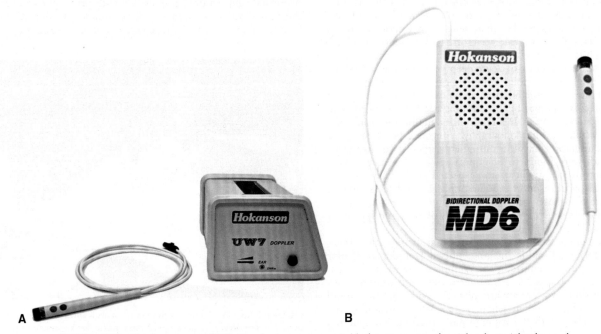

FIGURE 27.3. Continuous-wave (CW) Doppler instruments suitable for assessment of peripheral arterial pulses and measurement of ankle pressures. *A*, Portable Doppler. *B*, Pocket Doppler. Photos courtesy of D. E. Hokanson, Inc.

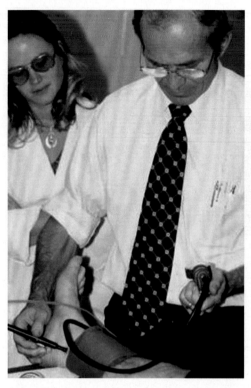

FIGURE 27.4. Dr. Strandness measuring an ankle pressure in the 1970s.

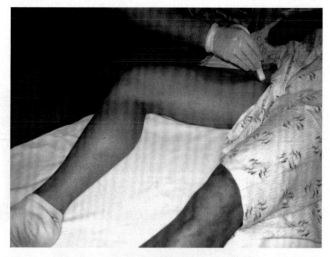

FIGURE 27.5. Patient positioning for the 2-point compression venous ultrasound examination. The leg is externally rotated, and the common femoral vein is imaged from the inguinal ligament to the confluence of the deep femoral and femoral veins in transverse view.

COMPRESSION ULTRASOUND FOR DEEP VEIN THROMBOSIS

Screening for Proximal Lower Extremity Deep Vein Thrombosis

As discussed in Chapter 19, a complete lower extremity venous duplex examination performed in the vascular laboratory includes evaluation of multiple anatomic sites from the inferior vena cava to the tibial veins with B-mode imaging, pulsed Doppler spectral waveforms, and color Doppler. Although this comprehensive approach has become the standard test for diagnosis of acute deep vein thrombosis (DVT), a relatively quick 2-point compression ultrasound examination of the common femoral and popliteal veins has been advocated as a point of care screening test for acute proximal lower extremity DVT.[9] In a randomized multicenter trial comparing whole-leg ultrasonography with the 2-point compression examination in 2465 outpatients, these two diagnostic strategies were found to be equivalent for the management of symptomatic patients with suspected DVT.[10] The 2-point compression ultrasound examination has also been shown to compare favorably with CT venography for the diagnosis of femoropopliteal DVT with a sensitivity of 86% and specificity of 100%.[11]

The 2-point compression ultrasound examination relies completely on B-mode imaging; pulsed Doppler and color Doppler are not required. The common femoral and popliteal veins are imaged in a transverse view, and compressions are performed by downward pressure with the ultrasound probe, as illustrated in Chapter 19. After positioning the patient supine with the leg externally rotated, the common femoral vein is imaged from the inguinal ligament to the confluence of the deep femoral and femoral veins (Fig. 27.5). Next, the popliteal vein is imaged using a posterior approach

from the adductor canal proximally to the confluence of the tibial veins distally (Fig. 27.6). The vein at both of these sites is compressed throughout its length in a transverse image. It is standard practice to point the indicator mark on the probe toward the right side of the patient for all transverse images, as shown in Figure 27.7, so the left side of the image will correspond to the patient's right side—similar to the conventional orientation of a transverse image from a CT scan. With the posterior approach to the popliteal vein, the vein is typically closer to the transducer (skin line) than the artery (Fig. 27.8).

In some patients, thrombus will be immediately visualized in the vein lumen (Fig. 27.9), and in those cases, probe compression may not be necessary and should be performed with caution. When thrombus is visualized, longitudinal views can be used to assess the extent of the thrombus (Fig. 27.10). A normal vein is fully compressible with probe pressure, and the vessel walls are seen to coapt completely (Fig. 27.11). Failure of the vein walls to coapt is abnormal and suggests

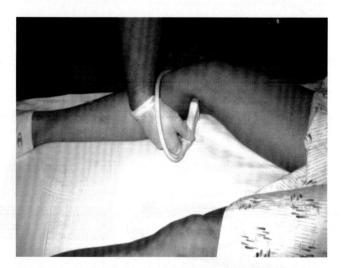

FIGURE 27.6. The 2-point compression venous ultrasound examination. The popliteal vein is imaged from a posterior approach in transverse view from the adductor canal proximally to the confluence of the tibial veins distally.

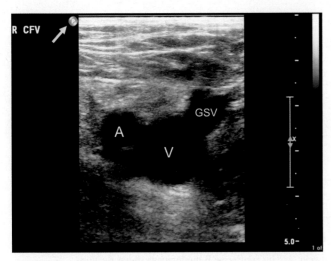

FIGURE 27.7. Transverse B-mode image of the right common femoral vein (*V*) in standard orientation. The indicator mark on the ultrasound probe (*yellow arrow*) is pointed toward the patient's right side, so the common femoral artery (*A*) is lateral and the great saphenous vein (*GSV*) is medial.

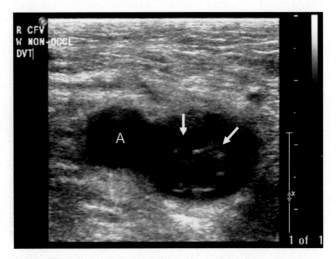

FIGURE 27.9. Transverse B-mode image of the right common femoral vein with thrombus visualized in the lumen (*white arrows*). The common femoral artery (*A*) is lateral to the vein.

that thrombus is present in the lumen. This is especially true for acute thrombus, which tends to be hypoechoic. In some cases, ultrasound visualization is poor, and the examination is considered as equivocal or nondiagnostic.

Most of the reported experience with the 2-point compression examination for detection lower extremity DVT has been in the emergency room setting. A systematic review was carried out to compare the results of the 2-point compression examination as performed by emergency physicians and a complete formal diagnostic ultrasound examination of the lower extremity.[12] Six eligible studies that included a total of 936 patients were analyzed, and the overall sensitivity and specificity of the 2-point compression examination were 95% and 96%, respectively. This review also identified a number of methodologic issues that could limit the generalizability of these favorable results. The main limitations of the 2-point compression examination are that it will not detect DVT limited to the inferior vena cava and iliac veins or distal DVT in the axial or muscular calf veins. However,

the results of published studies suggest that DVT isolated to these very proximal and distal segments is unusual in the outpatient setting, and the majority of patients with proximal lower extremity DVT will have abnormalities at the common femoral or popliteal vein levels that can be identified by ultrasound.[13]

When properly performed and interpreted, it is appropriate to begin or withhold anticoagulant treatment based on a positive or negative 2-point compression ultrasound examination for lower extremity DVT. Depending on the clinical probability and the results of d-dimer testing, a negative 2-point compression ultrasound examination may be sufficient to exclude a diagnosis of lower extremity DVT.[14] However, when the clinical probability is high, a complete diagnostic lower extremity venous duplex should be considered to identify isolated inferior vena cava, iliac, or calf DVT, even when the 2-point compression examination is negative. When the 2-point compression examination is positive, treatment for lower extremity DVT can be initiated; however, it is always prudent to obtain a complete diagnostic lower extremity venous duplex to confirm the findings and document the extent of the thrombotic process.

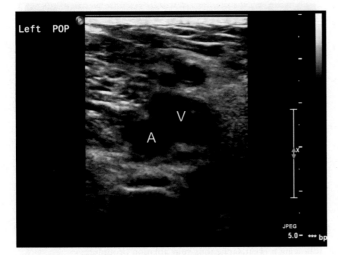

FIGURE 27.8. Transverse B-mode image of a left popliteal vein (*V*) taken from the posterior approach. The popliteal vein is closer to the skin line or transducer (top of the image) than the popliteal artery (*A*).

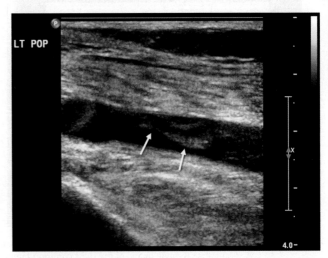

FIGURE 27.10. Longitudinal B-mode image of a left popliteal vein with thrombus visualized in the lumen (*white arrows*).

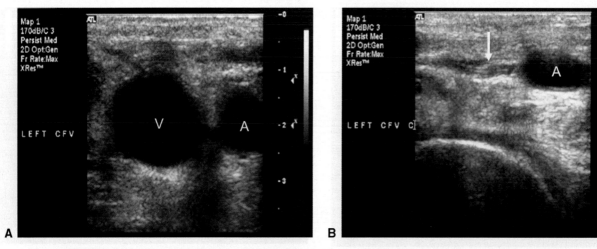

FIGURE 27.11. Normal compression of a common femoral vein. *A*, This transverse B-mode image shows the noncompressed left common femoral vein (*V*) located medial to the common femoral artery (*A*). *B*, The left common femoral vein is completely compressed (*white arrow*), while the common femoral artery lumen remains visible (*A*).

Assessment after Saphenous Vein Ablation

Although the prevalence of thrombus extension from the superficial veins into the deep veins following saphenous vein ablation procedures is relatively low, it is common practice to perform an ultrasound examination within the first week after the procedure in order to identify those patients who might require anticoagulant treatment (see Chapter 29). Since these follow-up examinations only require limited imaging of the superficial veins and saphenofemoral or saphenopopliteal junctions, this assessment can be performed as a point of care examination in an office or clinic setting. The scanning skills required for this examination are similar to those described for 2-point compression venous ultrasound.

Ablation of the superficial veins can be confirmed by obtaining a transverse B-mode image and performing probe compressions. In successfully ablated veins, echogenic material is visualized within the noncompressible superficial vein lumen. The proximal extent of superficial vein thrombus and any extension into the adjacent deep vein should be assessed by transverse and longitudinal B-mode imaging and probe

compression (Fig. 27.12). If the superficial vein thrombus extends into the deep vein by more than 50% of the deep vein diameter, then standard treatment for DVT is generally recommended. Lesser degrees of thrombus extension into the deep vein can be followed with serial ultrasound examinations or treated with anticoagulants, at the discretion of the physician.

SCREENING FOR VASCULAR COMPLICATIONS OF FEMORAL ACCESS

Arterial Pseudoaneurysm

With the increasing use of percutaneous femoral artery and vein access for diagnostic and therapeutic vascular procedures, there has been a corresponding increase in the incidence of access site complications (see Chapter 32). These complications typically involve the distal external iliac artery,

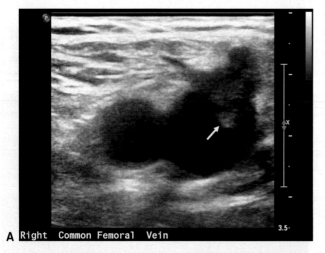
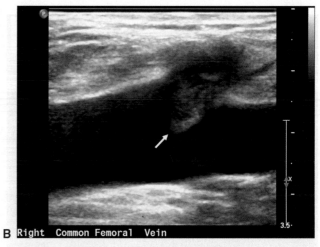

FIGURE 27.12. Thrombus at the saphenofemoral junction following a great saphenous vein ablation procedure. *A*, Transverse B-mode image of the right common femoral vein with thrombus visualized extending into the lumen from the great saphenous vein (*white arrow*). *B*, Longitudinal B-mode image of the same right common femoral vein with thrombus extending into the lumen (*white arrow*).

common femoral artery, or the proximal superficial and deep femoral arteries. The acute and focal nature of access site complications such as arterial pseudoaneurysms and arteriovenous fistulas are well suited for a point of care ultrasound examination. In addition, the presence of significant arterial stenosis or occlusion can be evaluated by measurement of ankle pressures and calculation of the ankle-brachial indices. The basic scanning skills required for this type of examination are similar to those already described for the 2-point compression ultrasound examination for suspected DVT and the assessment for complications after saphenous vein ablation.

A pseudoaneurysm most commonly presents as an enlarging pulsatile mass at a recent femoral access site. The arteries in the area of the puncture site are initially evaluated with B-mode imaging in transverse and longitudinal planes for any evidence of arterial wall defects or extraluminal masses. Color Doppler and Doppler spectral waveforms are then used to document the presence of flow within the visualized arteries as well as the local flow patterns. The presence of arterial flow outside the vessel lumen indicates the presence of a pseudoaneurysm, along with the typical "to-and-fro" flow pattern found in the neck between the arterial lumen and the active pseudoaneurysm cavity (Fig. 27.13). Once the presence of an arterial pseudoaneurysm has been established, treatment by percutaneous thrombin injection can be carried out under ultrasound guidance.

Arteriovenous Fistula

The presence of a palpable thrill or bruit associated with a recent femoral access site suggests the presence of an arteriovenous fistula. Definitive diagnosis of an arteriovenous fistula requires assessment of the flow patterns in the involved artery and vein with pulsed Doppler spectral waveforms. If the flow rate through the fistula is relatively large, the flow pattern in the proximal artery will be characterized by increased diastolic flow velocities, while the flow pattern in the adjacent vein will

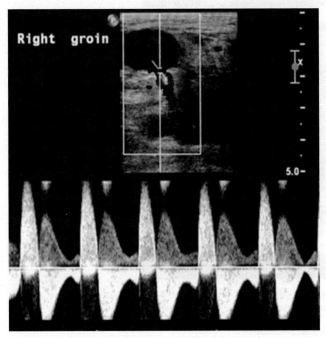

FIGURE 27.13. Color Doppler image and spectral waveform of a pseudoaneurysm neck in the right groin showing the typical "to-and-fro" flow pattern.

show high velocities and increased pulsatility (Fig. 27.14). A focal, high-velocity jet may be detected at the site of the fistula. The ankle-brachial index will also be decreased on the affected side if the fistula flow is sufficient to produce a pressure drop in the distal arterial circulation. These features are discussed in more detail in Chapter 32.

ULTRASOUND-GUIDED VASCULAR ACCESS

The use of ultrasound imaging to guide placement of needles and catheters into vascular structures is a technique that can be applied in a variety of medical settings, and it is not unique to vascular specialists. Experience has shown that the use of ultrasound guidance improves success rates and lowers the risk of complications associated with vascular access.[4,15,16] In 2001, the Agency for Healthcare Research and Quality recommended the use of ultrasound guidance for placement of central venous catheters as one of the top evidence-based practices that could improve patient safety.[17]

Ultrasound guidance can be used for vascular access in either a static or dynamic fashion. Static guidance involves identifying the vessel to be cannulated by ultrasound imaging and marking the intended access site on the skin. Vessel puncture is then performed with no additional imaging. With dynamic guidance, real-time B-mode ultrasound is used to visualize the needle as it penetrates the tissues and enters the intended vessel. Static guidance may be easier to perform, particularly for inexperienced users; however, dynamic guidance results in the highest rates of cannulation success. In a randomized trial comparing dynamic ultrasound, static ultrasound, and reliance on anatomic landmarks without ultrasound guidance for central venous cannulation, both ultrasound techniques were superior to use of landmarks alone.[18] Overall cannulation success rates were 98% for dynamic guidance, 82% for static guidance, and 64% for landmarks alone. The greatest benefit of ultrasound guidance appears to be for accessing the internal jugular vein compared to the femoral and subclavian vein sites. Training in the use of ultrasound guidance for insertion of central venous catheters can be facilitated by the use of a simulator (Fig. 27.15).

Dynamic ultrasound guidance can be performed using either an "in-plane" view with a longitudinal image of the vessel or an "out-of-plane" view with a transverse image of the vessel (Figs. 27.16 and 27.17). The in-plane or longitudinal approach is generally preferable because it allows visualization of the entire length of the needle, including the tip, as it approaches the target vessel. However, maintaining continuous visualization of the needle in the B-mode image requires considerable skill and coordination. With the out-of-plane approach, the needle will be perpendicular to the plane of the ultrasound image, and it is not possible to follow the tip of the needle as it moves through the tissue. The main advantage of the out-of-plane approach is that it shows the target vessel in cross-section and its relationship to adjacent structures. A combination of out-of-plane and in-plane views is often helpful during a cannulation attempt, with a transverse view used initially to define the important anatomic relationships and then changing to a longitudinal view in order to visualize the needle tip approaching and entering the vessel.

Although most of the published experience on ultrasound-guided vascular access has emphasized the insertion of central venous catheters, the same basic techniques can be used to assist with placement of catheters in peripheral veins, for insertion of radial artery lines, and during venous ablation procedures (see Chapter 29).

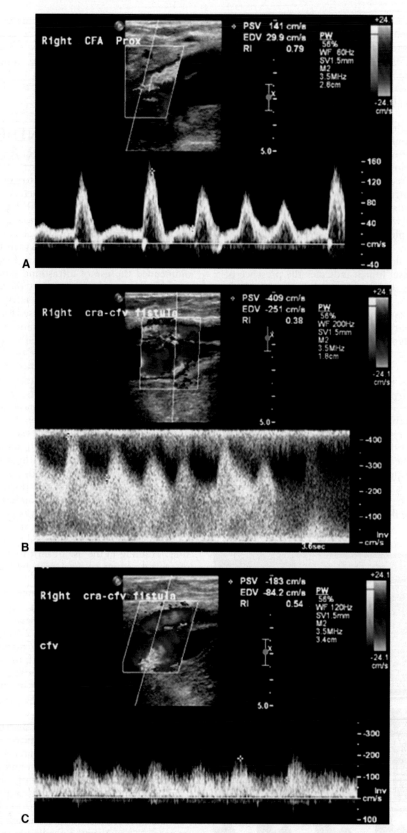

FIGURE 27.14. Flow patterns associated with an arteriovenous fistula between the right common femoral artery and common femoral vein. *A,* Spectral waveforms taken in the artery proximal to the fistula show increased diastolic velocities (low vascular resistance). *B,* A high-velocity jet is present at the site of the fistula. *C,* The flow pattern in the common femoral vein shows high velocities and increased pulsatility.

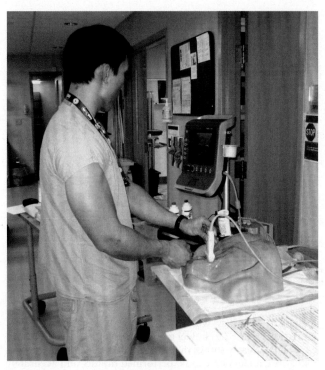

FIGURE 27.15. A simulator for training in the use of ultrasound guidance for insertion of central venous catheters.

SCREENING FOR ABDOMINAL AORTIC ANEURYSMS

In 2005, the U.S. Preventive Services Task Force (USPSTF) issued a statement recommending one-time abdominal aortic aneurysm screening with ultrasound in men 65 to 75 years of age who have ever smoked, with no recommendation for men in that age range who had never smoked, and a recommendation against screening in women.[19] Other groups have made similar recommendations.[20,21] The Society for Vascular Surgery recommended baseline ultrasound screening for abdominal aortic aneurysms in all men aged 60 to 85 years, women aged 60 to 85 years with cardiovascular risk factors, and both men and women over 50 years of age with a family history of abdominal aortic aneurysm; however, according to these guidelines, patients who are considered unfit for any intervention should not be screened.[21]

These recommendations are supported by the results of multiple randomized controlled trials. One such trial included 67,800 white men between the ages of 65 and 74 years who were randomized to undergo ultrasound screening (invited group, $n = 33,839$) or no ultrasound screening (control group, $n = 33,961$).[22] Those in the invited group who were found to have small abdominal aortic aneurysms (≥ 3 cm in diameter) received follow-up ultrasound scans for a mean of 4.1 years, and surgical repair was considered for symptomatic aneurysms, aneurysms ≥ 5.5 cm in diameter, and those that expanded at a rate of ≥ 1 cm per year. There were 65 aneurysm related deaths in the invited group compared to 113 in the control group, resulting in an overall risk reduction of 42% in the screened population. Longer-term follow-up indicates that the benefits of screening for abdominal aortic aneurysms are maintained and that this approach is also cost-effective.[23]

The ultrasound evaluation of abdominal aortic aneurysms is discussed in detail in Chapter 15. Technical guidelines for ultrasound screening are available from the Society for Vascular Ultrasound (SVU) and the American Institute for Ultrasound in Medicine (AIUM). The Intersocietal Accreditation Commission (IAC) also includes abdominal aortic aneurysm screening in its standards and guidelines for vascular testing accreditation (see Chapter 3). Although screening can be done in the vascular laboratory, the basic technique is relatively simple and can be readily performed by properly trained health care providers in a point of care setting. This involves scanning of the abdominal aorta from the diaphragmatic hiatus to the bifurcation in a transverse view using B-mode imaging alone. Diameter measurements are made with the electronic calipers in both the anterior-posterior and transverse dimensions from outer wall to outer wall. Representative images of the maximum measured diameter are recorded for documentation. In general, the anterior-posterior measurement is more accurate due to better visualization of the aortic walls which are approximately perpendicular to the ultrasound scan lines, compared to the transverse measurement in which the ultrasound scan lines encounter the vessel wall tangentially (Fig. 27.18). The normal diameter of an infrarenal aorta is typically 2.0 cm or less, and the commonly used threshold for an abdominal aortic aneurysm is a diameter of 3.0 cm.

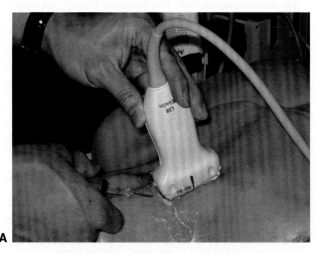

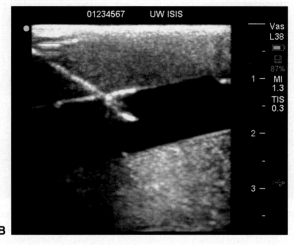

FIGURE 27.16. The "in-plane" or longitudinal image approach for ultrasound guidance using a simulator. *A,* Probe and needle position. *B,* B-mode image of the needle tip in the target vessel.

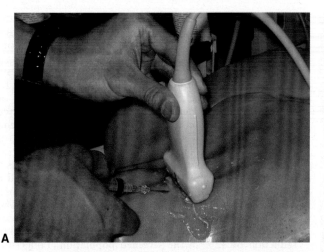

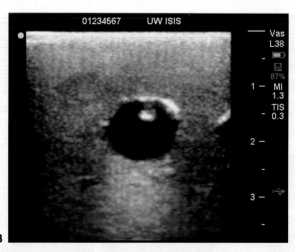

FIGURE 27.17. The "out-of-plane" or transverse image approach for ultrasound guidance using a simulator. *A*, Probe and needle position. *B*, B-mode image of the target vessel with the needle visualized in the lumen; the exact location of the needle tip is more difficult to determine in this view.

Ultrasound screening for abdominal aortic aneurysms is highly accurate, with a sensitivity and specificity of approximately 95% and 100%, respectively.[19,24] Point of care screening for abdominal aortic aneurysms has been successfully performed in the emergency department setting, with the results depending on the experience and training of the providers.[24,25] Lin et al[5] compared diameter measurements of the abdominal aorta obtained by physicians using a portable, hand-held ultrasound device to those from a formal abdominal duplex ultrasound examination performed by certified vascular sonographers. The portable ultrasound evaluation was carried out as part of the routine physical examination in a vascular surgery clinic. A total of 104 patients with a mean age of 67 years were evaluated, and the mean examination times for the portable ultrasound and formal duplex scan were 5.3 and 3.1 minutes, respectively. Considering the formal duplex scan as the reference test, the sensitivity and specificity of the portable ultrasound evaluation for detecting an abdominal aortic aneurysm were 93% and 97%, respectively. The positive and negative predictive values for the portable ultrasound evaluation were 89% and 98%, respectively, and the overall

diagnostic accuracy was 98%. Although there are technical limitations related to bowel gas and patient body habitus, this experience clearly shows that ultrasound screening for abdominal aortic aneurysm can be performed rapidly and accurately in a point of care setting.

CONCLUSIONS

The vascular applications of point of care ultrasound typically involve rapid, focused examinations that provide information that can be used immediately to facilitate patient care. Appropriate use of these techniques can increase the efficiency of care, supplement or direct more advanced imaging methods, and decrease medical errors. However, point of care ultrasound is not a substitute for a complete vascular laboratory ultrasound examination by a vascular sonographer. Traditional ultrasound practitioners are justifiably concerned about the quality of point of care examinations and the lack of necessary experience and training among some health care providers performing point of care ultrasound. The best way to assure quality is to set standards, provide training, and verify skills.

To address this need, some professional societies and academic institutions offer training in various applications of point of care ultrasound. The American Registry for Diagnostic Medical Sonography (ARDMS), which credentials sonographers and physicians in the established ultrasound specialties, is also looking at new approaches to assess competency in this rapidly expanding field. These educational and regulatory initiatives should help to define scopes of practice in point of care ultrasound and create formal pathways for training and certification. Finally, instruction in a variety of point of care ultrasound applications is now being introduced into medical school curricula, making it possible for students to acquire these skills during their medical training and to use point of care ultrasound as an integral part of their routine clinical practice.[26]

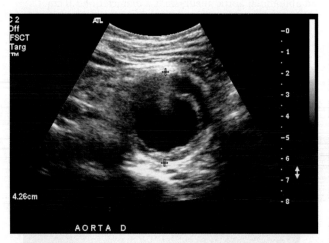

FIGURE 27.18. Diameter measurement of an abdominal aortic aneurysm using the electronic calipers. The anterior-posterior measurement of 4.26 cm from outer wall to outer wall is shown. The anterior and posterior aortic walls are visualized more clearly than are the lateral walls, making this measurement easier to obtain.

References

1. Goldberg BB. Obstetric US imaging: The past 40 years. *Radiology* 2000;215:622-629.
2. Strandness DE Jr, Schultz RD, Sumner DS, et al. Ultrasonic flow detection: A useful technique in the evaluation of peripheral arterial disease. *Am J Surg* 1967;113:311-320.
3. Strandness DE Jr. History of ultrasonic duplex scanning. *Cardiovasc Surg* 1996;4:273-280.

4. Moore CL, Copel JA. Current concepts: Point-of-care ultrasonography. *N Engl J Med* 2011;364:749-757.

5. Lin PH, Bush RL, McCoy SA, et al. A prospective study of a hand-held ultrasound device in abdominal aortic aneurysm evaluation. *Am J Surg* 2003;186:455-459.

6. Kimura BJ, Yogo N, O'Connell CW, et al. Cardiopulmonary limited ultrasound examination for "quick look" bedside application. *Am J Cardiol* 2011;108:586-590.

7. Cardim N, Golfin CF, Ferreira D, et al. Usefulness of a new miniaturized echocardiographic system in outpatient cardiology consultations as an extension of the physical examination. *J Am Soc Echocardiogr* 2011;24:117-124.

8. Volpicelli G, Elbarbary M, Blaivas M, et al. International evidence-based recommendations for point-of-care lung ultrasound. *Intensive Care Med* 2012;38:577-591.

9. Crisp JG, Lovato LM, Jang TB. Compression ultrasonography of the lower extremity with portable vascular ultrasonography can accurately detect deep vein thrombosis in the emergency department. *Ann Emerg Med* 2010;56:601-610.

10. Bernardi E, Camporese G, Buller HR, et al. Serial 2-point ultrasonography plus D-dimer vs whole-leg color-coded Doppler ultrasonography for diagnosing suspected symptomatic deep vein thrombosis. *JAMA* 2008;300:1653-1659.

11. Shiver SA, Lyon ML, Blaivas M, et al. Prospective comparison of emergency physician–performed venous ultrasound and CT venography for deep venous thrombosis. *Am J Emerg Med* 2010;28:354-358.

12. Burnside PR, Brown MD, Kline JA. Systematic review of emergency physician–performed ultrasonography for lower-extremity deep vein thrombosis. *Acad Emerg Med* 2008;15:493-498.

13. Blaivas M. Point-of-care ultrasonographic deep venous thrombosis evaluation after just ten minutes training: Is this offer too good to be true? *Ann Emerg Med* 2010;56:611-613.

14. Goldhaber SZ, Bounameaux H. Pulmonary embolism and deep vein thrombosis. *Lancet* 2012;379:1835-1846.

15. Revised statement on recommendations for use of real-time ultrasound guidance for placement of central venous catheters. *Bull Am Coll Surg* 2011;96:36-37.

16. Lamperti M, Bodenham AR, Pittiruti M, et al. International evidence-based recommendations on ultrasound-guided vascular access. *Intensive Care Med* 2012;38:1105-1117.

17. *Making Health Care Safer: A Critical Analysis of Patient Safety Practices.* Rockville: Agency for Healthcare Research and Quality. (AHRQ publication no. 01-E058.)

18. Truman JM, Rose J, Briggs WM, et al. Randomized, controlled clinical trial of point-of-care limited ultrasonography assistance of central venous cannulation: The Third Sonography Outcomes Assessment Program (SOAP-3) Trial. *Crit Care Med* 2005;33:1764-1769.

19. U.S. Preventive Services Task Force. Screening for abdominal aortic aneurysm: Recommendation statement. *Ann Intern Med* 2005;142:198-202.

20. Hirsch AT, Haskal ZJ, Hertzer NR, et al. ACC/AHA 2005 Practice guidelines for the management of patients with peripheral arterial disease (lower extremity, renal, mesenteric, and abdominal aortic). *Circulation* 2006;113:463-654.

21. Kent KC, Zwolak RM, Jaff MR, et al. Screening for abdominal aortic aneurysm: A consensus statement. *J Vasc Surg* 2004;39:267-269.

22. The Multicentre Aneurysm Screening Study Group. The multicentre aneurysm screening study (MASS) into the effect of abdominal aortic aneurysm screening on mortality in men: A randomised controlled trial. *Lancet* 2002;360:1531-1539.

23. Kim LG, Scott RAP, Ashton HA, et al. A sustained benefit from screening for abdominal aortic aneurysm. *Ann Intern Med* 2007;146:699-706.

24. Tayal VS, Graf CD, Gibbs MA. Prospective study of accuracy and outcome of emergency ultrasound for abdominal aortic aneurysm over two years. *Acad Emerg Med* 2003;10:867-871.

25. Hoffman B, Bessman ES, Um P, et al. Successful sonographic visualization of the abdominal aorta differs significantly among a diverse group of credentialed emergency department providers. *Emerg Med* 2011;28:472-476.

26. Hoppmann RA, Rao VV, Poston MB, et al. An integrated ultrasound curriculum (iUSC) for medical students: 4-yaer experience. *Crit Ultrasound J* 2011;3:1-12.

CHAPTER 28 ■ **PREOPERATIVE VEIN MAPPING**

KATHLEEN D. GIBSON AND AARON EBERT

Endovascular approaches for the treatment of infrainguinal arterial disease (angioplasty, stenting, and atherectomy) are increasingly being offered as initial procedures for patients with lower extremity ischemia.[1] Bypass grafting, however, remains the gold standard to which all other treatments are compared. The BASIL trial randomized 452 patients with critical limb ischemia to a "surgery first" or "angioplasty first" revascularization. That study demonstrated the superiority of bypass surgery over angioplasty for overall long-term survival and a trend toward decreased rates of amputation in patients with critical limb ischemia who survived for at least 2 years after randomization.[2] Both prosthetic grafts and autogenous veins are used as bypass conduits, but in most series, long-term patency rates for autogenous veins are superior.[3,4] This is particularly true when the distal anastomosis is below the knee.[5] While a multitude of studies have documented superior patency for autogenous vein grafts, it is also clear that a prosthetic graft is better than a poor-quality vein in terms of patency. As such, preoperative vein mapping is an important part of surgical planning for finding adequate vein to use as a conduit, both in diameter and in quality. In addition, vein mapping with skin marking can be an invaluable aid to the surgeon for planning incisions and identifying branches that will require ligation.

AUTOGENOUS CONDUITS: REVERSED VEIN, IN SITU VEIN, AND ALTERNATIVE VEIN

The two main techniques for utilizing autogenous conduit for infrainguinal arterial revascularization involve either removing and reversing the vein graft (taken from the same lower limb, the opposite lower limb, or the upper extremities) or leaving the vein graft in situ. The most common autogenous conduit used for bypass grafting is the great saphenous vein (GSV). Its proximity to arterial target vessels as well as its size and length make it the ideal conduit for lower extremity bypass. In the absence of an adequate GSV, the small saphenous vein (SSV), or arm veins (cephalic or basilic), can be used as alternative conduits.

The GSV can be dissected out and removed entirely from its normal anatomic location, reversed, and then tunneled along the anatomic course of the native arterial circulation. With a reversed vein graft, the proximal to distal reversal is necessary to allow blood to flow through the graft in the proper direction relative to the valves within the vein. Alternatively, the vein can be left in its anatomic position (an in situ graft). In this procedure, the saphenofemoral junction (SFJ) is divided, and the hood of the SFJ is used to create the proximal arterial anastomosis. The distal end of the vein is

then mobilized and swung over to the target artery to create the distal anastomosis. Because the normal valves would prohibit flow in the arterial direction through the in situ graft, the valve leaflets must be lysed with a device inserted into the vein called a valvulotome. Additionally, to prevent arteriovenous fistulae, all major venous side branches must be ligated.

Long-term patency rates of in situ vein grafts and reversed vein grafts are similar,[6,7] and the choice of bypass technique is largely dependent on the distal bypass target and surgeon's preference. In situ bypass grafts offer the advantages of fewer or shorter incisions, avoidance of the need for tunneling the vein anatomically, and better vein-to-artery size match for distal (tibial artery) anastomoses. Graft patency versus occlusion is readily apparent with in situ bypass grafts on physical examination, as the graft pulse is usually easily palpable in the thigh and calf. The superficial location of in situ bypass grafts also facilitates Doppler evaluation and duplex graft surveillance (see Chapter 17). In some cases, however, the SFJ is too low to allow an in situ bypass, as the vein simply will not reach the intended proximal anastomotic site. Reversed vein grafts avoid the need for valve lysis and allow visual examination of the entire vein at the time of surgery. The bypass graft is also less likely to become exposed if there is a wound problem as it is tunneled anatomically in the deeper tissue planes.

In the absence of an adequate GSV, alternative autogenous conduits can be used for infrainguinal bypasses. Arm veins (basilic or cephalic), the SSV, and spliced vein segments from various sources (a composite graft) can be used. Although patency and limb salvage rates are acceptable using alternative autogenous conduits, they are significantly inferior to bypasses utilizing a single segment of GSV.[8]

VEIN MAPPING

Vein mapping is an integral part of preoperative planning for infrainguinal arterial revascularization. It serves three important functions:

1. Identifying adequate venous conduit for bypass in terms of diameter, length, and vein quality
2. Locating major vein branches
3. Characterizing any anatomic anomalies along the course of the vein

Mapping is valuable even if the patient has a previous history of vein harvest or stripping, as dual saphenous trunks do occur, and it is possible that there will still be a GSV segment or a usable tributary vein present. Identifying adequate venous conduit includes assessing the diameter of the vein as well as identifying any vein segments that are abnormal. Despite having an adequate diameter, veins that show thickening and

414

phlebosclerosis make poor conduits. In general, veins must be a minimum of 2.0 mm in diameter to be adequate for use as a bypass conduit. Recent data have shown that veins less than 3.0 mm in diameter have more than double the risk of early failure compared to veins greater than 3.0 mm in diameter.[9]

In some circumstances, the GSV is inadequate in caliber, quality, or length or is absent from previous harvest for another arterial bypass procedure or due to a venous procedure (stripping or endothermal ablation). While often relatively short in length, the SSV is sometimes a usable conduit, as is the cephalic vein or basilic vein. The length of conduit needed for the bypass procedure should be anticipated prior to mapping. In a vein mapping procedure, if the GSV in the leg intended for bypass is not adequate, the contralateral GSV, the ipsilateral and contralateral SSV, and the arm veins should be assessed.

In addition to documenting the diameter, length, depth, and quality of the vein in a written report, the course of the vein is marked directly on the skin along with any identified side branches. Marking and identification of venous side branches off of the GSV has utility for both in situ and reversed grafts. For reversed grafts, the marking allows the surgeon to make an incision directly over the vein, avoiding skin flaps. In our practice, we make multiple small incisions over the GSV when harvesting for a reversed graft, leaving multiple "skin bridges." This technique makes lining up the skin for closure easier, and we believe healing is better. By having the branches marked, we can center an incision over the branch in order to divide it, rather than having the branch under one of the skin bridges. For in situ grafts, marking of the branches allows the surgeon to ligate them directly prior to the completion duplex ultrasound or angiogram, saving considerable time. With complete preoperative vein marking, the operation is often finished after the first completion angiogram as all of the arteriovenous fistulae have already been divided.

Scanning Technique

Preparation and Instrumentation

Vein mapping may be done at the time of the patient's initial arterial duplex evaluation; however, it is more often performed after the surgeon has met with the patient and a definite plan for a bypass graft has been made. If the vein mapping occurs more than a week before the anticipated surgery, the patient will usually need to come back for marking of the conduit on the skin, because the marks fade and wear off over time. We will sometimes send the patient home with an indelible marker to "redraw" the mapping marks daily if we are concerned that the marking will be gone prior to surgery. Prior to mapping, there should be written or verbal communication between the surgeon and the vascular technologist regarding the length of conduit needed for the bypass. If the single marked vein is not long enough for the proposed bypass graft, multiple vein segments may need to be marked in order to have enough conduit for a composite graft. If there are any concerns regarding the length or quality of the vein, these should be discussed with the surgeon during the examination so that alternative venous conduits can be located if necessary.

The vein mapping is performed with a high-frequency transducer. We typically use the intraoperative "hockey stick" 12-MHz transducer, although in obese patients, a medium-frequency transducer may be needed as well. The patient should change into an exam gown or loose athletic shorts so that the legs are exposed, and they should be warm, relaxed, and comfortable to avoid spasm of the veins. Both the examination room and the ultrasound gel should be warm to prevent vasospasm. The patient is tilted into a 45-degree reverse Trendelenburg (foot down) position, and for GSV mapping, the leg is externally rotated, while for SSV mapping, the patient is prone. A tourniquet may be used if desired.

Protocol and Documentation

The diameters of the vein along with any anatomic abnormalities are noted in the written report (Fig. 28.1). If the vein courses above the fascial layer, this is indicated. This is important information because the surgeon typically expects the vein to be under the fascia and could inadvertently damage the vein if it was not known that the vein is in a more superficial position. In some patients, adequate veins for conduit may be present both below and above the fascia, representing, in essence, a "duplicate" system in which either vein may be used. In this situation, both veins should be marked with diameters noted. This is of particular importance for in situ bypass procedures, as the surgeon could inadvertently use the "wrong branch" distally. An example of a duplicate system is shown in cross-sectional and longitudinal views in Figure 28.2. In most but not all cases, the deeper branch (underneath the saphenous fascia) will be larger, thicker walled, and have fewer branches.

Patency of the vein is determined by documenting spontaneous flow or flow with augmentation. Prior to recording of diameters, a sweep is made and compression of the vein is carried out over its entire length with the probe in transverse view to look for any wall thickening or intraluminal defects such as chronic phlebitis (Fig. 28.3). Scanning is then carried out from the SFJ, and cross-sectional measurements are documented incrementally at the SFJ, proximal, medial, and distal thigh, knee, and proximal, mid, and distal calf. Varicosities and incompetent segments are noted.

Documentation of vein diameter is performed from proximal to distal. The vein should be imaged in both cross-sectional and longitudinal views. Figure 28.4 shows a cephalic vein with an adequate diameter for bypass, and Figure 28.5 shows a cephalic vein with diameters too small to be used as conduit. Care must be taken to avoid compressing the vein with the probe and making the diameter falsely small. If the vein appears to be in spasm (with bright, thick walls), warming

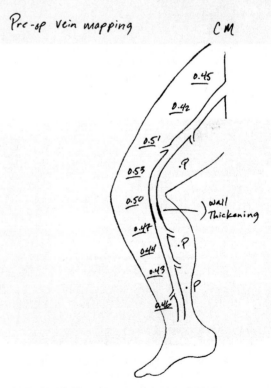

FIGURE 28.1. Report of a vein mapping.

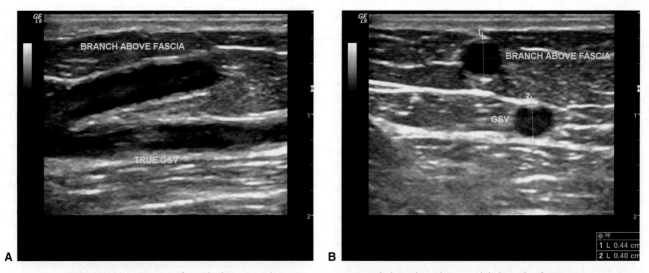

FIGURE 28.2. Images of a "duplicate" saphenous vein system with branches above and below the fascia in longitudinal (A) and cross-sectional (B) views.

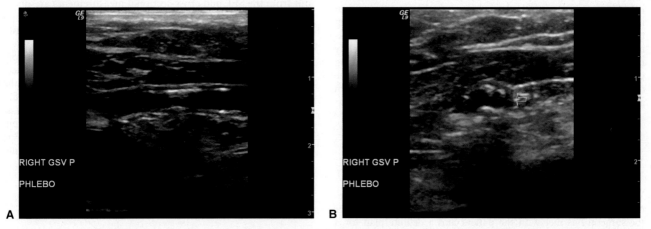

FIGURE 28.3. Images of phlebosclerosis in a vein in longitudinal (A) and cross-sectional (B) views.

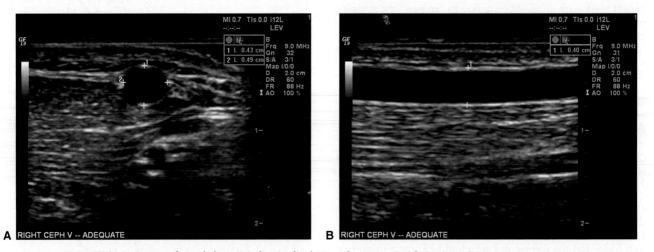

FIGURE 28.4. Images of a cephalic vein in longitudinal (A) and cross-sectional (B) views. Diameter measurements are indicated and are adequate for use as a bypass conduit.

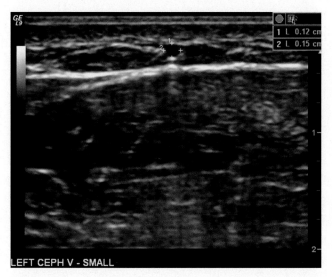

FIGURE 28.5. Cephalic vein in cross section with diameters of 0.12 cm and 0.15 cm, too small to use as a bypass conduit.

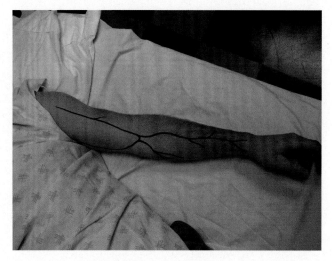

FIGURE 28.7. Arm vein mapping.

the limb with heated towels, increasing the degree of reverse Trendelenburg, or using a tourniquet may be helpful. If these measures do not change the appearance of the vein, it is likely that the vein is sclerotic rather than in spasm. If the vein diameter is inadequate or borderline, the surgeon should be notified during the examination. Any abnormalities such as intraluminal defects, varicose segments, or sclerosis should also be communicated to the surgeon.

Marking the course of the vein on the skin while scanning can be problematic, as pens typically will not mark through ultrasound gel. In our vascular laboratory, we make dashed lines along the course of the vein through the gel with a colored pencil. It is important to hold the transducer at a right angle to the patient's skin while marking in order to place

the mark directly over the vein. The locations of all branches and perforator veins are also marked (branches drawn on and perforators denoted by the letter "P"). The leg is then wiped clean of gel, and the dashed lines are connected with an indelible marker. Following this second stage of marking, the transducer is placed perpendicularly over the mark to ensure that it is directly over the vein. This spot check is performed over the length of the marked vein. This double check is important, as the surgeon relies intraoperatively on precise marking of the course and location of the vein and branch points. If the vein is marked "off center," the incision may be misplaced, causing a skin flap. Figures 28.6 and 28.7 show vein mapping of both a GSV and of arm veins. An alternative method of marking is to use the tip of a straw to gently make indentations in the skin over the vein and then use a pen to connect the indentations.

CONCLUSIONS

Proper planning is imperative for any successful operation, and for infrainguinal bypass procedures, vein mapping is critically important. Quality and anatomy of autogenous vein bypass conduit is highly variable; therefore, the vascular laboratory is an important partner with the surgeon in ensuring good patient care. Communication between the surgeon and the vascular technologist at all stages is also imperative in order for the appropriate information to be conveyed and to avoid the necessity for repeat studies to search for alternative conduit.

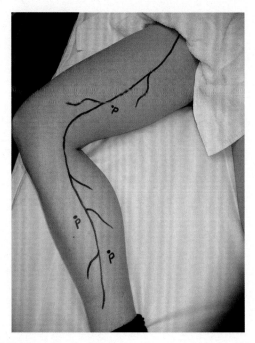

FIGURE 28.6. Great saphenous vein map with branches and perforators (P) indicated.

References

1. Kudo T, Chandra FA, Kwun WH, et al. Changing pattern of surgical revascularization for critical limb ischemia over 12 years: Endovascular vs. open bypass surgery. *J Vasc Surg* 2006;44(2):304-313.
2. Bradbury A, Adam D, Bell J, et al. Bypass versus angioplasty in severe ischaemia of the leg (BASIL) trial: An intention-to-treat analysis of amputation-free and overall survival in patients randomized to a bypass surgery-first or a balloon angioplasty-first revascularization strategy. *J Vasc Surg* 2010;51(5 Suppl):5S-17S.
3. Klinkert P, Schlepers A, Burger DH, et al. Vein versus polytetrafluoroethylene in above-knee femoropopliteal bypass grafting: Five-year results of a randomized controlled trial. *J Vasc Surg* 2003;37(1):149-155.
4. Ballotta E, Renon L, Toffano M, et al. Prospective randomized study on bilateral above-knee femoropopliteal revascularization: Polytetrafluoroethylene graft versus reversed saphenous vein. *J Vasc Surg* 2003;38(5):1051-1055.

PREOPERATIVE PLANNING, INTRAOPERATIVE ASSESSMENT AND PROCEDURAL GUIDANCE

5. Donker J, Ho G, Te Slaa A, et al. Midterm results of autologous saphenous vein and ePTFE pre-cuffed bypass surgery in peripheral arterial occlusive disease. *Vasc Endovascular Surg* 2011;45(7):598-603.

6. Davidovic LB, Markovic DM, Vojnovic BR, et al. Femoro-popliteal reconstructions: "In-situ" versus "reversed" technique. *Cardiovasc Surg* 2001;9(4):356-361.

7. Moody AP, Edwards PR, Harris PL. In-situ versus reversed femoropopliteal vein grafts: Long-term follow-up of a prospective randomized trial. *Br J Surg* 1992;79(8):750-752.

8. Arvela E, Venermo M, Soderstrom M, et al. Outcome of infrainguinal single-segment great saphenous vein bypass for critical limb ischemia is superior to alternative autologous vein bypass, especially in patients with high operative risk. *Ann Vasc Surg* 2012;26(3):396-403.

9. Schanzer A, Hevelone N, Owens CD, et al. Technical factors affecting autogenous vein graft failure: Observations from a large multicenter trial. *J Vasc Surg* 2007;46(6):1180-1190.

CHAPTER 29 ■ VENOUS ABLATION PROCEDURES

KATHLEEN D. GIBSON AND AARON EBERT

Venous insufficiency is arguably the most common condition evaluated in an outpatient vascular laboratory setting. Varicose veins and deep venous insufficiency cause leg fatigue, pain, and swelling in millions of patients and are two of the most common conditions treated by vascular surgeons. In Western populations, 20% to 34% of women and 7% to 28% of men have visible varicose veins.[1–3] The prevalence of varicose veins increases significantly with age.[4] Incompetence of the great saphenous vein (GSV) is the most common cause of varicose veins; however, the small saphenous vein (SSV) shows valvular incompetence in up to 20% of affected limbs.[5]

The most common treatment for truncal saphenous incompetence historically was high ligation and stripping. This surgical procedure required general or spinal anesthesia in a hospital-based setting. With the advent of the less invasive endovenous thermal ablation techniques utilizing radiofrequency (RF)[6] and laser (EVLT)[7,8] energy sources, patients are now treated with a relatively quick in-office procedure under local anesthesia. Advances in venous imaging and endovascular techniques made the application of this technology clinically successful, and endovenous techniques are now essentially the standard of care.

Ultrasound-guided foam sclerotherapy (UGFS) has been extensively used in Europe to treat both saphenous vein incompetence and tributary incompetence.[9–11] The use of UGFS to treat superficial venous insufficiency in the United States is increasingly being practiced,[12] and interdisciplinary quality improvement guidelines for the use of physician-created foam have been developed.[13] Phase III clinical trials using proprietary endovenous microfoam (BTG, West Conshohocken, PA) to treat GSV incompetence have been completed, and a new drug application has been recently submitted to the FDA.[14] Highly accurate ultrasound imaging is critical to the performance of successful UGFS. Ultrasound is used to guide venous access and to follow the progress of the foamed agent within the vein to ensure that it effectively treats the intended vein target and does not reach unintended veins in any significant volume.

A number of emerging technologies rely on duplex ultrasound imaging for safe and effective treatment of truncal superficial venous insufficiency. These include mechanical-chemical ablation (MOCA, Clarivein, Vascular Insights, Madison, CT),[15] steam ablation (Cermavein, Cerma, Archamps, France),[16] and ablation using cyanoacrylate glue (Venaseal, Sapheon Inc., Morrisville, NC).[17] All endovenous techniques require duplex ultrasound imaging for their successful application and therefore offer a unique opportunity to partner vascular technologists with physicians in the treatment of venous insufficiency. In our practice, each step in treating patients with varicose veins—from pretreatment imaging to treatment and postoperative follow-up—requires a close and rewarding partnership with the vascular laboratory.

PRETREATMENT EVALUATION

Preoperative planning is the key to successful treatment of varicose veins using any of the ablation techniques. Patients first undergo a thorough history and physical examination. They are queried regarding any previous vein procedures (sclerotherapy, ablation, or stripping), history of deep venous thrombosis (DVT), superficial thrombophlebitis, or personal or family history of thrombophilia. This information is passed on to the vascular laboratory prior to duplex scanning and can guide the vascular technologist on what to look out for while scanning. Patients with recurrent varicose veins after procedures such as stripping often do not have straightforward venous anatomy and may require additional time for their study. Because care must also be taken in performing venous procedures on patients with peripheral arterial disease, pedal pulses should always be palpated during the initial physical examination. If these pulses are abnormal, the vascular laboratory may be called upon to perform a concomitant arterial evaluation.

A meticulous duplex ultrasound examination is the next step in preprocedure planning. A detailed "roadmap" of incompetent saphenous trunks and other sources of varicose veins is important. Failure to address nonsaphenous sources of varicosities such as perforators, accessory branches, and pelvic veins can lead to immediate or early treatment failure and patient dissatisfaction (see Chapter 25). In our practice, along with the formal report, the vascular technologist draws a "map" of the varicose veins including the diameters of the GSV and the SSV and the presence of any relevant accessory branches and perforator veins (Fig. 29.1). Incompetent anterolateral and posteromedial branches from the GSV are common, and if untreated, these may be associated with an unsatisfactory clinical result. It is not uncommon for the GSV or the SSV to terminate in the distal thigh or calf, with continuation as a branch above the superficial fascia. Such a branch is referred to not as the GSV or the SSV but as a tributary.[18] Incompetent tributaries above the fascial layer in any part of the limb should be noted. Depth of the veins under the skin has potential ramifications for endovenous treatment. "Shallow" veins require more local anesthetic, and patients often have more discomfort after the procedure. Some suprafascial veins are close enough to the skin to preclude thermal ablation, and other techniques such as ambulatory phlebectomy or UGFS can be considered

419

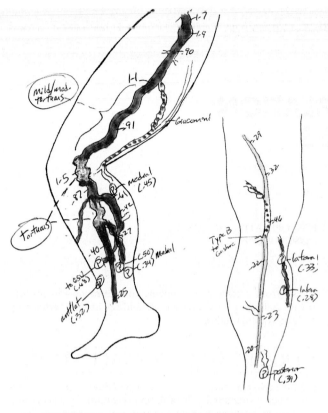

FIGURE 29.1. Preoperative varicose vein map report.

on these veins. An assessment of the deep system is particularly important in patients with a history of DVT, edema, skin changes, or ulceration or in young patients with severe varicosities and suspicion for Klippel-Trenaunay syndrome.

In patients presenting with groin, medial thigh, and upper posterior thigh varicose veins, a pelvic source from an incompetent internal iliac vein branch should be considered (Fig. 29.2). This varicose vein pattern is almost invariably seen only in female patients, and it is most often present during or after pregnancy. It is common in these cases that the terminal valve of the GSV is competent, and the GSV becomes incompetent when a varicose vein branch from the pelvic veins empties into it. When performing a varicose vein study, if the GSV is incompetent and yet the terminal valve is competent, an alternative source for the reflux should be investigated such as a perforator vein, a pelvic branch, or a branch from an incompetent accessory vein.

Precise near-field resolution is the most important feature for diagnostic imaging and treatment of varicose veins. In our practice, we use a GE Logic 9 machine with a 12-MHz "hockey stick" probe and a 10-MHz linear probe for preoperative mapping. Documentation of deep and superficial venous incompetence, as well as the presence of any clinically significant refluxing perforator veins, is noted.

TREATMENT

After the surgeon is provided with a report and a detailed vein map, a treatment plan can be made. Endovenous ablation techniques can be used to treat the GSV, SSV, accessory branches, and even perforator veins. An incompetent anterolateral branch from the saphenofemoral junction (SFJ) is a common cause of lateral thigh and calf varicosities, with the varicosities often terminating in an incompetent lateral calf perforator. Depending on the distribution and size of side branches, adjunctive treatments such as microphlebectomy, perforator ligation, and UGFS can be considered and performed at the same time as the EVLT or RF procedure.

The importance of good duplex imaging in ensuring the safety and efficacy of endovenous techniques cannot be overstated. Each step of the procedure from initial access of the vein to adequate tumescent anesthesia to proper placement of the laser or RF catheter requires accurate imaging. In many practices, the treating physician holds the ultrasound probe with one hand and accesses the vein with the other, and a vascular

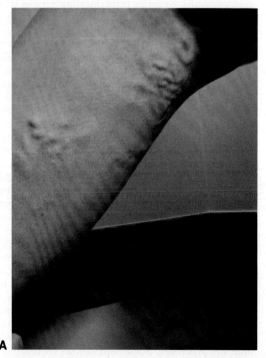

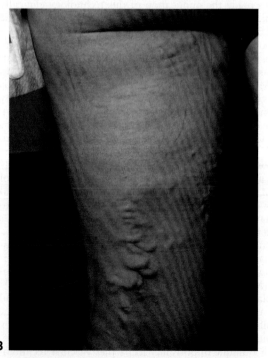

A   **B**

FIGURE 29.2. *A, B,* Nonsaphenous sources of varicose veins. A pelvic source of reflux should be considered in patients presenting with groin, medial thigh, or upper posterior thigh varicose veins.

technologist is either not involved or simply adjusts the controls on the ultrasound machine. Our team includes a registered vascular technologist (RVT) who holds the probe and plays an integral role in the procedure. We find this two-person approach increases the speed and efficiency of the procedure, and we also find it to be less ergonomically fatiguing for the surgeon. This team approach has been very rewarding in our practice, increasing collegiality between the RVT and physician, as well as improving the diagnostic skills of our vascular technologists. Being an active member of the treatment team helps the vascular technologist to think "like a surgeon" during venous examinations—anticipating what information will be needed for successful treatment of the venous abnormalities.

Scanning Technique

Many practices use compact or laptop-sized duplex ultrasound machines for endovenous ablation. We have found the near-field resolution of these machines to be suboptimal, particularly in the performance of UGFS, and we use the same machine for treatment as we do for preoperative veins mapping. To perform endovenous ablation, the patient is positioned supine for the GSV and either prone or supine for the SSV. A quick prescan is performed to ensure that there has been no change since the varicose vein mapping study. The vascular technologist scans through the saphenous trunks, identifies perforator veins and potential difficulties, and finds a good target site for cannulation. The limb is then prepped and draped in a sterile fashion.

Venous Access and Catheter Placement

Cannulation of the vein—obtaining needle and wire access—is the most critical step to a successful procedure. Venopuncture with failed wire access inevitably causes venospasm. If this occurs, a more proximal access site must be used, although occasionally a more distal access site will also work, as long as the introducer wire can traverse the area of spasm. The desired venous access site is identified by ultrasound imaging after prepping, and access can be accomplished using either a cross-sectional or longitudinal view. In our practice, we usually access the vein initially in cross section, and then switch to a longitudinal view for wire placement (Fig. 29.3). There may be multiple cannulation sites depending on how many venous segments need to be ablated.

The probe is positioned directly over the vein lumen, centered in a cross-sectional view, providing a clear image of the

vein lumen for the physician. Depth and gain are adjusted for maximal visualization of the target vein. A wheal of local anesthetic is placed in the dermis superficial to the vein to be accessed. Access is gained with a micropuncture kit (19 g reflective tip access needle, 0.018" short wire, and 4-Fr microsheath) for EVLT and with a proprietary access kit for an RF procedure, while visualizing the target vein with the 12-MHz "hockey stick" probe. The excellent near-field resolution of this probe makes access of even relatively small veins possible. Once the physician sees a "flash" of blood in the micropuncture needle, indicating that the vein has been cannulated, the probe is lifted (carefully, so as not to disturb the needle and puncture site) and turned to provide a longitudinal plane image. This view allows the physician to see the wire enter the lumen clearly. If there is blood return but the wire will not pass, it is possible that the needle may not have entered the lumen fully or the needle could have punctured through the lumen and is "back walled." The longitudinal view provides the best image for confirmation of wire placement, and often one can salvage a back-walled puncture with slow needle withdrawal using this view.

The sheath size for EVLT is 4 French (1.33 mm), and sheath size for RF is 7 French (2.3 mm). In practice, access of veins less than 2.0 mm in diameter is very difficult, and accessing veins greater than 3.0 mm in diameter is straightforward if using a 4 French sheath. If the veins are seen on imaging to be in spasm, and are smaller than they had been on the preoperative mapping, access may be difficult. Placing the patient in reverse Trendelenburg position, warming the limb with sterile towels, using a bed warmer, and sedating the patient can often enlarge the veins to a size that is accessible. Some practices use topical nitroglycerine to induce vasodilation and improve ease of access.

With laser ablation, after access with a micropuncture needle, a micropuncture sheath is advanced and proper placement is confirmed. A 0.035-mm wire is then passed into the desired position. The vascular technologist scans over the vein from the puncture site to the desired end point to ensure that the wire is coursing through the target vein and not entering the deep system through a perforator vein. The wire should be visualized to cross the SFJ into the common femoral vein for the GSV (unless there has been previous SFJ ligation) or through the saphenopopliteal junction (SPJ) for the SSV (if there is a connection between the SSV and the popliteal vein). A long sheath that has been flushed with heparinized saline is then passed over the wire, the wire is removed, and a laser fiber placed through the sheath. For RF ablation, the catheter is generally placed through the short 7 French sheath and passed directly to the SFJ or SPJ with direct ultrasound

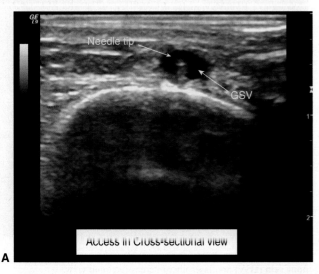

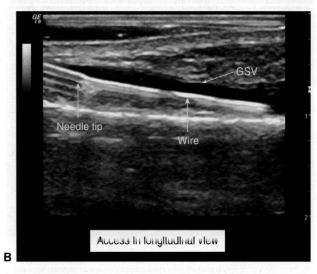

A   **B**

FIGURE 29.3. Vein cannulation in cross-sectional (*A*) and longitudinal views (*B*). (GSV, great saphenous vein).

visualization. If the target vein is tortuous or has dilated segments that "catch" the edge of the catheter, a 0.025 or smaller guidewire may be used to facilitate RF catheter placement.

The tip of the laser fiber or RF catheter should be positioned back at least 2.0 to 2.5 cm from the SFJ or SPJ. If a superficial epigastric or external pudendal vein or a competent thigh extension branch vein are present at the SFJ or SPJ, we recommend positioning the device tip distal (i.e., caudal) to these branches to keep them open (Fig. 29.4). Proper positioning may keep the junction patent and make thrombus extension into deep veins less likely. In our practice, the RVT and the surgeon must both agree that the tip is adequately distal (caudal) to the SFJ or SPJ before proceeding. Attention to leg position is important, since a fiber or catheter entering the GSV below the knee and positioned 2 cm caudal to the SFJ while the knee is in extension may easily protrude into the common femoral vein during knee flexion done to facilitate tumescent injections. Failure to appreciate and recognize this movement of the device tip could lead to injury of the common femoral vein with permanent serious consequences. The quality of ultrasound imaging and the expertise of the vascular technologist are of paramount importance in ensuring the safety of endovenous procedures.

Tumescent Anesthesia

Tumescent anesthesia—the injection of a saline and local anesthetic solution around the vein to be treated—is the next step in the procedure. Tumescent anesthesia has four purposes:

1. It helps to push blood out of the vein and collapse the vein wall onto the laser or RF catheter, thus preventing a layer of blood from "protecting" the vein wall from the intentional thermal injury.
2. It pushes the surrounding tissue away from the vein, including saphenous or sural nerve fibers.
3. The local anesthetic numbs the tissue surrounding the vein.
4. It provides a "heat sink" around the vein to dilute and dissipate the heat from the endothermal energy. The layer of tumescent solution should "push" the vein down so that it is at least 1 cm below the surface of the skin.

Ultrasound imaging guides the tumescence injection and ensures that an adequate "collar" of solution surrounds the vein. A micropuncture or spinal needle is used to inject the solution just above and parallel to the sheath to create a layer of

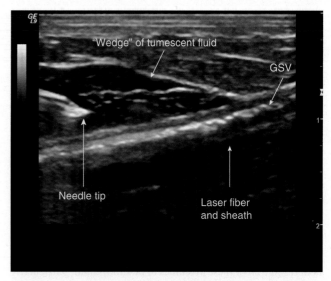

FIGURE 29.5. Tumescent fluid surrounding the great saphenous vein (GSV) and sheath with laser fiber in longitudinal view.

tumescence surrounding the sheath and laser or RF catheter. The tumescence lifts the fascia away from the vein creating a visible wedge of fluid above the vein (Fig. 29.5). The ultrasound probe is generally held in a longitudinal view during injection of tumescence, and a cross-sectional view will verify adequate tumescence around a collapsed vein. Placement of the probe directly perpendicular to the saphenous vein is essential to successful tumescence. This allows the surgeon to "come in" directly over the vein, with the tumescent needle in full view in the ultrasound image. This also ensures that the tumescent fluid is distributed evenly around the vein lumen and compresses all sides. If the vein is under a fascial layer, the cross-sectional view of the laser or RF catheter and sheath within the vein after tumescence should look like an "eye" (Fig. 29.6).

Activation of the Catheter

Prior to starting the actual ablation, the patient is placed in Trendelenburg position. Positioning and tumescence are utilized to empty as much blood as possible from the vein to

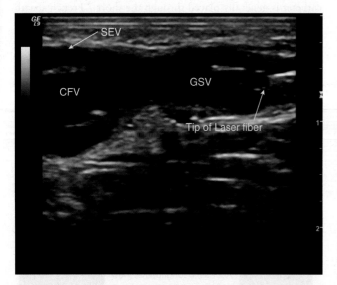

FIGURE 29.4. Position of a laser fiber tip distal to the superficial epigastric vein (SEV). (CFV, common femoral vein; GSV, great saphenous vein).

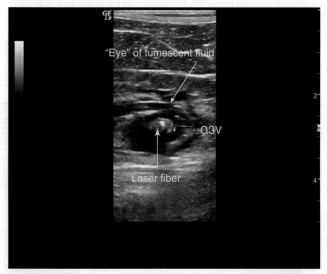

FIGURE 29.6. "Eye" of tumescent fluid surrounding the great saphenous vein (GSV) and laser fiber in cross-sectional view.

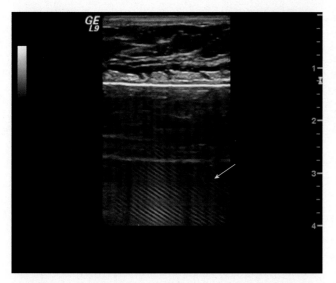

FIGURE 29.7. Ultrasound image during activation of the radiofrequency catheter with the typical linear diagonal artifact (*yellow arrow*).

FIGURE 29.8. An ablated great saphenous vein (GSV) appears bright and small on ultrasound imaging (*blue arrows*).

be treated. The vascular technologist positions the ultrasound probe over the catheter or device tip and reconfirms the distance from the tip to the deep vein confluence. After appropriate eyewear is placed on the patient and all personnel (for laser ablation only), the device is activated. For laser ablation, the catheter is slowly pulled back according to the manufacturer's instructions. With RF ablation, the vein is closed in 6.5 cm segments, with each segment ablated for 20 to 40 seconds. Ultrasound imaging should be used to verify that the laser or RF device is firing correctly, as steam bubbles should be visible, and with the RF device, a linear diagonal artifact will be seen (Fig. 29.7). In our practice, failure of the laser to fire has occurred, and this was only apparent on ultrasound as the laser console gave no indication of a problem. The vascular technologist follows the movement of the laser or RF catheter with ultrasound scanning as the surgeon pulls it back. This helps with accurate pullback speed and confirms a safe distance between the vein and the skin to prevent burns. With RF ablation, gentle pressure is held over the catheter as it is firing to compress the vein wall against the device.

The final step in the procedure is to verify closure of the target vein and to assess the SFJ or SPJ to make sure there is no thrombus extending into the common femoral vein or popliteal vein. An ablated vein appears bright and small on imaging (Fig. 29.8). The SFJ or SPJ is inspected for any thrombus protrusion from the superficial veins. On the day of the procedure, visualization of deep venous thrombus is rare. When seen, the extent of the thrombus should be measured, and treatment with anticoagulation is at the discretion of the treating physician. Significant DVT and pulmonary emboli are rare with endovenous thermal ablation.

For UGFS, access can either be obtained with a catheter as described for endothermal ablation when a large straight vein is the target, or with a butterfly or other needle for smaller and more tortuous veins. Once an intravenous position has been verified with ultrasound and blood return, foamed sclerosant can be injected. In order to avoid inadvertent placement of foam into the deep venous system, small volumes should be injected and the progress of the foam followed with ultrasound. The location of perforator veins in proximity to the veins being treated should be known in order to avoid large volumes of sclerosant entering the deep veins. With proper technique, the treated veins will promptly go into intense vasospasm and appear small and bright on ultrasound (Fig. 29.9).

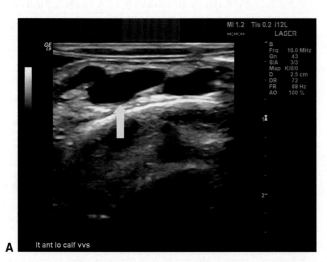
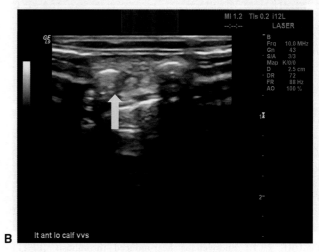

FIGURE 29.9. Varicose veins before *(A)* and after *(B)* ultrasound-guided foam sclerotherapy. The treated veins go into intense vasospasm and appear small and bright on ultrasound imaging (*yellow arrows*).

POSTOPERATIVE FOLLOW-UP

In many practices, patients return for a routine follow-up duplex within the first week after the procedure to assess for DVT. There is no consensus about the need for and the timing of duplex scans after ablation in asymptomatic patients, given the low likelihood of clinically significant findings. In our practice, while we have generally not seen thrombus protruding into deep veins on the day of the procedure, we do sometimes see such thrombi on our initial follow-up ultrasound. Many authors have noted thrombus protrusion into the deep veins with an incidence of 0% to 8% for the GSV[19-21] and 0% to 5.7% for the SSV.[20,22,23] Many practices refer to these thrombi as "endovenous heat-induced thrombosis" (EHIT) rather than DVT, as their etiology and natural history are certainly different than de novo DVT (Fig. 29.10). Other practices use the term "postablation superficial thrombus extension" (PASTE) to describe thrombus extensions that can occur with either heat ablation (RF or laser) or chemical ablation (sclerotherapy).

The treatment and follow-up of EHIT are controversial. We do not treat or follow thrombi that are flush with the SFJ or SPJ. Thrombi less than 5.0 mm in diameter are followed with serial duplex. Thrombi extending 5.0 mm or more into the SFJ or SPJ and filling less than 50% of the diameter of the deep vein are treated with low molecular weight heparin (LMWH) or fondaparinux until the thrombus recedes out of the deep vein. Thrombi filling greater than 50% of the diameter of the deep vein or occlusive thrombi are treated according to standard DVT guidelines. This is consistent with practices presented by other groups,[24] although there is no clear evidence that treatment is necessary in asymptomatic patients. We have found it helpful for our vascular technologists to sketch out a longitudinal and cross-sectional drawing of the EHIT for help in assessing whether this is merely a "tail" of the GSV or SSV thrombus, or a significant thrombus impeding venous return and threatening occlusion (Fig. 29.11). Follow-up duplex scans are performed at the discretion of the treating physician until the thrombus has resolved.

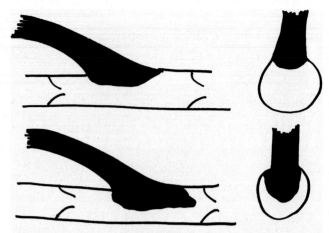

FIGURE 29.11. Vascular laboratory drawings of EHIT that include both longitudinal and cross-sectional views of the thrombus.

CONCLUSIONS

Endovenous techniques for the treatment of superficial venous incompetence offer the vascular laboratory a unique opportunity to participate in the therapy of venous disorders. Accurate ultrasound imaging ensures the safety and efficiency of these procedures. The active role of vascular technologists in endovenous ablation creates a rewarding interaction with the surgical team and has an additional benefit of improving diagnostic skills.

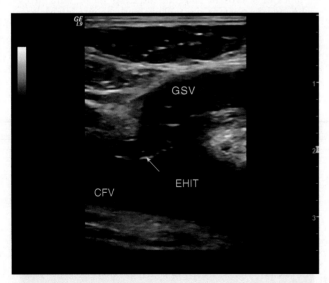

FIGURE 29.10. Endovenous heat-induced thrombosis (EHIT) (*yellow arrow*). (CFV, common femoral vein; GSV, great saphenous vein).

References

1. Sisto T, Reunanen A, Laurikka J, et al. Prevalence and risk factors of varicose veins in lower extremities: Mini-Finland health survey. *Eur J Surg* 1995;161(6):405-414.
2. Callam MJ. Epidemiology of varicose veins. *Br J Surg* 1994;81(2): 167-173.
3. Maurins U, Hoffman BH, Lösch C, et al. Distribution and prevalence of reflux in the superficial and deep venous system in the general population-results from the Bonn Vein Study, Germany. *J Vasc Surg* 2008;48(3): 680-687.
4. Clark A, Harvey I, Fowkes F. Epidemiology and risk factors for varicose veins among older people: Cross-sectional population study in the UK. *Phlebology* 2010;25(5):236-240.
5. Englehorn CA, Englehorn AL, Cassou MF, et al. Patterns of saphenous reflux in women with varicose veins. *J Vasc Surg* 2005;41(4):645-651.
6. Goldman MP. Closure of the greater saphenous vein with endoluminal radiofrequency thermal heating of the vein wall in combination with ambulatory phlebectomy: Preliminary 6-month follow-up. *Dermatol Surg* 2000;26(5): 452-456.
7. Navarro L, Min R, Boné C. Endovenous laser: A new minimally invasive treatment for varicose veins-preliminary observations using an 810 nm diode laser. *Dermatol Surg* 2001;27:117-122.
8. U.S. Food and Drug Administration. New device approval. http://www.fda.gov/cdrh/pdf/p990021a.pdf.
9. Hamel-Desnos C, Desnos P, Wollman JC, et al. Evaluation of the efficacy of polidocanol in the form of foam compared with liquid form in sclerotherapy of the great saphenous vein: Initial results. *Dermatol Surg* 2003;29: 1170-1175.
10. Rasmussen LR, Lawaetz M, Bjoern L, et al. Randomized clinical trial comparing endovenous laser ablation, radiofrequency ablation, foam sclerotherapy and surgical stripping for great saphenous varicose veins. *Br J Surg* 2011;98:1079-1087.
11. Bradbury AW, Bate G, Pang K, et al. Ultrasound-guided foam sclerotherapy is a safe and clinically effective treatment for superficial venous reflux. *J Vasc Surg* 2010;52:939-945.
12. Rathbun S, Norris A, Morrison N, et al. Performance of endovenous foam sclerotherapy in the USA. *Phlebology* 2012;27:59-66.
13. Rathbun S, Norris A, Morrison N, et al. Performance of endovenous foam sclerotherapy in the USA for the treatment of venous disorders: ACP/SVM/AVF/SIR quality improvement guidelines.. *Phlebology* 2014;29(2): 76-82.

14. BTG International Ltd. Press announcement. http://www.btgplc.com/development/our-programmes.
15. Elias S, Raines JK. Mechanochemical tumescentless endovenous ablation: Final results of the initial clinical trial. *Phlebology* 2012;27(2):67-72.
16. van den Bos RR, Milleret R, Neumann M, et al. Proof of principle study of steam ablation as a novel thermal therapy for saphenous veins. *J Vasc Surg* 2011;53:181-186.
17. Min RJ, Almeida JI, McLean DJ, et al. Novel vein closure procedure using a proprietary cyanoacrylate adhesive: 30 day swine model results. *Phlebology* 2012;27:398-403.
18. Eklof B, Perrin M, Delis KT, et al. Updated terminology of chronic venous disorders: The VEIN-TERM transatlantic interdisciplinary document. *J Vasc Surg* 2009;49:498-501.
19. Min RJ, Khilnani N, Zimmet SE. Endovenous laser treatment of saphenous vein reflux: Long-term results. *J Vasc Interv Radiol* 2003;14:991-996.
20. Ravi R, Rodriguez-Lopez JA, Traylor EA, et al. Endovenous ablation of incompetent saphenous veins: A large single-center experience. *J Endovasc Ther* 2006;13:244-248.
21. Mozes G, Kalra M, Carmo M, et al. Extension of saphenous thrombus into the femoral vein: A potential complication of new endovenous ablation techniques. *J Vasc Surg* 2005;41:130-135.
22. Gibson KD, Ferris BF, Polissar N, et al. Endovenous laser treatment of the small saphenous vein: Efficacy and complications. *J Vasc Surg* 2007;45(4):795-803.
23. Proebstle TM, Gul D, Kargl A, et al. Endovenous laser treatment of the lesser saphenous vein with a 940-nm diode laser: Early results. *Dermatol Surg* 2003;29(4):357-361.
24. Jimenez JC, Lawrence PF, Harlander-Locke M, et al. Segmental thermal ablation of the small saphenous vein (SSV) using an endovenous heat-induced thrombus (EHIT) classification system and treatment algorithm. Abstract presented at the 2012 Annual Meeting of the Western Vascular Society, Park City, UT. http://www.vascularweb.org/wvs/annualmeeting/Pages/2012-Annual-Meeting.aspx.

PREOPERATIVE PLANNING, INTRAOPERATIVE ASSESSMENT AND PROCEDURAL GUIDANCE

CHAPTER 30 ■ INTRAOPERATIVE DUPLEX EVALUATION OF ARTERIAL REPAIRS

DENNIS F. BANDYK AND KELLEY D. HODGKISS-HARLOW

Assurance of technical adequacy is a fundamental principle of vascular surgery whether performed by an open surgical or endovascular technique. Unrecognized repair site defects can result in thrombosis, embolization, and stenosis and contribute to early hemodynamic failure. Verifying that the arterial reconstruction is technically "normal" should be routine and a step central to quality patient care.

How to best accomplish the intraprocedural assessment depends on the type of arterial intervention as well as preferences and experience of the surgeon or interventionist. While arteriography is considered the standard for evaluation after an endovascular intervention, routine use of arteriography in the operating room (OR) after open arterial repair may require additional arterial access, and it is best done in a dedicated hybrid OR suite, which is expensive and not always available. It can be cumbersome for OR staff to wear protective lead garments throughout the operation or to rescrub after donning lead. Multiple angiography runs are needed for complete anatomic imaging to exclude a significant abnormality.

Duplex scanning provides both anatomic and hemodynamic assessment and has been used for intraoperative evaluation after carotid endarterectomy; for renal and visceral artery reconstructions; and to confirm functional (stenosis-free) patency of lower limb bypass grafts or sites of endovascular therapies.[1-7] Ultrasound imaging can be performed transcutaneously or by direct placement of the transducer on exposed vessels in the surgical field. Duplex scanning uses high-resolution B-mode imaging, both color and pulsed Doppler flow analysis to identify residual abnormalities, and the application of anatomic and velocity spectral criteria to confirm an acceptable technical result or to categorize the significance of residual abnormalities.[8]

Duplex ultrasound is a suitable alternative to arteriography in terms of accuracy, but it also has the advantages of being noninvasive and readily available in most vascular surgery suites. The diagnostic accuracy for excluding technical error is in the range of 90%. Importantly, a normal study is associated with a high negative predictive value for early repair site failure.[1-3,5,7] The principal limitation of duplex scanning is the need for hands-on skills and experience to perform vessel imaging and to acquire the necessary pulsed Doppler velocity spectral recordings.

The goal of this intraoperative assessment is to optimize the technical precision of the arterial intervention and, in the process, to modify open surgical and endovascular interventions to improve outcome.[7] Despite careful operative or endovascular technique, a variety of abnormalities (stenosis, plaque dissection, platelet-thrombus, occlusion, low-flow state) can persist after an arterial intervention (Table 30.1). If the altered anatomy and associated flow disturbance are severe, the defect can induce blood coagulation to form platelet aggregates that can embolize or induce repair site thrombosis. Even without thrombosis, a residual stenosis alters hemodynamics in a way that predisposes to repair site myointimal hyperplasia and early failure.[2,3,5] A secondary intervention in the immediate or early postprocedural period can often salvage this situation, but overall patient morbidity, health care costs, and the likelihood of reintervention are increased.

Intraoperative assessment with duplex scanning also provides a dynamic means to identify and characterize arterial pathology to be repaired. For example, intraoperative duplex scanning can find focal stenoses from extrinsic compression due to popliteal entrapment or median arcuate ligament compression, and then it can be used to verify normal hemodynamics after release of the compressive fibromuscular bands.[9-11]

Intraprocedural testing using duplex or intravascular ultrasound (IVUS) can be done in less than 10 minutes ultrasound is more convenient than arteriography; and study interpretation is based on straightforward criteria.[2-5,8]

TECHNIQUES FOR INTRAOPERATIVE ASSESSMENT

Duplex scanning is complementary to other intraoperative assessments such as visual inspection, pulse palpation, continuous-wave (CW) Doppler flow analysis, and angiography. Repair site imaging is typically performed after the intervention is completed but before the incision is closed or catheter access is terminated. At this point in the procedure, inspection and pulse assessment are considered to be normal or acceptable. In this setting, duplex scanning will identify an unsuspected problem in 3% to 15% of cases, with the nature of the problem dependent on the anatomic site of the arterial intervention.[1-5] When the initial clinical assessment or a completion angiogram is abnormal or equivocal, duplex testing can be helpful in further defining the residual abnormality based on anatomic and hemodynamic criteria. Application of duplex ultrasound is feasible for all

TABLE 30.1

INTRAOPERATIVE DUPLEX ULTRASOUND IDENTIFIED ABNORMALITIES RELATIVE TO ARTERIAL REPAIR, IN DECREASING ORDER OF FREQUENCY

Carotid artery bifurcation endarterectomy or stent angioplasty

Residual common carotid plaque/shelf
Suture stenosis or adventitial band across posterior wall of ICA
Stent deformation with residual lumen stenosis
Platelet thrombus within carotid repair site
Clamp injury (dissection) in proximal diseased CCA
ICA kink or lumen or dissection or distal to repair site
Abnormal ICA flow hemodynamics
   No or low diastolic flow indicating a distal occlusive lesion
   High systolic-diastolic flow velocity (reperfusion syndrome, ICA spasm)

Infrainguinal bypass/angioplasty

Conduit—angioplasty site stenosis
Anastomotic stenosis
Platelet thrombus within arterial repair
Graft entrapment or torsion
Low graft flow due to diseased runoff

Visceral endarterectomy or bypass

Anastomotic stenosis
Dissection
Platelet thrombus in repair or outflow artery

CCA, common carotid artery; ICA, internal carotid artery.

open surgical arterial repairs and transcutaneous imaging of peripheral angioplasty procedures (Table 30.2); however, carotid, iliac, and mesenteric or renal artery angioplasty procedures are better assessed for technical adequacy with angiography, pressure measurements, or IVUS findings.

Transducer Selection

A high-frequency (10 to 15 MHz) hockey stick–shaped, linear array transducer is preferred for detailed intraoperative imaging. Asepsis is maintained by placing the transducer in a sterile plastic sleeve, with gel for acoustic coupling (Fig 30.1). To image deeper vessels (carotid stent, lower limb angioplasty sites, anatomic tunneled bypass grafts), a 5- to 7-MHz linear array transducer is used to scan transcutaneously over the area of interest.

Scanning Technique

The assistance of a vascular technologist to optimize instrument settings facilitates testing, whether performed in the operating room or interventional angiography suite. The surgeon manipulates the transducer over the arterial repair, assessing the B-mode image and color Doppler display, and directs where velocity spectra should be recorded, including any identified abnormalities. Sterile saline is instilled into the operative wound for acoustic coupling, and the transducer is positioned over the artery for scanning in sagittal and transverse planes (Fig. 30.2). Pulsed Doppler velocity spectra should be recorded from a longitudinal image of the artery using an ultrasound beam angle of 60 degrees or less to the vessel wall. The entire arterial repair should be imaged to assess lumen caliber and identify major anatomic defects such as residual plaque, stenosis, or wall dissection. Color Doppler imaging is useful to detect and interrogate sites of flow disturbance produced by flaps, kinks, stenosis, and retained vein conduit valves.

The sequence of scanning should begin at the inflow artery of the repair and proceed distally with imaging of the entire reconstruction and outflow artery. For carotid endarterectomy or visceral artery repairs, only a 10 to 15 cm vessel segment needs to be imaged, while evaluation of an infrainguinal vein bypass requires additional time to image the vein conduit, anastomotic regions, and the inflow/outflow arteries. Testing should be performed when the patient's hemodynamic status is normal. If hypotension is present, the condition should be corrected before scanning commences. If arterial

TABLE 30.2

DIAGNOSTIC METHODS AND "NORMAL" THRESHOLD CRITERIA FOR INTRAPROCEDURAL ASSESSMENTS OF OPEN SURGICAL AND ENDOVASCULAR PERIPHERAL ARTERIAL REPAIRS

■ PROCEDURE	■ ANGIOGRAM[a]	■ ARTERY PRESSURE MEASUREMENTS/IVUS[b]	■ DUPLEX ULTRASOUND[c]
Open surgical repairs			
Carotid endarterectomy	<20% DR	Not used	PSV < 150 cm/s
Renal bypass	Not used	Not used	PSV < 180 cm/s
Mesenteric bypass	Not used	Not used	PSV < 180 cm/s
Infrainguinal bypass	<30% DR	Not used	PSV < 180 cm/s
Endovascular interventions			
Carotid PTA stent	<20% DR	IVUS	PSV < 150 cm/s
Renal PTA	<30% DR	<10-mm gradient	Not used
Mesenteric PTA	<30% DR	<10-mm gradient	Not used
Iliac PTA	<30% DR	<10-mm gradient	Not used
Infrainguinal PTA	<30% DR	Not used	PSV < 180 cm/s
Vein bypass PTA	<30% DR	Not used	PSV < 180 cm/s

[a]Criteria for acceptable residual stenosis, expressed as % DR.
[b]Measurement of systolic pressure gradient, expressed as mm Hg.
[c]PSV threshold for revision of residual stenosis, used in conjunction with B-mode imaging criteria of stenosis and PSV ratio of >2.0 at the site of abnormality.
DR, diameter reduction; IVUS, intravascular ultrasound; PSV, peak systolic velocity; PTA, percutaneous transluminal angioplasty.

FIGURE 30.1. A 12-MHz "hockey stick" linear array transducer is inserted in a sterile plastic sleeve filled with ultrasound gel for use in the operative field.

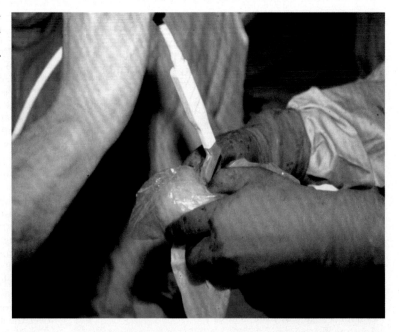

spasm, a high-resistance flow state, or low graft flow velocity is detected, direct intra-arterial injection of papaverine (30 to 60 mg) can augment flow by reducing peripheral vascular resistance, thereby enhancing diagnostic accuracy for stenosis detection. Of note, papaverine should *not* be injected into the cerebral circulation. (Intra-arterial nitroglycerine 100 to 200 μg can be used to reduce carotid vasospasm.)

Arteriographic imaging is already an integral part of most endovascular procedures, and many surgeons also utilize completion angiography after carotid endarterectomy or lower limb arterial intervention,[8,12-16] but duplex scanning is more sensitive for detecting some types of abnormalities.[12-14,17-19] Duplex scanning adds hemodynamic assessment of repair sites and the detection of subtle abnormalities such as vein valve stenosis and intimal flaps. The presence and severity of a lesion can be characterized using pulsed Doppler spectral recordings with measurement of peak systolic velocity (PSV) and the velocity ratio (Vr) across the stenosis. The clinical value of duplex testing is based on the rationale that if a residual lesion is identified,

additional intervention can be performed immediately with the goal of achieving normal repair site hemodynamics.

The vascular laboratory should allot approximately 30 minutes for intraoperative examinations, including instrument transport, setup, scanning, and image archiving. When intraoperative duplex scanning is routinely employed, most scans will be uncomplicated (i.e., associated with "normal" findings) and will typically require less than 10 minutes of hands-on scanning time.

Interpretation Criteria

The interpretation algorithm for intraoperative duplex ultrasonography is similar for all types of arterial interventions (Fig. 30.3). Testing is performed after clinical assessment indicates a patent repair and normal pressure pulsation. If B-mode imaging detects lumen abnormalities, velocity spectral recordings are used to document the presence and severity of

FIGURE 30.2. A vein patch carotid endarterectomy and placement of a small footprint 12-MHz linear array transducer (enclosed in a sterile plastic sleeve) in the neck wound for intraoperative assessment.

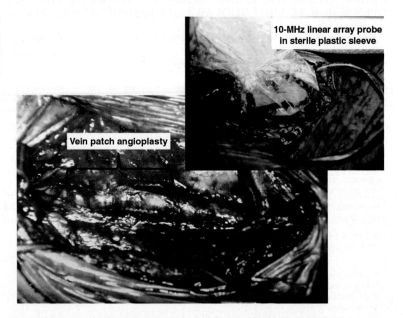

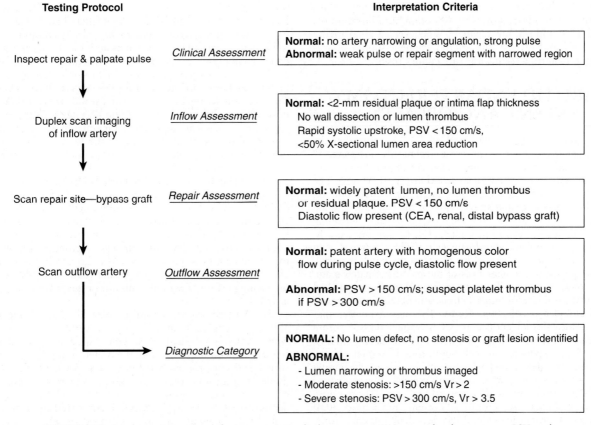

Testing Protocol

Inspect repair & palpate pulse — *Clinical Assessment*

Duplex scan imaging of inflow artery — *Inflow Assessment*

Scan repair site—bypass graft — *Repair Assessment*

Scan outflow artery — *Outflow Assessment*

Diagnostic Category

Interpretation Criteria

Normal: no artery narrowing or angulation, strong pulse
Abnormal: weak pulse or repair segment with narrowed region

Normal: <2-mm residual plaque or intima flap thickness
No wall dissection or lumen thrombus
Rapid systolic upstroke, PSV < 150 cm/s,
<50% X-sectional lumen area reduction

Normal: widely patent lumen, no lumen thrombus
or residual plaque. PSV < 150 cm/s
Diastolic flow present (CEA, renal, distal bypass graft)

Normal: patent artery with homogenous color
flow during pulse cycle, diastolic flow present

Abnormal: PSV > 150 cm/s; suspect platelet thrombus
if PSV > 300 cm/s

NORMAL: No lumen defect, no stenosis or graft lesion identified
ABNORMAL:
- Lumen narrowing or thrombus imaged
- Moderate stenosis: >150 cm/s Vr > 2
- Severe stenosis: PSV > 300 cm/s, Vr > 3.5

FIGURE 30.3. Interpretation pathway for intraoperative duplex scanning. CEA, carotid endarterectomy; PSV, peak systolic velocity; Vr, velocity ratio.

disturbed flow, that is, systolic velocity increase with spectral broadening. Anatomic defects with no or minimal flow disruption can be observed, but residual stenosis should be corrected. The interpretation criteria for repair site revision are similar for carotid, renal, and peripheral arterial interventions (Table 30.3). In general, an anatomic defect associated with a PSV greater than 150 to 180 cm/s and Vr across the site greater than 2.5 indicates a hemodynamically significant lesion with 50% or greater diameter reduction (DR). Velocity spectra with PSV greater than 300 cm/s signify a pressure-reducing, flow-reducing stenosis, and if lumen thrombus is imaged, platelet thrombus may have developed.[1,3]

The most common anatomic lesions identified by duplex testing consist of residual atherosclerotic plaque, stenosis, dissection, platelet-thrombus aggregates, intimal-media flaps, retained valve leaflets, and vessel kinks or compression.[1-5] When an anatomic defect is detected, Doppler spectral waveforms are recorded across the arterial segment with measurements of PSV and Vr. Spectral waveforms are also inspected for dampening (prolonged acceleration time), changes in phasicity,

PREOPERATIVE PLANNING, INTRAOPERATIVE ASSESSMENT AND PROCEDURAL GUIDANCE

TABLE 30.3

INTERPRETATION CRITERIA FOR CLINICALLY SIGNIFICANT ANATOMIC LESIONS AND RESIDUAL HEMODYNAMIC STENOSIS RELATIVE TO ARTERIAL REPAIR SITE AND TYPE

REPAIR SITE	TRANSDUCER	CRITERIA FOR ANATOMIC LESION	CRITERIA FOR RESIDUAL STENOSIS
Carotid			
CEA	10- to 15-MHz linear "hockey stick"	>2-mm residual plaque or mobile dissection/flap	PSV > 150 cm/s, Vr > 2, mobile lesion with >2 mm thickness
CAS	7- to 9-MHz linear array or 20-MHz IVUS	>30% diameter stent compression	
Visceral/renal	10- to 15-MHz linear array	>30% diameter reduction, lumen thrombus	PSV > 200 cm/s, Vr > 2, spectral broadening
Infrainguinal bypass	10- to 15-MHz linear "hockey stick"	>30% diameter reduction, thrombus	PSV > 150 cm/s or graft PSV <45 cm/s, Vr > 2.5, EDV > 15 cm/s
Lower limb Angioplasty	5- to 7-MHz linear array	>30% diameter reduction, extensive plaque dissection	PSV > 180 cm/s, Vr > 2.5, EDV > 15 cm/s

CEA, carotid endarterectomy; CAS, carotid stent angioplasty.

and spectral broadening that indicates turbulent flow. Flaps more than 2 mm in length, wall dissection, and intraluminal thrombus should prompt repair.[2,8] Whenever an abnormality is identified and revised, the arterial segment should be rescanned to confirm a technically satisfactory result.

CAROTID ENDARTERECTOMY/ STENT ANGIOPLASTY

Duplex ultrasound is the preferred method to verify that the carotid endarterectomy repair site is technically adequate.[2,18] Testing is performed immediately after closure of the arteriotomy and restoration of internal carotid artery (ICA) flow. The carotid repair is imaged beginning in the proximal common carotid artery (CCA) and slowly moving the transducer along the CCA and ICA to the most distal extent possible, including all sites of vascular clamp placement. Use of prosthetic patching, especially polytetrafluoroethylene (PTFE) material, can interfere with lumen imaging due to air in the patch material. Air may persist in the interstices of the prosthetic patch material for days, but it is still possible to scan through nonpatched artery wall, evaluate for lumen defects, and obtain center-stream pulsed Doppler velocity waveforms. The most common anatomic abnormalities identified are CCA plaque and ICA suture line stenosis. Plaques with greater than 2 mm thickness (that is, a "shelf"), focal dissection with flow around residual plaque, and clamp injuries should be repaired. Fronds of the intima that move with each cardiac cycle are typically not associated with a flow disturbance and do not require repair. The majority (>90%) of studies will confirm a "normal" repair (Fig. 30.4) with a widely patent lumen and PSV less than 150 cm/s in the ICA at the endarterectomy end point.[1,2] Interpretation criteria

for a "significant" stenosis include an anatomic defect with a PSV greater than 150 cm/s and Vr greater than 2 (Fig. 30.5). Exploration of the carotid repair will typically confirm an anatomic defect that can be corrected by additional endarterectomy, patch angioplasty, or patch extension. After revision, repeat duplex testing should be performed to verify that the abnormality has been corrected and no new defects have occurred. The decision to repair an external carotid artery (ECA) stenosis (PSV > 300 cm/s) or occlusion depends on surgeon bias regarding the clinical importance of maintaining patency in this branch. Typically, residual plaque in the ECA can be removed through a transverse incision at the origin of this vessel without clamping the CCA or ICA.

The prevalence of carotid reintervention based on intraoperative duplex scanning is in the range of 3% to 5% for repair of CCA or ICA defects, with an additional 3% to 5% if correction of residual ECA stenoses are included.[1,2,18] The likelihood that a "normal" carotid repair based on intraoperative duplex criteria will develop a clinically significant problem in the immediate postoperative period is extremely low (<1%), and the likelihood of finding a greater than 50% DR stenosis on testing performed within 3 months of the procedure is similarly low.[2,18]

The Vascular Study Group of New England found variable use completion imaging after carotid endarterectomy. Approximately one-half of surgeons used imaging at least selectively, with duplex testing the preferred modality.[18] Most surgeons do not routinely repair residual ECA plaque. When duplex testing was routinely used, 8% of repairs were reexplored, and these cases were associated with higher stroke and death rate (3.9% vs. 1.7%; $p = 0.3$) compared to cases where completion imaging was not performed or when it demonstrated a satisfactory result.

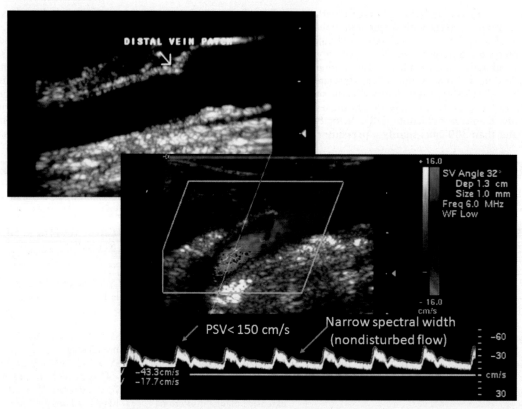

FIGURE 30.4. Duplex ultrasound of a vein patch carotid endarterectomy site with a normal B-mode image (*top*) and pulsed Doppler velocity spectral waveform (*bottom*) in the distal patch and internal carotid artery.

Proximal ICA after 1⁰ Closure   **Immediate Revision—Vein Patch**

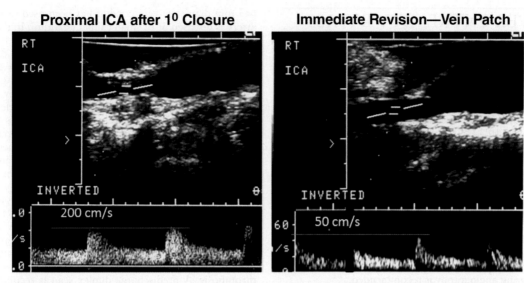

FIGURE 30.5. Abnormal duplex scan of a carotid endarterectomy site following primary arteriotomy closure. *Left,* Stenosis in the internal carotid artery (ICA) with peak systolic velocity (PSV) of 200 cm/s. *Right,* Following repair by patch angioplasty, no ICA stenosis is imaged and PSV is decreased to 50 cm/s, which is in the normal range.

Assessment of Carotid Stents Using Intravascular Ultrasound

Carotid stent angioplasty (CAS) has become more prevalent, and intraprocedural assessment of stent deployment can be performed using a 20-MHz IVUS catheter. High-resolution imaging of the extracranial carotid bifurcation and distal ICA is possible before and after CAS.[12,19] IVUS imaging provides accurate vessel lumen diameter measurements for appropriate stent sizing. Using a slow catheter pull-back technique after stent deployment, the entire stented artery segment can be imaged for stent wall apposition, verification of color flow, and assessment of stent deformation produced by calcified plaque (Fig. 30.6).

If greater than 50% cross-sectional lumen area reduction is identified, additional dilation of the stent can be performed. IVUS usage resulted in lower ($p < 0.05$) contrast agent volumes due to fewer angiogram runs for stent sizing and verification of adequate stent deployment and identified ($p < 0.01$) more residual stent abnormalities (N = 12, 11%) versus CAS with angiogram assessment alone (N = 2, 1.8%). Duplex ultrasound surveillance following CAS demonstrated a higher ($p < 0.01$) incidence of greater than 50% diameter-reducing in-stent stenosis in the angiography-alone group (11% vs. 7% at 1 month).[12] These authors concluded that the quality control of the CAS procedure was enhanced by IVUS imaging, which directed stent and balloon sizing, and IVUS was more accurate than angiography in confirming adequate stent expansion.

Circular deployment   **Elliptical Stent >20% stenosis**   **Increased Stent Lumen after Repeat Balloon Angioplasty**

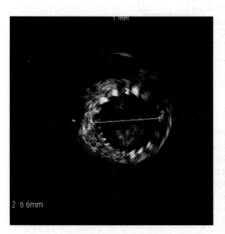
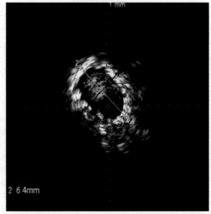
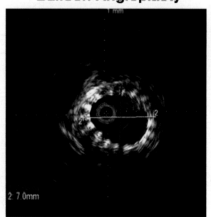

FIGURE 30.6. Intravascular ultrasound (IVUS) images following carotid stent angioplasty for greater than 70% internal carotid artery stenosis. Pullback of the IVUS catheter through the deployed stent allows imaging and measurement of stent diameters and assessment of circular stent expansion after balloon dilation.

PREOPERATIVE PLANNING, INTRAOPERATIVE ASSESSMENT AND PROCEDURAL GUIDANCE

LOWER EXTREMITY BYPASS GRAFTS

Intraoperative duplex scanning of infrainguinal vein bypass grafts has been shown to identify an anatomic defect that meets threshold criteria for revision in 10% to 27% of procedures (arm or spliced vein, 27%; in situ saphenous vein, 16%; translocated nonreversed saphenous vein, 13%; reversed saphenous vein, 10%).[3] The entire bypass graft should be scanned beginning at the distal anastomotic region. Injection of papaverine (30 to 60 mg) into the vein graft with a 27-gauge needle prior to scanning will vasodilate the arterial runoff bed and augment graft blood flow; this is referred to as "papaverine-augmented" duplex scanning (Figs. 30.7 and 30.8). The observation of a PSV greater than 45 cm/s and a low-resistance flow pattern (i.e., flow throughout diastole) in the distal graft and outflow artery is characteristic of a successful bypass graft. Low PSV or a high-resistance flow pattern with antegrade flow only during systole is abnormal, and a careful evaluation of the graft runoff using angiography is recommended.

After in situ saphenous vein bypass, color Doppler imaging can locate patent vein side branches for ligation and assess for adequacy of valve cusp lysis. Assessment of PTFE prosthetic bypass grafts is limited to imaging the anastomotic sites and the runoff artery, because conduit imaging is limited due to ultrasound attenuation by air within the graft wall. This limitation is not clinically important, as PTFE conduits should not be expected to have narrowing in the body of graft.

Duplex testing is classified as "normal" (no stenosis identified and graft PSV greater than 45 cm/s) or "abnormal" (a stenosis was identified or low graft flow state was found). Sites of color Doppler–detected stenosis are classified according to PSV and Vr as *moderate* (PSV > 150 cm/s, Vr > 2.5) or *severe* (PSV > 300 cm/s, Vr > 3.5). Although a PSV greater than 150 cm/s is the threshold for a bypass abnormality, a PSV in the range of 150 to 200 cm/s may be recorded when a small

(<3 mm diameter) vein conduit has been used or the outflow artery is diseased or of small caliber (<2 mm). In these circumstances, the Vr across this segment is less than 2.0, indicating hyperemic flow rather than a focal stenosis. When duplex scanning demonstrates an anastomotic stenosis or a graft defect (retained valve cusp, stricture, torsion) with PSV greater than 180 cm/s and Vr greater than 2.5, immediate revision of the site is recommended (Fig. 30.9). Intragraft platelet-thrombus formation is a lesion that develops in 3% of bypass graft procedures.[3] The duplex features include a velocity pattern for "high-grade" stenosis (PSV > 300 cm/s) and mobile lumen thrombus on real-time B-mode imaging. This graft lesion can be treated by segmental vein replacement and perfusion of the distal graft and runoff arteries with a thrombolytic agent.

If there is low graft velocity (PSV < 45 cm/s), assessment for a systemic cause (hypotension, cardiogenic shock) or outflow artery spasm should be made. If no such problem is identified, a postoperative regimen of heparin anticoagulation, dextran, and antiplatelet therapy is recommended, as grafts with this hemodynamic pattern are associated with a high risk of early thrombosis. A predischarge duplex scan is recommended for all bypass grafts with either an unrepaired stenosis or an intraoperative low-flow state to assess for persistent residual stenosis and to ensure that graft hemodynamics are adequate for continued patency.

Outcome of bypass grafting can be predicted by the intraoperative duplex findings. The incidence of early graft failure is low when intraoperative duplex testing is normal: only 1% at 30 days and 1.5% at 90 days. If a duplex-detected stenosis was not corrected or a low graft flow state was present, the incidence of graft failure within 30 to 90 days was found to increase to 8% to 30%. When intraoperative duplex assessment was used, the primary patency at 90 days was similar for in situ (94%), nonreversed (94%), and reversed (89%) saphenous vein bypasses but was lower for arm vein bypass grafts (82.5%, $p < 0.01$).[3,4] End-diastolic velocity recorded from the distal graft predicts bypass failure when less than

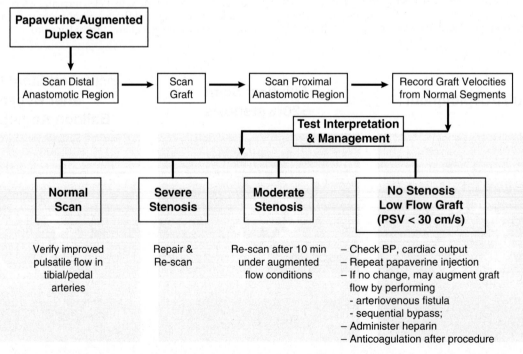

FIGURE 30.7. Algorithm for intraoperative scanning of an infrainguinal vein bypass graft. Following duplex assessment, the findings are used to classify the repair into one of four categories: normal scan, severe stenosis, moderate stenosis, and no stenosis but low-flow graft.

**BK Graft Segment Velocity Spectra
before Papaverine—High PVR**

**BK Graft Segment Velocity Spectra
after Papaverine—Low PVR**

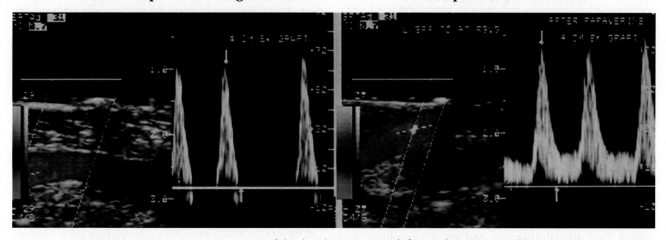

FIGURE 30.8. Papaverine augmentation of distal saphenous vein graft flow. *Left,* Prior to vasodilator injection. *Right,* Following injection. The velocity spectral waveform pattern changes from high resistance to low resistance with antegrade flow during the entire cardiac cycle. Note that peak systolic velocity does not change appreciably.

5 cm/s, (for example, when high peripheral arterial resistance to graft flow is present). When duplex testing identifies this type of bypass graft abnormality, measures to improve flow hemodynamics should be performed.[5,13]

DUPLEX-MONITORED ANGIOPLASTY

Duplex scanning is an efficient, cost-effective method to assess peripheral percutaneous transluminal angioplasty (PTA) site hemodynamics once angiography confirms an adequate anatomic result (<30% residual stenosis).[14-16] The goal of duplex-monitored angioplasty is to confirm normal hemodynamics (PSV < 180 cm/s, Vr < 2) at a time when arterial access is still available and additional interventions can be carried out.

Testing should be performed under "papaverine-augmented" flow conditions, and if a residual stenosis is identified, reintervention is recommended. Treatment options may include atherectomy, dilation with a larger balloon, stent placement, or more prolonged balloon dilation. A persistent duplex-detected stenosis correlates with early failure; after femoropopliteal balloon angioplasty, the 1-year primary patency was 85% when PTA site hemodynamics was normal versus 15% when a residual homodynamic stenosis (PSV > 180 cm/s, Vr > 2) was present.[15] Reported experience using duplex-monitored PTA resulted in reinterventions in 15% of native artery angioplasty procedures and 30% of angioplasty procedures performed for vein graft stenosis.[15,16] Technical advantages of this approach includes accurate selection of balloon and stent size and confirmation of angioplasty site hemodynamics with guide wire access still in place.

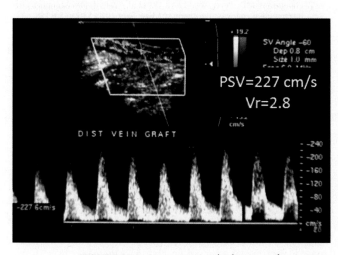

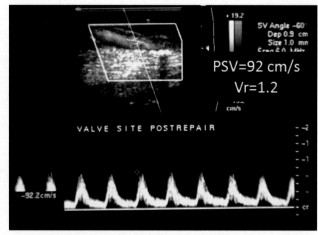

FIGURE 30.9. Intraoperative duplex scan of an in situ saphenous vein arterial bypass with stenosis. *Left,* Abnormal velocity waveform at a valve site (peak systolic velocity [PSV] = 227 cm/s; velocity ratio [Vr] = 2.8) indicating a retained valve leaflet. *Right,* After reintroduction of the valvulotome, the velocity waveform shows nondisturbed flow with a normal PSV of 92 cm/s and Vr of 1.2.

PREOPERATIVE PLANNING, INTRAOPERATIVE ASSESSMENT AND PROCEDURAL GUIDANCE

VISCERAL ARTERY RECONSTRUCTION

The clinical consequences of thrombosis after mesenteric and renal artery intervention can be catastrophic. A failed mesenteric bypass graft can produce intestinal infarction and is associated with high morbidity. Similarly, renal artery thrombosis can lead to renal ischemia and renal failure if the contralateral kidney is not functioning properly. A visceral artery repair or bypass graft can be imaged from the inflow artery origin (aorta, iliac, hepatic, splenic) to the distal artery in both longitudinal and transverse planes using B-mode and color Doppler imaging. Velocity spectra are recorded within the repair and in the distal visceral artery at a pulsed Doppler beam angle of 60 degrees or less. Having a low threshold to repair any abnormal duplex findings has been reported to improve early and late outcomes.[7]

The most common abnormalities identified in open surgical visceral artery reconstructions include suture stenosis, intimal flaps, arterial dissection, and low flow produced by distal thrombus formation. Residual anatomic defects with PSV greater than 180 to 200 cm/s and turbulent velocity spectra should be corrected. Minor lumen abnormalities with PSV less than 180 cm/s can be safely observed. If the significance of the duplex-detected abnormality is equivocal, angiography should be performed. Routine duplex assessment of mesenteric and renal artery repairs is associated with an 8% and an 11% immediate revision rate, respectively.[6,7] The appropriate management of minor defects remains unclear, but most reports favor a repair because a "normal" reconstruction based on duplex imaging is associated with excellent early and late outcomes.

ENDOVASCULAR AORTIC GRAFTS

Iatrogenic common femoral artery (CFA) and distal external iliac artery (EIA) defects after endovascular aneurysm repair (EVAR) can be detected with intraoperative duplex scanning. In one prospective series, 14% had abnormal findings that prompted arterial treatment with flap excision, tacking sutures, revision, or patch angioplasty.[20] Timely diagnosis and repair of these defects may decrease the incidence of early limb occlusion following endograft placement.

SUMMARY

Duplex ultrasound testing is an appropriate alternative to angiography for intraoperative assessment of arterial revascularization. Vascular surgeons can easily master the hands-on skills needed to perform the examination and identify clinically significant anatomic and residual stenosis.

Decisions about technical adequacy using objective criterion–based pulsed Doppler velocity spectral recordings can be made with a high degree of confidence. Routine application of intraoperative duplex testing is controversial[21] but is endorsed by vascular surgeons experienced with this technique to improve the technical precision of open and endovascular interventions.

References

1. Bandyk DF, Mills JL, Gahtan V, et al. Intraoperative duplex scanning of arterial reconstructions: Fate of repaired and unrepaired defects. *J Vasc Surg* 1994;20:426-433.
2. Ascher E, Markevich N, Kallakuri S, et al. Intraoperative carotid artery duplex scanning in a modern series of 650 consecutive primary endarterectomy procedures. *J Vasc Surg* 2004;39:416-420.
3. Bandyk DF, Johnson BL, Gupta AK, et al. Nature and management of duplex abnormalities encountered during infrainguinal vein bypass grafting. *J Vasc Surg* 1996;24:430-438.
4. Johnson BL, Bandyk DF, Back MR, et al. Intraoperative duplex monitoring of infrainguinal vein bypass procedures. *J Vasc Surg* 2000;31:678-690.
5. Rzucidlo EM, Walsh DB, Powell RJ, et al. Prediction of early graft failure with intraoperative completion duplex ultrasound scan. *J Vasc Surg* 2002;36:975-981.
6. Hansen KJ, O'Neil EA, Reavis SW, et al. Intraoperative duplex sonography during renal artery reconstruction. *J Vasc Surg* 1991;3:364-374.
7. Oderich GS, Panneton JM, Macedo TA, et al. Intraoperative duplex ultrasound of visceral revascularizations: Optimizing technical success and outcome. *J Vasc Surg* 2003;38:684-691.
8. Parsa P, Hodgkiss-Harlow K, Bandyk DF. Interpretation of intraoperative arterial duplex ultrasound testing. *Sem Vasc Surg* 2013;26:105-110.
9. Altintas U, Helgstrand UV, Hansen MA, et al. Popliteal artery entrapment syndrome: Ultrasound imaging, intraoperative findings, and clinical outcome. *Vasc Endovascular Surg* 2013;47(7):513-518.
10. Causey MW, Singh N, Miller S, et al. Intraoperative duplex and functional popliteal entrapment syndrome: Strategy for effective treatment. *Ann Vasc Surg* 2010;24(4):556-561.
11. Relles D, Moudgill N, Rao A, et al. Robotic-assisted median arcuate ligament release. *J Vasc Surg* 2012;56(2):500-503.
12. Bandyk DF, Armstrong PA. Use of intravascular ultrasound (IVUS) as a "quality control" technique during carotid stent-angioplasty: Are there risks to its use? *J Cardiovasc Surg* 2009;50:727-733.
13. Scali ST, Beck AW, Nolan BW, et al. Completion duplex ultrasound predicts early graft thrombosis after crural bypass in patients with critical limb ischemia. *J Vasc Surg* 2011;54:1001-1010.
14. Mewissen MW, Kinney EV, Bandyk DF, et al. The role of duplex scanning versus angiography in predicting outcome after balloon angioplasty in the femoropopliteal artery. *J Vasc Surg* 1992;15:860-864.
15. Johnson BL, Avino AJ, Bandyk DF. Duplex-monitored angioplasty of peripheral artery and infrainguinal vein graft stenosis. In Whittemore AD (ed). *Advances in Vascular Surgery*, Vol 8. St. Louis: CV Mosby, 2000, pp 83-95.
16. Ascher E, Marks NA, Hingorani AP, et al. Duplex guided endovascular treatment for occlusive and stenotic lesions of the femoral-popliteal arterial segment: A comparative study in the first 253 cases. *J Vasc Surg* 2006;44:1230-1237.
17. Humphries MD, Pevec WC, Laird JR, et al. Early duplex scanning after infrainguinal endovascular therapy. *J Vasc Surg* 2011;53(2):353-358.
18. Wallert JB, Goodney PP, Vignati JJ, et al. Completion imaging after carotid endarterectomy in the Vascular Study Group of New England. *J Vasc Surg* 2011;54:376-385.
19. Joan MM, Moya BG, Agustí FP, et al. Utility of intravascular ultrasound examination during carotid stenting. *Ann Vasc Surg* 2009;23(5):606-611.
20. Hingorani AP, Ascher E, Marks N, et al. Iatrogenic injuries of the common femoral artery (CFA) and external iliac artery (EIA) during endograft placement: An underdiagnosed entity. *J Vasc Surg* 2009;50(3):505-509.
21. Norgren L, Hiatt WR, Dormandy JA, et al. TASC II Working Group. Inter-Society Consensus for the Management of Peripheral Arterial Disease (TASC II). *J Vasc Surg* 2007;45(Suppl S):S5-S67.

CHAPTER 31 ■ INTRAVASCULAR IMAGING

MISTY HUMPHRIES

The ability to assess endovascular interventions by real-time means has historically been limited. Angiography provides only a two-dimensional representation of the cylindrical vessel lumen, and subtle plaque irregularities may be missed. Characterization of arterial plaque when imaged by angiography is frequently limited to identification of calcification. Although Ascher et al have advocated duplex ultrasound for guidance of endovascular procedures, it has not been widely accepted, in part due to the personnel support needed and the limited ability of ultrasound to visualize vessels deep in the pelvis and leg with adequate resolution.[1] Computed tomography (CT) and magnetic resonance imaging (MRI) are difficult to apply in the intraoperative realm because of equipment limitations, although further imaging refinements may make this easier in the future. Limitations in these modalities have stimulated interest in imaging within blood vessels.

Intravascular imaging is not a new concept. As early as the 1950s, angioscopy was developed in an attempt to determine intraluminal plaque characteristics. This technology requires complete cessation of blood flow, and the large size of the initial devices limited clinical utility. Newer devices are as small as 0.75 mm in outer diameter and can image approximately 1 to 5 mm in depth. They are also mounted with a proximal occlusion balloon to stop blood flow and permit clear imaging. Most of these smaller devices are still in development, and clinical use has been limited. Over the same time frame, intravascular ultrasound (IVUS) has been steadily refined. Not until the late 1980s were Yock et al able to reduce the size of a single ultrasound transducer system in order to image coronary arteries, making IVUS a clinically useful tool.[2] Since then, IVUS systems have undergone multiple refinements to make them the small easily applied imaging systems we have today.

Optical coherence tomography (OCT), a newer technology, is rapidly gaining momentum and is being incorporated into peripheral devices to improve endovascular capabilities. It uses near infrared light as opposed to ultrasound waves. This allows OCT devices to have a markedly improved resolution compared to IVUS, the trade-off being limited to evaluating vessels of relatively small diameter. Device improvement and development have allowed physicians who deliver vascular care to better understand intravascular pathology and the pitfalls of interventions.

VASCULAR WALL ANATOMY AND ATHEROSCLEROSIS

A complete discussion of arterial wall anatomy is beyond the scope of this chapter, but a simple understanding of basic anatomy and plaque characteristics warrants mentioning, given that the greatest advantage of intravascular imaging is the ability to define plaque composition and identify features that may affect procedural outcomes. The arterial wall is composed of three distinct layers: the tunica intima, media, and adventitia. The intima layer is closest to the flowing blood and consists of endothelial cells separated from the subendothelial space by the basal lamina. The subendothelial space is an extracellular matrix composed of proteoglycans and collagen that extends to the internal elastic lamina.

Atherosclerotic lesions develop as the endothelium increases expression of leukocyte adhesion molecules. A subsequent increase in endothelial permeability allows leukocytes and lipoproteins to move into the subendothelial space where macrophages and smooth muscle cells are located. With progression of the lesion, lipoproteins are taken up by macrophages and transformed into foam cells that form the lipid core of atherosclerotic lesions. Progressive inflammation in this area also stimulates smooth muscle cell proliferation in the subendothelial space. Activated smooth muscle cells continue the production of growth factors and stimulate further proliferation. As collagen and extracellular matrix are deposited, the fibrous cap becomes more developed. With increased levels of inflammatory mediators within the vessel wall, both smooth muscle cells and endothelial cells may undergo apoptosis causing thinning of the cap. This can lead to vulnerable or unstable plaque. With rupture of this plaque, the inner lipid core becomes exposed along with other prothrombotic elements and subsequent thrombosis may occur.[3] The ability to detect these histologic changes and treat lesions with targeted therapy based on plaque characteristics has been a long-term goal. IVUS offers a tool to improve outcomes and refine new therapeutic intravascular technology.

INTRAVASCULAR ULTRASOUND

Technical Considerations

There are two varieties of IVUS catheters: mechanical and phased array (Fig. 31.1). Mechanical transducers use electrical current generated through a piezoelectric crystal to produce and receive sound waves. Typically, mechanical transducers have a single transducer element that rotates circumferentially on a drive shaft at approximately 1900 rotations per minute to create a cross-sectional image. Phased array transducers are stationary. They have multiple transducer elements, typically 64 in current catheters, positioned in a radial fashion that fire in circumferential succession. This produces an array of

435

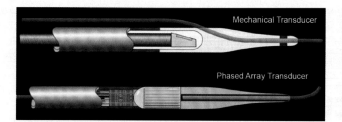

FIGURE 31.1. Mechanical and phased array transducers. Mechanical transducer images may have artifact related to the wire position. (Courtesy of Boston Scientific Corporation, Natick, MA.)

images, which are processed into a 360-degree cross-sectional image of the vessel lumen and wall.

Both types of transducers have limitations and generate artifacts that the user must be familiar with. Mechanical transducers typically have a wire channel that runs alongside the transducer that generates a wire artifact in the images (Fig. 31.2). In addition, mechanical transducers can trap small bubbles that result in air speckling if not flushed properly. Nonuniform rotational distortion (NURD) is a rotational distortion that occurs with mechanical transducers. This is typically seen in tortuous vessels, with kinking of guide catheters, or when hemostatic Tuohy-Borst valves are tightened excessively over the catheter. Excess stress on the IVUS catheter causes bending, and the rotational speed of the transducer varies, causing image acquisition to be distorted. Manufacturers of mechanical transducers have introduced corrective software to prevent this distortion. Phased array transducers can have ring-down artifacts. This represents an area immediately surrounding the catheter obscured by acoustic oscillations within the transducer. Adjustments in the gain of the transducer can be made once the catheter is outside of the sheath or guide catheter and not apposed to the arterial wall to minimize this artifact. Care must be taken to avoid adjusting too much, as true luminal signals can also be suppressed.[4]

IVUS catheters range in frequency from 8 to 50 MHz. As with all ultrasound probes, higher frequencies provide greater spatial resolution. The trade-off for using higher frequency probes is decreased depth of tissue penetration. Balancing

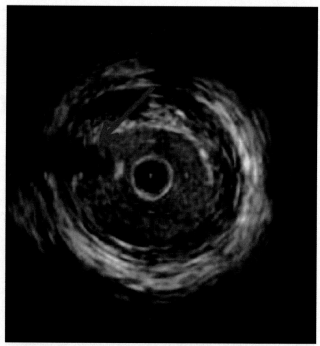

FIGURE 31.2. Wire artifact associated with mechanical IVUS transducers (*red arrow*).

these two factors is imperative when selecting the appropriate catheter for intravascular imaging. Catheters suitable for imaging the aorta and inferior vena cava (IVC) have a frequency range from 9 to 15 MHz. These catheters are typically able to image vessels with a maximum diameter of 5 to 6 cm, depending on the system. Optimal imaging of the iliac and common femoral arteries and veins can be obtained with catheters of 15 to 20 MHz. Smaller vessels, such as the superficial femoral, tibial, and renal arteries, are best imaged with transducers of 20 to 40 MHz (Table 31.1). Although vessel size may initially dictate the catheter used, other factors such as delivery system, sheath size, and wire access also factor into the selection of the appropriate catheter for the case at hand.

TABLE 31.1

CHARACTERISTICS OF CURRENT COMMERCIALLY AVAILABLE PHASED ARRAY AND MECHANICAL IVUS CATHETERS

	■ SMALL VESSEL PHASED ARRAY	■ MID-VESSEL PHASED ARRAY	■ LARGE VESSEL PHASED ARRAY	■ MID-VESSEL MECHANICAL	■ LARGE VESSEL MECHANICAL
Frequency	20 MHz	24 MHz	10 MHz	40 MHz	15 MHz
Vessel imaging diameter	20 mm	24 mm	60 mm	20 mm	60 mm
Minimum sheath size	5 F	6 F	8.5 F	6 F	8.5 F
Wire diameter	0.014″	0.018″	0.038″	0.018″	0.038″
Delivery system	Rapid exchange	Rapid exchange	Over the wire	Rapid exchange	Over the wire
ChromoFlo®	Yes	Yes	No	No	No
Appropriate vessels	Tibial Popliteal Renal	Femoral Iliac Subclavian	Aorta IVC Common Iliac	Femoral Iliac Subclavian	Aorta IVC Common Iliac

IVC, inferior vena cava.

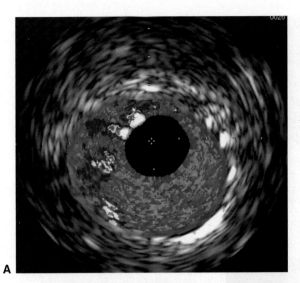 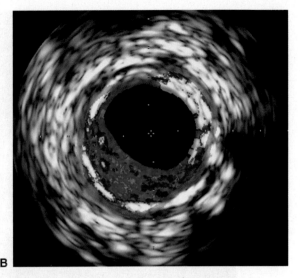

FIGURE 31.3. Virtual histology of peripheral plaque. *A,* Fibro-fatty plaque with small areas of necrotic core. *B,* Fibroatheroma with dense areas of calcification.

Interpretation of IVUS imaging can be aided by two specific technologies: virtual histology and ChromaFlo®. Virtual histology is a computer-generated color map created from the reflected ultrasound signals. This map is displayed on the screen superimposed over the gray-scale image. Each of the four colors used represents a different component of plaque (Fig. 31.3). Deep green represents fibrous plaque, lighter green is fibro-fatty plaque, white represents dense calcium, and red is necrotic core. In an attempt to better understand the ability of virtual histology to characterize plaque, the Virtual Histology Intravascular Ultrasound Assessment of Carotid Artery Disease: The Carotid Artery Plaque Virtual Histology Evaluation (CAPITAL) study used virtual histology to assess carotid plaque prior to

endarterectomy in 15 patients. Histologic composition of the plaques was compared to the virtual histology generated by IVUS. The authors found the diagnostic accuracy of virtual histology to range from 72.4% for calcified fibroatheroma to 99.4% for thin-cap fibroatheroma. The specificity ranged from 82% for intimal thickening to 100% for thin-cap fibroatheroma.

Small and mid-sized vessel phased array catheters are also able to offer color flow (ChromaFlo®) technology. When the location or patency of the vessel lumen is unclear, color flow imaging can be turned on to display the flow channel of the vessel (Fig. 31.4). Applications of this technology include evaluating the luminal irregularity of plaque and stent apposition. This technology has also been mounted on a reentry needle for use in sub-intimal angioplasty.

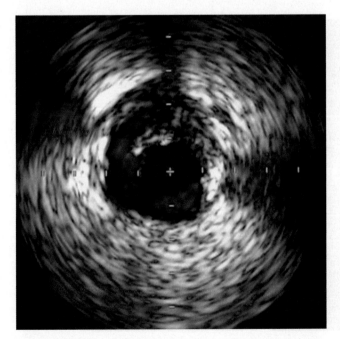

FIGURE 31.4. ChromaFlo® imaging showing delineation of an edge dissection after angioplasty. (Images courtesy of Volcano Corporation, San Diego, CA.)

Applications

Venous

IVUS has emerged as an important adjunct for endovascular venous procedures. When used during thrombolytic procedures, IVUS can identify residual thrombus. Acute thrombus is difficult to visualize completely with IVUS images (Fig. 31.5). Chronic thrombus, on the other hand, is usually devoid of red blood cells and contains a higher concentration of fibrin, making it more echogenic and easier to distinguish from the vessel wall. Bands, frozen valves, spurs, or venous webs as the cause of thrombosis may not be easily identified with venography. IVUS can delineate irregularities that may be amenable to simple angioplasty and can determine if stent placement is required.

Use of IVUS has become essential in the treatment of iliac vein obstruction or stenosis resulting from arterial compression, also known as May-Thurner syndrome. Classic May-Thurner is caused by compression of the left common iliac vein by the right common iliac artery. Two additional areas of possible compression are located where the right external iliac artery crosses the right external iliac vein and where the left hypogastric artery crosses the left external iliac vein. Venography may show a flattening of the vein where compressed, and chronic compression can lead to scarring and thrombosis (Fig. 31.6). Venography can also severely

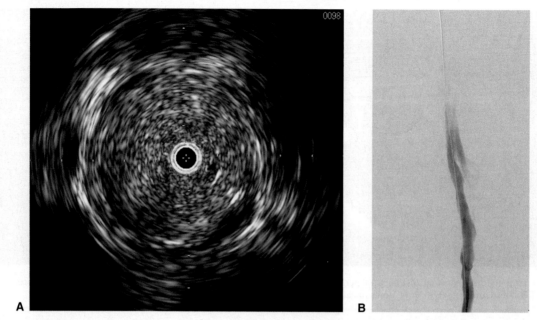

FIGURE 31.5. *A,* Intravascular ultrasound of acute thrombus filling the lumen of the external iliac vein. *B,* Venography demonstrating no flow of contrast through the external iliac vein due to acute deep venous thrombosis.

underestimate the degree of venous stenosis, and stent sizing after recanalization without IVUS can lead to significant undersizing. Therefore, IVUS has become the preferred method for identifying the area of greatest venous narrowing to ensure accurate stent placement.

IVUS can be used for placement of IVC filters. This avoids radiation, iodinated contrast, and often transport of the patient from the intensive care unit. The standard approach for IVUS-guided IVC filter placement is from a femoral access

site. The IVUS catheter is used to identify the left renal vein, which is anatomically lower than the right. Once the location of this vein is determined, the IVUS catheter is marked and removed so it can be used as a guide for the specific distance to insert the IVC filter for deployment. When transitioning to an IVUS-guided protocol for IVC filter placement, the general recommendation is to also use fluoroscopy for the first several procedures to ensure that the anatomy is clear and the filter placement is accurate.

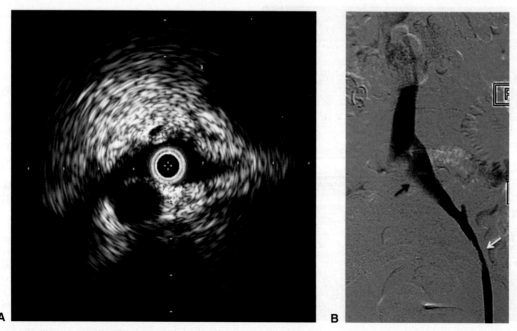

FIGURE 31.6. *A,* IVUS of the left common iliac vein compressed by the right common iliac artery. *B,* Venography showing the left common iliac vein flattened (*red arrow*). This is a classic sign for May-Thurner syndrome. Additionally, a residual chronic stenosis is seen in the external iliac vein (*white arrow*).

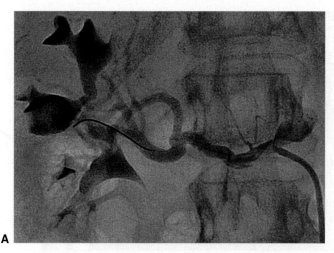
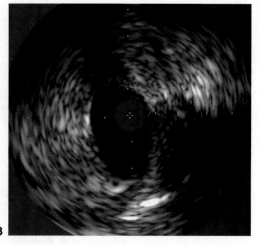

A   **B**

FIGURE 31.7. *A*, Renal angiography was unable to fully characterize this ostial right renal artery stenosis. *B*, IVUS and pressure gradient measurements showed a significant narrowing. After stent placement, the patient's renal artery flow improved and the antihypertensive medical regimen was decreased.

Arterial

PERIPHERAL ARTERIAL

Identification of ostial renal artery lesions can be challenging. Patients with renal artery stenosis (RAS) may have impaired renal function, and efforts are made to avoid large volumes of nephrotoxic contrast. The renal arteries typically branch off in a downward direction from the lateral aspects of the aorta, but this can vary. With age, the aorta can also become tortuous, and the lateral locations of the renal artery origins become more posterior or anterior. This makes optimization of angiographic views of the renal artery ostia difficult (Fig. 31.7). When RAS is confirmed or suspected based on preoperative duplex ultrasound or an ACE-inhibitor–induced creatinine elevation, but it cannot be adequately imaged with angiography, IVUS can assist with delineation of lesion length and location. Used in conjunction with pressure measurements taken across renal artery lesions, IVUS has been shown to more accurately estimate the true degree of RAS and assist with selection of patients that may benefit from renal artery stenting.[5]

Endovascular procedures have become first-line therapies for peripheral artery disease. Despite the evolution of these interventions, long-term patency rates vary widely depending on the arterial segment treated.[6] Two-dimensional angiography can lead to inaccurate calculation of the true degree of arterial stenosis due to the inability to image the arterial wall. IVUS can visualize both the arterial wall and lumen, adding valuable insight on the nature and true severity of arterial narrowing. The ability to determine the exact vessel diameter allows for more precise selection of balloons and stents (Fig. 31.8). In a study of iliac artery interventions by Buckley et al, IVUS demonstrated that 40% of the stents placed were initially under-expanded. By addressing this problem at the initial procedure, the authors were able to show improved 3- and 6-year outcomes.[7] Undersized stents cause early restenosis or lead to more limb-threatening thrombosis.

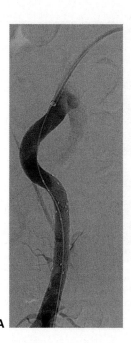
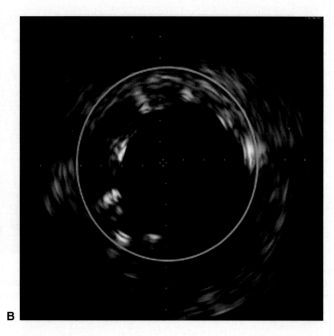

FIGURE 31.8. *A*, In this angiogram, the stent appears to be fully expanded and apposed to the arterial wall. *B*, Live IVUS imaging demonstrated that the stent was not apposed to the arterial wall during diastole.

A   **B**

FIGURE 31.9. *A,* Pioneer catheter with entry needle deployed. *B,* Relationship of the reentry needle and IVUS probe. (Images courtesy of Medtronic, Minneapolis, MN.)

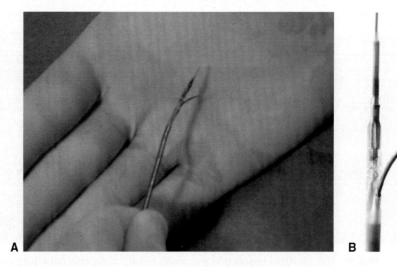

The information provided by IVUS may help to avoid these complications and lead to improved outcomes for de novo peripheral arterial interventions.

For those patients who do develop restenosis, IVUS can aid in identification of the cause. Neointimal hyperplasia is generally recognized as the main cause of stent failure, although studies in the coronary and carotid literature have shown that negative arterial remodeling may also play a role in restenosis.[8,9] The distinction between these two processes is essential to determine adequate treatment. Neointimal hyperplasia can reasonably be treated by endovascular means. Negative arterial remodeling may require consideration of alternative treatments such as bypass or interposition grafting.

By combining IVUS with a reentry device, the Pioneer catheter (Medtronic, Minneapolis, MN) is a valuable tool for treating chronic total arterial occlusions. The catheter is dual lumen with a phased array transducer located near the tip. Just proximal to the transducer is a deployable reentry needle (Fig. 31.9). If wire maneuvers fail to reenter the true lumen during subintimal angioplasty, the catheter is advanced in the subintimal space. Color flow imaging can identify the true lumen of the vessel (Fig. 31.10). The true lumen is oriented at the 12 o'clock position and the reentry needle is deployed. A second wire is advanced into the true lumen, and the needle is withdrawn before the catheter is removed. The small reentry track can then be dilated to accommodate subsequent stent placement.

AORTIC PATHOLOGY

Abdominal aortic aneurysm repair with endovascular stent grafts (EVAR) is now the preferred treatment in appropriately selected patients. Sizing for stent placement is typically performed with arterial timed contrast-enhanced CT. In patients with poor renal function, IVUS can limit nephrotoxic contrast administration, and when used in conjunction with carbon dioxide angiography, contrast may be avoided altogether. Additional techniques to limit contrast include the use of hybrid operating rooms with specialized image processing software. A rotational image can be merged with preoperative CT images to create a roadmap for the patient. IVUS can confirm the location of the celiac, superior mesenteric, and bilateral renal arteries (Fig. 31.11). Once the renal arteries are identified, subsequent aortic neck measurements

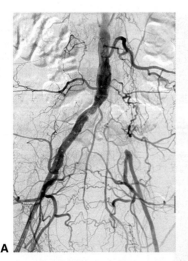
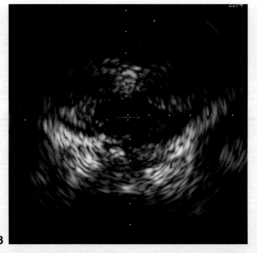
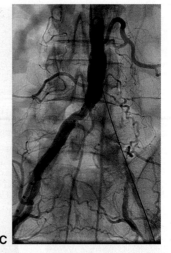

FIGURE 31.10. *A,* Chronic total occlusion of the left common iliac artery that could not be crossed with a catheter and wire alone. *B,* IVUS within the subintimal space. The true lumen is visualized with color flow imaging at the 12 o'clock position. *C,* Using the Pioneer catheter, the lesion was crossed and the true lumen reentered. Bilateral balloon expandable stents were then placed to restore the aortic bifurcation.

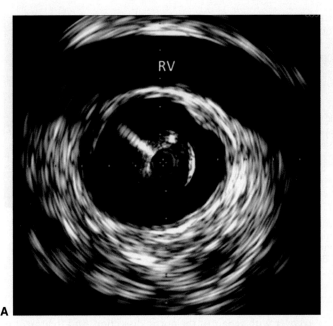

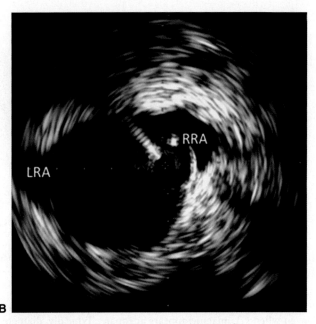

FIGURE 31.11. *A,* The renal vein (*RV*) is seen crossing the aorta anteriorly. This landmark can be used to identify and orient the left (*LRA*) and right (*RRA*) renal arteries (*B*) as they branch from the aorta.

can be obtained. A similar technique can be used to identify the aortic bifurcation and determine the size of the common iliac arteries (Fig. 31.12). After aortic diameter measurements are made and the graft is selected, a catheter can be left in the lowest renal artery as a marker while the graft is deployed. Graft limb length measurements can be made by identifying the bifurcation of the common iliac artery with IVUS and using a catheter with 1 cm marks to measure the precise limb length. Use of IVUS alone for EVAR measurements is an advanced skill and should be used with caution by those new to the technology.

In addition to abdominal aortic aneurysm measurements, IVUS should be used liberally for sizing of thoracic aortic grafts. Even with sophisticated reconstruction software, precise measurements of the thoracic aorta can be difficult. This is especially true in the region of the aortic arch. Traumatic aortic injuries (TAI) represent a challenging problem. The intimal tear in TAI is usually distal to the left subclavian artery, and subclavian revascularization is rarely needed after thoracic endovascular aortic repair (TEVAR) for TAI. The patient's initial imaging is likely to be done without arterial timed contrast, as these patients undergo extensive workup to evaluate for multiple traumatic injuries.[10] These images can underestimate the size of the aorta. Studies in traumatic porcine models have shown that the thoracic aortic diameter can be underestimated by as much as 40% prior to resuscitation.[11]

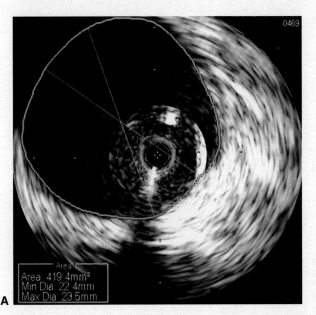

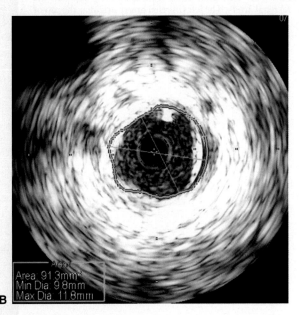

FIGURE 31.12. Aortic neck (*A*) and iliac artery (*B*) diameter measurements.

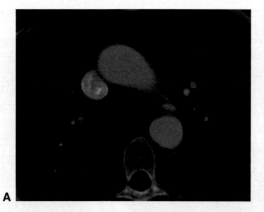
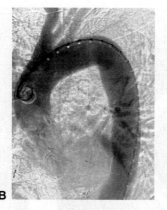
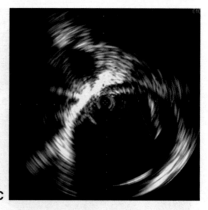

FIGURE 31.13. *A,* Traumatic aortic injury with pseudoaneurysm on CT of the chest in a patient with multiple injuries after a motor vehicle accident. *B,* Conventional angiography did not completely visualize the injury. *C,* IVUS demonstrates the intimal tear (*red arrow*) and most proximal aspect of the pseudoaneurysm. Complete coverage of the tear was documented on images obtained after stent deployment.

Diameter measurements should also be repeated with IVUS even when CT imaging appears adequate. Typically, diameter measurements are obtained just proximal to the intimal tear and within the descending aorta to ensure appropriate graft selection. Small traumatic pseudoaneurysms may not be visualized with conventional angiography despite adequate rotation of the image intensifier (Fig. 31.13). IVUS can accurately identify the exact location of the intimal tear, and this can be correlated with angiographic landmarks. This ensures complete coverage of the intimal tear while sparing the left subclavian artery.

As with other thoracic aortic pathology, endovascular repair of thoracic aortic dissection requires IVUS. Type B aortic dissections cause symptoms by either static or dynamic lumen compromise. With static obstruction, the dissection flap extends into the ostia of branch vessels and results in collapse of the vessel lumen and thrombosis of the vessel distally (Fig. 31.14). In this situation, flow is not likely to recover with repair of the aortic dissection, and treatment of the branch vessel with bypass or stent placement is required. Dynamic obstruction, on the other hand, results from collapse of the vessel lumen during systole. The degree of ischemia in dynamic obstruction can change depending on the extent of the intimal tear, systolic blood pressure, and heart rate. Treatment of symptomatic type B dissections with stent graft placement can seal the proximal entry tear and result in thrombosis of the false lumen (Fig. 31.15). Because of the potential for multiple reentry tears located along the dissection flap, IVUS is essential during endovascular treatment. Use of fluoroscopy alone cannot ensure that the wire does not pass from the true to false lumen along the flap. Endograft placement within the false lumen has been reported and may require urgent open operative conversion or subsequent aortic replacement.

FIGURE 31.14. Extension of an aortic dissection flap into the right (*R*) renal artery. The left (*L*) renal artery origin at the top of the screen is supplied by the false lumen.

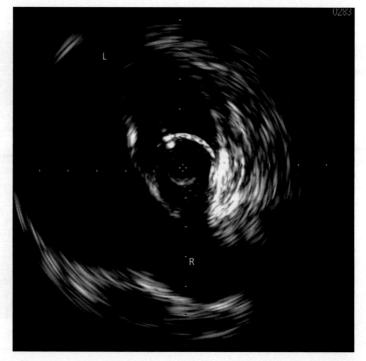

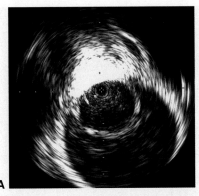 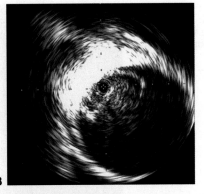 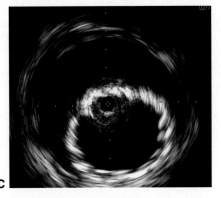

FIGURE 31.15. IVUS images of a dynamic aortic dissection. *A,* During diastole, the true lumen is widely patent. *B,* With systole, the true lumen is near completely collapsed. *C,* This patient had an endovascular stent placed to maintain the patency of the lumen and relieve symptoms of ischemia.

OPTICAL COHERENCE TOMOGRAPHY

Technical Considerations

OCT uses reflected near infrared light to create high-resolution images of the arterial wall. The optic lens is positioned within a flexible fiber optic catheter to allow for uninhibited rotation. The rapid exchange system utilizes a 0.014″ guidewire, and requires a 6-French sheath (Fig. 31.16). The current commercially available imaging device is approved for 2- to 3.5-mm vessels. The catheter is able to perform pullback image captures of 5-cm vessel lengths. It also requires preparation and continuous flushing with angiographic contrast. OCT has the distinct advantage of markedly improved resolution compared to IVUS, although this comes at the expense of limited tissue penetration (Table 31.2). In addition, OCT can capture 100 frames/s with pullback speeds of 20 mm/s. This allows for rapid image capture and limits ischemic time that may occur during imaging across high-grade lesions.

There are distinct artifacts with OCT that users need to be cognizant of prior to operating the system (Fig. 31.17). Because of the location of the optic lens in relation to the guidewire and the rotational image acquisition, images will contain a wire shadow. Additionally, blood located within the lumen can cause speckling or swirling. Speckling is caused by red blood cells not being fully removed from the lumen by the flushing agent; however, flushing with undiluted contrast can avoid this artifact. Swirling artifact may be seen when the flush runs out during the pullback or enters side branches. As with rotational

IVUS catheters, a form of nonuniform rotation distortion can occur. This can produce edge-type artifacts that mimic irregular plaque. Finally, metallic stents can cause various shadowing artifacts. These can be readily identified by the circumferential pattern, but may mask other plaque characteristics.

In contrast to IVUS which requires a histologic overlay, plaque composition can be more easily distinguished with OCT. Normal intima appears brighter compared with the media and adventitia but will not be as thick as the media. Intimal thickening and fibrous plaque can be seen in early atherosclerotic disease. OCT can identify early expansion of the intima and the homogenous bright fibrous plaque. Lipid, on the other hand, will appear bright near the lumen of the vessel, but the media will be darker with higher attenuation and diffusion of the edge signal (Fig. 31.18). As opposed to IVUS and conventional angiography, calcific plaque appears darker with a low attenuation and sharp edges in OCT imaging. The ability to distinguish plaque from thrombus with OCT has helped to guide treatment selection in the coronary and carotid literature.[12,13]

Applications

The majority of reported studies using OCT in the peripheral arterial circulation have evaluated the carotid arteries. In an early case report using OCT for evaluation of carotid

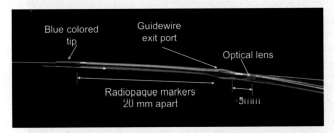

FIGURE 31.16. St. Jude optical coherence tomography catheter is inserted over a 0.014″ guidewire and requires a 6-French access sheath. (Image courtesy of St. Jude Medical, St. Paul, MN.)

TABLE 31.2

COMPARISON OF OPTICAL COHERENCE TOMOGRAPHY AND INTRAVASCULAR ULTRASOUND

	▪ OPTICAL COHERENCE TOMOGRAPHY	▪ INTRAVASCULAR ULTRASOUND
Axial resolution	12–15 μm	100–200 μm
Beam width	20–40 μm	200–300 μm
Frame rate	100 frames/s	30 frames/s
Pullback speed	20 mm/s	0.5–1.0 mm/s
Max. scan diameter	10 mm	15 mm
Tissue penetration	1.0–2.0 mm	10 mm

FIGURE 31.17. Artifacts with optical coherence tomography. Radial circumferential shadowing stent artifact is seen around the periphery of the vessel. Intraluminal swirling is also noted around the catheter. This can be cleared with contrast flushing during the pullback image acquisition.

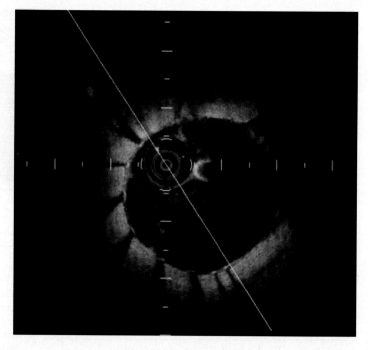

stenosis after a hemispheric stroke, Yoshimura et al were able to identify irregular intraluminal thrombus as opposed to more stable plaque. This prompted the authors to recommend carotid endarterectomy instead of carotid stent placement.[12] Further evaluation of 34 symptomatic and asymptomatic patients with IVUS and OCT found intraluminal thrombus in 15/34 (44%) patients with OCT versus 1/34 (2.9%) with IVUS. Symptomatic patients were more likely to have intraluminal thrombus than asymptomatic patients, 76% and 12%, respectively.[14] There were no procedure-related embolic complications in this study, which may reflect the technical skill of the interventionalists as well as the small size of the OCT catheter. Current work with carotid plaque characterization is underway using MRI to determine plaque composition and to guide treatment decisions in symptomatic and asymptomatic patients prior to endarterectomy or carotid stent placement. Although noninvasive, MRI cannot discern microscopic histologic characteristics of plaque.

Work in the lower extremity circulation has been limited by the inability of OCT to image vessels of larger size. Recent device development has combined the optic lens with technology to maneuver through chronic total occlusions of the lower extremity arteries (Fig. 31.19). This device offers the capacity to cross lesions while maintaining visualization. The catheter is available in 5- and 6-French sizes with working lengths that range from 110 to 150 cm. Once the chronic total occlusion is identified, the catheter is advanced to the proximal cap. Continuous flushing of the catheter with saline allows adequate visualization. Using three identifying markers, the catheter is advanced while maintaining orientation of the middle marker along the layered vessel wall. As the catheter moves beyond the chronic total occlusion and back into the vessel lumen, swirling artifact of the blood and contrast mixing will appear. This signals the operator to advance the guidewire. Angiography is used to confirm the wire is in the lumen of the vessel and appropriate treatment is selected.

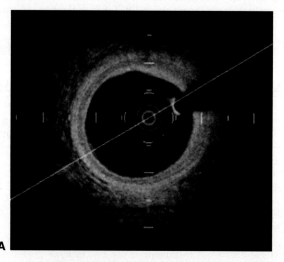 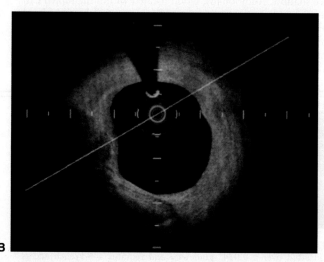

A   **B**

FIGURE 31.18. *A,* The layered arterial wall is easily visualized with a small amount of intraluminal fibrous plaque. *B,* Thickening of the media with areas of darker lipid plaque at the 6 o'clock to 9 o'clock positions.

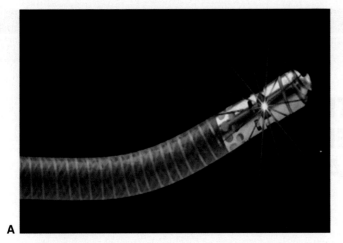
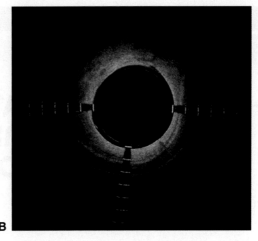

FIGURE 31.19. The ocelot catheter (*A*) combines optical coherence tomography technology with a catheter to cross chronic total occlusions. The catheter has three identifying markers (*B*). The middle marker (*red arrow*) is oriented along the vessel wall. (Images courtesy of Avinger, Redwood City, CA.)

CONCLUSIONS

Endovascular therapy continues to move to the forefront of treatment for peripheral artery disease, and intravascular imaging will play a larger role as practitioners attempt to improve outcomes while limiting radiation and nephrotoxic contrast administration. Although not required on every case, practitioners should become facile with these technologies on routine cases so they are able to interpret images during critical moments. Further research in this area should focus on how these new imaging techniques improve interventional patency and possibly reduce the need for reintervention.

References

1. Ascher E, Marks NA, Hingorani AP. Duplex-guided infrainguinal balloon angioplasty and stenting. A 4-year experience. *J Cardiovasc Surg (Torino)* 2008;49(2):151-158.
2. Yock PG, Linker DT, Angelsen BA. Two-dimensional intravascular ultrasound: technical development and initial clinical experience. *J Am Soc Echocardiogr* 1989;2(4):296-304.
3. Geng YJ. Progression of atheroma: a struggle between death and procreation. *Arterioscler Thromb Vasc Biol* 2002;22(9):1370-1380.
4. Mintz GS, Nissen SE, Anderson WD, et al. American College of Cardiology clinical expert consensus document on standards for acquisition, measurement and reporting of intravascular ultrasound studies (IVUS)33A report of the American College of Cardiology task force on clinical expert consensus documents developed in collaboration with the European Society of Cardiology endorsed by the Society of Cardiac Angiography and Interventions. *J Am Coll Cardiol* 2001;37(5):1478-1492.
5. Leesar MA, Varma J, Shapira A, et al. Prediction of hypertension improvement after stenting of renal artery stenosis: comparative accuracy of translesional pressure gradients, intravascular ultrasound, and angiography. *J Am Coll Cardiol* 2009;53(25):2363-2371.
6. Norgren L, Hiatt WR, Dormandy JA, et al. Inter-Society Consensus for the Management of Peripheral Arterial Disease (TASC II). *J Vasc Surg* 2007;45(Suppl S):S5-S67.
7. Buckley CJ, Arko FR, Lee S, et al. Intravascular ultrasound scanning improves long-term patency of iliac lesions treated with balloon angioplasty and primary stenting. *J Vasc Surg* 2002;35(2):316-323.
8. Berry C, L'Allier PL, Gregoire J, et al. Comparison of intravascular ultrasound and quantitative coronary angiography for the assessment of coronary artery disease progression. *Circulation* 2007;115(14):1851-1857.
9. Post MJ, de Smet BJ, van der Helm Y, et al. Arterial remodeling after balloon angioplasty or stenting in an atherosclerotic experimental model. *Circulation* 1997;96(3):996-1003.
10. Azizzadeh A, Valdes J, Miller CC III, et al. The utility of intravascular ultrasound compared to angiography in the diagnosis of blunt traumatic aortic injury. *J Vasc Surg* 2011;53(3):608-614.
11. Jonker FH, Mojibian H, Schlosser FJ, et al. The impact of hypovolaemic shock on the aortic diameter in a porcine model. *Eur J Vasc Endovasc Surg* 2010;40(5):564-571.
12. Yoshimura S, Kawasaki M, Hattori A, et al. Demonstration of intraluminal thrombus in the carotid artery by optical coherence tomography: technical case report. *Neurosurgery* 2010;67(3 Suppl Operative):onsE305; discussion onsE.
13. Tsimikas S, DeMaria AN. The clinical emergence of optical coherence tomography: defining a role in intravascular imaging. *J Am Coll Cardiol* 2012;59(12):1090-1092.
14. Yoshimura S, Kawasaki M, Yamada K, et al. Visualization of internal carotid artery atherosclerotic plaques in symptomatic and asymptomatic patients: a comparison of optical coherence tomography and intravascular ultrasound. *AJNR Am J Neuroradiol* 2012;33(2):308-313.

CHAPTER 32 ■ EVALUATION AND TREATMENT OF FEMORAL PSEUDOANEURYSMS

R. EUGENE ZIERLER AND WATSON B. SMITH

An *arterial aneurysm* is generally defined as a focal dilatation that involves either the whole or a part of the vessel circumference. In *true* aneurysms, the dilatation includes all layers of the arterial wall, and flowing blood is entirely contained within the vessel lumen. With *false* aneurysms or *pseudoaneurysms*, there is a defect in the arterial wall, and blood flows outside the arterial lumen but is contained by the perivascular tissues. A *dissecting* aneurysm is a dilatation of an artery associated with penetration of blood into the layers of the arterial wall. Table 32.1 presents a classification of arterial aneurysms by etiology. Pseudoaneurysms typically result from disruption of the arterial wall related to blunt or penetrating trauma, open surgical procedures, or percutaneous arterial interventions. One common mechanism for pseudoaneurysms is a gradual breakdown of the anastomosis between a prosthetic graft and a native artery. These *anastomotic pseudoaneurysms* typically involve the common femoral, deep femoral, or proximal superficial femoral arteries and have been found in 2% to 5% of patients undergoing aortofemoral or femoropopliteal bypass grafting.[1,2] The incidence of femoral pseudoaneurysms related to percutaneous arterial puncture is increasing owing to the use of groin artery catheterization for cardiac, peripheral arterial, and carotid interventions.

CLINICAL PRESENTATION

With the growing emphasis on "minimally invasive" treatment of cardiovascular diseases, there has been a marked increase in the use of percutaneous diagnostic and therapeutic procedures. The most frequently used arterial access site is the common femoral artery, and the reported prevalence of femoral pseudoaneurysms is in the range of 0.05% to 4%.[3-5] Some devices for catheter-based interventions require large sheath sizes as well as aggressive use of anticoagulants and antiplatelet agents; these factors appear to increase the risk for pseudoaneurysms. The method used to achieve hemostasis after sheath removal may also contribute to this risk. These developments have increased the incidence of other complications related to percutaneous femoral artery puncture, including groin hematomas, retroperitoneal bleeding, and arteriovenous fistulas.

Femoral pseudoaneurysms usually originate at the arterial puncture site from the wall of the artery closest to the skin surface. This is most often at the level of the common femoral artery but may involve any segment from the distal external iliac to the proximal superficial femoral or deep femoral artery. A pseudoaneurysm forms when the puncture site fails to seal and a cavity filled with arterial blood forms adjacent to the arterial wall. This cavity is connected to the arterial lumen by a "neck" of variable length and often contains both flowing blood and laminated thrombus (Fig. 32.1). Pseudoaneurysm cavities are typically in the range of 1 to 3 cm in diameter when first detected, and some consist of multiple interconnected lobes. Rarely, a femoral pseudoaneurysm is associated with an arteriovenous fistula originating from a separate puncture site. Although the natural history of femoral pseudoaneurysms is unpredictable, those with flow-filled cavities less than 2 cm in maximum diameter are more likely to thrombose spontaneously than are those with larger cavities.

A femoral pseudoaneurysm should be suspected whenever an enlarging hematoma is noted adjacent to a puncture site within hours to days after a percutaneous arterial procedure. Many patients report a "popping" sensation and pain in the catheterized groin. These signs and symptoms are typically accompanied by extensive ecchymosis of the overlying skin; however, bruising is common in this setting, even in the absence of a pseudoaneurysm. A palpable thrill or continuous bruit over the groin suggests the presence of an arteriovenous fistula, with or without an associated pseudoaneurysm. Palpation usually reveals a tender pulsatile mass, but it is often difficult to distinguish between true pulsatility and transmitted pulsation through a hematoma. Therefore, the diagnosis should always be confirmed by duplex ultrasound evaluation.

DIAGNOSIS

Scanning Technique

With the patient supine and the ipsilateral leg externally rotated, initially evaluate the distal external iliac, common femoral, deep femoral, and proximal superficial femoral arteries and veins in a standard fashion for stenosis, aneurysm, or thrombosis. This is typically done with a 5- to 7-MHz linear array

TABLE 32.1

CLASSIFICATION OF ARTERIAL ANEURYSMS BY ETIOLOGY

DEGENERATIVE	MECHANICAL
Nonspecific (atherosclerosis)	Pseudoaneurysms (traumatic, anastomotic)
Fibromuscular dysplasia	Poststenotic (coarctation)
INFLAMMATORY (ARTERITIS)	CONNECTIVE TISSUE DISORDER
Behçet's disease	Marfan's syndrome (dissecting)
Kawasaki's disease	Ehlers-Danlos syndrome
Giant cell	Cystic medial necrosis (dissecting)
Polyarteritis nodosa	CONGENITAL/INHERITED
INFECTIOUS (MYCOTIC)	Cerebral (Berry's)
Syphilis	Persistent sciatic artery
Bacterial	
Fungal	

transducer. However, B-mode resolution is often poor owing to extravasated blood in the tissue, and a lower-frequency transducer may be needed for adequate depth penetration. A curved array is useful if a large field of view is required, whereas a phased array is best if there is a small acoustic window or deep inguinal crease. After the native vessels have been assessed, scan the surrounding area for masses. Color-flow imaging is helpful for distinguishing between pseudoaneurysms and nonvascularized masses such as hematomas, seromas, or enlarged lymph nodes. Although pseudoaneurysms are the most frequently suspected postcatheterization vascular problem, other abnormalities that may be present include intimal flaps, arterial thrombosis, arterial dissections, arteriovenous fistulas, extrinsic compression of veins, and deep vein thrombosis.

Ultrasound Findings

The key features of a pseudoaneurysm on duplex ultrasound are a vascularized cavity connected to the adjacent artery by a neck that exhibits a characteristic "to-and-fro" spectral waveform pattern, representing arterial flow in and out of the pseudoaneurysm (Fig. 32.2). Radial pulsations are usually visible in or around the cavity on B-mode imaging, and arterial flow is detectable within the cavity by both pulsed and color-flow Doppler. A distinctive "yin-yang" pattern is often seen on the color-flow image (Fig. 32.3). Document the size and location of the pseudoaneurysm, and follow the neck to locate the exact point of origin. Also measure the length of the neck between the arterial defect and the vascularized cavity. Whereas the true size of a pseudoaneurysm includes both the active or vascularized portion and any surrounding thrombus, the most important feature is the size of the vascularized cavity. Images and reports should clearly distinguish between these measurements.

Arteriovenous fistulas occur when both the artery and the adjacent vein have been punctured, resulting in a persistent high-flow connection between the two vessels. These lesions usually produce a striking image on color-flow Doppler in the area of the communicating channel, with a prominent "color bruit" (Fig. 32.4). Elevated peak velocities and aliasing are typically found at the site of the fistula, with a characteristic high-velocity/low-pulsatility waveform (Fig. 32.5). Arteriovenous fistulas can also be located by identifying increased systolic and diastolic velocities in the artery proximal to the lesion that normalize distally (Fig. 32.6). Venous segments proximal (central) to the fistula contain turbulent and pulsatile flow patterns (Fig. 32.7).

APPROACHES TO TREATMENT

Based on the risk of progressive enlargement and rupture, most pseudoaneurysms should be treated at the time of diagnosis. However, small asymptomatic pseudoaneurysms with

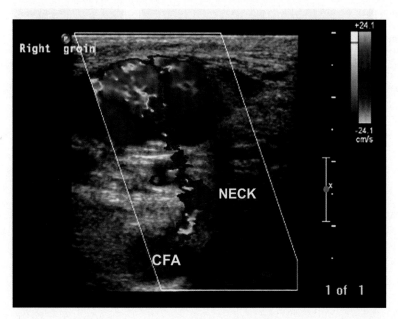

FIGURE 32.1. Transverse B-mode and color-flow image of a right femoral pseudoaneurysm shows the native common femoral artery (CFA) and pseudoaneurysm neck (NECK) connecting to the active pseudoaneurysm cavity (*upper left*). The cavity appears partially thrombosed with incomplete color filling.

PREOPERATIVE PLANNING, INTRAOPERATIVE ASSESSMENT AND PROCEDURAL GUIDANCE

FIGURE 32.2. Pulsed Doppler spectral waveform shows the typical "to-and-fro" flow pattern found in a pseudoaneurysm neck. Note both forward (positive) and reverse (negative) velocity components.

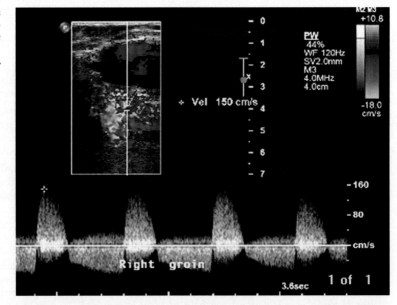

FIGURE 32.3. Ultrasound image of a femoral pseudoaneurysm shows the "yin-yang" color-flow pattern in the vascularized or active portion of the cavity.

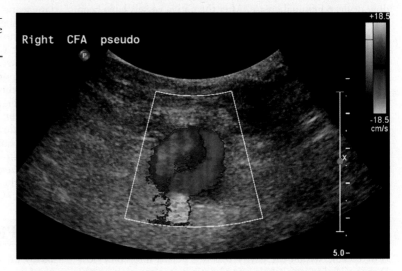

FIGURE 32.4. Prominent color-flow bruit associated with an arteriovenous fistula between the common femoral artery (CFA) and the common femoral vein (CFV). (From Smith WB, Zaccardi M, Zierler RE. Diagnosis and treatment of femoral pseudoaneurysms. *Vasc Ultrasound Today* 2005;10:199–220. Used with permission.)

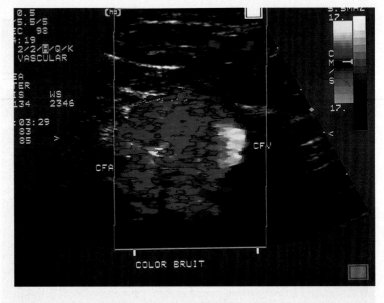

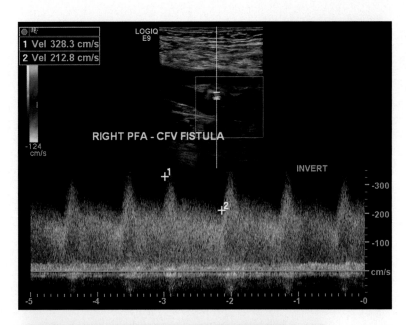

FIGURE 32.5. A high-velocity/low-pulsatility spectral waveform from a postcatheterization arteriovenous fistula between the right profunda femoris artery (PFA) and the common femoral vein (CFV). Note the very high diastolic flow velocity.

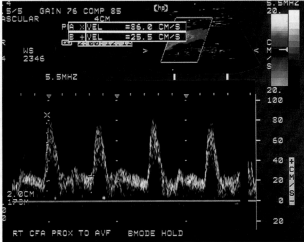

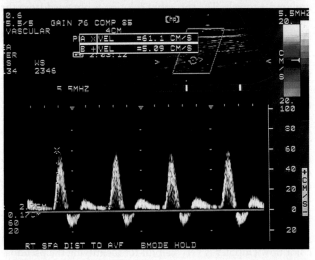

FIGURE 32.6. Changes in the arterial flow pattern proximal and distal to an arteriovenous fistula. *Top,* Common femoral artery spectral waveform taken proximal to the fistula shows increased systolic and diastolic velocities (low resistance pattern). *Bottom,* Superficial femoral artery spectral waveform taken distal to the same fistula shows decreased velocities and the return of a high-resistance triphasic flow pattern. (From Smith WB, Zaccardi M, Zierler RE. Diagnosis and treatment of femoral pseudoaneurysms. *Vasc Ultrasound Today* 2005;10:199-220. Used with permission.)

vascularized cavities less than 2 cm in diameter may be followed by serial ultrasound evaluations and treated if they do not thrombose spontaneously. Patients on antiplatelet agents or anticoagulants are less likely to show spontaneous thrombosis. Options for treatment include direct open surgical repair, ultrasound-guided compression, and ultrasound-guided thrombin injection. Open surgery requires exposure of the puncture site through a groin incision and direct repair of the arterial defect by simple suture or patch angioplasty. Any concomitant arterial defects such as intimal flaps or fistulas can also be repaired using this approach. Although direct surgical repair is highly effective and relatively safe, many patients with femoral pseudoaneurysm have significant medical comorbidities that make a less invasive approach preferable.

Permanent obliteration of a femoral pseudoaneurysm cavity by ultrasound-guided compression was first described in 1991.[6] This technique involves direct compression of the pseudoaneurysm cavity using the ultrasound probe, with the goal being to occlude the neck of the pseudoaneurysm without completely occluding the adjacent artery. Although success rates of up to 75% have been reported with ultrasound-guided compression, this approach has significant limitations.[7,8] Compression of a groin pseudoaneurysm is physically difficult for the operator and painful for the patient. In addition, prolonged periods of compression—up to 1 hour or more—are often required. For these reasons, ultrasound-guided thrombin injection is now clearly the preferred initial treatment for most femoral pseudoaneurysms.

Thrombin is an enzyme that converts fibrinogen to fibrin, a critical step in the process of blood coagulation. Although products containing human thrombin are now available for clinical use (Recothrom, ZymoGenetics, Inc.), most of the reported experience with ultrasound-guided thrombin injection for treatment of femoral pseudoaneurysms has been with thrombin preparations of bovine origin (Thrombin-JMI, King Pharmaceuticals, Inc.). These products are labeled "topical" thrombin, with the intended use being as a hemostatic agent on the surfaces of bleeding tissues. The instructions for use in the standard topical thrombin kit state that it should not be injected, so treatment of femoral pseudoaneurysms is considered to be an "off-label" use. Nevertheless, this approach is commonly practiced and is clearly safe and effective. In 2002, the American Medical Association created a specific CPT (current procedural terminology) code (36002) to cover "injection procedures (e.g., thrombin) for percutaneous treatment of extremity pseudoaneurysm."

FIGURE 32.7. Turbulent and pulsatile spectral waveform from the common femoral vein (CFV) proximal (central) to the arteriovenous fistula shown in Figure 32.5.

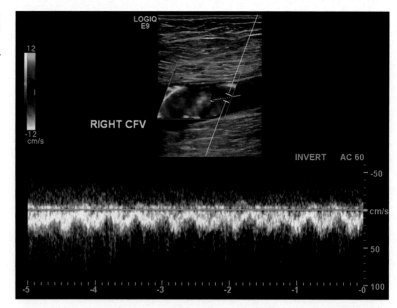

Although most patients with postcatheterization femoral pseudoaneurysms are good candidates for ultrasound-guided thrombin injection, some contraindications must be recognized (Table 32.2). These include any evidence of infection in the groin, ischemia (blistering) of the overlying skin, distal limb ischemia, and any history of allergic reaction to thrombin or bovine materials (when bovine thrombin is used). Rapid enlargement can be a sign of serious bleeding requiring immediate surgical repair. When ultrasound evaluation shows a short or absent pseudoaneurysm neck, or a very large arterial defect, the risk of propagation of thrombus into the native artery is higher, and surgical repair may be preferable. Small pseudoaneurysms, particularly those with active cavities less than 1 cm in diameter, can be difficult to inject and may thrombose spontaneously.

TECHNIQUE OF ULTRASOUND-GUIDED THROMBIN INJECTION

Preparation

As previously mentioned, ultrasound-guided thrombin injection for the treatment of femoral pseudoaneurysms is an off-label use, and informed consent should be obtained from the patient after explaining the risks, benefits, and alternative treatment options. The procedure is best done at the bedside

TABLE 32.2

CONTRAINDICATIONS TO ULTRASOUND-GUIDED THROMBIN INJECTION

Local infection (cellulites, abscess)
Rapid enlargement[a]
Ischemia (blistering) of overlying skin
Distal limb ischemia
History of allergy to thrombin
Short or absent pseudoaneurysm neck[a]
Large neck (arterial defect)[a]
Pseudoaneurysm cavity size ≤1 cm[a]

[a]Relative contraindications (see text).

rather than in the vascular laboratory to minimize patient movement after the injection. Discomfort from the skin puncture and injection is minimal, and local anesthesia is usually not necessary; however, it should be considered for pediatric patients and anxious adult patients.

Ultrasound-guided thrombin injection typically requires both a sonographer to operate the duplex scanner and a physician to perform the injection. However, some skilled physicians choose to do this on their own, scanning with one hand and injecting with the other. The use of a sterile sheath for the ultrasound probe and a biopsy guide for the needle has been described, but these are not essential. A 21- or 22-gauge spinal needle can be used for the injection. Use of an ECHOTIP needle (21G × 9 cm, COOK, Inc., Bloomington, IN) with an etched barrel facilitates ultrasound visualization of the needle in tissue, but a similar effect can be achieved by scratching the barrel of an ordinary spinal needle with a sterile scalpel blade. Other required supplies include sterile gloves, skin antiseptic, and sterile towels. The thrombin solution is obtained from the standard topical thrombin kit, which includes the thrombin in powder form and saline diluent to produce 5 mL of thrombin solution with a concentration of 1000 Units/mL. About 1 to 2 mL of this solution is drawn up into a small syringe, which is then fitted with the needle to be used for the injection.

Needle Insertion and Injection

The sonographer scans the patient and selects a probe orientation that provides clear visualization of the active pseudoaneurysm cavity, neck, and adjacent artery and vein as well as a convenient location for needle insertion. Ideally, this should allow the needle to enter the pseudoaneurysm cavity at a location as far away from the neck and native vessels as possible. This probe position is maintained while the adjacent skin is sterilely prepared and isolated with sterile towels. Although color-flow Doppler is very helpful for identifying the pseudoaneurysm cavity, it will interfere with visualization of the needle tip, so it should be turned off at the time of needle insertion.

Insert the needle in the plane of the B-mode image to provide maximum visualization of the entire length of the needle and location of the tip (Fig. 32.8). Hold the probe stationary during needle insertion to provide a clear "target." It is extremely important not to withdraw on the syringe plunger or allow blood to enter the needle, because this will result in

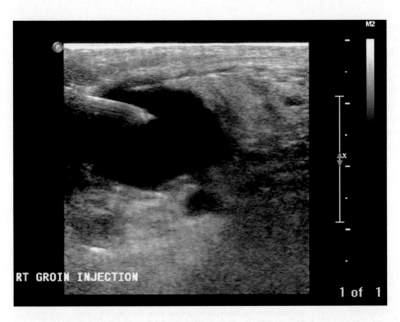

FIGURE 32.8. B-mode image of an ECHOTIP needle entering a pseudoaneurysm cavity from the upper left. The pseudoaneurysm neck and native artery are at the lower right.

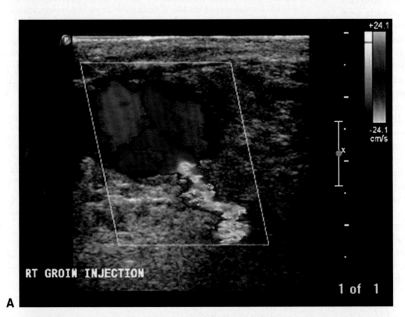

A

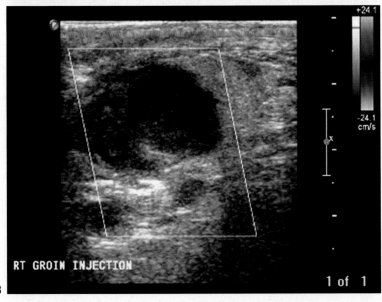

B

FIGURE 32.9. B-mode and color-flow image of a femoral pseudoaneurysm immediately before (A) and after (B) ultrasound-guided thrombin injection. Prior to injection flow is visualized in the active pseudoaneurysm cavity; following injection, the cavity appears thrombosed with diffuse echoes and no flow visualized.

PREOPERATIVE PLANNING,
INTRAOPERATIVE ASSESSMENT
AND PROCEDURAL GUIDANCE

clot formation within the needle. If this occurs, withdraw the needle and expel the clot or place a new needle on the syringe. Once the tip of the needle is clearly visualized in the active pseudoaneurysm cavity, slowly inject about 0.5 to 1.0 mL (500 to 1000 Units) of the topical thrombin solution. Thrombosis of the pseudoaneurysm cavity usually occurs within 5 to 10 seconds and can be confirmed using color-flow Doppler (Fig. 32.9). If any residual flow is noted, injection of another 0.5 to 1.0 mL is indicated. Multiple injections at several sites may be required in patients with complex, multiple-lobed pseudoaneurysms. Although there is no established limit on the total amount of thrombin that can be used, it is unusual to require more than 1.5 to 2.0 mL.

Postinjection Follow-up

When evaluating a pseudoaneurysm after an initially successful ultrasound-guided thrombin injection, it is important to maximize Doppler sensitivity to detect any areas of low flow that may be present within the thrombosed cavity. The transmitting frequency should be low enough to provide adequate depth penetration, with low-color pulse repetition frequency (PRF) and filter settings. Also, make sure there is adequate gain and confirm all color-flow findings with pulsed Doppler and spectral waveform analysis. In addition to confirming persistent thrombosis of the pseudoaneurysm cavity, it is important to look for other lesions that may have been masked by color bruits or poor B-mode resolution at the initial examination.

After successful ultrasound-guided thrombin injection, monitor the pseudoaneurysm for 10 to 15 minutes by duplex ultrasound to confirm complete and persistent obliteration of the active cavity. Also examine the adjacent femoral artery and vein to check for patency. Check lower extremity pulses and ankle-brachial indices to look for any evidence of arterial thrombosis or distal embolization. Deliberate compression of the groin after thrombin injection is not necessary and possibly dangerous, because it could displace thrombus from the pseudoaneurysm cavity into the native artery.

A period of strict bed rest (4 to 6 hours) is generally recommended after successful treatment of a femoral pseudoaneurysm by ultrasound-guided thrombin injection.[7,8] This is analogous to the period of bed rest used after removal of a femoral sheath to allow complete sealing of the puncture site. A follow-up duplex scan can be obtained 24 to 48 hours later to check for recurrence of the pseudoaneurysm; however, the need for a routine follow-up scan is controversial, because the rate of recurrence is very low.[9] Clinical experience suggests that follow-up scans can be reserved for patients with recurrent signs or symptoms.

RESULTS

The initial success rate for ultrasound-guided thrombin injection of femoral pseudoaneurysms in most reported series is in the range of 93% to 100%.[3,7,8,10-15] This approach is also effective in patients on anticoagulants. Recurrence of a pseudoaneurysm after successful thrombosis appears to be rare, occurring in about 3% of patients in one series.[9] Complications have been described in only 2% or less of patients and include thrombosis of the adjacent native artery, distal embolization, and allergic reactions.[3,7,8,12,13,16] Severe coagulopathy has been described after exposure to bovine thrombin, related to stimulation of antibodies to factor V.[17] Although rare, such reactions appear to be less frequent with thrombin derived from human sources.[18] Ischemic complications are usually due to inadvertent injection of thrombin solution into the artery or propagation of thrombus from the pseudoaneurysm cavity into the arterial lumen.

References

1. Nichols WK, Stanton M, Silver D, et al. Anastomotic aneurysms following lower extremity revascularization. *Surgery* 1980;8:366-374.
2. Satiani B, Kazmers M, Evans WE. Anastomotic arterial aneurysms: A continuing challenge. *Ann Surg* 1980;192:674-682.
3. Olsen DM, Rodriguez JA, Vranic M, et al. A prospective study of ultrasound scan-guided thrombin injection of femoral pseudoaneurysm: A trend toward minimal medication. *J Vasc Surg* 2002;6:779-782.
4. Messina LM, Brothers TF, Wakefield TW, et al. Clinical characteristics and surgical management of vascular complications in patients undergoing cardiac catheterization: Interventional versus diagnostic procedures. *J Vasc Surg* 1991;13:593-600.
5. Kresowik TF, Khoury MD, Miller BV, et al. A prospective study of the incidence and natural history of femoral vascular complications after percutaneous transluminal coronary angioplasty. *J Vasc Surg* 1991;13:328-336.
6. Fellmeth BD, Roberts AC, Bookstein JJ, et al. Postangiographic femoral artery injuries: Nonsurgical repair with US-guided compression. *Radiology* 1991;178:671-675.
7. Paulson EK, Sheafor DH, Kliewer MA, et al. Treatment of iatrogenic femoral arterial pseudoaneurysms: Comparison of US-guided thrombin injection with compression repair. *Radiology* 2000;215:403-408.
8. Friedman SG, Pellerito JS, Scher L, et al. Ultrasound-guided thrombin injection is the treatment of choice for femoral pseudoaneurysms. *Arch Surg* 2002;137:462-464.
9. Stone PA, AbuRahma AF, Hayes JD, et al. Selective use of duplex ultrasound after successful thrombin injection of pseudoaneurysms. *J Vasc Ultrasound* 2005;29:67-70.
10. Lonn L, Olmarker A, Geterud K, et al. Prospective randomized study comparing ultrasound-guided thrombin injection to compression in the treatment of femoral pseudoaneurysms. *J Endovasc Ther* 2004;11:570-576.
11. Taylor BS, Rhee RY, Muluk S, et al. Thrombin injection versus compression of femoral artery pseudoaneurysms. *J Vasc Surg* 1999;30:1052-1059.
12. Kang SS, Labropoulos N, Mansour MA, et al. Percutaneous ultrasound-guided thrombin injection: A new method for treating postcatheterization femoral pseudoaneurysms. *J Vasc Surg* 1998;28:1120-1121.
13. Calton WC, Franklin DP, Elmore JR, et al. Ultrasound-guided thrombin injection is a safe and durable treatment for femoral pseudoaneurysms. *Vasc Surg* 2001;35:379-383.
14. Sackett WR, Taylor SM, Coffey CB, et al. Ultrasound-guided thrombin injection of iatrogenic femoral pseudoaneurysms: A prospective analysis. *Am Surg* 2000;66:937-940.
15. Stone PA, AbuRahma AF, Flaherty SK. Reducing duplex examinations in patients with iatrogenic pseudoaneurysms. *J Vasc Surg* 2006;43: 1211-1215.
16. Gabrielli R, Rosati MS, Vitale S, et al. Fatal complication after thrombin injection for post-catheterization femoral pseudoaneurysm. *Thorac Cardiov Surg* 2011;59:370-377.
17. Sarfati MR, Dilorenzo DJ, Kraiss LW, et al. Severe coagulopathy following intraoperative use of topical thrombin. *Ann Vasc Surg* 2004;18:349-351.
18. Vasquez V, Reus M, Pinero A, et al. Human thrombin for treatment of pseudoaneurysms: Comparison of bovine human thrombin sonogram-guided injection. *AJR Am J Roentgenol* 2005;184:1665-1671.

CHAPTER 33 ■ DIALYSIS ACCESS PROCEDURES

TED R. KOHLER AND BRIDGET A. MRAZ

The incidence of end-stage renal disease (ESRD) has increased owing to the aging of our population and the increasing prevalence of diabetes. ESRD was a fatal illness until the establishment of chronic hemodialysis in the 1960s. Since then, the life expectancy of patients with ESRD has increased dramatically. As a result, there are nearly half a million ESRD patients in the United States today, the majority of whom are maintained by chronic hemodialysis (the remainder undergo peritoneal dialysis).[1] The lives of hemodialysis patients depend on functional access to their circulation that provides an adequate volume of blood flow for the dialysis process, approximately 600 mL/min. Creation and maintenance of dialysis access is the leading cause of hospitalizations of these patients and costs the health care system in excess of a billion dollars annually. These costs can be reduced by increased use of native veins for dialysis access fistulas and better approaches to maintenance of patency—areas in which duplex scanning can play a major role. Duplex ultrasound helps identify veins for fistula creation that may otherwise be overlooked, ensures adequacy of arterial inflow and venous outflow, and aids in determining adequacy of fistula maturation and identification of reasons for maturation failure. Duplex scanning can also diagnose problems related to maintenance of fistulas, including arterial steal, pseudoaneurysms, infections, and stenoses in the access or venous outflow. This chapter reviews dialysis access and the role that duplex scanning plays in this process.

TYPES OF DIALYSIS ACCESS

Maintenance hemodialysis was made possible by development of the Scribner shunt in 1960 by Scribner, Dillard, and Quinton in Seattle.[2] These expanded polytetrafluoroethylene (ePTFE) shunts were placed percutaneously into a peripheral artery and vein (typically at the wrist or ankle) with tubing exiting the skin (Fig. 33.1). This allowed direct connection of arterial flow into the dialysis machine and venous return back to the patient's circulation. When not in use, the two ePTFE tubes were connected to each other, creating a loop fistula outside the body. These devices were not suitable for long-term access because they were awkward, limited use of the extremity, and were plagued by frequent thrombosis and infection. The most common use of these devices was to support patients while recovering from acute renal failure. The later development of native arteriovenous fistulas by Cimino and Brescia,[3] who described surgical creation of a fistula between the radial artery and the cephalic vein in 1962, provided the first durable method that could support chronic dialysis access. When arterialized, the cephalic vein dilates and thickens, allowing high-flow access to the bloodstream by direct needle puncture of this vein. This process of maturation takes about 8 weeks or longer, although some centers have advocated earlier use in the case of larger veins. To this day, the Cimino-Brescia fistula remains the first choice for access owing to its durability, low morbidity, and freedom from infection. In the years since the original description of the radiocephalic fistula, surgeons have found that nearly any adequately sized upper extremity vein can be connected to an artery to create a similar fistula, and deep veins can be transposed to a superficial location to allow percutaneous access. Most patients, even those whose superficial veins are nearly all sclerotic from multiple phlebotomies during years of chronic illness, have an upper arm basilic or brachial vein that can be transposed for dialysis use. Veins less than 2.5 mm in diameter tend not to mature as fistulas, and those that are 4 mm or greater tend to function reliably, while those of intermediate diameter have variable results. Vein distensability has also been shown to affect maturation rates.[4] Common types of dialysis access are listed in Table 33.1.

When prosthetic grafts were developed for arterial bypass, it became obvious that these devices could substitute for veins as sites for access to the circulation. Most materials used for bypass grafts, such as Dacron, ePTFE, umbilical veins, and bovine carotid arteries, have been used for dialysis access. Of these, ePTFE has become the material of choice owing to its ease of placement and puncture and its relative durability.[5] Despite the many advantages of prosthetic grafts (Table 33.2), they are more prone to infection than native vessels and half fail within 1 year of placement. Native arteriovenous fistulas are preferred to prosthetic grafts not only because they have better patency rates and fewer infections but also because they require fewer secondary procedures to maintain patency. Traditionally, the United States has had particularly low rates for placement of

453

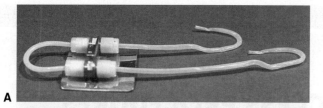

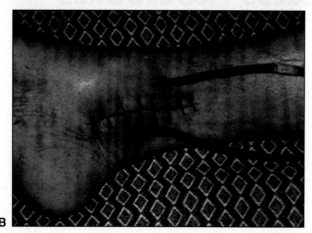

FIGURE 33.1. *A,* Polytetrafluoroethylene tubing used in early Scribner shunts. One side was placed in an artery (typically the radial or posterior tibial artery) and the other into an accompanying vein. The tubes exited the skin where they were connected to the dialysis machine or to each other when not in use. *B,* A Scribner shunt in place at the ankle.

Prosthetic grafts are favored in this situation because they do not require the lengthy maturation times of native fistulas; some of these devices can be accessed on the day of surgery. Reimbursement patterns also favor prosthetic grafts because their placement is reimbursed at a higher rate than creation of most arteriovenous fistulas. Prosthetic grafts are now being considered as a reasonable option in elderly patients and for use before resorting to the upper arm basilic vein transposition, which has increased morbidity compared with simpler native fistulas.[6]

For the reasons given previously, there has been a major initiative by the National Kidney Foundation (NKF) to encourage greater use of native arteriovenous fistulas for dialysis access in the United States. The Kidney Disease Outcomes Quality Initiative (KDOQI) by the NKF and the Fistula First initiative by the Centers for Medicaid and Medicare Services have been successful in improving these numbers. Their goal is at least 65% use of native arteriovenous fistulas. One of the prime components of this initiative is the use of preoperative duplex scanning. The use of native vessels for creation of dialysis access has improved in the United States from 31% in 2003 to 44% by the end of 2006, and some centers are reporting rates up to 90%. These improvements have been attributed to many practice and educational factors such as encouraging early referral of patients with kidney disease before their veins have been depleted by multiple phlebotomies, awareness of the advantages of native fistulas by surgeons, use of deep veins that require transposition to a more superficial location (primarily basilic vein transposition), and improved reimbursement for creation of complex arteriovenous fistulas. The use of preoperative duplex scanning has also facilitated the placement of native fistulas by identifying suitable veins that are not evident on physical examination, confirming the patency of the central veins, and ensuring the adequacy of arterial inflow.

native arteriovenous fistulas. In 2002, the percentage of new access sites that used native fistulas was only 32% in the United States whereas it was 80% in Japan and 70% in Europe. The factors that influenced the preference for ePTFE include a high rate of maturation failure in native fistulas, late referral to the surgeon, urgent need for dialysis, inadequacy of upper extremity veins, and reimbursement incentives.

Patients who are referred late in the course of their illness often need dialysis urgently and frequently do not have suitable veins for arteriovenous fistula creation because no one has thought to preserve their superficial upper extremity veins.

PREDIALYSIS ACCESS PLANNING

The main principle of access planning is to preserve as many veins as possible for subsequent use when the access fistula or device stops working, which inevitably will happen if the patient lives long enough. Thus, the surgeon works from the most distal location possible to more central locations, starting with the nondominant upper extremity, then the dominant upper extremity, then more unusual locations such as the femoral or axillary arteries. Native arteriovenous fistulas are used

TABLE 33.1

COMMON HEMODIALYSIS ACCESS TYPES

LOCATION	VESSELS	FISTULA (ONE ANASTOMOSIS)	GRAFT (TWO ANASTOMOSES)
1. Wrist (Brescia-Cimino)	Radial artery to cephalic vein	✓	
2. Forearm	Radial artery to basilic vein	✓	
3. Cubital space	Brachial artery to cephalic vein	✓	
4. Upper arm	Brachial artery to basilic vein (transposition)	✓	
5. Forearm	Radial artery to available vein		✓
6. Upper arm	Brachial artery to axillary vein		✓
7. Thigh	Femoral artery to saphenous vein	✓	

TABLE 33.2

ADVANTAGES OF PROSTHETIC GRAFTS FOR DIALYSIS ACCESS

Large surface area/length available for cannulation
Technically easy to cannulate
Short time from insertion to maturation
Multiple insertion sites available
Variety of shapes and configurations available to facilitate placement
Easy to handle and implant
Reliably high flow
Comparatively easy to repair surgically

first whenever possible, then prosthetic material at each level. The order of preferred access procedures is typically a wrist or snuffbox fistula between the radial artery and the cephalic vein (the snuffbox is the space between the extensor hallucis longus and the extensor pollicis brevis at the base of the thumb, where a distal branch of the radial artery and the cephalic vein lie in close proximity), a brachial artery-to-cephalic vein fistula at the elbow, and finally a transposition of the basilic vein in the arm to the brachial artery (note that the "arm" is the proper anatomic term for what is frequently referred to as the "upper arm"). There are many variations on this theme that can be used by the creative surgeon. For example, the basilic vein in the forearm, which runs too dorsally for use in dialysis, may be transposed and connected to the radial artery, or the median antebrachial vein may be connected in a side-to-side fashion in the upper forearm to the radial artery with lysis of vein valves allowing reverse flow through this vein into the forearm venous system.[7] These unusual procedures can produce complicated anatomy, which should be diagramed by the surgeon to allow the dialysis technicians and sonographers to understand the anatomy when placing the patient on dialysis or studying the fistula for possible abnormalities (Fig. 33.2).

The main purpose of preoperative duplex scanning is to confirm the patency and determine the size of the cephalic and basilic veins in the upper extremity. Many studies have shown that the main predictor of success for a new access is the size of the outflow vein. Most authors state that a minimum diameter of 2.5 mm is required for a reasonable chance

of successful maturation for a native arteriovenous fistula, although some now suggest that the failure rate is unacceptable for veins below 3 mm. A vein diameter of at least 3 mm, and preferably 4 mm or greater, is required for a prosthetic graft. In addition to having an adequate caliber, veins must be superficial enough for ease of puncture. Veins deeper than 6 mm from the skin surface are difficult to access unless they are exceptionally large. Thus, depth is an important consideration. Excessive depth does not preclude use of the vein but often requires the surgeon to "superficialize" it—surgically transposing it to a more superficial location. Patency of the central veins should also be assessed, especially in patients who have had prior access through central venous catheters.

A complete evaluation must include the arterial supply to the extremity. Renal failure patients are particularly prone to develop calcification of their arteries due to secondary hyperparathyroidism and an imbalance of calcium and phosphate. Heavily calcified arteries may not be suitable for access use owing to the difficulty in suturing these vessels. These patients develop occlusive disease in arteries from the aortic branches all the way to the digital vessels, which can result in inadequate flow for successful dialysis. Arterial occlusive disease also places patients at increased risk for clinically significant steal that can cause irreversible pain, loss of sensation, and weakness in the hand, as discussed later in this chapter. A preoperative digit-brachial pressure index of less than 0.6 should raise concern for the risk of steal. Some examiners check the response to hyperemia created by simple fist clenching. There should be an increase in diastolic flow with release of the clenched fist. Absence of this response suggests lack of reserve and increased risk for steal.

As described in Table 33.3, a predialysis access duplex mapping examination consists of three main components: (1) central venous mapping, (2) superficial venous mapping, and (3) arterial mapping. Specific mapping protocols should be developed at each facility by the local vascular technologists and access surgeons. Some consider an examination complete if the duplex of the nondominant arm is "normal." Most often, the nondominant arm is used first; however, the referring physician or surgeon may want to use the patient's dominant arm in unusual circumstances such as stroke affecting the dominant side. In general, if "right only" or "left only" is not specified, the vessels are evaluated bilaterally (this applies to the

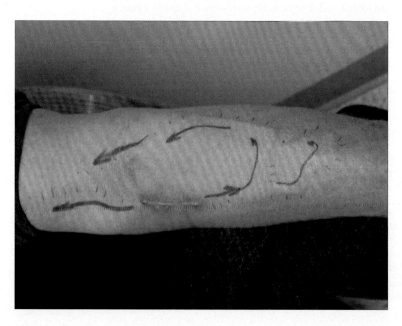

FIGURE 33.2. A proximal radial artery arteriovenous fistula with skin markings to indicate the path of flow, which is bidirectional in this case. Such diagrams are useful for both the dialysis technicians who access the fistula and the sonographers who scan them. (Courtesy of William C. Jennings, M.D.)

upper or lower extremities) to ensure that all possible critical information is obtained. Adequate communication with the referring physician is particularly important prior to revision of an existing dialysis access fistula or graft to make sure that questions about anatomy, outflow veins, potential substitute veins, or arterial inflow are answered.

A standard duplex ultrasound system is required for this examination with high-resolution B-mode imaging, color Doppler, and spectral waveform analysis. A selection of transducers with a choice of operating frequencies and "footprints" is necessary for scanning of the central and peripheral extremity vessels. These include a midrange-frequency linear array transducer (e.g., L7-4) for general applications and a high-frequency transducer (e.g., L12-5, L10-5 intraoperative, L15-7 intraoperative) for assessing the superficial veins. A small curved array transducer (e.g., C8-5), such as one designed for scanning neonatal heads, is excellent when scanning around the clavicle.

The examination begins with the patient in the supine position for bilateral brachial artery pressures and with the head slightly turned away from the limb being examined for evaluation of the subclavian and axillary veins. For evaluation of the arm veins, the head of the bed may be elevated 45 degrees with the arm dependent. Warming and a tourniquet, as described later in this chapter, may promote distention of the superficial veins. Several examiner positions can be utilized to scan the arms. Whenever possible, the examiner is positioned closest to the limb being evaluated (e.g., scan the right arm from the patient's right side). Reaching across the patient's body with one arm and operating the controls on the ultrasound system with the other arm causes muscle strain for the sonographer and can lead to musculoskeletal injuries. Thus, for a bilateral examination, after scanning the first arm, the machine may be moved to the contralateral side. Alternatively, if the examiner prefers to scan with one hand but still avoid reaching across to the contralateral side, the patient may be turned 180 degrees.

Central Venous Mapping

The normal anatomy of the upper extremity central veins is illustrated in Figure 33.3. Patency of the central veins should be ensured as far as possible, particularly in patients who have had prior venous access through puncture of these veins. Patency is compromised in about 20% of patients who have had indwelling central catheters for dialysis or other purposes. For these reasons, the central veins should be scanned first when performing a predialysis access mapping examination. The two main forms of central venous obstruction are stenosis and thrombosis. Stenosis in the innominate or subclavian vein is particularly common in patients with prior central venous catheters for short-term dialysis. Doppler findings with subclavian vein stenosis include a focal increase in Doppler flow velocity with poststenotic turbulence centrally and a continuous flow pattern peripherally. The duplex evaluation for upper extremity deep vein thrombosis is discussed in Chapter 20. Doppler waveforms from the innominate (brachiocephalic), subclavian, and axillary veins are all assessed for patency, normal flow pattern, and symmetry with the contralateral side.

The supraclavicular subclavian vein is a common location for venous stenosis where the subclavian vein curves to join the internal jugular vein. This segment often contains a valve that can become stenotic due to fibrosis of the leaflets. The infraclavicular subclavian vein is more easily imaged but is less likely to be stenotic. Doppler waveform analysis of flow in the infraclavicular subclavian vein can provide clues to the presence of a more proximal obstruction.

The axillary vein is a less common location for obstruction but may be a site of numerous collateral flow channels when a more central stenosis or occlusion exists. Subclavian vein obstruction may cause reversed flow in the axillary vein, which drains into chest wall collaterals. These prominent subcutaneous chest wall veins may be visible.

TABLE 33.3

PREDIALYSIS ACCESS MAPPING

1. Central venous mapping

- Scan the innominate, subclavian, and axillary veins to evaluate for patency and flow pattern.

2. Superficial venous mapping

- Scan the cephalic vein from wrist to shoulder, noting any anatomic anomalies and evidence of phlebosclerosis. Diameter should be carefully documented throughout the entire course of the vein. Map and mark the vein.
- Scan the basilic vein from its origin to its confluence with the brachial vein near the axilla, noting any anatomic anomalies and evidence of phlebosclerosis. Diameter should be carefully documented throughout the entire course of the vein. Map and mark the vein.
- Document patency and size of the median cubital vein. Map and mark the vein.

3. Arterial mapping

- Obtain bilateral brachial systolic blood pressures and Doppler waveforms.
- Scan the brachial, radial, and ulnar arteries, documenting any evidence of atherosclerosis, abnormalities, or anomalies (e.g., high bifurcation of the brachial), and any stenosis, which must be confirmed with spectral waveform analysis.
- Allen's test may be performed if the veins are acceptable.
  - If abnormal (digit pressure drops to <80 mm Hg or a >30% drop with compression of the radial artery), proceed to the next limb area.
  - If normal, measure ipsilateral first and third finger pressures (if not already done).

If no acceptable vein is found, proceed to contralateral arm.
If neither upper extremity is acceptable, proceed to lower extremity.

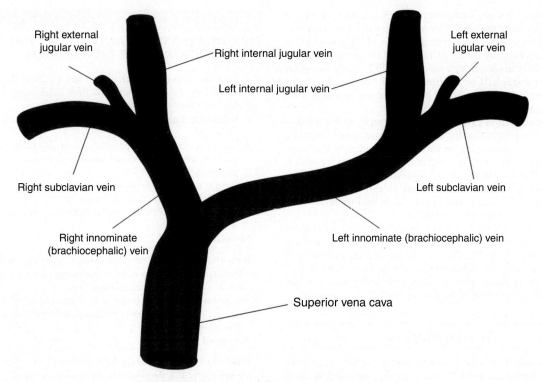

FIGURE 33.3. Anatomy of the upper extremity central veins.

Superficial Venous Mapping

The entire cephalic vein (from the wrist to its confluence with the subclavian vein) should be scanned noting any branching, wall thickening, or thrombosis (Fig. 33.4). The diameter of the cephalic vein is measured along its entire course. A tourniquet can also be useful. Some examiners advocate use of two tourniquets, one above the elbow to occlude the deep veins and one below to occlude more superficial veins. The examination may begin without the use of a tourniquet. A diameter of 3 mm or greater is generally adequate. A tourniquet should be used if vein diameter is less than 3 mm. Diameter should be recorded with a note regarding use or nonuse of a tourniquet. Vein measurements can be obtained using either a long-axis

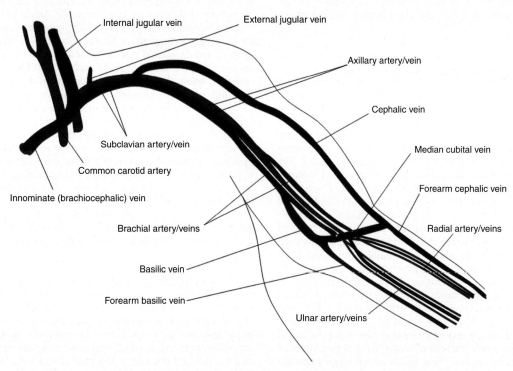

FIGURE 33.4. Anatomy of the upper extremity arteries and veins.

or a transverse image, with minimal pressure on the skin to avoid compressing the vein. The long-axis view has been recommended to avoid inadvertent use of an oblique transverse image, which can cause overestimation of the diameter. If the cephalic vein is inadequate, a survey should be done for other veins in the distal half of the forearm. If other forearm veins are 3 mm or larger, they should be mapped and marked from the wrist to the antecubital fossa.

The basilic vein is examined from the wrist to the confluence with the brachial vein, noting the confluence location, branching, wall thickening or thrombosis, and vein diameter. Because the brachial vein is sometimes used for a transposition fistula, the diameter of this vessel should also be obtained. The anatomy of the basilic vein is quite variable; it may confluence with the brachial vein at the proximal or mid upper arm or with the axillary vein more centrally.

The median cubital is a short superficial vein that passes across the anterior aspect of the elbow between the cephalic and the basilic veins. The anatomy of the median cubital vein is extremely variable. Whenever it is associated with a patent basilic or cephalic vein, the diameter and patency of the median cubital vein should be documented.

Arterial Mapping

Bilateral brachial systolic blood pressures are obtained with the patient supine to assess for occlusive disease in the innominate, subclavian, and axillary arteries. Doppler velocity waveforms are also obtained from the brachial arteries in both arms. However, blood pressures generally should not be taken in arms with a patent fistula or graft, to avoid inadvertent thrombosis of the access. The subclavian and axillary arteries are scanned, with particular attention to these segments if the brachial systolic blood pressures are unequal. Normal velocity waveforms in the upper extremity arteries are triphasic with no significant focal velocity increases. Upper extremity arterial duplex scanning is discussed in Chapter 14. The brachial, radial, and ulnar arteries are scanned throughout their entire course, noting any atherosclerosis, tortuosity, medial calcification, or anatomic variants such as a high bifurcation of the brachial artery into the radial and ulnar branches in the proximal arm.

Palmar Arch (Allen's Test)

If the forearm arteries and veins appear adequate for creation of a forearm fistula or graft, the palmar arch is evaluated to determine whether the blood supply to the hand is dependent on either the radial or the ulnar artery alone. The ulnar artery is often the dominant of the two forearm arteries and, therefore, is usually preserved for arterial supply to the hand. The radial artery is often nondominant and can be utilized for arterial inflow to the access site with little risk of hand ischemia. Patency of the palmar arch, which connects the radial and ulnar artery circulations, is evaluated with Allen's test. In the classic, less reliable form, this test uses simple observation of the return of pink color to the palm after clenching the fist with either the radial or the ulnar artery manually compressed. Slow return of color with one or the other artery manually occluded suggests that the hand is reliant on the occluded artery for its primary blood supply. A more quantitative version of Allen's test can be performed using photoplethysmography (PPG), as outlined in Table 33.4. Duplex scanning of the palmar arch can also be used for a direct evaluation of flow from the radial and ulnar arteries into the palm, using manual occlusion of these arteries at the wrist. These variations of Allen's test are described in more detail in Chapter 34.

TABLE 33.4

PHOTOPLETHYSMOGRAPHY ALLEN'S TEST FOR COMPLETENESS OF THE PALMAR ARCH

1. Place the PPG cell on the thumb and a 2.5-cm digital cuff around the base of the thumb of the hand being examined.
2. Record the PPG waveform.
3. Inflate the digital cuff to higher than the systolic blood pressure.
4. Slowly release the cuff pressure while observing the point at which the PPG pulsations return and record that pressure.
5. Repeat the thumb pressure while occluding the radial artery at the wrist with your fingers.
6. Also record the PPG waveform with the radial artery occluded.

Normal Allen's test:

If the thumb pressure remains above 80 mm Hg, or if there is less than a 30% drop with compression of the radial artery, this is a negative (normal) Allen's test.
The normal PPG waveform is a "volume pulse" with a quick systolic upstroke, a sharp peak, and a dicrotic notch on the downslope.

Abnormal Allen's test:

If the thumb pressure drops below 80 mm Hg, or if there is a more than 30% drop with compression of the radial artery, call this a positive (abnormal) Allen's test.
An abnormal PPG waveform is "dampened" with a slowed systolic upstroke, a rounded peak, and a downslope that is bowed away from the baseline without a dicrotic notch.

PPG, photoplethysmography.

Lower Extremity Mapping

Lower extremity sites may be considered for dialysis if there is no upper extremity alternative. The first step in the lower extremity evaluation is obtaining the ankle-brachial index bilaterally, being careful to avoid applying pressure cuffs over an existing patent graft or fistula. Generally, a dialysis access graft or fistula should not be placed in an extremity with an abnormally low ankle-brachial index or ankle pressure. The common femoral and proximal superficial femoral arteries in the thigh should be scanned to evaluate for stenosis and extent of calcification. Focal velocity increases of greater than 1.5-fold are suggestive of a significant stenosis. Duplex evaluation of the lower extremity arteries is discussed in Chapter 12. If vein mapping of the lower extremity is requested, the approach is similar to mapping these veins for use in arterial bypass surgery (see Chapter 28). Evaluation of the saphenofemoral junction and great saphenous vein is performed to the level of the knee for thrombosis, wall thickening, chronic webbing, varicosity, branching, and diameter. The common femoral, deep femoral, and femoral veins are evaluated for patency and velocity waveform patterns, as discussed in Chapter 19.

Pitfalls of Predialysis Access Mapping

A cold environment (cold room or cold gel) may cause the superficial veins to vasoconstrict and appear smaller on B-mode image than in their normal state. Furthermore, superficial veins are easily compressed, which makes accurate diameter measurements a delicate procedure. Optimal results are obtained if the patient is in a warm environment for at least 30 minutes prior to scanning. Directly warming the extremity with a heating pad and exercise of the extremity may also be helpful, as is gentle repeated slapping over the vein, as is done prior to phlebotomy. In some cases, it may be necessary to bring the patient back on another day for a repeat examination.

Patients with ESRD commonly present to the vascular laboratory with a history of multiple prior dialysis access procedures and revisions. There may be patent or occluded access sites, which complicate ultrasound evaluation and mapping. In these cases, obtaining as much detailed surgical history as possible is very helpful. Operative notes or diagrams are particularly helpful in this setting.

INTRAOPERATIVE EVALUATION

There are several ways for the surgeon to assess the adequacy of a new access site in the operating room. Simple palpation can often determine whether the access is functioning well. There should be a strong palpable thrill along the course of a fistula and in the draining vein of a graft. Absence of a thrill indicates inadequate flow, often due to impaired arterial inflow. Problems with outflow result in a strong pulse in the fistula or graft due to increased pressure resulting from restricted outflow. A normal access will have an obvious thrill that disappears and is replaced by a strong pulse when the outflow is manually occluded. If a sterile flow meter is available, this can be used to ensure that initial flow through the new fistula is at least 200 mL/min. Sterile continuous-wave Doppler examination should indicate low-resistance flow (high velocities with significant forward flow during diastole) in the fistula and in the artery just proximal to it. The artery distal to the anastomosis may also have this velocity pattern if it carries retrograde flow into the fistula from collateral vessels (such as flow from the ulnar artery through the palmar arch to the radial artery).

The surgeon should make sure that the circulation to the hand is adequate by listening to continuous-wave Doppler arterial signals at the wrist and palm as well as at the base of the fingers. Unfortunately, it is difficult to quantitate this examination to ensure that flow to the hand is sufficient to prevent a clinically significant steal. Even with adequate distal perfusion, it is common for these signals to be slightly diminished by the fistula and augmented when it is occluded. Digit pressures of at least 60 mm Hg are reassuring but are difficult to obtain at the time of surgery. Intraoperative angiography can also be helpful when there is doubt about fistula function. Central vein stenosis or occlusion is best studied with computerized tomography or magnetic resonance angiography.

Duplex scanning also can be a useful tool in the operating room. When a new arteriovenous fistula is created, the vein should have a diameter of at least 2.5 to 3.0 mm and should have flows of 200 mL/min or more. The vein should also be within 6 mm of the skin surface, although the surgeon may choose to superficialize the vein at a separate procedure after it has matured to a larger, thicker, and sometimes slightly elongated vessel that is more easily manipulated. The intraoperative duplex assessment is described in Chapter 30.

ACCESS MATURATION

Adequacy of access for hemodialysis can be judged by the rule of sixes: 6 weeks after placement, there should be a length of at least 6 cm for cannulation, the access should be no more than 6 mm below the skin surface for ease of puncture, and blood flow should be at least 600 mL/min for adequate filtration. These parameters can be assessed with duplex scanning, which can evaluate problems that may be interfering with vein maturation such as the presence of large side branches

that divert flow, narrowing of the outflow vein or more central venous outflow obstruction, and stenosis of the arterial anastomosis. It is helpful to scan new fistulas 4 to 6 weeks after surgery to ensure that they are maturing or determine the cause of nonmaturation.[8] Aggressive intervention soon after access creation may speed maturation and even salvage some fistulas that may not otherwise have matured. Possible interventions include ligation of venous side branches, repair of venous or arterial stenoses, vein angioplasty (balloon-assisted maturation), and vein superficialization.[9]

Volume Flow Measurements for Maturation

Access monitoring has typically relied on anatomic imaging (i.e., angiography) to evaluate access function and maturity. However, current recommendations support the addition of physiologic testing using Doppler measurements to identify low volume flow, a hemodynamic parameter predictive of impending thrombosis or difficult hemodialysis. Volume flow rates are typically in the range of 800 to 1200 mL/min in functioning fistulas and grafts. Flow rates of less than 500 mL/min are generally considered indicative of possible impending failure. Native vein fistulas tend to require less flow to remain patent than do prosthetic grafts. Table 33.5 lists some threshold volume flow criteria for dialysis access sites. Volume flow is more predictive of access failure than increased velocity, whereas velocity is better for detecting stenosis. Volume flow calculations also can help determine failure to mature (decreased volume flow) or cardiac volume overload (increased volume flow).

Most current duplex ultrasound systems include software to calculate volume flow based on the relationship between flow, velocity, lumen diameter, and cross-sectional area:

$$Q = v \times A \times 60 \, \text{seconds} = v \times \pi \left(d^2 \right)/4 \times 60 \, \text{seconds}$$

where Q = volume flow (mL/min), v = time-averaged and spatially averaged velocity across the lumen (cm/s), A = cross-sectional area at the site of velocity measurement (cm^2), and d = lumen diameter (cm). Multiplying by 60 seconds is necessary to obtain Q in mL/min. The pulsed Doppler sample volume is expanded to include the entire vessel diameter in long axis, and velocity spectral waveforms are recorded with a Doppler angle of 60 degrees. The time-averaged velocity is measured over at least two or three cardiac cycles and assumes laminar flow and a circular conduit. Measurements are obtained at several locations along the access graft or fistula outflow vein, approximately 3 to 4 vessel diameters away from the arterial anastomosis (Fig. 33.5). In the case of a tortuous fistula with variable diameters, it may be useful to measure the volume flow in the inflow artery rather than the fistula, as measurements are meant to be obtained in a straight vessel segment. Testing should not be performed during or immediately after dialysis, because reduction in blood pressure is a potential source of error. Dialysis access duplex is best performed in the vascular laboratory on a nondialysis day.[10,11]

TABLE 33.5

DIALYSIS ACCESS VOLUME FLOW CRITERIA

<450 mL/min	Poor dialysis, limited patency for prosthetic grafts (native fistulas may remain patent)
>500 mL/min	Normal native arteriovenous fistula
>700 mL/min	Normal prosthetic graft
>1400 mL/min	Possible congestive heart failure

FIGURE 33.5. *A,* Adequate volume flow in an expanded polytetrafluoroethylene (ePTFE) access graft calculated by duplex scanning. The display indicates a conduit diameter of 0.616 cm, time-averaged mean velocity (TAMV) of 67.0 cm/s, lumen area of 0.298 cm^2, and volume flow of 1197 mL/min. *B,* Poor volume flow of 418 mL/min is demonstrated by duplex scanning in another patient with a cephalic vein fistula.

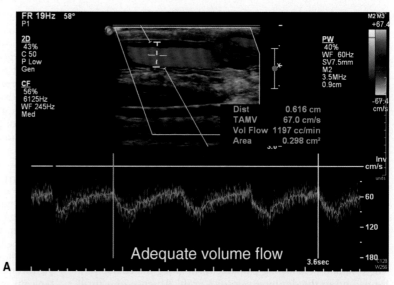

A

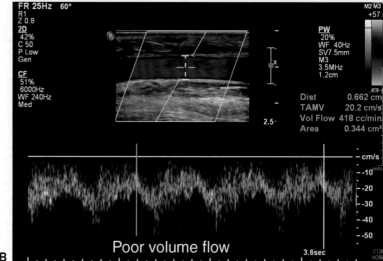

B

LONG-TERM MONITORING

Duplex scanning is one of several methods used to monitor dialysis access function. Some others include measurements of flows and pressures during dialysis and looking at trends in these values over time. There have been many randomized trials of duplex surveillance, but its efficacy in improving access site survival is dubious, particularly in the case of grafts.[12] However, there is general agreement that duplex scanning is indicated when there are signs or symptoms of access complications or decreased function.

The most common mode of failure for dialysis access sites is narrowing of venous outflow by intimal hyperplasia at or within a few centimeters of the venous anastomosis, but stenosis can occur anywhere in the circuit, from the donor artery (which may narrow from atherosclerosis) to the central veins (Fig. 33.6).[13] Locations particularly prone to intimal hyperplasia include vein valve and puncture sites, the transposed basilic vein where it turns down into the brachial vein, the cephalic vein where it joins the deep venous system, and the central veins (Fig. 33.7). Venous stenosis causes reduced flow and increased upstream pressure, which can be appreciated as a reduced thrill and increased pulsation in the fistula or graft. The vein may collapse during dialysis when more blood is extracted from the arterial side than is entering the fistula on the venous side. Venous outflow obstruction, at any level, causes blood returning

from the dialysis machine to recirculate in the fistula, thus making dialysis inefficient, as indicated by calculation of blood urea nitrogen clearance during dialysis. Increasing venous outflow obstruction may also be detected by elevation of pressure in the venous circuit of the dialysis machine. A pattern of increasing venous pressures over time is particularly concerning. Increased fistula pressure causes lengthening of the bleeding time at puncture sites after needle withdrawal. Some indications of a failing access site are listed in Table 33.6.

Duplex scanning often can identify the cause of access failure, particularly when it is due to arterial or venous stenosis (either in the fistula or centrally), and it can determine if flow is significantly reduced. With increasing limitations on scanning time, it may be tempting for the vascular technologists to immediately begin scanning. However, a brief patient interview and physical examination are well worth the time and help guide the examination.

Patient Interview and Physical Examination

The following questions can help guide the assessment of a dialysis access site:

1. Is the current hemodialysis access a native fistula or a graft?
2. Where is it located and what material was used?

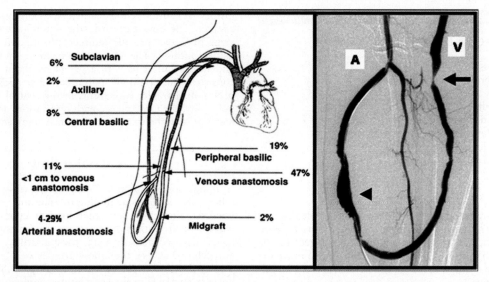

FIGURE 33.6. *Left*, Distribution of sites of narrowing in dialysis access grafts. *Right*, Angiogram of a loop ePTFE forearm access graft shows an area of dilatation (*triangle*) and a stenosis at the venous anastomosis (*arrow*). A, arterial anastomosis; V, venous anastomosis. (From Roy-Chaudhury P, Sukhatme VP, Cheung AK. Hemodialysis vascular access dysfunction: A cellular and molecular viewpoint. *J Am Soc Nephrol* 2006;17:1112-1127., used with permission.)

3. Is it currently being used for dialysis but is not working well?
4. Is it thrombosed?
5. Has it been ligated?
6. Has the patient had any prior access complications requiring catheter-based interventions or open surgical revisions?
7. Does the patient have any signs or symptoms of hand ischemia?

The fistula or graft should be palpated to identify the presence or absence of a thrill—the normal "buzzing" felt over a site with high-velocity fistula flow. Using the thrill as a guide, follow the fistula or graft by palpation to identify its course. This will provide a mental image and help direct the duplex examination. A diagram of the access site is also helpful. A stethoscope may be used to detect a bruit over the course of the fistula or graft. As previously discussed,

the presence of a strong pulse without a thrill suggests an outflow obstruction.

The dialysis access duplex evaluation consists of three main components: (1) central venous outflow, (2) arterial inflow, and (3) conduit surveillance (Table 33.7). Conduit surveillance is somewhat different for native vein fistulas and grafts. For a fistula, the access conduit is the superficial vein to which the artery is connected by a single anastomosis; with grafts, the access conduit is the graft itself, and there are two anastomoses to evaluate. Documentation of location and flow direction with regard to access fistulas and grafts can be confusing, especially if the terms "proximal" and "distal" are used; it is best to replace these terms with the unambiguous "central" and "peripheral."

Begin the examination with the patient in the supine position with the head slightly turned away from the limb being examined. The limb being examined should always be closest to the sonographer. In other words, scan the patient's left

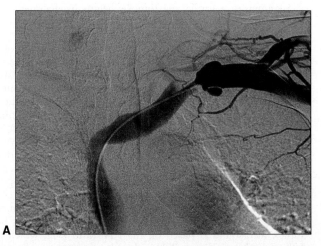

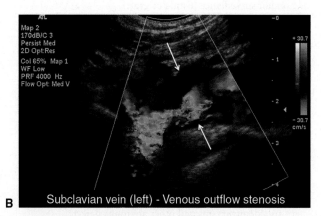

FIGURE 33.7. *A*, Venogram shows a subclavian vein stenosis in a dialysis access patient. This is typical of lesions that form after central venous catheter placement. *B*, Duplex image of a subclavian vein stenosis (*arrows*).

INDICATIONS OF A FAILING ACCESS SITE

Decreased access flow
Rising venous pressures during dialysis
Recirculation
Diminished thrill
Increased pulsation
Increased bleeding time after needle withdrawal
Swelling of the limb
Development of venous collaterals

arm with the ultrasound machine on the patient's left side and scan the patient's right arm with the ultrasound machine on the patient's right side. In this setting, it is advantageous to be able to scan with both hands, and taking the time to move the equipment when evaluating the contralateral arm is ergonomically advantageous.

Central Venous Outflow

The central veins are a vital component of a dialysis access duplex evaluation. There are two aspects to consider: (1) the presence or absence of central venous obstruction and (2) flow patterns that may suggest a problem within the fistula or graft. Central venous outflow obstruction is a common finding in long-term dialysis access patients, particularly those with a

DUPLEX EVALUATION OF DIALYSIS ACCESS

1. Central venous outflow

- Scan the innominate, subclavian (supra- and infraclavicular), and axillary veins, evaluating for central venous outflow obstruction (thrombosis or venous stenosis).

2. Arterial inflow

- Scan the subclavian and axillary arteries, documenting the presence of atherosclerosis or other abnormalities.
- Scan the brachial, radial, and ulnar inflow arteries, documenting the PSV prior to the anastomosis.
- Record the velocity in the artery peripheral to the anastomosis to evaluate for steal.

3. Conduit surveillance (fistula or graft)

A. Fistula anastomosis and superficial venous outflow
- Document the level of the fistula anastomosis and identify the involved artery and vein.
- Measure the diameter of the anastomosis.
- Record peak systolic velocities at the anastomosis.
- Evaluate the forearm and/or upper arm outflow vein throughout its course for evidence of venous stenosis (especially at valve sites) and for thrombosis.

B. Graft
- Identify the arterial anastomosis. Record peak systolic velocities at the anastomosis.
- Scan the proximal, mid, and distal segments of the graft, evaluating for patency and stenosis with spectral waveform analysis. Use B-mode and color Doppler imaging to look for pseudoaneurysms and other anatomic defects.
- Identify the venous anastomosis and evaluate for venous stenosis.

history of central venous catheters, as discussed later in this chapter. The flow pattern in the innominate and subclavian veins may also provide indirect information about graft or fistula outflow. The Doppler waveform in the innominate and subclavian veins with a patent fistula or graft will have consistent "arterialized" pulsatility (Fig. 33.8A). With graft occlusion, Doppler waveforms in the central veins lack such pulsatility, are more phasic with respiration, and may be symmetrical with the veins on the contralateral side.

Arterial Inflow

Although a less common location for obstruction, arterial inflow may be inadequate due to anatomic variants, atherosclerosis, dissection, or other arterial conditions. Doppler waveforms from the inflow arteries to a patent fistula or graft have increased velocity with low pulsatility. However, with an occluded access, the inflow arteries will "normalize" and display a typical triphasic waveform (Fig. 33.8B). Arterial stenosis at any level in the vasculature supplying the access may reduce the pulsatility and velocity of flow within the graft or fistula and lead to access failure.

The brachial, radial, and ulnar arteries all should be evaluated central to the level of the anastomosis. Flow patterns in the native arteries are also evaluated 2 to 4 cm peripheral to the anastomosis to document distal perfusion to the hand. Peripheral to the anastomosis, the arterial waveform may return to a high-resistance pattern, as is normally seen in an extremity artery, or it may show alternating or retrograde flow direction suggestive of a steal, as discussed later in this chapter.

Conduit Surveillance (Native Vein Fistula)

An access fistula is a direct surgical connection between an artery and a vein. This requires a single anastomosis, which is most commonly created at the wrist (radiocephalic fistula), cubital space (brachiocephalic fistula), or the upper arm (basilic vein transposition fistula). The cephalic vein is preferred because it is more superficial than the basilic vein. If the basilic vein is used, it is transposed and brought closer to the surface for accessibility. The various anastomotic configurations are illustrated in Figure 33.9. After first scanning the central veins and the arterial inflow, evaluation of a fistula continues with the anastomosis, followed by the superficial venous outflow vessel that is typically either the cephalic or the basilic vein.

Scanning of a fistula anastomosis begins by documenting the level of the fistula and identifying the involved artery and vein, evaluating both the arterial inflow and distal perfusion to the hand. The diameter of the arteriovenous anastomosis is measured and is often only 4 or 5 mm, since larger diameters have a higher risk of causing a steal. Measurement of the fistula anastomosis may help the vascular surgeon determine whether banding or a distal revascularization–interval ligation (DRIL) procedure is possible to decrease symptomatic arterial steal. The peak systolic velocity (PSV) at the anastomosis is measured, keeping in mind that it is common to see relatively high velocities at anastomotic sites followed by turbulence due to caliber change and angulation. Doppler spectral velocity waveform and color Doppler scales should be set appropriately to compensate for aliasing.

Because increased velocities are common at a fistula anastomosis, one method of quantifying anastomotic stenosis by duplex ultrasound is based on the PSV ratio (Vr), which is defined as the maximum PSV within the anastomosis divided by the PSV of the inflow artery measured approximately 2 cm proximal to the anastomosis. A Vr of 3.0 or greater and a PSV

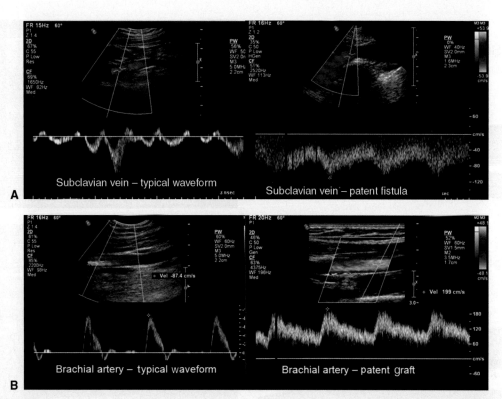

FIGURE 33.8. *A,* Normal subclavian vein Doppler waveform (*left*) contrasts with the subclavian vein waveform associated with outflow from a patent fistula or graft (*right*). *B,* The triphasic high resistance waveform (*left*) is seen in a normal brachial artery; the continuous, low-resistance waveform (*right*) represents inflow to a patent dialysis access fistula or graft.

of 400 cm/s or greater are suggestive of a stenosis of at least 50% diameter reduction. However, B-mode confirmation of an intraluminal defect at the anastomosis is necessary since the geometry of the vessels may cause a velocity increase without true stenosis (Fig. 33.10).[14]

The main superficial venous outflow from a fistula is usually through the cephalic or basilic vein. Failure of the venous conduit to mature may be due to the presence of large venous side branches. Slow or failed maturation may occur if fistula flow is diminished by flow through these side branches, and ligation of these vessels can direct flow back into the main fistula, allowing it to mature.

The entire length of the outflow vein is evaluated with B-mode, color Doppler, and Doppler spectral waveforms. B-mode imaging in long-axis and transverse views will help identify intraluminal defects such as thrombus, chronic webbing, a fibrotic valve, or caliber change. Color Doppler is useful in the detection of aliasing along the length of the outflow vein, which may help to quickly identify sites of stenosis. Doppler spectral waveforms are also assessed along the length of the outflow vein. Within the venous outflow of the fistula, PSVs should be in the range of 150 to 300 cm/s. Some laboratories use a two-fold focal velocity increase (Vr of 2.0) with associated poststenotic turbulence as a threshold to indicate a significant stenosis within the fistula. Occlusion is identified by the presence of intraluminal echoes with no obtainable color Doppler flow or velocity waveforms.

Conduit Surveillance (Prosthetic Graft)

Grafts have two anastomotic sites (arterial and venous) and may be created from a variety of materials, with ePTFE being the most common. The evaluation of a graft includes three segments: (1) the arterial anastomosis, (2) the central, mid, and peripheral graft, and (3) the venous anastomosis. A loop graft is often created to provide more access site length. The inflow artery is anastomosed to the graft at one end with the graft directed peripherally; the graft then makes a loop coursing back toward the heart and is anastomosed to an outflow vein. With a straight graft configuration, the inflow artery is anastomosed to a graft that courses directly back toward the heart and is then anastomosed to an outflow vein (Fig. 33.11).

Continue the duplex evaluation of a graft from the arterial system, measuring the diameter and velocity at the arterial anastomosis. As previously discussed, high velocities at an arterial anastomosis are common; however, diameters of graft anastomoses are less variable than those of fistula anastomoses. As with the evaluation of a fistula, also document the Doppler flow pattern in the artery beyond the arterial anastomosis to look for evidence of a steal (retrograde flow with low resistance). Although velocities at anastomotic sites of access grafts are extremely variable, the general criteria for stenosis listed previously for native fistulas can be applied to grafts. A PSV of 400 cm/s or greater and a focal velocity increase with a Vr of 3.0 or greater are suggestive of a significant (≥50% diameter reduction) stenosis.

An initial B-mode evaluation of the graft in transverse and long axis will identify any intraluminal abnormalities that may be masked by the color Doppler display. When scanning the graft, annotate "central" (arterial side if scanning a loop graft), "mid," and "peripheral" (venous side if scanning a loop graft). Interrogate the graft with the pulsed Doppler for focal velocity increases that may be due to intraluminal thrombus, neointimal hyperplasia, chronic webbing, clamp injury, or stenosis at a revision site. Velocities along the graft are variable; however, some general criteria for significant (≥50% diameter reduction) stenosis that have been applied to arterial inflow,

Side of artery to side of vein

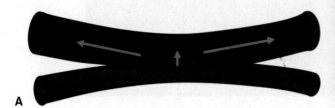

Side of artery to end of vein

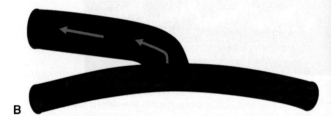

End of artery to side of vein

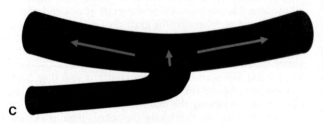

End of Artery to End Vein

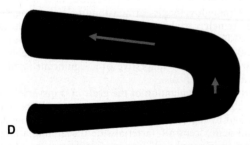

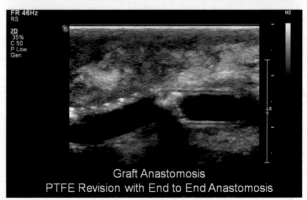

FIGURE 33.9. Anastomotic configurations for direct native arteriovenous fistulas. *A*, Side-to-side anastomosis between artery and vein. Example: radial artery to basilic vein fistula in the proximal forearm. *B*, End-to-side anastomosis (side of artery to end of vein). Example: end of cephalic vein to side of radial artery fistula just beyond the cubital space. *C*, End-to-side anastomosis (end of artery to side of vein). Example: end of distal radial artery to side of basilic vein fistula at the wrist. *D*, End-to-end anastomosis. Example: not a fistula (artery to vein), but a graft revision with an ePTFE-to-ePTFE anastomosis.

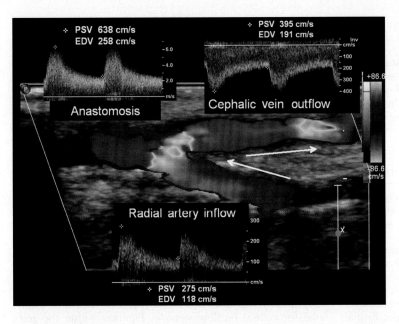

FIGURE 33.10. Color Doppler image and Doppler spectral waveforms show increased velocity at a widely patent fistula anastomosis. Although the peak systolic velocity (PSV) is greater than 400 cm/s, the velocity ratio is less than 3.0.

graft/fistula, and venous outflow segments include a PSV of 300 to 400 cm/s or greater, end-diastolic velocity (EDV) of 240 cm/s or greater, and Vr of 2.0 or greater.

Graft occlusion is often identified by the absence of a palpable thrill before the patient comes to the vascular laboratory. In these cases, the patient may go directly to the interventional suite for a salvage procedure. Duplex confirmation of graft occlusion is based on the presence of intraluminal echoes, absence of flow on Doppler spectral waveforms, and lack of

color Doppler flow using low velocity and color scales. An exception is synthetic graft materials (such as polyurethane) that do not allow ultrasound penetration, causing complete shadowing across the lumen of the graft and preventing any direct interrogation with Doppler. In this case, Doppler waveforms in the artery upstream and downstream from the graft provide indirect evidence of graft patency. With a patent graft, the upstream Doppler waveform has increased velocity with a low-resistance flow pattern; downstream, the flow pattern may

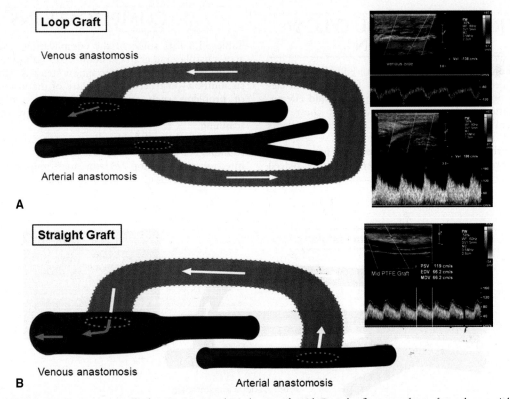

FIGURE 33.11. *A,* A normally functioning prosthetic loop graft with Doppler flow waveforms from the arterial and venous sides. The arterial waveform (*bottom*) shows increased velocity with a low-resistance flow pattern; the venous waveform (*top*) shows high velocities and arterial pulsatility. *B,* A normally functioning straight prosthetic graft with Doppler flow waveforms from the mid–graft segment. *Arrows* indicate direction of flow.

return to a typical high-resistance peripheral artery waveform. The graft may be collapsed if chronically occluded or previously ligated.

The venous outflow anastomosis should be identified and its diameter measured. Synthetic grafts may be anastomosed to a vein cuff rather than directly to the deep vein. It is common to have a venous outflow stenosis at or just beyond the venous anastomosis, as identified by a focal velocity increase with an audible Doppler bruit and poststenotic turbulence.

Lower Extremity Dialysis Access Surveillance

Lower extremity arteriovenous fistulas are generally a last resort when all upper extremity options have been exhausted. Choices for conduit include prosthetic grafts, the great saphenous vein, or the femoral vein (formerly called the superficial femoral vein), placed between the common or superficial femoral artery and a deep vein in the thigh. The great saphenous vein may be mobilized and anastomosed to the superficial femoral artery at the mid-thigh (Fig. 33.12). Duplex evaluation is similar to that for a fistula in the upper extremity: evaluate the arterial inflow, the anastomosis, the fistula outflow conduit (usually the great saphenous vein), and the deep venous outflow in the common femoral vein for stenosis or intraluminal thrombosis. One difference from the upper extremity fistula evaluation is the measurement of ankle pressures and the ankle-brachial index. The ankle pressure will normally decrease after creation of a lower extremity fistula, but this is unlikely to be clinically significant unless arterial occlusive disease is present. Additionally, in this patient population, medial calcification is common and can result in falsely elevated ankle pressures. When this occurs, toe pressures should be taken (see Chapter 13).

CENTRAL VENOUS OUTFLOW OBSTRUCTION

Extremity venous hypertension may be caused by high fistula flow rates or central venous obstruction. This results in elevated venous pressure and ipsilateral arm and hand edema, skin discoloration (red-purple), and prominent chest wall venous collaterals. This condition is more common in patients who have had intravenous lines placed in these vessels, particularly when the subclavian vein has been used for tunneled dialysis catheters. For this reason, catheters should be placed in the internal jugular vein whenever practical. Venous outflow obstruction is particularly prone to cause venous hypertension and edema in limbs with a dialysis access fistula or graft, since a functioning access site can increase flow by a liter or more per minute.

The Doppler flow pattern in the outflow veins of a patent dialysis access fistula or graft is characterized by regular pulsatility without the respiratory phasicity, dynamic vein wall motion, or the random velocity changes typically seen in normal upper extremity veins (Fig. 33.8A). Obstruction may occur at any location from the venous anastomosis of the fistula to the superior vena cava. With venous outflow stenosis, a focal velocity increase is seen in an otherwise "arterialized" vein segment. In one study, a PSV ratio across the vein segment of greater than 2.5 was associated with critical narrowing in central veins.[15] Some central venous occlusions may be difficult to visualize with duplex scanning. The presence of abundant, well-developed venous collaterals is a clue to the presence of a central vein stenosis or occlusion.

Patients who are referred to the vascular laboratory because of increased venous pressures during dialysis or prolonged dialyzing times due to recirculation should be evaluated for venous outflow stenosis. Findings within the graft may be normal, but a significant venous stenosis may be found beyond the venous anastomosis. The most common locations for venous outflow stenoses are as follows: directly beyond the venous anastomosis in the native outflow vein (often the axillary vein in the case of an upper extremity graft); the transposed basilic vein where it turns down into the brachial vein; the cephalic vein where it joins the deep venous system; and within the proximal subclavian or innominate veins due to intraluminal scarring from prior central venous lines (Fig. 33.13).

COMPLICATIONS

Table 33.8 lists some of the complications associated with access fistulas and grafts in addition to failure to provide adequate flow for dialysis due to inflow stenosis, access thrombosis, outflow obstruction, or failure of maturation. Diagnosis of problems such as fluid collections, pseudoaneurysms, and steal phenomenon is fairly straightforward with duplex scanning.

Nonvascularized fluid collections are commonly seen surrounding or adjacent to a dialysis access site (Fig. 33.14). Infection may develop near the anastomoses or at the puncture sites and result in perigraft fluid or an abscess cavity.

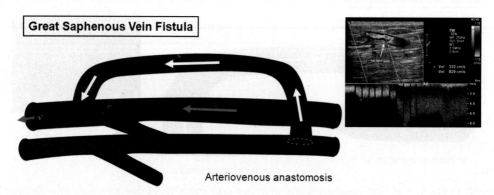

FIGURE 33.12. Lower extremity fistula using the great saphenous vein as the conduit with the anastomosis to the superficial femoral artery. *Arrows* indicate direction of flow. The duplex image shows a stenosis related to a valve site in the great saphenous outflow vein with a peak systolic velocity (PSV) of 829 cm/s.

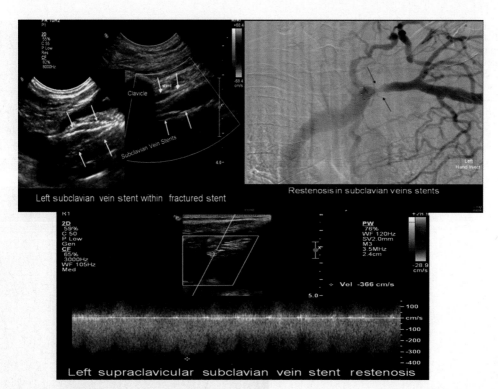

FIGURE 33.13. Case of subclavian vein obstruction. The patient presented 3 days after a transaxillary rib resection and multiple venous stents for a left subclavian vein stenosis causing increased venous pressures during dialysis. *Bottom*, Doppler spectral waveform with increased peak systolic velocity (PSV) of 366 cm/s, consistent with a severe, focal restenosis of the stented subclavian vein. *Upper left*, B-mode images show a stent fracture in the left subclavian vein *(arrows)*. *Upper right*, contrast venogram shows the left subclavian vein in-stent restenosis and extensive collateral veins due to the patent access graft in the left arm.

Perigraft fluid is apparent on B-mode imaging as an irregular hypoechoic area surrounding the graft. A *seroma* is a pocket of clear fluid that sometimes develops after surgery whereas *abscesses* that contain pus may have internal septations and debris. A *hematoma* is a static collection of blood outside of a blood vessel; on duplex scanning, a hematoma appears as a hypoechoic or heterogeneous mass. A *lymphocele* is a fluid collection containing lymph that forms when the lymphatic channels are disrupted. On B-mode imaging, a lymphocele appears as a well-circumscribed hypoechoic structure and is most often found at the groin.

A *pseudoaneurysm* is a cavity with active flow outside the wall of a blood vessel or graft. Unlike a hematoma, a pseudoaneurysm has a direct communication with the blood vessel lumen. This communication is referred to as the "neck" of the pseudoaneurysm and will display a "to-and-fro" flow pattern in the spectral waveform. On the color Doppler display, a

pseudoaneurysm has a swirling appearance as the arterial flow enters the pseudoaneurysm sac through the neck to create a "hot air balloon" appearance. With dialysis access sites, pseudoaneurysms may develop if the puncture site does not seal when the needle is removed (Fig. 33.15). In rare instances, a pseudoaneurysm may develop if an artery is inadvertently punctured during cannulation.

Steal Phenomenon

A steal develops when the artery supplying the fistula or graft is unable to provide adequate flow into both the fistula and the distal arterial circulation. In this situation, flow preferentially follows the path of least resistance through the fistula, resulting in decreased arterial pressure and flow in the distal extremity. Flow may even be reversed in the distal artery and move toward the low-resistance fistula. Clinically significant steal rarely occurs unless there is occlusive disease in the arterial system proximal or distal to the access site. Upstream stenosis reduces flow; downstream stenosis makes the hand more susceptible to ischemia when flow is decreased. Steal is more common in diabetic patients who are particularly prone to occlusive disease in the upper extremity arteries.

Reduced arterial flow to the hand causes pain, weakness, numbness, and, in extreme cases, gangrene and loss of digits. This phenomenon must be recognized and treated immediately, because permanent damage to the hand occurs rapidly. Treatment options include narrowing the arterial inflow with banding or clipping, creating a bypass graft from the artery above the fistula to the hand and ligating

TABLE 33.8

ACCESS SITE COMPLICATIONS

Infection
Seroma
Lymphocele
Hematoma
Pseudoaneurysm
Steal phenomenon
Venous hypertension
Edema

PREOPERATIVE PLANNING, INTRAOPERATIVE ASSESSMENT AND PROCEDURAL GUIDANCE

FIGURE 33.14. *A*, B-mode image shows perigraft fluid around an ePTFE access graft. *B*, B-mode and color Doppler image of a hematoma adjacent to an ePTFE graft anastomosis. *C*, B-mode and color Doppler image of a groin lymphocele causing extrinsic compression of a lower extremity access fistula.

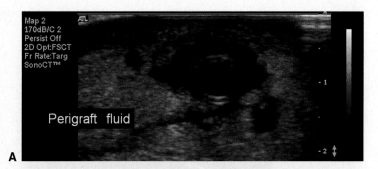

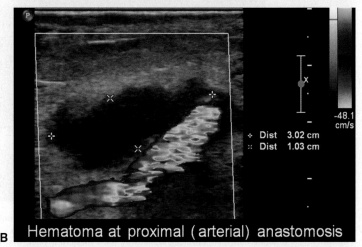

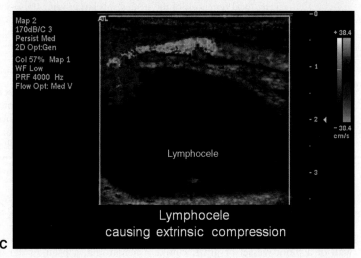

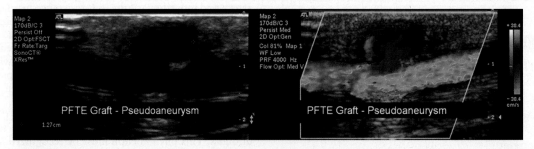

FIGURE 33.15. A small pseudoaneurysm in an ePTFE access graft. *Left*, B-mode image. *Right*, Color Doppler image. Note the area of flow outside the graft wall between the graft and the skin surface.

the artery just distal to the fistula to prevent reversed flow (the previously mentioned DRIL procedure), proximalization of the inflow (providing flow to the graft or fistula from a more proximal artery), and ligation of the access site. Various ePTFE grafts are now on the market with configurations designed to narrow the arterial inflow segment in an attempt to prevent excessive flow through the graft. Most common among these is the tapered graft that has a short 4-mm diameter segment for the arterial anastomosis and a longer 7-mm diameter segment for the area to be cannulated.

On duplex examination, the direction of flow should be noted in the arteries peripheral to the fistula, particularly when reversed flow is present. A careful search should be carried out for arterial stenosis, which is particularly common in diabetic patients. A steal is characterized by retrograde flow (away from the hand) in the radial or ulnar artery peripheral to the anastomosis (Fig. 33.16).

Patients may present with a cold, painful hand, especially while dialyzing. Extremely high-flow fistulas (>900 mL/min/1.73 m^2 body surface area) are more likely to be associated with steal phenomenon. Measurement of digit pressures with an appropriate-sized cuff and flow detection with PPG is a useful diagnostic test, as described in Chapter 14. A digit pressure of 60 mm Hg or greater or a digit-brachial index of 0.6 or greater is generally indicative of adequate perfusion. Measurements obtained with and without manual compression of the fistula will give the clinician an indication of the response to treatment. This provocative examination is best carried out by two technologists, with one technologist performing manual compression of the fistula or graft and the second obtaining PPG pressures on the symptomatic finger.

CONCLUSION

Dialysis access grafts and fistulas are the lifeline for patients with ESRD. Creation and maintenance of these access sites is the main cause of hospitalization and costly complications in these patients. Duplex scanning is an invaluable asset for preoperative planning to choose the correct procedure with the best long-term performance, to evaluate fistula maturation, and to diagnose complications such as steal or access failure. The ease of duplex scanning, its noninvasive nature, and relatively low cost, along with the detailed information it provides, make it an essential component of the care of this challenging patient population.

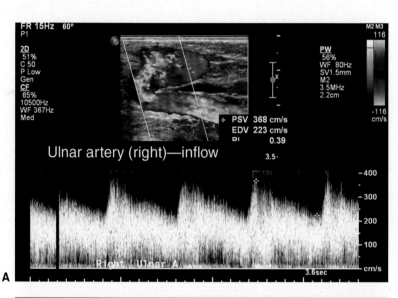

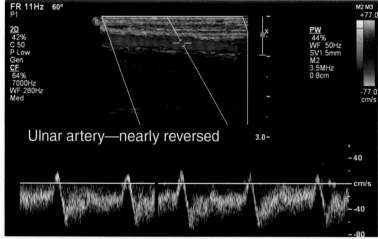

FIGURE 33.16. *A,* The flow pattern just central to the ulnar artery anastomosis of a patent access site displays increased peak velocities with low resistance. *B,* This abnormal, mostly retrograde flow pattern indicates a complete steal in the ulnar artery beyond the anastomosis.

PREOPERATIVE PLANNING, INTRAOPERATIVE ASSESSMENT AND PROCEDURAL GUIDANCE

References

1. Foley RN, Collins AJ. End-stage renal disease in the United States: An update from the United States Renal Data System. *J Am Soc Nephrol* 2007;18:2644-2648.
2. Quinton W, Dillard D, Scribner BH. Cannulation of blood vessels for prolonged hemodialysis. *Trans Am Soc Artif Intern Organs* 1960;6:104-113.
3. Cimino JE, Brescia MJ. Simple venipuncture for hemodialysis. *N Engl J Med* 1962;267:608-609.
4. van der Linden J, Lameris TW, van den Meiracker AH, et al. Forearm venous distensibility predicts successful arteriovenous fistula. *Am J Kidney Dis* 2006;47:1013-1019.
5. Scher LA. Strategies for hemodialysis access graft: Where to start and where to go next. Presented at the American College of Surgeons 32nd Annual Spring Meeting, April 2004, Boston, Massachusetts.
6. Chan MR, Sanchez RJ, Young HN, et al. Vascular access outcomes in the elderly hemodialysis population: A USRDS study. *Semin Dial* 2007;20:606-610.
7. Bruns SD, Jennings WC. Proximal radial artery as inflow site for native arteriovenous fistula. *J Am Coll Surg* 2003;197:58-63.
8. Grogan J, Castilla M, Lozanski L, et al. Frequency of critical stenosis in primary arteriovenous fistulae before hemodialysis access: Should duplex ultrasound surveillance be the standard of care? *J Vasc Surg* 2005;41:1000-1006.
9. De Marco Garcia LP, Davila-Santini LR, Feng Q, et al. Primary balloon angioplasty plus balloon angioplasty maturation to upgrade small-caliber veins (<3 mm) for arteriovenous fistulas. *J Vasc Surg* 2010;52:139-144.
10. Bandyk DF. Expected flow parameters within hemodialysis access selection for remedial intervention of non-maturing conduits. *Vasc Endovasc Surg* 2008;42:150-157.
11. Sands JJ, Glidden D, Miranda C. Hemodialysis access flow measurement—comparison of ultrasound dilution and duplex ultrasonography. *ASAIO J* 1996;42:899-901.
12. Tonelli M, James M, Wiebe N, et al. Ultrasound monitoring to detect access stenosis in hemodialysis patients: A systematic review. *Am J Kidney Dis* 2008;51:630-640.
13. Roy-Chaudhury P, Sukhatme VP, Cheung AK. Hemodialysis vascular access dysfunction: A cellular and molecular viewpoint. *J Am Soc Nephrol* 2006;17:1112-1127.
14. Lockhart ME, Robbin ML. Doppler of hemodialysis fistula. In Mohler ER, Gerhard-Herman M, Jaff MR (eds). *Essentials of Vascular Laboratory Diagnosis*. Malden: Blackwell Publishing, pp 160-172.
15. Labropoulos N, Borge M, Pierce K, et al. Criteria for defining significant central vein stenosis with duplex ultrasound. *J Vasc Surg* 2007;46:101-107.

CHAPTER 34 ■ RADIAL ARTERY EVALUATION BEFORE CORONARY ARTERY BYPASS GRAFTS

MOLLY J. ZACCARDI AND NAHUSH A. MOKADAM

ROLE OF THE VASCULAR LABORATORY
NONINVASIVE DIAGNOSTIC APPROACHES
UNIVERSITY OF WASHINGTON PROTOCOL

Patient Preparation
Equipment
Examination Technique
Interpretation Criteria and Reporting

The choice of conduit in coronary artery bypass grafting is often surgeon and institution specific. Nonetheless, the general consensus is that this choice can play a crucial role in the outcomes of patients undergoing coronary revascularization. Increased attention has been paid to the use of multiple arterial conduits for coronary artery bypass, including the left internal mammary artery, the right internal mammary artery, and the radial artery. The radial artery was first introduced in 1973 for aortocoronary bypass.[1] However, initial enthusiasm faded quickly, because the radial artery was prone to premature graft occlusion and spasm. The development of pharmacologic therapy to minimize arterial spasm, along with new techniques for arterial harvest, rejuvenated interest in the radial artery as a conduit for coronary artery bypass.[2] Although long-term outcomes data comparing the radial artery with the saphenous vein are fraught with bias, there is a suggestion that the use of a radial artery graft improves survival or, at the very least, is equivalent to the use of saphenous vein grafts.[3,4] For these reasons, the routine and widespread use of the radial artery has not gained a major foothold in the cardiac surgery community, but it does remain a very good option in many patients.

The radial artery is one of the two end arteries supplying the hand. The ability to safely harvest the radial artery depends on adequate ulnar artery inflow and an intact palmar arch. The traditional and most simplistic evaluation of the arterial supply to the hand has been Allen's test. However, the adequacy of Allen's test has been questioned, leading to the practice of relying on more objective criteria to prevent hand ischemia after harvesting the radial artery.[5]

ROLE OF THE VASCULAR LABORATORY

When the radial artery is being considered for use as a conduit, the vascular laboratory can provide important preoperative information regarding collateral circulation to the hand and the size and patency of the radial artery to answer the key questions listed below:

1. **Will the collateral circulation be adequate to ensure perfusion of the hand following removal of the radial artery?**
   In most patients, the deep and superficial palmar arches of the hand provide collateral routes between the radial and the ulnar arteries and allow safe harvesting of the radial artery. The classic superficial palmar arch connects the ulnar artery and the superficial palmar branch of the radial artery. The classic deep palmar arch connects the radial artery and the deep branch of the ulnar artery (Fig. 34.1). However, cadaver studies have reported that up to 34% of hands have an incomplete deep or superficial palmar arch.[6-10] Table 34.1 summarizes five such studies. In these cases, removal of the radial artery could lead to digital ischemia. In addition, it has been suggested that a complete arch may be present in the hand but that collateral flow might still be inadequate. Examples of complete and incomplete superficial palmar arches are demonstrated in Figure 34.2 from a report by Gellman et al.[11]

2. **Is the radial artery size (diameter and length) adequate for use as a coronary artery bypass graft?**
   Ideally, the length of the radial artery conduit should be sufficient to reach from the aorta to the lateral wall of the heart (15 to 18 cm) for an obtuse marginal bypass. The diameter should be at least 2 mm, but preferably larger. The cadaver study of Gellman et al[11] reported radial artery lumen diameters ranging from 2.3 to 5 mm, with an average of approximately 2.6 mm. Anatomic variants such as ulnar artery dominance may be associated with a smaller radial artery diameter. Early or late bifurcations can also reduce the usable length of the radial artery. In a study of 192 cadavers (384 arms), Rodriguez-Niedenfuhr et al[12] found anatomic variants in 24% of the upper arm (brachial) arteries and 19% of the forearm (radial and/or ulnar) arteries. A summary of this report is presented in Table 34.2.

3. **Is the radial artery obstructed or calcified?**
   Stenosis or calcification of the radial artery can reduce the long-term patency of a coronary artery bypass graft. These abnormalities are common in this patient population, as noted by Ruengsakulrach et al.[13] These authors examined 73 patients preoperatively with ultrasound and found an overall 31.5% incidence of radial artery calcification or echogenic plaques.

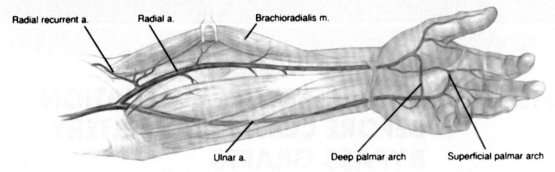

FIGURE 34.1. Normal anatomy of the forearm and hand arteries, including the deep and superficial palmar arches of the hand.

TABLE 34.1

PREVALENCE OF INCOMPLETE SUPERFICIAL AND DEEP PALMAR ARCHES FROM CADAVER STUDIES

	NUMBER OF CADAVER HANDS	INCOMPLETE SUPERFICIAL PALMAR ARCH (%)	INCOMPLETE DEEP PALMAR ARCH (%)
Coleman and Anson (1961)[7]	650	21.5	3
Ikeda et al (1988)[8]	220	3.6	23.1
Mezzogiorno et al (1994)[9]	60	—	33.3
Orzkus et al (1998)[10]	80	20	—
Ruengsakulrach et al (2001)[6]	50	34	10

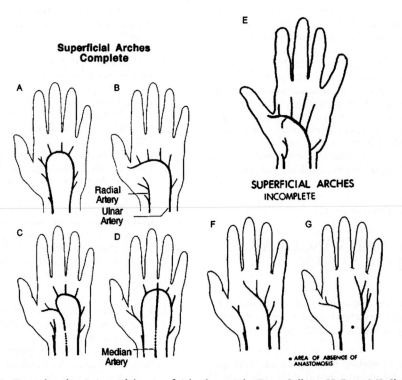

FIGURE 34.2. Examples of variations of the superficial palmar arch. (From Gellman H, Botte MJ, Shankweiler J, et al. Arterial patterns of the deep and superficial palmar arches. *Clin Orthop* 2001;383:41-46, used with permission.)

TABLE 34.2

SUMMARY OF ANATOMICAL VARIANTS FOUND IN A CADAVER STUDY
OF 384 LIMBS

	■ ARTERIAL PATTERNS	■ DESCRIPTION	■ INCIDENCE
Arm			
1 artery	**Brachial (Normal)**		76.06%
	Superficial brachial	Brachial artery is superficial to the nerve	4.9
2 arteries	Brachial and accessory brachial	Brachial artery branches in the upper arm and rejoins above the elbow	0.26
	Brachial and brachioradial	Radial artery with high origin	13.8
	Brachial and superficial brachioradial	Radial with high origin and superficial to the nerve	<0.26
	Brachial and brachioulnar	Ulnar artery with a high origin	0.26
	Brachial and superficial brachioulnar	Ulnar with high origin and superficial to the nerve	4.2
	Brachial and superficial brachioulnoradial	Brachial has radial and ulnar branches but continues into interosseus	0.52
	Brachial and superficial brachiomedian	High origin of the median artery, which is superficial to muscles	<0.26
	Brachial and brachiointerosseus	High origin of the interosseus artery coexisting with brachial artery	<0.26
Forearm			
1 artery	Ulnar and radial absent		<0.26
	Radial and ulnar absent		<0.26
2 arteries	**Ulnar and radial (Normal)**		**81.22%**
	Ulnar and brachioradial	High origin of the radial artery	13.8
	Ulnar and superficial brachioradial	High origin of the radial artery and superficial to muscle/tendons	<0.26
	Ulnar and superficial radial	Radial artery superficial to muscle	0.52
	Radial and brachioulnar	High origin of the ulnar artery	0.26
	Radial and superficial brachioulnar	Ulnar has a high origin and is superficial to muscle	4.2
3 arteries	Ulnar and radial and brachiomedian	High origin of the median artery	<0.26
	Ulnar, radial, and superficial brachioradial	Radial duplication	<0.26
	Radial, ulnar, and superficial brachioulnar	Ulnar duplication	<0.26

Adapted from Rodriguez-Niedenfuhr M, Vazquez T, Nearn L, et al. Variations of the arterial pattern in the upper limb revisited: A morphological and statistical study, with a review of the literature. *J Anat* 2001;199:547-566.

NONINVASIVE DIAGNOSTIC APPROACHES

Several protocols, with varying equipment and algorithms, have been described in an attempt to provide information on the upper extremity arterial circulation needed by the cardiac surgeon.[14] The simplest method is Allen's test. Allen's test, first described in 1929, was originally performed by first having the patient make a tight fist to empty blood from the hand.[15] The radial and ulnar arteries were then digitally compressed and the hand was opened, resulting in blanching of the palm (Fig. 34.3). After a few seconds, compression on the ulnar artery was released, and the length of time required for color to return to the palm was recorded (Fig. 34.4). In 2000, Jarvis et al[5] described the limitations of this method. There was

disagreement on the cutoff point between positive and negative tests, which varied between 5 and 10 seconds. They also reported observer bias in deciding when the normal palmar rubor had returned and found that false-negative results could occur if the wrist was hyperextended. Kamienski and Barnes[16] reported a 73% false-positive rate due to subjectivity of the test or observer bias.

Prior to the report of Jarvis et al,[5] Starnes et al[17] compared a "modified" Allen's test with direct digit pressure measurement. This modified Allen's test was considered positive if radial artery compression caused a decrease in the audible Doppler flow signal from the superficial palmar arch. The change in the Doppler flow signal was compared with the digit pressure difference before and after radial artery compression (Fig. 34.5). A pressure drop in the first or second digit of 40 mm Hg or more suggested an inadequate collateral pathway in the hand.

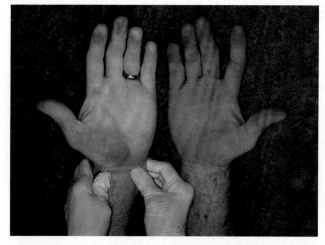

FIGURE 34.3. Allen's test shows open left hand with radial and ulnar artery compression producing pallor of the hand and fingers.

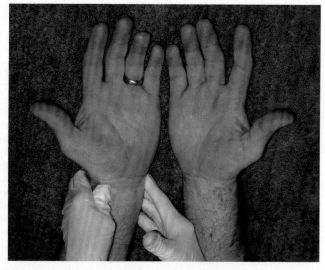

FIGURE 34.4. Allen's test shows open left hand with release of ulnar artery compression while radial artery compression is maintained. Note return of normal color to the hand.

Both of these tests attempted to reduce the subjectivity noted by Jarvis et al[5] and Kamienski and Barnes.[16] Starnes et al[17] reported a high false-positive rate of 50% with the modified Allen's test and concluded that the change in digit pressure was more effective in avoiding complications after radial artery harvest. However, neither Starnes et al[17] nor Jarvis et al[5] were able to address specific anatomic variants or vessel diameters.

In 2003, Sullivan et al[18] compared changes in peak systolic velocity in the ulnar artery at the wrist with changes in digit pressures in response to radial artery compression. This study showed a poor correlation between ulnar artery velocities and digit pressures. For this reason, they favor the use of digit pressure measurement with and without radial artery compression. Their protocol includes segmental arm blood pressure measurements to identify arterial obstruction of the major arteries of the arm. The normal values for pressure measurements in the upper extremity were established by Sumner et al in 1979.[19] Brachial, radial, and ulnar artery systolic pressures should differ by less than 15 mm Hg from side to side.

A brachial artery systolic pressure difference of greater than 15 mm Hg suggests an obstruction involving the proximal arteries (brachial, axillary, subclavian, or innominate) on the side with the lower pressure. In addition, a gradient between adjacent levels in the same extremity (upper arm and forearm) of greater than 15 mm Hg is suggestive of obstruction between those two levels.

In 2004, Agrifoglio et al[20] compared the modified Allen's test with the snuffbox test using color duplex scanning. This was based on the theory that the region of the anatomic snuffbox is a junction between the dorsal branch of the radial artery and the deep palmar arch (Fig. 34.6). Duplex ultrasound with color flow allowed them to identify the dorsal branch. The snuffbox test included scanning of the radial artery in the snuffbox with and without ulnar artery compression. Radial artery flow was evaluated with compression,

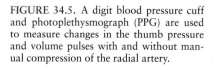

FIGURE 34.5. A digit blood pressure cuff and photoplethysmograph (PPG) are used to measure changes in the thumb pressure and volume pulses with and without manual compression of the radial artery.

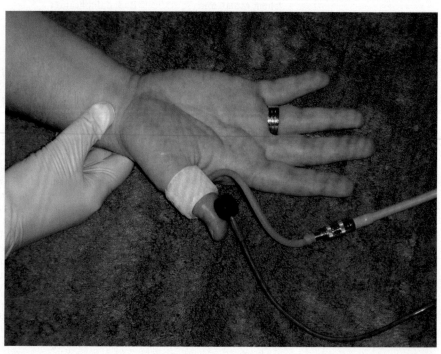

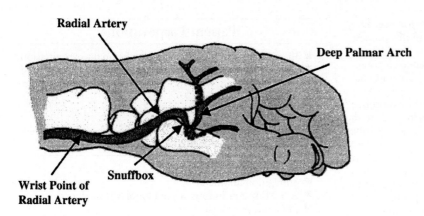

Radial Artery

Deep Palmar Arch

Snuffbox

**Wrist Point of
Radial Artery**

FIGURE 34.6. The arteries in the region of the anatomic snuffbox.

and reverse flow was considered evidence of good collateral circulation. Next, flow was measured in the palmar arch with radial artery compression; reverse flow in this artery indicated good perfusion of the superficial palmar arch. Lastly, the radial artery was scanned to rule out calcification or stenosis and to assess the diameter. In this study of 150 patients being evaluated for radial artery harvest, Allen's test did not detect any abnormalities, whereas the snuffbox test detected inadequate collateral flow in 8 (5%). The radial artery was harvested in the remaining 142 patients without ischemic hand complications.

Abu-Omar et al[21] were able to use 99% of all radial arteries in a group of 287 patients examined for bypass graft conduit. In their study, if Allen's test was normal, they proceeded to surgery. If Allen's test was abnormal, they performed a duplex scan to assess the radial and ulnar arteries. Only 15% of their

patients had an abnormal Allen's test. Of these 43 patients, 38 had normal duplex scans of the radial and ulnar arteries and went on to radial artery harvest. In the five remaining patients with an abnormal Allen's test, the duplex examination identified stenosis or occlusion in either the radial or the ulnar arteries or both. These patients were not considered candidates for radial artery harvest. No postoperative ischemic complications occurred in any of the patients who underwent radial artery harvest in this study.

UNIVERSITY OF WASHINGTON PROTOCOL

The testing algorithm shown in Figure 34.7 is used to guide the vascular technologist through a three step process for

PREOPERATIVE PLANNING, INTRAOPERATIVE ASSESSMENT AND PROCEDURAL GUIDANCE

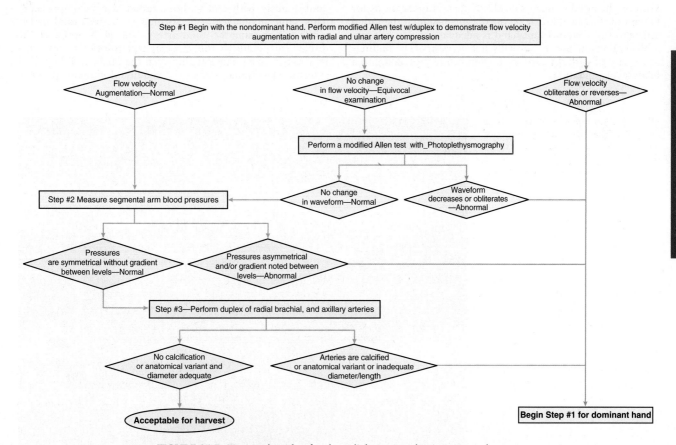

FIGURE 34.7. Testing algorithm for the radial artery evaluation prior to harvest.

determining the suitability of the radial artery for use as a coronary artery bypass graft conduit. The goals of this process are to assess the adequacy of collateral flow to the hand, detect significant occlusive lesions in the upper extremity arteries, and examine the radial artery to identify calcification and anatomic anomalies.

Collateral flow in the hand is assessed with a modified Allen's test. The modified Allen's test is performed with duplex ultrasound by measuring ulnar artery peak systolic velocities with and without radial artery compression and radial artery peak systolic velocities with and without ulnar artery compression. Augmentation of velocities in the radial and ulnar arteries with the corresponding compression indicates adequate collateral flow and an intact palmar arch. We find this modification for assessing collateral flow to be effective in most patients. However, in equivocal cases, or if an increase in velocities is not detected, we perform the modified Allen's test using a photoplethysmograph (PPG). This approach assesses changes in volume pulse waveforms in the thumb during radial artery compression, as shown in Figure 34.5. The PPG examination is not the initial method of choice for assessing the palmar arch because it requires additional equipment, time, and is less convenient for bedside examinations.

Significant upper extremity arterial obstruction is assessed with segmental limb blood pressures, and duplex scanning is used to measure the radial artery diameter and identify any anatomic anomalies of the upper extremity arteries. Calcification is identified with B-mode imaging and is recognized by highly echogenic vessel walls. The examination begins with the nondominant hand. Kohonen et al[22] evaluated 33 patients with contraindications to radial artery harvest on the nondominant side using Doppler ultrasonography and PPG. They found that 73% of patients with contraindications on the nondominant side also had contraindications for harvest of the radial artery on the dominant side. If the radial artery to the nondominant hand is adequate by our criteria, a bilateral examination is usually not necessary. The findings are discussed with the cardiac surgeon before proceeding to a bilateral examination.

Patient Preparation

- Identify the nondominant hand to begin the examination.
- Query the length of conduit or number of grafts needed.
- Perform testing with the patient in the resting, supine position.

Equipment

- Blood pressure cuffs 10 and 12 cm in width
- Sphygmomanometer
- A 5-MHz continuous-wave Doppler transducer
- PPG and photocell
- Strip chart recorder
- Duplex ultrasound system
- Mid to superficial range linear array transducer (5 to 15 MHz)

Examination Technique

Step 1: Assess Collateral Flow in the Hand

ALLEN'S TEST WITH DUPLEX SCANNING

Evaluate collateral circulation to the hand with a duplex ultrasound system and a linear array transducer (Fig. 34.8). Place the transducer longitudinally along the lateral aspect of the wrist to locate the ulnar artery. Color flow is helpful for quickly visualizing small vessels; however, arterial pulsations can also be used for vessel identification. Obtain Doppler spectral waveforms using an insonation angle of 60 degrees to the vessel wall. Record ulnar artery waveforms continuously with and without radial artery compression. This same maneuver is performed with the radial artery while compressing the ulnar artery. During this process, the duplex image allows the vascular technologist to note differences in size (diameter) between the ulnar and the radial arteries. The ulnar artery is usually dominant (larger).

FIGURE 34.8. Step 1 of the testing algorithm. The Allen's test is performed with the duplex scanner (see text for details).

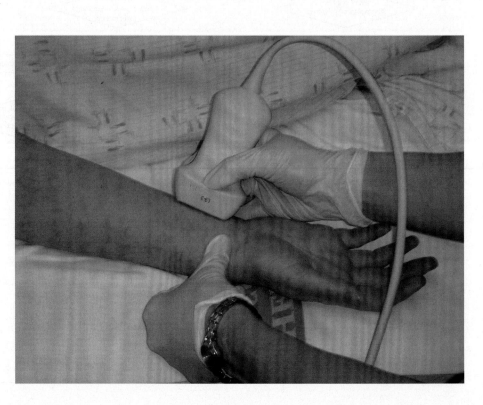

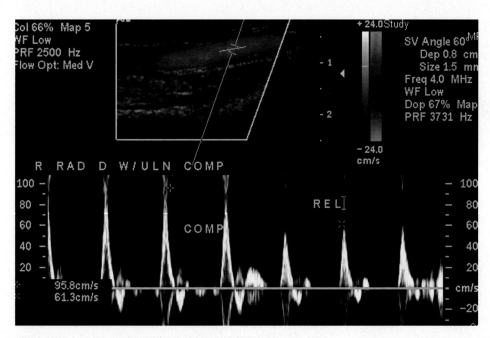

FIGURE 34.9. Doppler spectral waveforms show the normal flow response of a radial artery to ulnar artery compression (COMP) and release (REL). Ulnar artery compression results in an increase (augmentation) in radial artery flow (peak velocity).

If the ulnar artery appears small, diameter measurements are documented in the proximal, mid, and distal segments. In the case of a small ulnar artery, the surgeon may be reluctant to remove the radial artery. The peak systolic velocity response to compression maneuvers can be interpreted as follows.

1. Augmentation indicates that the palmar arch is intact (Fig. 34.9). Proceed to step 2.
2. Lack of augmentation suggests an equivocal result. Proceed to Allen's test with PPG.
3. Obliteration indicates inadequate collateral pathways in the hand. Do not continue with the nondominant hand. Proceed to evaluation of the dominant hand. If the dominant hand reveals inadequate collateral circulation, do not continue the examination and contact the cardiac surgery team.

ALLEN'S TEST WITH PPG

Place double-stick tape on the thumb pad and attach the PPG photocell. Use a strip chart recorder (AC-coupled) to document the amplitude and shape of the volume pulse waveform recorded from the thumb (Figs. 34.10 and 34.11). Compress the radial artery and observe the effect on the waveform. Interpret the response as follows.

1. An increase or no change in the amplitude of the PPG volume pulse waveform indicates adequate collateral flow. Proceed to step 2.
2. A decrease in amplitude or obliteration of the PPG volume pulse waveform indicates inadequate collateral flow. Do not continue with the nondominant hand. Proceed to evaluation of the dominant hand. If the dominant hand reveals inadequate collateral circulation, do not continue the examination and contact the cardiac surgery team.

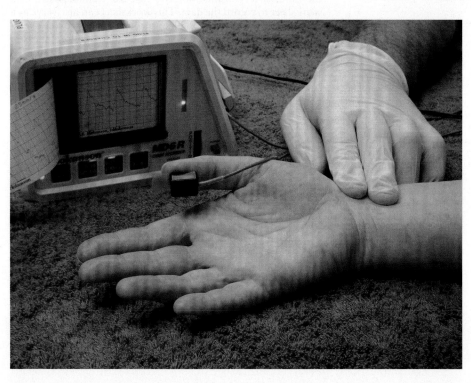

FIGURE 34.10. The Allen's test performed with a photoplethysmograph (PPG). The PPG photocell sensor is attached to the pad of the thumb with double-stick tape. Changes in the volume pulse waveforms are monitored during manual radial artery compression.

PREOPERATIVE PLANNING, INTRAOPERATIVE ASSESSMENT AND PROCEDURAL GUIDANCE

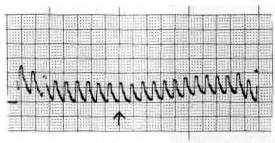

No Change

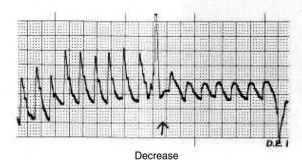

Decrease

Obliteration

FIGURE 34.11. The various responses of the photoplethysmograph (PPG) volume pulse waveforms recorded from the thumb when the radial artery is compressed. The *Arrows* indicate the point in time of radial artery compression.

Step 2: Measure Segmental Arm Blood Pressures

Wrap blood pressure cuffs around the upper arm (12 cm width) and the forearm (10 cm width) as shown in Figure 34.12. Record systolic blood pressures from the brachial, radial, and ulnar arteries using a 5-MHz continuous-wave Doppler transducer. Record the brachial artery pressure by placing the transducer at the level of the brachial artery just distal to the upper arm cuff. Obtain the radial and ulnar artery pressures by positioning the transducer at the appropriate sites on the wrist (Fig. 34.12). If the pressures are within the normal range according to the Sumner criteria, go to step 3.[19] If the segmental pressure measurements suggest obstruction, do not continue examining the nondominant side.

Step 3: Perform a Duplex Scan of the Radial, Brachial, and Axillary Arteries

Begin by placing the linear array transducer longitudinally on the radial artery at the wrist as shown in Figure 34.8. Record a Doppler flow signal at an angle of 60 degrees to the vessel, and note any evidence of arterial wall calcification (Fig. 34.13). Calcification appears in the B-mode image as highly echogenic (bright) areas in the vessel walls. Rotate the transducer for a transverse view to measure the diameter of the radial artery (Fig. 34.14). Continue scanning proximally on the arm along the entire radial artery using a longitudinal view to document any velocity changes indicating a stenosis and a transverse view to document diameter measurements for uniformity and sizing. It is important to note the location of the origin of the radial artery from the brachial artery, as this is one of the most common sources for anatomic anomalies. Continue scanning proximally through the axillary artery for calcification, stenosis, and atypical anatomy. Document diameter and velocity measurements in the proximal, mid, and distal segments of the radial artery, as well as the mid segments of the brachial, and axillary arteries. Flow velocities may be recorded from the subclavian artery as well.

Interpretation Criteria and Reporting

Table 34.3 summarizes the interpretation criteria that apply to the radial artery evaluation. The vascular technologist uses a worksheet to record the data. This worksheet can also serve as a preliminary report. Figures 34.15 through 34.18 provide examples of worksheets and reports for normal and abnormal cases.

FIGURE 34.12. Step 2 of the testing algorithm (segmental pressure measurements). Cuffs are positioned at upper arm and forearm levels. The Doppler transducer is shown recording the radial artery flow signal.

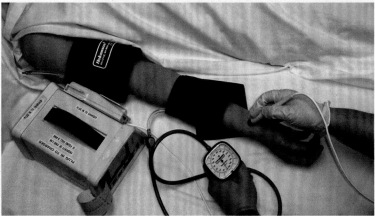

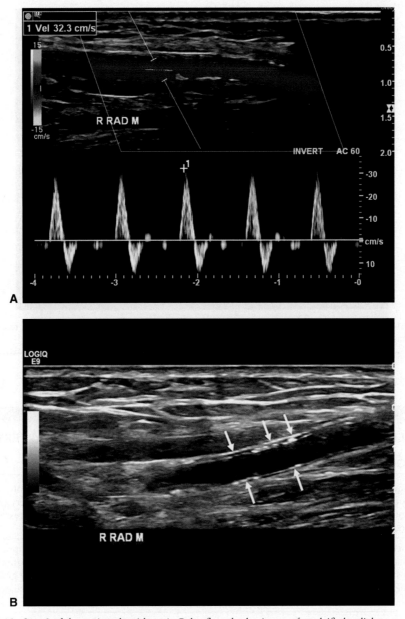

FIGURE 34.13. Step 3 of the testing algorithm. *A,* Color-flow duplex image of a calcified radial artery with a peak velocity of 32 cm/s and normal multiphasic spectral waveforms. *B,* B-mode image of the same radial artery showing a calcified segment with brightly echogenic walls (*arrows*).

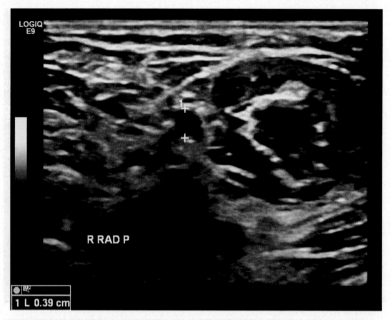

FIGURE 34.14. Step 3 of the testing algorithm. B-mode image of a radial artery in transverse view to document the diameter measurement of 3.9 mm.

TABLE 34.3

CRITERIA USED TO ESTABLISH SAFE HARVESTING OF THE RADIAL ARTERY

■ NORMAL	■ ABNORMAL
Augmentation of the ulnar artery peak systolic velocities with radial artery compression and augmentation of the radial artery peak systolic velocities with ulnar artery compression	No evidence of augmentation of either the radial or ulnar artery peak systolic velocities with compression maneuvers
Segmental pressures—symmetrical arm (brachial, radial, and ulnar) systolic pressures bilaterally. No significant blood pressure gradients between upper arm and lower arm levels	Segmental pressures—brachial pressure >15 mm Hg lower than opposite arm Radial or ulnar artery pressure gradient >15 mm Hg compared to ipsilateral brachial artery
Duplex—no evidence of radial artery stenosis, calcification, dilatations, or anatomical variants of the radial artery	Duplex—radial artery stenosis, calcification, dilatation, or diameter measurement <2 mm.
Duplex—no anatomical variants	Duplex—anatomical variants *Brachial artery* High or low bifurcation Missing brachial artery *Radial artery* Origin low in the forearm Deep to pronator teres muscle *Ulnar artery* Congenital arteriovenous malformations Anomalous superficial ulnar artery Ulnar artery dominance

UPPER EXTREMITY ARTERIAL DUPLEX – VASCULAR DIAGNOSTIC SERVICE

NORMAL EXAMPLE

-PRELIMINARY REPORT-
STUDY WILL BE REVIEWED BY
VASCULAR SURGERY DIVISION

HISTORY/INDICATION: 58 yo male
pre op CABG for
radial artery eval

.23 cm *.24 cm* *.25 cm*

.31 cm

.21 cm

.27 cm

RIGHT	SYSTOLIC PRESSURES	LEFT
142	BRACHIAL	138
140	RADIAL	136
136	ULNAR	144

PRELIMINARY INTERPRETATION
DISCUSSED WITH:

PATIENT ✓

MD ✓

IMPRESSION:

① – Radial artery augments w/ ulnar compression
   – Ulnar artery "   " Radial "
       on RIGHT & LEFT suggests
       complete arch

② No significant upper extremity arterial obstruction

③ No anatomical variants in Radial arteries
                        bilaterally

DATE: TIME: SIGNATURE:

PT NO

NAME

DOB

UW Medicine
Harborview Medical Center – UW Medical Center
University of Washington Physicians
Seattle, Washington

VASCULAR EXAMINATIONS
UPPER EXTREMITY ARTERIAL DUPLEX NOTES

UH1831 REV AUG 05

PROGRESS — BLUE

PREOPERATIVE PLANNING, INTRAOPERATIVE ASSESSMENT AND PROCEDURAL GUIDANCE

FIGURE 34.15. Example of a worksheet from a normal examination.

VASCULAR DIAGNOSTIC SERVICE

This is a 58 year old male who is referred for non-invasive upper extremity arterial evaluation. The patient presents with coronary artery disease, pre-operative for a CABG.

RADIAL ARTERY EVALUATION

MODIFIED ALLENS TEST

Manual compressions of the ipsilateral radial and ulnar arteries are performed while Duplex Doppler waveforms are obtained from the ulnar and radial arteries.
-Right: Augmentation in Doppler waveform during radial or ulnar arterial compression.
-Left: Augmentation in Doppler waveform during radial or ulnar arterial compression.

SEGMENTAL PRESSURES (mmHg)

Brachial Artery........Right-142	Left-138	
Radial Artery	140	136
Ulnar artery	136	144

-Continuous-wave Doppler waveforms were recorded:
Triphasic arterial Doppler waveforms noted on the right
Triphasic arterial Doppler waveforms noted on the left

UPPER EXTREMITY ARTERIAL DUPLEX (COMPLETE)
Doppler peak systolic velocities (cm/sec)
Doppler angles are 60-degrees unless noted

	RIGHT	LEFT
BRACHIAL	100	100
RADIAL PROXIMAL	90	60
RADIAL MID	100	50
RADIAL DISTAL	85	90
ULNAR PROXIMAL	90	50
ULNAR MID	100	100
ULNAR DISTAL	85	100

B-mode image: unremarkable; no visual anatomical variations.

RADIAL ARTERY DIAMETER (cm)

	RIGHT	LEFT
PROXIMAL	0.31	0.23
MID	0.21	0.24
DISTAL	0.27	0.25

IMPRESSION:

1. No evidence of significant arterial obstruction or anatomical variation within the right or left upper extremities.
2. Indirect evidence suggests complete palmar arches bilaterally.
3. The right and left radial arteries are of uniform, normal caliber (diameter measurements listed above).

FIGURE 34.16. Example of a final report from a normal examination.

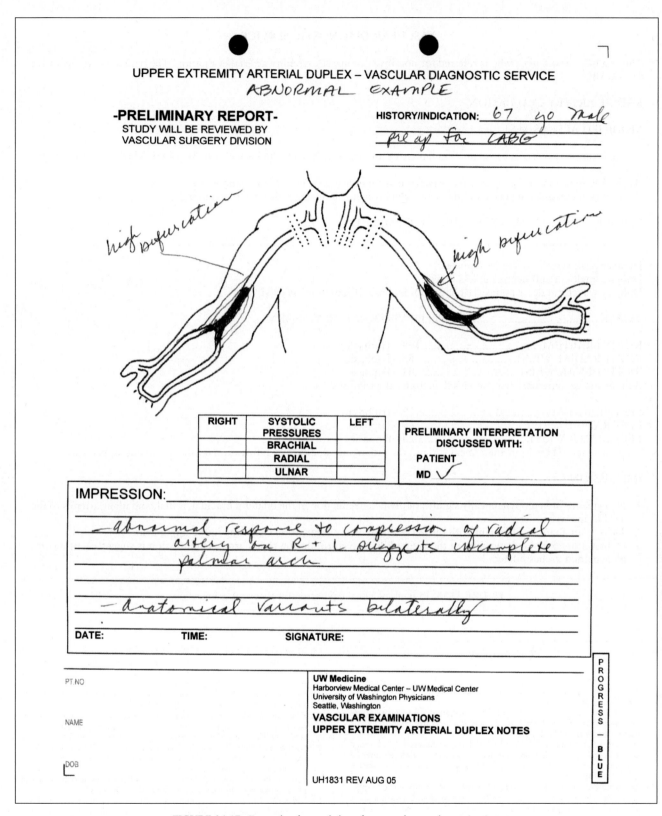

FIGURE 34.17. Example of a worksheet from an abnormal examination.

VASCULAR DIAGNOSTIC SERVICE

This is a 67 year old male who is referred for non-invasive upper extremity arterial evaluation. The patient is pre-operative for a CABG.

RADIAL ARTERY EVALUATION

MODIFIED ALLENS TEST

Manual compressions of the ipsilateral radial artery are performed while PPG waveforms are obtained from the thumb and little finger.
-Right: Obliteration of the digital PPG waveform occurs during radial arterial compression.
-Left: Extreme dampening occurs in the digital PPG waveform during radial arterial compression.

UPPER EXTREMITY ARTERIAL DUPLEX (COMPLETE)

Doppler peak systolic velocities (cm/sec)
Doppler angles are 60-degrees unless noted
Doppler waveform descriptions: Triphasic (T), Biphasic (B), monophasic (M)

VESSEL...DOPPLER VELOCITY - WAVEFORM

RIGHT BRACHIAL ....108 -Triphasic
RIGHT RADIAL WRIST...............................83 -Triphasic
RIGHT ULNAR WRIST...............................41 -Triphasic
B-mode image: unremarkable; no visual anatomical variations.

LEFT BRACHIAL ....79 -Triphasic
LEFT RADIAL WRIST.................................69 -Triphasic
LEFT ULNAR WRIST..................................24 -Biphasic
B-mode image: There is an anatomical variant; the radial and ulnar artery bifurcation occurs in the mid upper arm.

IMPRESSION:

1. No evidence of hemodynamically significant diameter reduction in the bilateral brachial, radial, and ulnar arteries to the level of the wrist.
2. There is an anatomical variant with the left brachial artery bifurcation occurring in the upper arm.
3. Obliteration/extreme dampening of the digital PPG waveform during radial artery compression is suggestive of incomplete palmar arches bilaterally.

FIGURE 34.18. Example of a final report from an abnormal examination.

References

1. Carpentier A, Guermonprez JL, Doloche A, et al. The aorta-to-coronary radial bypass graft: A technique avoiding pathological changes in grafts. *Ann Thorac Surg* 1973;16:111-121.
2. Acar C, Ramsheyi A, Pagny JY, et al. The radial artery for coronary artery bypass grafting: Clinical and angiographic results at five years. *J Thorac Cardiovasc Surg* 1998;116:981-989.
3. Zacharias A, Habib RH, Schwann RA, et al. Improved survival with radial artery versus vein conduits in coronary bypass surgery with left internal thoracic artery to left anterior descending artery grafting. *Circulation* 2004;109:1489-1496.
4. Hayward PAR, Hare DL, Gordon I, et al. Effect of radial artery or saphenous vein conduit for the second graft on 6-year clinical outcome after coronary artery bypass grafting. Results of a randomized trial. *Eur J Cardiothorac Surg* 2008;34:113-117.
5. Jarvis MA, Jarvis CL, Jones PRM, et al. Reliability of Allen's test in selection of patients for radial artery harvest. *Ann Thorac Surg* 2000;70:1362-1365.
6. Ruengsakulrach P, Eizenberg N, Fahrer C, et al. Surgical implications of variations in hand collateral circulation: Anatomy revisited. *J Thorac Cardiovasc Surg* 2001;122:682-686.
7. Coleman SS, Anson BJ. Arterial patterns in the hand based upon a study of 650 specimens. *Surg Gynecol Obstet* 1961;113:409-424.
8. Ikeda A, Ugawa A, Kazihari Y, et al. Arterial patterns in the hand based on a three-dimensional analysis of 220 cadaver hands. *J Hand Surg* 1988;13:501-509.
9. Mezzogiorno A, Passiatore C, Mezzogiorno V. Anatomic variations of the deep palmar arteries in man. *Acta Anat* 1994;149:221-224.
10. Orzkus K, Pestelmace T, Soyluoglu AI, et al. Variations of the superficial palmar arch. *Folia Morphol* 1998;57:251-255.
11. Gellman H, Botte MJ, Shankweiler J, et al. Arterial patterns of the deep and superficial palmar arches. *Clin Orthop* 2001;383:41-46.
12. Rodriguez-Niedenfuhr M, Vazquez T, Nearn L, et al. Variations of the arterial pattern in the upper limb revisited: A morphological and statistical study, with a review of the literature. *J Anat* 2001;199:547-566.
13. Ruengsakulrach P, Brooks M, Sinclair R, et al. Prevalence and prediction of calcification and plaques in radial artery grafts by ultrasound. *J Thorac Cardiovasc Surg* 2001;122:398-399.
14. Habib J, Baetz L, Satiani B. Assessment of collateral circulation to the hand prior to radial artery harvest. *Vasc Med* 2012;17:352-361.
15. Allen EV. Thromboangiitis obliterans: Methods of diagnosis of chronic occlusive arterial lesions distal to the wrist with illustrative cases. *Am J Med Sci* 1929;178:237-244.
16. Kamienski RW, Barnes RW. Critique of the Allen test for continuity of the palmar arch assessed by Doppler ultrasound. *Surg Gynecol Obstet* 1976;142:861-864.
17. Starnes SL, Wolk SW, Lampman RM, et al. Noninvasive evaluation of hand circulation before radial artery harvest for coronary artery bypass grafting. *J Thorac Cardiovasc Surg* 1999;117:261-266.
18. Sullivan VV, Higgenbotham C, Shanley CJ, et al. Can ulnar artery velocity changes be used as a preoperative screening tool for radial artery grafting in coronary artery bypass graft? *Ann Vasc Surg* 2003;17:253-259.

19. Sumner DS, Lambeth A, Russell JB. Diagnosis of upper extremity obstructive and vasospastic syndromes by Doppler ultrasound, plethysmography, and temperature profiles. In Puel P, Boccalon H, Enjalbert A (eds). *Hemodynamics of the Limbs*. Toulouse, France: GEPESC, 1979, pp 365-373.
20. Agrifoglio M, Dainese L, Pasotti S, et al. Preoperative assessment of the radial artery for coronary artery bypass grafting: Is the clinical Allen test adequate? *Ann Thorac Surg* 2005;79:570-572.
21. Abu-Omar Y, Mussa S, Anastasiadis K, et al. Duplex ultrasonography predicts safety of radial artery harvest in the presence of an abnormal Allen test. *Ann Thorac Surg* 2004;77:116-119.
22. Kohonen M, Teerenhovi O, Terho T, et al. Non-harvestable radial artery. A bilateral problem? *Interact Cardiovasc Thorac Surg* 2008;7: 797-800.

CHAPTER 35 ■ DUPLEX SCANNING PRIOR TO FIBULA FREE FLAP TRANSFERS

MOLLY J. ZACCARDI AND NEAL FUTRAN

Microvascular free tissue transfer is commonly used for reconstruction of complex head and neck defects. Many options exist for transfer of free vascularized bone, but the fibula free flap is the most widely used for reconstruction of ablative, posttraumatic, or congenital mandibular and maxillary deformities. This approach provides excellent restoration of mandibular and maxillary form and the potential for further oral rehabilitation.[1,2] The combination of bone, muscle, and skin available in this flap makes it well suited for the reconstruction of these composite defects. The blood supply of the fibula and overlying skin is based on the peroneal artery and its accompanying veins (Fig. 35.1). Up to 25 cm of bone is available for harvest, which allows for the reconstruction of angle-to-angle defects. Fibula bone is dense medullary bone that can readily accept osseointegrated implants. The segmental periosteal blood supply allows for multiple osteotomies without flap ischemia, and this property permits maximum contouring of the donor bone to the recipient site. A principle advantage of the fibula free flap is the ability to incorporate a skin paddle with the harvest. The fibula skin paddle has the potential to become sensate by including the lateral sural cutaneous nerve in the flap harvest. The donor site is usually closed primarily, and morbidity is minimal (Figs. 35.2 and 35.3).

The most feared donor site complication in fibula flap harvest is foot ischemia secondary to sacrifice of the peroneal artery. In most people, the peroneal artery does not supply a significant amount of the pedal circulation, but there are particular features of the vascular anatomy of the lower leg that may preclude the fibula from being transferred as a vascularized free flap.[2,3] Because the peroneal artery is almost always present, the fibula flap has a dependable pedicle; however, its removal may jeopardize the vascular supply to the leg if the posterior tibial or anterior tibial arteries are diseased, absent, or aberrantly originating from the peroneal artery. The peroneal artery usually terminates above the ankle joint, whereas the anterior and posterior tibial arteries continue across this joint to supply the dorsal and plantar surfaces of the foot, respectively. Congenital anomalies or acquired disease of the infrageniculate vessels is estimated to result in a dominant peroneal artery in 7% to 12% of the population.[4] An uncommon but important anatomic variant is that of *arteria peronea magna*, a congenital anomaly in which the peroneal artery is the sole vessel to the foot, with patients having normal distal pulses and no associated ischemic symptoms. This condition has been described as occurring in 0.2% to 0.9% of the population.[5,6] These observations have led Urken et al[3] to state that the most serious consequence of fibula flap transfer is the lack of collateral circulation to the foot, leading to ischemia following interruption of the peroneal artery.

PREOPERATIVE ASSESSMENT

Controversy exists regarding the extent of evaluation that is required in the preoperative assessment of fibula free flap donor sites. Large series have been reported without the benefit of a preoperative vascular assessment of any kind and with no adverse sequelae.[1,2] Some reconstructive surgeons believe that a thorough history and physical examination should be the primary screening tools and that imaging should be used only for the small percentage of patients who have abnormal pedal pulses, a history of trauma, or symptoms suggestive of claudication.[4,6] Others believe that vascular imaging is necessary in the preoperative assessment of all potential fibula free flap candidates.[7,8] Many head and neck cancer patients are elderly and have a history of smoking as well as a higher prevalence of peripheral vascular disease than is found in the general population. In a survey of 206 vascular surgeons in the United Kingdom, 88% of respondents indicated that not performing presurgical vascular imaging bordered on clinical negligence.[9] Our opinion is that it is essential that patients be safely and comprehensively evaluated for vascular disease or significant anatomic variants before surgery. Defining the length and branching pattern of the peroneal artery preoperatively also provides the surgeon with a "roadmap" that aids and shortens the time required for peroneal artery dissection. The viability of such flaps is entirely dependent on the integrity of their vascular supply, making the detection of peroneal artery disease or anomaly of paramount importance.[10]

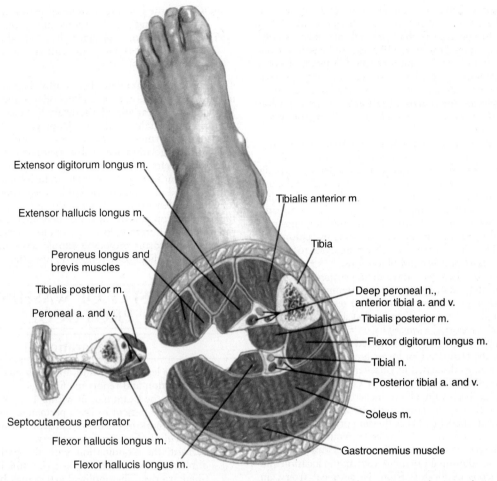

Extensor digitorum longus m.

Extensor hallucis longus m.

Peroneus longus and brevis muscles

Tibialis posterior m.

Peroneal a. and v.

Septocutaneous perforator

Flexor hallucis longus m.

Flexor hallucis longus m.

Tibialis anterior m.

Tibia

Deep peroneal n., anterior tibial a. and v.

Tibialis posterior m.

Flexor digitorum longus m.

Tibial n.

Posterior tibial a. and v.

Soleus m.

Gastrocnemius muscle

FIGURE 35.1. The composite flap as shown consists of a segment of the peroneal artery, peroneal vein, and a portion of the fibula with the perforating arteries supplying the overlying skin. (From Urken ML, Sullivan MJ. Fibular osteocutaneous free flaps. In Urken ML, Cheney ML, Sullivan MJ, et al (eds). *Atlas of Regional and Free Flaps for the Head and Neck Reconstruction.* New York: Raven, 1995, pp 291-206, with permission.)

Standard catheter angiography has long been the "gold standard" for the evaluation of lower extremity vascular patency, allowing high-resolution imaging of the trifurcation vessels, including assessment for the presence of significant stenoses or congenital branch anomalies. Numerous investigators have reported angiographically detected abnormalities that altered the operative plan in up to 25% of cases.[8,11] However, this technique is invasive and involves considerable ionizing radiation exposure for the patient, and it also suffers from the shortcomings of high cost and potential morbidities (hematoma, thrombosis, vessel injury, and contrast reactions). Less invasive tests, such as magnetic resonance angiography (MRA) and computed tomography angiography (CTA), have been reported to be equally effective in peripheral vascular mapping without arterial catheterization. MRA offers the capability of reliable noninvasive vascular imaging

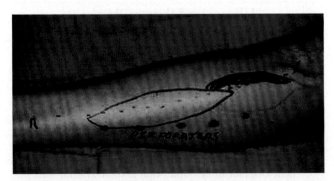

FIGURE 35.2. Preoperative marking for a fibula osteocutaneous free flap dissection. Note the location of the peroneal perforators.

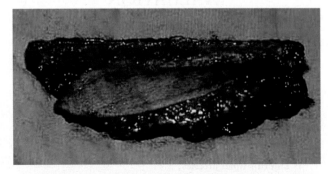

FIGURE 35.3. A harvested fibula osteocutaneous free flap.

PREOPERATIVE PLANNING, INTRAOPERATIVE ASSESSMENT AND PROCEDURAL GUIDANCE

in the absence of ionizing radiation exposure and without the use of iodine-based contrast media.[12] Furthermore, MRA has the advantage of costing less than one-half as much as conventional angiography. However, MRA is problematic for the claustrophobic patient and requires special hardware (surface coil) to enhance imaging. CTA involves considerable ionizing radiation exposure, administration of iodine-based contrast media, and potential for nonvisualization of the trifurcation vessels due to the presence of "blooming" artifact from adjacent calcified plaque.[13,14]

These limitations have prompted the application of less invasive and less expensive imaging techniques in the routine preoperative assessment of patients being considered for fibula free flap procedures. Significant interest has focused on the use of color-flow duplex (CFD) ultrasound in this clinical setting because of its accuracy in mapping the vascular anatomy and relative cost savings when compared with both angiography and MRA.[7,10,15] CFD combines B-mode imaging, color-flow Doppler, and Doppler spectral waveform analysis to noninvasively assess vessel patency and blood flow.[16-18] Hatsukami et al[19] and Kerr and Bandyk[20] have demonstrated the ability of CFD to accurately examine the lower extremity vasculature and diagnose arterial occlusive disease. CFD resolution of flow in vessels as small as 1 mm in diameter has also been demonstrated. Aly et al[21] reported a sensitivity of 92% and specificity of 99% for duplex sonography compared with conventional angiography in the evaluation of lower limb arterial occlusive disease. Moreover, as discussed in Chapter 36, vascular mapping of the rectus abdominis muscle by CFD prior to breast reconstruction has been valuable for incision planning.[22]

These facts served as a catalyst to design a clinical protocol to study the effectiveness of CFD evaluation prior to fibula free flap harvest. Examination of the lower extremity vasculature with CFD can be completed within 60 minutes. Doppler sonography affords the additional capability to map the location and extent of cutaneous perforators from the peroneal artery, an important determinant of skin-paddle viability in the osteocutaneous fibula flap. Futran et al[15] applied this technique to the assessment of 38 patients in preparation for fibula free flap harvesting, and the results of the vascular evaluation precluded flap transfer in 4 (10.5%). In a similar study, Futran et al[23] further described the use of the ankle-brachial index (ABI) in the preoperative evaluation of potential fibula free flap candidates. They found good correlation between an ABI of less than 1.0 and subsequent arterial occlusive disease confirmed by angiography. However, they also found an unacceptable number of patients with an ABI greater than 1.0 who had arterial disease. Thus, they concluded that an ABI of less than 1.0 can exclude lower extremities as donor sites, but a lower extremity with an ABI of greater than 1.0 requires further evaluation by CFD.

VASCULAR LABORATORY EVALUATION

Lower extremity arterial duplex scanning is covered in detail in Chapter 12, and lower extremity venous scanning is described in Chapter 19. The techniques and basic concepts of these examinations are applied to the preoperative vascular laboratory assessment prior to fibula free flap transfer in order to achieve the following goals.

1. Rule out significant obstructions in the lower extremity arteries.
2. Identify significant anatomic variants (branching patterns) and arterial disease of the posterior tibial and anterior tibial arteries.
3. Provide a roadmap for the surgeon, documenting anatomy and patency of the peroneal artery.

4. Obtain the size and number of peroneal artery perforators, marking their locations on the leg.
5. Rule out chronic or acute deep vein thrombosis in the popliteal and tibial veins with special attention to the peroneal veins.

The testing algorithm described in this chapter was developed in the 1990s by Dr. Futran et al in collaboration with the D.E. Strandness, Jr, Vascular Laboratory.[15] Since that time, the overall image quality and color Doppler sensitivity of duplex ultrasound instruments has improved significantly. The original Futran algorithm was subsequently modified to include Doppler waveforms from the tibial arteries at the ankle. This provides identification of arterial occlusive disease in patients with calcified and noncompressible tibial arteries. We believe these improvements have reduced the time required to perform the examination and the operator dependence to obtain accurate results. In addition, lower extremity arterial pressures and Doppler waveforms provide a simple screening method that other forms of diagnostic testing do not offer.

UNIVERSITY OF WASHINGTON PROTOCOL

Preparation

- Allow at least 1 hour and up to 2 hours to perform the examination and report the findings.
- Schedule the examination within 1 week of surgery and instruct the patient to use a permanent ink pen to maintain the markings if the ones made during the examination begin to fade prior to surgery.
- Perform the examination with the patient supine for duplex assessment of the anterior tibial and posterior tibial arteries. The popliteal artery may be better visualized with the patient in the prone position. The peroneal artery and perforators are easily visualized with the patient in the lateral decubitus position.

Equipment

- Duplex ultrasound system (B-mode, color Doppler, and spectral waveform analysis)
- Midrange transducer (4 to 10 MHz)
- Blood pressure cuffs (10 cm wide for the ankle and 12 cm wide for the arms; two of each)
- Sphygmomanometer
- Permanent marking pen
- Measuring tape or ruler

Ultrasound System Presets

- Color Doppler settings (mean flow) are adjusted to approximately 30 cm/s for the popliteal artery and 15 cm/s for the tibial arteries. The range may be reduced for lower flow velocities in the perforator arteries.
- Doppler settings for arterial spectral waveforms are optimized for peak flow velocities ranging from 60 to 140 cm/s in the popliteal artery and 25 to 110 cm/s in the tibial arteries. Angle correction is utilized for all arterial velocity measurements, including the perforators. This requires an angle of 60 degrees or less between the incident Doppler ultrasound beam and the arterial wall.
- Doppler settings for venous spectral waveforms are lower than for arterial spectral waveforms and are optimized for velocities ranging from 10 to 20 cm/s.

EXAMINATION TECHNIQUE

Step 1. Rule Out Atherosclerotic Disease in the Lower Extremity with the ABI and Doppler Waveforms

Documentation of the ABI is the first step in the modified Futran algorithm shown in Figure 35.4. As discussed in Chapter 13, in most patients, the ABI measurement will detect any significant arterial occlusive disease in the lower extremity. Systolic pressures are recorded with Doppler using all three tibial arteries (anterior tibial/dorsalis pedis, posterior tibial, and peroneal) at the level of the ankle. When different pressures are obtained in the various tibial arteries, the *highest* value should be used to calculate the ABI. A ratio of this ankle pressure to the highest brachial systolic pressure of less than 1.0 indicates the presence of lower extremity arterial obstruction. If the ABI is clearly abnormal (<0.95), it is our custom to contact the referring provider, and the examination of that limb is likely to be discontinued. Calcification of the vessel

walls is reported when arterial pressures cannot be measured at the ankle owing to vessel noncompressibility (ankle pressures >250 mm Hg) or when the ABI is >1.40. In these cases, we rely on Doppler waveform analysis of flow in the tibial arteries at the ankle. If the Doppler waveforms are normally multiphasic (Fig. 35.5A) as opposed to abnormally monophasic (Fig. 35.5B), and the ABI is ≥1.0 but ≤1.40, the protocol proceeds to the next step.

Step 2. Identify Atherosclerosis, Calcification, and Anatomic Variants of the Posterior Tibial and Anterior Tibial Arteries

Normally, the anterior tibial artery is the first branch of the popliteal artery. The popliteal artery then continues as the tibioperoneal trunk. The posterior tibial and peroneal arteries usually arise at the bifurcation of the tibioperoneal trunk within 2 to 3 cm from the origin of anterior tibial artery. Anatomic variants are common in this arterial segment and may appear as illustrated in Figure 35.6.

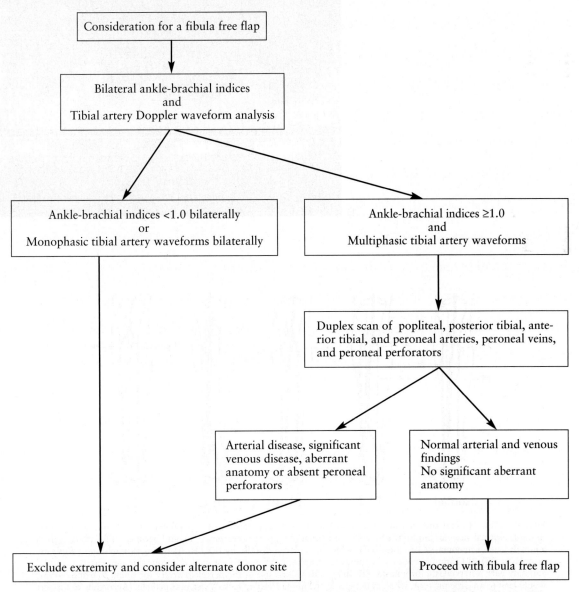

FIGURE 35.4. Algorithm for preoperative assessment of fibula free flap donor sites. (Modified from Futran ND, Stack BC Jr, Zachariah AP. Ankle-arm index as a screening examination for fibula free tissue transfer. *Ann Otol Rhinol Laryngol* 1999;108:777-780.)

PREOPERATIVE PLANNING, INTRAOPERATIVE ASSESSMENT AND PROCEDURAL GUIDANCE

FIGURE 35.5. *A*, Normal, multiphasic tibial artery Doppler spectral waveform. *B*, Abnormal, monophasic tibial artery Doppler spectral waveform.

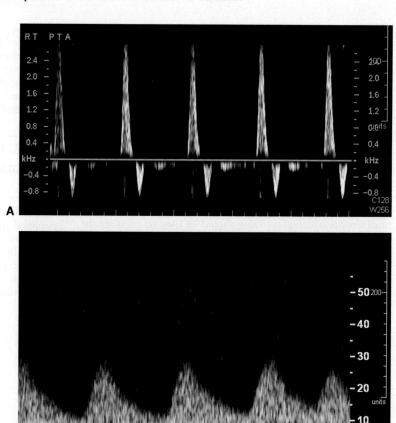

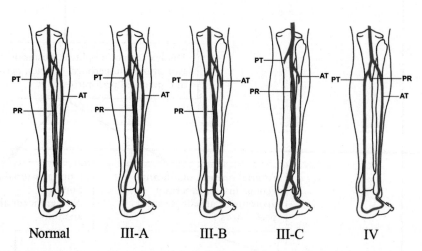

FIGURE 35.6. Normal and anatomic variants of the branching patterns at the popliteal artery "trifurcation." *Left to right*, Normal vascular anatomy of the anterior tibial (AT), posterior tibial (PT), and peroneal (PR) arteries; III-A anomaly with a hypoplastic or aplastic PT, which is replaced distally by the PR; III-B anomaly with a hypoplastic or aplastic AT; III-C anomaly with a hypoplastic or aplastic AT and PT (so-called peroneal magna artery); and IV anomaly with a hypoplastic or aplastic PR. In type III-C legs, use of the peroneal artery for fibula free flap harvest would lead to an ischemic foot, whereas in type IV, the fibula free flap lacks a vascular pedicle. (According to Lippert H, Pabst R. Arteries of the lower leg. In Lippert H, Pabst R (eds). *Arterial Variations in Man: Classifications and Frequency*. Munich: Bergmann Verlag, 1985, pp 63-64; and Kim D, Orron DE, Skillman JJ. Surgical significance of popliteal artery variants: A unified angiographic classification. *Ann Surg* 1989;210:776, used with permission.)

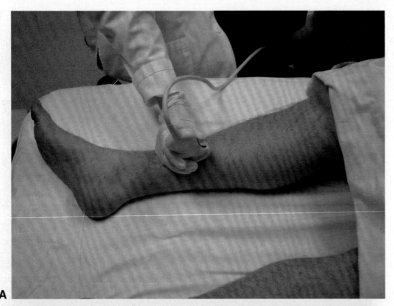

A

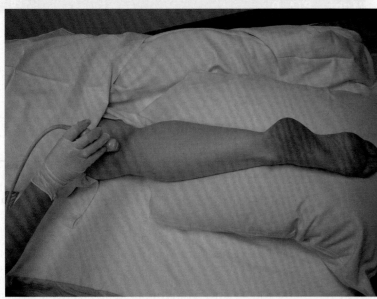

B

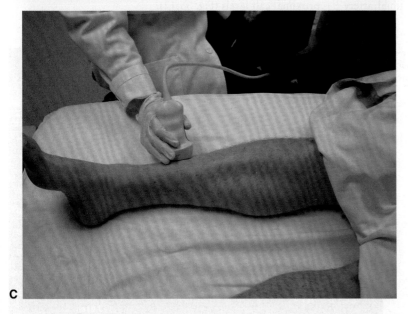

C

FIGURE 35.7. *A,* Placement of the transducer for scanning of the posterior tibial artery. *B,* Scanning of the popliteal artery with the patient prone. This approach may also be advantageous for locating the origins of the tibial and peroneal arteries. *C,* Placement of the transducer for scanning of the anterior tibial artery.

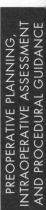

PREOPERATIVE PLANNING, INTRAOPERATIVE ASSESSMENT AND PROCEDURAL GUIDANCE

FIGURE 35.8. Color Doppler image of a posterior tibial artery (PTA) shows dense calcification of the arterial walls (*arrows*). The Doppler spectral waveform is abnormally monophasic.

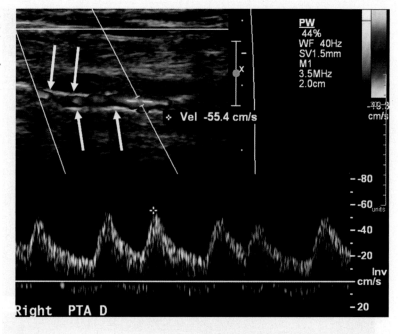

With the patient supine, a midrange transducer is placed posterior to and slightly proximal to the medial malleolus (Fig. 35.7A), and the posterior tibial and peroneal arteries are identified by their proximity to the adjacent paired veins. The posterior tibial artery is evaluated longitudinally by sliding the transducer proximally on the calf to its origin. The popliteal artery is also evaluated for disease or abnormalities of the branching pattern. In some patients, the popliteal artery may be better visualized with the patient in the prone position (Fig. 35.7B). Doppler spectral waveforms are recorded along the visualized arteries to document normal patency or the presence of stenosis or occlusion. This process is repeated for the anterior tibial artery by placing the transducer anterior and lateral to the tibia at the ankle and scanning proximally to the level of the origin (Fig. 35.7C). B-mode images are recorded to document the presence or absence of calcification (Fig. 35.8). A focal velocity increase (at least a doubling of the peak systolic velocity) followed by poststenotic turbulence indicates a significant stenosis ($\geq$50% diameter reduction), as demonstrated in Figure 35.9. Identification of a tibial artery

that is stenotic, absent, or originates from the peroneal artery (aberrant) precludes the fibula on that side from being used as the donor site for a flap.

Step 3. Assess the Anatomy and Patency of the Peroneal Artery

The normal peroneal artery anatomy is shown in Figure 35.10. The transducer is placed posterior and slightly proximal to the lateral malleolus, and the peroneal artery is followed longitudinally toward its origin (Fig. 35.11). Scanning of the peroneal artery is performed in the same manner as for the anterior and posterior tibial arteries. The length and branching pattern of the peroneal artery are recorded as a roadmap for the referring provider. In addition, the peroneal artery is visualized in long-axis (longitudinal) and short-axis (transverse) view to document diameter measurements at the ankle, mid-calf, and proximal calf levels (Fig. 35.12).

FIGURE 35.9. Color Doppler image and spectral waveform show a significant velocity increase in this anterior tibial artery (ATA), consistent with a severe stenosis. The peak systolic velocity is 458 cm/s.

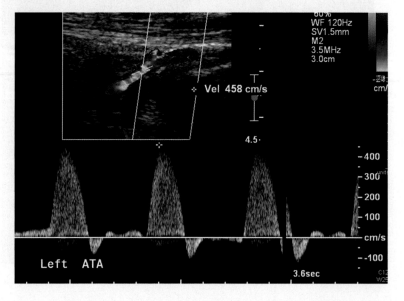

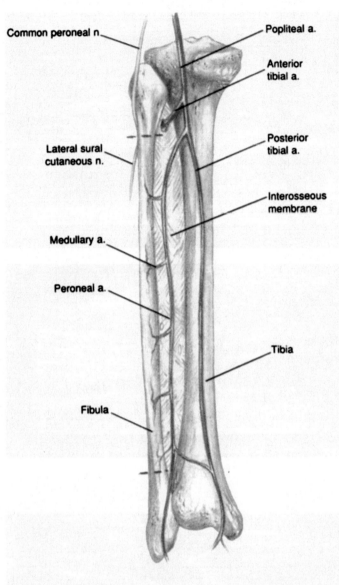

FIGURE 35.10. Relationship between the peroneal artery and the fibula. The perforating arteries are also shown. (From Urken ML, Sullivan MJ. Fibular osteocutaneous free flaps. In Urken ML, Cheney ML, Sullivan MJ, et al (eds). *Atlas of Regional and Free Flaps for the Head and Neck Reconstruction*. New York: Raven, 1995, pp 291-206, with permission.)

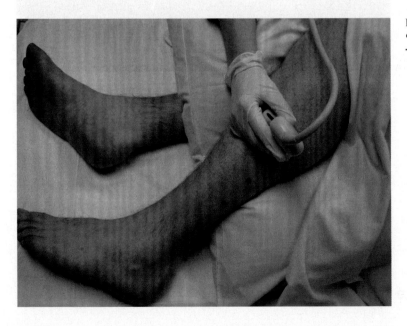

FIGURE 35.11. Placement of the transducer for scanning of the peroneal artery.

PREOPERATIVE PLANNING,
INTRAOPERATIVE ASSESSMENT
AND PROCEDURAL GUIDANCE

FIGURE 35.12. Peroneal artery diameter measurements. *A,* Longitudinal color Doppler image with a diameter measurement of 0.20 cm. *B,* Longitudinal B-mode image with a diameter measurement of 0.17 cm.

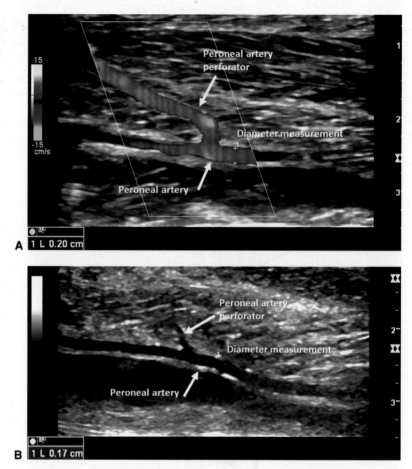

FIGURE 35.13. *A,* Color Doppler long-axis (longitudinal) view of a peroneal artery and peroneal artery perforator. *B,* Short-axis (transverse) view of the same vessels.

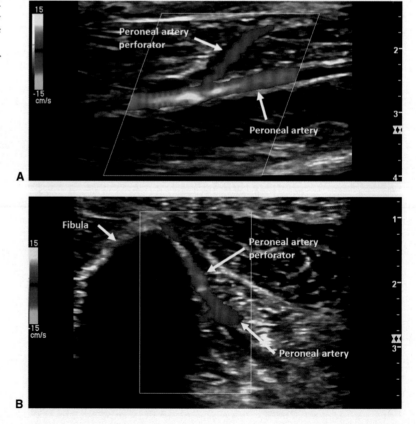

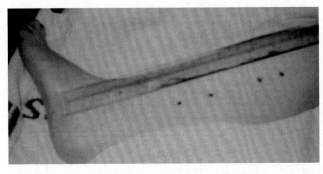

FIGURE 35.14. The peroneal perforators are marked on the skin, and the location of each perforating artery is recorded by measuring the distance from a landmark such as the fibular head or the lateral malleolus.

Step 4. Document and Mark the Size, Number, and Location of the Peroneal Artery Perforators

The perforators are branches of the peroneal artery that travel toward the skin. Perforators are described as "musculocutaneous" (coursing through the muscle) or "septocutaneous" (coursing around the fibula). Recognizing these anatomic details will make it easier for the technologist to locate the perforators. The peroneal perforators can be identified with

the peroneal artery in long-axis (Fig. 35.13A) or short-axis (Fig. 35.13B) view. Beginning at the ankle, slide the transducer proximally until a perforator is visualized. Center each perforator in the middle of the transducer field, remove gel, and mark the location on the skin using a permanent ink pen. After all perforators have been identified and marked, measure the distance of each perforator from a landmark such as the lateral malleolus or fibular head (Fig. 35.14).

Step 5. Assess the Patency of the Peroneal Veins

Beginning again at the ankle, identify the paired peroneal veins in short-axis or long-axis view (Fig. 35.15). Perform compression maneuvers in a short-axis view and document complete vein wall collapse on B-mode image throughout the paired veins. Noncompressibility of the veins indicates acute or chronic deep vein thrombosis, and the length and location of the obstruction is reported. The peroneal veins may be difficult to visualize in short-axis view and are often more easily seen with color Doppler in long-axis view (Fig. 35.15B).

Diagnostic Criteria and Reporting

A specifically designed worksheet is used to record the data and to guide the examination (Fig. 35.16). Examples of final reports are shown in Figure 35.17. The diagnostic criteria

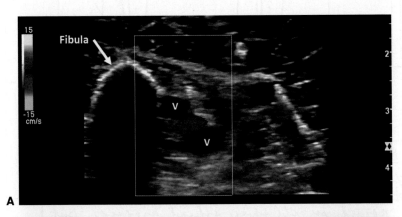

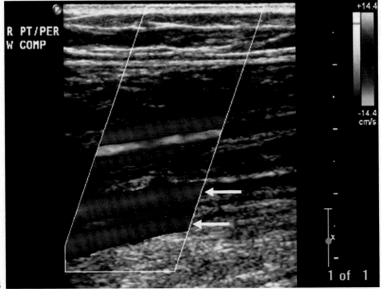

FIGURE 35.15. A, Color Doppler image of the paired peroneal veins in a short-axis (transverse) view. There is acoustic shadowing from the fibula (arrow). The peroneal artery is in the center (red) with the paired peroneal veins (V) on each side. B, Color Doppler image of the paired posterior tibial veins and peroneal veins in long-axis (longitudinal) view along with the accompanying arteries. The peroneal vessels are located more deeply in this view with the artery shown in red and the accompanying paired veins in blue (arrows).

PRE FIBULA FLAP VASCULAR DUPLEX – VASCULAR DIAGNOSTIC SERVICE

-PRELIMINARY REPORT-
STUDY WILL BE REVIEWED BY
VASCULAR SURGERY DIVISION

HISTORY/INDICATION: 72 year old man pre-op for reconstructive surgery

SYSTOLIC PRESSURES (mmHg)

	RIGHT	LEFT
BRACHIAL	134	136
POST-TIB	136	94
ANT-TIB	138	68
PERONEAL	136	82
ABI (INDEX)	>1.0	.69

PERONEAL VELOCITY (cm/sec)

	RIGHT	LEFT
PROXIMAL	28	
MIDDLE	61	
DISTAL	31	

PERONEAL SPECTRAL WAVEFORM

	RIGHT	LEFT
PROXIMAL	Biphasic	
MIDDLE	"	
DISTAL	"	

PERONEAL DIAMETER (cm)

	RIGHT	LEFT
PROXIMAL	.81	
MIDDLE	.30	
DISTAL	.23	

PERONEAL ARTERY DUPLEX

	R	L
CALCIFICATION	++	
ANATOMICAL VARIANT	no	
# of Perforators	6	
(Distance from malleolus) cm.	33.5	
	31	
	28	
	23	
	18	
	11.5	

PERONEAL VEIN DUPLEX

COMPRESSION

	R	L
Proximal	nl	
Middle	nl	
Distal	nl	

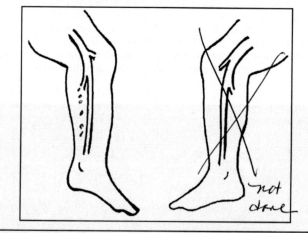

not done

PRELIMINARY INTERPRETATION DISCUSSED WITH:

PATIENT ✓

MD ✓

IMPRESSION: Left leg not evaluated due to abnormal ABI's. Right leg: - No evidence of stenosis or anatomical variants in the posterior/anterior tibial or peroneal arteries. - Calcification noted in all three tibial arteries but waveforms and pressures are within normal limits - Peroneal veins patent - 6 perforators (peroneal) marked.

DATE: 1/14/2008   TIME: 1430   SIGNATURE:

PT.NO

NAME

DOB

UW Medicine
Harborview Medical Center – UW Medical Center
University of Washington Physicians
Seattle, Washington

VASCULAR EXAMINATIONS
PRE FIBULA FLAP VASCULAR DUPLEX NOTES

UH1832 REV AUG 05

P
R
O
G
R
E
S
S
—
B
L
U
E

FIGURE 35.16. A technologist worksheet specifically designed for the fibula free flap examination.

UNIVERSITY OF WASHINGTON MEDICAL CENTER

D.E. Strandness, Jr. Vascular Laboratory
Accredited by the Intersocietal Accreditation Commission (IAC Vascular Testing)

This is a 50 year old woman who is being evaluated preoperatively for mandibular reconstructive surgery utilizing a fibula free flap. We are asked to perform lower extremity arterial and venous duplex evaluations to assess for tissue vascular patency.

ANKLE/BRACHIAL INDEX (mmHg)

```
-----------------------------------Right-----Left
Brachial Artery-----------------124-----122
Posterior Tibial Artery--------154-----146
Anterior Tibial Artery---------142-----134
Peroneal Artery----------------142-----140
Ankle-Brachial Index (ABI)--1.24-----1.18
```

Doppler flow waveforms were recorded: Normal triphasic waveforms are obtained on the right and left.

LOWER EXTREMITY ARTERIAL DUPLEX (LIMITED)

```
Velocities-----------------------------Right----------Left
Popliteal Artery Proximal-------36 cm/s----45 cm/s
Popliteal Artery Distal-----------60 cm/s----66 cm/s

Posterior Tibial Artery Prox----84 cm/s----73 cm/s
Posterior Tibial Artery Mid-----92 cm/s----124 cm/s
Posterior Tibial Artery Distal---79 cm/s----103 cm/s
B-mode image: unremarkable

Anterior Tibial Artery Prox-----94 cm/s----86 cm/s
Anterior Tibial Artery Mid------74 cm/s----102 cm/s
Anterior Tibial Artery Distal----70 cm/s----47 cm/s
B-mode image: unremarkable

Peroneal Proximal----------------51 cm/s----71 cm/s
Peroneal Mid----------------------50 cm/s----65 cm/s
Peroneal Distal--------------------43 cm/s----52 cm/s
B-mode image: unremarkable

Peroneal Diameters-----------------Right-------Left
Peroneal Proximal----------------0.54 cm------0.39 cm
Peroneal Mid----------------------0.28 cm------0.28 cm
Peroneal Distal--------------------0.29 cm------0.21 cm
B-mode image: unremarkable
```

Peroneal Artery Perforators:
Distance measured in cm from the lateral malleolus at their most superficial aspect

```
----------------------------------Right--------Left
#1----------------------------8.0 cm -----10.0 cm
#2----------------------------15.0 cm -----18.0 cm
#3----------------------------18.5 cm -----20.5 cm
#4----------------------------21.0 cm -----26.0 cm
#5----------------------------25.0 cm -----30.0 cm
#6----------------------------33.0 cm
```

LOWER EXTREMITY VENOUS DUPLEX (LIMITED)

Deep System:
Doppler flow signals obtained in the right and left popliteal veins are spontaneous, phasic and augmentable. The right and left paired posterior tibial and peroneal veins demonstrate augmentable color-Doppler flow signals.

Complete vein wall compression is noted on B-mode image throughout the imaged deep venous system, including gastrocnemius and soleal muscular branches where applicable.

FINAL PHYSICIAN INTERPRETATION

1. Ankle brachial indices are normal at rest bilaterally: 1.24 on the right and 1.18 on the left. Normal triphasic tibial artery flow waveforms are obtained bilaterally.

2. Right
-No evidence of peroneal artery focal stenosis, intimal-medial calcification, or anatomical variation.
-Six right peroneal artery perforators are mapped and marked.
-No deep vein thrombosis in the popliteal, tibial, or peroneal veins.

3. Left
-No evidence of peroneal artery focal stenosis, intimal-medial calcification, or anatomical variation.
-Five left peroneal artery perforators are mapped and marked.
-No deep vein thrombosis in the popliteal, tibial, or peroneal veins.

A

FIGURE 35.17. *A*, Example of a normal final report from a fibula free flap examination.

UNIVERSITY OF WASHINGTON MEDICAL CENTER

D.E. Strandness, Jr. Vascular Laboratory
Accredited by the Intersocietal Accreditation Commission (IAC Vascular Testing)

This is a 67 year old male with a history of stroke who is being evaluated preoperatively for reconstructive surgery utilizing a fibula free flap. We are asked to perform lower extremity arterial and venous duplex evaluations to assess for tissue vascular patency.

ANKLE/BRACHIAL INDEX (mmHg)

```
-------------------------------Right-----Left
Brachial Artery------------------108-----112
Posterior Tibial Artery----------62-----80
Anterior Tibial Artery-----------NI-----*68
Peroneal Artery------------------62-----NI
Ankle-Brachial Index (ABI)---0.55----0.71
```

*Waveforms from the left anterior tibial artery are retrograde, suggesting collateral flow.
NI = Not identified

Doppler flow waveforms were recorded: Monophasic tibial artery waveforms were obtained on the right and left.

LOWER EXTREMITY ARTERIAL DUPLEX (LIMITED)

```
Velocities----------------------------Right----------Left
Popliteal Artery Proximal--------16 cm/s-----0 cm/s
Popliteal Artery Distal-------------11 cm/s----35 cm/s
B-mode image: Visible calcific plaque

Posterior Tibial Artery Prox-------19 cm/s----31 cm/s
Posterior Tibial Artery Mid--------26 cm/s----24 cm/s
Posterior Tibial Artery Distal------17 cm/s----26 cm/s
B-mode image: Visible calcific plaque

Anterior Tibial Artery Prox--------14 cm/s-----0 cm/s
Anterior Tibial Artery Mid----------9 cm/s-----0 cm/s
Anterior Tibial Artery Distal--------0 cm/s-----0 cm/s
B-mode image: Visible calcific plaque

Peroneal Proximal------------------10 cm/s----21 cm/s
Peroneal Mid------------------------11 cm/s---20 cm/s
Peroneal Distal-----------------------11 cm/s---19 cm/s (mid-distal)
B-mode image: Visible calcific plaque
```

The venous portion of this exam was not done due to the presence of significant arterial disease.

FINAL PHYSICIAN INTERPRETATION

1. Ankle brachial indices are abnormal at rest bilaterally: 0.55 on the right and 0.71 on the left. Distal tibial artery flow waveforms are abnormally monophasic bilaterally.

2. Right
-Flow waveforms in the popliteal artery are consistent with a significant proximal arterial obstruction.
-Calcific plaque is visible in the popliteal and tibial arteries; cannot rule out segmental tibial artery occlusion. The distal anterior tibial artery is occluded.

3. Left
-The proximal popliteal artery is occluded with reconstitution of flow in the proximal to mid segment.
-Calcific plaque is visible in the popliteal and tibial arteries; cannot rule out segmental tibial occlusion. The anterior tibial artery is occluded.

B

FIGURE 35.17. (*Continued*) B, Example of an abnormal final report. Notice that the venous portion of the examination was not done due to the abnormal ankle-brachial indices and the presence of significant arterial occlusive disease.

used in the donor site selection process for fibula flap free transfer are listed in Table 35.1.

UNIVERSITY OF WASHINGTON EXPERIENCE

In 2007 and 2008, we performed the fibula flap CFD examination on 52 limbs of 27 patients (14 males, 13 females; mean age 61 years). One limb in each of two patients was not evaluated owing to previous limb surgery or fracture. Calcified tibial arteries were noted bilaterally in 10 patients (37%). An abnormal ABI or abnormal tibial artery Doppler waveforms were detected in 3 patients (11%). The tibial veins were patent in all patients. Peak systolic velocities in patent anterior tibial, posterior tibial, and peroneal arteries ranged from 25 to 114 cm/s, with a mean of 63 cm/s. Peroneal artery diameter measurements ranged from 0.14 to 0.49 cm, with a mean of 0.30 cm. An average of four peroneal perforators was identified in each limb. One patient (4%) was noted to have an anatomic variant

TABLE 35.1

DIAGNOSTIC CRITERIA USED TO SCREEN FOR ARTERIAL DISEASE AND AID IN PATIENT/LIMB SELECTION FOR FIBULA FLAP FREE TRANSFER

	■ NORMAL	■ ABNORMAL
ABI	≥ 1.0	< 1.0
Tibial and peroneal artery Doppler waveforms	Multiphasic	Monophasic or absent
Anterior and posterior tibial arteries	Uniform PSVs	Stenosis or occlusion
	Originate from the popliteal artery or tibioperoneal trunk	Absent Originate from the peroneal artery
Peroneal artery	Uniform PSVs	Stenosis or occlusion Calcification
Perforators	One or more large perforators	Absent or small perforators
Peroneal vein	Patent	Obstructed

ABI, ankle-brachial index; PSV, peak systolic velocity.

in one limb—the anterior tibial artery was absent distally and the dorsalis pedis artery arose from the peroneal artery.

In a recent 52-month period beginning in 2009, we evaluated 109 patients (212 legs) being considered for a fibula free flap transfer procedure, and the results are summarized in Table 35.2. Abnormalities were detected in 132 or 63% of the limbs, suggesting that the vascular laboratory plays an important role in screening prior to these procedures.

VALIDATION STUDIES

In 1992, Moneta et al[24] found that CFD studies could accurately map 94% of anterior tibial arteries, 96% of posterior tibial arteries, and 83% of peroneal arteries. The sensitivity of CFD in identifying abnormal arteries is reported to be 87.5% for stenotic lesions and 95% for occlusions.[25] The

reliability of normal CFD study results in predicting uncomplicated fibula free flap harvest has also been documented. In 1998, Futran et al[7,15] reported a 100% success rate of flap transfer and no distal extremity complications in patients with normal results on preoperative CFD studies. In addition, CFD accurately identified vascular anomalies and was considered to be extremely effective in imaging the peroneal vessels. In 2003, Smith et al[10] found that patients with normal angiographic findings had corresponding normal CFD studies. Furthermore, patients with a normal CFD examination underwent fibula free flap transfer without complications. These authors also concluded that CFD is accurate in predicting poor fibula free flap donor sites in patients without strong histories of peripheral arterial disease. Among 18 lower extremities in which the results of CFD were abnormal, angiography revealed anatomy that was considered high risk for fibula free flap harvest in 16 and safe in 2.

TABLE 35.2

ABNORMALITIES IDENTIFIED BY NONINVASIVE VASCULAR TESTING IN 212 LIMBS BEING EVALUATED FOR FIBULA FREE FLAP TRANSFER

■ NO. OF LIMBS	■ % OF LIMBS	■ ABNORMAL FINDINGS
30	14	Abnormal ankle pressure or Doppler waveforms in a tibial artery (anterior, posterior tibial, or peroneal artery).
14	7	Anatomical variant involving the tibial or peroneal arteries (an absent or ectatic tibial artery, a peroneal artery filling via the anterior tibial artery, or a long tibioperoneal trunk).
28	13	Arterial obstruction ranging from 20% diameter reduction to occlusion or plaque in the distal femoral, popliteal, or tibial/peroneal arteries (nine of these limbs had normal ankle pressures or Doppler waveforms).
4	2	Only one peroneal perforator detected.
50	24	Evidence of medial calcification by B-mode imaging.
6	3	Chronic venous disease or an absent peroneal vein.

CONCLUSION

Based on this experience, patients with normal CFD studies can safely undergo fibula free flap harvest. CFD studies that demonstrate either monophasic Doppler waveforms or absence of flow in any of the trifurcation vessels identify high-risk extremities, and potential fibula free flap candidates with these findings can be excluded without the need for angiography as a secondary assessment. The main limitations of CFD are that it is still somewhat operator dependent, allows only segmental views of vascular anatomy, and may be difficult to interpret in the presence of arterial wall calcification.

References

1. Hidalgo DA, Rekow A. A review of 60 consecutive fibula free flap mandibular reconstructions. *Plast Reconstr Surg* 1995;96:585-596.
2. Wei F, Seah C, Tsai Y, et al. Fibula osteoseptocutaneous flap for reconstruction of composite mandibular defects. *Plast Reconstr Surg* 1994;93:294-304.
3. Urken ML, Sullivan MJ. Fibular osteocutaneous free flaps. In Urken ML, Cheney ML, Sullivan MJ, et al (eds). *Atlas of Regional and Free Flaps for the Head and Neck Reconstruction.* New York: Raven, 1995, pp 291-206.
4. Lutz BS, Wei FC, Ng SH, et al. Routine donor leg angiography before vascularized free fibula transplantation is not necessary: A prospective study in 120 clinical cases. *Plast Reconstr Surg* 1999;103:121-127.
5. Griswold MA, Jakob PM, Heidemann RM, et al. Generalized autocalibrating partially parallel acquisitions (GRAPPA). *Magn Reson Med* 2002;47:1202-1210.
6. Disa JJ, Cordeiro PG. The current role of preoperative arteriography in fibula free flaps. *Plast Reconstr Surg* 1998;102:1083-1088.
7. Futran ND, Stack BC Jr, Payne LP. Use of color Doppler flow imaging for preoperative assessment in fibular osteoseptocutaneous free tissue transfer. *Otolaryngol Head Neck Surg* 1997;117:660-663.
8. Blackwell KE. Donor site evaluation for fibula free flap transfer. *Am J Otolaryngol* 1998;19:89-95.
9. Whitley SP, Sandhu S, Cardozo A. Preoperative vascular assessment of the lower limb for harvest of a fibular flap: The views of vascular surgeons in the United Kingdom. *Br J Oral Maxillofac Surg* 2004;42:307-310.
10. Smith RB, Thomas RD, Funk GF. Fibula free flaps: The role of angiography in patients with abnormal results on preoperative color flow Doppler studies. *Arch Otolaryngol Head Neck Surg* 2003;129:712-715.
11. Carroll WR, Esclamado R. Preoperative vascular imaging for the fibular osteocutaneous flap. *Arch Otolaryngol Head Neck Surg* 1996;122:708-712.
12. Kelly AM, Cronin P, Hussain HK, et al. Preoperative MR angiography in free fibula flap transfer for head and neck cancer: Clinical application and influence on surgical decision making. *AJR Am J Roentgenol* 2007;188:268-274.
13. Chow LC, Napoli A, Klein MB, et al. Vascular mapping of the leg with multi-detector row CT angiography prior to free-flap transplantation. *Radiology* 2005;237:353-360.
14. Jin KN, Lee W, Yin YH, et al. Preoperative evaluation of lower extremity arteries for free fibular transfer using MDCT angiography. *J Comput Assist Tomogr* 2007;31:820-825
15. Futran ND, Stack BC Jr, Zaccardi MJ. Preoperative color flow Doppler imaging for fibula free tissue transfers. *Ann Vasc Surg* 1998;12:445-450.
16. Sumner DS. Evaluation of noninvasive testing procedures: Data analysis and interpretation. In Bernstein EF (ed). *Vascular Diagnosis.* St. Louis: CV Mosby, 1993, pp 39-63.
17. Merrit CRB. Vascular imaging. In Bernstein EF (ed). *Vascular Diagnosis.* St. Louis: CV Mosby, 1993, pp 235-240.
18. Merrit CRB. Real time Doppler color imaging. In Bernstein EF (ed). *Vascular Diagnosis.* St. Louis: CV Mosby, 1993, pp 241-248.
19. Hatsukami TS, Primozich JF, Zierler RE, et al. Color Doppler imaging of the infrainguinal arterial occlusive disease. *J Vasc Surg* 1992;16:527-533.
20. Kerr TM, Bandyk DF. Color Doppler imaging of peripheral arterial disease before angioplasty or surgical intervention. In Bernstein EF (ed). *Vascular Diagnosis.* St. Louis: CV Mosby, 1993, pp 527-533.
21. Aly S, Sommerville K, Adiseshiah M, et al. Comparison of duplex imaging and arteriography in the evaluation of lower limb arteries. *Br J Surg* 1998;85:1099-1102.
22. Rand RP, Cramer BS, Strandness ED. Color flow duplex scanning in the preoperative assessment of TRAM flap perforators: A report of 32 consecutive patients. *Plast Reconstr Surg* 1994;93:453-459.
23. Futran ND, Stack BC Jr, Zachariah AP. Ankle-arm index as a screening examination for fibula free tissue transfer. *Ann Otol Rhinol Laryngol* 1999;108:777-780.
24. Moneta GL, Yeager RA, Antonovic R, et al. Accuracy of lower extremity arterial duplex mapping. *J Vasc Surg* 1992;15:275-283.
25. Polak JF. Peripheral arterial disease: Evaluation with color flow and duplex sonography. *Radiol Clin North Am* 1995;33:71-90.

CHAPTER 36 ■ DUPLEX SCANNING PRIOR TO FLAP PROCEDURES FOR BREAST RECONSTRUCTION

MOLLY J. ZACCARDI, JEAN HADLOCK, AND RICHARD P. RAND

There have been substantial advances over the past four decades in the area of postmastectomy breast reconstruction. At the present time, it is usually possible to provide most patients with a high-quality reconstruction using either alloplastic implant products or autogenous tissue flaps. In some cases, a combination of the two techniques is required. However, most plastic surgeons would agree that the best reconstructions come from a patient's own tissue. Using the patient's tissue provides a natural-feeling breast that can be sculpted by the surgeon to match the opposite breast. For those patients requiring unilateral reconstruction, an implant is much more limited in its ability to match the opposite natural breast. In addition, the frequent use of radiation therapy in modern breast cancer treatment has a significant impact on reconstructive options. Radiated tissues will not generally allow for tissue expansion and implant reconstruction without a high risk of developing a hard and misshapen breast mound. For that reason, autogenous tissue flap reconstructions are best in radiated patients because they bring their own healthy blood supply and replace much of the damaged tissue with nonradiated skin and fat.

FLAP PROCEDURES FOR BREAST RECONSTRUCTION

The most common source of tissue used to restore the breast comes from the lower abdomen. In the early 1980s, surgeons discovered that the same tissue that is disposed of in a tummy tuck could be transferred to the chest to create a breast mound. The patient benefits by receiving the most natural reconstruction of the breast while also obtaining a flat, tighter abdomen. There are multiple ways to transfer the vascularized tissue from the abdomen based on various blood flow options, as listed in Table 36.1.

The blood supply to the transverse rectus abdominis myocutaneous (TRAM) flap travels down through the rectus muscle from the continuation of the internal mammary vessels in the chest as the superior epigastric artery and vein. Maintaining this blood supply allows the surgeon to elevate and rotate the flap and transfer it to the chest through a tunnel made over the xiphoid. Once on the chest, it is shaped into the breast mound. Using only one rectus abdominis muscle is called a "single-pedicle flap"; using both muscles is the "double-pedicle flap." Both of the muscles are used in unilateral reconstruction cases when there is a midline scar in the lower abdomen that blocks blood flow across the scar or when the surgeon feels the need to use all of the tissue from the abdomen to make the appropriate breast size. The disadvantage of this approach is the significant sacrifice in abdominal wall integrity and function. In bilateral pedicled TRAM flap cases, both muscles must be used to supply blood to each side independently.

Pedicled TRAM flaps, particularly the single-pedicled variety, have the least robust blood flow because of the long distance from the origin of the blood supply to the flap. As a result, flaps based on the more dominant perfusion from the inferior epigastric artery system have been developed. However, because the origin of this pedicle is in the pelvis, it tethers the flap in that region and requires that it be disconnected and transferred. This is referred to as a "free flap" because it is temporarily separated from the body before being reattached in a new location. This requires the use of microsurgical techniques to reestablish blood flow to the flap in the area of the breast. The two most common recipient vessels for the free flap are the internal mammary artery and vein adjacent to the sternum and the thoracodorsal pedicle in the axilla.

In order to minimize the functional compromise to the abdominal wall, surgeons have continued to devise new methods to provide the flap with blood flow with little or no muscle sacrifice. These are all microsurgical procedures and include "muscle-sparing" free TRAM flaps in which only a small cuff of muscle is taken with the flap. Also, the deep inferior epigastric perforator (DIEP) and superficial inferior

501

TABLE 36.1

MULTIPLE APPROACHES TO TRANSFER OF TISSUE FROM THE ABDOMEN FOR BREAST RECONSTRUCTION BASED ON VARIOUS BLOOD FLOW OPTIONS

TRAM flap
    Single pedicle
    Double pedicle
    Free microsurgical
DIEP flap
SIEA flap

epigastric artery (SIEA) flaps take no muscle with them at all. There has been much discussion among surgeons as to which of these microsurgical options is best. Fundamentally, it comes down to a balance between providing sufficient blood flow to the flap for its complete survival and minimizing the functional insult to the abdominal wall. Each of these operations is a one-time-only proposition and cannot be redone if the tissue does not survive. Consequently, all efforts must be made to maximize the blood flow to the flap, and the risk of outright flap loss should be less than 1%. Marginal blood flow leading to fat necrosis also needs to be rare, because fat necrosis creates hard lumps in the flap that may mimic recurrent cancer. To address these issues, we developed the technique of using color-flow duplex imaging to assess the blood supply of potential flaps for breast reconstruction. The ability to preoperatively map (locate and mark) the arterial perforators on the abdominal wall assists the surgeon in planning the procedure to ensure that the dominant vessels are included in the flap. This evaluation is useful for all of the flaps described in this chapter, but it is most important in those flaps that depend on fewer perforators for their perfusion.

THE VASCULAR LABORATORY AND TRAM FLAP SURGERY

In the 1980s, a series of reports described the intraoperative use of a continuous-wave Doppler device to map the perforator arteries for TRAM flap surgery.[1-5] These authors were primarily concerned with identifying variations in the anatomy of the blood vessels and selecting the flap segment most likely to have adequate perfusion. Michelow et al[5] evaluated 66 patients undergoing breast reconstruction and found that approximately 80% had a single vascular axis coursing through the rectus abdominis muscle, while nearly 20% displayed two axes (Fig. 36.1). In this patient population, the majority of vascularity was found in the middle third of the rectus abdominis muscle; however, in approximately 28% of the patients, the blood supply was located in the medial or lateral third of the muscle. Many surgeons prefer not to use the entire rectus abdominis muscle in an effort to reduce complications such as postoperative hernias. The goal in a muscle-sparing procedure is to harvest a segment of muscle that has adequate perfusion. Rozen et al[6] performed computed tomography angiography (CTA) in eight consecutive patients undergoing flap surgery for breast reconstruction. The CTA results revealed three distinct patterns of deep inferior epigastric artery branching (Fig. 36.2). The majority of perforators are in the region of the umbilicus, but the locations are rarely symmetrical from side to side. The anatomy of the rectus abdominis muscle and perforating arteries is shown in Figure 36.3.

In 1990, Miles Cramer from the vascular laboratory at the University of Washington and Dr. Richard Rand from the University of Washington Division of Plastic Surgery set out to improve on the intraoperative examinations of the early 1980s and introduced preoperative duplex ultrasound imaging to further reduce the risk of tissue loss in breast reconstruction surgery.[7] They performed duplex scanning (B-mode imaging, pulsed Doppler spectral analysis, and color-flow Doppler) in 13 patients and 2 normal volunteers (all female)

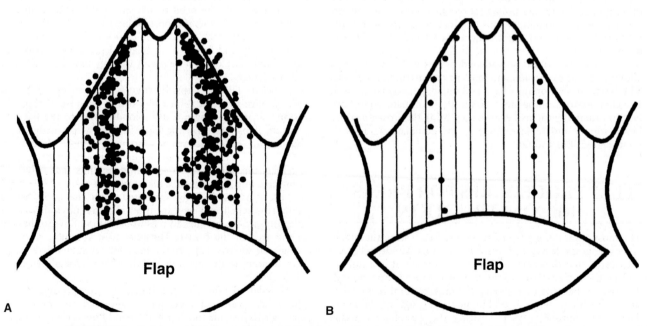

FIGURE 36.1. *A,* Accumulated scatter diagram of Doppler sound points shows the location of the arterial supply to the rectus abdominis muscles in 66 patients. *B,* Plotted Doppler sound points indicate the vascular axis of the flap in 129 rectus abdominis muscles. (From Michelow BJ, Hartrampf CR Jr, Bennett GK. TRAM flap safety optimized with intraoperative Doppler. *Plast Reconstr Surg* 1990;86:143-146, with permission.)

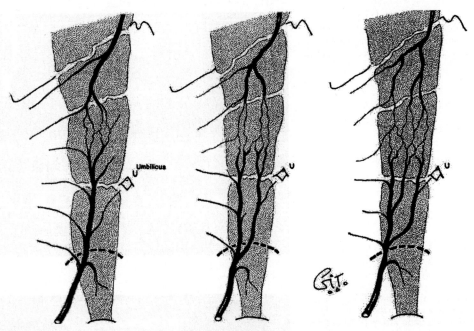

FIGURE 36.2. Three patterns of branching for the deep inferior epigastric artery. (From Rozen WM, Phillips TJ, Ashton MW, et al. Preoperative imaging for DIEA perforator flaps: A comparative study of computed tomographic angiography and Doppler ultrasound. *Plast Reconstr Surg* 2008;121:1-8, with permission.)

between March and November 1991. Their hypothesis was that duplex scanning would provide more detailed anatomic and physiologic information than the continuous-wave Doppler examinations performed by others. In addition, this critical information could be obtained preoperatively to aid in

surgical planning. Cramer et al[7] were successful in documenting the following features:

- Patency and continuity of the deep inferior epigastric arteries (Figs. 36.4 and 36.5)
- Patency and continuity of the internal mammary arteries (Fig. 36.6)
- Peak systolic velocities and diameter measurements for the perforator arteries (Fig. 36.7)
- Locations of perforator arteries by zone and side, with reference to the umbilicus
- Ability to mark each perforator artery on the skin with a high level of accuracy (Fig. 36.8)

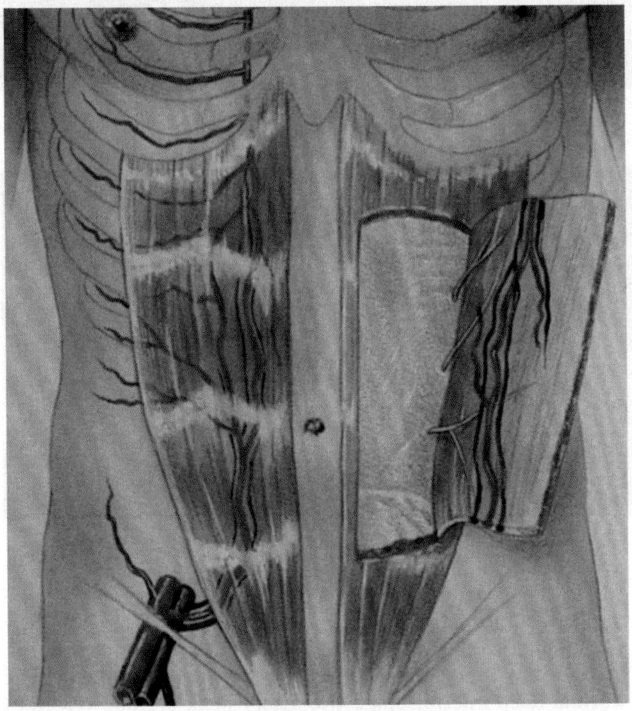

They concluded that the preoperative duplex examination allows the surgeon to incorporate a greater number of perforators into the flap and provides reliable information to identify any abnormal or unusual anatomy. The approach described by Cramer et al[7] has been the protocol at the University of Washington prior to flap procedures for breast reconstruction until recently when CTA has also been used to visualize and evaluate perforator vessels.[8]

VASCULAR EVALUATION PRIOR TO FLAP SURGERY

The duplex evaluation performed in the vascular laboratory prior to flap procedures for breast reconstruction can be divided into three parts. First, patency of the inflow vessels to the perforator arteries of the rectus abdominis muscle must be documented. Second, the perforator arteries are assessed for flow (peak systolic velocity), size (diameter), and number. The locations of the perforator arteries are also marked on the skin preoperatively. Third, patency of the internal mammary, subclavian, and axillary arteries is documented. Depending on the type of surgical procedure to be done, one of these arteries may become the sole source of perfusion to the flap.

FIGURE 36.3. Origin of the deep inferior epigastric artery from the external iliac artery. It courses up the posterior aspect of the rectus abdominis muscle to anastomose with branches of the superior epigastric artery.

FIGURE 36.4. Color-flow image and Doppler spectral waveform from a common femoral artery (CFA) showing the origin of the deep inferior epigastric artery (IEA).

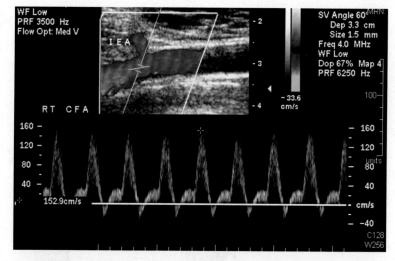

FIGURE 36.5. Duplex evaluation of the deep inferior epigastric artery (*red*) as it courses deep to the rectus abdominis muscle. The inferior epigastric artery (IEA) spectral waveform is also shown with a peak systolic velocity of about 43 cm/s.

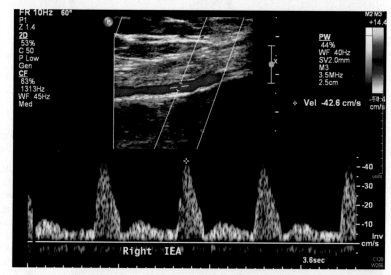

FIGURE 36.6. Duplex evaluation of the internal mammary artery. Ultrasound reflections from the pleura of the lung (*dashed arrow*) can create a mirror-image artifact that appears as two internal mammary arteries (*solid arrows*), one on each side of the pleura. The real internal mammary artery is on top (*yellow arrow*).

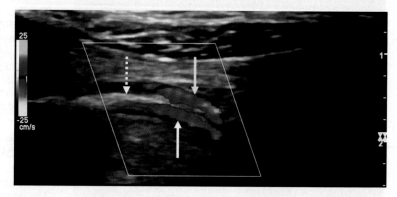

Evaluate Inflow to the Flap Tissue

The inflow vessel to the perforator arteries of the rectus abdominis muscle is the deep inferior epigastric artery, which originates from the distal external iliac or proximal common femoral artery. The iliac and common femoral arteries are evaluated by duplex scanning, using the B-mode image to locate the vessels and pulsed Doppler waveforms to document the peak systolic velocities and flow patterns. The velocity criteria for lower extremity arteries established by Jager et al[9] are applied. A normal external iliac or common femoral artery is characterized by a triphasic flow pattern and uniform peak systolic flow velocities in the range of 80 to 120 cm/s. The normal deep inferior epigastric artery peak systolic velocities were noted by Cramer et al[7] to range from approximately 40 to 45 cm/s. Stenosis is suspected if there is a focal velocity increase followed by a turbulent, poststenotic flow pattern. Lower extremity arterial duplex scanning is discussed in detail in Chapter 12.

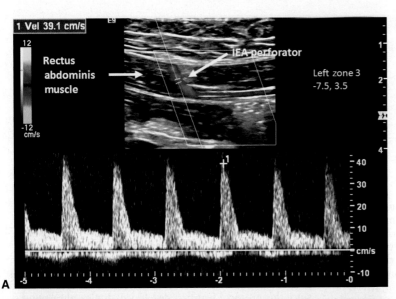

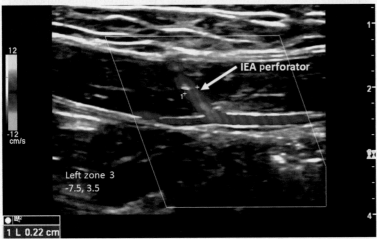

FIGURE 36.7. *A,* Peak systolic velocity measurement of 39 cm/s from an inferior epigastric artery (IEA) perforator in zone III on the left side. The perforator is located 7.5 cm below the umbilicus and 3.5 cm to the left of the midline. *B,* Diameter measurement of the same IEA perforator (0.22 cm).

Evaluate the Perforator Arteries

In 1994, Rand et al[10] published their experience with 32 consecutive patients undergoing TRAM flap surgery and reported nearly 98% complete flap survival. One patient with a significant smoking history had a failed unilateral flap owing to venous occlusion. The preference in this series was to incorporate a

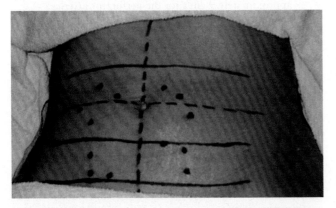

FIGURE 36.8. Markings from a preoperative TRAM flap duplex study show perforator locations on both sides for zones I, II, and III (zone IV not shown).

minimum of three perforators with flow velocities greater than 20 cm/s into the flap. If the velocities were lower than 20 cm/s in three perforators, an effort was made to include additional perforators into the flap. One false-positive duplex assessment was reported in this study, but there were no false negatives.

Further validation for the role of duplex scanning prior to TRAM flap surgery was reported by Meunier et al.[11] In this study, 20 patients were evaluated preoperatively using the protocol described by Rand et al.[9] Four patients were rejected for the flap procedure after the duplex examination revealed an insufficient number of perforator arteries or perforator arteries that were small with low flow; the remaining 16 patients were considered candidates for surgery. These authors found two false negatives intraoperatively, and there were no false positives. Flap survival without revision was approximately 90%. This study did reveal two limitations of duplex scanning prior to flap procedures. First, the venous network of the muscle could not be evaluated, and venous congestion is one of the causes of complications after free flap surgery.[12] Second, obesity (with increased depth of vessels) and abdominal scar tissue may interfere with ultrasound imaging.[8]

The clinical experience described previously and a study in cadavers by Heitmann et al[13] provide a range of measurements and other parameters that can serve as guidelines. Any findings that fall outside these measurements should be brought to the attention of the surgeon. Table 36.2 lists the expected number of perforators per side and zone on the abdomen, and Table 36.3 gives the range of flow velocities normally found in

TABLE 36.2

AVERAGE NUMBER OF RECTUS ABDOMINIS MUSCLE ARTERIAL PERFORATORS PER SIDE AND PER ZONE

	■ ZONE I	■ ZONE II	■ ZONE III	■ ZONE IV	■ TOTAL
Mean	1.30	1.80	2.40	1.10	6.60

From Cramer MM, Rand RP, Strandness DE. Color flow duplex scanning: A technique to improve transverse rectus abdominis myocutaneous (TRAM) viability. *J Vasc Technol* 1993;17:7-16, with permission.

the perforator and deep inferior epigastric arteries. Meunier et al[11] reported average diameters for the deep inferior epigastric and perforator arteries. These diameter measurements are compared with the cadaver study performed by Heitmann et al[13] in Table 36.4. According to Rand et al,[10] the absence of at least one perforator per zone measuring a minimum of 1 mm, velocities of less than 13 cm/s in a perforator artery, or velocities of less than 40 cm/s in the deep inferior epigastric artery should be brought to the attention of the surgeon.

Evaluate the New Source of Perfusion to the Flap

The last part of the preoperative evaluation is to assess the proposed inflow vessels for the new flap. A TRAM flap is dependent on perfusion from the internal mammary artery, which originates from the subclavian artery, but a free flap is perfused by the thoracodorsal pedicle, which relies on the subscapular branch of the axillary artery. For these reasons, a bilateral upper extremity duplex examination of the subclavian and axillary arteries and veins is performed to rule out stenosis and obstruction. This part of the examination is especially important, because many of these patients have had radiation to their breast that may cause damage to the internal mammary vessels, or previous surgery with lymph node dissection that may interfere with the thoracodorsal pedicle. Duplex scanning is used to document that the internal mammary artery has uniform peak systolic flow velocities and that the accompanying vein is patent. Schwabegger et al[14] used power Doppler imaging to compare diameter measurements and flow velocities in the internal mammary arteries and veins preoperatively and intraoperatively and found a good correlation between the studies. The criteria used to assess the subclavian, axillary, and internal mammary arteries are summarized in Table 36.5. Upper extremity arterial duplex scanning is discussed in Chapter 14.

EXAMINATION PROTOCOL

Preparation

We originally reserved 2 to 3 hours for a duplex examination prior to flap procedures for breast reconstruction. However, since this protocol was first developed, duplex ultrasound systems have improved significantly, with better B-mode image resolution and color-flow Doppler capabilities. This provides much finer detail in soft tissue images and easier documentation of flow velocities in small vessels. As a result, we currently allow 1.5 to 2 hours to perform the examination and report the findings. Patients should be scheduled as close to the surgery date as possible so the locations of arterial perforators can be marked on the abdominal wall. If necessary, the patient can be given a permanent ink pen to "refresh" the marks and keep them visible until the operation is performed. It is also helpful to have the patient refrain from eating for at least 3 hours prior to the duplex scan to reduce peristalsis and motion artifact.

Equipment

- Duplex ultrasound system (B-mode, color-flow Doppler, and spectral waveform analysis)
- Transducer range of 4 to 15 MHz
- Permanent marking pen
- Ruler

Ultrasound System Presets

- Color-flow Doppler settings (mean flow) are adjusted to approximately 80 cm/s for the iliac artery and reduced to approximately 9 cm/s for the perforator arteries.
- Settings for Doppler spectral waveforms are optimized for peak flow velocities ranging from 60 to 140 cm/s in the external iliac and common femoral arteries and

TABLE 36.3

PEAK SYSTOLIC FLOW VELOCITIES IN THE PERFORATOR AND DEEP INFERIOR EPIGASTRIC ARTERIES

Perforator artery velocity range	13-22 cm/s
Deep inferior epigastric artery mean velocity	42 cm/s

From Cramer MM, Rand RP, Strandness DE. Color flow duplex scanning: A technique to improve transverse rectus abdominis myocutaneous (TRAM) viability. *J Vasc Technol* 1993;17:7-16, with permission.

TABLE 36.4

DIAMETER MEASUREMENTS OF THE DEEP INFERIOR EPIGASTRIC AND PERFORATOR ARTERIES

	■ MEUNIER ET AL[11]	■ HEITMANN ET AL[13]
Deep inferior epigastric artery	2.8-3.6 mm	2.8-5.0 mm
Perforator artery	0.5-1.0 mm	≤1 mm

TABLE 36.5

DUPLEX CRITERIA FOR OBSTRUCTION OF THE SUBCLAVIAN, AXILLARY, AND INTERNAL MAMMARY ARTERIES

	■ NORMAL WAVEFORM	■ NORMAL PEAK SYSTOLIC VELOCITIES	■ ABNORMAL WAVEFORM	■ ABNORMAL PEAK SYSTOLIC VELOCITIES
Subclavian artery	Triphasic	80-120 cm/s	Stenosis—focal velocity increase with poststenotic turbulent flow, loss of triphasic waveform Occlusion—absent Doppler signal	Ratio of >2 from prestenotic segment to stenotic segment
Axillary artery	Triphasic	60-80 cm/s	Same as above	Same as above
Internal mammary artery	Triphasic	15-95 cm/s (average 85 cm/s)	Same as above	Not applicable

approximately 20 cm/s for the inferior epigastric and perforator arteries. Doppler angle correction is used for all arterial velocity measurements. This requires an angle of 60 degrees or less between the incident Doppler ultrasound beam and the arterial wall.

Step 1. Mark the Four Zones

The patient is positioned supine with the abdomen exposed. A grid is drawn on the patient's abdomen with a ruler and marking pen, starting with vertical and horizontal lines through the umbilicus (Fig. 36.9). Another horizontal line is drawn parallel to and 4 cm above the first line, and zone I is located between these two lines. Three more horizontal lines are drawn at 4-, 8-, and 12-cm intervals below the umbilicus to define zones II, III, and IV. Each perforator artery can now be identified by zone and side. This allows the surgeon to select specific zones to be used for the flap.

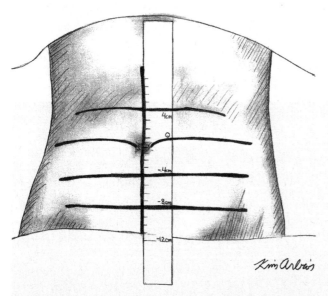

FIGURE 36.9. Grid drawn on the patient's abdomen to record the locations of the rectus abdominis perforator arteries by zone and side (also see Fig. 36.8).

Step 2. Scan the Distal External Iliac, Common Femoral, and Inferior Epigastric Arteries

The distal external iliac and proximal common femoral arteries are evaluated in a longitudinal view at the inguinal crease. These vessels are important because they provide the inflow to the inferior epigastric and perforator arteries. Using a midrange-frequency transducer and the recommended Doppler settings for peripheral arteries, spectral waveforms are recorded with the Doppler beam at a 60-degree angle to the long axis of the vessels. Areas of narrowing, atherosclerotic plaque, or occlusion are noted. The transducer is then angled slightly medially to visualize the origin of the inferior epigastric artery from the distal external iliac or proximal common femoral artery. The Doppler sample volume is swept through the origin of the inferior epigastric artery, and spectral waveforms are recorded. Normal parameters for these vessels are given in Tables 36.3 and 36.4. The origin of the inferior epigastric artery and its relationship to the common femoral artery are shown in Figures 36.4 and 36.10.

Step 3. Assess the Size, Number, and Location of Inferior Epigastric Perforators

The inferior epigastric perforator arteries are identified with the inferior epigastric artery in transverse view (Fig. 36.11). Perforator arteries are evaluated one side at a time. Starting in zone IV, optimize the image of the epigastric artery and rectus abdominis muscle in transverse view and slide superiorly. The inferior epigastric artery and vein will be visualized posterior to the rectus abdominis muscle (Fig. 36.5). Move the transducer slowly throughout zone IV in search of the perforator arteries. The perforators will arise from the inferior epigastric artery and pass anteriorly through the muscle (Fig. 36.12). As each perforator is identified, it should be followed to its most superficial location on the muscle. Record a Doppler spectral waveform and obtain a B-mode image for diameter measurement (Fig. 36.7). Note whether a perforator divides or is tortuous through the facial layer. Center the perforator under the transducer as it enters the facial layer, remove the gel, and mark the location on the skin using a permanent marker. Continue in zone IV until all the perforators are located, evaluated, and marked. This procedure is then repeated for zones

FIGURE 36.10. Color-flow image shows the origin of the inferior epigastric artery from the common femoral artery (also see Fig. 36.4).

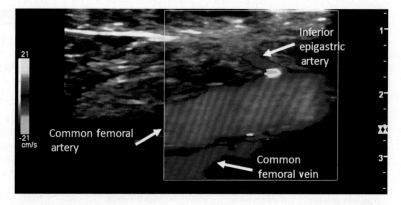

FIGURE 36.11. An inferior epigastric perforator artery is identified in this color-flow image (*red*), with the inferior epigastric artery (IEA) in transverse view (*blue*).

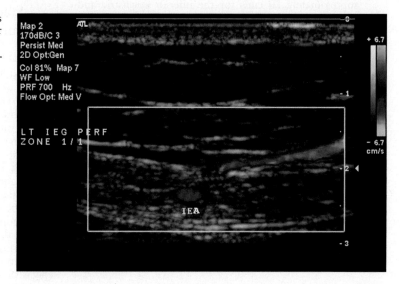

FIGURE 36.12. Color-flow image of a tortuous inferior epigastric perforator artery passing anteriorly through the rectus abdominis muscle. The inferior epigastric artery (IEA) is located toward the bottom of the image.

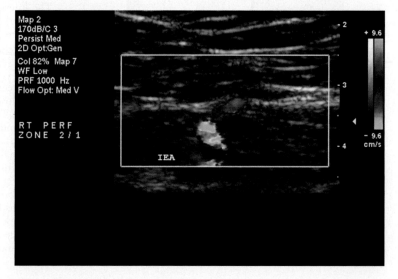

UNIVERSITY OF WASHINGTON MEDICAL CENTER – VASCULAR DIAGNOSTIC SERVICE

TRAM FLAP PERFORATOR DUPLEX
-PRELIMINARY REPORT-
STUDY WILL BE REVIEWED BY
VASCULAR SURGERY DIVISION

HISTORY/INDICATION: _52 yo ♀_

pre-op breast reconstruction

VESSEL	VELOCITY cm/sec	DIAMETER cm	VERT +/- cm	HORIZ +/- cm
RIGHT				
ZONE I	56	0.11	+2.0	4.0
	51	0.11	+1.0	5.5
ZONE II	30	0.10	-0.5	1.5
	63	0.11	-1.0	3.5
ZONE III	26	0.10	-5.5	2.0
ZONE IV				
LEFT				
ZONE I	87	0.13	+2.5	1.5
	17	0.12	+0.5	5.0
ZONE II	16	0.10	-1.5	2.0
	13	0.10	-3.5	2.0
ZONE III				
ZONE IV				

EPIGASTRIC ARTERIES:
Continuous to ZONE ___2___ RIGHT   ZONE ___2___ LEFT

PERFORATORS ___5___ RIGHT   ___4___ LEFT

IMA	RIGHT	LEFT
	99 cm/sec Vein patent	84 cm/sec Vein patent

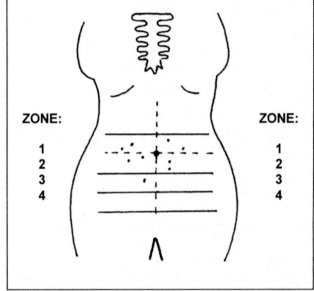

ZONE:
1
2
3
4

ZONE:
1
2
3
4

IMPRESSION: _1. A total of nine inferior epigastric perforating arteries are mapped and marked on the skin._
2. The right and left internal mammary arteries and associated veins are patent with no evidence or obstruction.

DATE AND HOUR:

PT.NO

NAME

DOB

University of Washington Academic Medical Center
Harborview Medical Center – UW Medical Center
University of Washington Physicians
Seattle, Washington
VASCULAR EXAMINATIONS
TRAM FLAP PERFORATOR DUPLEX NOTE

UH1830 REV NOV 02

PROGRESS — BLUE

PREOPERATIVE PLANNING, INTRAOPERATIVE ASSESSMENT AND PROCEDURAL GUIDANCE

A

FIGURE 36.13. *A,* Example of a technologist worksheet for recording data during the TRAM flap evaluation.

UNIVERSITY OF WASHINGTON MEDICAL CENTER

D.E. Strandness, Jr. Vascular Laboratory
Accredited by the Intersocietal Accreditation Commission (IAC Vascular Testing)
==

TRAM/DIEP FREE FLAP PERFORATOR ARTERIAL DUPLEX:

==

INDICATIONS: This is a 33 year old female who is referred for TRAM arterial perforator duplex evaluation. The patient presents with breast cancer and requires a free DIEP flap for reconstruction.

==

A total of 3-right and 4-left epigastric perforators were identified and marked on the skin.

Peak Systolic Velocities:

RIGHT
------------Velocity----Diameter------Horizontal----Vertical
Zone I
------------ 25 cm/s----- 0.14 cm------- −4.5 cm------- +0.5
 Zone II
------------ 29 cm/s----- 0.13 cm------- −3.5 cm------- −3.0
Zone III
------------ 36 cm/s----- 0.18 cm------- −4.0 cm------- −5.5
Zone IV
None identified

LEFT
------------Velocity----Diameter------Horizontal----Vertical
Zone I
------------ 19 cm/s----- 0.14 cm------- +4.5 cm------- +1.5 cm
Zone II
------------ 19 cm/s----- 0.13 cm------- +2.5 cm------- −0.5 cm
Zone III
------------ 32 cm/s----- 0.14 cm------- +2.5 cm------- −4.5 cm
------------ 18 cm/s----- 0.13 cm------- +4.0 cm------- −5.0 cm
Zone IV
None identified

Peak systolic velocities---------Right---------Left
Inferior epigastric artery------42 cm/s------46 cm/s
Internal mammary artery-----79 cm/-------69 cm/s

Doppler waveforms are non-damped and triphasic.

==

FINAL PHYSICIAN INTERPRETATION

1. 3-Right and 4-Left inferior epigastric artery perforators were located, mapped, and marked on the skin.
2. Right and Left internal mammary arteries are patent without evidence of significant focal stenosis.

==

B

FIGURE 36.13. (*Continued*) *B* and *C*, Examples of reports describing the results of the TRAM/DIEP free flap perforator arterial duplex.

UNIVERSITY OF WASHINGTON MEDICAL CENTER

D.E. Strandness, Jr. Vascular Laboratory
Accredited by the Intersocietal Accreditation Commission (IAC Vascular Testing)
===

TRAM/DIEP FREE FLAP PERFORATOR ARTERIAL DUPLEX:
===

INDICATIONS: This is a 47 year old female who is referred for TRAM arterial perforator duplex evaluation. The patient presents with breast cancer and requires a free DIEP flap for reconstruction.

===

A total of 7-right and 3-left epigastric perforators were identified and marked on the skin.

Peak Systolic Velocities:

```
-------Velocity---Diameter---Vertical---Horizontal
-------(cm/s)------(cm)--------(cm)---------(cm)
```

RIGHT
Zone I
```
---------24 cm/s----0.14 cm----- +3.0 cm---- 8.0 cm
```
Zone II
```
---------60 cm/s----0.21 cm----- −1.5 cm---- 8.0 cm
---------22 cm/s----0.12 cm----- −0.5 cm---- 4.5 cm
```
Zone III
```
---------32 cm/s----0.17 cm----- −6.5 cm---- 6.0 cm
---------54 cm/s----0.21 cm----- −5.0 cm---- 3.5 cm
```
Zone IV
```
---------52 cm/s----0.15 cm----- −10.5 cm--- 5.0 cm
---------28 cm/s----0.19 cm----- −10.0 cm--- 2.0 cm
```

LEFT
Zone I
```
---------40 cm/s----0.17 cm----- +0.5 cm---- 3.5 cm
```
Zone II
```
---------33 cm/s----0.18 cm----- −3.5 cm---- 3.0 cm
```
Zone III
```
---------39 cm/s----0.14 cm----- −7.5 cm---- 4.0 cm
```
Zone IV
```
---------none-----------------------------
```

The left inferior epigastric artery courses within the muscle throughout zones 4, 3, and 2.
Peak systolic velocities in the internal mammary artery are 109 cm/s on the right and 93 cm/s on the left
Doppler waveforms are non-damped and triphasic.

===

FINAL PHYSICIAN INTERPRETATION

1. 7-right and 3- left inferior epigastric artery perforators were located, mapped, and marked on the skin.
2. Right and left internal mammary arteries are patent without evidence of significant focal stenosis.

C

FIGURE 36.13. (*Continued*).

III, II, and I. The average number of perforators per zone is listed in Table 36.2.

Step 4. Assess the Internal Mammary Artery and Accompanying Veins

Using duplex ultrasound settings appropriate for peripheral artery studies, place the transducer parallel and adjacent to the sternum between the second and the third ribs. Identify the internal mammary artery and accompanying veins in a longitudinal view and record a Doppler spectral waveform. The vessels may be visible only between areas of shadowing produced by the ribs. It is also common to observe a mirror-image or reflection artifact due to the pleura of the lung, which appears as a duplicate vessel (Fig. 36.6). Document any areas of arterial stenosis or occlusion as well as venous patency and flow direction. Repeat this study sequence on the opposite side.

Step 5. Measure the Location of the Perforator Arteries

Using a ruler, measure the location of the perforators in relation to the umbilicus, and record the data on the preliminary worksheet (Fig. 36.13).

CONCLUSIONS

Reported experience indicates that preoperative duplex mapping improves overall outcomes for breast reconstruction.[15-17] Noninvasive techniques for evaluating blood flow can also be used to compare perfusion and aid in selection among the various types of flap procedures.[18,19] A systematic review by Pratt et al[20] evaluated the role of five imaging techniques prior to reconstructive flap procedures: CTA, magnetic resonance angiography (MRA), handheld Doppler, color duplex scanning, and catheter angiography. Although high

PREOPERATIVE PLANNING, INTRAOPERATIVE ASSESSMENT AND PROCEDURAL GUIDANCE

level evidence is lacking for some of these techniques, this review concluded that CTA and MRA were the most accurate and had the least interobserver variation. Uppal et al[15] also found that both duplex ultrasound and CTA mapping reduced operating time for flap breast reconstructions, but that CTA was superior. However, when the expertise is available, duplex scanning has clear cost advantages over CTA and can avoid patient exposure to radiation and iodinated contrast.[21,22]

References

1. Boyd JB, Taylor GI, Corlett R. The vascular territories of the superior epigastric and the deep inferior epigastric systems. *Plast Reconstr Surg* 1984;73:15-16.
2. Hartrampf CR. Abdominal wall competence in transverse abdominal island flap operations. *Ann Plast Surg* 1984;12:139-146.
3. Hartrampf CR, Bennett GK. Autogenous tissue reconstruction in the mastectomy patient: A critical review of 300 patients. *Ann Surg* 1987;205: 508-518.
4. Miller LB, Bostwick J, Hartramp CR, et al. The superiorly based rectus abdominis flap: Predicting and enhancing its blood supply based on an anatomic and clinical study. *Plast Reconstr Surg* 1988;81:721-724.
5. Michelow BJ, Hartrampf CR Jr, Bennett GK. TRAM flap safety optimized with intraoperative Doppler. *Plast Reconstr Surg* 1990;86:143-146.
6. Rozen WM, Phillips TJ, Ashton MW, et al. Preoperative imaging for DIEA perforator flaps: A comparative study of computed tomographic angiography and Doppler ultrasound. *Plast Reconstr Surg* 2008;121: 1-8.
7. Cramer MM, Rand RP, Strandness DE. Color flow duplex scanning: A technique to improve transverse rectus abdominis myocutaneous (TRAM) viability. *J Vasc Technol* 1993;17:7-16.
8. Aubry A, Pauchot J, Kastler A, et al. Preoperative imaging in the planning of deep inferior epigastric artery perforator flap surgery. *Skeletol Radiol* 2013:42:319-327.
9. Jager KA, Phillips DJ, Martin RL, et al. Non-invasive mapping of lower limb arterial lesions. *Ultrasound Med Biol* 1985;11:515-521.
10. Rand RP, Cramer MM, Strandness DE Jr. Color flow duplex scanning in the preoperative assessment of TRAM flap perforators: A report of 32 consecutive patients. *Plast Reconstr Surg* 1994;93:453-459.
11. Meunier B, Waiter E, Roshe G, et al. Preoperative color-Doppler assessment of vascularisation of the rectus abdominis: Anatomic basis of breast reconstruction with a transverse rectus abdominis myocutaneous flap—a prospective study. *Surg Radiol Anat* 1997;19:35-40.
12. Blondeel PN, Arnstein M, Verstraete K, et al. Venous congestion and blood flow in free transverse rectus abdominis myocutaneous and deep inferior epigastric perforator flaps. *Plast Reconstr Surg* 2000;106:1295-1299.
13. Heitmann C, Felmerer G, Durmus C, et al. Anatomical features of perforator blood vessels in the deep inferior epigastric perforator flap. *Br J Plast Surg* 2000;53:205-208.
14. Schwabegger AH, Bodner G, Reiger M, et al. Internal mammary vessels as a model for power Doppler imaging of recipient vessels in microsurgery. *Plast Reconstr Surg* 1999;104:1656-1661.
15. Uppal RS, Casaer B, Van Landuyt K, et al. The efficacy of preoperative mapping of perforators in reducing operative times and complications in perforator flap breast reconstruction. *J Plast Reconstr Aesthet Surg* 2009;62:859-864. Epub May 1, 2008.
16. Berg WA, Chang BW, DeJong MR, et al. Color Doppler flow mapping of abdominal wall perforating arteries for transverse rectus abdominis myocutaneous flap in breast reconstruction: Method and preliminary results. *Radiology* 1994;192.447-450.
17. Chang BW, Luethke R, Berg WA, et al. Two-dimensional color Doppler imaging for precision preoperative mapping and size determination of TRAM flap perforators. *Plast Reconstr Surg* 1994;93:197-200.
18. Heitland AS, Markowitz M, Koellensperger E, et al. Duplex ultrasound imaging in free transverse rectus abdominis muscle, deep inferior epigastric artery perforator, and superior gluteal artery perforator maps. *Ann Plast Surg* 2005;55:117-121.
19. Loh N, Ch'en IY, Olcott E, et al. Power Doppler imaging in preoperative planning and postoperative monitoring of muscle flaps. *J Clin Ultrasound* 1997;25:465-471.
20. Pratt G, Rozen W, Chubb D, et al. Preoperative imaging for perforator flaps in reconstructive surgery. *Ann Plast Surg* 2012;69:3-9.
21. Cina A, Barone-Adesi L, Cipriani A, et al. Planning deep interior epigastric perforator flaps for breast reconstruction: a comparison between multidetector computed tomography and magnetic resonance angiography. *Eur Radiol* 2013:23:2333-2343.
22. Saba L, Atzeni M, Rozen W, et al. Non-invasive vascular imaging in perforator flap surgery. *Acta Radiol* 2013;54:89-98.

VASCULAR LABORATORY TESTING PROTOCOLS

MELISSA LOJA, EDWARD RONNINGEN, AND MOLLY ZACCARDI

Vascular laboratories must have specific, written protocols for each test performed. These protocols describe the indications for testing, equipment needed, and the elements of proper technique, including patient positioning and preparation, the anatomic extent of the examination, whether a bilateral examination is necessary, and variations in technique that may be used. There should also be a description of the documentation required for each examination.

The Intersocietal Accreditation Commission (IAC) accredits facilities performing vascular testing (www.intersocietal.org/vascular/). The accreditation process provides a means for facilities to evaluate and improve the quality of patient care they provide. The IAC publishes detailed Standards and Guidelines for vascular testing facilities which define the minimum requirements for laboratory organization and examinations in the areas of extracranial cerebrovascular, intracranial cerebrovascular, peripheral arterial, peripheral venous, visceral vascular, and screening. To receive IAC accreditation, each facility must submit the protocols it uses and case studies that provide examples of tests that are in compliance with its own protocols.

The protocols included in this appendix are based on the practices of the D. E. Strandness Jr Vascular Laboratory at the University of Washington and the University of California Davis Vascular Laboratory and were compiled by Melissa Loja, MD, with the assistance of Edward Ronningen, BS, RVT, and Molly Zaccardi, MHA, RVT. These comprehensive protocols were created to conform to the general requirements of the 2015 IAC Standards and Guidelines. However, to improve the usefulness or thoroughness of testing in a particular laboratory, examination steps or documentation components may be added at the discretion of the Medical Director and Technical Director.

Cerebrovascular
Extracranial Cerebrovascular
Transcranial Doppler (Duplex)

Peripheral Arterial
Lower Extremity Arterial Physiologic Testing
Lower Extremity Exercise Testing
Lower Extremity Arterial Duplex
Upper Extremity Arterial Physiologic Testing
Upper Extremity Arterial Duplex

Venous
Lower Extremity Venous Duplex
Lower Extremity Venous Reflux Evaluation
Vein Mapping: Lower Extremity
Upper Extremity Venous Duplex
Vein Mapping: Upper Extremity

Abdominal Vascular
Aortoiliac Arterial Duplex
Visceral Duplex: Mesenteric
Visceral Duplex: Renal Arteries

EXTRACRANIAL CEREBROVASCULAR

Purpose:
To evaluate the extracranial carotid, vertebral, and subclavian arteries with duplex ultrasound for the presence and severity of stenosis or other abnormalities.

Indications:
- Stroke
- Transient ischemic attack
- Aphasia, hemiparesis, or unilateral sensory loss
- Visual disturbances, including amaurosis fugax
- Carotid bruit
- Preoperative assessment
- Intraoperative assessment of a repaired carotid artery
- Postoperative or poststenting evaluation
- Follow-up of a known stenosis
- Trauma
- Vertebral insufficiency
- Subclavian steal syndrome

Extent of Examination:
- Examinations should be bilateral, unless unilateral examination is specifically requested.
- A complete bilateral study (CPT® 93880) evaluates the following:
  - Common carotid artery (CCA), internal carotid artery (ICA), and external carotid artery (ECA)
  - Vertebral artery
  - Subclavian artery
- The carotid arteries are evaluated from the level of the proximal common carotid artery to the distal cervical segment of the internal carotid artery (~4 cm from the bifurcation).
- Bilateral arm blood pressure measurements are indicated when vertebral or subclavian artery stenosis is suspected (based on history, physical examination, or by velocity increases within the vertebral or subclavian arteries).
- Indications for a unilateral or limited examination (CPT® 93882) may include surveillance after intervention, intraoperative examination, or when specifically requested.

Equipment and Supplies:
- System capabilities: Duplex ultrasound with B-mode, color, and spectral Doppler capabilities
- Transducers:
  - Linear 5- to 10-MHz probe
  - L10–L5 intraoperative linear array ("hockey stick") probe for intraoperative evaluation

■ Sterile probe covers for intraoperative examinations
■ 10-cm or 12-cm blood pressure cuff for brachial blood pressure measurement

Patient Positioning and Preparation:

1. Confirm study requested, patient identity, and examination indication.
2. Review pertinent patient medical history and symptoms.
3. Expose the patient's neck; place towels to avoid gel on the patient's clothing.
4. Place the patient in supine position, with head turned approximately 45 degrees to the contralateral side.

Scanning Steps:

1. If indicated, obtain bilateral arm systolic blood pressures.
2. Begin the examination with the right side.
3. Record a cine-loop transverse scan through the CCA, bifurcation, and ICA.
4. B-mode imaging is used to depict the anatomy and the presence of intraluminal echoes, plaque formation, or other abnormalities within the extracranial carotid arteries.
5. Color flow Doppler (CFD) is used when needed to document vessel patency and flow direction.
6. Spectral Doppler is used to interrogate arterial flow velocities within the common carotid, internal carotid, external carotid and vertebral and subclavian arteries, bilaterally. Spectral Doppler velocities are obtained from specified levels throughout all arteries evaluated to determine presence of, location, and severity of stenosis.
7. If indicated, calculate the ICA: CCA velocity ratio using the highest ICA velocity and a velocity from an unobstructed segment of the mid- to distal CCA 2 cm proximal to the bifurcation as a reference point.
   a. Indicated when examination suggests greater than 50% stenosis of the ICA

Documentation Requirements: Normal Examination

■ B-mode images
  ● Cine-loop transverse scan through the common carotid artery, bifurcation, and internal carotid artery
  ● Long-axis (and short axis if beneficial) views of the following:
    ❑ Common carotid artery
    ❑ Bifurcation
    ❑ Proximal internal carotid artery
    ❑ Proximal external carotid artery
■ Spectral Doppler analysis
  ● Record Doppler signals at an angle of 60 degrees, when possible.
  ● Obtain waveforms and measure peak systolic velocities at the following:
    ❑ Common carotid artery:
      ○ Proximal
      ○ Distal (~2 cm proximal to the bifurcation)
    ❑ Internal carotid artery (also document end-diastolic velocity):
      ○ Proximal
      ○ Mid
      ○ Distal (at least 4 cm from the bifurcation)
    ❑ External carotid artery
      ○ Proximal
    ❑ Vertebral artery (also document direction of flow):
      ○ Mid
      ○ Origin, if indicated
    ❑ Subclavian artery:
      ○ Proximal
■ Color flow Doppler

● Example of flow separation at the bifurcation (if visualized)
■ ICA: CCA ratio (when indicated)

Documentation Requirements: Additional Findings or Abnormal Examination

■ Bilateral brachial blood pressures must be documented when vertebral or subclavian artery stenosis is found.
■ Document any regions of plaque or other abnormalities with additional B-mode and spectral Doppler imaging.
■ Demonstrate velocities immediately proximal and distal to any vessel segment with a focal velocity increase.
■ Documentation after carotid endarterectomy or carotid stenting must include representative B-mode imaging and spectral Doppler waveforms with velocity measurements recorded at the proximal, mid-, and distal sites.
■ For symptomatic stenosis of greater than 50% diameter reduction or any stenosis greater than 80% diameter reduction, the following may be measured:
  ● The distance from the angle of the mandible to the carotid bifurcation
  ● The distance the plaque extends into the internal carotid artery
  ● The diameter of the native distal (normal segment) internal carotid artery
  ● The diameter of the mid- (normal segment) common carotid artery

TRANSCRANIAL DOPPLER (DUPLEX)

Purpose:

To evaluate the circulation of the brain for intracranial arterial stenosis, vasospasm, occlusion, collateralization, and emboli.

Indications:

■ Screening children aged 2 to 16 years with sickle cell disease to assess stroke risk
■ Detection and evaluation of vasospasm after traumatic brain injury or subarachnoid hemorrhage
■ Evaluation of intracranial hemodynamics in the presence of extracranial cerebrovascular disease
■ Intraoperative and postoperative monitoring of intracranial flow
■ Assessment of the vertebrobasilar circulation for collateralization or stenosis

Extent of Examination:

■ Examinations should be bilateral, unless unilateral examination specifically requested.
■ If the status of the extracranial arteries is unknown, first perform an Extracranial Cerebrovascular study (carotid and vertebral artery duplex scan), per protocol.
■ A complete bilateral study (CPT® 93886) evaluates the following:
  ● Anterior cerebral artery (ACA), middle cerebral artery (MCA), and posterior cerebral artery (PCA)
  ● Terminal segment and siphon of the internal carotid artery
  ● Anterior communicating (ACom) and posterior communicating artery (PCom), when identified as a collateral pathway
  ● Ophthalmic artery (when indicated)
  ● Vertebral and basilar arteries
■ Indications for a unilateral or limited examination (CPT® 93888) may include intraoperative and postoperative transcranial Doppler.

- Emboli detection studies without venous microbubble injection (CPT® 92892) may be done intraoperatively during carotid endarterectomy or for the diagnosis of atheroembolization from proximal sources.

Equipment:

- System capabilities: B mode and color and spectral Doppler
- Transducers:
  - 2- to 3-MHz pulsed Doppler transducer
  - Nonimaging probe for intraoperative examination
- Headgear for attaching transducer during intraoperative monitoring

Patient Positioning and Preparation:

1. Confirm study requested, patient identity, and examination indication.
2. Review pertinent patient medical history and symptoms.
3. Place the patient in supine position, with head to one side to evaluate the transtemporal, orbital, and transoccipital windows.
4. Vertebral and basilar arteries are best assessed from sitting position.
5. Place the patient in a lateral decubitus position, with neck flexed, to image the suboccipital window.
6. The patient should remain awake for the duration of the examination.

Procedural Steps:

- Settings:
  - For patient safety, output power must not exceed 10% of maximum emitted power or 17 mW/cm² or equivalent measurements.
  - Enlarge sample volume for intraoperative emboli monitoring.
  - Decrease power output to minimal levels to evaluate the ophthalmic arteries.
- Color flow Doppler is used to determine vessel location, patency, and flow direction.
- Pulsed wave Doppler is used to evaluate flow velocities at specified depth levels and segments within each vessel.
- Criteria based on Doppler findings (mean velocity and flow direction) are used to determine the presence, location, and severity of stenosis.
- The pulsatility index (PI) may be used as an indication of resistance distal to the insonated site. It is usually calculated by the Gosling equation: PI = (peak systolic velocity – end-diastolic velocity)/mean velocity.

TRANSCRANIAL DUPLEX:

Transtemporal window:

- Place the transducer above the ear and angle the probe inferiorly, superiorly, anteriorly, and posteriorly to locate the transtemporal window.
- Identify the MCA running adjacent to the sphenoid bone, with flow toward the transducer from depths of 3 to 6 cm.
  - Record Doppler signals from proximal, mid-, and distal segments; note flow direction.
- Increase the depth to 6 to 7 cm and angle the transducer anteriorly to locate and evaluate the ACA. The ACA runs toward the midline, away from the transducer (A1 segment). Follow the vessel as it turns superiorly (A2).
  - Sweep through the vessel and record the highest velocity Doppler signal, noting flow direction.

- At the level of the ACA, angle the transducer posteriorly to locate and evaluate the PCA. Visualize the P1 and P2 segments of the PCA.
  - Sweep through the vessel and record the highest velocity Doppler signal, noting flow direction.
- Angle the transducer inferiorly at the level of the MCA/ACA bifurcation (depth of ~6 to 7 cm) to locate and evaluate the terminal internal carotid artery.
  - Record the highest Doppler flow velocity and note flow direction of the terminal internal carotid artery.
- Record and identify any collateral pathways, including the anterior or posterior communicating arteries.

Transorbital window:

- Use the nonimaging transducer and decrease power output to 10%.
- Locate the ophthalmic artery at a depth of 4 to 6 cm.
  - Sweep through the vessel and record the highest velocity Doppler signal, noting flow direction.
- Using the nonimaging transducer, the siphon of the internal carotid artery can be evaluated (if not adequately evaluated through the transtemporal window).
- The carotid artery siphon is best evaluated with this approach at a depth of 6.5 to 7 cm.

Transoccipital window:

- With the patient sitting, head tilted down, place the transducer at the base of the skull, angled superiorly.
- At a depth of 7 to 8 cm, locate the vertebral arteries.
  - Sweep through the vessel and record the highest velocity Doppler signal, noting flow direction.
- Using the same approach, at a depth of 8 to 10 cm, identify the basilar artery.
  - Sweep through the vessel and record the highest velocity Doppler signal, noting flow direction.

Submandibular window:

- Use the submandibular approach to image the distal internal carotid artery if not able to image through the transtemporal or transorbital windows.
- The carotid artery is best evaluated via the submandibular approach at a depth of 4.5 to 7 cm.

Notes

- Calculate mean velocities for all insonated arteries using the following equation:

$$\text{mean velocity} = \frac{(\text{PSV} - \text{EDV})}{3} + \text{EDV}$$

- Record the depths at which the artery of interest is insonated.
- Depths listed are for adults.

INTRAOPERATIVE EMBOLI MONITORING:

- Position headgear and mark the location of the temporal window.
- Set headgear and fix monitor to the ipsilateral MCA at a depth of 4.5 to 5.5 cm.
- Perform baseline examination, noting MCA velocities prior to induction of anesthesia.
- Document events (e.g., changes in mean velocities, emboli rate) during cross-clamping, shunt placement, plaque dissection, clamp removal, and arterial closure.
- Monitor the ipsilateral MCA in the recovery room for 20 minutes.
- Emboli rate is calculated and reported per hour.

NORMAL TCD FINDINGS

■ ARTERY	■ WINDOW	■ DEPTH (mm)	■ DIRECTION	■ MEAN FLOW VELOCITY
MCA	Temporal	30–60	Toward the probe	55 ± 12 cm/s
ACA	Temporal	60–85	Away	50 ± 11 cm/s
PCA	Temporal	60–70	Bidirectional	40 ± 10 cm/s
TICA	Temporal	55–65	Toward	39 ± 09 cm/s
ICA (siphon)	Orbital	60–80	Bidirectional	45 ± 15 cm/s
OA	Orbital	40–60	Toward	20 ± 10 cm/s
VA	Occipital	60–80	Away	38 ± 10 cm/s
BA	Occipital	80–110	Away	41 ± 10 cm/s

ACA, anterior cerebral artery; BA, basilar artery; ICA, internal carotid artery; MCA, middle cerebral artery; OA, ophthalmic artery; PCA, posterior cerebral artery; TCD, transcranial Doppler; TICA, terminal internal carotid artery; VA, vertebral artery.

Documentation Requirements: Normal Examination

- Record all Doppler signals at an angle of zero degrees, when possible.
- Record mean velocity for all arteries insonated.
- Record the depth ranges for each artery insonated.

Transtemporal window:
- Spectral Doppler analysis, velocity measurements, and flow direction from the following:
  - Middle cerebral artery (3 to 6 cm depth)
    - ❏ Proximal
    - ❏ Mid
    - ❏ Distal
  - Anterior cerebral artery (6 to 7 cm depth)
  - Posterior cerebral artery (6 to 7 cm depth)
  - Terminal segment of the internal carotid artery (6 to 7 cm depth)
  - Anterior communicating artery (when identified as a collateral pathway)
  - Posterior communicating artery (when identified as a collateral pathway)

Transorbital window:
- Spectral Doppler recordings and velocity measurements from the following:
  - Ophthalmic artery (4 to 6 cm depth), when appropriate
  - Terminal segment or siphon of the internal carotid artery (if not imaged in the transtemporal window)

Transoccipital window:
- Spectral Doppler recordings and velocity measurements from the following:
  - Terminal vertebral artery (6 to 8 cm depth)
  - Basilar artery (8 to 12 cm depth)
    - ❏ Proximal
    - ❏ Distal

Documentation Requirements: Additional Findings or Abnormal Examination

- Document any regions of bruits, plaque, turbulence, delayed systolic upstroke, side-to-side asymmetry, or other abnormalities.
- Document signs of collateralization or vasospasm.
- Demonstrate velocities immediately proximal and distal to any region with a focal velocity increase.
- Documentation after intervention, including stenting, must include representative B-mode imaging and spectral Doppler waveforms with velocity measurements recorded at the proximal, mid-, and distal sites.

- For emboli monitoring, hold the probe on the vessel of interest for 10 to 15 minutes and record the number of emboli during that time period (Table A1.1).

LOWER EXTREMITY ARTERIAL PHYSIOLOGIC TESTING

Purpose:

To detect, diagnose, and characterize the severity of lower extremity arterial occlusive disease.

Indications:

- Diminished lower extremity pulses
- Claudication
- Lower extremity rest pain, ulceration, or gangrene
- Surveillance after intervention
- Prognosis for tissue healing
- Screening for peripheral arterial disease
- Screening for or evaluation of arterial injury

Extent of Examination:

- Examinations should be bilateral.
- Single-level physiologic testing (CPT® 93922) must include waveform recording; the examination includes the following:
  - Ankle-brachial index (ABI) and toe-brachial index (TBI), with pressures measured from the following:
    - ❏ Anterior tibial or dorsalis pedis artery
    - ❏ Posterior tibial artery (PT)
    - ❏ Peroneal artery (when indicated)
    - ❏ Digit (typically great toe or second toe)
- Multilevel physiologic testing (CPT® 93923) includes the following:
  - Segmental pressures
    - ❏ Doppler waveform analysis of the following:
      - ○ Brachial arteries
      - ○ Common femoral arteries
      - ○ Popliteal arteries
      - ○ Posterior tibial arteries
      - ○ Dorsalis pedis or anterior tibial arteries
    - ❏ Bilateral systolic pressure measurements:
      - ○ High thigh
      - ○ Low thigh
      - ○ Calf
      - ○ Ankle (posterior tibial artery)
      - ○ Ankle (dorsalis pedis or anterior tibial artery)
    - ❏ TBI

- Pulse volume recordings (PVR)—plethysmography
  - ❑ High thigh
  - ❑ Low thigh
  - ❑ Calf
  - ❑ Ankle
- The segmental pressures with Doppler waveforms and PVR give similar information about the level of arterial occlusive disease; performing one or both may follow institution-specific guidelines.
- Indications for performing a PVR or segmental pressure examination include an abnormal ABI found at an initial evaluation, or when ABIs are changed in a follow-up examination, as is demonstrated in Figure A1.1.
- Screen patients for treadmill testing if the patient's pain is related to exercise. Screening criteria for treadmill testing can be found in the Exercise Testing protocol.
- No pressure measurements are to be made with cuffs applied over bypass grafts, stents, dialysis access, central catheter lines, or other devices.
- Perform a TBI in lieu of ABI in patients with infrapopliteal interventions.

Equipment:

- Capabilities: continuous-wave Doppler, photoplethysmograph (PPG) for TBI, and air plethysmograph for PVR
- Transducers:
  - 5- to 10-MHz continuous-wave Doppler
  - Photoplethysmograph
- Blood pressure cuffs:
  - 10- to 12-cm cuffs for brachial and ankle pressures for ABI
  - 2.5-cm digit cuffs and PPG probes for TBI
  - High-thigh, low-thigh, below-knee, and ankle cuffs for PVR (four-cuff method, tapered cuffs).
  - High-thigh, low-thigh, below-knee, and ankle cuffs for segmental pressures (four-cuff method).
    - ❑ The width of the cuff should be 20% greater than the diameter of the limb at the site of cuff application.

Patient Positioning and Preparation:

1. Confirm study requested, patient identity, and examination indication.

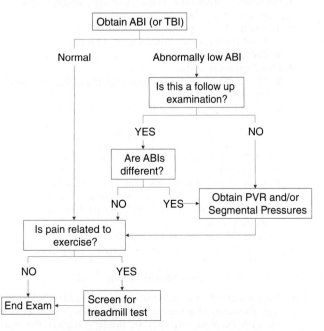

FIGURE A1.1 Indications for physiologic tests.

2. Review pertinent patient medical history and symptoms, including the presence and locations of any wounds or ulceration.
3. The patient should be in a resting supine position for 5 to 10 minutes prior to starting the examination.
4. Expose the patient's lower extremities as needed, using a gown to preserve privacy; use a gown or towels to avoid gel on the patient's clothing.

Evaluation Steps:

ANKLE-BRACHIAL INDEX (ABI):
1. Obtain bilateral brachial artery systolic blood pressures using continuous-wave Doppler techniques.
2. Begin examination with the right lower extremity.
3. Obtain bilateral posterior tibial and dorsalis pedis (or anterior tibial) artery systolic blood pressures using continuous-wave Doppler techniques.
   a. Insonate the artery of interest with a continuous-wave Doppler.
   b. Inflate the cuff 20 mm Hg above the last audible signal.
   c. Deflate the cuff slowly by 2 to 3 mm Hg increments until the first audible signals are heard.
   d. Record the pressure and Doppler waveform.
4. Obtain a systolic pressure from the peroneal artery if neither the anterior tibial nor posterior tibial artery signal is audible.
5. Evaluate the left lower extremity.
6. Calculate ABI:

   a. $\text{Right ABI} = \dfrac{\text{higher systolic pressure right ankle}}{\text{higher brachial pressure}}$

   b. $\text{Left ABI} = \dfrac{\text{higher systolic pressure left ankle}}{\text{higher brachial pressure}}$

   c. The higher of the two brachial artery pressures is used for both denominators.

TOE-BRACHIAL INDEX (TBI):
1. Evaluate the right side and then the left side.
2. Photoplethysmography is used to obtain systolic pressures from the great toes.
   a. Inflate the toe cuff 20 mm Hg above the level that flattens the PPG waveform.
   b. Deflate the cuff slowly by 2 to 3 mm Hg increments until a pulsatile PPG signal is detected.
   c. Record the pressure and plethysmographic waveform.
3. Obtain bilateral systolic brachial artery blood pressures using continuous-wave Doppler techniques (if not already done).
4. Calculate TBI:

   a. $\text{Right TBI} = \dfrac{\text{systolic pressure right toe}}{\text{higher brachial pressure}}$

   b. $\text{Left TBI} = \dfrac{\text{systolic pressure left toe}}{\text{higher brachial pressure}}$

   c. The higher of the two brachial artery pressures is used for both denominators.

PULSE VOLUME RECORDINGS:
1. For the four-cuff method, tapered pneumatic cuffs are placed at the high thigh, low thigh, below knee, and proximal to the ankle.
2. A standardized quantity of air is used to inflate the cuffs to a supravenous pressure (~60 mm Hg).
3. Volume changes that occur in the limb at the level of the cuffs are detected and displayed as pulsatile (volume pulse)

waveforms. These waveforms are evaluated for differences between consecutive cuff segments and between extremities.

SEGMENTAL PRESSURE MEASUREMENT:

1. Pneumatic cuffs are placed at the high thigh, low thigh, below knee, and proximal to the ankle.
2. Segmental systolic arterial pressures are obtained from both lower extremities at the high-thigh, low-thigh, below-knee, and ankle levels. Pressure gradients and lower extremity: arm ratios are used to assess the presence, level, and severity of peripheral arterial disease.
3. Proceed distal to proximal, sequentially inflating the ankle, below-knee, low-thigh, and high-thigh cuffs in the following fashion:
   a. Inflate the cuff 20 mm Hg above the last audible signal in the ankle.
   b. Deflate the cuff slowly by 2 to 3 mm Hg increments until the first audible signal is heard.
   c. Record the pressure and Doppler waveform.
4. Obtain ankle pressures for both the pedal arteries and in the bilateral brachial arteries to calculate an ABI.
5. Perform a TBI.
6. Record Doppler waveforms at the common femoral, popliteal, posterior tibial, and anterior tibial arteries.
7. Calculate lower extremity: arm indices at each level, using the higher of the two brachial artery pressures for the denominator at all levels.

Documentation Requirements:

ANKLE-BRACHIAL INDEX (ABI):
- Bilateral brachial artery systolic pressures
- Doppler waveform and systolic pressure measurement of the bilateral:
  - Posterior tibial arteries
  - Dorsalis pedis or anterior tibial arteries
  - Peroneal arteries (when indicated)
- ABI calculation

TOE-BRACHIAL INDEX (TBI):
- Bilateral brachial artery systolic pressures
- Photoplethysmographic (volume pulse) waveform and systolic pressure measurement from the bilateral toes.
  - The first (great) toe is typically used, but other toes may be used if the first toe is deformed, absent, or otherwise unusable for pressure measurements.
- Toe PPG waveform
- TBI calculation

PULSE VOLUME RECORDINGS:
- For the four-cuff method, PVR (volume pulse) waveforms at the bilateral:
  - High thigh
  - Low thigh
  - Below knee (calf)
  - Ankle
- For the three-cuff method, only one PVR waveform at the thigh level is obtained.

SEGMENTAL PRESSURES:
- Doppler waveform from the bilateral:
  - Common femoral arteries
  - Popliteal arteries
  - Posterior tibial arteries
  - Dorsalis pedis or anterior tibial arteries
- Bilateral systolic pressure measurements:
  - High thigh
  - Low thigh

- Below knee (calf)
- Ankle (posterior tibial artery)
- Ankle (dorsalis pedis or anterior tibial artery)
- TBI measurement is included.
- Lower extremity: arm indices are reported at each level tested.

LOWER EXTREMITY EXERCISE TESTING

Purpose:

To identify arterial occlusive disease that may not be hemodynamically significant at rest, to characterize the severity of intermittent claudication, and to distinguish true (vasculogenic) intermittent claudication from other causes of lower extremity symptoms caused by walking.

Indications:

- Claudication symptoms
- Evaluation after intervention

Extent of Examination:

- All testing should be bilateral.
- No pressures are to be measured over bypass grafts or stents.
- A complete examination (CPT® 93924) includes the following:
  - Ankle-brachial index (ABI) at rest.
  - ABI immediately after—and at timed intervals after—exercise on a treadmill.
  - Record walking time to onset of symptoms (pain-free walking time) and maximum walking time.
  - Toe-brachial index (TBI) may be used if the ankle pressure cannot be accurately measured.

Equipment:

- Treadmill (calibrated for speed and incline)
- Measurement capabilities: continuous-wave Doppler, photoplethysmograph (PPG) for TBI, and air plethysmography for PVR
- Transducers:
  - 5- to 10-MHz continuous-wave Doppler
  - Photoplethysmograph
- Blood pressure cuffs:
  - 10- to 12-cm cuffs for brachial pressures and ankle pressures for ABI
  - 2.5-cm digit cuffs and PPG probes for TBI

Patient Positioning and Preparation:

1. Confirm study requested, patient identity, and examination indication.
2. Review pertinent patient symptoms and medical history, and in particular the nature of lower extremity symptoms and conditions that might be contraindications to exercise testing.
3. Expose the patient's lower legs as needed.
4. Shoes should be worn if appropriate for the examination.

Procedural Steps:

1. Screen patients for contraindications to treadmill testing, including shortness of breath or chest pain at rest or with exercise, inability to safely complete the test, confusion, or systemic blood pressure greater than 200 mm Hg (Table A1.2 and Figure A1.2).

TABLE A1.2

EXERCISE TREADMILL TESTING: CONTRAINDICATIONS AND SAFETY GUIDELINES

■ CONTRAINDICATIONS TO TESTING	■ SAFETY GUIDELINES
• History of unstable angina or myocardial infarction within the last 6 mo • Patient required to carry nitroglycerin • Shortness of breath, chest or arm pain at rest or with walking • Limited walking ability due to arthritis, neuropathy, joint disease, gangrene, age, stroke, prosthesis, or critical limb ischemia • Instability, dizziness, confusion • Systolic blood pressure exceeding 200 mm Hg	• Use the auto-off safety clip. • The patient should wear shoes. • Testing in bare feet should be done with caution. • The patient should step on and off from the side of the treadmill at its lowest point. • The patient should remain in front of safety line while walking. • The test may be terminated at any time at the discretion of the technologist.

2. Obtain resting ankle and brachial pressures, per protocol.
3. Leave both ankle cuffs and one brachial cuff (on higher pressure side) on the patient.
4. Attach the safety auto-off clip to the patient.
5. Instruct the patient to use front handrail and walk in front of the safety line at all times.
6. Start the patient waking on the treadmill with the following settings (Figure A1.2):
   a. Speed: 2.0 mph.
   b. Grade: 0% initial grade. Increase grade by 2% every 2 minutes.
   c. Duration: 10 minutes, or until patient's maximum walking ability.
   d. If the patient cannot tolerate the settings, the speed or grade may be decreased as needed. Document the speed and grade used.

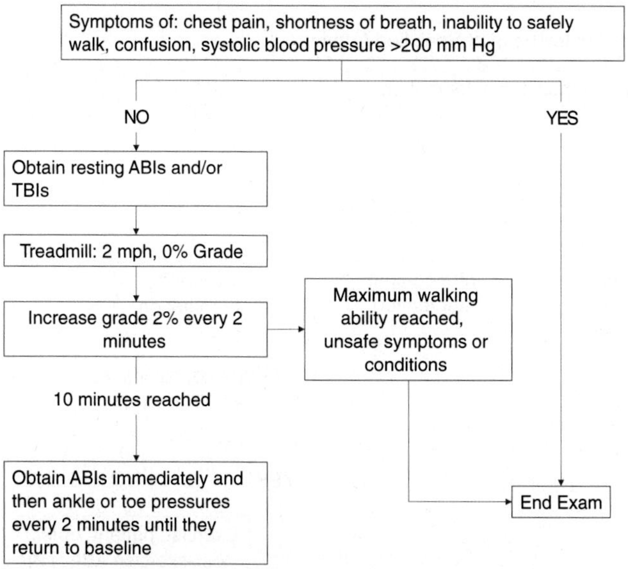

FIGURE A1.2 Protocol for treadmill testing.

7. Monitor patient at all times for safety (steadiness) as well as symptoms of chest pain, shortness of breath, and leg, thigh, or hip pain.
8. Document the symptoms the patient develops during exercise, including time of onset, severity, and location.
9. Have the patient lie supine immediately on completion of treadmill walking.
10. Measure brachial and bilateral ankle pressures at completion of treadmill walking (within 1 minute of stopping walking).
11. Repeat ankle pressure measurements at 2-minute intervals until the pressures are within 10 mm Hg of the baseline measurement.

Documentation Requirements:

■ Ankle-brachial index, per protocol:
  ● At rest (baseline)
  ● Immediately after exercise
■ Ankle pressure measurements:
  ● At 2-minute intervals until the pressures are normalized or within 10 mm Hg of the baseline measurement
■ Toe-brachial index per protocol, when indicated
■ Documentation of the following:
  ● Time of onset of symptoms, severity, and location
  ● Maximal walking time
  ● Total time to recovery

LOWER EXTREMITY ARTERIAL DUPLEX

Purpose:

To evaluate lower extremity arteries for stenosis or other abnormalities. Lower extremity duplex examinations are typically performed to detect, diagnose, and characterize the severity of arterial occlusive disease. Specialized examinations include evaluation of bypass grafts, follow-up of endovascular therapies, suitability of the lower extremity arteries for the purpose of autologous transplantation, and other purposes.

Indications:

■ Abnormal lower extremity pulse examination
■ Intermittent claudication
■ Ischemic rest pain
■ Lower extremity ulceration or gangrene
■ Trauma, suspected arterial occlusion, pseudoaneurysm, or arteriovenous fistula
■ Surveillance after endovascular intervention or peripheral arterial bypass
■ Follow-up of a known arterial stenosis
■ New onset of lower extremity symptoms after an intervention
■ Intraoperative evaluation of a peripheral arterial bypass graft
■ Preoperative evaluation of the peroneal artery prior to fibula free flap

Extent of Examination:

■ A complete bilateral study (CPT® 93925) evaluates the following:
  ● Aorta and bilateral common, internal, and external iliac arteries (see Aorto-iliac for protocol) when the examination suggests a proximal stenosis
  ● Common femoral artery (CFA), deep femoral artery, and superficial femoral artery (SFA)

- Popliteal artery
- Tibioperoneal trunk
- Posterior tibial artery (PT), anterior tibial artery (AT), and peroneal artery
- Bypass graft or stent, when present

■ A prefibula free-flap arterial assessment (CPT® 93925 bilateral, 93926 unilateral) evaluates the following:
- Popliteal artery
- Posterior tibial artery (PT), anterior tibial artery (AT), and peroneal artery
- Perforators from the peroneal artery
- Popliteal vein
- Posterior tibial veins and peroneal veins

■ An ankle-brachial index (ABI) should be included with all examinations, except in the case of infrapopliteal interventions:
- Include a toe-brachial index (TBI) when tibial vessels are calcified, in the setting of infrapopliteal intervention, when specifically requested, or when the ABI is suspected to unreliable.
- Include a treadmill test, if indicated after aortoiliac intervention, or when symptoms are associated with exercise, as shown in Figure A1.3.
- Cuffs should not be applied for pressure measurement over bypass grafts, stents, dialysis access, central catheter lines, or other devices.
- See Lower Extremity: Arterial Physiologic Testing for protocol.

■ Indications for a unilateral or limited examination (CPT® 93926) may include surveillance after intervention, intraoperative examination, or arterial injury.

■ For suspected vessel injury, including pseudoaneurysm, traumatic injury, and suspected arteriovenous fistula, the native arteries (CPT® 93926) proximal and distal to the injury, as well as the surrounding veins of interest (CPT® 93971), are evaluated.

Equipment and Supplies:

■ System capabilities: B-mode, color, and spectral Doppler and continuous-wave Doppler (for ABI)
■ Transducers:
- 5- to 10-MHz linear probe
- Curved 2- to 5-MHz probe for increased depths, if needed

- 5-MHz continuous-wave Doppler for ABI measurement
- L15 to L7 MHz compact linear array probe for intraoperative examination

■ Sterile probe covers for intraoperative examinations
■ Photoplethysmograph (PPG) for TBI measurements
■ 10- to 12-cm blood pressure cuff for ABI measurement
■ 2.5-cm digit cuffs for TBI measurement

Patient Positioning and Preparation:

1. Confirm study requested, patient identity, and examination indication.
2. Review pertinent patient medical history and symptoms.
3. The patient should fast 4 hours prior to the examination if the abdominal aorta or iliac vessels are included in the evaluation.
4. Expose the patient's lower extremity, using a gown to preserve privacy; use a gown or towels to avoid getting gel on the patient's clothing.
5. Position the patient supine with the leg bent slightly at the knee and externally rotated.
6. For a preoperative assessment of the peroneal artery, the patient should lie in the lateral decubitus position with the knee bent.

Evaluation Steps:

COMPLETE EVALUATION:
1. Begin the examination with the right lower extremity.
2. Doppler sampling should occur at intervals that approximate the length of the transducer.
3. Record Doppler signals at an angle of 60 degrees when possible.
4. Sample volume should be small (unless documenting an occlusion or trying to obtain a signal through plaque).
5. B-mode imaging is used to depict vessel anatomy from the level of the external iliac artery to the calf; assess for presence of intraluminal echoes, plaque, or other abnormalities.
6. Color flow Doppler can be used to assess vessel patency.
7. Spectral Doppler flow velocity measurements and velocity ratios are applied to determine presence and severity of stenoses.
8. Record Doppler spectra (at approximately probe length intervals, or less) through any graft body or

FIGURE A1.3 Algorithm for examination after lower extremity intervention.

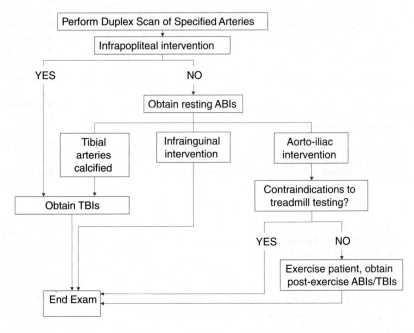

stent; the inflow and outflow vessels of any stent or graft should be identified.

9. If indicated, perform an Aorto-iliac study per protocol.
10. Perform an ABI per protocol, except after infrapopliteal intervention.
11. If indicated, perform a TBI.
12. If indicated, perform treadmill testing.

LIMITED EVALUATION:

1. Evaluate the native arteries proximal to, distal to, and in the area of interest using B-mode imaging and spectral Doppler.
2. For evaluation of arterial injury, also evaluate the veins above, below, and at the area of interest using B-mode and spectral Doppler imaging to assess for patency and flow characteristics; evaluate for vein compressibility.
3. Perform an ABI per protocol (or when requested), or if it is expected that arterial flow to the distal limb is affected.
4. If a pseudoaneurysm is evaluated, demonstrate the following:
   a. Flow characteristics within the pseudoaneurysm and within the neck.
   b. Measure the size of the pseudoaneurysm and the length of the neck.
5. If a graft is present, image the proximal and distal anastomoses as well as the proximal, mid-, and distal graft.
6. If a stent is present, image the vessel proximal and distal to the ends of the stent as well as the proximal, mid-, and distal stent.

PREOPERATIVE ARTERIAL EVALUATION (PERONEAL ARTERY BASED FLAP):

1. Obtain bilateral resting ABIs using the anterior tibial artery or dorsalis pedis artery, posterior tibial artery, and peroneal arteries.
   a. If the ABI is abnormal: contact the ordering physician before proceeding.
   a. If the ABI is normal: proceed with the examination.
2. Assess the popliteal, tibial, and peroneal arteries with spectral Doppler.
3. Identify all perforator arteries.
   a. Perforator arteries arise from the peroneal artery and course toward the fibula or may course parallel to the peroneal artery before coursing toward the fibula.
   b. Mark the skin to indicate the perforators with a dashed line and dots to indicate the origin and termination points.
   c. Measure the location (distance in cm from the malleolus) for each perforator.
4. Assess the popliteal, posterior tibial, and peroneal veins for patency.

Documentation Requirements: Normal Examination

COMPLETE EVALUATION:

- ■ B-mode imaging
  - ● Representative images from the following:
    - ❑ Aorta, common, and external iliac arteries (when indicated)
    - ❑ Common femoral artery
    - ❑ Superficial femoral artery
    - ❑ Proximal deep femoral artery
    - ❑ Popliteal artery
    - ❑ Tibioperoneal trunk, posterior tibial artery, anterior tibial artery, and peroneal artery (when indicated)
- ■ Spectral Doppler analysis
  - ● Obtain waveforms and measure peak systolic velocities at the following:
    - ❑ Aorta and common and external iliac artery (when indicated)
    - ❑ Common femoral artery
    - ❑ Deep femoral artery origin
    - ❑ Superficial femoral artery
      - ○ Proximal
      - ○ Mid
      - ○ Distal
    - ❑ Popliteal artery
      - ○ Proximal
      - ○ Mid
      - ○ Distal
    - ❑ Anterior tibial artery
    - ❑ Tibioperoneal trunk
    - ❑ Posterior tibial artery
    - ❑ Peroneal artery
- ■ Ankle-brachial index
- ■ Toe-brachial index (when indicated)

LIMITED EVALUATION:

- ■ B-mode and spectral Doppler imaging of the following:
  - ● Arterial segment of interest
  - ● Arterial segments:
    - ❑ Proximal to injury
    - ❑ Distal to injury
  - ● Veins (trauma or iatrogenic injury)
    - ❑ Proximal to injury
    - ❑ Adjacent to injury
    - ❑ Distal to injury
- ■ Ankle-brachial index

PREOPERATIVE ARTERIAL EVALUATION:

- ■ B-mode imaging
  - ● Representative images of the following:
    - ❑ Posterior tibial
    - ❑ Popliteal artery
  - ● Representative images, diameter measurements, and distance from the lateral malleolus:
    - ❑ Peroneal artery
      - ○ Proximal
      - ○ Mid
      - ○ Distal
  - ● Complete vein wall coaptation of the following:
    - ❑ Popliteal vein
    - ❑ Posterior tibial and peroneal veins
- ■ Spectral Doppler analysis
  - ● Obtain waveforms and measure peak systolic velocities at the following:
    - ❑ Popliteal artery
    - ❑ Anterior tibial artery
      - ○ Proximal
      - ○ Mid
      - ○ Distal
    - ❑ Posterior tibial artery
      - ○ Proximal
      - ○ Mid
      - ○ Distal
    - ❑ Peroneal artery
      - ○ Proximal
      - ○ Mid
      - ○ Distal
  - ● Demonstrate phasicity and augmentation at the following:
    - ❑ Popliteal vein
- ■ Color Doppler analysis
  - ● Identify and mark:
    - ❑ Perforator arteries from the peroneal artery
  - ● Demonstrate patency of the following:
    - ❑ Posterior tibial and peroneal vein
- ■ Ankle-brachial index

Documentation Requirements: Additional Findings or Abnormal Examination

- Document any regions of concern (plaque or other abnormalities) with both B-mode imaging and spectral Doppler.
- Demonstrate velocities immediately proximal and distal to any region with a focal velocity increase.
- Documentation after bypass or stenting must include representative B-mode image and spectral Doppler waveforms with velocity measurements recorded at the proximal, mid-, and distal sites.
  - Spectral Doppler evaluation of the inflow and outflow arteries must be included as well as waveforms from throughout the graft or stent.
  - If a bypass graft is identified without detectable flow (suggesting occlusion), it is important to evaluate medially and laterally to ensure that there is not more than one graft present. An occluded graft may be a prior failed bypass graft.
  - Changes in velocities may occur at the anastomoses if the graft and native arteries differ in diameter. Size discrepancy should be described.
- Images with color flow Doppler alone or power Doppler may be used to help demonstrate regions of concern or stenosis to better display abnormalities.
  - It should be recognized that this feature alone can falsely over- or underestimate stenosis severity.
- For a pseudoaneurysm, note the following:
  - Flow characteristics
  - Size of the following:
    - Pseudoaneurysm
    - Neck
  - Perform the same protocol for a postprocedure evaluation of a pseudoaneurysm after thrombin injection as for the preprocedure evaluation.
- Two images in the region of interest should be obtained with B mode from different views to demonstrate the absence of a structure, pseudoaneurysm, or mass.

UPPER EXTREMITY ARTERIAL PHYSIOLOGIC TESTING

Purpose:

To evaluate the upper extremity for the presence and location of arterial occlusive disease, including evaluations after provocative maneuvers.

Indications:

- Sensitivity to cold or suspected vasospastic disease
- Symptoms of thoracic outlet syndrome
- Upper extremity arterial insufficiency, including ischemia of the fingers
- Postoperative or postintervention evaluation
- Follow-up after aortic debranching procedures

Extent of Examination:

- Examinations should be bilateral.
- Multilevel physiologic testing (CPT® 93923) includes the following:
  - Upper extremity segmental pressures
    - Doppler waveform analysis of the bilateral:
      - Subclavian arteries
      - Axillary arteries
      - Brachial arteries
      - Radial arteries
      - Ulnar arteries
    - Systolic pressure measurements:
      - Arm
      - Forearm
      - Wrist (ulnar artery)
      - Wrist (radial artery)
    - Plethysmographic waveforms (PPG) from digits of interest
  - Thoracic outlet syndrome evaluation
    - PPG waveforms from the bilateral index fingers are recorded before and after provocative maneuvers.
  - Digit ischemia evaluations
    - PPG waveforms from all digits are recorded before and after provocative maneuvers.
- No pressure measurements are to be made with cuffs applied over bypass grafts, stents, or dialysis access.

Equipment:

- Capabilities: continuous-wave (or pulsed) Doppler, photoplethysmograph (PPG)
- Transducers:
  - 5- to 10-MHz continuous wave Doppler
  - Photoplethysmograph
- Blood pressure cuffs:
  - 10- and 7-cm cuffs for brachial and forearm segmental blood pressures
  - 2.5-cm digit cuff for digit pressures

Patient Positioning and Preparation:

1. The examination room should have a controlled temperature.
2. Confirm study requested, patient identity, and examination indication.
3. Review pertinent patient medical history and symptoms, including the presence and locations of any wounds or ulceration.
4. The patient should rest supine position for 5 to 10 minutes prior to starting the examination.
5. Expose the patient's upper extremities as needed, using a gown to preserve privacy; use a gown or towels to avoid gel on the patient's clothing.

Evaluation Steps:

1. Evaluate the right upper extremity and then the left.
2. Place cuffs on the arm, forearm, and wrist to measure systolic blood pressures from the arm, forearm, and wrist using both radial and ulnar arteries.
3. Record spectral Doppler waveforms from the subclavian, axillary, brachial, radial, and ulnar arteries.
4. Obtain photoplethysmographic waveforms from the digit(s) of interest.
5. Perform provocative maneuvers:
   a. Cold sensitivity:
      i. Place the photoplethysmographic probe on the symptomatic finger or index finger of each hand, and record the PPG waveform.
      ii. Place the hand in a small plastic bag to protect the probe.
      iii. Have the patient immerse hands in ice water for 3 minutes.
      iv. Record arterial waveform after immersion, and if abnormal at 5 and 10 minutes.
   b. Thoracic outlet syndrome:
      i. Place photoplethysmographic probe on the symptomatic finger or index finger of each hand.

ii. Record PPG waveforms while the patient performs coordinated arm movements. For each maneuver, record the PPG waveform with the patient's head turned to the left and to the right:
1. Resting
2. Arm abducted to 90 degrees
3. Arm abducted to 180 degrees
4. Military position (shoulders back, chest out)
5. Any specific position(s) associated with the patient's symptoms

Documentation Requirements:

DOPPLER WAVEFORM ANALYSIS
- Obtain waveforms from the following:
  - Subclavian artery
  - Axillary artery
  - Brachial artery
  - Radial artery
  - Ulnar artery

PHOTOPLETHYSMOGRAPHIC (PPG) WAVEFORM ANALYSIS
- Index finger or symptomatic finger(s)

SEGMENTAL PRESSURE MEASUREMENT:
- Arm
- Forearm
  - Wrist
  - Radial artery
  - Ulnar artery
- Digits of interest (plethysmography)

PROVOCATIVE MANEUVERS (WHEN APPLICABLE):
- Pre- and post-ice water immersion
  - PPG waveforms are obtained (and systolic blood pressures may be measured) from the symptomatic digit(s) in each hand at the following intervals:
    - Resting.
    - Immediately postimmersion.
    - 5 minutes' postimmersion.
    - 10 minutes' postimmersion.
    - If immediate postimmersion pressures are unchanged from baseline, the 5- and 10-minute postimmersion evaluations are not required.
- Thoracic outlet syndrome evaluation
  - PPG waveforms will be obtained during all maneuvers. During each maneuver, the patient will turn head to the left and to the right and the resulting findings will be appropriately recorded:
    - Resting
    - Arm elevated to 90 degrees
    - Arm elevated to 180 degrees
    - Military position (shoulders back, chest out)

UPPER EXTREMITY ARTERIAL DUPLEX

Purpose:

To evaluate upper extremity arteries for stenosis or other abnormalities. Upper extremity duplex examinations may be performed to detect, diagnose, and characterize the severity of arterial occlusive disease, but are often performed to evaluate the suitability of the upper extremity arteries prior to dialysis access creation or radial artery harvesting for autologous transplantation.

Indications:

- Diminished or absent upper extremity pulses
- Exertional arm pain (arm claudication)
- Finger ulceration or gangrene
- Follow-up after endovascular intervention or bypass graft
- Upper extremity trauma, suspected pseudoaneurysm, or arteriovenous fistula
- Preoperative evaluation for patients needing hemodialysis access
- Preoperative evaluation prior to radial artery harvesting for coronary artery bypass grafting (CABG)
- Preoperative evaluation of the radial artery prior to forearm free flap

Extent of Examination:

- A complete upper extremity arterial examination (CPT® 93930) evaluates the arteries of both upper extremities (bilateral):
  - Innominate artery (evaluate when proximal stenosis is suspected)
  - Subclavian arteries
  - Axillary arteries
  - Brachial arteries
  - Radial and ulnar arteries
- Indications for a unilateral or limited examination (CPT® 93931) include surveillance after intervention, suspected vessel injury, and when specifically requested.
- Pre-CABG arterial assessment (CPT® 93930 bilateral, 93931 unilateral) includes the following:
  - Bilateral complete (or unilateral limited) upper extremity arterial examination
  - Diameter measurements of the radial artery
  - Assessment of the radial artery with ulnar artery compression
  - Assessment of the ulnar artery with radial artery compression
  - Allen test
- Preforearm free-flap arterial assessment (CPT® 93930 bilateral, 93931 unilateral) includes the following:
  - Bilateral complete (or unilateral limited) upper extremity arterial examination
  - Diameter measurements of the radial artery
  - Assessment of the radial artery with ulnar artery compression
  - Assessment of the ulnar artery with radial artery compression
  - Assessment of the radial veins
  - Allen test
- For suspected vessel injury (including pseudoaneurysm, traumatic injury, and suspected arteriovenous fistula), the native arteries (CPT® 93931) proximal and distal to the injury, as well as the surrounding veins of interest (CPT® 93971), are evaluated.
- Examinations should include bilateral brachial blood pressures.
  - Pressure measurements should not be made with cuffs placed over bypass grafts, stents, dialysis access, central catheter lines, or other devices.

Equipment and Supplies:

- System capabilities: B-mode, color, and spectral Doppler and continuous-wave Doppler (for brachial artery pressure measurement)
- Transducer:
  - 5- to 10-MHz linear probe
  - Curved 2 to 5 MHz (to examine the origin of the subclavian arteries, if needed)

- Photoplethysmograph for digit pressure evaluation with Allen test
- 10- to 12-cm blood pressure cuff for bilateral brachial blood pressure measurements
- 2.5-cm digit cuffs for digit pressure measurements

Patient Positioning and Preparation:

1. Confirm study requested, patient identity, and examination indication.
2. Review pertinent patient medical history and symptoms.
3. Expose the patient's upper extremity, using a gown to preserve privacy; use a gown or towels to avoid getting gel on the patient's clothing.
4. The patient should lie in a supine position with the arm slightly bent at the elbow and the palm turned upward (anterior) with the arm in a relaxed position, abducted laterally.

Evaluation Steps:

COMPLETE EVALUATION:

1. Begin the bilateral examination with the right upper extremity.
2. Duplex ultrasound is used to evaluate the upper extremity arteries. B-mode imaging is used to depict vessel anatomy and to identify intraluminal echoes, plaque formation, or other abnormalities.
3. Color flow Doppler is used to assess vessel patency.
4. Spectral Doppler flow velocity measurements and ratios are used to determine the presence and severity of stenoses.
5. Measure bilateral brachial artery blood pressures.

LIMITED EVALUATION:

1. Evaluate the arteries proximal to, distal to, and at the area of interest using B-mode imaging and spectral Doppler.
2. For the evaluation of arterial injury, also evaluate the veins above, below, and at the area of interest using B-mode and spectral Doppler imaging to assess for patency and flow characteristics; evaluate for vein compressibility.
3. Measure bilateral brachial artery blood pressures.
4. If a pseudoaneurysm is evaluated, demonstrate the following:
   a. Flow characteristics within the pseudoaneurysm and within the neck.
   b. Measure the size of the pseudoaneurysm and the length of the neck.
5. If a graft is present, image the proximal and distal anastomoses as well as the proximal, mid-, and distal graft.
6. If a stent is present, image the vessel proximal and distal to the ends of the stent as well as the proximal, mid-, and distal stent.

PREOPERATIVE ARTERIAL EVALUATION:

1. Perform a complete upper extremity arterial evaluation, as described above.
2. Assess the ulnar artery flow velocities, with and without radial artery compression.
3. Assess the radial artery flow velocities, with and without ulnar artery compression.
4. Perform an Allen test:
   a. Attach a photoplethysmographic (PPG) probe to the first and fifth digits of the hand.
   b. Record representative PPG waveforms and digit pressures with the following maneuvers:
      i. No arterial compression
      ii. Ulnar artery compression
      iii. Radial artery compression

5. Obtain bilateral brachial artery systolic pressures measurements.
6. For evaluations prior to forearm free-flap procedures, assess the radial veins for patency.

Documentation Requirements: Normal Examination

COMPLETE EXAMINATION:

- B-mode imaging
  - Representative images from the following:
    - Innominate artery (when indicated)
    - Subclavian artery
    - Axillary artery
    - Brachial artery
    - Radial and ulnar arteries
- Spectral Doppler analysis
  - Record all Doppler signals at an angle of 60 degrees, when possible.
  - Obtain waveforms and measure peak systolic velocities at the following:
    - Innominate artery (when indicated)
    - Subclavian arteries
    - Axillary arteries
      - Proximal
      - Distal
    - Brachial arteries
      - Proximal
      - Mid
      - Distal
    - Radial arteries
      - Proximal
      - Mid
      - Distal
    - Ulnar arteries
      - Proximal
      - Mid
      - Distal
- Measure and record bilateral systolic brachial blood pressures.

LIMITED EVALUATION:

- B-mode imaging and spectral Doppler of the following:
  - Arterial segment of interest
  - Arterial segments
    - Proximal to injury
    - Distal to injury
  - Veins (when indicated)
    - Proximal to injury
    - Adjacent to injury
    - Distal to injury
- Measure and record bilateral systolic brachial blood pressures.

PREOPERATIVE ARTERIAL EVALUATION:

- Document complete upper extremity arterial study.
- Additional B-mode imaging.
  - Vein wall coaptation with compression:
    - Radial veins (for forearm free flap)
  - Diameter measurements
    - Radial artery
      - Proximal
      - Mid
      - Distal
- Additional color Doppler imaging.
  - Demonstrate patency of the radial veins
- Additional spectral Doppler analysis.
  - Obtain waveforms and measure peak systolic velocities at the following:
    - Radial artery with ulnar artery compression
    - Ulnar artery with radial artery compression

- Photoplethysmographic waveforms and pressure measurements from digits (Allen test) with the following:
  - No arterial compression
  - Ulnar artery compression
  - Radial artery compression
- Measure and record bilateral systolic brachial blood pressures.

Documentation Requirements: Additional Findings or Abnormal Examination

- Document any regions of plaque or other abnormalities with both B-mode and spectral Doppler imaging.
- Demonstrate velocities immediately proximal and distal to any region with a focal velocity increase.
- Documentation after bypass or stenting must include representative B-mode imaging and spectral Doppler waveforms with velocity measurements recorded at the proximal, mid-, and distal sites.
  - Spectral Doppler evaluation of the inflow and outflow arteries must be included as well as waveforms from throughout the graft or stent.
  - Increase velocities may occur at anastomoses if the vessels differ in diameter. Size discrepancy should be described.
- For a pseudoaneurysm, note the following:
  - Flow characteristics
  - Size of pseudoaneurysm
  - Length of neck
- Perform the same protocol for a postprocedure evaluation of a pseudoaneurysm as the preprocedure evaluation.
- Two images in the region of interest should be obtained with B mode from different views to demonstrate the absence of any abnormal structure, pseudoaneurysm, or mass.

LOWER EXTREMITY VENOUS DUPLEX

Purpose:

To evaluate the lower extremity veins for patency, presence of acute thrombus, postthrombotic changes, or other abnormalities.

Indications:

- Concern for deep vein thrombosis (DVT) due to swelling, calf tenderness, or erythema
- Concern for or confirmed pulmonary embolism (PE)
- Follow-up of previously diagnosed DVT
- Part of a complete venous reflux examination
- Following up after endoluminal thermal ablation of superficial lower extremity veins, including RF ablation and laser procedures

Extent of Examination:

- Veins evaluated in the lower extremity venous examination include the following:
  - Inferior vena cava (IVC) and common iliac and external iliac veins (when indicated)
    - Indications for IVC evaluation include presence of a femoral catheter, pelvic pathology, prior IVC filter placement, or abnormal common femoral vein (CFV) waveforms.
  - Common femoral vein (CFV), deep femoral vein, femoral vein, and popliteal vein
  - Posterior tibial (PTV) veins and peroneal veins
  - Gastrocnemius and soleal veins (when indicated, for example, with calf symptoms)
  - Great and small saphenous veins (when indicated)
- A bilateral (CPT® 93970) or unilateral (CPT® 93971) examination may be requested.
- Perform a bilateral examination on all inpatients, patients with systemic symptoms or concern for pulmonary embolism (PE), patients with a positive unilateral examination, or if specifically requested. This is specified in Figure A1.4. If the indications are uncertain for a unilateral examination, then a bilateral examination should be done.
- An examination after endovenous ablation (CPT® 93971) includes the following:
  - After great saphenous vein ablation, assess the following:
    - Common femoral vein
    - Saphenofemoral junction
    - Deep femoral vein

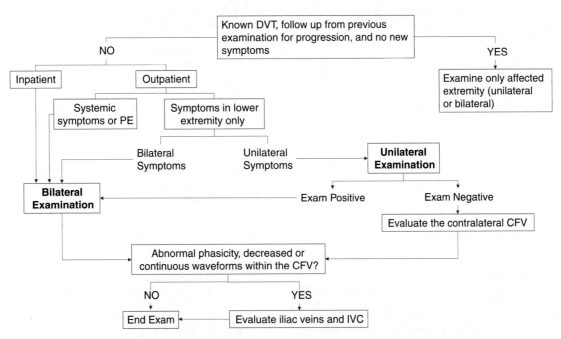

FIGURE A1.4 Algorithm depicting indications for determining the extent of a lower extremity venous duplex.

❏ Femoral vein
❏ Great saphenous vein
● After small saphenous vein ablation, assess the following:
  ❏ Femoral vein
  ❏ Popliteal vein
  ❏ Posterior tibial and peroneal veins
  ❏ Small saphenous vein

Equipment:

■ System capabilities: B mode, color Doppler, and spectral Doppler
■ Transducers:
  ● 5- to 10-MHz linear probe
  ● Curved 2- to 5-MHz probe for increased depths, if needed

Patient Positioning and Preparation:

1. Confirm study requested, patient identity, and examination indication.
2. Review pertinent patient medical history and symptoms.
3. Place the examination table or bed in reverse Trendelenburg position.
4. Position the patient supine with the leg bent at the knee and externally rotated in a relaxed position.
   a. The popliteal vein may also be visualized with the patient prone.
   b. The peroneal veins may be better visualized from the lateral malleolus.
5. Expose the patient's lower extremity, using a gown to preserve privacy; use a gown or towels to avoid getting gel on the patient's clothing.

Evaluation Steps:

COMPLETE EXAMINATION:

1. Begin the examination with the right lower extremity or the extremity of interest in a unilateral examination.
2. B-mode imaging is used from the inguinal ligament to the ankle to evaluate the venous anatomy and to look for the presence of intraluminal echoes in the deep and superficial veins.
3. Sequential probe compressions are performed in a transverse view throughout all segments to evaluate for complete vein wall coaptation.
4. Color flow and spectral Doppler are used to evaluate vessel patency and venous flow characteristics including spontaneity, respiratory phasicity, and response to augmentation.
5. If performing a unilateral examination, a spectral Doppler waveform must be obtained from the contralateral common femoral vein.
   a. If there is an abnormal waveform or loss of respiratory phasicity in a common femoral vein, an iliac vein and IVC evaluation should be completed.
6. If indicated by symptoms or clinical findings, obtain representative B-mode images of compression in the great saphenous vein at the femoral confluence and midthigh as well as the small saphenous vein.
   a. Perform when specifically requested, or with suspicion of thrombosis.

POST-RFA EXAMINATION:

1. B-mode imaging is used to depict the anatomy and the presence of intraluminal echoes in the deep veins of the lower extremity 10 cm proximal and distal to the junction of the superficial veins and the deep veins of interest.
2. Sequential probe compressions are performed throughout all segments to evaluate for complete wall coaptation.

3. Color flow and spectral Doppler are used to evaluate vessel patency and venous flow characteristics including spontaneity, respiratory phasicity, and response to augmentation.
4. Document patency or occlusion of the superficial vein of interest.
5. Document maximum and minimum great saphenous vein diameters, when applicable (prior to intervention).

Documentation Requirements: Normal Examination

COMPLETE EXAMINATION:

■ B-mode imaging
  ● Transverse (axial) images demonstrating vein wall coaptation at the level of the following:
    ❏ Common femoral vein at the saphenofemoral junction
    ❏ Femoral vein in the proximal thigh with the deep femoral vein
    ❏ Femoral vein in the distal thigh
    ❏ Popliteal vein
    ❏ Posterior tibial veins
    ❏ Peroneal veins
■ Spectral Doppler analysis
  ● Record all Doppler signals at an angle of 60 degrees, when possible.
  ● Demonstrate respiratory phasicity and responses to distal augmentation maneuvers in the following:
    ❏ Common femoral vein
    ❏ Femoral vein
    ❏ Popliteal vein
  ● For unilateral examinations, a spectral Doppler waveform will be obtained from the contralateral common femoral vein.
■ Color flow Doppler:
  ● Document patency of posterior tibial veins and peroneal veins.

Documentation Requirements: Additional Findings or Abnormal Examination

■ IVC and iliac veins (when indicated):
  ● B-mode imaging
    ❏ Inferior vena cava
    ❏ Common iliac vein
      ○ Proximal
      ○ Distal
    ❏ External iliac vein
  ● Spectral Doppler waveforms:
    ❏ Common iliac vein
    ❏ External iliac vein
  ● Color Doppler demonstrating patency
    ❏ Inferior vena cava
■ Calf veins (when indicated):
  ● B-mode transverse images demonstrating vein wall coaptation, color Doppler demonstrating patency of muscular veins:
    ❏ Gastrocnemius veins
    ❏ Soleal veins
■ Superficial veins (when indicated):
  ● B-mode transverse images demonstrating vein wall coaptation:
    ❏ Great saphenous vein
      ○ At the saphenofemoral junction
      ○ Midthigh
    ❏ Small saphenous vein
  ● Color Doppler
    ❏ Great saphenous vein
    ❏ Small saphenous vein

POST-RFA EXAMINATION:

- B-mode images
  - Treated great saphenous vein, evaluate for the following:
    - ❏ Incompressibility
    - ❏ Vein wall thickening
    - ❏ Increased echogenicity
  - Transverse images demonstrating vein wall coaptation of the following:
    - ❏ Common femoral vein at the saphenofemoral junction (SFJ)
      - ○ Femoral vein in the proximal thigh with the deep femoral vein
      - ○ Femoral vein and midthigh
  - After small saphenous vein ablation, assess the following:
    - ❏ Femoral vein
    - ❏ Popliteal vein
    - ❏ Posterior tibial and peroneal veins
    - ❏ Small saphenous vein
- Spectral Doppler examination
  - Demonstrate respiratory phasicity and responses to distal augmentation maneuvers:
    - ❏ After great saphenous vein ablation:
      - ○ Common femoral vein at the level of the SFJ
    - ❏ After small saphenous vein ablation, assess the following:
      - ○ Popliteal vein
- Use color flow or spectral Doppler analysis to evaluate great saphenous or small saphenous vein patency.
- Document maximum and minimum great or small saphenous vein diameters, when applicable.
- Document any regions of abnormalities with both B-mode imaging and spectral Doppler.
- Document presence of any additional tributaries, as needed.

LOWER EXTREMITY VENOUS REFLUX EVALUATION

Purpose:

To evaluate the lower extremity veins for venous obstruction and valvular function.

Indications:

- Varicose veins
- Venous stasis ulceration
- Venous claudication
- Leg swelling or pain
- History of deep vein thrombosis
- Pre- or postoperative evaluation for patients treated with endovenous thermal ablation

Extent of Examination:

- Examinations should be bilateral, unless specifically requested (CPT® 93965).
- A complete examination includes the following:
  - Lower extremity venous duplex examination to assess for thrombosis, chronic occlusion, or post-thrombotic changes
    - ❏ See Lower Extremity Venous Duplex for protocol.
  - Venous reflux evaluation
    - ❏ Common femoral vein
    - ❏ Femoral vein
    - ❏ Popliteal vein
    - ❏ Great saphenous vein
    - ❏ Small saphenous vein

Equipment:

- System capabilities: B mode, color Doppler, and spectral Doppler
- Transducers:
  - 5- to 10-MHz linear probe
  - Curved 2- to 5-MHz probe for increased depths, if needed
- Rapid cuff inflator and deflator
- Tapered thigh cuff with large diameter tubing for venous reflux testing
- 12-cm cuffs (these cuffs also have large diameter tubing and are designed for venous reflux testing)

Patient Positioning and Preparation:

1. Confirm study requested, patient identity, and examination indication.
2. Review pertinent patient medical history and symptoms.
3. Place the examination table or bed in reverse Trendelenburg position for the evaluation for venous thrombosis or obstruction.
4. Position the patient supine with the leg bent at the knee and externally rotated in a relaxed position.
   a. The popliteal vein may also be visualized with the patient prone.
   b. The peroneal veins may be better visualized from the lateral malleolus.
5. Expose the patient's lower extremity, using a gown to preserve privacy; use a gown or towels to avoid getting gel on the patient's clothing.
6. Testing for venous valvular function is performed with the patient standing; reflux-provoking test maneuvers are standardized by the use of pneumatic cuffs, which are automatically inflated and deflated.
   a. The patient is evaluated in a supported standing position.
   b. The limb to be evaluated is relaxed and nonweight bearing by having the patient stand on a platform designed to allow the leg to dangle or with the patient standing with support from an orthopedic frame.
   c. Thigh and calf cuffs are positioned:
      i. For reliable compression of deep veins in the thigh, the width of the cuff should approximate the diameter of the limb.
      ii. Preset the pressure on the rapid cuff inflator to 80 mmHg.

Evaluation Steps:

1. Perform a lower extremity venous duplex, per protocol.
2. The deep and superficial veins of the lower extremity are evaluated with duplex scanning to determine the presence of reflux with the standing distal cuff deflation technique.
   a. The patient stands, using a stepstool or other support, as described above.
   b. Weight is carried on the contralateral lower extremity; the extremity to be examined is kept in a relaxed, slightly knee-bent position.
   c. Evaluation is first done with the thigh cuff.
      i. Identify the common femoral vein in long axis (above the thigh cuff) and obtain a Doppler spectral waveform.
      ii. Using the automatic cuff inflator, inflate the cuff to a pressure of 80 mm Hg for 3.0 seconds.
      iii. The cuff is then rapidly deflated.
      iv. Pulsed Doppler is used to detect and measure the duration of venous reflux in the common femoral vein (retrograde venous flow).
   d. Evaluation is then done with the 12-cm calf cuff, after removing the thigh cuff.

i. Identify the popliteal vein in long axis (above the calf cuff) and obtain a Doppler spectral waveform.
ii. The cuff inflator inflates the cuff to a pressure of 100 mm Hg for 3.0 seconds.
iii. The cuff is then rapidly deflated.
iv. Pulsed Doppler is used to detect and measure the duration of venous reflux in the popliteal vein (retrograde venous flow).
e. The great saphenous vein should be evaluated in a similar fashion in the proximal, mid-, and distal thigh with the use of the calf cuff.

Documentation Requirements: Normal Examination

- B-mode images
  - Vein compression in transverse views (per lower extremity venous duplex protocol)
    - ❏ Common femoral vein at the saphenofemoral junction
    - ❏ Femoral vein in the proximal thigh (with the deep femoral vein)
    - ❏ Femoral vein and distal thigh
    - ❏ Popliteal vein
    - ❏ Posterior tibial veins
    - ❏ Peroneal veins
  - Vein wall compression and diameter measurements (maximum and minimum)
    - ❏ Great saphenous vein
    - ❏ Small saphenous vein
- Spectral Doppler analysis
  - Record all Doppler signals at an angle of 60 degrees, when possible.
  - Demonstrate respiratory phasicity and responses to distal augmentation maneuvers (per lower extremity venous duplex protocol) in the following:
    - ❏ Common femoral vein
    - ❏ Femoral vein
    - ❏ Popliteal vein
  - Reflux evaluation is done at multiple deep and superficial vein sites:
    - ❏ Common femoral vein
    - ❏ Great saphenous vein
      - ○ Saphenofemoral junction
      - ○ Midthigh
      - ○ Knee
    - ❏ Femoral vein
    - ❏ Popliteal vein
    - ❏ Small saphenous vein
- Color flow Doppler (per lower extremity venous duplex protocol):
  - Posterior tibial veins and peroneal veins

Documentation Requirements: Additional Findings or Abnormal Examination

- Document tortuous segments, perforators, or accessory saphenous vein tributaries.
- Document any regions of concern or other abnormalities with both B-mode and spectral Doppler imaging.
- Document any additional tributaries, as needed.

VEIN MAPPING: LOWER EXTREMITY

Purpose:

To evaluate the great and small saphenous veins prior to harvesting for use as bypass conduit.

Indication:

- Preoperative examination prior to bypass or dialysis access procedures

Extent of Examination:

- A bilateral (CPT® 93970) examination should be done in most cases, although a unilateral (CPT® 93971) examination may be requested.
- A complete examination includes the evaluation of the following:
  - Great saphenous veins.
  - Accessory saphenous veins, when identified.
  - The small saphenous vein is evaluated when the great saphenous vein is found to be inadequate for use, as shown in Figure A1.5.
- The upper extremity superficial veins are evaluated if there are no adequate veins in the lower extremities.
- Vein diameter measurements must be obtained anterior to posterior and inner wall to inner wall.

Equipment:

- System capabilities: B mode, color Doppler, and spectral Doppler
- Transducers:
  - 5- to 10-MHz linear probe
- Gentian violet dispensed from a vial, syringe, and cotton swab
- Tape measure

Patient Positioning and Preparation:

1. Confirm study requested, patient identity, and examination indication.
2. Review pertinent patient medical history and symptoms.
3. Expose the patient's lower extremity, using a gown to preserve privacy; use a gown or towels to avoid getting gel or dye on the patient's clothing.
4. The patient should lie in supine position with the lower extremity bent slightly at the knee, externally rotated in a relaxed position.
5. Place the examination table or bed in reverse Trendelenburg position.

Evaluation Steps:

1. Begin the examination with the right lower extremity, or the extremity of interest in a unilateral examination.

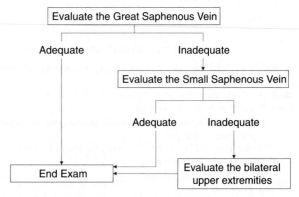

FIGURE A1.5 Evaluation of superficial lower extremity veins prior to harvest for bypass grafting.

2. B-mode imaging is used to depict the anatomy, patency, and appearance of the superficial veins of the lower extremity, from the inguinal ligament to the ankle.
3. Sequential probe compressions are performed in transverse view throughout all segments to evaluate for complete wall coaptation.
4. If a vein segment appears abnormal, color flow and spectral Doppler may be used to confirm vein patency.
5. Measurements are recorded along the great saphenous vein in the proximal, mid-, and distal thigh, knee level, midcalf, and at the ankle.
6. Scanning the vein in a transverse plane, the location of the vein is marked on the patient's skin using Gentian violet, if requested.
7. The length of the vein is measured, when indicated.
8. Evaluate any accessory great saphenous veins.
9. Image the ipsilateral small saphenous vein, if indicated.
   a. Record images at the knee, midcalf, and ankle.
   b. Only mark the small saphenous vein when the great saphenous vein appears inadequate for use.

Documentation Requirements:

- B-mode images
  - Transverse images demonstrating vein wall coaptation and diameter measurements (inner wall to inner wall) of the following:
    - ❑ Great saphenous vein at the following:
      - ○ Proximal thigh
      - ○ Midthigh
      - ○ Distal thigh
      - ○ Knee level
      - ○ Midcalf
      - ○ Ankle
    - ❑ Small saphenous vein (when indicated)
      - ○ Ankle
      - ○ Midcalf
      - ○ Knee
    - ❑ Any accessory great saphenous veins identified
- Doppler analysis
  - At least one image documenting patency of the great saphenous vein (either color or spectral Doppler)
- If requested, measure the length of the veins.
- If requested, mark the course of the vein on the leg.

UPPER EXTREMITY VENOUS DUPLEX

Purpose:

To evaluate the upper extremity veins for patency, presence of acute thrombus, postthrombotic changes, or other abnormalities.

Indications:

- Concern for deep venous thrombosis (DVT): swelling, tenderness, or erythema
- Concern for or confirmed pulmonary embolism (PE)
- Suspicion of venous thoracic outlet obstruction
- Follow-up of previously diagnosed DVT
- As part of preprocedural assessment

Extent of Examination:

- Veins evaluated in the upper extremity venous examination include the following:
  - Internal jugular vein
  - Subclavian vein (when possible)
  - Axillary vein
  - Brachial vein
  - Cephalic and basilic veins
- A bilateral (CPT® 93970) or unilateral (CPT® 93971) examination may be requested.
- Complete a bilateral examination on patients with systemic symptoms or concern for PE, patients with a positive unilateral examination, or if specifically requested. This is demonstrated in Figure A1.6. If the indications for a bilateral versus a unilateral examination are uncertain, then a bilateral examination should be done.

Equipment:

- System capabilities: B mode, color Doppler, and spectral Doppler
- Transducers:
  - 5- to 10-MHz linear probe
  - Phased array 2- to 4-MHz probe for increased depths, if needed

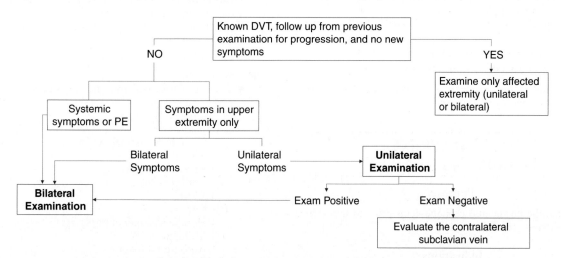

FIGURE A1.6 Algorithm for determining the extent of an upper extremity venous duplex.

Patient Positioning and Preparation:

1. Confirm study requested, patient identity, and examination indication.
2. Review pertinent patient medical history and symptoms.
3. Expose the patient's upper extremity, using a gown to preserve privacy; use a gown or towels to avoid getting gel on the patient's clothing.
4. The patient should lie supine with the arm slightly bent and rotated outward in a relaxed position.

Evaluation Steps:

- Begin the examination with the right upper extremity, or the extremity of interest in a unilateral examination.
- B-mode imaging is used to depict the anatomy and the presence of intraluminal echoes in the deep veins of the upper extremity from the neck to the wrist.
- Sequential probe compressions are performed throughout all segments to determine complete wall coaptation.
- Color flow and spectral Doppler are used to evaluate vessel patency and venous flow characteristics including spontaneity, respiratory phasicity, cardiac pulsatility, and response to augmentation.
- If performing a unilateral examination, a spectral Doppler waveform must be obtained from the contralateral subclavian vein.

Documentation Requirements: Normal Examination

- B-mode imaging
  - Transverse images demonstrating vein wall coaptations of the following:
    - ❑ Internal jugular vein
    - ❑ Subclavian vein (when possible)
    - ❑ Axillary vein
    - ❑ Brachial veins
    - ❑ Cephalic and basilic veins
- Spectral Doppler analysis
  - Record all Doppler signals at an angle of 60 degrees, when possible.
  - Demonstrate respiratory and cardiac phasicity in the following:
    - ❑ Internal jugular vein
    - ❑ Innominate vein (when possible)
    - ❑ Subclavian vein
    - ❑ Axillary vein
  - For unilateral examinations: A spectral Doppler waveform will be obtained from the contralateral subclavian vein.
- Color flow Doppler:
  - Cephalic, basilic, and brachial veins (when necessary)

Documentation Requirements: Additional Findings or Abnormal Examination

- Document any regions of abnormalities with both B-mode imaging and spectral Doppler.

VEIN MAPPING: UPPER EXTREMITY

Purpose:

To evaluate the basilic and cephalic veins prior to harvesting for use as bypass conduit.

Indications:

- Preoperative examination prior to bypass procedure

- As part of a preoperative assessment prior to a dialysis access procedure

Extent of Examination:

- A bilateral (CPT® 93970) examination should be done in most cases, although a unilateral (CPT® 93971) examination may be requested.
- A complete examination includes the evaluation of the following:
  - Cephalic vein
  - Basilic vein

Equipment:

- System capabilities: B mode, color Doppler, and spectral Doppler
- Transducers:
  - 5- to 10-MHz linear probe
- Gentian violet dispensed from a vial, syringe, and cotton swab
- Tape measure

Patient Positioning and Preparation:

1. Confirm study requested, patient identity, and examination indication.
2. Review pertinent patient medical history and symptoms.
3. Expose the patient's upper extremity, using a gown to preserve privacy; use a gown or towels to avoid getting gel or dye on the patient's clothing.
4. The patient should lie in supine position with the upper extremity bent slightly at the elbow and externally rotated in a relaxed position.

Procedural Steps:

1. Begin the examination with the right lower extremity, or the extremity of interest in a unilateral examination.
2. Evaluate patency of the veins with color or spectral Doppler.
3. Evaluate the veins with probe compressions in transverse view to identify areas of thickening, thrombus, or other abnormalities.
4. Record measurements along the veins in the proximal and midarm, antecubital fossa, midforearm, and at the wrist.
5. Scan through the vein in a transverse plane and mark the location of the vein on the patient's skin using Gentian violet, if requested.
6. The length of the veins is measured, if indicated.

Documentation Requirements:

- B-mode images
  - Transverse images demonstrating vein wall coaptation and diameter measurements (inner wall to inner wall) of the following:
    - ❑ Cephalic vein
      - ○ Shoulder/proximal upper arm
      - ○ Midupper arm
      - ○ Antecubital fossa
      - ○ Midforearm
      - ○ Wrist
    - ❑ Basilic vein
      - ○ Shoulder/proximal upper arm
      - ○ Midupper arm
      - ○ Antecubital fossa
      - ○ Midforearm
      - ○ Wrist

- Doppler analysis
  - At least one image will be obtained to show patency of the vessel (either spectral Doppler or color flow image).
- If requested, measure the length of the veins.
- If requested, mark the course of the vein on the arm.

AORTOILIAC ARTERIAL DUPLEX

Purpose:

To evaluate for stenosis, occlusion, or other abnormalities (including aneurysms) of the abdominal aorta and iliac arteries. Additional roles for aortoiliac duplex scanning include surveillance after endovascular aneurysm repair (EVAR) and follow-up after surgical bypass or stenting.

Indications:

- Aneurysm screening (age >55 years, family history of aneurysm, history of smoking, concomitant aneurysms, or inability to evaluate by physical examination due to obesity or other factors)
- Pulsatile mass on abdominal examination
- Follow-up of known iliac artery or abdominal aortic aneurysms
- Evidence of lower extremity occlusive inflow disease after the evaluation of the lower extremity arteries
- Claudication, diminished pulses, ischemic rest pain, lower extremity ulceration, or gangrene
- Follow-up of a known aortoiliac stenosis
- Surveillance after endovascular intervention or arterial bypass
- New onset of symptoms after an intervention
- Aortic coarctation
- Distal emboli

Extent of Examination:

- Indications for a complete study (CPT® 93978) include an initial abdominal aorta or iliac artery evaluation as well as an initial inflow bypass graft evaluation.
  - The examination evaluates the flow characteristics and diameter of the following:
    - ❏ Aorta from the suprarenal aorta to the bifurcation
    - ❏ Bilateral common iliac artery (CIA), internal iliac artery (IIA), and external iliac artery (EIA)
    - ❏ Bypass graft or stent, when present
  - After endovascular aneurysm repair (CPT® 93971), surveillance duplex examination evaluates the following:
    - ❏ From the suprarenal aorta to the distal fixation sites within the iliac arteries
    - ❏ Celiac artery, superior mesenteric artery (SMA), renal arteries, and inferior mesenteric artery (IMA)
    - ❏ Any patent lumbar artery branches
    - ❏ Internal iliac arteries
- Indications for a limited study (CPT® 93979) include follow-up after intervention as well as follow-up of a known abdominal aortic or iliac artery aneurysm, stenosis, or other pathologies.
  - The limited examination evaluates the flow characteristics and diameter of the following:
    - ❏ Aorta from the suprarenal aorta to the bifurcation
    - ❏ Bilateral common iliac arteries
    - ❏ Bilateral internal and external iliac arteries, when specifically indicated
    - ❏ Bypass graft or stent, when present
    - ❏ Excluded aneurysm sac diameter and flow characteristics

- An ankle-brachial index (ABI) should be included with all examinations, except in the case of infrapopliteal interventions.
  - Include a toe-brachial index (TBI) when tibial vessels are calcified, in the setting of infrapopliteal intervention, when specifically requested, or when the ABI measurement is greater than 1.40 or otherwise suspected to be unreliable.
  - Include a treadmill test, if indicated, after aortoiliac intervention or when symptoms are associated with leg exercise.
  - No systolic pressures are to be obtained over bypass grafts, stents, dialysis access, central catheter lines, or other devices.
  - See Lower Extremity: Arterial Physiologic Testing for protocol.

Equipment:

- System capabilities: B-mode imaging and color and spectral Doppler
- Transducer:
  - 2- to 5-MHz curved array probe
  - 5- to 10-MHz continuous-wave Doppler for ABI measurement
  - Photoplethysmograph probe for TBI measurements
- 10- to 12-cm blood pressure cuffs for ABI measurement
- 2.5-cm digit cuffs and PPG for TBI measurement

Patient Positioning and Preparation:

1. Confirm examination requisition, patient identity, and examination indication.
2. Obtain pertinent patient medical history and current symptoms.
3. The patient should fast overnight or for at least 4 hours prior to the examination.
4. Expose the patient's abdomen, using a gown to preserve privacy; use gown or towels to avoid gel on the patient's clothing.
5. The patient should lie in supine position.
6. The lateral decubitus position may be used in patients with a large abdominal girth or when bowel gas interferes with imaging in the supine position.

Procedural Steps:

COMPLETE EXAMINATION

1. B-mode imaging is used to depict vessel anatomy, diameter, and intraluminal abnormalities.
2. Obtain longitudinal images of the abdominal aorta from the suprarenal aorta to the bifurcation.
3. Using B-mode imaging in a lateral and anteroposterior planes, record maximal diameters of the abdominal aorta.
4. Color flow Doppler is used to assess vessel patency.
5. Spectral Doppler flow velocity measurements and ratios are applied to determine the presence and severity of stenoses.
6. The common iliac, external iliac, and internal iliac arteries are evaluated in the same fashion, bilaterally.
7. Perform an ABI, per protocol.

LIMITED EXAMINATION:

1. Evaluate the abdominal aorta as in a complete examination.
2. When indicated, the common iliac, external iliac, and internal iliac arteries are evaluated.
3. Perform an ABI, per protocol.

POST-EVAR EXAMINATION:

1. Evaluate the abdominal aorta in a similar fashion as in a complete examination.
2. Measure the size of the excluded aneurysm sac; measure the largest diameter and circumference and note the location of the measurement.
3. Measure the diameter and flow velocities within the graft limbs and iliac arteries.
4. Use spectral Doppler to note the velocity of flow within the celiac artery, SMA, and renal arteries.
5. Use color Doppler to assess for flow within the aneurysm sac; if detected, evaluate further with pulsed Doppler.
6. Assess for any patent lumbar branches.
7. Perform an ABI, per protocol.

Documentation Requirements: Normal Examination

COMPLETE EVALUATION:

- B-mode imaging
  - Longitudinal images of the abdominal aorta:
    - Proximal
    - Mid
    - Distal
  - Axial (transverse) views with maximum diameter measurements:
    - Aorta
      - Suprarenal (at the level of the celiac artery/SMA origins)
      - Pararenal (at the level of the renal arteries)
      - Infrarenal
      - Terminal (at the bifurcation)
    - Common iliac artery
      - Origin or proximal
      - Distal
    - Bilateral external iliac arteries
      - Proximal
      - Distal
    - Bilateral internal iliac arteries
      - Proximal (when visualized)
- Spectral Doppler analysis
  - Record all Doppler signals at an angle of 60 degrees, when possible.
  - Obtain waveforms and measure peak systolic and end-diastolic velocities:
    - Aorta
      - Proximal to or at level of SMA origin
      - Midinfrarenal segment
      - Distal
    - Visceral artery origins
      - Celiac artery
      - SMA
      - Renal arteries
    - Bilateral common iliac arteries
      - Origin
    - Bilateral external iliac arteries
    - Bilateral internal iliac arteries (when visualized)
- Ankle-brachial index
  - Toe-brachial index (when indicated)

LIMITED EVALUATION:

- B-mode imaging
  - Longitudinal images of the aorta:
    - Proximal
    - Mid
    - Distal
  - Axial views of the abdominal aorta at the following locations with maximum diameters measurements:
    - Aorta
      - Suprarenal (at the level of celiac artery/SMA origins)
      - Pararenal (at the level of renal arteries)

- Infrarenal
- Terminal (at the bifurcation)
  - Common iliac arteries, when indicated
  - Other iliac artery dimensions, when indicated
- Spectral Doppler analysis
  - Obtain waveforms and measure peak systolic and end-diastolic velocities of the following:
    - Aorta
      - SMA origin
      - Mid
      - Distal
    - Bilateral common iliac arteries
      - Origin
- Ankle-brachial index
  - Toe-brachial index (when indicated)

POST-EVAR EVALUATION:

- B-mode imaging
  - Longitudinal images of the aorta:
    - Proximal
    - Mid
    - Distal
  - Axial views of the abdominal aorta at the following locations with maximum diameters measurements:
    - Aorta
      - Suprarenal (at the level of the celiac artery/SMA origins)
      - Pararenal (at the level of the renal arteries)
      - Largest segment of the aneurysm sac; measure diameter and circumference
      - Proximal fixation site
    - Distal fixation sites
    - Internal iliac artery
      - Proximal
- Spectral Doppler analysis
  - Obtain waveforms and measure peak systolic and end-diastolic velocities, and note flow direction when pertinent in the following:
    - Aorta
      - Celiac axis
      - SMA origin
      - Proximal renal arteries
      - Inferior mesenteric artery origin (when present)
      - Proximal fixation site
      - Midendograft, proximal to the bifurcation
      - Right and left graft limbs
        - Proximal
        - Mid
        - Distal
    - Common iliac arteries
    - External iliac arteries
    - Internal iliac arteries
    - Patent lumbar branches
- Color flow Doppler analysis
  - Evaluate for flow within the aneurysm sac.
- Ankle-brachial index
  - Toe-brachial index (when indicated)

Documentation Requirements: Additional Findings or Abnormal Examination

- Document any regions of plaque, aneurysm, or other abnormalities with both B-mode imaging and spectral Doppler.
- Demonstrate velocities immediately proximal and distal to any region with a focal velocity increase.
- Documentation after bypass or stenting must include representative B-mode imaging and spectral Doppler

waveforms with velocity measurements recorded at the proximal, mid-, and distal sites.

- Spectral Doppler waveforms from inflow and outflow arteries must be included as well as waveforms from throughout a graft or stent.
- Increased velocities may occur at anastomoses if the vessels differ in diameter; size discrepancies should be described.
- Images with color flow Doppler (CFD) alone or color power Doppler (CPD) may be used. Color may help to characterize abnormalities, demonstrate stenoses, or better display flow abnormalities. CFD and CPD alone can falsely over- or underestimate stenosis severity.
- The residual lumen size is measured when mural thrombus is present.

VISCERAL DUPLEX: MESENTERIC

Purpose:

To evaluate for stenosis, occlusion, or other abnormalities within the mesenteric arteries and their branches.

Indications:

- Epigastric bruit
- Concern for mesenteric artery stenosis: postprandial abdominal pain, weight loss, food fear, and persistent diarrhea
- Suspected celiac artery compression syndrome
- Follow-up after aortic dissection
- Follow-up after mesenteric artery stenting or bypass graft
- Follow-up of known stenosis

Extent of Examination:

- A complete study (CPT® 93975) includes evaluation of the following:
  - Aorta
  - Celiac axis
  - Common hepatic artery
  - Splenic artery
  - Superior mesenteric artery (SMA)
  - Inferior mesenteric artery (IMA)
  - Bilateral renal arteries
  - Superior mesenteric vein (SMV) and inferior vena cava (IVC), when indicated
- A limited study (CPT® 93976) does not evaluate all of the arteries required in a complete study, for example, a renal artery ultrasound duplex scan.

Equipment:

- System capabilities: B-mode imaging and color and spectral Doppler
- Transducer:
  - 2- to 5-MHz curved array probe

Patient Positioning and Preparation:

1. Confirm examination requisition, patient identity, and examination indication.
2. Obtain pertinent patient medical history and current symptoms.
3. The patient should fast overnight or for at least 4 hours prior to the examination.
4. Expose the patient's abdomen, using a gown to preserve privacy; use gown or towels to avoid gel on the patient's clothing.
5. The patient should lie in supine position; reverse Trendelenburg may be used.
6. The lateral decubitus position may be used in patients with a large abdominal girth or when bowel gas interferes with imaging with the patient supine.

Procedural Steps:

1. B mode is used, scanning transversely through the length of the abdominal aorta for maximum size and presence of plaque to the level of the bifurcation.
2. Pulsed Doppler is then used to sample velocities in the abdominal aorta in the longitudinal plane.
3. Color flow Doppler is used, scanning transversely through the abdominal aorta, beginning just below the xiphoid process; sweeping distally, the celiac artery is identified arising anteriorly from the abdominal aorta.
4. The superior mesenteric artery (SMA) is then identified arising anteriorly from the abdominal aorta, with the left renal vein traversing between the SMA and aorta.
5. Moving the probe distally, the right and left renal arteries are identified, often arising approximately at the 10 o'clock and 4 o'clock positions, respectively.
6. Continuing to scan in the transverse plane, the inferior mesenteric artery is identified distal to the renal arteries at about the 2 o'clock position, just proximal to the aortic bifurcation.
7. Doppler flow velocity measurements should include a sample in the celiac artery origin in the transverse plane at a zero-degree Doppler angle.
8. The splenic and common hepatic arteries are evaluated for poststenotic turbulence.
9. Doppler flow velocity measurements at the origin of the SMA are made in the sagittal plane with a 60-degree Doppler angle.
10. Doppler interrogation should include a 60-degree sample at the origins of the right and left renal arteries.
11. A Doppler flow velocity measurement is made at the origin of the inferior mesenteric artery.

Documentation Requirements: Normal Examination

- B-mode imaging:
  - Axial or sagittal views as indicated at the following locations:
    - ❏ Suprarenal aorta
    - ❏ Celiac axis
    - ❏ Origin of the superior mesenteric artery
    - ❏ Origin of the common hepatic artery and splenic artery
    - ❏ Origin of the inferior mesenteric artery
    - ❏ Renal artery origins
    - ❏ Infrarenal aorta (with maximum diameter measurement)
- Spectral Doppler analysis
  - Record all Doppler signals at an angle of 60 degrees, when possible.
  - Obtain waveforms and measure peak systolic and end-diastolic velocities of the following:
    - ❏ Aorta
      - ○ At the SMA origin
      - ○ Mid
      - ○ Distal
    - ❏ Celiac artery, at the following locations:
      - ○ Origin
      - ○ Proximal
      - ○ Mid (when possible)
      - ○ Distal (when possible)
    - ❏ Common hepatic artery
    - ❏ Splenic artery

- Superior mesenteric artery, at the following locations:
  - Origin
  - Proximal
  - Mid
  - Distal
- Inferior mesenteric artery, at the following locations:
  - Origin
  - Proximal
- Bilateral renal arteries
  - Origin
  - Proximal
  - Mid
  - Distal
- Document patency of the superior mesenteric vein and inferior vena cava, if indicated.

Documentation Requirements: Additional Findings or Abnormal Examination

- Document any regions of plaque or other abnormalities with both B-mode imaging and spectral Doppler.
- Demonstrate velocities immediately proximal and distal to any region with a focal velocity increase.
- Document any areas of abnormal flow direction within the mesenteric arteries.
- Documentation after bypass or stenting must include representative B-mode imaging and spectral Doppler waveforms with velocity measurements recorded at the proximal, mid-, and distal sites.
  - Spectral Doppler waveforms of the inflow and outflow arteries must be included as well as waveforms from throughout the graft or stent.
  - Increased velocities may occur at anastomoses if the vessels differ in diameter; size discrepancies should be described.
- To evaluate for possible transient or reversible median arcuate ligament compression of the celiac artery, record waveforms in the celiac artery with and without deep inspiration.
- If the celiac artery is occluded, the gastroduodenal artery (GDA) should be evaluated for patency and flow direction.
- Images with color flow Doppler or power Doppler may be used to help demonstrate regions of concern or stenosis to better display abnormalities.

VISCERAL DUPLEX: RENAL ARTERIES

Purpose:

To evaluate for stenosis, occlusion, or other abnormalities of the renal arteries.

Indications:

- Resistant hypertension (persistent on multiple antihypertensive medications)
- Progressive renal insufficiency of unknown etiology
- Concern for renal artery stenosis
- Epigastric bruit
- Evaluation for fibromuscular dysplasia or renal artery aneurysm
- Follow-up after renal artery stenting or bypass graft
- Follow-up of known stenosis

Extent of Examination:

- A renal arterial duplex scan (CPT® 93976) includes evaluation of the bilateral:
  - Renal arteries, including superior and inferior segmental arteries

- Renal veins
- Kidney length measurements and parenchymal flow evaluation
- All examinations are bilateral, unless requested otherwise.

Equipment:

- System capabilities: B-mode imaging and color and spectral Doppler
- Transducer:
  - 2- to 5-MHz curved array probe

Patient Positioning and Preparation:

1. Confirm examination requisition, patient identity, and examination indication.
2. Obtain pertinent patient medical history and current symptoms.
3. The patient should fast overnight or for at least 4 hours prior to the examination.
4. Expose the patient's abdomen, using a gown to preserve privacy; use gown or towels to avoid gel on the patient's clothing.
5. The patient should start in a supine position for evaluation of the aorta and renal arteries, moving to lateral decubitus positions with arm raised above the head to evaluate the kidneys and distal renal arteries.

Procedural Steps:

1. From an anterior approach, the abdominal aorta is identified in transverse view just below the xiphoid process.
2. B mode is utilized to sweep through the abdominal aorta to evaluate for maximum size and presence of plaque.
3. Doppler flow velocity measurements are then made within the abdominal aorta in a longitudinal plane, with a peak systolic velocity recorded at the level of the superior mesenteric artery (SMA).
4. The pulsed Doppler sample volume should be as small as possible during the renal artery duplex examination.
5. Color flow Doppler is used to scan the aorta in the transverse plane beginning at the level of the xiphoid process.
6. Scanning distally, the celiac artery is first identified arising anteriorly from the abdominal aorta.
7. The superior mesenteric artery (SMA) is then be identified arising anteriorly from the abdominal aorta with the left renal vein traversing between the SMA and aorta.
8. Moving the probe distally, the right and left main renal arteries are identified arising approximately at the 10 o'clock and 4 o'clock positions, respectively.
9. Doppler spectral waveforms are obtained using a 60-degree angle at the origins of the right and left renal arteries.
10. The proximal and midrenal arteries are interrogated with a 60-degree Doppler angle from the anterior approach.
11. The patient is turned to the left lateral decubitus position.
12. The right kidney is evaluated in B mode and in long axis for length measurements; three measurements are obtained and averaged.
13. Color flow Doppler is used to demonstrate parenchymal flow.
14. The superior and inferior segmental arteries are evaluated with spectral Doppler.
15. The renal artery is evaluated at the hilum and the distal segment.

16. The renal vein is evaluated with Doppler at the hilum.
17. Repeat with the patient in the right lateral decubitus position to evaluate the left kidney.
18. Calculate the renal: aortic ratio (RAR) in the renal artery segment with the highest peak systolic velocity for each side with the following equation:

$$RAR = \frac{\text{Renal artery peak systolic velocity}}{\text{Aortic peak systolic velocity}}$$

Documentation Requirements: Normal Examination

- B-mode imaging
  - Longitudinal view of the aorta
  - Axial views at the following locations:
    - ❏ Infrarenal aorta (with maximum diameter measurement)
    - ❏ Origins of the renal arteries
    - ❏ Two sagittal views of both kidneys in long axis with pole-to-pole length measurements
- Color flow Doppler
  - Demonstrate flow in the parenchyma of the bilateral kidneys
  - Demonstrate patency of the renal veins at the hilum (color flow or spectral Doppler)
- Spectral Doppler analysis
  - Record Doppler signals at an angle of 60 degrees whenever possible and at zero degrees in the renal parenchyma.
  - Obtain waveforms and measure peak systolic and end-diastolic velocities of the following:
    - ❏ Aorta at the SMA origin
    - ❏ Renal arteries at the following locations:
      - ○ Origin
      - ○ Proximal
      - ○ Mid
      - ○ Distal
      - ○ Terminus at the hilum
  - Obtain waveforms and measure peak systolic velocity, end-diastolic velocity, and resistive index (RI) of the following:
    - ❏ Superior segmental branch arteries
    - ❏ Inferior segmental branch arteries

Documentation Requirements: Additional Findings or Abnormal Examination

- Document any regions of plaque or other abnormalities with both B-mode imaging and spectral Doppler.
- Demonstrate velocities immediately proximal and distal to any region with a focal velocity increase.
- Document any areas of abnormal flow direction within the mesenteric arteries.
- Documentation after bypass or stenting must include representative B-mode imaging and spectral Doppler waveforms with velocity measurements recorded at the proximal, mid-, and distal sites.
  - Spectral Doppler waveforms of the inflow and outflow arteries must be included as well as waveforms from throughout the graft or stent.
  - Increased velocities may occur at anastomoses if the vessels differ in diameter; size discrepancies should be described.

Resources

1. Society for Vascular Ultrasound. Professional Performance Guidelines. 2014. http://www.svunet.org/practicemanagement/professionalperformance guidelines
2. Intersocietal Accreditation Commission. IAC Standards and Guidelines for Vascular Testing Accreditation. February 1, 2015. http://www.intersocietal. org/vascular/main/standards.htm
3. American Medical Association. *CPT® 2015 Professional Edition*. Chicago, IL: American Medical Association.

VASCULAR LABORATORY EDUCATION AND TRAINING

Vascular laboratory professionals—technologists/sonographers and physicians—have specific knowledge and expertise in the use of noninvasive vascular testing. Entering the profession requires relevant education, training, and clinical experience. There are numerous pathways for meeting these requirements, but for individuals initially entering the field, a formal training program is the most common.

VASCULAR TECHNOLOGIST EDUCATION AND TRAINING

Training of vascular technologists (sonographers) can follow any of several different pathways. While it was common in the early days of vascular laboratories to recruit staff from nursing or other health care professions and then to provide on-the-job training, most vascular technologists now enter the field after completion of a prescribed course of study, typically in a degree program.

Educational standards for curriculum content have been established through consensus with input from multiple medical organizations and are outlined in the National Educational Curriculum (NEC) (http:\\www.jrcdms.org). These organizations include the American Registry for Diagnostic Medical Sonography (ARDMS) (http:\\www.ardms.org), Cardiovascular Credentialing International (CCI) (http:\\www.cci-online.org), the Commission on Accreditation of Allied Health Education Programs (CAAHEP) (http:\\www.caahep.org), the Joint Review Committee on Education in Diagnostic Medical Sonography (JRC-DMS) (http:\\www.jrcdms.org), the Joint Review Committee on Education in Cardiovascular Technology (JRC-CVT) (http:\\www.jrccvt.org), and several professional specialty societies.

Goals and essential elements of undergraduate educational programs have been outlined in a position paper from the Society for Vascular Ultrasound (SVU): Guidelines for Undergraduate Educational Programs in Vascular Ultrasound (http:\\www.svunet.org/advocacy/svupositionpapers). Programs need to prepare students with the cognitive, psychomotor, and affective skills and experience necessary to perform patient examinations, assess information from ultrasound images and related vascular testing, report summary findings, and use independent judgment and systematic problem solving. Vascular ultrasound programs may be based in a hospital or clinic, a community college or junior college, a 4-year college or university, or some other type of postsecondary vocational, technical, or proprietary school. Programmatic accreditation through CAAHEP is desirable.

Vascular ultrasound education takes 18 months or more of full-time study in a program that includes classroom education, student laboratories, and clinical experience. The curriculum will cover the range of noninvasive vascular examinations in sufficient detail for graduates to competently and independently perform complete examinations on a variety of patients as well as successfully pass their certification examinations.

Twelve months of supervised clinical experience (~1600 hours) performing vascular testing is typical. Clinical sites should be accredited by the Intersocietal Accreditation Commission (IAC) or the American College of Radiology (ACR).

PHYSICIAN EDUCATION AND TRAINING

There are several education and training pathways that physicians may follow to become vascular laboratory professionals. In the past, practicing physicians learned about vascular laboratory topics and acquired interpretation experience through a combination of self-directed learning, continuing medical education (CME) programs, and supervised practical and interpretive experience in an established vascular laboratory.

As the vascular laboratory developed and assumed an integral role in the care of vascular patients, learning about the use and interpretation of noninvasive vascular tests was incorporated into the curriculum of certain graduate medical education programs, including cardiology, vascular medicine, radiology, and other specialties. For vascular surgery residencies and fellowships in the United States and Canada, vascular laboratory training is a curriculum requirement, and the Registered Physician in Vascular Interpretation (RPVI) credential from the ARDMS is required by the Vascular Surgery Board of the American Board of Surgery (VSB-ABS) before a vascular surgeon may be considered for certification.

For their graduates to meet the RPVI prerequisites, graduate medical education and other training programs must provide didactic instruction and clinical experience with vascular testing. This includes a course of study that covers the techniques, limitations, accuracies, and methods of interpretation for the noninvasive vascular examinations that the physician will interpret. The physician must also acquire supervised practical experience in each testing area that includes observing or participating in testing procedures, and the physician must document experience with supervised interpretation of at least 500 studies that represent a broad range of tests and pathology. In the early phases of this experience, direct supervision by a clinical educator is needed.

CURRICULUM OUTLINE

Some of what a vascular laboratory physician is expected to know is general information learned in medical school, including anatomy, physiology, and the pathophysiology of vascular diseases. Much of the knowledge needed, however, is technical or specific to the evaluation of vascular disorders and is beyond the level taught in undergraduate medical education. For this, a curriculum covering core vascular laboratory competencies is needed. The Accreditation Council for Graduate Medical Education (ACGME) core competencies are described in Table A2-1.

TABLE A2-1

ACCREDITATION COUNCIL FOR GRADUATE MEDICAL EDUCATION (ACGME) CORE COMPETENCIES

Patient Care	Identify, respect, and care about patients' differences, values, preferences, and expressed needs; listen to, clearly inform, communicate with and educate patients; share decision-making and management; and continuously advocate disease prevention, wellness, and promotion of healthy lifestyles, including a focus on population health
Medical Knowledge	Established and evolving biomedical, clinical, and cognate sciences and the application of knowledge to patient care
Practice-Based Learning and Improvement	Investigation and evaluation of patient care provided, appraisal and assimilation of scientific evidence, and improvements in patient care
Interpersonal and Communication Skills	Effective information exchange and teaming with patients, families, and other health professionals
Professionalism	Carrying out professional responsibilities, adherence to ethical principles, and sensitivity to a diverse patient population
Systems-Based Practice	Awareness of and responsiveness to the larger context and system of health care and the ability to effectively use resources to provide care of optimal value

TABLE A2-2

MEDICAL KNOWLEDGE

■ PATIENT AND DISEASE STATES	■ ULTRASOUND PHYSICS	■ INSTRUMENTATION AND EQUIPMENT	■ TESTING PROTOCOLS AND INTERPRETATION CRITERIA
Normal anatomy, physiology, and hemodynamics (cerebrovascular, venous, peripheral arterial, abdominal/visceral)	Continuous wave and pulsed-wave Doppler	Examination facilities and patient care equipment	Transducer selection
	Pressure measurements	Duplex ultrasound scanner	Patient safety and bioeffects
Vascular pathology and pathophysiology (cerebrovascular, venous, peripheral arterial, abdominal/visceral)	B-mode imaging	Continuous-wave and pulsed-wave Doppler	Image assessment of vascular anatomy and pathology
	Color Doppler	Photoplethysmography (PPG)	Vessel measurement
	Power Doppler	Plethysmography	Velocity and velocity ratio criteria
	Ultrasound contrast agents	Laser Doppler	Waveform assessment
		Transcutaneous PO_2	Pressure indices
			Waveform indices (resistive index, pulsatility index)
			Provocative maneuvers
			Volume flow measurements
			Reflux testing

TABLE A2-3

PATIENT CARE (ELEMENTS OF INTERPRETATION OF VASCULAR LABORATORY EXAMINATIONS)

■ COMMON ELEMENTS	■ INDIVIDUAL EXAMINATION EVALUATION
Incorporate clinical indications in study interpretation	Identify and report on incidental findings
Incorporate physiologic and anatomic findings in interpretation	Incorporate comparison of present study with prior testing
Assess examination quality, accuracy, and completeness	Modify interpretation of tests due to anatomic or medical conditions
	Modify interpretation of tests due to technical limitations (e.g., artifacts)

TABLE A2-4

PATIENT CARE (TYPES OF VASCULAR LABORATORY EXAMINATIONS)

■ BASIC EXAMINATIONS	■ ADVANCED DIAGNOSTIC EXAMINATIONS	■ PROCEDURE PLANNING, GUIDANCE, MONITORING AND ASSESSMENT	■ SURVEILLANCE AND FOLLOW-UP EXAMINATIONS
Extracranial carotid and vertebral arteries	Transcranial Doppler (TCD) and transcranial duplex	Transcranial Doppler monitoring for carotid interventions	Carotid endarterectomy and stenting
Aortoiliac and lower extremity arterial—duplex scanning	Mesenteric, portal, and hepatic veins	Cardiovascular risk assessment	Infrainguinal bypass grafts
Lower extremity arteries— indirect physiologic assessment	Pelvic venous insufficiency	Vascular access	Peripheral artery interventions
Noninvasive diagnosis of upper extremity arterial disease	Trauma	Preoperative vein mapping	Aortic endografts
Aortic and peripheral artery aneurysms		Venous ablation	Dialysis access
Lower extremity venous thrombosis		Intraoperative evaluation of arterial repairs	Organ transplantation
Upper extremity venous thrombosis		Intravascular ultrasound and physiologic assessment	
Chronic venous insufficiency		Evaluation and treatment of femoral pseudoaneurysms	
Mesenteric arteries		Dialysis access planning	
Renal arteries		Radial artery evaluation prior to coronary artery bypass grafts	
		Duplex scanning prior to fibula free flap transfers	
		Duplex scanning prior to flap procedures for breast reconstruction	

Vascular laboratory competence requires physicians to gain specific **medical knowledge** in three domains: (1) patient and disease states, (2) physics and instrumentation, and (3) protocols and interpretation criteria (Table A2-2). While medical school curricula may address vascular anatomy, hemodynamic principles, physiology and pathophysiology, and clinical presentations of vascular diseases, a more advanced level of knowledge is required for vascular laboratory physicians. Topics such as ultrasound physics, operation of vascular laboratory equipment, and Doppler principles are not part of general knowledge for most physicians but must be understood to be able to interpret vascular examinations. In addition, specific knowledge of how vascular laboratory studies are performed and reported is needed.

With this foundational knowledge, the vascular laboratory physician provides a **patient care** service by interpreting vascular laboratory studies. In most cases, this professional service requires evaluation of examination findings, recognition of artifacts, consideration of patient-specific circumstances, and contextual integration of the available data (Tables A2-3 and A2-4). This patient care service is provided in each of the testing areas offered by the vascular laboratory (extracranial cerebrovascular, intracranial cerebrovascular, peripheral arterial, peripheral venous, visceral vascular, and screening).

The vascular laboratory physician and vascular technologist have a shared responsibility. The physician should understand the technologist's scope of practice and technical expertise; the technologist needs to provide the physician with appropriate images and documentation of examination findings. Ideally, the organization of the vascular laboratory should promote effective information exchange between team members and subsequent **communication** of the findings and interpretation to the requesting provider (Table A2-5).

Quality assurance (QA) and quality improvement (QI) require the participation and commitment of both the vascular laboratory's medical staff and technical personnel. Patient care can be improved by staff collaboration in performance reviews and outcomes assessments to confirm the quality and accuracy of the reported data. From the results of internal reviews, as well as recognition of scientific evidence and practice standards, vascular laboratories can implement new testing protocols or revise existing ones. This **practice-based learning and improvement** leads to better patient care (Table A2-6).

TABLE A2-5

COMMUNICATION AND REPORTING

Preliminary and final reports
Communicate critical findings to referring practitioner

TABLE A2-6

PRACTICE-BASED LEARNING AND IMPROVEMENT

Quality assurance
Quality improvement
Outcomes reporting
Test validation and revision
Facility accreditation
Credentialing and certification of personnel

TABLE A2-7

PROFESSIONALISM

Compliance with vascular laboratory and institutional policies

Protection of private health information (PHI)

TABLE A2-8

SYSTEMS-BASED PRACTICE

Evidence-based practice

Use of practice guidelines

Use of picture archiving and communication system (PACS)

Use of electronic health record and reporting

Physicians are expected to learn and practice **professionalism** in their vascular laboratory roles, including protection of private health information (PHI), prompt reporting of critical findings, and compliance with professional behavioral and performance standards (Table A2-7). It is also important to learn the important role of the vascular laboratory in **systems-based practice**. This can include systems of information management as well as systems of care. Modern vascular laboratory practices use informatics systems that function within larger networks and interface with other systems and users. Understanding how to effectively use these data management systems is essential (Table A2-8). Because vascular laboratories often function within health care systems, effective use of noninvasive vascular testing can provide benefits to patient care with concomitant reductions in the costs of care.

INSTRUCTIONAL METHODS

Reading, didactic instruction, and use of online courses can provide important background information, but practical in-person experience in the vascular laboratory is essential. The interpreting physician needs to know the details of the laboratory's work flow, how examination protocols are implemented, how testing equipment is used, and the steps for creating, modifying, and finalizing reports. In addition, participating in the vascular laboratory provides case-based learning opportunities. While vascular laboratory interpreting physicians do not need to be experts in *performing* diagnostic studies, a structured experience with 40 or more hours of time observing and assisting in examinations can provide a suitable technical introduction. The educational value of this time will be maximized if there are specific expectations established for instructor and student.

A curriculum example is provided in Table A2-9. This curriculum outlines a series of practical experiences in the vascular laboratory that provides the physician with an understanding of vascular laboratory operations, the scope of practice for the technical staff, how commonly requested studies are performed, and an introduction to the techniques used in the conduct of specific examinations. Educational program directors and vascular laboratories may use this, or a similar curriculum, to specify their goals and objectives for learners as well as the specific actions expected of the instructor and learner in each session.

TABLE A2-9

VASCULAR LABORATORY PRACTICAL INSTRUCTION PROGRAM FOR PHYSICIANS

■ LEARNING OBJECTIVES	■ INSTRUCTOR RESPONSIBILITIES	■ LEARNER RESPONSIBILITIES	■ COMPLETION STANDARDS
1. Vascular Laboratory Operations and Instrumentation			
Identify steps in ordering, conducting, and reporting vascular laboratory examinations Use appropriate steps to ensure patient and staff safety Become familiar with basic principles and operation of an ultrasound duplex scanner Know required and expected elements and format for vascular laboratory reports	Provide orientation to vascular laboratory facilities and equipment Describe vascular laboratory staffing Discuss training and scope of practice of vascular technologists List roles and responsibilities of vascular laboratory technologists and support staff Demonstrate steps in vascular examination workflow Identify and describe components of duplex scanner, including user interfaces, transducers, and displays Guide learner in setup of duplex scanner, including loading correct patient and examination from work list, selection of appropriate transducer and presets, and initiation of appropriate protocol (if applicable) Direct learner through steps required to send images to PACS and create preliminary report	Demonstrate professionalism interacting with patients and vascular laboratory staff Use appropriate hand hygiene and Universal Precautions With assistance, set up duplex scanner and prepare patient for vascular study With assistance, send images to picture archiving and communication system (PACS) and create preliminary report Learn the steps required to open preliminary report, add interpretation, finalize, and create addenda	Use electronic entry to submit an order for an examination in the vascular laboratory Demonstrate the steps to create an addendum to a final report Access a preliminary report Demonstrate the steps to add a physician impression to a preliminary report Complete all tasks according to vascular laboratory standards

VASCULAR LABORATORY PRACTICAL INSTRUCTION PROGRAM FOR PHYSICIANS (*Continued*)

■ LEARNING OBJECTIVES	■ INSTRUCTOR RESPONSIBILITIES	■ LEARNER RESPONSIBILITIES	■ COMPLETION STANDARDS
	Show steps for adding impressions to preliminary reports and adding an addendum to a final report Discuss procedures for final review of reported examinations used to identify errors or discrepancies		

2. Cerebrovascular: Extracranial

■ LEARNING OBJECTIVES	■ INSTRUCTOR RESPONSIBILITIES	■ LEARNER RESPONSIBILITIES	■ COMPLETION STANDARDS
Understand steps to evaluate patients referred for cerebrovascular examinations Learn methods of carotid artery and vertebral artery evaluation with duplex scanning Identify primary adjustments in displayed B-mode images, color Doppler images, and Doppler velocity waveforms	Demonstrate duplex scanner setup for cerebrovascular evaluation Discuss patient and examiner positioning for proper ergonomics Demonstrate transducer orientation and use Guide learner in basic system operation to optimize depth, focal zones, gain, and other imaging controls Demonstrate color Doppler and power Doppler use and adjustments Guide learner in adjusting Doppler sample volume positioning, Doppler gain, pulse repetition frequency, baseline position, and other Doppler controls Discuss common imaging artifacts and pitfalls encountered	Review history and indications for examination of patients to be evaluated Measure and record bilateral brachial blood pressures Evaluate for carotid and supraclavicular bruits With assistance, prepare and position patient for duplex scan Observe basic imaging techniques for cerebrovascular examination As directed, adjust imaging and Doppler controls With direct guidance, perform unilateral examination of carotid artery, vertebral, and subclavian arteries With assistance, send images to PACS and create preliminary report of extracranial cerebrovascular examination	Set up duplex scanner for extracranial cerebrovascular examination Acquire and record cine loop of sweep of carotid artery in transverse view Acquire and record B-mode images of common, external, and internal carotid arteries, vertebral artery, subclavian artery With assistance, acquire and record color Doppler images and velocity waveforms from common, external, and internal carotid arteries, vertebral artery, subclavian artery Transmit images from duplex scanner to PACS Generate preliminary report Complete all tasks according to vascular laboratory standards for cerebrovascular testing

3. Peripheral Venous: Deep Vein Thrombosis

■ LEARNING OBJECTIVES	■ INSTRUCTOR RESPONSIBILITIES	■ LEARNER RESPONSIBILITIES	■ COMPLETION STANDARDS
Identify normal and abnormal venous anatomy Describe venous hemodynamic principles Recognize the clinical significance of venous thromboembolism (VTE) Understand the role of ultrasound duplex scanning for diagnosis of deep vein thrombosis	Supervise learner's preparation and patient positioning for venous examination Guide learner though steps for setting up of duplex scanner for venous evaluation Discuss transducer selection for superficial and deep vessel examinations Demonstrate transducer orientation and use Guide learner in basics system operation, image adjustment, use of color and pulsed Doppler controls Review additional duplex scan controls that alter preset image acquisition and image processing Demonstrate performance of lower extremity venous duplex scan Demonstrate imaging of the inferior vena cava and iliac veins Guide learner in acquisition of venous images Discuss pitfalls and technical limitations of venous duplex scanning	Review history and indications for examination of patients to be evaluated Evaluate extremities for signs of venous disease Prepare and position patient for duplex scan Observe basic imaging techniques for venous duplex scan examination As directed, adjust imaging and Doppler controls With assistance, measure vessel diameter using system measurement tools With direct guidance, perform unilateral examination of femoral and popliteal veins and great saphenous vein With assistance, send images to PACS and create preliminary report of venous examination	Set up duplex scanner for extremity venous examination Identify vessels on recorded B-mode images of iliac veins and the inferior vena cava and use system tools to measure inferior vena cava diameter Acquire and record cine loop images of deep and superficial veins, with and without compression Acquire and record color Doppler images and velocity waveforms from deep and superficial veins without and with augmentation maneuvers Transmit images from duplex scanner to PACS Generate preliminary report Complete all tasks according to vascular laboratory standards for venous testing

(*Continued*)

TABLE A2-9

VASCULAR LABORATORY PRACTICAL INSTRUCTION PROGRAM FOR PHYSICIANS (*Continued*)

■ LEARNING OBJECTIVES	■ INSTRUCTOR RESPONSIBILITIES	■ LEARNER RESPONSIBILITIES	■ COMPLETION STANDARDS
4. Peripheral Venous: Evaluation of Venous Insufficiency			
Characterize chronic venous disease using clinical, etiologic, anatomic, and pathophysiologic classification (CEAP) reporting criteria Understand the role of venous duplex scanning for the evaluation of venous insufficiency and the testing methods used for assessing competence of venous valves Use standing reflux examination with automated release of limb cuffs to evaluated venous segments for valvular competence	Assist learner in preparation and positioning of patient for venous reflux examination Guide learner though steps of positioning, applying, and using pneumatic cuffs Guide learner in basics system operation, image adjustment, use of color and pulsed Doppler controls Demonstrate performance of lower extremity venous reflux examination Discuss worksheet use and record preliminary observations and findings Guide learner in recording of venous images Discuss pitfalls and technical limitations of venous reflux examination	Review history and indications for examination of patients to be evaluated Evaluate extremities for signs of venous disease Prepare and position patient recumbent and upright for duplex scan to evaluate for venous reflux Observe basic imaging techniques for venous duplex scan examination As directed, adjust imaging and Doppler controls With assistance, measure vein valve closure time (reflux time) using system measurement tools With direct guidance, perform unilateral reflux examination of femoral and popliteal veins and great saphenous vein at the saphenofemoral junction and in the midthigh With assistance, send images to PACS and create preliminary report of venous examination	Acquire and record cine loop and static images of deep and superficial veins, prior to and after cuff release Measure reflux time for each segment evaluated Transmit images from duplex scanner to PACS Generate preliminary report Correctly classify lower extremity venous disease using CEAP classification Complete all tasks according to vascular laboratory standard
5. Peripheral Arterial: Physiologic Testing			
Understand physiologic (indirect) testing methods used for evaluation of lower extremity arterial disease Use results of physiologic testing, in combination with history and physical examination findings, to diagnose and assess the severity of peripheral artery disease (PAD) Recognize artifacts in measurements of limb blood pressure that result from medial calcinosis or other test limitations Distinguish ischemic symptoms from nonvascular causes of lower extremity pain	Review the diagnostic equipment used in the vascular laboratory for arterial testing, including physiologic testing system (segmental pressures), treadmill, and laser Doppler skin perfusion pressure measurement system Demonstrate use of Doppler flow detector (and settings), pneumoplethysmograph, photoplethysmograph, chart recorder, cuff inflator, and remote control Supervise learner's preparation and positioning of patient for lower extremity arterial examination Assist learner in the application of cuffs for examination and demonstrate setup of system Direct learner in acquisition of Doppler waveforms Demonstrate operation of treadmill and instruct patient in conduct of treadmill test Perform treadmill exercise test, with learner assisting Demonstrate, if applicable, use of laser Doppler skin perfusion measurement system Discuss pitfalls and technical limitations of arterial indirect testing	Review patient history, indications for examination, and performed complete lower extremity pulse examination and assess for bruits Measure ankle-brachial indices As directed, apply segmental cuffs to both lower extremities Use continuous wave Doppler probe to obtain Doppler waveforms at each level With assistance, perform segmental pressure measurement With assistance, acquire segmental pulse volume recordings Measure limb pressures prior to and after exercise on treadmill With assistance, send study to PACS and create preliminary report of arterial examination	Obtain Doppler signals from lower extremity arteries at multiple levels Measure pressures and calculate ankle-brachial indices Generate preliminary report Complete all tasks according to vascular laboratory standards for peripheral arterial physiologic testing

VASCULAR LABORATORY PRACTICAL INSTRUCTION PROGRAM FOR PHYSICIANS (Continued)

■ LEARNING OBJECTIVES	■ INSTRUCTOR RESPONSIBILITIES	■ LEARNER RESPONSIBILITIES	■ COMPLETION STANDARDS
6. Peripheral Arterial: Native Vessel and Graft Duplex Scanning			
Understand the role of duplex scanning for evaluation of peripheral arteries and grafts Learn the methods of peripheral artery and graft evaluation with duplex scanning Use system controls to adjust displayed B-mode images, color Doppler images, and Doppler velocity waveforms	Demonstrate duplex scanner setup for peripheral arterial evaluation Discuss patient and examiner positioning for proper ergonomics Demonstrate transducer orientation and use Provide direction, as required, for learner to operate system controls to optimize depth, focal zones, gain, and other imaging controls Guide learner's adjustments of color Doppler Guide learner in adjusting Doppler sample volume positioning, Doppler gain, pulse repetition frequency, baseline position, and other Doppler controls Discuss common imaging artifacts and pitfalls encountered with peripheral arterial examinations	Review history and indications for examination of patients to be evaluated Examine extremity pulses, auscultate for bruits, evaluate extremities for signs of arterial disease and prior operations Prepare and position patient recumbent and upright for arterial duplex scan Observe scanning techniques used for peripheral artery duplex scan examination With assistance, adjust imaging and Doppler controls With assistance, measure arterial diameters using system measurement tools With assistance, send images to PACS and create preliminary report of peripheral arterial examination	Set up duplex scanner for peripheral arterial examination Acquire and record images of common femoral, deep femoral, superficial femoral, popliteal, and tibioperoneal arteries If applicable, acquire and record images of graft anastomoses and conduit Complete all tasks according to vascular laboratory standards
7. Abdominal Vascular Evaluation: Aorta and Iliac Testing			
Understand the relationships between transducer frequency and imaging depth and the effects of depth on spatial and temporal resolution, imaging frame rate, and ultrasound focus Use ultrasound B-mode imaging to identify abdominal vascular and anatomic landmarks Describe the role of ultrasound screening and techniques used for detection of abdominal aortic aneurysms Use ultrasound duplex scanning to detect and characterize the severity of arterial occlusive disease Understand the role of duplex scanning for follow-up after endovascular aortic aneurysm repair (EVAR)	Discuss patient and examiner positioning for proper ergonomics Demonstrate duplex scanner setup for abdominal vascular testing Demonstrate transducer selection, orientation, and use Compare imaging characteristics of high-frequency transducer for imaging of superficial structures and low-frequency transducer for deeper structures Guide learner in performing imaging survey of the abdomen Guide learner's adjustments of color Doppler controls Guide learner in adjusting Doppler sample volume positioning, Doppler gain, pulse repetition frequency, baseline position, and other pulsed Doppler controls Discuss common imaging artifacts and pitfalls encountered with abdominal arterial examinations Review protocol for post-EVAR examination	Evaluate the patient prior to performing ultrasound examination Review previous studies, if available to make comparisons to the current study Review patient history, including prior operations or endovascular procedures, arterial disease risk factors, smoking status Review for symptoms of aortoiliac disease, aneurysmal or occlusive disease, including back pain, increased pulsation of abdomen, groin, or popliteal fossa; signs of distal emboli, claudication Examine extremity pulses, auscultate for bruits, evaluate extremities for signs of arterial disease and prior operations Measure and record ankle-brachial index (ABI) Verify the requested examination is appropriate for the patient With guidance, perform imaging survey of the abdomen Image and measure the abdominal aorta Assist technologist's conduct of aortoiliac or post-EVAR examination, adjusting imaging and Doppler settings, as directed With assistance, measure the aorta and iliac artery diameters using measurement tools	Set up duplex scanner for abdominal vascular examination Acquire and record images of the liver, gall bladder, hepatorenal fossa, spleen, right kidney, and left kidney Acquire and record images of the aorta, including longitudinal view and transverse views at the level of the renal arteries, midabdominal aorta, and aortic bifurcation As directed, acquire and record color Doppler images and velocity waveforms from representative aortoiliac segments Transmit images from duplex scanner to PACS Generate preliminary report Complete all tasks according to vascular laboratory standards for abdominal vascular testing

(Continued)

VASCULAR LABORATORY PRACTICAL INSTRUCTION PROGRAM FOR PHYSICIANS (*Continued*)

■ LEARNING OBJECTIVES	■ INSTRUCTOR RESPONSIBILITIES	■ LEARNER RESPONSIBILITIES	■ COMPLETION STANDARDS
8. Abdominal Vascular: Renal and Mesenteric			
Understand the role of the vascular laboratory for diagnosis and follow-up of renal and mesenteric artery occlusive disease Use ultrasound duplex scanning to detect and characterize the severity of visceral arterial occlusive disease Understand the role of duplex scanning for follow-up after endovascular and surgical treatment of branches of the abdominal aorta Recognize limitations inherent in use of ultrasound for evaluation of visceral vessels	Discuss patient and examiner positioning for proper ergonomics Assist in transducer selection and duplex scanner setup for abdominal vascular testing Review protocol for visceral arterial studies Perform renal and mesenteric duplex scan, describing observational features of the examination Guide learner in performing the imaging survey of the abdomen Guide learner's adjustments of image, color Doppler, and pulsed Doppler Guide learner in adjusting Doppler sample volume positioning, Doppler gain, pulse repetition frequency, baseline position, and other Doppler controls Discuss common imaging artifacts and pitfalls encountered with visceral arterial examinations	Evaluate the patient prior to performing ultrasound examination Verify if the requested examination is appropriate for the patient With guidance, perform imaging survey of the abdomen Image and measure the abdominal aorta Assist technologist's conduct of renal and mesenteric examination, adjusting imaging and Doppler settings, as directed With assistance, measure the length of the kidneys using measurement tools	Set up duplex scanner for visceral vascular examination Acquire and record images of the renal and mesenteric arteries as the technologist scans As directed, acquire and record color Doppler images and velocity waveforms from representative aortoiliac segments Transmit images from duplex scanner to PACS Generate preliminary report Complete all tasks according to vascular laboratory standards for visceral artery evaluation
9. Peripheral Vascular Evaluation: Specialized Applications—Preoperative Vessel Mapping			
Understand the role of the vascular laboratory for preoperative assessment and procedure planning Identify superficial and deep vessels for preoperative assessment (vein bypass, dialysis access procedures, radial artery evaluation prior to coronary artery bypass, fibular free flap, or breast reconstruction)	Review specialized testing applications offered in the vascular laboratory and discuss the importance of communication with the surgeon Discuss techniques for surface marking and documentation of findings in preliminary report Review details of protocol to be used for specific test Assist learner, as needed, in measurement of pressures and recording of plethysmographic waveforms, if these are part of the examination to be performed Demonstrate imaging components of specialized testing application	Evaluate the patient prior to performing ultrasound examination Confirm that the requested examination is appropriate for the patient Determine tests needed for patient evaluation and review applicable vascular laboratory policy and procedure documents With assistance, perform physiologic (indirect) tests, if these are required components of the evaluation to be performed Assist technologist in the conduct and documentation of imaging components of the examination	Set up testing equipment to be used for specified examination If indicated, complete indirect components of the examination If indicated, mark surface of skin to localize mapped vascular structures Transmit images from duplex scanner to PACS Complete all tasks according to vascular laboratory standards

TABLE A2-9

VASCULAR LABORATORY PRACTICAL INSTRUCTION PROGRAM FOR PHYSICIANS (*Continued*)

■ LEARNING OBJECTIVES	■ INSTRUCTOR RESPONSIBILITIES	■ LEARNER RESPONSIBILITIES	■ COMPLETION STANDARDS
10. Vascular Laboratory Accreditation and Quality Assurance			
Understand the purpose of vascular laboratory accreditation and the requirements to gain and maintain accreditation Identify methods used to maintain consistency in reporting, identify and correct errors, and confirm accuracy of vascular laboratory exams Use calculations of specificity, sensitivity, predictive value, and accuracy to describe the results of a diagnostic test in comparison with a reference standard Understand the ARDMS certification processes for vascular technologists and interpreting physicians, including prerequisites for RPVI application	Review the vascular laboratory quality control (QC) policies for ultrasound imaging and physiologic testing systems Review the vascular laboratory quality assurance (QA) processes Review the vascular laboratory continuous quality improvement (CQI) processes	Perform quality assurance steps on a minimum of ten examinations Assist in preparation of cases for vascular laboratory CQI meeting Review ARDMS PVI examination application requirements and content outline	Complete all tasks according to vascular laboratory standards

EDUCATIONAL MILESTONES FOR LEARNERS

Milestones based on the concepts used by the ACGME for assessing progression through residency training can be developed to evaluate a physician's progression through training in the vascular laboratory (Table A2-10). Milestones are knowledge, skills, attitudes, and other attributes for each of the ACGME core competencies, organized in a developmental framework from less to more advanced. They are descriptors and targets for performance as trainees move from entry level through completion of their educational program. Tracking from Level 1 to Level 5 is synonymous with moving from novice to expert, although these levels do not correspond with specific periods of education. Milestones for progression from novice (medical school graduate) to advanced vascular laboratory physician (appropriate for medical director of an accredited vascular laboratory) are listed in Table A2-11, which provides a summary of milestones specific to vascular laboratory subcompetencies.

TABLE A2-10

MILESTONES FOR PHYSICIAN EDUCATION IN VASCULAR LABORATORY COMPETENCIES

Level 1: The physician demonstrates milestones expected of medical school graduate with basic knowledge of vascular anatomy and physiology.

Level 2: The physician is advancing and demonstrates additional milestones, but with performance less than expected for midlevel trainee.

Level 3: The physician continues to advance and demonstrate additional milestones, consistently including the majority of milestones targeted for training.

Level 4: The physician has advanced so that he or she now substantially demonstrates the milestones targeted for training. A minimally competent vascular laboratory physician is at this level (e.g., new medical staff of an accredited vascular laboratory).

Level 5: The physician has advanced beyond performance targets set for initial vascular laboratory training and is demonstrating "aspirational" goals, which might describe the performance of someone who has been in practice at an advanced level (medical director of a vascular laboratory). It is expected that only a few exceptional physicians will reach this level during training.

TABLE A2-11

VASCULAR LABORATORY MILESTONES

LEVEL 1	LEVEL 2	LEVEL 3	LEVEL 4	LEVEL 5
Medical Knowledge: Vascular Anatomy and Pathologic Anatomy				
Demonstrates general knowledge of normal anatomy	Demonstrates knowledge of pathologic anatomy	Understands anatomic and physiologic contributions to clinical presentations	Describes impact of patient-specific anatomy on treatment plans	Demonstrates knowledge of uncommon or rare variants
Medical Knowledge: Hemodynamics and Vascular Physiology				
Demonstrates knowledge of blood pressure, flow, and regulation of vascular resistance	Demonstrates knowledge of fluid dynamics, laminar and turbulent flow, fluid energy, and effects of stenoses; Understands venous physiology, muscle pump function, role of vein valves; Understands Poiseuille's law and Bernoulli's principle in hemodynamics	Understands physiology of special vascular beds, including splanchnic circulation, hepatoportal venous system, and cerebral autoregulation	Uses knowledge vascular physiology and hemodynamics in patient care, procedural planning, and outcome assessment	Recognizes effects of drugs, devices, and vascular pathophysiology on hemodynamic patterns; Recognizes significant of changes seen with longitudinal surveillance
Medical Knowledge: Ultrasound Physics				
Demonstrates knowledge of pressure measurements methods and limitations	Understands basic acoustic principles; Demonstrates knowledge of continuous wave and pulsed wave Doppler, B-mode imaging, color Doppler, power Doppler principles	Ability to recognize artifacts and technically limited examinations and to account for these in the interpretation of the vascular laboratory studies; Understands causes of ultrasound imaging and Doppler artifacts	Understands mechanical and thermal bioeffects of ultrasound	Recognizes effects of transducer design and image processing systems
Medical Knowledge: Instrumentation and Equipment				
Demonstrates familiarity with examination facilities, patient care equipment, and types of vascular laboratory instrumentation	Understands operational principles of the duplex ultrasound scanner, continuous wave and pulsed wave Doppler, photoplethysmography (PPG), plethysmography, laser Doppler, and transcutaneous PO_2	Understands principles of transducer design, ultrasound focus, resolution, factors that affect signal-to-noise ratio	Applies knowledge of ultrasound physics and instrumentation as it relates to operation of image pre- and postprocessing, harmonic imaging, specialized imaging modalities	Uses and programs scanning protocol and other functions of advanced duplex ultrasound imaging systems
Medical Knowledge: Testing Protocols and Interpretation Criteria				
Knowledge of the testing principles and laboratory interpretation guidelines; Familiarity with the indications for vascular laboratory testing and applicable reporting standards	Identifies appropriate transducer for examination; Understands interpretation criteria using vessel measurements, velocities, and velocity ratio criteria; Understands methods for assessment of venous valvular competence with duplex scanning	Recognizes need to modify imaging protocols based on patient comorbidities; Understands calculation of and use of volume flow measurements; Understands calculation of and use of waveform indices (resistive index, pulsatility index); Demonstrates knowledge of provocative maneuvers	Deviates from established criteria in situations where standard criteria may not be appropriate, explaining in the report any discrepancies between the findings and interpretation	Demonstrates knowledge of ultrasound contrast agent use

Patient Care				
Measures pressures and calculates ankle-brachial indices	Interprets basic examinations	Interprets advanced diagnostic examinations	Observes and interprets subtle findings	Implements innovative imaging technology to enhance the care of the patient
Identifies normal anatomy on B-mode images	Incorporates clinical indications in study interpretation	Interprets surveillance and follow-up examinations	Provides interpretation of imaging findings for operative planning for intermediate and advanced procedures	
	Image assessment of vascular anatomy and pathology	Reviews the indications for the examination, technologist's reported findings, saved images, and other supporting documentation and then enters a clear and concise interpretation of the exam result in a draft report	Identifies and reports on incidental findings	
	Differentiates normal from abnormal findings	Interprets waveforms for indirect assessment of vascular diseases	Modifies interpretation of tests due to anatomic or medical conditions	
	Incorporates physiologic and anatomic findings in interpretation	Makes core observations, formulates differential diagnoses, and recognizes critical findings	Modifies interpretation of tests due to technical limitations (e.g., artifacts)	
	Makes secondary observations and prioritizes differential diagnoses	Interprets vascular laboratory studies exams in accordance with laboratory policies, using established protocols and diagnostic criteria	Incorporates comparison of present study with prior testing	
	Modifies imaging protocol to optimize data acquisition	Uses imaging findings in operative planning for basic procedures		
Communication and Reporting				
Understands use and report generation functions of the electronic record systems and review functions of the PACS	With direct supervision, generates an accurate, concise, and organized report of imaging findings	Independently generates an accurate, concise, and organized report of imaging findings	Communicates critical findings to referring practitioners	Manages reporting systems
Recognizes essential elements of preliminary and final reports				Develops reporting standards
Practice-Based Learning and Improvement				
Understand the purpose of vascular laboratory accreditation and the requirements to gain and maintain accreditation	Assesses examination quality, accuracy, and completeness	Participates in quality assurance and quality improvement programs	Participates in facility accreditation or reaccreditation process	Teaches imaging interpretation to other learners
Identify methods used to maintain consistency in reporting, identify and correct errors, and confirm accuracy of vascular laboratory exams	Use calculations of specificity, sensitivity, predictive value, and accuracy to describe the results of a diagnostic test in comparison with a reference standard	Meets prerequisites for RPVI credential		Implements new testing protocols or revises existing ones based on the results of reviews of scientific evidence
Understand the ARDMS certification processes for vascular technologists and interpreting physicians, including prerequisites for Registered Physician in Vascular Interpretation (RPVI) application				

(Continued)

TABLE A2-11

VASCULAR LABORATORY MILESTONES (*Continued*)

LEVEL 1	LEVEL 2	LEVEL 3	LEVEL 4	LEVEL 5
Professionalism				
Protects private health information (PHI)	Complies with professional behavioral and performance standards	Understands causes and means to avoid work-related musculoskeletal disorders in the vascular laboratory	Acquires RPVI credential Demonstrates leadership in vascular laboratory operations	Assumes leadership role in vascular laboratory Actively participates and contributes to the programs of vascular ultrasound professional societies and organizations
Recognizes roles and scope of practice of vascular laboratory staff and technologists				
Systems-Based Practice				
Demonstrates basic knowledge of how health systems operate	Describes how patient care is provided in the system and recognizes specific system failures that can affect patient care	Follows vascular laboratory protocols and guidelines for patient care	Demonstrates knowledge of system factors that contribute to reporting errors and is aware that variations in care occur	Implements new or revised standards for reporting or diagnosis
Accesses and uses informatics systems used by the vascular laboratory	Understands communication and informatics standards used in the vascular laboratory (DICOM, HL7, etc.)	Understands principles of billing and coding	Assigns appropriate diagnostic and billing codes for vascular laboratory services	
	Understands operations and interactions of informatics systems			

Note: Page numbers followed by *f* and *t* indicate figures and tables, respectively.